FISCHBACH'S MANUAL OF Laboratory and Diagnostic Tests

TENTH EDITION

FISCHBACH'S MANUAL OF Laboratory and Diagnostic Tests

TENTH EDITION

Frances Talaska Fischbach, RN, BSN, MSN

Associate Professor of Nursing (Ret)
School of Nursing
University of Wisconsin-Milwaukee
Milwaukee, Wisconsin

Margaret A. Fischbach, RN, JD

Vice President - Legal & Compliance
Milwaukee Center for Independence
Milwaukee, Wisconsin

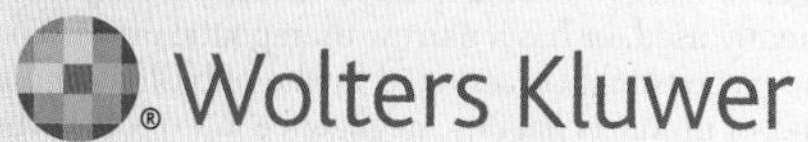

Philadelphia • Baltimore • New York • London
Buenos Aires • Hong Kong • Sydney • Tokyo

Acquisitions Editor: Natasha McIntyre
Supervising Development Editor: Heather A. Rybacki
Editorial Coordinator: Annette Ferran
Marketing Manager: Katie Schlesinger
Production Project Manager: Marian Bellus
Design Coordinator: Stephen Druding
Art Director: Jennifer Clements
Manufacturing Coordinator: Karin Duffield
Prepress Vendor: Absolute Service, Inc.

10th Edition

9 8 7 6 5 4 3 2 1

Printed in China

Library of Congress Cataloging-in-Publication Data

Names: Fischbach, Frances Talaska, author. | Fischbach, Margaret A., author.
Title: Fischbach's manual of laboratory and diagnostic tests / Frances Talaska Fischbach, Margaret A. Fischbach.
Other titles: Manual of laboratory and diagnostic tests
Description: Tenth edition. | Philadelphia : Wolters Kluwer, [2018] | Preceded by A manual of laboratory and diagnostic tests / Frances Talaska Fischback, Marshall Barnett Dunning III. Ninth edition. 2015. | Includes bibliographical references and index.
Identifiers: LCCN 2017036850 | ISBN 9781496377128
Subjects: | MESH: Clinical Laboratory Techniques | Diagnostic Techniques and Procedures | Laboratory Manuals
Classification: LCC RB38.2 | NLM QY 25 | DDC 616.07/5—dc23 LC record available at https://lccn.loc.gov/2017036850

LWW.com

RRS1709

Dedicated to the memory of John E. Fischbach
1926–2012

Contributors, Consultants, and Research Assistants

Mei W. Baker, MD, FACMG
Co-Director, Newborn Screening Laboratory
Wisconsin State Laboratory of Hygiene
University of Wisconsin–Madison
Associate Professor, Department of Pediatrics
University of Wisconsin School of Medicine and Public Health
Madison, Wisconsin

Patti Cobb, RD, CD
Chief Clinical Dietitian
Food and Nutrition Services
Froedtert Hospital
Milwaukee, Wisconsin

Ann Shafranski Fischbach, RN, BSN, CAOHC, CPID
Case Manager
Restore Wheaton Franciscan Health Care
Milwaukee, Wisconsin

Dina Iskander, OD
Primary Care
West Park Opthalmology
New York, New York

Paul J. Jannetto, PhD, DABCC, FACB, MT (ASCP)
Director, Toxicology and Drug Monitoring Laboratory
Director, Metals Laboratory
Mayo Clinic
Rochester, Minnesota

Jennifer M. Johnson, BA, RN, BSN
Cardiothoracic Procurement Coordinator
Thoracic Transplant Programs
Loyola University Medical Center
Maywood, Illinois

Mary Fischbach Johnson, BA, MS
Research Assistant
New York, New York

Stanley F. Lo, PhD, DABCC, FACB
Associate Professor, Pathology
Children's Hospital of Wisconsin
Medical College of Wisconsin
Milwaukee, Wisconsin

Tammy Mack, RN, BSN
Imaging Services Manager
Education, Nursing and Quality
Froedtert Hospital
Milwaukee, Wisconsin

Charles R. Myers, PhD
Professor of Pharmacology and Toxicology
Medical College of Wisconsin
Milwaukee, Wisconsin

Christine Naczek, MT (ASCP)
Manager, Blood Banking and Pre-Transfusion Testing
Dynacare Laboratories, LLC
Milwaukee, Wisconsin

Anne Witkowiak Nezworski, RN, BSN
Maternity and Newborn Specialist
Marshfield Clinic, Eau Claire Center
Eau Claire, Wisconsin

Hershel Raff, PhD
Professor of Medicine, Surgery and Physiology
Medical College of Wisconsin
Aurora St. Luke's Medical Center Research Institute
Milwaukee, Wisconsin

Jeffrey W. Schneider, RN, BSN
Staff Nurse
Froedtert Hospital
Milwaukee, Wisconsin

Frank G. Steffel, BS, CNMT
Program Director–Nuclear Medicine/PET Technology
Froedtert Hospital
Milwaukee, Wisconsin

Patricia A. Van Kampen, RN
Milwaukee County Behavioral Health Division
Research Assistant
Milwaukee, Wisconsin

Patti Wilson BSN, RN, CIC
Infection Control Coordinator
Froedtert Hospital
Milwaukee, Wisconsin

Michael Zacharisen, MD
Professor of Pediatrics
Children's Hospital of Wisconsin
Milwaukee, Wisconsin

Reviewers

Tamella Livengood, MSN, FNP
Nursing Faculty
Northwestern Michigan College
Traverse City, Michigan

Jodi Orm, MSN, RN, CNE
Nurse Educator and Guest Lecturer
Founder and Principal Consultant
iNurseEd Consulting

Preface

PURPOSE

The purpose of *Fischbach's Manual of Laboratory and Diagnostic Tests,* in this tenth edition, is to promote the delivery of safe, effective, and informed care for patients undergoing diagnostic tests and procedures and also to provide students, educators, researchers, healthcare providers, and others with a unique resource. This comprehensive manual provides a foundation for understanding diagnostic tests, from the relatively simple to the most complex, that are delivered to varied populations in varied settings. It describes in depth the healthcare provider's role by providing the information necessary for quality care planning, individualized patient assessment, analysis of patient needs, appropriate interventions, patient education, patient follow-up, and outcome evaluation.

Potential risks and complications of diagnostic testing mandate that proper test protocols, interfering factors, follow-up testing, and collaboration among those involved in the testing process be a significant part of the information included in this text.

ORGANIZATION

This book is organized into 16 chapters and 5 appendices. Chapter 1 outlines the clinician's role in diagnostic testing and includes interventions for safe, effective, informed pre-, intra-, and posttest care. This chapter includes a patient's bill of rights and patient responsibilities, a model for the role of the clinical team in providing diagnostic care and services, and descriptions of different test environments, and it emphasizes the importance of communication as the key to desired outcomes. The intratest section includes information about collaborative approaches facilitating family presence during invasive procedures; risk management; the collection, handling, and transport of specimens; infection control; controlling pain; comfort measures; administration of drugs and solutions; monitoring fluid intake and loss; using required equipment kits and supplies; properly positioning the patient for the procedure; managing the environment; and patient monitoring. The reader is referred back to Chapter 1, Diagnostic Testing, throughout the text for information about the clinician's role and diagnostic services. Chapters 2 through 16 focus on specific categories of studies.

CHAPTER CONTENT AND FEATURES

Studies are organized in a similar way for ease of use and include:

Introductory Information

- Background rationale
- Test purpose
- Interfering factors
- Description and method of the procedure and laboratory test completion
- Evidence-based outcomes
- Patient involvement

Normal Findings

- Normal reference values
- Conventional and SI units
- Age-related values and critical values when applicable

Procedures

- Process of intratest care
- Method of specimen collection and handling for laboratory tests
- Method of diagnostic procedures

Clinical Implications

- Interpretation of abnormal findings
- Unexpected outcomes
- Disease patterns
- Clinical considerations for newborn, infant, child, adolescent, and older adult groups when appropriate

Interventions

- Pre- and posttest patient care
- Specific guidelines for each test phase

Special **Clinical Alerts**, **Procedural Alerts**, and **Notes** NOTE appear frequently throughout to signal special cautions.

A fully updated bibliography at the end of each chapter, representing a composite of selected references from various disciplines, directs the clinician to information available beyond the scope of this book, and extensive appendices provide additional data for everyday practice.

REVISIONS AND ADDITIONS TO THE TENTH EDITION

The new edition includes:

- Updated HIV testing guidelines
- Simplified and standardized patient preparation instructions
- Consistent phrasing used for nursing interventions throughout the text so that users encounter the same verbiage to explain similar actions
- Revised and expanded art program

CURRENT DEVELOPMENTS IN LABORATORY AND DIAGNOSTIC TESTING

New technologies foster new scientific modalities for patient assessment and clinical interventions. Thus, the clinician is provided a greater understanding of the long chain of events from diagnosis through treatment and outcomes. In a brief span of years, new and improved technologies have led to developments in x-ray scanners, digital and enhanced imaging, magnetic resonance (MR), positron emission tomography (PET) scans of the heart and brain, enhanced ultrasound and nuclear medicine procedures, newly discovered genetic mutation studies, new cancer markers for diagnosis and prognosis, technology for fetal testing before birth, and postmortem testing after death. Many new technologies are faster, more patient-friendly, and more comfortable and provide an equivalent or higher degree of accuracy (i.e., HIV or hepatitis detection, monitoring for drug abuse or managing therapeutic drug levels). Saliva and breath testing is gaining ground as a mirror of body function; DNA; and emotional, hormonal, immune, and neurologic status as well as providing clues about faulty metabolism. Noninvasive and minimally invasive testing (e.g., using a swab to collect saliva from the mouth, procedures that require only one drop of blood), which is better suited for testing in environments such as the workplace, private home, and other nontraditional healthcare settings such as churches, is made possible by better collection methods and standardized collection techniques. The newest diagnostic laboratory technologies include handheld nucleic acid detectors for specific bacteria and viruses, handheld miniaturized chip-based DNA analyzers, reagentless diagnostics that introduce the sample (e.g., hand, finger, earlobe) to magnetic fields, and magnetic resonance spectroscopy (MRS). Noninvasive and minimally invasive diagnostics include infrared light to estimate glucose, rapid oral screen for HIV, proteomics, and functional and molecular techniques.

A resurgence in the use of traditional, trusted diagnostic modalities, such as electroencephalogram (EEG), is being seen in certain areas. Diseases such as HIV, antibiotic-resistant strains of pathologic organisms (e.g., tuberculosis [TB]), and type 2 diabetes are becoming more prevalent. In the workplace, thorough diagnostic testing is more common as applications are made for employment and disability benefits. Also, requirements for periodic monitoring of exposures to potentially hazardous workplace substances (chemicals, heavy metals), breathing and hearing tests, and TB and latex allergy testing require skill in administering and procuring specimens. The number of forensic DNA identity tests being performed has increased tremendously. Concurrently, consumer perceptions have shifted from implicit faith in the healthcare system to concerns regarding less control over choices for health care and more distrust of the system in general.

Managed care and its drive for control of costs for diagnostic services exert a tremendous effect on consumers' ability to access testing services care. This results in mixed access to services, depending on approval or denial of coverage.

These trends—combined with a shift in diagnostic care from acute care hospital settings to outpatient departments, physicians' offices, clinics, community-based centers, nursing homes, and, sometimes, even churches, stores, and pharmacies—challenge clinicians to provide standards-based, safe, effective, and informed care. Because the healthcare system is becoming a community-based model, the clinician's role is also changing. Updated knowledge and skills, flexibility, and a heightened awareness of the testing environment (point-of-care testing) are needed to provide diagnostic services in these settings.

Clinicians must also adapt their practice to changes in other areas. This includes developing, coordinating, and following policies and standards set forth by institutions, governmental bodies, and regulatory agencies. Being informed regarding ethical and legal implications such as informed consent, privacy, patient safety, the right to refuse tests, the right to truthful diagnoses and prognoses, end-of-life decisions, standards for quarantine to control infection, and trends in diagnostic research procedures adds another dimension to the clinician's accountability and responsibility. The consequences of certain types of testing (e.g., HIV, genetic) and the implications of confidential versus anonymous testing must also be kept in mind. For example, anonymous tests do not require the individual to give his or her name, whereas confidential tests do require a name. This difference has implications in the requirements and process of agency reporting for all patients as well as for select groups of infectious disease incidence, such as HIV.

Responding to these trends, the tenth edition of *Fischbach's Manual of Laboratory and Diagnostic Tests* is a comprehensive, up-to-date diagnostic reference source that includes information about newer technologies together with the time-honored, classic tests that continue to be an important component of diagnostic work. It meets the needs of students, educators, researchers, healthcare providers, and others whose work and study require this type of resource or reference manual.

Frances Talaska Fischbach
Margaret A. Fischbach

Acknowledgments

We acknowledge with sincere gratitude the contributions made by all of those individuals who participated in the revisions for the tenth edition of this book as well as prior editions.

Our special thanks go to Mary Fischbach Johnson and Patricia Van Kampen for their research and administrative support. We especially thank the contributors, consultants, and reviewers for their diligence and hard work to ensure the quality, completeness, and most up-to-date information contained herein. Our gratitude is extended to the entire staff at Wolters-Kluwer, especially Natasha McIntyre, Annette Ferran, and Heather A. Rybacki and to Don Famularcano, project manager at Absolute Service, Inc. Special recognition is also due to the editors, contributors, and staff who have worked on all prior editions of this work.

Finally, we thank our family, friends, and special people in our lives, too numerous to mention, on whom we relied for support and encouragement.

Frances Talaska Fischbach
Margaret A. Fischbach

Contents

Diagnostic Testing

1

OVERVIEW OF LABORATORY AND DIAGNOSTIC TESTING

Healthcare delivery is a complex system that involves many different disciplines and specialties, with care provided in a variety of settings. Consequently, healthcare providers must have an understanding and working knowledge of modalities beyond their own area of expertise. This includes diagnostic evaluation and diagnostic services.

Laboratory and diagnostic tests are tools to gain additional information about the patient. By themselves, these tests are not therapeutic; however, when used in conjunction with a thorough history and physical examination, these tests may confirm a diagnosis or provide valuable information about a patient's status and response to therapy that may not be apparent from the history and physical examination alone.

Table 1.1 lists the reasons for laboratory and diagnostic testing and examples of tests selected for each purpose. As an integral part of their practice, healthcare providers support patients and their family members in meeting the demands and challenges incumbent in the simplest to the most complex diagnostic testing. This testing begins before birth in the form of prenatal ultrasounds, genetic testing, and amniocentesis and frequently continues after death in the case of postmortem testing for evidentiary or forensic purposes, organ transplantation, or death reporting (autopsy).

The healthcare provider who provides diagnostic services must have basic requisite knowledge to plan patient care and an understanding of psychoneuroimmunology (effects of stress on health status). He or she must be able to make careful judgments and gather vital information about the patient and the testing process to diagnose appropriately within the parameters of the healthcare provider's professional standards.

The Diagnostic Testing Model

The diagnostic testing model incorporates three phases: pretest, intratest, and posttest. Figure 1.1 provides an overview of the responsibilities of the healthcare provider before, during, and after testing.

NOTE The three phases are termed *preanalytical, analytical,* and *postanalytical* in laboratory terminology.

The later parts of this chapter address the interventions and knowledge required by healthcare providers in each phase of the test process.

Standards and Guidelines

To ensure accurate, optimal test results, each phase of testing requires a specific set of guidelines and standards to be followed. Patient care standards and standards of professional practice are key points in developing a collaborative approach to patient care during diagnostic evaluation. Standards of care provide clinical guidelines and set minimum requirements for professional practice and patient care (Table 1.2).

Test Selection and Evidence-Based Guidelines

Test selections are based on subjective clinical judgment, evaluation of risks and benefits, guidelines and recommendations (refer to Table 1.2), and evidence-based health care.

Evidence-based guidelines grade the quality of scientific evidence for a specific test or procedure based on published reports of clinical trials, expert consensus, or clinical expertise. Levels of evidence are A, B, C, and E, with A indicating that a test or procedure is supported by the best scientific evidence and E referring to expert opinion or consensus (Chart 1.1).

TABLE 1.1 Goals of Test Selection with Examples

Intended Purpose of Test	Example(s) of Diagnostic Test(s)	Indication
Screening	Stool occult blood, fecal occult blood testing	Yearly screening after 50 yr of age
Monitoring	Serum potassium	Yearly in patients taking diuretic agents or potassium supplements; in cases of some cardiac arrhythmias
Monitoring	Liver enzyme levels	Monitor patient taking hepatotoxic drugs; establish baseline values
Diagnosis	Serum amylase	In the presence of abdominal pain, suspect pancreatitis
Diagnosis	Thyroid-stimulating hormone (TSH) test	Suspicion of hypothyroidism, hyperthyroidism, or thyroid dysfunction in patients ≥50 yr of age
Diagnosis & monitoring	Chlamydia and gonorrhea	In sexually active persons with multiple partners; monitor for pelvic inflammatory disease
Detecting	Hematocrit and hemoglobin	Baseline study; abnormal bleeding; detection of anemia (use complete blood count [CBC] results if they are recent)
Screening & diagnosis	Cervical Papanicolaou (Pap) test	Yearly for all women ≥18 yr of age; more often with high-risk factors (e.g., dysplasia, HIV, herpes simplex); check for human papillomavirus (HPV), chlamydia, and gonorrhea using DNA
Diagnosis	Urine culture	Bladder infection
Screening	Tuberculosis (TB) skin test	Easiest test to use for TB screening of individuals <35 yr of age or those with history of negative TB skin tests; for persons in resident homes
Detecting	TB blood test QuantiFERON Gold TB	Blood test to assess TB exposure in risk population
Screening & monitoring	Fasting blood glucose (FBG)	Every 3 yr starting at 45 yr of age; hemoglobin A_{1c} to monitor diabetes control
Diagnosis	Urinalysis (UA)	Signs or history of recurrent urinary tract disease; incontinence; pregnant women; men with prostatic hypertrophy
Monitoring	Prothrombin time (PT)/International normalized ratio (INR)	Monitoring anticoagulant treatment
Screening	Prostate-specific antigen (PSA) and digital rectal examination	Screen men ≥50 yr of age for prostate cancer yearly
Evaluating, diagnosing & monitoring	Chest x-ray	Monitor for lung lesions and infiltrates; congestive heart failure; anatomic deformities, after trauma, before surgery, follow-up for positive TB skin test and monitor treatment

table continues on pg. 4 >

TABLE 1.1, continued

Intended Purpose of Test	Example(s) of Diagnostic Test(s)	Indication
Screening	Mammogram	Screen by 40 yr of age in women and then every 12–18 mo between 40 and 49 yr of age, annually at ≥50 yr of age; follow-up for history and treatment of breast cancer; routine screening when strong family history of breast carcinoma
Screening	Colon x-rays, flexible sigmoidoscopy after 5 yr, and colonoscopy after 10 yr	Screen adults for colon cancer beginning at age 50 yr; follow for presence of hemoglobin- or guaiac-positive stools, polyps, diverticulosis
Evaluation, diagnosing & monitoring	Computed tomography (CT) scans	Before and after treatment for certain cancers, injuries, illness (e.g., suspected transient ischemic attack, cerebrovascular accident; diagnostic evaluation of certain signs and symptoms)
Diagnosing & screening	Other genetic tests	Assist in establishing or ruling out familial inheritable diseases

Some tests are mandated by government agencies (e.g., U.S. Preventive Services Task Force) or clinical practice guidelines of professional societies (e.g., American Congress of Obstetricians and Gynecologists); others are deemed part of necessary care based on the individual practitioner's judgment and expertise, primary healthcare provider, or a group practitioner consensus. There is not a consensus as to the frequency of testing (e.g., annually or after a certain age). Some will commonly be ordered at point of care.

Use of these guidelines for selecting or eliminating diagnostic tests may aid in effective case management and cost containment. Selecting tests based on evidence-based guidelines can overcome "blanket testing"—in which the provider orders unwarranted tests, often in response to pressure from patients—which has resulted in significant costs to the healthcare system. It can also identify when multiplex testing (conducting multiple tests on a single sample) can be beneficial, such as with autoimmune disorders or genetically inherited disease, producing cost savings in the long run.

Clinical Value of a Test

The clinical value of a test is related to its *sensitivity*, its *specificity*, and the *incidence of the disease* in the population tested.

- *Specificity* refers to the ability of a test to correctly identify individuals who do not have the disease. The formula for specificity is as follows:

$$\text{Specificity (\%)} = \frac{\text{number of true negatives}}{\text{number of true negatives} + \text{number of false positives}} \times 100$$

NOTE *One-hundred percent specificity would indicate there are no false positives—that is, the test identifies all individuals who do not have the disease.*

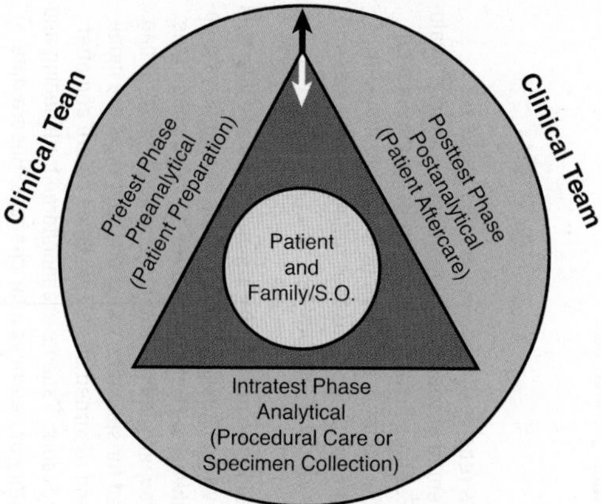

Pretest Interventions

Know test terminology.
Translate into language patient understands.
Assess for test indications, interferences, contraindications; identify risk-prone patients and modify care plan.
Obtain informed consent.
Order appropriate tests correctly.
Prepare and educate patient and family.
Consider ethical and legal aspects.
Support patient and/or family.
Document, report, and maintain proper records.

Intratest Interventions

Follow regulatory standards and institutional policies.
Perform/assist with procedure.
Collect and transport specimens.
Observe standard/universal precautions.
Provide physical support and reassure patient.
Provide comfort; medicate and sedate as necessary.
Facilitate family presence during diagnostic procedures.
Monitor appropriately.
Prevent and/or treat complications.
Report, document, and maintain proper records.

Posttest Interventions

Interpret test results; if abnormal, assess pretest compliance.
Know and treat critical values.
Monitor for posttest sedation and complications.
Follow infection control guidelines.
Provide social support and counsel for unexpected outcomes.
Order follow-up tests at appropriate intervals and inform patient.
Re-educate patient for future testing.
Evaluate the effectiveness of managed care outcomes.
Summarize diagnostic care.
Document and maintain proper records and report results to the patient and clinician as mandated by government.
Help patient integrate test results into lifestyle.

FIGURE 1.1. A model for the role of the clinical team in diagnostic care and services. Diagnostic care and services are performed safely and effectively in all three phases. S.O., significant others.

TABLE 1.2 Standards for Diagnostic Evaluation

Source of Standards for Diagnostic Service	Standards for Diagnostic Testing	Examples of Applied Standards for Diagnostic Testing
Professional practice parameters of American Nurses Association (ANA), American Medical Association (AMA), American Society for Clinical Pathology (ASCP), American College of Radiology, Centers for Disease Control and Prevention (CDC), and The Joint Commission healthcare practice requirements	Use a model as a framework for choosing the proper test or procedure and to interpret test results. Use laboratory and diagnostic procedures for screening, differential diagnoses, follow-up, and case management.	Test strategies include single tests or combinations or panels of tests. Panels can be performed in parallel, as a series, or both. Patient education and proper patient preparation are involved.
The guidelines of the major agencies, such as American Heart Association (e.g., stress tests after abnormal electrocardiogram [ECG]), American Cancer Society (e.g., colonoscopy for colon cancer), and American Diabetes Association (e.g., hemoglobin A_{1c} <7% for diabetes)	Order the correct test; appropriately collect and transport specimens. Properly perform tests in an accredited laboratory or diagnostic facility. Accurately report test results. Communicate and interpret test findings. Treat or monitor the disease and the course of therapy. Provide diagnosis as well as prognosis.	Patients receive diagnostic services based on a documented assessment of need for diagnostic evaluation. Patients have the right to receive information about the benefits and risks of testing so they can make informed decisions that reflect their needs and desires for diagnostic care.
Individual agency and institution standards: • Policies, procedures, and quality control criteria for specimen collection • Procedure statement for monitoring the patient after an invasive procedure • Policy for universal witnessed consent situations • Statements on quality improvement standards • Standards of professional practice and standards of patient care • Policy for obtaining informed consent or witnessed consent • Policies for unusual situations	Observe standard precautions (formerly known as universal precautions). Use latex allergy protocols and required methodology of specimen collection. Use standards and statements for monitoring patients who receive sedation and analgesia. Vital signs are monitored and recorded at specific times before and after the procedure. Patients are monitored for bleeding and respiratory or neurovascular changes. Record data regarding outcomes when defined care criteria are implemented and practiced. Protocols to obtain appropriate consents are employed, and deviations from basic consent policies are documented and reported to the proper individual.	The healthcare provider wears protective eyewear and gloves when handling all body fluids and employs proper handwashing before and after handling specimens and between patient contacts. Labeled biohazard bags are used for specimen transport. Vital signs are monitored and recorded at specific times before and after the procedure. Patients are monitored for bleeding and respiratory or neurovascular changes. Record data regarding outcomes when defined care criteria are implemented and practiced. Protocols to obtain appropriate consents are employed, and deviations from basic consent policies are documented and reported to the proper individual.

State and federal government communicable disease reporting regulations: Centers for Disease Control and Prevention (CDC), U.S. Department of Health & Human Services, Agency for Healthcare Research and Quality (AHRQ), and Clinical Laboratory Improvement Act (CLIA)	Clinical laboratory personnel and other healthcare providers follow regulations to control the spread of communicable diseases by reporting certain disease conditions, outbreaks, and unusual manifestations, morbidity, and mortality data. Findings from research studies provide healthcare policy makers with evidence-based guidelines for appropriate selection of tests and procedures.	The healthcare provider reports laboratory evidence of certain disease classes (e.g., sexually transmitted diseases, diphtheria, Lyme disease, symptomatic HIV infection; see list of reportable diseases). Personnel with hepatitis A may not handle food or care for patients, young children, or elderly people for a specific period of time. Federal government regulates shipment of diagnostic specimens. Magnetic resonance imaging and computed tomography are used to evaluate persistent low back pain according to AHRQ guidelines.
U.S. Department of Transportation	Alcohol testing is done in emergency departments in special situations (e.g., following a motor vehicle crash, homicide, or suicide or in an unconscious individual).	Properly trained personnel perform blood, saliva, and breath alcohol testing and use required kits as referenced by federal law.
Occupational Safety and Health Administration (OSHA)	The healthcare provider is properly trained, under mandated guidelines, to administer employee medical surveillance.	Properly trained personnel perform respirator qualification, fit testing, and monitoring for toxic exposure.
Clinical and Laboratory Standards Institute (CLSI)	Develops standards and guidelines for laboratory testing. Standards define specific materials, methods, and practices as they relate to laboratory specimen tests. Guidelines describe essential criteria for a procedure that can be modified by the user to fit his or her needs.	Provides healthcare professionals with practical guidelines for consistency in procedural methods in laboratory testing.

CHART 1.1 Grading Guidelines for Scientific Evidence

Grade	Guideline	Example
A	Clear evidence from all appropriately conducted trials	Measure plasma glucose through an accredited lab to diagnose or screen for diabetes
B	Supportive evidence from well-conducted studies or registries	Draw fasting blood plasma specimens for glucose analysis
C	No published evidence; or only case, observational, or historical evidence	Self-monitoring of blood glucose may help to achieve better control
E	Expert consensus or clinical experience or Internet polls	Measure ketones in urine or blood to monitor and diagnose diabetic keto acidosis (DKA) (in home or clinic)

- *Sensitivity* refers to the ability of a test to correctly identify individuals who have the disease. The formula for sensitivity is as follows:

$$\text{Sensitivity (\%)} = \frac{\text{number of true positives}}{\text{number of true positives} + \text{number of false negatives}} \times 100$$

NOTE *One-hundred percent sensitivity would indicate there are no false negatives—that is, the test identifies all individuals with the disease as having the disease.*

- *True positive*: positive test result in a person with the disease
- *True negative*: negative test result in a person without the disease
- *False positive*: positive test result in a person without the disease
- *False negative*: negative test result in a person with the disease

Sensitivity and specificity do not change with different populations of ill and healthy patients.

- *Incidence* refers to the number of new cases of a disease, during a specified period of time, in a specified population or community.
- *Prevalence* refers to the number of existing cases of a disease, at a specific period of time, in a given population.
- *Predictive values* refer to the ability of a screening test result to correctly identify the disease state. The predictive value of a test can be very different when applied to people of differing ages, gender, geographic locations, and cultures. *True-positive results* correctly identify individuals who actually have the disease, and *true-negative results* correctly identify individuals who do not actually have the disease. *Positive predictive value* equals the percentage of positive tests with true-positive results (i.e., the individual does have the disease). *Negative predictive value* refers to the percentage of negative tests with true-negative results (i.e., the individual does not have the disease).

$$\text{Positive predictive value} = \frac{\text{number of true positives}}{\text{number of true positives} + \text{number of false positives}} \times 100$$

$$\text{Negative predictive value} = \frac{\text{number of true negatives}}{\text{number of true negatives} + \text{number of false negatives}} \times 100$$

See Table 1.3 for an example that demonstrates the specificity, sensitivity, and predictive values for a screening test to identify the cystic fibrosis gene.

$$\text{Specificity (\%)} = \frac{341}{346} \times 100 = 98.5\%$$

TABLE 1.3 Sample Test Results

Test Result	Have Gene for Cystic Fibrosis	Do Not Have Gene for Cystic Fibrosis	Total
Positive	62	5	67
Negative	15	341	356
TOTAL	77	346	423

$$\text{Sensitivity (\%)} = \frac{62}{77} \times 100 = 80.5\%$$

Thus, this screening test will give a false-negative result about 20% of the time (e.g., the person does have the cystic fibrosis gene but his or her test results are negative).

$$\text{Positive predictive value} = \frac{62}{67} \times 100 = 92.5\%$$

Thus, there is an 8% chance that the person will test positive for the cystic fibrosis gene but does not have it.

$$\text{Negative predictive value} = \frac{341}{356} \times 100 = 95.7\%$$

Thus, there is a 5% chance that the person will test negative for the cystic fibrosis gene but actually does have it.

Test Results

It is important to understand normal or reference values/intervals and ranges.

1. Normal ranges can vary to some degree from laboratory to laboratory. Frequently, this is because of the particular type of equipment used. Theoretically, *normal* can refer to the ideal health state, to average reference values or intervals, or to types of statistical distribution. Normal values are those that fall within two standard deviations of the mean value for the normal population. The reference interval typically represents the upper and lower limits wherein 95% of healthy people would fall. Although establishing normal or reference values is complex, it is much more so in the pediatric population. There are many challenges related to gender- and age-specific reference intervals in the pediatric population.
2. The reported reference range for a test can vary according to the laboratory used, the method employed, the population tested, and methods of specimen collection and preservation.
3. Most normal blood test values are determined by measuring fasting specimens.
4. Specific factors can influence test results. For example, patient posture can significantly alter the values for plasma volume, hemoglobin, hematocrit, and a number of other laboratory values.

Laboratories must specify their own normal ranges. Many factors affect laboratory test values and influence ranges. Thus, values may be normal under one set of prevailing conditions but may exhibit different limits in other circumstances. Age, gender, race, environment, posture, diurnal and other cyclic variations, foods, beverages, fasting or postprandial state, drugs, and exercise can affect derived values. Interpretation of laboratory results must always be in the context of the patient's state of being. Circumstances such as hydration, nutrition, fasting state, mental status, or compliance with test protocols are only a few of the situations that can influence test outcomes.

Units of Measurement

Scientific publications and many professional organizations are changing clinical laboratory data values from conventional U.S. units (also referred to as U.S. customary units) to Système International (SI) units. Currently, many data are reported in both units.

The SI system uses seven dimensionally independent units of measurement to provide logical and consistent measurements. For example, SI concentrations are written as amount per volume (moles or millimoles per liter) rather than as mass per volume (grams, milligrams, or milliequivalents per deciliter, 100 milliliters, or liter). Numerical values may differ between systems or may be the same. For example, chloride is the same in both systems: 95 to 105 mEq/L (conventional) and 95 to 105 mmol/L (SI).

Converting to Système International Units

Clinical laboratory data may be reported in conventional U.S. units, SI units, or both. Examples of conversion of data from the two systems are included in Table 1.4. To convert SI units to conventional U.S. units, *divide* by the factor; to convert conventional U.S. units to SI units, *multiply* by the factor.

Example:

To convert a digoxin (drug management) level of 0.6 nmol/L (SI units), *divide* by the factor 1.281 to obtain conventional units of 0.5 ng/dL.

To convert a Ca^{2+} (electrolyte) value of 8.6 mg/dL (conventional units), *multiply* by the factor 0.2495 to obtain the SI units of 2.15 mmol/L.

Margins of Error

Recognize margins of error. For example, if a patient has a battery of chemistry tests, the possibility exists that some tests will be abnormal owing purely to chance. This occurs because a significant margin of error arises from the arbitrary setting of limits. Moreover, if a laboratory test is considered normal up to the 95th percentile, then 5 times out of 100, the test will show an abnormality even though a patient is not ill. A second test performed on the same sample will probably yield the following: 0.95 × 0.95, or 90.25%. This means that 9.75 times out of 100, a test will show an abnormality even though the person has no underlying health disorder. Each successive testing will produce a higher percentage of abnormal results. If the patient has a group of tests performed on one blood sample, the possibility that some of the tests will read abnormal due purely to chance is not uncommon.

DIAGNOSTIC TESTING AND THE HEALTHCARE DELIVERY SYSTEM

Testing Environments

Diagnostic testing occurs in many different environments. Many test sites have shifted into community settings and away from hospitals and clinics.

- *Point-of-care testing* (POCT) refers to medical testing done in close proximity to the site of patient care (e.g., in the primary care setting or acute care settings [emergency department, critical care units, ambulances]), thus moving toward decentralized testing. POCT is convenient for the patient, produces rapid reporting of test results, and allows for more timely assessment, management, and treatment.
- Testing in the home care environment requires skill in procedures such as drawing blood samples, collecting specimens from retention catheters, proper labeling, handling, and transporting of specimens, and documentation. Moreover, teaching the patient and family members how to collect specimens is an important part of the process.

TABLE 1.4 Examples of Conversions to Système International (SI) Units

Component	System	Conventional U.S. Reference Intervals	Conventional U.S. Unit	Conversion Factor	SI Reference Intervals	SI Unit Symbol
Alanine aminotransferase (ALT)	Serum	5–40	U/L	1.00	5–40	U/L
Albumin	Serum	3.9–5.0	g/dL	10	39–50	g/L
Alkaline phosphatase	Serum	35–110	U/L	0.01667	0.6–1.8	μkat/L
Aspartate aminotransferase (AST)	Serum	5–40	U/L	0.01667	0.08–0.67	μkat/L
Bilirubin	Serum					
Direct		0–0.2	mg/dL	17.10	0–4	μmol/L
Total		0.1–1.2	mg/dL	17.10	2–20	μmol/L
Calcium	Serum	8.6–10.3	mg/dL	0.2495	2.15–2.57	mmol/L
Carbon dioxide, total	Serum	22–30	mEq/L	1.00	22–30	mmol/L
Chloride	Serum	98–108	mEq/L	1.00	98–108	mmol/L
Cholesterol	Serum					
Age <29 yr		<200	mg/dL	0.02586	<5.15	mmol/L
30–39 yr		<225	mg/dL	0.02586	<5.80	mmol/L
40–49 yr		<245	mg/dL	0.02586	<6.35	mmol/L
>50 yr		<265	mg/dL	0.02586	<6.85	mmol/L
Complete blood count	Blood					
Hematocrit						
Men		42–52	%	0.01	0.42–0.52	1
Women		37–47	%	0.01	0.37–0.47	1
Red cell count	Blood					
Men		4.6–6.2 × 10^6	/mm^3	10^6	4.6–6.2 × 10^{12}/L	
Women		4.2–5.4 × 10^6	/mm^3	10^6	4.2–5.4 × 10^{12}/L	
White cell count		4.5–11.0 × 10^3	/mm^3	10^6	4.5–11.0 × 10^9/L	
Platelet count		150–300 × 10^3	/mm^3	10^6	150–300 × 10^9/L	
Cortisol	Serum					
8 AM		5–25	μ/dL	27.59	140–690	nmol/L
8 PM		3–13	μg/dL	27.59	80–360	nmol/L

table continues on pg. 12 >

TABLE 1.4, continued

Component	System	Conventional U.S. Reference Intervals	Conventional U.S. Unit	Conversion Factor	SI Reference Intervals	SI Unit Symbol
Cortisol	Urine	20–90	μg/24 hr	2.759	55–250	nmol/24 hr
Creatine kinase (CK)	Serum					
High CK group (black men)		50–250	U/L	1.00	50–250	U/L
Intermediate CK group (nonblack men, black women)		35–345	U/L	1.00	35–345	U/L
Low CK group (nonblack women)		25–145	U/L	1.00	25–145	U/L
Creatinine kinase isoenzyme, MB fraction	Serum	>5	%	0.01	>0.05	1
Creatinine	Serum	0.4–1.3	mg/dL	88.40	35–115	μmol/L
Men		0.7–1.3	mg/dL	88.40	62–115	μmol/L
Women		0.4–1.1	mg/dL	88.40	35–97	μmol/L
Digoxin, therapeutic	Serum	0.5–2.0	ng/mL	1.281	0.6–2.6	nmol/L
Erythrocyte indices	Blood					
Mean corpuscular volume (MCV)		80–100	$microns^3$	1.00	80–100	fL
Mean corpuscular hemoglobin (MCH)		27–31	pg	1.00	27–31	pg
Mean corpuscular hemoglobin concentration (MCHC)		32–36	%	0.01	0.32–0.36	1
Ferritin	Serum					
Men		29–438	ng/mL	1.00	29–438	μg/L
Women		9–219	ng/mL	1.00	9–219	μg/L
Folate	Serum	2.5–20.0	ng/mL	2.266	6–46	nmol/L
Follicle-stimulating hormone (FSH)	Serum					
Children		≤12	mIU/mL	1.00	≤12	IU/L
Men		2.0–10.0	mIU/mL	1.00	2.0–10.0	IU/L
Women, follicular		3.2–9.0	mIU/mL	1.00	3.2–9.0	IU/L
Women, midcycle		3.2–9.0	mIU/mL	1.00	3.2–9.0	IU/L
Women, luteal		2.0–6.2	mIU/mL	1.00	2.0–6.2	IU/L
Gases, arterial	Blood					
PO_2		80–95	mm Hg	0.1333	10.7–12.7	kPa
PCO_2		37–43	mm Hg	0.1333	4.9–5.7	kPa

Glucose	Serum	62–110	mg/dL	0.05551	3.4–6.1	mmol/L
Iron	Serum	50–160	μg/dL	0.1791	9–29	μmol/L
Iron-binding capacity	Serum					
Total iron-binding capacity		230–410	μg/dL	0.1791	41–73	μmol/L
Saturation		15–55	%	0.01	0.15–0.55	1
Lactate dehydrogenase	Serum	120–300	U/L	1.00	120–300	U/L
Luteinizing hormone	Serum					
Men		4.9–15.0	mIU/mL	1.00	4.9–15.0	IU/L
Women, follicular		5.0–25	mIU/mL	1.00	5.0–25	IU/L
Women, luteal		3.1–13	mIU/mL	1.00	3.1–13	IU/L
Magnesium	Serum	1.2–1.9	mEq/L	0.4114	0.50–0.78	mmol/L
Osmolality	Serum	278–300	mOsm/kg	1.00	278–300	mmol/kg
Osmolality	Urine	None defined	mOsm/kg	1.00	None defined	mmol/kg
Phenobarbital, therapeutic	Serum	15–40	μg/mL	4.306	65–175	μmol/L
Phenytoin, therapeutic	Serum	10–20	μg/mL	3.964	40–80	μmol/L
Phosphate (phosphorus, inorganic)	Serum	2.3–4.1	mg/dL	0.3229	0.75–1.35	mmol/L
Potassium	Serum	3.7–5.1	mEq/L g/mL	1.00	3.7–5.1	mmol/L
Protein, total	Serum	6.5–8.3	g/dL	10.0	65–83	g/L
Sodium	Serum	134–142	mEq/L	1.00	134–142	mmol/L
Theophylline, therapeutic	Serum	5–20	μg/mL	5.550	28–110	μmol/L
Thyroid-stimulating hormone (TSH)	Serum	0–5	μIU/mL	1.00	0–5	mIU/L
Thyroxine	Serum	4.5–13.2	μg/dL	12.87	58–170	nmol/L
T_3-uptake ratio	Serum	0.88–1.19	1	1.00	0.88–1.19	1
Triiodothyronine (T_3)	Serum	70–235	ng/mL	0.01536	1.1–3.6	nmol/L
Triglycerides	Serum	50–200	mg/dL	0.01129	0.55–2.25	mmol/L
Urate (uric acid)	Serum					
Men		2.9–8.5	mg/dL	59.48	170–510	μmol/L
Women		2.2–6.5	mg/dL	59.48	130–390	μmol/L
Urea nitrogen	Serum	6–25	mg/dL	0.3570	2.1–8.9	mmol/L
Vitamin B_{12}	Serum	250–1000	pg/mL	0.7378	180–740	pmol/L

Source: Blair ER (ed.): Damon Clinical Laboratories Handbook. Stow, OH, Lexi-Comp, 1989.

- In occupational environments, testing may be done to reduce or prevent known workplace hazards (e.g., exposure to lead) and to monitor identified health problems. This can include preemployment baseline screening, periodic monitoring of exposure to potentially hazardous workplace substances, and drug screening. Skill is required in drawing blood samples, performing breathing tests, monitoring and documenting chain of custody, and obtaining properly signed and witnessed consent forms for drug, genetic, and HIV testing.
- Nursing homes and long-term care facilities tend to produce more routine pretest, posttest, and follow-up testing because patients are frequently taken or transferred to hospitals for more complex procedures (e.g., computed tomography [CT] scans, endoscopies). Increasing numbers of full code (i.e., resuscitation) orders lead to greater numbers and varieties of tests. In addition, confused, combative, or uncooperative behaviors are seen more frequently in these settings. Understanding patient behaviors and using appropriate communication strategies and interventions for this patient population are necessary skills.
- In the realm of public health, diagnostic test responsibilities focus on wellness screenings, preventive services, disease control, counseling, and treatment of individuals with problems. Case finding frequently occurs at health fairs, outreach centers, homeless shelters, municipal health departments, mobile health vans, and church settings. Responsibilities vary according to setting and may include providing test information, procuring specimens, and recommending referrals to appropriate caregivers. These responsibilities may even extend to transporting and preparing specimens for analysis or actually performing specimen analysis (e.g., stool tests for occult blood, tuberculosis (TB) skin testing, and procuring blood or saliva samples for HIV/AIDS testing).

The type of setting may also be determined by the type of test. Certain tests (e.g., cholesterol screening, blood glucose, electrocardiogram [ECG], lipid profiles, TB skin tests) can be done in the field, meaning that the service is brought to the patient's environment. Other tests (e.g., x-rays using contrast media and those that require special patient preparation, invasive procedures, nuclear medicine procedures, hormone levels, and 24-hour urine testing panels) must be done in a healthcare setting. Magnetic resonance imaging (MRI) and ultrasound procedures are commonly performed in freestanding or specialty diagnostic centers. Complex tests such as endoscopic retrograde cholangiopancreatography (ERCP), cardiac catheterization, and bronchoscopy may require hospital admission or at minimum outpatient status. As testing equipment becomes more technologically sophisticated and risks associated with testing are reduced, the environment in which diagnostic procedures take place will also shift.

Although patient populations and testing environments vary, the potential contagions are universal and of concern for both the patient and the healthcare provider. *Standard precautions must be used in all testing environments to ensure safety for patients and healthcare providers.* Refer to Appendix A for an in-depth discussion of standard precautions.

Reimbursement for Diagnostic Services

Differences in both diagnostic care services and reimbursement may vary between private and government insurance. Nonetheless, quality of care should not be compromised in favor of cost reduction. Advocate for patients regarding insurance coverage for diagnostic services by informing the patient and his or her family or significant others that it may be necessary to check with their insurance company before laboratory and diagnostic testing to make certain that costs are covered. Coordinate with other healthcare team members, such as social workers and facility billing staff, for resources regarding insurance reimbursement.

Many insurance companies employ case managers to monitor costs, diagnostic tests ordered, and other care. As a result, the insurance company or third-party payer may reimburse only for certain tests or procedures or may not cover tests they consider to be not medically necessary. To help facilitate reimbursement for diagnostic services, be sure to include proper documentation (e.g., date of laboratory

CHART 1.2 Tests Covered by Most Insurance Carriers

α-Fetoprotein
Blood counts
Blood glucose testing
Carcinoembryonic antigen
Collagen crosslinks, any method (urine osteoporosis)
Digoxin therapeutic drug assay
Fecal occult blood
γ-Glutamyltransferase
Glycated hemoglobin/glycated protein
Hepatitis panel
HIV testing (diagnosis)
HIV testing (prognosis including monitoring)
Human chorionic gonadotropin
Lipids
Partial thromboplastin time
Prostate-specific antigen
Prothrombin time
Serum iron studies
Thyroid testing
Tumor antigen by immunoassay—CA125
Tumor antigen by immunoassay—CA15-3/CA27
Tumor antigen by immunoassay—CA19-9
Urine culture

service and specimen collected) and proper current procedural terminology (CPT) codes. Chart 1.2 lists laboratory tests that are covered by most insurance carriers, both private and government, which should be taken into consideration by the healthcare provider when selecting an appropriate test.

THE HEALTHCARE PROVIDER'S ROLE IN LABORATORY AND DIAGNOSTIC TESTING

Understanding the basics of safe, effective, and informed care is important. These basics include assessing risk factors and modifying care accordingly, using a collaborative approach, following proper guidelines for procedures and specimen collection, and delivering appropriate care throughout the process. Providing reassurance and support to the patient and his or her significant others, intervening appropriately, and clearly documenting patient teaching, observations, and outcomes during the entire process are necessary (refer to Fig. 1.1).

NOTE *Eighty-seven percent of adults in the United States use the Internet, and 72% of those adults use the Internet for health information. However, not all information on the Internet is complete or accurate; therefore, the healthcare provider plays a vital role in educating and supporting the patient about laboratory tests and diagnostic procedures.*

Preparing patients for diagnostic or therapeutic procedures, collecting specimens, carrying out and assisting with procedures, and providing follow-up care have long been requisite activities of professional practice. If test results are inconclusive or negative and no definitive medical diagnosis can be established, other tests and procedures may be ordered. Thus, testing can become an involved and lengthy process. This care may continue even after the patient's death. Diagnostic postmortem services include death reporting, possible postmortem investigations, and sensitive communication with grieving families and significant others regarding autopsies, unexplained death, other postmortem testing, and organ donation.

Healthcare providers need to work as a team to meet diverse patient needs, to facilitate certain decisions, to develop comprehensive plans of care, and to help patients modify their daily activities to meet test requirements in all three phases.

Insurance reimbursement for testing also influences trends. Managed care and case management, together with collaboration among the diverse healthcare disciplines and the patient, are key factors in determining how and to what degree optimal diagnostic services are used.

As societies become more culturally blended, the need to appreciate and work within the realm of cultural diversity becomes imperative. Interacting with patients and directing them through diagnostic testing can present certain challenges if one is not familiar with and sensitive to the healthcare belief system of the patient and his or her significant others. When facing language differences, it may be necessary for a translator to be present during all phases of the process to ensure clear communication. Special attention and communication skills are necessary for these situations as well as when caring for children and for comatose, confused, or frail patients. Consideration of these issues will significantly influence compliance, outcomes, and positive responses to the procedure. To be most effective, healthcare providers must be open to a holistic perspective and attitude that affects their caregiving, communication, and patient-empowering behaviors. Healthcare providers who understand the patient's basic needs and expectations and strive to accommodate those as much as possible are truly acting as patient advocates.

ELEMENTS OF SAFE, EFFECTIVE, INFORMED CARE THROUGHOUT THE TESTING PROCESS

There are several key elements that must be considered and applied in order to ensure safe, effective informed care throughout the pretest, intratest, and posttest phases.

Communication

At the heart of informed patient-centered care is the ability to communicate effectively. Frequently, communication must take place within a compressed time frame because of time constraints. Thus, the importance of communicating effectively cannot be emphasized enough. Effective communication is the key to achieving desired outcomes, preventing misunderstanding and errors, and helping patients feel that they are secure, informed partners and are connected to the diagnostic process. One must always keep in mind that the human person is an integration of body, mind, and spirit and that these three entities are intimately bound together to make each person unique. Skillful assessment of physical, emotional, psychosocial, and spiritual dimensions provides a sound database from which to plan communication and teaching or instruction strategies.

Individuals have different needs and changing capacities for learning as they progress from child to adult to older adult. It is important for the healthcare provider to know the different developmental levels and stages and the ways in which clear communication can be achieved at any level.

For the pediatric patient, teaching tools might include tours of the diagnostic area, play therapy, films or videos, models of equipment that the child can touch or manipulate, and written materials and pictures appropriate to the child's developmental stage. Shorter attention spans and the unpredictable nature of children can make teaching a challenge in this population. Mentally retarded or mentally ill patients may need significant others close by who can guide communication between caregiver and patient. Gentle, simple, nurturing behaviors usually work well with children and developmentally challenged individuals.

Adolescents may be at the stage of developing their own unique identity as they move toward adulthood. Teaching may be more effective without parents present; however, it is important to include parents at some point. Drawings, illustrations, or videos are helpful. Because body image is very important at this stage, honest, supportive behaviors are necessary, especially if some alteration in physical appearance will be necessary (e.g., removal of jewelry, no makeup allowed).

The opportunity to participate actively and to ask questions is important for adults. They bring to the communication process their lifetime of perceptions and experiences. This can be a proverbial double-edged sword. Listening well to verbal cues, as well as paying attention to nonverbal messages, cannot be overemphasized. For example, interacting with patients who have Alzheimer's disease can present special challenges. The presence of a significant other who has experience communicating with this patient can be the key to performing a successful procedure.

Provide an environment that is quiet, private, and free of distractions to promote dialogue and communication. Ask by what name or title the patient wishes to be addressed. Referring to a patient as a room number, a procedure, or a disease is demeaning and inexcusable—it reduces the patient to the level of an object rather than a person.

Nonverbal communication behaviors such as proper eye contact, firm handshake, sense of respect, and *appropriate* humor can reduce anxiety. Do not dismiss the power of touch, the sense of making time for the patient, and the use of appropriate and positive verbal cues. The greater part of communication (>70%) is perceived through body language. If words do not match body language and behaviors, patients will react to the body language they observe as their primary frame of reference. Negative communication by caregivers often is experienced by patients as an uncaring attitude and results in a sense of discouragement.

Every person engaged in the *entire* process of testing is a link in the ongoing communication continuum. This continuum is only as effective as the weakest link that joins all activities and all communication together.

Testing Protocols

Develop consistent protocols for teaching and testing that encompass comprehensive pretest, intratest, and posttest care modalities. Prepare patients for those aspects of the procedure experienced by most patients. Healthcare providers can collaborate to collect data and to develop a list of common patient experiences, responses, and reactions.

Interfering Factors

Minimize test outcome deviations by following proper test protocols. Make certain the patient and his or her significant others know what is expected of them. Written instructions are very helpful to remind patients of expectations.

Reasons for deviations may include the following:

1. Incorrect specimen collection, handling, storage, or labeling
2. Wrong preservative or lack of preservative
3. Delayed specimen delivery resulting in old or deteriorating specimens
4. Incorrect or incomplete patient preparation
5. Hemolyzed blood samples
6. Incomplete sample collection, especially of timed samples

Patient factors that can alter test results may include the following:

1. Incorrect pretest diet
2. Current drug therapy
3. Type of illness

4. Dehydration
5. Position or activity at time of specimen collection
6. Postprandial status
7. Time of day
8. Pregnancy
9. Level of patient knowledge and understanding of and cooperation with the testing process
10. Stress
11. Nonadherence or noncompliance with instructions and pretest preparation
12. Undisclosed drug or alcohol use
13. Age and gender

Avoidance of Errors

To avoid mistakes that affect safety, quality, and cost, know what equipment and supplies are needed and how the test is performed. Communication errors account for more incorrect results than do technical errors. Properly identify and label every specimen as soon as it is obtained. Bar code technology reduces transcription error rates and data entry is faster and more accurate. Determine the type of sample needed and the collection method to be used.

In addition, the following should also be considered:

- Is the test invasive or noninvasive?
- Are contrast media injected or swallowed?
- Is there a need to fast?
- Are fluids restricted or forced?
- Are medications administered or withheld?
- What is the approximate length of the procedure?
- Are consent forms properly completed?
- Is a local anesthetic, conscious sedation, oxygen, analgesia, or anesthesia required?

Report test results as soon as possible. Critical values must be reported immediately (STAT, *Latin*: *statim*, instantly/immediately) to the appropriate healthcare provider (e.g., physician, nurse practitioner, nurse, or physician assistant [PA]), depending on institutional policy.

Instruct patients and their significant others regarding their responsibilities. Accurately outline the steps of the testing process and any restrictions that may apply. Conscientious, clear, timely communication among healthcare departments can reduce errors and inconvenience to both staff and patients.

Patient Independence

Allow the patient to maintain as much control as possible during the diagnostic phases to reduce stress and anxiety. Include the patient and his or her significant others in decision making.

Ethics and the Law

Consider legal and ethical implications. These include the patient's right to information, correct diagnosis and prognosis, properly signed and witnessed consent forms, and explanations and instructions regarding chain-of-custody requirements and risks as well as benefits of tests.

1. *Chain of custody* is a legal term descriptive of a procedure to ensure specimen integrity from collection, to transport, to receipt, to analysis and specimen storage. A special form is used to provide a written record. The right to informed consent before certain tests and procedures pertains to patient autonomy, the ethical right of self-determination, the legal right to be free of procedures

to which one does not consent, and the right to determine what will be done to one's own body. Risks, benefits, and alternatives are explained and written consent should be obtained well in advance of the procedure.

2. The patient must demonstrate appropriate cognitive and reasoning faculties to sign a legally valid consent. Conversely, a patient may not legally give consent while under the immediate influence of sedation, anesthetic agents, or certain classes of analgesics and tranquilizers. If the patient cannot validly and legally sign a consent form, an appropriately qualified individual may give consent for the patient.
3. Guidelines and wishes set forth in advance directives or living will documents must be honored, especially in life-threatening situations. Such directives may prevent more sophisticated invasive procedures from being performed. Some states have legislated that patients can procure do-not-resuscitate (DNR) orders and medical DNR bracelets that indicate their wishes. A copy of a patient's advance directives should be in the healthcare record.
4. A collaborative team approach is essential for responsible, lawful, and ethical patient-focused care. The healthcare provider who orders the test has a responsibility to inform the patient about risks and test results and to discuss alternatives for follow-up care. Other healthcare providers can provide additional information and clarification and can support the patient and family in achieving the best possible outcomes. The duty to maintain confidentiality, to provide freedom of choice, and to report infectious diseases may result in ethical dilemmas.
5. When faced with ethical dilemmas, choosing the correct course of action is a challenge. The responsibility to provide safe, effective care may conflict with the ethics of privacy, confidentiality, quality of life, and patient safety. The Health Insurance Portability and Accountability Act (HIPAA) of 1996 has set forth regulations regarding patient confidentiality. Protected health information (PHI) is addressed under HIPAA regulations and includes any information—whether oral, written, electronic, or recorded in any manner—that is created or received by a healthcare provider; relates to the patient's past, present, or future healthcare management; identifies the patient (e.g., Social Security number, medical record number); or can be used to identify a patient. HIPAA also provides rights to patients (e.g., the right to request, amend, correct, or limit their PHI).

Respect for the dignity of the individual reflects basic ethical considerations. Patients and family have a right to consent, to question, to request other opinions, and to refuse diagnostic tests. Conversely, caregivers have the right to know the diagnoses of the patients they care for so that they can minimize the risks to themselves.

Patient's Bill of Rights and Patient Responsibilities

Patients have a right to expect that an agency's or institution's policies and procedures will ensure certain rights and responsibilities for them. At all times, the patient has the right to the following:

1. To considerate, honest, respectful care, with attention given to privacy and maintenance of personal dignity, cultural and personal values and beliefs, and physical and developmental needs, regardless of the setting.
2. To be involved in decision making and to participate actively, if so desired, in the testing process, assuming the patient is competent to make these choices.
3. To participate in the informed consent process before testing and to be told of the benefits, risks, and reasonable alternative approaches to tests ordered.
4. To be informed regarding test costs and reimbursement responsibility.
5. To refuse diagnostic testing.
6. To have ease in making an appointment.
7. To expect to have the support and presence of family or significant others, if so desired and appropriate, during the testing process.

8. To expect that standards of care will be followed by all personnel involved in the testing process and to eliminate duplication of testing and information.
9. To expect safe, skilled, quality care provided by trained personnel with expertise in their field.
10. To expect patient and family education and instructions regarding all phases of the testing process and procedure, including the nature and purpose of the test, pretest preparation, actual testing, posttest care benefits, risks, side effects, and complications. Information is provided in a sensitive and objective manner.
11. To expect to have access to test results and to be informed in a timely manner of test results and implications, treatment, and future testing if necessary.
12. To expect to be counseled appropriately regarding abnormal test outcomes as well as alternative options and available treatments.
13. To expect to have acceptable pain control and comfort measures provided throughout the testing process.
14. To expect that all verbal, written, and electronic communication; medical records; and healthcare record transfers will be accurate and confidential. *Exception: when reporting of situation is required by law (e.g., certain infectious diseases, child abuse).*

The patient has the following responsibilities:

1. To comply with test requirements (e.g., fasting, special preparations, medications, enemas) and to inform the healthcare provider if they are unable to do so.
2. To report active or chronic disease conditions that may alter test outcomes, be adversely affected by the testing process, or pose a risk to healthcare providers.
3. To keep appointments for diagnostic procedures and follow-up testing.
4. To disclose drug and alcohol use as well as use of supplements and herbal products despite being informed that these products could affect test outcomes (e.g., erroneous test results).
5. To disclose allergies and past history of sensitivity and complications or adverse reactions to tests (e.g., reaction to contrast materials or latex allergy).
6. To report any adverse effects attributed to tests and procedures after being advised regarding signs and symptoms of such.
7. To supply specimens that are their own.
8. To report visual or hearing impairments or inability to read, write, or understand English.
9. To report use of performance-enhancing drugs.
10. To inform tester if he or she does not understand testing, the necessity of the test, and his or her involvement in test process.

Cultural Sensitivity

Preserving the cultural well-being of any individual or group promotes compliance with testing and easier recovery from routine as well as more invasive and complex procedures. Sensitive questioning and observation may provide information about certain cultural traditions, concerns, and practices related to health. For example, the Hmong people believe the soul resides in the head and that no one should touch an adult's head without permission. Patting a Hmong child on the head may violate this belief. Healthcare personnel should make an effort to understand the cultural differences of populations they serve without passing judgment. Most people of other cultures are willing to share this information if they feel it will be respected. Sometimes, a translator is necessary for accurate communication.

Many cultures have diverse beliefs about diagnostic testing that requires blood sampling. For example, alarm about having blood specimens drawn or concerns regarding the disposal of body fluids or tissue may require healthcare providers to demonstrate the utmost patience, sensitivity, and tact when communicating information about blood tests. Using ethnographic interviewing helps to access meaningful patient cultural values, increases patient and family acceptance of diagnostic care, and shows respect for the social aspects of the diagnosis.

PRETEST PHASE: ELEMENTS OF SAFE, EFFECTIVE, INFORMED CARE

Pretest care involves appropriate test selection, obtaining and documenting consent, proper patient preparation, individualized patient education, emotional support, and effective communication. These interventions are essential to achieve the desired outcomes and prevent misunderstandings and errors.

Basic Knowledge and Necessary Skills

Know the test terminology and the purpose, process, procedure, and normal reference values or results of the test. Understand the diagnostic process, which begins with assessment of signs and symptoms, involves diagnostic testing and knowledge of normal and pathologic structure and function, and often ends with the labeling of a condition or disease. Be able to describe the test in language the patient understands.

The environments in which diagnostic services are provided, the degree of cultural diversity present in the community, and the physical, emotional, social, and spiritual state of the patient all influence the patient's response to the procedure. Including the patient's significant others is a vital component of the entire process and must not be taken lightly or casually dismissed.

History and Assessment

Obtain a relevant, current health history; perform a physical assessment if indicated. Identify conditions that could influence the actual testing process or test outcomes (e.g., pregnancy, diabetes, cultural needs, language barrier, physical impairment, or altered mental state).

1. Perform a risk assessment for potential injury, adverse event, or noncompliance. A risk assessment before testing identifies risk-prone patients and helps to prevent complications. Factors that increase a patient's risk for complications and may affect test outcomes are listed in Chart 1.3.
2. Identify contraindications to testing such as allergies (e.g., iodine, latex, medications, contrast media). Records of previous diagnostic procedures may provide pertinent information.
3. Assess for coping styles, knowledge deficit, and teaching needs.
4. Assess fears and phobias (e.g., claustrophobia, panic attack, fear of needles and blood). Ascertain what strategies the patient uses to deal with these reactions and try to accommodate these.
5. Observe standard precautions with every patient (see Appendix A).
6. Document relevant data. Address patient concerns and questions. This information adds to the database for collaborative problem-solving activities among the medical, laboratory-diagnostic, and nursing disciplines.

CLINICAL ALERT

Laboratory tests are used to assess a patient's wellness or establish a diagnosis. For example, type 2 diabetes mellitus affects an estimated 28 million Americans, and many of these cases are preventable with a healthy lifestyle. Therefore, monitoring fasting serum glucose levels in at-risk groups (older adults and obese individuals) is indicated. Furthermore, if the serum level is 100 to 125 mg/dL (6.1 to 6.9 mmol/L), a test for glycosylated hemoglobin (HbA_{1c}) would be considered.

Methodology of Testing

1. Verify orders and document them with complete, accurate, and legible information.
2. Document all drugs the patient is taking because these may influence test outcomes (see Appendix E).
3. Follow testing procedures accurately. Ensure that specimens are correctly obtained, preserved, handled, labeled, and delivered to the appropriate department.

CHART 1.3 Factors That Increase a Patient's Risk for Complications and May Affect Test Outcomes

Age ≥65 yr: decrease/increase for expected test outcomes
History of falls
History of chronic illness
History of allergies (e.g., latex, contrast iodine, radiopharmaceuticals, and other medications)
Infection or increased risk for infection (e.g., HIV, organ transplantation, chemotherapy, radiation therapy)
Behavior issues that may affect the patient's ability to follow instructions or participate in the testing procedures
Seizure disorders
Uncontrolled pain
Gastric motility dysfunction
Use of assistive devices for activities of daily living
Unsteady gait, balance problems
Neuromuscular conditions
Weakness, fatigability
Paresthesias
Impaired judgment or illogical thinking
Severe visual problems
Hearing impairment
Use of diuretics, sedatives, analgesics, or other prescription or over-the-counter (OTC) drugs
Alcohol or illegal drug use or addiction

4. Observe precautions for patients in isolation. Use standard precautions or other transmission-based precautions as dictated by infection control policies of the institution.
5. Use personal protective equipment (PPE) as appropriate. PPE standards aim to prevent the transmission of bloodborne pathogens from patients to healthcare providers, and protect patients and healthcare providers alike.
6. As much as possible, coordinate patient activities with testing schedules to avoid conflicts with meal times and administration of medications, treatments, or other diagnostic tests and travel time.
   a. Maintain NPO (i.e., Latin: *non per os*, nothing by mouth) status when necessary.
   b. Administer the proper medications in a timely manner. Schedule tests requiring contrast substances in the proper sequence so as not to invalidate succeeding tests.

Patient Preparation

Prepare the patient correctly. This preparation begins at the time of scheduling and extends to the testing facility.

1. Provide information about the testing site and give directions for locating the facility.
2. Tell the patient to plan to be at the department 15 minutes before testing if the test is scheduled for a specific time. Upon his or her arrival, properly identify the patient by at least two identifiers (e.g., ask the patient to state his or her full name and spell the last name and provide their date of birth). Once the patient's identity has been confirmed, have the patient review any preprinted labels that may be used to label lab specimens and/or wristband if appropriate. Review and clearly explain all pretest instructions with the patient (e.g., if the patient is given fasting directions for a test, explain what *fasting* actually means).

3. Be cognizant of special needs of the patient with physical limitations or disabilities, ostomies, or diabetes; children; elderly patients; and patients with diverse cultural needs or limited health literacy.
4. Give simple, accurate, precise instructions (scripted) according to the patient's level of understanding. For example, the patient needs to know when and what to eat and drink or how long to fast.
5. Encourage dialogue about fears and apprehensions. Walking a patient through the procedure using imagery and relaxation techniques may help the patient to cope with anxieties. Never underestimate the value of a caring, supportive presence.
6. Assess for the patient's ability to read and understand instructions. Poor eyesight or hearing difficulties may impair understanding and compliance. Speak slowly and clearly. Do not bombard the patient with information. Instruct the patient to use assistive devices such as eyeglasses and hearing aids if necessary. Clear, written instructions can reinforce verbal instructions and should be used whenever possible. In some cases, a translator, sign language interpreter, or legal representative may be necessary.
7. Assess for language and cultural barriers. Patients behave according to personal values, perceptions, beliefs, traditions, and cultural and ethnic influences. Take these into consideration and value the patient's uniqueness to the highest degree possible.
8. Document accurately in all testing phases.

Patient Education

Educate the patient and family regarding the testing process and what will be expected of them. Record the date, time, type of teaching, information given, and person(s) to whom the information was given.

1. Provide sensory and objective information that relates to what the patient will likely physically feel and the equipment that will be used. This will allow the patient to envision a realistic representation of what will occur. Avoid technical and medical jargon and adapt information to the patient's level of understanding.
2. Encourage questions and verbalization of feelings, fears, and concerns. Do not dismiss, minimize, or invalidate the patient's anxiety through trivial remarks such as "Don't worry." Develop listening skills and be aware of nonverbal signals (i.e., body language) because these frequently provide a more accurate picture of what the patient really feels than what he or she says. Use therapeutic communication skills to support the patient.
3. Emphasize that there is usually a waiting period (i.e., turnaround time) before test results are relayed back to the healthcare providers and nursing unit. The patient may have to wait several days for results. Offer listening, presence, and support during this time of great concern and anxiety.
4. Record test result information. Include the patient's response. The possibility that a diagnosis will require a patient to make significant lifestyle changes (e.g., diabetes) requires intense support, understanding, education, and motivation. Document specific names of audiovisual and reading materials to be used for audit, reimbursement, and accreditation purposes.

Factors such as anxiety, language barriers, and physical or emotional impairments may impact the patient's ability to fully understand and assimilate instructions and explanations. To validate the patient's understanding of what is presented, ask the patient to repeat instructions given to evaluate assimilation and understanding of presented information.

Include and reinforce information about the diagnostic plan, the procedure, time frames, and the patient's role in the testing process.

INTRATEST PHASE: ELEMENTS OF SAFE, EFFECTIVE, INFORMED CARE

Intratest care focuses on specimen or tissue collection, monitoring the testing environment, performing or assisting with procedures, providing emotional and physical comfort and reassurance, administering analgesics and sedatives, and monitoring vital signs and other parameters during testing.

Basic Knowledge and Necessary Skills

The healthcare provider needs basic knowledge about the procedure and test and should have the required skills to perform testing or to assist in the process. Safe practices, proper collection of specimens, minimizing delays, providing support to the patient, preparing or administering analgesia and sedatives, monitoring various bio-parameters as necessary, and being alert to potential side effects or complications are integral activities of the intratest phase. Invasive procedures place patients at greater risk for complications and adverse events and require ongoing vigilance and observation. Monitoring fluid intake and loss, body temperature, and respiratory and cardiovascular systems and treating problems in these domains require critical thinking and quick responses.

Infection Prevention

Follow accepted infection prevention and control protocols. Observe special measures and sterile techniques as appropriate. Identify patients at risk for infection, such as immunocompromised patients. Initiate strict respiratory and contact isolation as necessary. Quality assurance requires proper collection, transport, and receipt of specimens and use of properly cleaned and prepared instruments and equipment. Refer to Appendix A for additional information on standard precautions for safe practice, infection control, isolation, quarantine surveillance, and reporting. The term *standard precautions* refers to a system of disease control that presupposes that each direct contact with body fluids or tissues is potentially infectious and that every person exposed to these must protect him- or herself. Consequently, healthcare providers must be both informed and conscientious about adhering to standard precautions and strict infection control guidelines.

Healthcare providers must be scrupulous about proper hand hygiene. According to the Centers for Disease Control and Prevention (CDC), proper hand hygiene must be practiced before patient contact and before donning gloves, when inserting catheters or other devices that do not require surgery, and after contact with a patient's skin, body fluids, or wound dressings and after removing gloves. Proper protective clothing and other devices, or PPE, must be worn as necessary.

Procurement and disposal of specimens according to U.S. Occupational Safety and Health Administration (OSHA) standards must be followed. Moreover, institutions may have procedures and policies of their own to ensure compliance (e.g., specimens are to be placed directly into biohazard bags).

NOTE *Standard precautions prevail in all situations in which risk for exposure to blood, tissue, and other body fluids is even remotely possible.*

NOTE *Communicable diseases subject to quarantine include cholera, diphtheria, infectious TB, plague, yellow fever, smallpox, viral hemorrhagic fevers (e.g., Lassa, Marburg, Ebola), and severe acute respiratory syndrome (SARS). Individuals are quarantined in an effort to reduce the transmission or spread of communicable diseases.*

Collaborative Approaches

A collaborative team approach is necessary for most procedures. Healthcare providers must assist and understand each other's roles in the procedure. Invasive procedures (e.g., lumbar punctures, cystoscopy) place patients at greater risk for complications and usually require closer monitoring during the test. Frequently, administration of intravenous (IV) sedation and other drugs is part of the procedure. Astute ongoing observation of the patient and critical thinking and quick decision-making skills during intense situations are requisites for healthcare providers in these settings.

TABLE 1.5 Classification of Risk Factors for a Higher Incidence of Adverse Reactions When Contrast Agents and Radiopharmaceuticals Are Used

Preexisting Disorders	Other Contributing Elements
Asthma	Allergy
Diabetes	Age-related (newborn and older adults)
Liver insufficiency	Dehydration
Multiple myeloma	Frequent use of contrast agents
Pheochromocytoma	High dosage of contrast and radiopharmaceuticals
Renal failure	Previous reaction to contrast agents
Seizure history	

Risk Management

Assess for and provide a safe environment for the patient at all times. Identify patients at risk and environments that may pose a risk. Previous falls, cerebrovascular accident (CVA), neuromuscular disorders, loss of balance, and use of ambulatory and other assistive devices are contributory risk factors (see Chart 1.3). Prevention of complications and management of risk factors are an important part of the intratest phase. As part of risk management, observe standard precautions and infection control protocols as necessary (see Appendix A).

Use special care during procedures that require iodine and barium contrasts, radiopharmaceuticals, latex products, sedation, and analgesia. Certain risk factors contribute to a higher incidence of adverse reactions when contrast agents and radiopharmaceuticals are used (Table 1.5). Remove jewelry, false teeth, and other prosthetic devices as necessary. Check for NPO or fasting status if appropriate.

Specimens and Procedures

The healthcare provider conducts or assists with certain diagnostic procedures. Examples of the types of assisted procedures include endoscopy, lumbar puncture, and cardiac catheterization. Diagnostic procedures often performed independently of other healthcare providers include Papanicolaou (Pap) test, centrifugation of blood samples, ECG, breathing tests, and pulse oximetry.

Collecting specimens and conducting procedures are the main interventions in the diagnostic pretest and intratest phases. Procure, process, transport, and store specimens properly. The community environment and healthcare settings in which testing takes place dictate protocols for doing this. Everyone involved in the process must have a thorough understanding of testing principles and protocols and must adhere to them to ensure accurate results.

Determine specimen type needed and method of sample procurement. Special equipment and supplies may be necessary (e.g., sterile containers, special kits).

There are three methods of collection: collection by the patient, supervised collection, and collection by the healthcare provider. Collection by the patient requires patient cooperation, understanding, and instruction. It does not always require direct supervision, as in a routine urine sample collected by the patient privately. Supervised collection requires supervision of the patient by trained personnel during specimen collection, as in a urine sample procured in a supervised setting for drug screening. An example of the third method of collection, in which the healthcare provider performs the entire collection, is aspirating a urine sample from an indwelling catheter.

Time of collection is also important. For example, results from a fasting blood glucose test versus results from a glucose tolerance test are significantly different as diagnostic parameters.

TABLE 1.6 Errors in Collection

Specimen Errors	Collector Errors
Insufficient volume	Transport delay
Improper type	Improper collection method
Insufficient number of samples	Wrong specimen container
Wrong transport medium or wrong or absent preservative	Incorrect documentation; wrong date or time
Storage at incorrect temperature	Incorrect storage
Incorrect order of draw	Air bubbles in tube
Improper centrifugation time	Unlabeled or mislabeled specimen and/or wrong patient identification information
Clotted sample	Improperly completed forms or computer data entry
Hemolyzed sample	Test tapes cut in half
Diluted sample	Discrepancies between test ordered and specimen collected
	Failure to properly transcribe and process orders

Note: Observing institutional protocols can prevent mishaps. Large-scale (affecting many patients) testing errors can result from improperly maintained or calibrated equipment at the site of sample analysis. There should be policies/procedures in place to address specimen, collection, and/or large-scale errors to include who should be notified and remedial action.

Specimens can be rejected for analysis because of factors related to the specimen itself or to the collection process (Table 1.6).

Blood collection is normally done by trained persons. (An exception is the self-test for blood glucose using equipment designed specifically for that purpose.) The time of collection is an important factor (e.g., a sequence of samples for a cardiac panel). For example, a peak drug level blood specimen is collected when highest drug concentration in the blood is expected. This type of test is used for therapeutic drug management and dosing. Conversely, a trough sample is collected when lowest drug concentration is expected. These types of tests are used for therapeutic drug monitoring, and specimens are collected and results reported before the next scheduled dose of medication.

Legal and forensic specimens are collected as evidence in legal proceedings, for criminal investigations, and after death. Examples include DNA samples and drug and alcohol levels. Factors such as chain-of-custody situations and witnessed collections may be involved.

The following list addresses some general comments about specimen collections:

1. Stool and urine collection requires clean, dry containers and kits.
2. Timed urine collection requires refrigeration or containers with special additives (preservatives).
3. Sterile, dry containers and special kits are needed for midstream clean-catch urine specimens.
4. Oral, saliva, and sputum specimens require specific techniques and kits and, sometimes, special preservatives.
5. Blood collection equipment includes gloves, needles, collection tubes, syringes, tourniquets, needle disposal containers, lancets for skin puncture, cleansing agents or antimicrobial skin preparations, gauze, and adhesive bandages.
6. Color-coded stoppers and tubes indicate the type of additive present in the collection tube (Table 1.7).
7. Additives preserve the specimen, prevent deterioration and coagulation, or block action of certain enzymes in blood cells.
8. Tubes with anticoagulants should be gently and completely inverted (end-over-end) 7 to 10 times after collection. This process ensures complete mixing of anticoagulants with the blood sample and prevents clot formation.

TABLE 1.7 Blood Specimen Collection Tube Colors

Collection Tube Color and Additives[a]	Use and Precautions
Yellow-topped tube: sodium polyethylene sulfonate (SPS)	For collection of blood cultures; aseptic technique for blood draw. Invert tube 8–10 times to prevent clot formation.
Light blue–topped tube: with sodium citrate as anticoagulant (removes calcium to prevent clotting)	For plasma-coagulation studies (e.g., prothrombin time [PT]; PT/partial thromboplastin time [PTT] and factor assays). The tube *must* be allowed to fill to its capacity or an improper blood/anticoagulant ratio will invalidate coagulation test results. Invert tube 3–4 times to prevent clotting.
Red or gold serum separator tubes (SSTs); no anticoagulant	For collecting serum samples such as chemistry analysis. SST tubes should be gently inverted (completely, end over end) 5 times after collection to ensure mixing of clot activator with blood and clotting within 30 min. After the 30-min period, centrifuge promptly at designated relative centrifugal force (rcf) for 15 ± 5 min to separate serum from cells. Serum can be stored in gel separator tubes after centrifugation for up to 48 hr. Do not freeze SST tubes. If frozen specimen is needed, separate serum into a labeled plastic transfer vial. Serum separation tubes must not be used to obtain therapeutic drug levels because the gel may lower the values.
Red-topped (plain) tube: no anticoagulant, no additive	For serum chemistry, serology, blood bank, collection of clotted blood specimens. Mix by inverting 5 times.
Royal blue–topped tube: without ethylenediaminetetraacetic acid (EDTA) or sodium heparin (no anticoagulant—blood will clot)	For aluminum, arsenic, chromium, copper, nickel, and zinc levels; tube free of trace elements
Gold or red marbled–topped tube: gel serum separator tube (SST)	For serum, used for most chemistry tests; these tubes should be gently inverted 5 times after collection to ensure mixing of clot activator with blood and clotting within 30 min. After 30-min period, centrifuge promptly at designated rcf for 15 ± 5 min to separate serum from cells. Serum can be stored in gel separator tubes after centrifugation for up to 48 hr. Do not freeze SST tubes. If frozen specimen is needed, separate serum into a labeled plastic transfer vial. Serum separation tubes must not be used for therapeutic drug levels. The gel may lower values. Not for blood bank use.
Light green marbled–topped tube: gel separator/lithium; heparin as anticoagulant	For potassium determination. Mix by inverting 8–10 times.

table continues on pg. 28 >

TABLE 1.7, continued

Collection Tube Color and Additives[a]	Use and Precautions
Tan/brown-topped tube: with heparin as anticoagulant	For heparinized plasma specimens for testing lead levels (i.e., lead-free tube). Invert tube 8–10 times.
Lavender-topped tube: with EDTA; removes calcium to prevent clotting	For whole blood and plasma, for hematology and complete blood counts (CBCs); prevents the filled tube from clotting. If the tube is less than half-filled, the proportion of anticoagulant to blood may be sufficiently altered to produce unreliable laboratory test results. Invert tube 8–10 times.
Royal blue–topped tube: no additive, with EDTA, or sodium heparin anticoagulant	For toxicology, cadmium and mercury: tube free of trace elements. Invert tube 8–10 times.
Gray-topped tube: with potassium oxalate and sodium fluoride	For glucose levels, glucose tolerance levels, and alcohol levels. Mix by inverting 8–10 times.
Plain pink tube: no additive or anticoagulant	For blood bank. Mix by inverting 8–10 times.
Black tube: with sodium citrate (binds calcium)	For Westergren sedimentation rate
Green-topped tube: with anticoagulant heparin (sodium, lithium, and ammonium heparin)	For heparinized plasma specimens, plasma chemistries, arterial blood gases, and special tests such as ammonia levels, hormones, and electrolytes. Invert 8–10 times to prevent clot formation.

List is arranged in sequence of draw according to Clinical and Laboratory Standards Institute (CLSI) guidelines.

[a]Clinical and Laboratory Standards Institute (formerly the National Committee for Clinical Laboratory Standards): Procedures for the Collection of Diagnostic Blood Specimens by Venipuncture: Approved Standard, 6th ed., H3-A6. Wayne, PA, Clinical and Laboratory Standards Institute, 2007.

9. Store specimens properly after collecting or transport them to the laboratory immediately for processing and analysis if possible. Failure to do so may result in specimen deterioration. STAT-ordered tests should always be hand-delivered to the laboratory and then processed as STAT.
10. Unacceptable specimens lead to increased costs and time wasted in getting results to the healthcare provider, patient, institution, and third-party payer. Exposure to sunlight, air, or other substances and warming or cooling can alter specimen integrity. Check with the laboratory for proper storage (e.g., ice, ice water, separate from ice), transport, and time limits.
11. As environments for specimen collection become more variable, modified procedures and protocols require the healthcare provider to keep abreast of the latest information related to these factors.

Equipment and Supplies

1. Use required kits, equipment, and supplies. Special kits are used for obtaining heel sticks and finger sticks, blood alcohol samples, saliva or oral fluid specimens, and urine specimens.
2. Do not use the kit if you notice a defect (e.g., moisture, pinholes, tears). In cases of sexual assault, special rape kits are required and a strict procedure, consisting of several steps, is followed.
3. Operating special equipment such as video monitors for endoscopic procedures may be required in some instances. Familiarity or training with current audiovisual and digital technology is necessary.
4. Use barrier drapes as directed. For example, arthroscopy drapes are positioned with the fluid control pouch at the knee.
5. Maintain aseptic technique during certain procedures (e.g., cystoscopy, bone marrow biopsy).

Presence of Family or Significant Others

Involving family members or significant others in the diagnostic care process makes them active participants in providing care and support to the patient. Facilitating family or significant other presence during invasive procedures may provide the opportunity to calm the patient, offer additional comfort, and reduce anxiety and fear. However, some individuals may find the option of observing procedures to be distressing or uncomfortable. Other patients may not want family members present. Healthcare providers acting as patient advocates recognize the importance of supporting the patient's need for reassurance and the family's need and right to be present during diagnostic procedures. The goal is to achieve an acceptable balance between all parties. Family or significant other presence should be documented in the healthcare record.

Positioning for Procedures

Proper body positioning and alignment involves placing the patient in the best possible position for the procedure and aligning the body correctly for optimal respiratory and circulatory function. Positions include prone, lithotomy, sitting, supine, jackknife, and Trendelenburg. Use positioning devices, arrange padding, and reposition as needed to prevent skin pressure and skin breakdown. The potential adverse effects of various positions, especially during lengthy procedures, include skin breakdown, venous compression, sciatic nerve injury, muscle injury, and low back strain. Necessary positioning skills include ensuring that the patient's airway, IV lines, skin integrity, and monitoring devices are not compromised and identifying those persons at potential risk for injury (e.g., elderly, thin, frail, sedated, or unconscious patients) before positioning. If wounds, skin breakdown, abrasions, or bruises are present before the procedure, accurately document their presence and location.

Administration of Drugs and Solutions

All drugs and solutions administered during diagnostic procedures are given according to established protocols. Drugs can be given by mouth, inhalation, intubation, parenterally (intramuscularly, intravenously, or subcutaneously), rectally, and by local or topical skin applications. IV fluids and endoscopic irrigating fluids are commonly administered.

Be cognizant of the potential for adverse reactions to drugs. Assess for previous drug problems with the patient before the procedure. Risks for injury are related to hypersensitivity, allergic or toxic reactions, impaired drug tolerance due to liver or kidney malfunction, extravasation of IV fluids, and absorption of irrigating fluids into the systemic circulation. Required skills include managing airways and breathing patterns; monitoring fluid intake and loss; monitoring body, skin, and core temperature; and observing the effects of sedation and analgesia (e.g., vital signs, rashes, edema). Use tape with caution, especially when skin integrity can be easily compromised, as in frail elderly patients.

Management of Environment

The main goal of environmental control is safe practice to ensure that the patient is free from injury related to environmental hazards and is free from discomfort. Be attentive to temperature and air quality; the patient's body temperature; exposure to noise, radiation, latex, and noxious odors; sanitation; and cleanliness.

1. Eliminate or modify sensory stimuli (e.g., noise, odors, sounds).
2. Post a PATIENT AWAKE sign if the patient is awake during a procedure or PATIENT ASLEEP for sleep studies.
3. Be sensitive to conversation among team members in the presence of the patient. At best, it can be annoying to the patient; at worst, it may be misinterpreted and have negative effects and consequences, such as stress and anxiety.

Latex Sensitivity and Allergy

The rise in incidence of latex allergy may be attributed not only to increased use of latex products in patient care but also to the manner in which raw latex was collected and aged. Allergic reactions are caused by latex proteins retained in the finished products, which can show great variations in latex allergen levels. The greatest environmental hazard exposure is produced by latex gloves and the powder from the gloves that becomes airborne.

The U.S. Food and Drug Administration (FDA) now requires that all medical devices containing natural rubber latex that may directly or indirectly contact the patient display the following statement: "Caution: This product contains natural rubber latex which may cause allergic reactions."

Increased or continued exposure increases sensitivity to latex allergens and worsens allergic reactions. Patients and healthcare providers can become sensitized to latex through repeated skin or mucous membrane contact or by inhaling aerosolized glove allergens.

Latex allergy often begins with a rash on the hands (from gloves).

Latex Allergy Precautions to Protect the Patient

Strategies and protocols include the following:

1. Identify allergic patients (those with a history of problems related to catheters, tubes, drains, household items, condoms, latex gloves, balloons, toys, and so on); allergy testing (see Chapter 8) may be desirable. Communicate and document data appropriately.
2. *Never* wear powdered latex gloves when caring for a sensitized patient.
3. Avoid contact of latex with tissue (e.g., wounds, mucous membranes, vaginal skin). *Practice proper handwashing.*
4. Use latex-free products. Examples include the following:
   Gloves
   Endotracheal tubes
   Suction and wound drainage tubes and reservoir systems
   Catheters
   Blood pressure cuffs
   Stethoscopes
   Temperature probe covers, tape, dressings, Ace wraps
   Monitoring equipment and supplies (leads, pulse oximeter probes, and cables)
5. Remove rubber stoppers from vials before withdrawing or reconstituting contents. Rinse syringes with sterile water or saline before use.
6. Remove latex ports from IV tubing and replace with stopcocks or nonlatex plugs. Tape ports shut if no other alternative is available. Replace ports on IV therapy bags with nonlatex ports.
7. Keep resuscitation equipment and emergency supplies and medications readily accessible at all times in the event that anaphylaxis occurs. (*Caution: Some resuscitation supplies and equipment may contain latex.*)
8. Instruct the patient about latex-containing supplies, both medical and nonmedical, that could pose problems (Chart 1.4).
9. Stay current in knowing which products contain latex. The Spina Bifida Association of America routinely publishes updated lists of latex-containing products (see www.spinabifidaassociation.org).

CLINICAL ALERT

Sensitive persons should carry autoinjectable epinephrine (e.g., EpiPen), nonlatex gloves, and emergency medical instructions; should wear a medical alert bracelet; should avoid *all* forms of latex; and should alert healthcare providers, family, friends, and employers of the diagnosis and need to avoid latex.

CHART 1.4 Items Containing Latex

Medical Supply Items That Frequently Contain Latex	Home and Community Items That Frequently Contain Latex
Anesthesia equipment, endotracheal tubes, airways	Appliance cords
Appliqués (clothing), spandex	Art supplies (paint, glue, rubber bands, erasers, ink)
Bandages, tapes	Balloons, toys, water toys, and equipment
Bed protectors	Balls (tennis, Koosh)
Blood pressure tubing, cuffs	Carpet backing, rubber floors, cushions
Bulb syringes	Condoms, diaphragms
Catheters (many and varied types)	Crutch accessories (tips, grips)
Dressings, elastic wraps	Dental braces, chewing gum
G-tubes, drains	Diapers, incontinence products
IV access (Y-sites, tourniquets, adapters, etc.)	Elastic in socks, underwear, etc.
Operating room masks, hats, shoe covers	Feeding nipples, pacifiers
Oxygen masks, cannula, resuscitation devices	Handles on garden and sporting equipment
Reflex hammers, syringes	Kitchen gloves
Stethoscopes	Tires, hoses
Suction equipment	
Surgical masks	

Note: These lists are not all-inclusive. If latex content is unknown, checking with the manufacturer or supplier before use is strongly advised.

NOTE *Assembling and maintaining a cart with latex-free supplies and equipment may be desirable to facilitate safe patient care.*

CLINICAL ALERT

If latex-free blood pressure cuffs and stethoscopes are not available, shield the patient's arm with stockinette and apply the cuff over it. Small-diameter (finger-sized) stockinette can be used to cover stethoscope tubing, leads, and so on.

CLINICAL ALERT

Symptoms of anaphylaxis include a dangerous drop in blood pressure, dyspnea, flushed facial appearance, swelling (of throat, tongue, and nose), a feeling of impending doom, and loss of consciousness.

CLINICAL ALERT

Protocols for management of an allergic reaction:

1. Airway maintenance
2. Administration of oxygen
3. Volume expansion (IV lactated Ringer's or normal saline solution)
4. Epinephrine IV
5. Steroids (orally or IV)
6. Diphenhydramine (orally or IV)
7. Aminophylline IV

Pain Control, Comfort Measures, and Patient Monitoring

Provide proper information, reassurance, and support throughout the entire procedure to allay anxiety and fear. Administer sedatives, pain medication, or antiemetics as ordered. Uphold the dignity of each patient, provide privacy, and minimize any situation that might cause embarrassment or stress. Continue monitoring throughout procedures as well as after completion if indicated.

1. Do not require the patient to remain disrobed any longer than necessary. Allow personal clothing and other accessories such as rings or religious medals, provided they do not pose a risk or interfere with the procedure. Ensure a reasonable degree of privacy.
2. Control pain and provide comfort measures. IV conscious sedation and drugs given to reverse the effects of test medications are part of this scenario. Allow the patient to maintain as much control as possible during all testing phases without compromising safety, the process and procedure, and test integrity. If possible, plan ahead to accommodate persons with special needs such as learning disabilities, visual or hearing impairment, ostomy, or diabetes management.
3. Monitor and document vital signs and other relevant parameters (e.g., pulse oximetry, ECG) throughout the procedure. Observe for problems and abnormal reactions and take appropriate measures to correct such situations. Make sure emergency equipment is readily available and functional.
4. Document the patient's response to the procedure during all phases. Also document significant events or situations that occur during testing. Record disposition of specimens.

Sedation and Analgesia

Increasing numbers of patients are receiving short-term moderate sedation and analgesia (also referred to as *conscious sedation*) for invasive diagnostic procedures. Even though the anesthesiologist or attending physician assumes responsibility for IV moderate sedation, other healthcare providers may administer the drugs and monitor the patient's response to these drugs. Advantages of moderate sedation and analgesia include short, rapid recovery; early ambulation; patient preference for light sleep and amnesia; patient cooperation during the procedure; protective reflexes remain intact; vital signs remain stable; and infrequent complications.

The American Society of Anesthesiologists Task Force on Sedation and Analgesia by Non-Anesthesiologists (2002) recommends using the term *moderate sedation and analgesia* rather than *conscious sedation* because it is a more accurate description of the goal of administering these drugs. Moderate sedation and analgesia is defined as a drug-induced depression of consciousness during which patients respond purposefully to verbal commands, either alone or accompanied by light tactile stimulation. No interventions are required to maintain a patent airway and spontaneous ventilation is adequate. Cardiovascular function is usually maintained. There are two goals of moderate sedation and analgesia: (1) to allow the patient to undergo unpleasant procedures by diminishing his or her discomfort, pain, and anxiety (while maintaining adequate cardiorespiratory factors and response to verbal commands and stimulation) and (2) to immobilize the patient to expedite complex procedures that require that the patient not move, especially children and uncooperative adults. Because it is not always possible to predict how a specific patient will respond to sedative and analgesic medications, practitioners intending to produce a given level of sedation should be able to rescue patients whose level of sedation becomes deeper than initially intended.

The primary drugs used for moderate sedation and analgesia are benzodiazepines and opiates, which are central nervous system (CNS) depressants. Opiates are also used for sedation, as are some tranquilizers (droperidol [Inapsine]); for pain relief, fentanyl (Sublimaze), morphine, and meperidine are used (Chart 1.5). Combinations of drugs may be more effective than single agents in some instances. Agents must then be appropriately reduced, and there is a greater need to monitor respiratory function. IV sedative and analgesic drugs are to be given in small incremental doses. When the drug is administered orally, rectally, intranasally, intramuscularly, or subcutaneously, allow time for drug absorption before giving another dose.

CHART 1.5 Examples of Sedatives and Analgesic Drugs Used

Diazepam (Valium)

CNS depressant, amnestic, lacks analgesia. Duration: 2–8 hr.

Dosage guidelines: 2–5 mg to maximum of 10 mg. No more than 5 mg/min. Give additional doses in 2.5 mg increments. Wait 3 min before redosing. Onset: 5–10 min; IV, 15–30 min. Reduce dose by ⅓ when an opiate is being used concomitantly.

Precautions: Increased effects if taking CNS depressants, alcohol, cimetidine, or disulfiram. Avoid in patients with renal disease.

Midazolam (Versed)

CNS depressant; 3–4 times as potent as diazepam. Provides sedation, amnesia, and decreases anxiety. Lacks analgesia. Duration: 60–90 min.

IV dosage guidelines: Initial dose: 0.1–0.2 mg/kg. 0.5–1.0 mg given slowly over at least 2–3 min; not to exceed 4 mg. Wait at least 2 min before redosing. Give in small increments after initial dose. Onset: 1–2 min (IV), 10–20 min (IM), 10–15 min (intranasally), 10–30 min (orally), and 10–30 min (rectally). Decrease dose if given with narcotics (by 25%–30% in healthy adult, by 55%–60% in elderly or debilitated). Duration: 30–60 min (IV), 1–2 hr (IM), 45–60 min (intranasally), and 60–90 min (orally or rectally).

Precautions: Watch for respiratory depression, especially in children. Contraindicated in patients with narrow-angle glaucoma.

Lorazepam (Ativan)

CNS depressant; lacks analgesia. Duration: 4–6 hr.

Dosage guidelines: 0.5–2 mg IV, given slowly; maximum 4 mg. Onset: 5–10 min. Decrease dose in elderly.

Precautions: Increased effects with monoamine oxidase inhibitors (MAOIs), barbiturates, narcotics, hypnotics, tricyclic antidepressants, alcohol; decreased effects with oral anticoagulants and heparin. Use with great caution in children. Owing to anticholinergic actions, use with caution in patients with asthma, narrow-angle glaucoma, prostatic hypertrophy, or bladder neck outlet obstruction.

Meperidine (Demerol)

Opiate narcotic analgesic sedative; 60–80 mg meperidine = 10 mg morphine. Duration: 2–4 hr.

IV dosage guidelines: 10 mg IV. Give increments slowly; 25–50 mg IV over 2 min; repeat at 5-min intervals; 10–15 mg maximum; 150 mg over total period of procedure. Decrease dose in elderly or debilitated; use caution with renal disease.

Precautions: Contraindicated if patient has had a MAOI in last 14 d; may precipitate severe and irreversible reaction and death; decrease dose if given with other narcotic, barbiturate, tranquilizer, tricyclic antidepressant, or sedative. Use with caution in patients with supraventricular tachycardia; may cause increased ventricular response.

Droperidol (Inapsine)

Major tranquilizer; no analgesic properties. Produces cognitive dissociation—a sense of detachment; antiemetic. Duration: Varies over several hours.

IV dosage guidelines: 0.625–1.25 mg; decrease dose in elderly. Onset: 3–10 min. Peak action: 30 min.

Precautions: Potentiates narcotics and other CNS depressants. Produces mild α-adrenergic block.

continues on pg. 34 >

CHART 1.5, continued

Fentanyl (Sublimaze)
Opiate narcotic analgesic sedative; much more powerful than morphine. Duration: 30–60 min.

IV dosage guidelines: 1.0–2.0 μg/kg. 25–50 mg IV at 5-min intervals, titrating time to patient response. May also be given by transdermal patch, or as a "lollipop" for children. Onset of sedation: 1–2 min; onset of analgesia: may not be noted for several minutes. Maximum dosage: 500 mg/5 hr.

Precautions: Potentiates narcotics and other CNS and respiratory depressants. Produces mild adrenergic block. Reversal with Narcan: Rapid IV administration may cause chest wall rigidity; treat with chemical paralytics, intubation, and ventilatory support.

Morphine
Opiate narcotic analgesic. Duration: 1–3 hr.

IV dosage guidelines: 2–15 mg IV over a 5-min period; maximum of 20 mg over total procedure time.

Precautions: Causes analgesia and respiratory depression; check respiratory status.

Ketamine (Ketalar)
A derivative of phencyclidine (PCP) used in pediatrics: analgesic, sedative, and amnestic. Duration: 10–30 min (IV), 60–90 min (IM).

Dosage guidelines: Rapid onset with both IV and IM (1 min IV and 5–6 min IM); longer if given orally or rectally.

Precautions: Causes copious saliva production and airway secretions (treated with atropine or Robinul). Does not cause respiratory depression. Associated with nightmares (rare in children) and not with oral or rectal routes.

Sufentanil (Sufenta)
Analgesic more potent than fentanyl; used in pediatrics. Duration: 1–2 hr.

Dosage guidelines: Onset: 5–15 min, intranasally; may be administered with Versed.

Precautions: Reversal with Narcan. Precautions same as for fentanyl (Sublimaze).

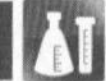
CLINICAL ALERT

Record ventilatory and oxygen status and hemodynamics *before* the procedure begins, after administration of sedative and analgesia, on completion of procedure, during initial recovery, and at time of discharge.

Interventions for Adult Patients Receiving Moderate Sedation and Analgesia

Preadministration

1. Explain the purpose of moderate sedation and analgesia before administering the medications. It is most commonly used for these diagnostic procedures: biopsies, bronchoscopy, ERCP, colonoscopy, gastroscopy, angiogram, cardiac catheterization, electrophysiologic studies, and cystoscopy. Medications may be administered intravenously or by mouth.
2. Assess the patient's health status, history of chronic or acute conditions, drug allergies, current medications and potential drug interactions, previous diagnostic test results, level of understanding,

orientation, mental status, and ability to cooperate with the procedure. Screen and identify patients who are at high risk for development of complications: the very young; the very old; and those with heart, lung, liver, kidney, or CNS disease, marked obesity, sleep apnea, pregnancy, or drug or alcohol abuse. Patients presenting for moderate sedation and analgesia should undergo a focused physical examination, including vital signs, auscultation of the heart and lungs, and evaluation of the airway.

3. Explain the process and procedure and what the patient may experience (feel sleepy, relaxed, no anxiety). Use a calm, caring manner. Not all providers agree on the fasting time frames, but there is an agreement that preprocedure fasting decreases risks during moderate sedation. Check your agency policy. For adults, no food or liquid should be taken for 2 to 6 hours before the procedure to allow for gastric emptying. For infants younger than 6 months of age, fast 4 to 6 hours (this includes milk, formula, and breast milk); clear liquids should be avoided for 2 hours before the procedure.
4. Before beginning the procedure, establish an IV line and keep it open with the ordered IV solution. Monitor patency of the line.
5. Monitor pulmonary ventilation (exhaled carbon dioxide) and apply pulse oximeter sensor especially if the patient is unable to be observed during moderate sedation. Monitor ECG, pulse oximetry, and patient response to verbal commands according to established guidelines before administering moderate sedation. Patient's vital signs should be documented (before, during, and after the procedure).
6. Provide a safe and caring environment. A designated individual, other than the healthcare provider performing the procedure, should be present to monitor the patient throughout the procedure. In anticipation of emergency situations, have resuscitation equipment and supplies of appropriate size readily available (oxygen therapy, IV fluid, reversal agents, and vasopressors).

Intra-Administration

1. Continuously assess pain or discomfort and sedation levels at frequent established intervals.
2. Administer sedation and analgesics as ordered, often in incremental doses.
3. Recognize physiologic effects of agents used for moderate sedation. These medications include the following, among others:
   a. Meperidine hydrochloride (Demerol)
   b. Diazepam hydrochloride (Valium)
   c. Midazolam hydrochloride (Versed)
   d. Lorazepam (Ativan)
   e. Droperidol (Inapsine) (Check with your pharmacy or institutional policy regarding use of this drug.)
   f. Fentanyl citrate (Sublimaze)
   g. Morphine sulfate
4. Monitor the IV site for infiltration and the general effects of the medication as well as the local analgesia site. Local anesthesia and sedation may cause adverse reactions.
5. Assess level of consciousness—responses of patients to commands during the procedure serve as a guide to their level of consciousness. If reflex withdrawal from painful stimulation is the only response, the patient is likely to be deeply sedated, approaching the state of general anesthesia.
6. Monitor pulmonary ventilation by auscultation of breath and observation of spontaneous respiration. Automated apnea monitoring (detection of exhaled CO_2) may be used but is not a substitute for monitoring ventilatory function.
7. Be cognizant that detecting changes in heart rate and blood pressure for hemodynamics reduces the risk for cardiovascular collapse and hypoedema.
8. Use pulse oximetry to detect hypoxemia and decrease adverse outcomes such as cardiac arrest and death.
9. Anticipate and monitor for potential complications. Arrhythmias should be promptly reported and treated if necessary. Many of these medications are respiratory depressants, mandating frequent

respiratory assessments. If oxygen saturation drops below acceptable levels (≤90%), sedation may need to be held or reversed. Have IV reversal agents such as naloxone (Narcan) and flumazenil (Romazicon) readily available. Supplemental oxygen therapy may be necessary until oxygen saturation levels, vital signs, neurologic response, and cardiac rhythms are at acceptable levels.

10. Respond to emergencies rapidly and appropriately during administration of, or recovery from, moderate sedation and analgesia.
11. Document carefully and completely all observations, including medications and dosages. Record unexpected outcomes and follow-up care.

Postadministration

1. Monitor vital signs, ECG, pulse oximetry, ventilation, neurologic signs, level of consciousness, and patient response to verbal commands according to established guidelines.
2. Monitor the patient after the procedure until the patient is stable and reactive to preprocedure levels.
3. Provide both verbal and written posttest instructions. Moderate sedation may not completely wear off for several hours. Patients should *not*
   a. Drive or operate power machinery or tools for at least 24 hours.
   b. Consume alcoholic beverages or make legal decisions for 24 hours.
   c. Smoke—if the patient is a smoker, emphasize the risks of smoking in the postsedation state (i.e., falling asleep).
   d. Take tranquilizers, pain medications, or other medications that may interact with drugs used for sedation without first contacting the healthcare provider.
4. Provide instructions for posttest care and the need for contacting the healthcare provider if any unexpected outcomes should occur.
5. Evaluate the patient for readiness for discharge. Patients should be alert and oriented or, if altered mental status was initially present, should have returned to baseline. Vital signs should be stable and within acceptable limits. Provide a safe transport or discharge in the presence of a responsible adult.
6. Allow sufficient time (up to 2 hours) to elapse after the last administration of reversal agents to ensure that patients do not become re-sedated after reversal effects have worn off.

POSTTEST PHASE: ELEMENTS OF SAFE, EFFECTIVE, INFORMED CARE

The focus of the posttest phase is on patient aftercare and the follow-up activities, observations, and monitoring necessary to prevent or minimize complications.

Basic Knowledge and Necessary Skills

The healthcare provider needs to be able to effectively evaluate outcomes and effectiveness of care and conduct follow-up counseling, discharge planning, and appropriate posttest referrals in this phase.

Abnormal Test Results

Review test results promptly. Report and interpret test outcomes correctly. Abnormal test patterns or trends can sometimes provide more useful information than single test outcome deviations. Conversely, single test results can be normal in patients with a proven disease or illness.

1. Look at both current and previous test results and review the most recent laboratory data first and then work sequentially backward to evaluate trends or changes from previous data. The patient's plan of care may need to be modified because of test results and changes in medical management.
2. Recognize abnormal test results and consider the implications for the patient in both the acute and the chronic stages of the disease as well as during screening.

3. The greater the degree of test abnormality, the more likely the outcome will be more serious.
4. Consider the impact of medications when tests are abnormal. Use of over-the-counter (OTC) drugs, vitamins, iron, and other minerals may produce false-positive or false-negative test results. Patients often do not disclose all medications they use, either unintentionally or deliberately. Commonly prescribed drugs that most often affect laboratory test outcomes include anticoagulants, anticonvulsants, antibiotic or antiviral agents, oral hypoglycemics, hormones, and psychotropic drugs. Consult a pharmacist or *Physicians' Desk Reference* (*PDR*) source about drugs the patient is taking. Be aware that patients who are addicted to drugs or alcohol may not provide accurate, reliable information about their use of these agents. In the same vein, sometimes athletes may not disclose their use of performance-enhancing drugs.
5. Consider biocultural variations when interpreting test results. See Table 1.8 for examples of some common variations.
6. Evaluate age-related variables and test outcomes; consider changes in physiology as the various body organs age (e.g., heart, lungs, kidneys).

CLINICAL ALERT

1. Correct test interpretation requires knowledge of all medications the patient is taking.
2. Support the patient and his or her significant others in understanding and coping with positive or negative test outcomes.
3. Recognize that critical values may pose an immediate threat to the patient's health status. Report these findings to the attending physician or other designated healthcare provider immediately. Carefully document results and actions taken as soon as possible.
4. Nearly all tests have limitations. Some tests cannot predict future outcomes or events. For example, an ECG cannot predict a future myocardial infarction; it can merely tell what has already occurred.
5. Devastating physical, psychological, and social consequences can result from being misdiagnosed with a serious disease because of false-positive or false-negative test results. Major alterations in lifestyles and relationships without just cause can be a consequence of these clinical aberrations (e.g., misdiagnosis of HIV or syphilis).

Follow-Up Counseling

1. Counsel the patient regarding test outcomes and their implications for further testing, treatment, and possible lifestyle changes. Provide time for the patient to ask questions and voice concerns about the entire testing process.
2. Test outcome interpretation involves reassessment of interfering factors and patient compliance if the results significantly deviate from normal and previous results.
3. No test is perfect; however, the greater the degree of abnormality indicated by the test result, the more likely it is that this outcome deviation is significant or represents a real disorder.
4. Notify the patient about test results after consultation with the healthcare provider. Treatment may be delayed if test results are misplaced or not communicated in a timely manner.
5. Help patients interpret the results of community-based testing.
6. Identify differences in the patient's view of the situation, the healthcare provider's views about tests and disease, and the healthcare team's perceptions.
7. When providing genetic counseling, the healthcare provider needs to be sensitive to the implications of genetic or metabolic disorders. Informing the patient or family about the genetic defect

TABLE 1.8 Biocultural Considerations

Diagnostic Test	Biocultural Variation
Orthopedic x-rays	Body proportions and tendencies: African American people exhibit longer arms and legs and shorter trunks than Caucasians. African American women tend to have wider shoulders and more narrow hips but with more abdominal adipose tissue than Caucasian women. Caucasian men tend to exhibit more abdominal adipose tissue than do African American men. Native Americans and Asian Americans have larger trunks and shorter limbs than do African American and Caucasian people. Asian American people tend to have wider hips and more narrow shoulders than do other peoples.
Bone density measurements	African American men have the densest bones, followed by African American women and Caucasian men, who have similar bone densities. Caucasian women have the least dense bones. Chinese, Japanese, and Inuit bone density is less than that of Caucasian Americans. Additionally, bone density decreases with age.
Test for glucose-6-phosphate dehydrogenase (G6PD) deficiency	G6PD deficiency may be the cause of hemolytic disease of newborns in Asian Americans and those of Mediterranean descent. Three G6PD variants occur frequently: Type A is common in African Americans (10% of males); the Mediterranean type is common in Iraqis, Kurds, Lebanese, and Sephardic Jews; and the Mahedial type is common in Southeast Asians (22% of males).
Cholesterol levels	African American and Caucasian ethnic groups have similar cholesterol levels at birth. During childhood, African American people develop higher levels than do Caucasian people; however, African American adults have lower cholesterol levels than do Caucasian adults.
Hemoglobin/hematocrit levels	The normal hemoglobin level for African American people is 1 g lower than that for other groups. Given similar socioeconomic conditions, Asian Americans and Mexican Americans have hemoglobin/hematocrit levels higher than those of Caucasian people.
Sickle cell anemia	Sickle cell anemia (or sickle cell disease) affects millions of people throughout the world. It is particularly common among people whose ancestors come from sub-Saharan Africa, Spanish-speaking regions (South America, Cuba, Central America), Saudi Arabia, India, and Mediterranean countries such as Turkey, Greece, and Italy. In the United States, it affects approximately 70,000–100,000 people, most of whose ancestors come from Africa. The disease occurs in approximately 1 in every 16,000 Hispanic American births. Approximately 1 in 13 African American babies has the sickle cell trait at birth.

requires special training in genetic science, family coping skills, and an understanding of legal and ethical issues. Confidentiality and privacy of information are vital.

8. Be familiar with crisis intervention skills for patients who experience difficulty dealing with the posttest phase.
9. Encourage the patient to take as much control of the situation as possible.
10. Recognize that the different stages of behavioral responses may last several weeks.
11. Provide social and emotional support as needed. Social support is a context-specific interpersonal process centered on the exchange of information between all parties involved. Emotional social support is centered on feelings of anxiousness, depression, and hopelessness, whereas instrumental social support deals with the more tangible needs, such as child care, transportation, food, and shelter.

Monitoring for Complications and Sedation Effects

Observe for complications or other risks, such as effects of sedation and analgesia, and take appropriate measures to prevent or deal with them in a safe patient environment.

1. The most common complications after invasive procedures are bleeding, infection (frequently a later complication), respiratory difficulties, perforation of organs, and adverse effects of conscious sedation and local anesthesia. Watch for related signs and symptoms such as redness, swelling, skin irritation, pain or tenderness, dyspnea, abnormal breath sounds, cyanosis, decreased or increased pulse rate, blood pressure deviations (e.g., hypertension, hypotension), laryngospasm, agitation or combative behavior, pallor, and complaints of dizziness. If adverse reactions or events occur, contact the healthcare provider immediately and initiate treatment as soon as possible.
2. Posttest assessments include evaluation of patient behaviors, complaints, activities, and compliance within the emotional, physical, psychosocial, and spiritual dimensions. Alterations in any of these domains may indicate a need for interventions appropriate to the dimension affected.
3. Older patients and children may require closer, more lengthy monitoring and observation. For example, invasive procedure sites should be observed and assessed for potential bleeding and circulatory problems in the immediate postprocedure phase and for infection as a later event (possibly several days later).
4. Patients who receive sedation, drugs, contrast media (e.g., iodine, barium), or radioactive substances must be evaluated and treated according to established protocols (see Chapters 9 and 10).
5. Infection control measures with standard precautions (see Appendix A) and aseptic techniques must be observed.

Test Result Availability

Collaborate with other disciplines to ensure that test results are made available to the healthcare provider, patient, and staff as soon as possible. Time-critical information is of limited value if it is delayed or not received. Even though computerized communication technologies contribute to faster information delivery, healthcare providers are often left waiting for crucial clinical data. Using facsimile (fax) machines, computers, and wireless networks properly can expedite the reporting of vital patient data to the healthcare provider so that treatment can begin without delay.

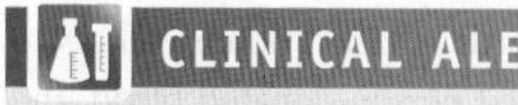

The issue of confidentiality demands that access to records and information should be on a strict need-to-know basis with secure and protected access available to select individuals.

Integration

Integration is a phase related to diagnosis, subsequent acceptance, healing, and health-promoting behavior. Interventions to promote integration include provision of coaching, promotion of self-care, behavior change, and expression of grief or loss.

Referral and Treatment

Referrals for further testing and beginning treatment are a part of the collaborative process. For example, the healthcare provider refers patients with abnormal Pap test results to the specialist for colposcopy, loop electrocautery excision procedure (LEEP), or cervical or endometrial biopsy. The healthcare provider refers the patient for genetic counseling and dietary therapy for genetic disorders such as phenylketonuria (PKU) cholesterol in the newborn.

Follow-Up Care

Posttest care should be consistent and should provide clearly understood discharge instructions. Emphasize the importance of and protocols for additional visits if these are ordered. Schedule ordered follow-up visits as appropriate. Use established protocols for discharge to home after testing is completed. For complex procedures that are invasive or require sedation, be certain that a responsible individual escorts the patient home. Provide specific instructions regarding infection control, barium elimination, iodine sensitivity, and resuming pretest activities. Have the patient repeat this information back to the person providing the information to ensure that it has been understood. Plan time for listening, support, discussion, and problem solving according to the patient's needs and requests. Follow-up by phone may be done after discharge if indicated.

Documentation, Record Keeping, and Reporting

Record information about all phases of the diagnostic testing process in the patient's healthcare record. Accurately document diagnostic activities and procedures during the pretest, intratest, and posttest phases because of legal, budgetary, reimbursement, and diagnosis-related group (DRG) and CPT code implications and constraints. Standardized forms are becoming more common.

The patient's healthcare record is the only way to validate the need for diagnostic care, the quality and type of care given, and the patient's response to the care and to ensure that current standards of medical and nursing care and diagnostic testing are being met. The medical record may also be the basis for reimbursement for diagnostic tests by Medicare (government) or private insurance programs. Accuracy, completeness, objectivity, and legibility are of utmost importance in the documentation process. Documentation of laboratory and diagnostic testing includes recording all pretest, intratest, and posttest care:

1. Document that the purpose, side effects, risks, and expected results and benefits, as well as alternative methods, have been explained to the patient and note who gave the explanation. Include information about medications, IV conscious sedation, start and end times, and patient responses. Describe allergic or adverse reactions. Record data regarding disposition of specimens as well as information about follow-up care and discharge instructions.
2. Document the patient's reasons for refusing a test along with any other pertinent information about the situation and who was given this report.
3. Maintain records of laboratory and diagnostic test data. Frequently, these records are transferred onto compact record storage systems such as microfilm or computer disks. For example, when an individual tests positive for HIV, it is necessary to review donor records at blood donor centers to determine whether the individual ever donated blood. If the infected person donated blood, the recipients of those blood components must be contacted and informed of the situation. This process is called *look back*. Because many years may pass between donation and transfusion and the time the donor tests HIV positive, medical history records of blood donors must be stored indefinitely.

4. Documentation should reflect the time, day, month, and year, either by date/time stamp in the electronic health record or handwritten on paper documents. This information can assume great importance in the office or clinic setting when charts become very lengthy. Enter appropriate assessment data and note the patient's concerns and questions that help to define the nursing diagnosis and focus for care planning. Document specific teaching and preparation of the patient before the procedure. Avoid generalizations.
5. When an interpreter is present, document the name and relationship to the patient. Record that patient consent to give confidential test information through an interpreter was obtained before revealing the information. Record any deviations from basic witnessed consent policies (e.g., illiteracy, non–English-speaking client, sedation immediately before the request for consent signature, consent per telephone); include nurse measures employed to obtain appropriate consent for the procedure.
6. Keep a record of all printed and written instructions. Record medications, treatments, food and fluids, intake status, beginning and end of specimen collection and procedure times, outcomes, and the patient's condition during all phases of diagnostic care. If the patient does not appear for testing, document this fact; include any follow-up discussion with the patient. Completely and clearly describe side effects, symptoms, adverse reactions, and complications along with follow-up care and instructions for posttest care and monitoring.
7. Document significant noncompliant behaviors such as refusal or inability to fast or to restrict or increase fluid or food intake, incomplete timed specimens, inadequate or improperly self-collected specimens, and missed or canceled test appointments. Place copies of letters sent in the patient's chart.
8. Reporting includes patient notification regarding test outcomes in a timely fashion and documentation that the patient or family has been notified regarding test results. Document follow-up patient education and counseling.
9. Report results to designated professionals. Report critical values immediately and document to whom results were reported, orders received, and urgent treatments initiated.
10. Report all communicable diseases to appropriate agencies.
11. Report and document situations that are mandatory by state statute (e.g., suspected elder abuse, child abuse as evidenced by x-rays).

CLINICAL ALERT

New reporting requirements are based on a syndrome recognition surveillance system for disease outbreaks, reservoirs for bacteria, for the highest illnesses, and risk bioterrorism diseases (botulism [food-borne illnesses], anthrax, smallpox, hemorrhagic fever, Hantaan virus, Ebola virus, yellow fever, and plague [bubonic and primary septicemia]). This system recognizes that animals (zoonotic) may be the primary source of diseases. It also highlights collaboration by desiring input from physicians, PAs, nurse practitioners, school nurses, emergency medical technicians (EMTs), veterinarians, laboratory technologists, and animal control (severe illness wildlife).

Reporting of infectious diseases and outbreaks and toxins to state and federal governments is part of record keeping. Charts 1.6 and 1.7 are examples of required reporting to the CDC and the state of Maryland, respectively. Check with your individual state or province for specific guidelines.

Guidelines for Disclosure

Follow agency guidelines for disclosure. Ethical standards may be a source of conflict and anxiety when the professional healthcare provider is acting in the role of patient advocate. Recommended guidelines for telling a patient about test results can alleviate some of this frustration. Under normal circumstances, the patient has the right to be informed of test results. Although the healthcare provider who orders the test is responsible for providing initial test result information, other designated individuals may need to facilitate and support the patient's right to know information about his or her health status.

CHART 1.6 Agents and Toxins Reportable to the APHIS or CDC

African horse sickness virus
African swine fever virus
Avian influenza virus (highly pathogenic)
Bacillus anthracis
Botulinum neurotoxins
Bovine spongiform encephalopathy agent
Brucella melitensis
Classical swine fever virus
Ebola virus
Foot-and-mouth disease virus
Francisella tularensis
Hendra virus
Lassa fever virus
Marburg virus
Nipah virus
Peronosclerospora philippinensis (*Peronosclerospora sacchari*)
Phoma glycinicola (formerly *Pyrenochaeta glycines*)
Ralstonia solanacearum race 3, biovar 2
Rathayibacter toxicus
Rift Valley fever virus
Rinderpest virus
Sclerophthora rayssiae var *zeae*
South American hemorrhagic fever viruses (Junin, Machupo, Sabia, Flexal, Guanarito)
Swine vesicular disease virus
Synchytrium endobioticum
Variola major virus (smallpox virus)
Variola minor (alastrim)
Venezuelan equine encephalitis virus
Virulent Newcastle disease virus
Xanthomonas oryzae
Xylella fastidiosa (citrus variegated chlorosis strain)
Yersinia pestis

APHIS, Animal and Plant Health Inspection Service; CDC, Centers for Disease Control and Prevention.
Source: U.S. Department of Agriculture: Guidance document for reporting the identification of a select agent or toxin. Updated October 11, 2012. Available at: www.selectagents.gov

In cases in which the patient brings family and significant others together to inform them about test results, communication becomes open and shared. This prevents the so-called conspiracy of silence, in which individuals in the scenario withhold information because they feel they are protecting the patient or family or because they do not know how to deal with the situation.

Patient Responses to Diagnosis

Develop crisis intervention skills to use when communicating with the patient who experiences difficulty dealing with abnormal test results or confirmation of disease or illness.

1. Encourage the patient to take as much control of the situation as possible.
2. Recognize that the different stages of behavioral responses to negative results may last several weeks or longer (Table 1.9).
3. Monitor changes in patient affect, mood, behaviors, and motivation. Do not assume that persons who initially have a negative perception of their health (e.g., denial of diabetes) will not be able to integrate better health behaviors into daily life once they accept the diagnosis.
4. Use the following strategies to lessen the impact of a threatening situation:
    a. Offer appropriate comfort measures.
    b. Allow patients to work through feelings of anxiety and depression. At the appropriate time, reassure them that these feelings and emotions are normal initially. Be more of a therapeutic listener than a talker.
    c. Assist the patient and family in making necessary lifestyle and self-concept adjustments through education, support groups, and other means. Emphasize that risk factors associated with certain diseases can be reduced through lifestyle changes. Be realistic. It is better to introduce change slowly rather than trying to promote adjustments on a grand scale in a short period of time.

CHART 1.7 Diseases and Conditions Reportable by Laboratory Directors and Healthcare Providers

AIDS[a]
Amebiasis
Anaplasmosis
Anthrax
Arbovirus infections (all types)
Babesiosis
Botulism
Brucellosis
Campylobacteriosis
Chlamydia trachomatis infection
Cholera
Coccidioidomycosis
Creutzfeldt-Jakob disease
Cryptosporidiosis
Cyclosporiasis
Dengue fever
Diphtheria
Eastern equine encephalitis
Ehrlichiosis
Encephalitis, infectious
Epsilon toxin of *Clostridium perfringens*
Escherichia coli O157:H7 infection
Giardiasis
Glanders
Gonococcal infection
Haemophilus influenzae, invasive disease
Hantavirus infection
Harmful algal bloom–related illness
Hemolytic uremic syndrome
Hepatitis, viral, types A, B, C, D, E, G, and other types
HIV infection[a]
Influenza-associated pediatric mortality
Influenza: novel influenza A virus infection
Isosporiasis
Kawasaki syndrome
LaCrosse virus infection[b]
Legionellosis
Leprosy
Leptospirosis
Listeriosis
Lyme disease
Malaria
Measles (rubeola)
Melioidosis
Meningitis, infectious
Meningococcal invasive disease
Microsporidiosis
Mumps (infectious parotitis)
Pertussis and pertussis vaccine adverse reactions
Pesticide-related illness
Plague
Pneumonia in a healthcare provider resulting in hospitalization
Poliomyelitis
Psittacosis
Q fever
Rabies (human)
Ricin toxin poisoning
Rocky Mountain spotted fever
Rubella (German measles) and congenital rubella syndrome
Saint Louis encephalitis[b]
Salmonellosis (nontyphoid fever types)
Severe acute respiratory syndrome (SARS)
Shiga-like toxin–producing enteric bacterial infections
Shigellosis
Smallpox and other orthopoxvirus infections
Staphylococcal enterotoxin B poisoning
Streptococcal invasive disease, group A and group B
Streptococcus pneumoniae, invasive disease
Syphilis
Tetanus
Trichinosis
Tuberculosis and suspected tuberculosis[c]
Tularemia
Typhoid fever (case, carrier, or both)
Vancomycin-resistant *Staphylococcus aureus*
Varicella (chickenpox), fatal cases only
Vibriosis, noncholera[d]
Viral hemorrhagic fever (all types)
Western equine encephalitis[b]
Yersiniosis

[a]AIDS and HIV, including $CD4^+$ lymphocyte count and viral load, are reportable.
[b]Reportable by laboratories only.
[c]TB confirmed by culture and suspected TB as indicated by the following:

1. A lab-confirmed acid-fast bacillus smear or biopsy report consistent with active TB
2. An abnormal chest x-ray
3. Initiation of two or more anti-TB medications

[d]Is not reportable if identified in any specimen taken from teeth, gingival tissues, or oral mucosa.

TABLE 1.9 Behavioral Responses

Immediate Response	Secondary Response
Acute emotional turmoil, shock, disbelief about diagnosis, denial	Insomnia, anorexia, difficulty concentrating, depression, difficulty in performing work-related responsibilities and tasks
Anxiety lasting several days until the person assimilates the information	Depression lasting several weeks as the person begins to incorporate the information and to participate realistically in a treatment plan and lifestyle adaptation

Expected and Unexpected Outcomes

Evaluate outcomes using the following steps:

1. Learn the normal or reference values and expected outcomes of the test. The patient or his or her significant others should be able to describe the purpose of the test and the testing process and should properly perform expected activities associated with testing. Offer assistance if necessary. If test outcomes are abnormal, the patient should be encouraged to comply with repeat testing and to introduce appropriate lifestyle changes realistically. Deal with anxiety and fears in a timely manner. Refer the patient to appropriate counseling resources if indicated. Above all, do not dismiss the patient's feelings and concerns casually.
2. Compare normal values with abnormal results and apply these comparisons to the patient's situation. Sometimes, desired outcomes cannot be achieved. For example, the patient cannot, for various reasons, fully participate in the teaching and learning process or the actual testing. Recommendations for follow-up care and lifestyle changes may not be able to be followed. Verbal and nonverbal cues can sometimes provide reasons (e.g., Alzheimer's disease, physical limitations) for this inability. In another instance, the patient might be noncompliant with pretest preparations and posttest activities. Denial of the situation is frequently a reason, although there are many other causes for noncompliance. Patients may refuse diagnostic testing because they feel the results may confirm their worst suspicions and fears.
3. Numerous and varied responses can be related to lack of appropriate problem-solving behaviors, inappropriate behaviors, fears or denial, concern about potential complications, inability to cope with or take control of the situation, depression or abnormal emotional patterns of response, and lack of support from significant others and family. Perceptions of having experienced uncaring acts can lead to frustration, despair, and hopelessness on the patient's part.
4. Adverse events (e.g., perforation, anaphylaxis, death) and health hazards may occur as a result of diagnostic procedures or problems with a medical device or product (e.g., reactions to latex gloves or other latex-containing medical devices). Health professionals are asked to monitor and voluntarily report faulty medical devices to the FDA so that action can be taken to protect the public. Reporting does not necessarily constitute an admission that medical personnel or the product caused or contributed to the adverse event.
5. Prompt action is necessary when results are abnormally high or low and are indicative of a serious situation (e.g., positive blood culture, abnormally elevated potassium level).
6. Modify, report, and collaborate with other healthcare providers when unexpected or abnormal values occur and when changes in medical care may be necessary as a result of test outcomes.
7. Examples of expected and unexpected test outcomes appear in Table 1.10.

TABLE 1.10 Test Outcomes

Expected Outcomes	Unexpected Outcomes
Anticipated outcomes will be achieved.	Some anticipated outcomes may not be achieved, possibly because of specific patient behaviors that interfere with care interventions (e.g., patient does not appear for testing appointment, patient did not fast or withhold medication when directed before testing).
Patient, family, and significant others should be able to describe the testing process and purpose and be able to properly perform expected activities. Information contributes to empowerment.	Inability of patient to fully participate in teaching or learning process is evidenced by verbal and nonverbal cues. Patient cannot properly perform expected activities. Misinterpretation and misinformation of diagnostic process results in panic, avoidance behaviors, and refusal to have tests done.
If test outcomes are abnormal, the appropriate lifestyle changes will be made, and the patient will adopt healthy behaviors.	Patient does not comply with test preparation guidelines and posttest recommended lifestyle changes, hides test results, and minimizes or exaggerates meaning of test outcomes.
With help, the patient is able to integrate the life event, diagnosis of illness, compromised health, and associated life changes and will be able to develop new life patterns.	Patient experiences frustration, anger, and feelings of loss and grief, even after learning new information or skills.
The patient does not develop complications and remains free from injury.	Patient exhibits untoward signs and symptoms (e.g., allergic response, shock, bleeding, nausea, vomiting, retention of barium).
If complications occur, they will be optimally resolved. Signs of infection are treated immediately, and infection is resolved.	Complications are not fully resolved, health state is compromised, and more extensive testing and care are needed.
Anxiety and fears will be alleviated and will not interfere with the testing process. The patient is helped to balance fears with the recognition of the potential for developing coping skills.	Because of anxiety, fear, or uncertainty, the patient is unable to collect specimens properly or to accurately comply with procedural steps. The nurse is unable to calm and reassure the patient. Invasive tests may be canceled if the patient is too anxious or fearful.
With support and education, the patient is able to cope with test outcomes revealing a chronic or life-threatening disease. Hope is inspired or generated, and the patient feels cared for.	There may be a lack of appropriate problem-solving behaviors, uncertainty or denial about test outcomes, inability to cope with test outcomes, extreme depression and abnormal patterns of responses, and refusal to take control of the situation or to cooperate with prescribed regimens. Anxiety, grief, guilt, or sense of social stigma about the illness persists. The patient uses alcohol or drugs. Caregivers are seen as uncaring.

RECOVERED MEDICAL ERRORS

Recovered medical errors can be defined as errors prevented through surveillance. In essence, a nurse or other paramedical personnel has identified, interrupted, and corrected a potential error, preventing an adverse reaction. Recovered medical errors can be divided into two major categories: (1) mistakes (e.g., laboratory findings used incorrectly, protocol not being followed in a technical procedure) and (2) poor judgment (e.g., a delay in a diagnostic test, unstable clinical signs/conditions not recognized). Being cognizant of the aforementioned can protect patients from harm.

LABORATORY RESPONSE NETWORK

The Laboratory Response Network (LRN), established by the CDC in 1999, is a network of local, state, and federal laboratories throughout the United States and internationally as well. These accredited labs have the capability to detect biologic and chemical terrorism agents and emerging infectious diseases, working together in response to public health emergencies. The LRN is made up of three levels (i.e., sentinel, reference, and national laboratories), each with a specific role. The sentinel labs collect, handle, and process specimens for biologic and chemical terrorism analyses; report their findings to the appropriate agency; and refer specimens to the appropriate lab for analysis. The reference labs perform tests to detect and confirm the presence of a threat. The national labs handle infectious agents and can identify specific agent strains.

BIOSAFETY

Biosafety is a major concern in laboratories handling pathogens. Containing hazardous agents in an effort to reduce or even eliminate the possible exposure of laboratory workers and others is a goal of biosafety. As such, there are four levels of biosafety for laboratories:

1. BSL-1 labs study agents not known to cause disease in otherwise healthy adults, whereby no special equipment is required and basic safety protocols are followed.
2. BSL-2 labs test for moderate-risk agents that pose a risk if swallowed, inhaled, or come in contact with the skin, whereby gloves, eyewear, handwashing, and decontamination facilities are used.
3. In BSL-3 labs, airborne, potentially lethal agents are studied. In these labs, gas-tight enclosures, specialized ventilation, and sealed windows are employed as well as clothing decontamination procedures.
4. The BSL-4 labs are used for high-risk life-threatening diseases for which there are no vaccines or treatment. In BSL-4 labs, personnel are required to wear full-body, air-supplied suits and shower when leaving the lab.

CONCLUSION

As professionals, we need to remember that patients are people just like us. These individuals present with their perceptions, worries, and anxieties regarding the diagnostic process and what their illness means to them and their loved ones; what strategies they use for coping; what resources are available for their use; and what other knowledge they have about themselves. As healthcare providers and patient advocates, we must be willing to "take on the mind" of another—that is, to identify with the patient's point of view as much as possible and to show empathy. Once we reach that point, we can then begin to understand and communicate with each other at the deeper levels necessary for a therapeutic relationship to occur.

BIBLIOGRAPHY

Ambruster D, Miller RR: The Joint Commission for Traceability in Laboratory Medicine (JCTLM): A global approach to promote the standardization of clinical laboratory test results. Clin Biochem Rev 42:236–240, 2007

American Medical Association: CPT 2017: Current Procedural Terminology. Chicago, AMA, 2017

American Society of Anesthesiologists Task Force on Sedation and Analgesia by Non-Anesthesiologists: Practice guidelines for sedation and analgesia by non-anesthesiologists. Anesthesiology 96(4):1004–1017, 2002

Auxter SF: Identifying inappropriate laboratory testing strategies. What testing procedures should be eliminated or updated? Clin Lab News 27(6), 2001

Bennett A, Fritsma GA: Quick Guide to Venipuncture. Washington, DC, AACC Press, 2010

Biesheuvel C, Irwig L, Bossuyt P: Observed differences in diagnostic test accuracy between patient subgroups: Is it real or due to reference standard misclassification? Clin Chem 53(10):1725–1729, 2007

Bonini P, Plebani M, Ceriotti F, Rubboli F: Errors in laboratory medicine. Clin Chem 48(5):691–698, 2002

Centers for Disease Control and Prevention: Guideline for hand hygiene in health-care settings. MMWR Recomm Rep 51(RR-16):1–44, 2002; and Hand Hygiene in Healthcare Settings; updated March 25, 2016

Centers for Disease Control and Prevention: Guidelines for environmental infection control in health-care facilities: Recommendations of CDC and the Healthcare Infection Control Advisory Committee. MMWR Recomm Rep 52(RR10):1–42, 2003; updates to Known or Suspected Ebola Vaccine effective August 1, 2015

Chizek M: Following JCAHO's lead on clinical safety in acute-care and LTC settings portends positive patient outcomes. Advance for Nurses. King of Prussia, PA, Merion Publishers, 2005

Clinical and Laboratory Standards Institute (formerly the National Committee for Clinical Laboratory Standards): Clinical Laboratory Safety; Approved Guideline, 3rd ed., GP19-A3, vol. 32 no. 9. Wayne, PA, Clinical and Laboratory Standards Institute, 2012

Clinical and Laboratory Standards Institute (formerly the National Committee for Clinical Laboratory Standards): Procedures for the Collection of Diagnostic Blood Specimens by Venipuncture: Approved Standard, 6th ed., vol. 27 no. 26, H3-A6. Wayne, PA, Clinical and Laboratory Standards Institute, 2007

Clinical and Laboratory Standards Institute (formerly the National Committee for Clinical Laboratory Standards): Protection of Laboratory Workers from Occupationally Acquired Infections; Approved Guideline, 4th ed., vol. 25, no. 10, M29-A3. Wayne, PA, Clinical and Laboratory Standards Institute, 2014

Cohn E, Larson E: Improving participant comprehension in the informed consent process. J Nurs Scholarsh 39(3):273–279, 2007

Davis K, Schoenbaum S, Audet AM: A 2020 vision of patient-centered primary care. J Gen Intern Med 20:953–957, 2005

Donovan HS, Ward SE, Song MK, et al: An update in the representational approach to patient education. J Nurs Scholarsh 39(3):259, 2007

Downer K: The debate on HIV screening: Should it be risk-based or routine? Clin Lab News, 31(8), 2005

Dykes PC, Rothschild JM, Hurley AC: Recovered medical error inventory. J Nurs Scholarsh 42(3):314–318, 2010

Engram BW: Consider the value of nationwide standardized hospital-based nursing documentation forms. Advance for Nurses. King of Prussia, PA, Merion Publishers, 2005

Enzman-Hagedorn MI: Caring practices in the 21st century: The emerging role of nurse practitioners. Topics in Advanced Practice Nursing eJournal 4(4), 2005

Finfgeld-Connett D: Clarification of social support. J Nurs Scholarsh 37(1):4–9, 2005

Fischbach FT: Documenting Care: Communication; Nursing Process; Documentation Standards. Philadelphia, FA Davis, 1991

Fischbach FT, Dunning MB: Nurses' Quick Reference to Common Laboratory and Diagnostic Tests, 6th ed. Philadelphia, Lippincott Williams & Wilkins, 2015

Galanti GA: Caring for Patients from Different Cultures, 4th ed. Philadelphia, University of Pennsylvania Press, 2008

Goroll AH, Mulley AG: Primary Care Medicine: Office Evaluation and Management of the Adult Patient, 7th ed. Philadelphia, Lippincott Williams & Wilkins, 2014

Gutman P: Occupational health nurses have a critical role in reducing needlestick incidence. Advance for Nurses. King of Prussia, PA, Merion Publishers, 2005

Keefe S: Nurses are employing innovative infection control approaches to combat hospital-acquired infections and save lives. Advance for Nurses. King of Prussia, PA, Merion Publishers, 2005

Kiechle FL: An Introduction to Phlebotomy, 14th ed. Northfield, IL, College of American Pathologists, 2013

Kline MV, Huff RM: Health Promotion in Multicultural Populations: A Handbook for Practitioners and Students. Thousand Oaks, CA, Sage Publications, 2008

Lauver DR, Ward, SE, Heidrich SM, et al: Patient-centered interventions. Res Nurs Health 25:246–255, 2002

Lipson GL, Dibble SL: Culture and Clinical Care. San Francisco, UCSF Nursing Press, 2005

Lorenz JM: 2007 patient safety goals: Encouraging patients and family members to partner with nurses in providing safe care is a win-win situation for everyone. Advance for Nurses. King of Prussia, PA, Merion Publishers, 15–17, 2007

Mangurten JA, Scott SH, Guzzetta CE, et al: Family presence: Making room. Am J Nurs 105(5), 2005

Martin RH: Incident reports: Documentation of unexpected or unusual events is crucial to promote quality, safety and risk management. Advance for Nurses. King of Prussia, PA, Merion Publishers, 25–27, 2006

McPhee SJ, Papadakis MA, Rabow, MW: Current Medical Diagnosis and Treatment, 56th ed. New York, Lange Medical Books/McGraw-Hill, 2016

Narayanan S, Young DS: Effects of Herbs and Natural Products on Clinical Laboratory Tests. Washington, DC, AACC Press, 2007

Nichols JH: Point-of-care testing: Moving toward evidence-based practice. Clin Lab News 31(10), 2005

Odom-Forren J, Watson DS: Practical Guide to Moderate Sedation/Analgesia, 2nd ed. St. Louis, MO, Mosby, 2005

Pizzi R: How attitudes, expectations, and knowledge influence testing trends. Clin Lab News 31(9), 2005

Powers BA: Nursing home ethics. Reflections on Nursing Leadership, 3rd Quarter, 23–25, 2005

Price CP, St John A, Kricka LJ: Point-of-Care Testing: Needs, Opportunity, and Innovation, 3rd ed. Washington, DC, AACC Press, 2010

Price CP, Glenn JL, Christenson RH: Applying Evidence-Based Laboratory Medicine: A Step-by-Step Guide. Washington, DC, AACC Press, 2009

Sacks DB, Bruns DE, Goldstein DE, et al: Evidence-based laboratory medicine and test utilization guidelines and recommendations for laboratory analysis or diagnoses and management of diabetes mellitus. Clin Chem 48(3):436–447, 2002

Shifren K: Women with heart disease: Can the common-sense model of illness help? Health Care for Women International 24:355–368, 2003

Smith RA, Cokkinides V, Eyre HJ: American Cancer Society guidelines for the early detection of cancer, 2006. CA Cancer J Clin 56:11–25, 2006

Tente JL, Anderson AL: Rapid assessment of agents of biological terrorism: Defining the differential diagnosis of inhalational anthrax using electronic communication in a practice-based research network. Ann Fam Med 2:434–437, 2004

The Joint Commission: 2017 National Patient Safety Goals. Available at: http://www.jointcommission.org

Tierney LM, Saint S, Whooley MA: Current Essentials of Medicine, 4th ed. New York, McGraw-Hill, 2010

U.S. Department of Health and Human Services: Healthy People 2020: National Health Promotion and Disease Prevention Objectives. Washington, DC, U.S. Government Printing Office, 2011

U.S. Preventive Services Task Force: Guide to Clinical Preventive Services. Rockville, MD, Agency for Healthcare Research and Quality, 2014

Vo-Dinh T: Nanotechnology in Biology and Medicine: Methods, Devices, and Applications. Boca Raton, FL, CRC Press Taylor & Francis Group, 2007

Whittemore R: Analysis of integration in nursing science and practice. J Nurs Scholarsh 37(3):261–267, 2005

Williamson M, Snyder M: Wallach's Interpretation of Diagnostic Tests, 10th ed. Philadelphia, Lippincott Williams & Wilkins, 2014

Wu AHB: Tietz Clinical Guide to Laboratory Tests, 4th ed. Philadelphia, Saunders Elsevier, 2006

Young DS: Effects of Drugs on Clinical Laboratory Tests, 5th ed. Washington, DC, AACC Press, 2000

Young DS: Effects of Preanalytical Variables on Clinical Laboratory Tests, 3rd ed. Washington DC, AACC Press, 2007

Young DS, Friedman RB: Effects of Disease on Clinical Laboratory Tests, 4th ed. Washington, DC, AACC Press, 2001

2 Blood Studies: Hematology and Coagulation

OVERVIEW OF BASIC BLOOD, HEMATOLOGY, AND COAGULATION TESTS

Composition of Blood

The average person circulates about 5 L of blood (1/13 of total body weight), of which 3 L is plasma and 2 L is cells. Plasma fluid derives from the intestines and lymphatic systems and provides a vehicle for cell movement. The cells are produced primarily by the bone marrow and account for blood "solids." Blood cells are classified as white cells (leukocytes), red cells (erythrocytes), and platelets (thrombocytes). White cells are further categorized as granulocytes (neutrophils, basophils, and eosinophils), lymphocytes, and monocytes.

Before birth, hematopoiesis occurs in the liver. In midfetal life, the spleen and lymph nodes play a minor role in cell production. Shortly after birth, hematopoiesis in the liver ceases and the bone marrow is the only site of production of erythrocytes, granulocytes, and platelets. B lymphocytes are produced in the marrow and in the secondary lymphoid organs; T lymphocytes are produced in the thymus.

Blood Tests

Tests in this chapter are basic screening tests that address disorders of hemoglobin (Hb) and hematopoiesis, synthesis, and function. Blood and bone marrow examinations constitute the major means of determining certain blood disorders (anemia, leukemia and porphyria disorders, abnormal bleeding and clotting); inflammation; infection; and inherited disorders of red blood cells (RBCs), white blood cells (WBCs), and platelets. Specimens are obtained through capillary skin punctures (finger, toe, heel), dried blood samples, arterial or venous sampling, or bone marrow aspiration. Specimens may be tested by automated or manual hematology instrumentation and evaluation.

BLOOD SPECIMEN COLLECTION PROCEDURES

Proper specimen collection presumes correct technique and accurate timing when necessary. Although blood tests are common procedures for many patients, fear of needles or sight of blood may cause fear or anxiety. Always assess the patient for these factors and provide patient education, reassurance, and support. Most hematology tests use liquid ethylenediaminetetraacetic acid (EDTA) as an anticoagulant. Tubes with anticoagulants should be gently but completely inverted end-over-end 7 to 10 times after collection. This action ensures complete mixing of anticoagulants with blood to prevent clot formation. Even slightly clotted blood invalidates the test, and the sample must be redrawn.

For plasma coagulation studies, such as prothrombin time (PT) and partial thromboplastin time (PTT), the tube must be allowed to fill to its capacity or an improper blood-to-anticoagulant ratio will invalidate coagulator results. Invert the tube end-over-end 7 to 10 times to prevent clotting.

• Capillary Puncture (Skin Puncture)

Capillary blood is preferred for a peripheral blood smear and can also be used for other hematology studies. Adult capillary blood samples require a skin puncture, usually of the fingertip or earlobe. For children over 1 year of age, the tip of the finger is often used. Under 1 year of age, the best sample is obtained from the great toe or side of the heel.

Procedure

Capillary Blood

1. Observe standard precautions (see Appendix A). Check for latex allergy. If allergy is present, do not use latex-containing products.
2. Obtain capillary blood from fingertips or earlobes (adults) or from the great toe or heel (newborns and infants younger than 1 year). Avoid using the lateral aspect of the heel where the plantar artery is located.
3. Disinfect puncture site, let it dry, and puncture skin with sterile disposable lancet, perpendicular to the lines of the patient's fingers, no deeper than 2 mm. If chlorhexidine is used, allow to dry thoroughly.
4. Wipe away the initial drop of blood. Collect subsequent drops in a microtube or prepare a smear directly from a drop of blood.
5. After collection, apply a small amount of pressure briefly to the puncture site to prevent painful extravasation of blood into the subcutaneous tissues.

PROCEDURAL ALERT

1. Do not squeeze the site to obtain blood because this alters blood composition and invalidates test values.
2. Warming the extremity or placing it in a dependent position may facilitate specimen collection.

Dried Blood Spot

1. In this method, a lancet is used, and the resulting droplets of blood are collected by blotting them with filter paper directly.
2. Check the stability of equipment and integrity of supplies when doing a finger stick. If provided, check the humidity indicator patch on the filter paper card. If the humidity circle is pink, do not use the filter paper card. The humidity indicator must be blue to ensure specimen integrity.
3. After wiping the first drop of blood on the gauze pad, fill and saturate each of the circles in numerical order by blotting the blood droplet with the filter paper. Do not touch the patient's skin to the filter paper; only the blood droplet should come in contact with the filter paper.
4. If an adult has a cold hand, run warm water over it for approximately 3 minutes. The best flow occurs when the arm is held downward, with the hand below heart level, making effective use of gravity. If there is a problem with proper blood flow, milk the finger with gentle pressure to stimulate blood flow or attempt a second finger stick; do not attempt more than two times.
5. When the blood circles penetrate through to the other side of the filter paper, the circles are fully saturated.

Interventions

Pretest Patient Care

1. Instruct the patient about purpose and procedure of test.
2. Follow guidelines in Chapter 1 for safe, effective, informed *pretest* care.

Posttest Patient Care

1. Apply small dressing or adhesive bandage to site.
2. Evaluate puncture site for bleeding or oozing.
3. Apply compression or pressure to the site if it continues to bleed.
4. Evaluate patient's medication history for anticoagulation, nonsteroidal anti-inflammatory drugs (NSAIDs), or acetylsalicylic acid (ASA)-type drug ingestion.
5. Review test results; report and record findings. Modify the nursing care plan as needed.
6. Follow guidelines in Chapter 1 for safe, effective, informed *posttest* care.

● Venipuncture

Venipuncture allows procurement of larger quantities of blood for testing. Care must be taken to avoid sample hemolysis or hemoconcentration and to prevent hematoma, vein damage, infection, and discomfort. Usually, the antecubital veins are the veins of choice because of ease of access. Blood values remain constant no matter which venipuncture site is selected, so long as it is venous and not arterial blood. Sometimes, the wrist area, forearm, or dorsum of the hand or foot must be used. Blood values remain consistent for all of these venipuncture sites.

1. Observe standard precautions (see Appendix A). If latex allergy is known or suspected, use latex-free supplies and equipment.
2. Assess the patient for fear or anxiety related to the procedure. Provide education, reassurance, and a supportive presence.
3. Position and tighten a tourniquet on the upper arm to produce venous distention (congestion). For elderly persons, a tourniquet is not always recommended because of possible rupture of capillaries. Large, distended, and highly visible veins increase the risk for hematoma.
4. Ask the patient to close the fist in the designated arm. Do not ask patient to pump the fist because this may increase plasma potassium levels by as much as 1 to 2 mEq/L (mmol/L). Select an accessible vein.

5. Cleanse the puncture site, working in a circular motion from the center outward, and dry it properly with sterile gauze. Chlorhexidine must dry thoroughly.
6. To anchor the vein, draw the skin taut over the vein and press the thumb below the puncture site. Hold the distal end of the vein during the puncture to decrease the possibility of rolling veins.
7. Puncture the vein according to accepted technique. Usually, for an adult, anything smaller than a 21-gauge needle might make blood withdrawal more difficult. A Vacutainer system syringe or butterfly system may be used.
8. Once the vein has been entered by the collecting needle, blood will fill the attached vacuum tubes automatically because of negative pressure within the collection tube.
9. Remove the tourniquet before removing the needle from the puncture site or bruising will occur.
10. Remove needle. Apply pressure and sterile dressing strip to puncture site.
11. The preservative or anticoagulant added to the collection tube depends on the test ordered. In general, most hematology tests use EDTA anticoagulant. Even slightly clotted blood invalidates the test, and the sample must be redrawn.
12. Take action to prevent these venipuncture errors:
    a. Pretest errors
        (1) Improper patient identification
        (2) Failure to check patient compliance with dietary restrictions
        (3) Failure to calm patient before blood collection
        (4) Use of wrong equipment and supplies
        (5) Inappropriate method of blood collection
    b. Procedure errors
        (1) Failure to dry site completely after cleansing with alcohol or chlorhexidine
        (2) Inserting needle with bevel side down
        (3) Using too small a needle, causing hemolysis of specimen
        (4) Venipuncture in unacceptable area (e.g., above an intravenous [IV] line)
        (5) Prolonged tourniquet application
        (6) Wrong order of tube draw
        (7) Failure to mix blood immediately that is collected in additive-containing tubes
        (8) Pulling back on syringe plunger too forcefully
        (9) Failure to release tourniquet before needle withdrawal
    c. Posttest errors
        (1) Failure to apply pressure immediately to venipuncture site
        (2) Vigorous shaking of anticoagulated blood specimens
        (3) Forcing blood through a syringe needle into tube
        (4) Mislabeling of tubes
        (5) Failure to label specimens with infectious disease precautions as required
        (6) Failure to put date, time, and initials on requisition
        (7) Slow or delayed transport of specimens to the laboratory

NOTE *A blood pressure cuff inflated to a point between systolic and diastolic pressure values can be used in place of a tourniquet.*

NOTE *The Vacutainer system consists of vacuum tubes (Vacutainer tubes), a tube holder, and a disposable multisample collecting needle* (Fig. 2.1).

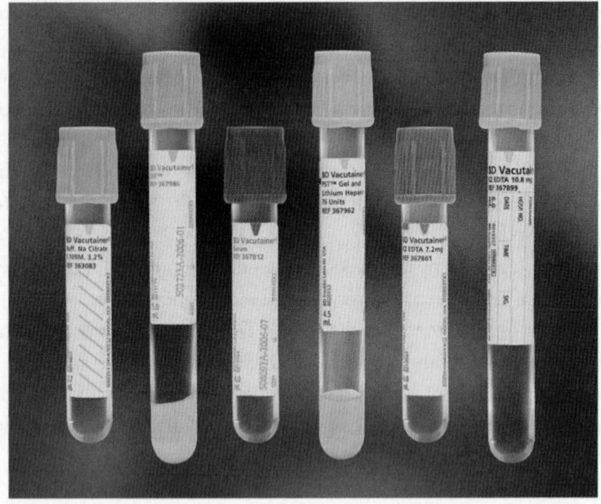

FIGURE 2.1. Evacuated tubes. Vacutainer Plus Plastic brand evacuated tubes. (Becton Dickinson, Franklin Lakes, NJ.)

Interventions

Pretest Patient Care

1. Instruct patient regarding sampling procedure. Assess for circulation or bleeding problems and allergy to latex. Verify with the patient any fasting requirements. Diagnostic blood tests may require certain dietary restrictions of fasting for 8 to 12 hours before test. Drugs taken by the patient should be documented because they may affect results.
2. Reassure patient that only mild discomfort may be felt when the needle is inserted.
3. Place the arm in a fully extended position with palmar surface facing upward (for antecubital access).
4. If withdrawal of the sample is difficult, warm the extremity with warm towels or blankets. Allow the extremity to remain in a dependent position for several minutes before venipuncture. For young children, warming the draw site should be routine to distend small veins.
5. Be alert to provide assistance should the patient become lightheaded or faint.
6. Prescribed local anesthetic creams may be applied to the area before venipuncture; wait 60 seconds for light-skinned persons and 120 seconds for dark-skinned persons after application of the cream before performing the procedure.

Posttest Patient Care

1. If oozing or bleeding from the puncture site continues for more than a few minutes, elevate the area and apply a pressure dressing. Observe the patient closely. Check for anticoagulant or ASA-type ingestion. If venous bleeding is excessive and persists for longer than 10 minutes, notify the healthcare provider.
2. Be aware that the patient occasionally becomes dizzy, faint, or nauseated during the venipuncture. The phlebotomist must be constantly aware of the patient's condition. If a patient feels faint, immediately remove the tourniquet and terminate the procedure. Place the patient in a supine position if possible. If the patient is sitting, lower the head between the legs and instruct the patient to breathe deeply. A cool, wet towel may be applied to the forehead and back of the neck, and, if necessary, ammonia inhalant may be applied briefly. Watch for signs of shock, such as increased heart rate and decreased blood pressure. If the patient becomes unconscious, notify the healthcare provider immediately.

3. Prevent hematomas by using proper technique (do not allow the needle to pass through the vein), releasing the tourniquet before the needle is withdrawn, applying sufficient pressure over the puncture site, and maintaining an extended extremity until bleeding stops. If a hematoma develops, apply a warm compress.
4. Assess the puncture site for signs and symptoms of infection, subcutaneous redness, pain, swelling, and tenderness.
5. Follow guidelines in Chapter 1 for safe, effective, informed *posttest* care.

CLINICAL ALERT

1. In patients with leukemia, agranulocytosis, or lowered resistance, finger stick and earlobe punctures are more likely to cause infection and bleeding than venipunctures. Should a capillary sample be necessary, the cleansing agent should remain in contact with the skin for at least 5–10 min. Chlorhexidine is a topical antimicrobial. It should be allowed to dry. It may then be wiped off with alcohol and the site dried with sterile gauze before puncture.
2. Do not draw blood from the same extremity being used for IV medications, fluids, or transfusions. If no other site is available, make sure the venipuncture site is below the IV site. Avoid areas that are edematous, are paralyzed, are on the same side as a mastectomy, or have infections or skin conditions present. Venipuncture may cause infection or circulatory impairment or impaired healing.
3. Prolonged tourniquet application causes stasis and hemoconcentration and will alter test results. If a vein cannot be found within a minute, release the tourniquet temporarily to avoid tissue necrosis.
4. Strenuous activity immediately before a blood sample draw can alter results because body fluids shift from the vascular bed to the tissue spaces and produce circulatory blood hemoconcentration. It may take 20–30 min of rest and reduced stress to reestablish fluid equilibrium.
5. Assess for interfering factors, including cellulitis, phlebitis, venous obstruction, lymphangitis, or arteriovenous fistulas or shunts.
6. To avoid spurious test results due to infusion of solutions, do not draw above an IV catheter. Choose a site distal to the IV line site.
7. After two unsuccessful attempts, another trained member of the healthcare team should be called.
8. Blood samples may be drawn off central lines. The lines must be flushed with saline before the blood draw.

● Arterial Puncture

Arterial blood samples are necessary for arterial blood gas (ABG) determinations or when it is not possible to obtain a venous blood sample. Arterial sticks are usually performed by a physician or a specially trained nurse or technician because of the potential risks inherent in this procedure. Samples are normally collected directly from the radial, brachial, or femoral arteries. If the patient has an arterial line in place (most frequently in the radial artery), samples can be drawn from the line. Be sure to record the amounts of blood withdrawn in order to track and total the amounts that are removed when frequent samples are required.

ABG determinations are used to assess the status of oxygenation and ventilation, to evaluate the acid–base status by measuring the respiratory and nonrespiratory components, and to monitor effectiveness of therapy. ABGs are also used to monitor critically ill patients, to establish baseline laboratory values, to detect and treat electrolyte imbalances, to titrate appropriate oxygen therapy, to qualify a patient for home oxygen use, and to assess the patient's status in conjunction with pulmonary function testing.

Arterial puncture sites must satisfy the following requirements:

- Sites must have available collateral blood flow.
- Sites must be easily accessible.
- Sites must be relatively nonsensitive as periarterial tissues.

For patients requiring frequent arterial monitoring, an indwelling arterial catheter (line) may be inserted. Follow agency protocols for obtaining arterial line blood samples. The procedure varies for neonate, pediatric, and adult patients (see Arterial Blood Gas Tests in Chapter 14).

Interventions

Pretest Patient Care

- Assess patient for the following contraindications to an arterial stick or indwelling arterial line in a particular area:
    - Absence of a palpable radial artery pulse
    - Positive Allen's test result, which shows only one artery supplying blood to the hand
    - Negative modified Allen's test result, which indicates obstruction in the ulnar artery (i.e., compromised collateral circulation)
    - Cellulitis or infection at the potential site
    - Presence of arteriovenous fistula or shunt
    - Severe thrombocytopenia (platelet count 20,000/mm^3)
    - Prolonged PT or PTT (>1.5 times the control is a relative contraindication)
- A Doppler probe or finger pulse transducer may be used to assess circulation and perfusion in dark-skinned or uncooperative patients.
- Before drawing an arterial blood sample, record the patient's most recent Hb concentration, mode and flow rate of oxygen, and temperature. If the patient has recently undergone suction or been placed on a ventilator or if delivered oxygen concentrations have been changed, wait at least 15 minutes before drawing the sample. This waiting period allows circulating blood levels to return to baseline levels. Hyperthermia and hypothermia also influence oxygen release from Hb at the tissue level.

Intratest Patient Care

- Observe standard precautions and follow agency protocols for the procedure.
- Place the patient in a sitting or supine position.
- Perform a modified Allen's test by encircling the wrist area and using pressure to obliterate the radial and ulnar pulses. Watch for the hand to blanch and then release pressure only over the ulnar artery. If the result is positive, flushing of the hand is immediately noticed, indicating circulation to the hand is adequate. The radial artery can then be used for arterial puncture. If collateral circulation from the ulnar artery is inadequate (i.e., negative test result) and flushing of the hand is absent or slow, then another site must be chosen. An abnormal Allen's test result may be caused by a thrombus, an arterial spasm, or a systemic problem such as shock or poor cardiac output.
- Elevate the wrist area by placing a small pillow or rolled towel under the dorsal wrist area. With the patient's palm facing upward, ask the patient to extend the fingers downward, which flexes the wrist and positions the radial artery closer to the surface.
- Palpate for the artery and maneuver the patient's hand back and forth until a satisfactory pulse is felt.

- Swab the area liberally with an antiseptic agent such as ChloraPrep.
- *OPTIONAL:* Inject the area with a small amount (<0.25 mL) of 1% plain Xylocaine (Lidocaine), if necessary, to anesthetize site. Assess for allergy first. This allows for a second attempt without undue pain.
- Prepare a 20- or 21-gauge needle on a preheparinized, self-filling syringe; puncture the artery; and collect a 3- to 5-mL sample. The arterial pressure pushes the plunger out as the syringe fills with blood. (Venous blood does not have enough pressure to fill the syringe without drawing back on the plunger.) Air bubbles in the blood sample must be expelled as quickly as possible because residual air alters ABG values. The syringe should then be capped and gently rotated to mix heparin with the blood.
- When the draw is completed, withdraw the needle, and place a 4- × 4-inch absorbent bandage over the puncture site. Do not recap needles; if necessary, use the one-handed mechanical, recapping, or scoop technique, or commercially available needles (e.g., BD SafetyGlide [BD, Franklin Lakes, NJ] or Sims Portex Pro-Vent [Smiths Medical, Keene, NH]). Maintain firm finger pressure over the puncture site for a minimum of 5 minutes or until there is no active bleeding evident. After the bleeding stops, apply a firm pressure dressing but do not encircle the entire limb, which can restrict circulation. Leave this dressing in place for at least 24 hours. Instruct the patient to report any signs of bleeding from the site promptly and apply finger pressure if necessary.
- Label the specimen with the patient's name, date and time of collection, and test(s) ordered. Indicate the type and flow rate of O_2 therapy or if the patient was on room air. Place the sample in an ice slurry and transport to the laboratory in a biohazard bag. Do not use blood for ABGs if the sample is more than 1 hour old.
- In clinical settings such as the perioperative or intensive care environment, ABG studies usually include pH, PCO_2, SO_2, total CO_2 content (TCO_2), O_2 content, PO_2, base excess or deficit, HCO_3, Hb, hematocrit (Hct), and levels of chloride, sodium, and potassium.

NOTE *Do not use Xylocaine that contains epinephrine; it causes blood vessel constriction and makes the arterial puncture difficult.*

NOTE *Putting the sample in an ice slurry prevents alterations in gas tensions because metabolic processes within the sample otherwise continue after blood is drawn.*

CLINICAL ALERT

Metabolizing blood cells can quickly alter blood gas values (primarily PaO_2) at normal body temperature (37°C). This occurs much slower at 0°C (i.e., temperature of ice water). An iced sample should remain stable for at least 1 hour. Any sample not placed in ice should be tested within minutes after it is drawn or else discarded. The main effect of cellular metabolism decreases PO_2. Several studies have shown a remarkable fall in PaO_2 if the blood contains >100,000 WBCs/mm^3 (i.e., leukocyte larceny), even when the sample is on ice. A WBC count of this magnitude (usually in leukemia) should mandate special handling, such as testing the sample immediately. Alternatively, check the patient's oxygen saturation by pulse oximetry, which is not affected by extreme leukocytosis.

CLINICAL ALERT

Some patients may experience light-headedness, nausea, or vasovagal syncope during the arterial puncture. Treat according to established protocols.

Posttest Patient Care

Posttest assessment of the puncture site and extremity includes color, movement, sensation, degree of warmth, capillary refill time, and quality of the pulse.

- The arterial puncture site must have a pressure dressing applied and should be frequently assessed for bleeding for several hours. Instruct the patient to report any bleeding from the site and to apply direct pressure to the site if bleeding occurs.
- Frequently monitor the puncture site and dressing for arterial bleeding for several hours. Instruct the patient not to use the extremity for any vigorous activity for at least 24 hours.
- Monitor the patient's vital signs and mental function to determine adequacy of tissue oxygenation and perfusion.
- Follow guidelines in Chapter 1 for safe, effective, informed *posttest* care.

Bone Marrow Aspiration

Bone marrow is located within cancellous bone and long-bone cavities. It consists of a pattern of vessels and nerves, differentiated and undifferentiated hematopoietic cells, reticuloendothelial cells, and fatty tissue. All of these are encased by endosteum, the membrane lining the bone marrow cavity. After proliferation and maturation have occurred in the marrow, blood cells gain entrance to the blood through or between the endothelial cells of the sinus wall.

A bone marrow specimen is obtained through aspiration or biopsy or needle biopsy aspiration. A bone marrow examination is important in the evaluation of a number of hematologic disorders and infectious diseases. The presence or suspicion of a blood disorder is not always an indication for bone marrow studies. A decision to use this procedure is made on an individual basis.

Sometimes, the bone marrow aspirate does not contain hematopoietic cells. This is known as a *dry tap*, which occurs when hematopoietic activity is so sparse that there are no cells to be withdrawn or when the marrow contains so many tightly packed cells that they cannot be suctioned out of the marrow. In such cases, a bone marrow biopsy would be advantageous. Before the bone marrow procedure is started, a peripheral blood smear should be obtained from the patient and a differential leukocyte count done.

Normal Findings

See Table 2.1.

Procedure

1. Assess the patient for fear or anxiety related to the procedure. Provide education, reassurance, and a supportive presence.
2. Follow standard precautions. Check for latex allergy; if allergy is present, do not use latex-containing products. Position the patient on the back or side according to site selected. The posterior iliac crest is the preferred site in all patients older than 12 to 18 months. Alternate sites include the anterior iliac crest, sternum, spinous vertebral processes T10 through L4, ribs, and tibia in children. The sternum is not generally used in children because the bone cavity is too shallow, the risk for mediastinal and cardiac perforation is too great, and the child may be uncooperative.
3. Clip hair if necessary and cleanse and drape the site as for any minor surgical procedure.
4. Inject a local anesthetic (procaine or lidocaine). This may cause a burning sensation. At this time, a skin incision of 3 mm is often made.
5. The healthcare provider introduces a short, rigid, sharp-pointed needle with stylet through the periosteum into the marrow cavity.

TABLE 2.1 Normal Values for Bone Marrow[a]

Formed Cell Elements	Normal Mean (%)	Range (%)
Undifferentiated cells	0.0	0.0–1.0
Reticulum cells	0.4	0.0–1.3
Myeloblasts	2.0	0.3–5.0
Promyelocytes	5.0	1.0–8.0
Myelocytes		
Neutrophilic	12.0	5.0–19.0
Eosinophilic	1.5	0.5–3.0
Basophilic	0.3	0.0–0.5
Metamyelocytes	25.6	17.5–33.7
Neutrophilic	0.4	0.0–1.0
Eosinophilic	0.0	0.0–0.2
Segmented granulocytes		
Neutrophilic	20.0	11.6–30.0
Eosinophilic	2.0	0.5–4.0
Basophilic	0.2	0.0–3.0
Monocytes	2.0	0–3
Lymphocytes	10.0	8–20
Megakaryocytes	0.4	0.0–3.0
Plasma cells	0.9	0.0–2.0
Erythroid series		
Pronormoblasts	0.5	0.2–4.2
Basophilic normoblasts	1.6	0.24–4.8
Polychromatic normoblasts	10.4	3.5–20.5
Orthochromatic normoblasts	6.4	3.0–25
Promegaloblasts	0	0
Basophilic megaloblasts	0	0
Polychromatic megaloblasts	0	0
Orthochromatic megaloblasts	0	0
Myeloid-to-erythroid ratio (ratio of WBC to nucleated RBC)	2:1–4:1	(Slightly higher in infants)

[a]These values are only for adults and should be used as a guideline. Normal values vary greatly; check with your reference laboratory.

6. Pass the needle–stylet combination through the incision, subcutaneous tissue, and bone cortex. The stylet is removed, and 1 to 3 mL of marrow fluid is aspirated. Alert the patient that when the stylet needle enters the marrow, he or she may experience a feeling of pressure. The patient may also feel moderate discomfort as aspiration is done, especially in the iliac crest. Use a Jamshidi needle for biopsy, although you can also use the Westerman-Jensen modification of the Vim-Silverman needle.
7. Remove the stylet and advance the biopsy needle with a twisting motion toward the anterosuperior iliac spine.
8. Rotate or "rock" the needle in several directions several times after adequate penetration of the base (3 cm) has been achieved. This frees up the specimen. Slowly withdraw the needle once this is done.
9. Push the biopsy specimen out backward from the needle. Use the specimen to make touch preparations or immediately place in fixative. Make slide smears at the bedside.
10. Apply pressure to the puncture site until bleeding ceases. Apply a sterile dressing to the site.
11. Label the specimen with the patient's name, date and time of collection, and test(s) ordered.

Clinical Implications

1. A specific and diagnostic bone marrow picture provides clues to many diseases. The presence, absence, and ratio of cells are characteristic of the suspected disease.
2. Bone marrow examination may reveal the following abnormal cell patterns:
   a. Multiple myeloma, plasma cell myeloma, macroglobulinemia
   b. Chronic or acute leukemias
   c. Anemia, including megaloblastic, macrocytic, and normocytic anemias
   d. Toxic states that produce bone marrow depression or destruction
   e. Neoplastic diseases in which the marrow is invaded by tumor cells (metastatic carcinoma, myeloproliferative and lymphoproliferative diseases)
   f. Agranulocytosis, which occurs when bone marrow activity is severely depressed, usually is a result of radiation therapy or chemotherapeutic drugs.
   g. Platelet dysfunction
   h. Some types of infectious diseases, especially histoplasmosis and tuberculosis
   i. Deficiency of body iron stores, microcytic anemia
   j. Lipid or glycogen storage disease
   k. Myelodysplastic syndrome is the name of a group of conditions that occur when blood-forming cells in the bone marrow are damaged.

Interventions

Pretest Patient Care

1. Observe standard precautions.
2. Instruct the patient about test procedure, purpose, benefits, and risks.
3. Ensure that a legal consent form is properly signed and witnessed. Bone marrow aspiration is usually contraindicated in the presence of hemophilia and other bleeding dyscrasias.
4. Reassure the patient that analgesics will be available if needed. Administer moderate sedation and analgesia, if ordered. Use an oxygen monitor to evaluate breathing effectiveness.
5. Bone marrow biopsies or aspirations can be uncomfortable. Tell the patient that squeezing a pillow may be helpful as a distraction technique. Offer emotional support.
6. Sites used for bone marrow aspiration or biopsy affect pretest, intratest, and posttest care. Sites used include the posterosuperior iliac crest, anterior iliac crest (if the patient is very obese), sternum (not used as often with children because cavity is too shallow, danger of mediastinal and cardiac perforation is too great, and observation of procedure is associated with apprehension and lack of cooperation), vertebral spinous processes T10 through L4 and ribs, tibia (often in children), and ribs. Position the patient according to the site selected.
7. Explain to the patient the importance of remaining still during the procedure.
8. Follow guidelines in Chapter 1 for safe, effective, informed *pretest* care.

Posttest Patient Care

1. Monitor vital signs until stable and assess site for excess drainage or bleeding.
2. Recommend bed rest for 30 to 60 minutes; then, normal activities can be resumed.
3. Monitor for signs and symptoms of shock (increased heart rate and decreased blood pressure).
4. Assess for signs and symptoms of infections (redness, swelling, pain, and tenderness).
5. Administer analgesics or sedatives as necessary. Soreness over the puncture site for 3 to 4 days after the procedure is normal. Continued or severe pain may indicate fracture.
6. Review test results; report and record findings. Modify the nursing care plan as needed. Counsel the patient regarding abnormal findings; explain the need for possible follow-up testing and treatment.
7. Follow guidelines in Chapter 1 for safe, effective, informed *posttest* care.

CLINICAL ALERT

1. Complications can include bleeding and sternal fractures. Osteomyelitis or injury to heart or great vessels is rare but can occur if the sternal site is used.
2. Manual and pressure dressings over the puncture site usually control excessive bleeding. Remove dressing in 24 hr. Redress site if necessary.
3. Fever, headache, unusual pain, or redness or pus at biopsy site may indicate infection (later event). Instruct patients to report these symptoms to their healthcare provider immediately.
4. The patient must remain still throughout this procedure.

BASIC BLOOD TEST

● Complete Blood Count (CBC)/Hemogram

A complete blood count (CBC), also referred to as a *hemogram*, consists of a WBC count, RBC count, Hb, Hct, RBC indices, and a platelet count. Table 2.2 contains the normal values for a CBC.

The CBC is a basic screening test and is one of the most frequently ordered laboratory procedures. The findings in the CBC give valuable diagnostic information about the hematologic and other body systems, prognosis, response to treatment, and recovery. The CBC consists of

TABLE 2.2 Normal Values for Hemogram

Age	WBC Count ($\times 10^3/mm^3$)	RBC Count ($\times 10^6/mm^3$)	Hb (g/dL)	Hct (%)	MCV (fL)
Birth–2 wk	9.0–30.0	4.1–6.1	14.5–24.5	44–64	98–112
2–8 wk	5.0–21.0	4.0–6.0	12.5–20.5	39–59	98–112
2–6 mo	5.0–19.0	3.8–5.6	10.7–17.3	35–49	83–97
6 mo–1 yr	5.0–19.0	3.8–5.2	9.9–14.5	29–43	73–87
1–6 yr	5.0–19.0	3.9–5.3	9.5–14.1	30–40	70–84
6–16 yr	4.8–10.8	4.0–5.2	10.3–14.9	32–42	73–87
16–18 yr	4.8–10.8	4.2–5.4	11.1–15.7	34–44	75–89
>18 yr (males)	5.0–10.0	4.5–5.5	14.0–17.4	42–52	84–96
>18 yr (females)	5.0–10.0	4.0–5.0	12.0–16.0	36–48	84–96
Age	**MCH (pg/cell)**	**MCHC (g/dL)**	**Platelets ($\times 10^3/mm^3$)**	**RDW (%)**	**MPV (fL)**
Birth–2 wk	34–40	33–37	150–450	—	—
2–8 wk	30–36	32–36	—	—	—
2–6 mo	27–33	31–35	—	—	—
6 mo–1 yr	24–30	32–36	—	—	—
1–6 yr	23–29	31–35	—	—	—
6–16 yr	24–30	32–36	—	—	—
16–18 yr	25–31	32–36	—	—	—
>18 yr	28–34	32–36	140–400	11.5–14.5	7.4–10.4

Hct, hematocrit; MCHC, mean corpuscular hemoglobin concentration; MCV, mean corpuscular volume; MPV, mean platelet volume; RBC, red blood cell; RDW, RBC distribution width; WBC, white blood cell.

a series of tests that determine number, variety, percentage, concentrations, and quality of blood cells:

1. WBC count: reports the total number of WBCs (leukocytes), which fight infection
2. Differential WBC count (Diff): identifies specific patterns of WBCs by percentage of each cell type (see Differential White Blood Cell Count [Diff; Differential Leukocyte Count] on page 67)
3. RBC count: reports the total number of RBCs, which carry O_2 from lungs to blood tissues and CO_2 from tissue to lungs
4. Hct: percentage of RBCs' mass compared to the total volume of blood
5. Hb: main component of RBCs and transports O_2 and CO_2
6. RBC indices: calculated values of size and Hb content of RBCs; important in anemia evaluations
7. Mean corpuscular volume (MCV)
8. MCHC
9. Mean corpuscular hemoglobin (MCH)
10. Stained red cell examination (film or peripheral blood smear)
11. Platelet count (often included in CBC): Thrombocytes are necessary for clotting and control of bleeding
12. RBC distribution width (RDW): indicates degree variability and abnormal cell size
13. Mean platelet volume (MPV): index of platelet production

These tests are described in detail in the following pages.

CLINICAL ALERT

Hct of <20% can lead to cardiac failure and death.
Hct of >60% is associated with spontaneous clotting of blood.
Hb value of <5.0 g/dL (<50 g/L) leads to heart failure and death.
Hb value of >20.0 g/dL (>200 g/L) results in hemoconcentration and clogging of capillaries.
A critical decrease in platelet value to $<20 \times 10^3/mm^3$ ($<20 \times 10^9/L$) is associated with a tendency for spontaneous bleeding, prolonged bleeding time, petechiae, and ecchymosis.

Normal Findings

See Table 2.2.

Interfering Factors

RBC Count

- Many physiologic variants affect outcomes: posture, exercise, age, altitude, pregnancy, and many drugs.

Hematocrit

- Physiologic variants affect Hct outcomes: age, gender, and physiologic hydremia of pregnancy.

Hemoglobin

- Physiologic variations affect test outcomes: high altitude, excessive fluid intake, age, pregnancy, and many drugs.

Mean Corpuscular Hemoglobin Concentration

- High values may occur in newborns and infants.
- Presence of leukemia or cold agglutinins may increase levels. Mean corpuscular hemoglobin concentration (MCHC) is falsely elevated with a high blood concentration of heparin.

MCH

- Hyperlipidemia and high heparin concentrations falsely elevate MCH values.
- WBC counts >50,000/mm^3 falsely elevate Hb values and falsely elevate the MCH.

WBC Count

- Hourly variation, age, exercise, pain, temperature, and anesthesia affect test results.

Neutrophils and Eosinophils

- Physiologic conditions such as stress, excitement, exercise, and obstetric labor increase neutrophil levels. Steroid administration affects levels for up to 24 hours.
- The eosinophil count is lowest in the morning and then rises from noon until after midnight. Do repeat tests at the same time every day. Stressful states such as burns, postoperative states, and obstetric labor decrease the count. Drugs such as steroids, epinephrine, and thyroxine affect eosinophil levels.

Platelets

- Physiologic factors include high altitudes, strenuous exercise, excitement, and premenstrual and postpartum effects.
- A partially clotted blood specimen affects the test outcome.

Interventions

Pretest Patient Care for Hemogram, CBC, and Differential (Diff) Count (All Components)

1. Explain test procedure. Explain that slight discomfort may be felt when skin is punctured. Refer to procedure for Venipuncture on page 52 for additional information.
2. Avoid stress, if possible, because altered physiologic status influences and changes normal hemogram values.
3. Select hemogram components ordered at regular intervals (e.g., daily, every other day). These should be drawn consistently at the same time of day for reasons of accurate comparison; natural body rhythms cause fluctuations in laboratory values at certain times of the day.
4. Dehydration or overhydration can dramatically alter values; for example, large volumes of IV fluids can "dilute" the blood, and values will appear as lower counts. The presence of either of these states should be communicated to the laboratory.
5. Fasting is not necessary. However, fat-laden meals may alter some test results because of lipidemia.
6. Some medications and other substances can alter results. Obtain a current medication history from the patient.
7. A high WBC count or diseases that cause RBCs to agglutinate may alter test results.

Posttest Patient Care for Hemogram, CBC, and Differential (Diff) Count (All Components)

1. Apply manual pressure and dressing to the puncture site on removal of the needle.
2. Monitor the puncture site for oozing. Maintain pressure dressings on the site if necessary. Notify the healthcare provider of unusual problems with bleeding. If a hematoma develops, apply a compress. If the hematoma is large, assess pulses distal to the phlebotomy site.
3. Resume normal activities and diet.
4. Bruising at the puncture site is not uncommon. Signs of inflammation are unusual and should be reported if the inflamed area appears large, if red streaks develop, or if drainage occurs.
5. Evaluate the outcome and counsel the patient appropriately about anemia, polycythemia, risk for infection, and related blood disorders.
6. Monitor patients with serious platelet defects for signs and symptoms of gastrointestinal bleeding, hemolysis, hematuria, petechiae, vaginal bleeding, epistaxis, and bleeding from gums.
7. Follow guidelines in Chapter 1 for safe, effective, informed *posttest* care.

CLINICAL ALERT

Never apply a total circumferential dressing and wrap because this may compromise circulation and nerve function if constriction, from whatever cause, occurs.

TESTS OF WHITE BLOOD CELLS

White Blood Cell (WBC) Count (Leukocyte Count)

WBCs (leukocytes) are divided into two main groups: granulocytes and agranulocytes. The granulocytes receive their name from the distinctive granules that are present in the cytoplasm of neutrophils, basophils, and eosinophils. However, each of these cells also contains a multilobed nucleus, which accounts for their also being called *polymorphonuclear (PMN) leukocytes*. In laboratory terminology, they are often called "polys" or PMNs. The agranulocytes, which consist of the lymphocytes and monocytes, do not contain distinctive granules and have nonlobular nuclei that are not necessarily spherical. The term *mononuclear leukocytes* is applied to these cells.

The endocrine system is an important regulator of the number of leukocytes in the blood. Hormones affect the production of leukocytes in the blood-forming organs, their storage and release from the tissue, and their disintegration. A local inflammatory process exerts a definite chemical effect on the mobilization of leukocytes. The life span of leukocytes varies from 13 to 20 days, after which the cells are destroyed in the lymphatic system; many are excreted from the body in fecal matter.

Leukocytes fight infection and defend the body by a process called *phagocytosis*, in which the leukocytes actually encapsulate foreign organisms and destroy them. Leukocytes also produce, transport, and distribute antibodies as part of the immune response to a foreign substance (antigen).

The WBC count serves as a useful guide to the severity of a disease process. Specific patterns of leukocyte response can be expected in various types of diseases as determined by the differential count (showing percentages of each of the different types of leukocytes). Leukocyte and differential counts, by themselves, are of little value as aids to diagnosis unless the results are related to the clinical condition of the patient—only then is a correct and useful interpretation possible. Signs and symptoms of increased WBCs include fever, bruising, petechiae, fatigue, anemia, bleeding of mucous membranes, weight loss, and frequent infections.

Normal Findings

Black adults: 3.2 to 10.0 × 10^3 cells/mm^3 or × 10^9/L or 3200 to 10,000 cells/mm^3
Adults: 4.5 to 10.5 × 10^3 cells/mm^3 or × 10^9/L or 4500 to 10,500 cells/mm^3
Children:
- 0 to 2 weeks: 9.0 to 30.0 × 10^3 cells/mm^3 or × 10^9/L or 9000 to 30,000 cells/mm^3
- 2 to 8 weeks: 5.0 to 21.0 × 10^3 cells/mm^3 or × 10^9/L or 5000 to 21,000 cells/mm^3
- 2 months to 6 years: 5.0 to 19.0 × 10^3 cells/mm^3 or × 10^9/L or 5000 to 19,000 cells/mm^3
- 6 to 18 years: 4.8 to 10.8 × 10^3 cells/mm^3 or × 10^9/L or 4800 to 10,800 cells/mm^3

CLINICAL ALERT

1. WBC count $<500/mm^3$ or $<0.5 \times 10^3/mm^3$ (or $\times 10^9/L$) is extremely serious and can be fatal.
2. WBC count $<2.0 \times 10^9/L$ represents a critical value.
3. WBC count $>30{,}000/mm^3$ or $>30.0 \times 10^3/mm^3$ (or $\times 10^9/L$) is a critical value.

NOTE *Normal values vary greatly; check with your reference laboratory.*

Procedure

1. Obtain a venous anticoagulated EDTA (lavender-topped tube) whole blood sample of 5 mL or a finger stick sample.
2. Label the specimen with the patient's name, date and time of collection, and test(s) ordered.
3. Blood is processed either manually or automatically, using an electronic counting instrument such as the Coulter Counter® or Abbott CELL-DYN®.

Clinical Implications

1. *Leukocytosis*: WBC count $>11,000/mm^3$ or $>11.0 \times 10^3/mm^3$ (or $>11 \times 10^9/L$)
   a. Leukocytosis is usually caused by an increase of only one type of leukocyte, and it is given the name of the type of cell that shows the main increase:
      (1) Neutrophilic leukocytosis or neutrophilia
      (2) Lymphocytic leukocytosis or lymphocytosis
      (3) Monocytic leukocytosis or monocytosis
      (4) Basophilic leukocytosis or basophilia
      (5) Eosinophilic leukocytosis or eosinophilia
   b. An increase in circulating leukocytes is rarely caused by a proportional increase in leukocytes of all types. When this does occur, it is usually a result of hemoconcentration.
   c. In certain diseases (e.g., measles, pertussis, sepsis), the increase of leukocytes is so great that the blood picture suggests leukemia. Leukocytosis of a temporary nature (leukemoid reaction) must be distinguished from leukemia. In leukemia, the leukocytosis is chronic and progressive.
   d. Leukocytosis occurs in acute infections, in which the degree of increase of leukocytes depends on severity of the infection, patient's resistance, patient's age, and marrow efficiency and reserve.
   e. Other causes of leukocytosis include the following:
      (1) Leukemia, myeloproliferative disorders
      (2) Trauma or tissue injury (e.g., surgery)
      (3) Malignant neoplasms, especially bronchogenic carcinoma
      (4) Toxins, uremia, coma, eclampsia, thyroid storm
      (5) Drugs, especially ether, chloroform, quinine, epinephrine (adrenaline), colony-stimulating factors
      (6) Acute hemolysis
      (7) Hemorrhage (acute)
      (8) After splenectomy
      (9) Polycythemia vera
      (10) Tissue necrosis
   f. Occasionally, leukocytosis is found when there is no evidence of clinical disease. Such findings suggest the presence of:
      (1) Sunlight, ultraviolet irradiation
      (2) Physiologic leukocytosis resulting from excitement, stress, exercise, pain, cold or heat, anesthesia
      (3) Nausea, vomiting, seizures
   g. Steroid therapy modifies the leukocyte response.
      (1) When corticotropin (adrenocorticotropic hormone [ACTH]) is given to a healthy person, leukocytosis occurs.
      (2) When ACTH is given to a patient with severe infection, the infection can spread rapidly without producing the expected leukocytosis; therefore, what would normally be an important sign is obscured.

2. *Leukopenia*: WBC count <4000/mm^3 or <4.0 × 10^3/mm^3 or <4.0 cells × 10^9/L occurs during and following:
   a. Viral infections, some bacterial infections, overwhelming bacterial infections
   b. Hypersplenism
   c. Bone marrow depression caused by heavy metal intoxication, ionizing radiation, drugs:
      (1) Antimetabolites
      (2) Barbiturates
      (3) Benzene
      (4) Antibiotics
      (5) Antihistamines
      (6) Anticonvulsants
      (7) Antithyroid drugs
      (8) Arsenicals
      (9) Cancer chemotherapy (causes a decrease in leukocytes; leukocyte count is used as a link to disease)
      (10) Cardiovascular drugs
      (11) Diuretics
      (12) Analgesics and anti-inflammatory drugs
   d. Primary bone marrow disorders
      (1) Leukemia (aleukemic)
      (2) Pernicious anemia
      (3) Aplastic anemia
      (4) Myelodysplastic syndromes
      (5) Congenital disorders
      (6) Kostmann's syndrome
      (7) Reticular agenesis
      (8) Cartilage-hair hypoplasia
      (9) Shwachman-Diamond syndrome
      (10) Chédiak-Higashi syndrome
   e. Immune-associated neutropenia
   f. Marrow-occupying diseases (fungal infection, metastatic tumor)
   g. Pernicious anemia

Interfering Factors

1. Hourly rhythm: There is an early-morning low level and late-afternoon peak. Age, gender, exercise, medications, pregnancy, pain, temperature, altitude, and anesthesia affect test results.
2. Age: In newborns and infants, the WBC count is high (10,000/mm^3 to 20,000/mm^3 or 10 × 10^9/L to 20 × 10^9/L); the count gradually decreases in children until the adult values are reached between 18 and 21 years of age.
3. Any stressful situation that leads to an increase in endogenous epinephrine production and a rapid rise in the leukocyte count

Interventions

Pretest Patient Care

1. Explain test purpose and procedure. Assess for signs and symptoms of increased WBCs (e.g., fever, bruising, petechiae, fatigue, anemia, bleeding of mucous membranes, weight loss, history of infections).
2. Refer to standard *pretest* care for hemogram, CBC, and differential count on page 63. Also, follow guidelines in Chapter 1 for safe, effective, informed *pretest* care.

3. Select hemogram components ordered at regular intervals (e.g., daily, every other day). These should be drawn consistently at the same time of day for reasons of accurate comparison; natural body rhythms cause fluctuations in laboratory values at certain times of the day.
4. Dehydration or overhydration can dramatically alter values; for example, large volumes of IV fluids can "dilute" the blood, and values will appear as lower counts. The presence of either of these states should be communicated to the laboratory.
5. Fasting is not necessary. However, fat-laden meals may alter some test results as a result of lipidemia.

Posttest Patient Care

1. Review test results; report and record findings. Modify the nursing care plan as needed. Counsel the patient regarding abnormal findings; explain the need for possible follow-up testing and treatment.
2. Refer to standard *posttest* care for hemogram, CBC, and differential count on page 67. Also, follow guidelines in Chapter 1 for safe, effective, informed *posttest* care.
3. In prolonged severe granulocytopenia or pancytopenia:
   - Give no fresh fruits or vegetables because the kitchen, especially in a hospital, may be a source of food contamination.
   - When the WBC count is low, a person can get a bacterial, pseudomonal, or fungal infection from fresh fruits and vegetables.
   - Use a minimal-bacteria or commercially sterile diet. All food must be served from a new or single-serving package.
   - Consider a leukemia diet. See dietary department for restrictions (e.g., cooked food only) and careful food preparation.
   - Do not give intramuscular injections.
   - Do not take rectal temperature, give suppositories, give enemas, or perform rectal exams.
   - Do not allow patients to floss their teeth.
   - Do not use razor blades.
   - Do not give aspirin or NSAIDs, which cause platelet dysfunction.
   - Observe closely for signs or symptoms of infection; often, patients have only a fever. Without leukocytes to produce inflammation, serious infections can have very subtle findings.
4. Possible treatments include administration of blood products as ordered, assisting the patient with activities of daily living to decrease fatigue, and close monitoring for signs of infections. Also, provide frequent mouth care and promote hygiene.

● Differential White Blood Cell Count (Diff; Differential Leukocyte Count)

The total count of circulating WBCs is differentiated according to the five types of leukocytes, each of which performs a specific function.

The differential count is expressed as a percentage of the total number of leukocytes (WBCs). The distribution (number and type) of cells and the degree of increase or decrease are diagnostically significant. The percentages indicate the *relative* number of each type of leukocyte in the blood. The *absolute* count of each type of leukocyte is obtained mathematically by multiplying its relative percentage by the total leukocyte count. The formula is:

Relative value (%) × WBC (cells/mm^3) = Absolute value (cells/mm^3)

NOTE *This is the preferred way of reporting.*

Function of Circulating White Blood Cells According to Leukocyte Type

Cell	These Cells Function to Combat
Neutrophils	Pyogenic infections (bacterial)
Eosinophils	Allergic disorders and parasitic infestations
Basophils	Parasitic infections, some allergic disorders
Lymphocytes	Viral infections (measles, rubella, chickenpox, infectious mononucleosis)
Monocytes	Severe infections, by phagocytosis

Differential For Leukocyte Count

Age	Bands/ Stab (%)	Segs/ Polys (%)	Eos (%)	Basos (%)	Lymphs (%)	Monos (%)	Metas (%)
Birth–1 wk	10–18	32–62	0–2	0–1	26–36	0–6	—
1–2 wk	8–16	19–49	0–4	0–0	38–46	0–9	—
2–4 wk	7–15	14–34	0–3	0–0	43–53	0–9	—
4–8 wk	7–13	15–35	0–3	0–1	41–71	0–7	—
2–6 mo	5–11	15–35	0–3	0–1	42–72	0–6	—
6 mo–1 yr	6–12	13–33	0–3	0–0	46–76	0–5	—
1–6 yr	5–11	13–33	0–3	0–0	46–76	0–5	—
6–16 yr	5–11	32–54	0–3	0–1	27–57	0–5	—
16–18 yr	5–11	34–64	0–3	0–1	25–45	0–5	—
>18 yr	3–6	50–62	0–3	0–1	25–40	3–7	0–1

Bands or stab cells, immature forms of neutrophils; Segs, segmented neutrophils; Polys, polymorphonuclear neutrophils; Eos, eosinophils; Basos, basophils; Lymphs, lymphocytes; Monos, monocytes; Metas, metamyelocytes.

The differential count alone has limited value; it must always be interpreted in relation to the WBC count. If the percentage of one type of cell is increased, it can be inferred that cells of that type are relatively more numerous than normal, but it is not known whether this reflects an actual increase in the (absolute) number of cells that are relatively increased or an absolute decrease in cells of another type. On the other hand, if the relative (percentage) values of the differential count and the total WBC count are both known, it is possible to calculate absolute values that are not subject to misinterpretation.

Historically, a differential count was done manually, but current hematology instruments do an automated differential count. The count is based on a combination of hydrodynamic focusing and fluorescent dyes in newer instrumentation. However, not all samples can be evaluated by automated methods. When a leukocyte count is extremely low or high, a manual count may be necessary. Extremely abnormal leukocytes, such as those in leukemia, also have to be counted by hand. The automated instrument has built-in quality control that senses abnormal cells and flags the differential. A microscopic count must then be done.

● Segmented Neutrophils (Polymorphonuclear Neutrophils, PMNs, Segs, Polys)

Neutrophils, the most numerous and important type of leukocytes in the body's reaction to inflammation, constitute a primary defense against microbial invasion through the process of phagocytosis. These cells can also cause some body tissue damage by their release of enzymes and endogenous pyogens. In their immature stage of development, neutrophils are referred to as "stab" or "band" cells. The term *band* stems from the appearance of the nucleus, which has not yet assumed the lobed shape of the mature cell.

This test determines the presence of neutrophilia or neutropenia. Neutrophilia is an increase in the absolute number of neutrophils in response to invading organisms and tumor cells. Neutropenia occurs when too few neutrophils are produced in the marrow, too many are stored in the blood vessel margin, or too many have been called to action and used up.

Normal Findings

Absolute count: 3000 to 7000/mm^3 or 3 to 7 $\times$ 10^9/L
African American adults: 1.2 to 6.6 $\times$ 10^9/L
Differential: 50% of total WBC count
0% to 3% of total PMNs are stab or band cells

NOTE *All references use this SI unit for reporting.*

Procedure

1. Obtain a 5-mL blood sample in a lavender-topped tube (with EDTA); label the specimen with the patient's name, date and time of collection, and test(s) ordered and place it in a biohazard bag.
2. Count as part of the differential.

Clinical Implications

1. Neutrophilia (increased absolute number and relative percentage of neutrophils) >8.0 $\times$ 10^9/L or 8000/mm^3; for African Americans: >7.0 $\times$ 10^9/L or 7000/mm^3
   a. Acute, localized, and general bacterial infections. Also, fungal and spirochetal and some parasitic and rickettsial infections.
   b. Inflammation (e.g., vasculitis, rheumatoid arthritis, pancreatitis, gout) and tissue necrosis (myocardial infarction, burns, tumors)
   c. Metabolic intoxications (e.g., diabetes mellitus, uremia, hepatic necrosis)
   d. Chemicals and drugs causing tissue destruction (e.g., lead, mercury, digitalis, venoms)
   e. Acute hemorrhage, hemolytic anemia, hemolytic transfusion reaction
   f. Myeloproliferative disease (e.g., myeloid leukemia, polycythemia vera, myelofibrosis)
   g. Malignant neoplasms—carcinoma
   h. Some viral infections (noted in early stages) and some parasitic infections
2. *Ratio* of segmented neutrophils to band neutrophils: normally, 1% to 3% of PMNs are band forms (immature neutrophils).
   a. Degenerative shift to left: In some overwhelming infections, there is an increase in band (immature) forms with no leukocytosis (poor prognosis).
   b. Regenerative shift to left: There is an increase in band (immature) forms with leukocytosis (good prognosis) in bacterial infections.
   c. Shift to right: Decreased band (immature) cells with increased segmented neutrophils can occur in liver disease, megaloblastic anemia, hemolysis, drugs, cancer, and allergies.
   d. Hypersegmentation of neutrophils with no band (immature) cells is found in megaloblastic anemias (e.g., pernicious anemia) and chronic morphine addiction.
3. Neutropenia (decreased neutrophils)
   a. <1800/mm^3 or <1.8 $\times$ 10^9/L
   b. African Americans: <1000/mm^3 or <40% of differential count

c. Causes associated with decreased or ineffective production
   (1) Inherited stem cell disorders and genetic disorders of cellular development
   (2) Acute overwhelming bacterial infections (poor prognosis) and septicemia
   (3) Viral infections (e.g., mononucleosis, hepatitis, influenza, measles)
   (4) Some rickettsial and parasitical (protozoan) diseases (malaria)
   (5) Drugs, chemicals, ionizing radiation, venoms
   (6) Hematopoietic diseases (e.g., aplastic anemia, megaloblastic anemias, iron-deficiency anemia, aleukemic leukemia, myeloproliferative diseases)
d. Causes associated with decreased survival
   (1) Infections mainly in persons with little or no marrow reserves, elderly people, and infants
   (2) Collagen vascular diseases with antineutrophil antibodies (e.g., systemic lupus erythematosus [SLE] and Felty's syndrome)
   (3) Autoimmune and isoimmune causes
   (4) Drug hypersensitivity (There is an extensive list of drugs that continues to grow. Women are more likely than men to have a drug sensitivity. Removal of offending drug results in return to normal.)
   (5) Splenic sequestration
e. Neutropenia in neonates (<5000/mm^3 or <5.0 × 10^9/L or <1000/mm^3 or <1.0 × 10^9/L after first week of life)
   (1) Maternal neutropenia, maternal drug ingestion, maternal isoimmunization to fetal leukocytes (maternal immunoglobulin G [IgG] antibodies to fetal neutrophils)
   (2) Inborn errors of metabolism (e.g., maple syrup urine disease)
   (3) Immune deficits—acquired
   (4) Deficits and disorders of myeloid stem cell (e.g., Kostmann's agranulocytosis, benign chronic granulocytopenia of childhood)
   (5) Congenital neutropenia
f. Pregnancy—progressive decrease until labor

4. Other leukocyte abnormalities and corresponding diseases are listed in Table 2.3.

NOTE *An ethnic difference exists only in neutrophils.*

Interfering Factors

1. Physiologic conditions such as stress, excitement, fear, vomiting, electric shock, anger, joy, and exercise temporarily cause increased neutrophils. Crying babies have neutrophilia.
2. Obstetric labor and delivery cause neutrophilia. Menstruation causes neutrophilia.
3. Steroid administration: Neutrophilia peaks in 4 to 6 hours and returns to normal by 24 hours (in severe infection, expected neutrophilia does not occur).
4. Exposure to extreme heat or cold
5. Age
   a. Children respond to infection with a greater degree of neutrophilic leukocytosis than adults do.
   b. Some elderly patients respond weakly or not at all, even when infection is severe.
6. Resistance
   a. People of any age who are weak and debilitated may fail to respond with a significant neutrophilia.
   b. When an infection becomes overwhelming, the patient's resistance is exhausted and, as death approaches, the number of neutrophils decreases greatly.
7. Myelosuppressive chemotherapy
8. Many drugs cause increases or decreases in neutrophils.

TABLE 2.3 Leukocyte Abnormalities and Diseases

Abnormality	Description	Associated Diseases
Toxic granulation	Coarse, black or purple, cytoplasmic granules	Infections or inflammatory diseases; acute reactive state
Döhle bodies	Small (1–2 μm), blue, cytoplasmic inclusions in neutrophils	Infections or inflammatory diseases, burns
Pelger-Huët anomalies	Neutrophil with bilobed nucleus or no segmentation of nucleus; chromatin is coarse, and cytoplasm is pink with normal granulation	Hereditary (congenital), myelogenous leukemia
May-Hegglin anomaly	Basophilic, cytoplasmic inclusions of leukocytes; similar to Döhle bodies	May-Hegglin syndrome (hereditary), includes thrombocytopenia and giant platelets
Alder-Reilly anomaly	Prominent azurophilic granulation in leukocytes; similar to toxic granulation; granulation is seen better with Giemsa stain	Hereditary, mucopolysaccharidosis
Chédiak-Higashi anomaly	Gray-green, large cytoplasmic inclusions that are fused giant lysosomes (phospholipids)	Chédiak-Higashi syndrome; few cases of acute myeloid leukemia
Lupus erythematosus (LE) cells	Neutrophilic leukocyte with a *homogeneous* red-purple inclusion that distends the cell's cytoplasm	LE and other collagen diseases, chronic hepatitis, drug reactions, serum sickness (not naturally occurring in the body—must be induced to form by mechanical trauma in vitro)
Tart cell	Neutrophilic leukocyte with a phagocytized nucleus of a granulocyte that retains some nuclear structure	Drug reactions (e.g., penicillin, procainamide) or actual phagocytosis
Myeloid "shift to left"	Presence of bands, myelocytes, metamyelocytes, or promyelocytes	Infections, intoxications, tissue necrosis, myeloproliferative syndrome, leukemia (chronic myelocytic), leukemoid reaction, pernicious anemia, hyposplenism
Hypersegmented neutrophil	Mature neutrophil with more than five distinct lobes	Megaloblastic anemia, hereditary constitutional hypersegmentation of neutrophils; long-term chronic infection
Leukemic cells (e.g., lymphoblasts, myeloblasts)	Presence of lymphoblasts, myeloblasts, monoblasts, myelomonoblasts, promyelocytes (none normally present in peripheral blood)	Leukemia (acute or chronic), leukemoid reaction, severe infectious or inflammatory diseases, myeloproliferative syndrome, intoxications, malignancies, recovery from bone marrow suppression
Auer bodies	Rodlike, 1–6 μm long, red-purple, refractile inclusions in neutrophils	Acute myelocytic leukemia or myelomonocytic leukemia
Smudge cell	Disintegrating nucleus of a ruptured leukocyte	Increased numbers in leukemic blood, particularly in acute lymphocytic leukemia or chronic lymphocytic leukemia when WBC count is $>10{,}000/mm^3$ or $>10 \times 10^9/L$

Interventions

Pretest Patient Care

1. Explain test purpose and procedure.
2. Refer to standard *pretest* care for hemogram, CBC, and differential count on page 63. Also, follow guidelines in Chapter 1 for safe, effective, informed *pretest* care.

Posttest Patient Care

1. Review test results; report and record findings. Modify the nursing care plan as needed. Counsel the patient regarding abnormal findings; explain the need for possible follow-up testing and treatment.
2. Monitor for neutrophilia or neutropenia.
3. Refer to standard *posttest* care for hemogram, CBC, and differential count on page 63. Also, follow guidelines in Chapter 1 for safe, effective, informed *posttest* care.

CLINICAL ALERT

Agranulocytosis (marked neutropenia and leukopenia) is extremely dangerous and is often fatal because the body is unprotected against invading agents. Patients with agranulocytosis must be protected from infection by means of reverse isolation techniques with strictest emphasis on handwashing technique.

● Eosinophils

Eosinophils, capable of phagocytosis, ingest antigen–antibody complexes and become active in the later stages of inflammation. Eosinophils respond to allergic and parasitic diseases. Eosinophilic granules contain histamine (one third of all the histamine in the body).

This test is used to diagnose allergic infections, assess severity of infestations with worms and other large parasites, and monitor response to treatment.

Normal Findings

Absolute count: 0 to 0.7×10^9/L
Differential: 0% to 3% of total WBC count

Procedure

1. Obtain a 5-mL blood sample in a lavender-topped tube (with EDTA). Label the specimen with the patient's name, date and time of collection (e.g., 3:00 p.m.), and test(s) ordered. Place it in a biohazard bag.
2. Perform a total WBC count, make a blood smear, count 100 cells, and report the percentage of eosinophils.
3. Be aware that an absolute eosinophil count is also available. It is done with a special eosinophil stain and manual counting on a hemacytometer. It must be done within 4 hours after collection or, if refrigerated, within 24 hours.

Clinical Implications

1. *Eosinophilia* (increased circulating eosinophils) >5% or >500 cells/mm^3 or >0.5×10^9/L occurs in:
   a. Allergies, hay fever, asthma
   b. Parasitic disease and trichinosis tapeworm, especially with tissue invasion

c. Some endocrine disorders, Addison's disease, hypopituitarism
d. Hodgkin's disease and myeloproliferative disorders, chronic myeloid leukemia, polycythemia vera
e. Chronic skin diseases (e.g., pemphigus, eczema, dermatitis herpetiformis)
f. Systemic eosinophilia associated with pulmonary infiltrates (PIE)
g. Some infections (scarlet fever, chorea), convalescent stage of other infections
h. Familial eosinophilia (rare), hypereosinophilic syndrome
i. Polyarteritis nodosa, collagen vascular diseases (e.g., SLE), connective tissue disorders
j. Eosinophilic gastrointestinal diseases (e.g., ulcerative colitis, Crohn's disease)
k. Immunodeficiency disorders (Wiskott-Aldrich syndrome, immunoglobulin A deficiency)
l. Aspirin sensitivity, allergic drug reactions
m. Löffler's syndrome (related to *Ascaris* species infestation), tropical eosinophilia (related to filariasis)
n. Poisons (e.g., black widow spider, phosphorus)
o. Hypereosinophilic syndrome ($>1.5 \times 10^9$/L), persistent extreme eosinophilia with eosinophilic infiltration of tissues causing tissue damage and organ dysfunction
   (1) Eosinophilic leukemia
   (2) Trichinosis invasion
   (3) Dermatitis herpetiformis
   (4) Idiopathic

2. *Eosinopenia* (decreased circulating eosinophils) is usually caused by an increased adrenal steroid production that accompanies most conditions of bodily stress and is associated with:
   a. Cushing's syndrome (acute adrenal failure): <50/mm^3
   b. Use of certain drugs such as ACTH, epinephrine, thyroxine, prostaglandins
   c. Acute bacterial infections with a marked shift to the left (increase in immature leukocytes)
3. *Eosinophilic myelocytes* are counted separately because they have a greater significance, being found only in leukemia or leukemoid blood pictures.

Interfering Factors

1. Daily rhythm: Normal eosinophil count is lowest in the morning and then rises from noon until after midnight. For this reason, serial eosinophil counts should be repeated at the same time each day.
2. Stressful situations, such as burns, postoperative states, electroshock, and labor, cause a decreased count.
3. After administration of corticosteroids, eosinophils disappear.
4. See Appendix E for drugs that affect test outcomes.

Interventions

Pretest Patient Care

1. Explain test purpose and procedure.
2. Refer to standard patient care for hemogram, CBC, and differential count on page 63. Also, follow guidelines in Chapter 1 for safe, effective, informed *pretest* care.

Posttest Patient Care

1. Review test results; report and record findings. Modify the nursing care plan as needed. Counsel the patient regarding abnormal findings; explain the need for possible follow-up testing and treatment.
2. Use special precautions if patient is receiving steroid therapy, epinephrine, thyroxine, or prostaglandins. Eosinophilia can be masked by steroid use.
3. Refer to standard *posttest* care for hemogram, CBC, and differential count on page 63. Also, follow guidelines in Chapter 1 for safe, effective, informed *posttest* care.

Basophils

Basophils, which constitute a small percentage of the total leukocyte count, are considered phagocytic. The basophilic granules contain heparin, histamines, and serotonin. Tissue basophils are called *mast cells* and are similar to blood basophils. Normally, mast cells are not found in peripheral blood and are rarely seen in healthy bone marrow.

Basophil counts are used to study chronic inflammation. There is a positive correlation between high basophil counts and high concentrations of blood histamines, although this correlation does not imply cause and effect. It is extremely difficult to diagnose basopenia because a 1000 to 10,000 count differential would have to be done to get an absolute count.

Normal Findings

Absolute count: 15 to 50/mm^3 or 0.02 to 0.05 $\times$ 10^9/L
Differential: 0% to 1.0% of total WBC count

Procedure

1. Obtain a 5-mL venous whole blood sample in a lavender-topped tube (with EDTA) and label the specimen with the patient's name, date and time of collection, and test(s) ordered.
2. Count as part of the differential.

Clinical Implications

1. *Basophilia* (increased count) >50/mm^3 or >0.05 $\times$ 10^9/L is commonly associated with the following:
    a. Granulocytic (myelocytic) leukemia
    b. Acute basophilic leukemia
    c. Myeloid metaplasia, myeloproliferative disorders
    d. Hodgkin's disease
2. It is less commonly associated with the following:
    a. Inflammation, allergy, or sinusitis
    b. Polycythemia vera
    c. Chronic hemolytic anemia
    d. After splenectomy
    e. After ionizing radiation
    f. Hypothyroidism
    g. Infections, including tuberculosis, smallpox, chickenpox, influenza
    h. Foreign protein injection
3. *Basopenia* (decreased count) <20/mm^3 or <0.02 $\times$ 10^9/L is associated with the following:
    a. Acute phase of infection
    b. Hyperthyroidism
    c. Stress reactions (e.g., pregnancy, myocardial infarction)
    d. After prolonged steroid therapy, chemotherapy, radiation
    e. Hereditary absence of basophils
    f. Acute rheumatic fever in children
4. *Presence of numbers of tissue mast cells* (tissue basophils) is associated with the following:
    a. Rheumatoid arthritis
    b. Urticaria, asthma
    c. Anaphylactic shock
    d. Hypoadrenalism
    e. Lymphoma

f. Macroglobulinemia
g. Mast cell leukemia
h. Lymphoma invading bone marrow
i. Urticaria pigmentosa
j. Asthma
k. Chronic liver or renal disease
l. Osteoporosis
m. Systemic mastocytosis

Interfering Factors

See Appendix E for drugs that affect test outcomes.

Interventions

Pretest Patient Care

1. Explain test purpose and procedure.
2. Refer to standard patient care for hemogram, CBC, and differential count on page 63. Also, follow guidelines in Chapter 1 for safe, effective, informed *pretest* care.

Posttest Patient Care

1. Review test results; report and record findings. Modify the nursing care plan as needed. Counsel the patient regarding abnormal findings; explain the need for possible follow-up testing and treatment.
2. Use special precautions if patient is receiving steroid therapy, epinephrine, thyroxine, or prostaglandins. Eosinophilia can be masked by steroid use.
3. Refer to standard *posttest* care for hemogram, CBC, and differential count on page 63. Also, follow guidelines in Chapter 1 for safe, effective, informed *posttest* care.

● Monocytes (Monomorphonuclear Monocytes)

These agranulocytes, the largest cells of normal blood, are the body's second line of defense against infection. Histiocytes, which are large macrophagic phagocytes, are classified as *monocytes* in a differential leukocyte count. Histiocytes and monocytes are capable of reversible transformation from one to the other.

These phagocytic cells of varying size and mobility remove injured and dead cells, microorganisms, and insoluble particles from the circulating blood. Monocytes escaping from the upper and lower respiratory tracts and the gastrointestinal and genitourinary organs perform a scavenger function, clearing the body of debris. These phagocytic cells produce the antiviral agent called *interferon*.

This test counts monocytes, which circulate in certain specific conditions such as tuberculosis, subacute bacterial endocarditis, and the recovery phase of acute infections.

Normal Findings

Absolute count: 100 to 500/mm^3 or 0.1 to 0.5 $\times$ 10^9/L
Differential: 3% to 7% of total WBC count, or 0.03 to 0.07 of total WBC count

Procedure

1. Obtain a 5-mL whole blood sample in a lavender-topped tube (with EDTA) and label the specimen with the patient's name, date and time of collection, and test(s) ordered.
2. Observe standard precautions.
3. Count as part of the differential.

Clinical Implications

1. In *monocytosis*: a monocyte increase of >500 cells/mm^3 or >0.5 × 10^9/L or >10%. The most common causes are bacterial infections, tuberculosis, subacute bacterial endocarditis, and syphilis.
2. Other causes of monocytosis
    a. Monocytic leukemia and myeloproliferative disorders
    b. Carcinoma of stomach, breast, or ovary
    c. Hodgkin's disease and other lymphomas
    d. Recovery state of neutropenia (favorable sign)
    e. Lipid storage diseases (e.g., Gaucher's disease)
    f. Some parasitic, mycotic, and rickettsial diseases
    g. Surgical trauma
    h. Chronic ulcerative colitis, enteritis, and sprue
    i. Collagen diseases and sarcoidosis
    j. Tetrachloroethane poisoning
3. Phagocytic monocytes (macrophages) may be found in small numbers in the blood in many conditions:
    a. Severe infections (sepsis)
    b. Lupus erythematosus
    c. Hemolytic anemias
4. Decreased monocyte count (<100 cells/mm^3 or <0.1 × 10^9/L) is not usually identified with specific diseases:
    a. Prednisone treatment
    b. Hairy cell leukemia
    c. Overwhelming infection that also causes neutropenia
    d. HIV infection
    e. Aplastic anemia (bone marrow injury)

Interfering Factors

See Appendix E for drugs that affect test outcomes.

Interventions

Pretest Patient Care

1. Explain test purpose and procedure.
2. Refer to standard *pretest* care for hemogram, CBC, and differential count on page 63. Also, follow guidelines in Chapter 1 for safe, effective, informed *pretest* care.

Posttest Patient Care

1. Review test results; report and record findings. Modify the nursing care plan as needed. Counsel the patient regarding abnormal findings; explain the need for possible follow-up testing and treatment. Monitor for leukemia and infection.
2. Refer to standard *posttest* care for hemogram, CBC, and differential count on page 63. Also, follow guidelines in Chapter 1 for safe, effective, informed *posttest* care.

● Lymphocytes (Monomorphonuclear Lymphocytes); CD4, CD8 Count; Plasma Cells

Lymphocytes are small mononuclear cells without specific granules. These agranulocytes are motile cells that migrate to areas of inflammation in both early and late stages of the process. These cells are the source of serum immunoglobulins and of cellular immune response and play an important role in immunologic reactions. All lymphocytes are manufactured in the bone marrow. B lymphocytes mature in the bone marrow, and T lymphocytes mature in the thymus gland. B cells control the antigen–antibody response that is specific to the offending antigen and is said to have "memory." The T cells, the master immune cells, include $CD4^+$ helper T cells, killer cells, cytotoxic cells, and $CD8^+$ suppressor T cells.

Plasma cells (fully differentiated B cells) are similar in appearance to lymphocytes. They have abundant blue cytoplasm and an eccentric, round nucleus. Plasma cells are not normally present in blood.

This test measures the number of lymphocytes in the peripheral blood. Lymphocytosis is present in various diseases and is especially prominent in viral disorders. Lymphocytes and their derivatives, the plasma cells, operate in the immune defenses of the body.

Normal Findings

Lymphocytes: 25% to 40% of total leukocyte count (relative value) or 1500 to 4000 cells/mm^3 or 1.5 to 4.0 × 10^9/L
Plasma cells: 0% or none
CD4 count: total WBC count × lymphocytes (%) × lymphocytes (%) stained with CD4
CD4/CD8 ratio: >1.0

Procedure

1. Obtain 5 mL of whole blood in a lavender-topped tube (with EDTA). Label the specimen with the patient's name, date and time of collection, and test(s) ordered.
2. Count lymphocytes as part of the differential count.

Clinical Implications

1. *Lymphocytosis*: >4000/mm^3 or >4.0 × 10^9/L in adults; >7200/mm^3 or >7.2 × 10^9 in children; and >9000/mm^3 or >9.0 × 10^9/L in infants occurs in:
   a. Lymphatic leukemia (acute and chronic) lymphoma
   b. Infectious lymphocytosis (occurs mainly in children)
   c. Infectious mononucleosis
      (1) Caused by Epstein-Barr virus
      (2) Most common in adolescents and young adults
      (3) Characterized by atypical lymphocytes (Downey cells) that are large and deeply indented, with deep blue (basophilic) cytoplasm
      (4) Differential diagnosis—positive heterophil test
   d. Other viral diseases
      (1) Viral infections of the upper respiratory tract (pneumonia)
      (2) Cytomegalovirus
      (3) Measles, mumps, chickenpox
      (4) Acute HIV infection
      (5) Infectious hepatitis (acute viral hepatitis)
      (6) Toxoplasmosis
   e. Some bacterial diseases such as tuberculosis, brucellosis (undulant fever), and pertussis
   f. Crohn's disease, ulcerative colitis (rare)
   g. Serum sickness, drug hypersensitivity
   h. Hypoadrenalism, Addison's disease
   i. Thyrotoxicosis (relative lymphocytosis)
   j. Neutropenia with relative lymphocytosis
2. *Lymphopenia*: <1000 cells/mm^3 or <1.0 × 10^9/L in adults; <2500 cells/mm^3 or <2.5 × 10^9/L in children occurs in:
   a. Chemotherapy, radiation treatment, immunosuppressive medications
   b. After administration of ACTH or cortisone (steroids); with ACTH-producing pituitary tumors

c. Increased loss through gastrointestinal tract owing to obstruction of lymphatic drainage (e.g., tumor, Whipple's disease, intestinal lymphectasia)
d. Aplastic anemia
e. Hodgkin's disease and other malignancies
f. Inherited immune disorders, AIDS, and AIDS immune dysfunction
g. Advanced tuberculosis ("miliary" tuberculosis), renal failure, SLE
h. Severe debilitating illness of any kind
i. Congestive heart failure

3. *CD4 count*: The number of $CD4^+$ lymphocytes is equal to the absolute number of lymphocytes (total WBC count × differential [%] of lymphocytes) times the percentage of lymphocytes staining positively for CD4. A severely depressed CD4 count is the single best indicator of imminent opportunistic infection.
   a. *Decreased* CD4 lymphocytes
      (1) Immune dysfunction, especially AIDS. For the CD4, the diagnosis of AIDS is made for counts <200. There is a 1:3 ratio between Hb and Hct.
      (2) Acute minor viral infections
   b. *Increased* CD4 lymphocytes
      (1) Therapeutic effect of drugs
      (2) Diurnal variation: Peak evening values may be two times morning values.
4. *Plasma cells* (not normally present in blood) are increased in:
   a. Plasma cell leukemia
   b. Multiple myeloma
   c. Hodgkin's disease
   d. Chronic lymphatic leukemia
   e. Cancer of liver, breast, prostate
   f. Cirrhosis
   g. Rheumatoid arthritis, SLE
   h. Serum reaction
   i. Some bacterial, viral, and parasitic infections

Abnormal Lymphocytes

Abnormality	Description	Associated Diseases
Atypical lymphocytes Reactive lymphocytes Downey cells Turk cells	Lymphocytes, some with vacuolated cytoplasm, irregularly shaped nucleus, increased numbers of cytoplasmic azurophilic granules, and peripheral basophilia; or some with more abundant basophilic cytoplasm, grossly indented cytoplasm	Infectious mononucleosis, viral hepatitis, other viral infections, tuberculosis, drug (e.g., penicillin) sensitivity, posttransfusion syndrome

Interfering Factors

1. Physiologic pediatric lymphocytosis is a condition in newborns that includes an elevated WBC count and abnormal-appearing lymphocytes that can be mistaken for malignant cells.
2. Exercise, emotional stress, and menstruation can cause an increase in lymphocytes.
3. African Americans normally have a relative (not absolute) increase in lymphocytes.
4. See Appendix E for drugs that affect outcomes.

Interventions

Pretest Patient Care

1. Explain test purpose and procedure.
2. Refer to standard *pretest* care for hemogram, CBC, and differential count. Also, follow guidelines in Chapter 1 for safe, effective, informed *pretest* care.

Posttest Patient Care

1. Review test results; report and record findings. Modify the nursing care plan as needed. Counsel the patient regarding abnormal findings; explain the need for possible follow-up testing and treatment. Monitor for lymphocytosis or lymphopenia.
2. Refer to standard *posttest* care for hemogram, CBC, and differential count. Also, follow guidelines in Chapter 1 for safe, effective, informed *posttest* care.

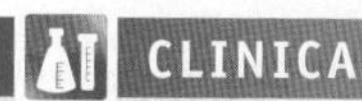

CLINICAL ALERT

A decreased lymphocyte count of <500/mm^3 (<0.5 × 10^9/L) means that a patient is dangerously susceptible to infection, especially viral infections. Institute measures to protect the patient from infection.

● Lymphocyte Immunophenotyping (T and B Cells)

Lymphocytes are divided into two categories, T and B cells, according to their primary function within the immune system. In the body, T and B cells work together to help provide protection against infections, oncogenic agents, and foreign tissue, and they play a vital role in regulating self-destruction or autoimmunity.

Most circulating lymphocytes are T cells with a life span of months to years. The life span of B cells is measured in days. *B cells (antibody)* are considered bursa or bone marrow dependent and are responsible for humoral immunity (in which antibodies are present in the serum). *T cells (cellular)* are thymus derived and are responsible for cellular immunity. T cells are further divided into helper T (CD3$^+$, CD4$^+$) cells and suppressor T (CD3$^+$, CD8$^+$) cells.

Evaluation of lymphocytes in the clinical laboratory is performed by quantitation of the lymphocytes and their subpopulations and by assessment of their functional activity. These laboratory analyses have become an essential component of the clinical assessment of two major disease states: *lymphoproliferative* states (e.g., leukemia, lymphoma), in which characterization of the malignant cell in terms of lineage and stage of differentiation provides valuable information to the oncologist to guide prognosis and appropriate therapy; and *immunodeficient* states (e.g., HIV infection, organ transplantation), in which the alterations in the immune system that occur secondary to infection are evaluated.

The method of lymphocyte quantitation and characterization is based on the detection of cell surface markers by very specific monoclonal antibodies. For cell surface immunophenotyping, flow cytometry has become the method of choice. Cell surface phenotyping is accomplished by reacting cells from an appropriate specimen with one or more labeled monoclonal antibodies and passing them through a flow cytometer, which counts the proportion of labeled cells.

Normal Findings for Adult Peripheral Blood by Flow Cytometry

T and B surface markers:
Total T cells (CD3$^+$): 53% to 88%
Helper T cells (CD3$^+$, CD4$^+$): 32% to 61%

Suppressor T cells ($CD3^+$, $CD8^+$): 18% to 42%
B cells ($CD19^+$): 5% to 20%
Natural killer cells ($CD16^+$): 4% to 32%
Absolute counts (based on pathologist's interpretation):
Total lymphocytes: 660 to 4600/mm^3 (0.6 to 4.6 × 10^9/L)
Total T cells ($CD3^+$): 812 to 2318/mm^3
Helper T cells ($CD3^+$, $CD4^+$): 589 to 1505/mm^3
Suppressor T cells ($CD3^+$, CD8+): 325 to 997/mm^3
B cells ($CD19^+$): 92 to 426/mm^3
Natural killer cells ($CD16^+$): 78 to 602/mm^3
Lymphocyte ratio:
Helper-to-suppressor T-cell ratio >1.0

Procedure

1. Obtain 5 mL of whole blood in a lavender-topped tube (with EDTA). Label the specimen with the patient's name, date and time of collection, and test(s) ordered.
2. Do not refrigerate or freeze the sample; it should remain at room temperature until testing is performed. Collect a separate 5-mL venous EDTA-anticoagulated blood sample for hematology at the same time. Because the interpretation of data is based on absolute values, it is imperative that a WBC count and differential count also be performed so that the appropriate data can be obtained.

Clinical Implications

1. Standard immunosuppressive drug therapy usually *decreases* lymphocyte totals.
2. Patients with an absolute helper T-lymphocyte count of <200/mm^3 are at greatest risk for developing clinical AIDS.
3. *Decreased T cells* occur in congenital immunodeficiency diseases (e.g., DiGeorge's syndrome, thymic hypoplasia).
4. *Decreased T cells* occur in kidney and heart transplant recipients receiving OKT-3, an immunomodulatory drug used to prevent rejection.
5. A marked *increase* in B cells occurs in lymphoproliferative disorders (e.g., chronic lymphocytic leukemia). In the typical case of chronic lymphocytic leukemia, the B cells would be positive for either κ or λ light chains (indicating monoclonality) and would express CD19 (a B-cell antigen).

Interventions

Pretest Patient Care

1. Explain purpose and specimen collection procedure. A recent viral cold can cause a decrease in total T cells, as can medications such as corticosteroids. Nicotine and strenuous exercise have also been shown to decrease lymphocyte counts.
2. Follow guidelines in Chapter 1 for safe, effective, informed *pretest* care.

Posttest Patient Care

1. Review test results; report and record findings. Modify the nursing care plan as needed.
2. Counsel the patient regarding abnormal findings; explain the need for possible follow-up testing and treatment. Lymphocyte immunophenotyping is performed to monitor patients who are HIV positive and have begun medication treatment. Transplantation patients are also retested at regular intervals to assess the threat of organ rejection or host infection. Also, see Chapter 8 for discussion of CD4 and CD8 cells.
3. Follow guidelines in Chapter 1 for safe, effective, informed *posttest* care.

STAINS FOR LEUKEMIAS

Several special WBC staining methods are used to diagnose leukemia, amyloid disease, lymphoma, and erythroleukemia; to differentiate erythema myelosis from sideroblastic anemia; to monitor progress and response to therapy; and to detect early relapse. *Amyloid* refers to starchlike substances deposited in certain diseases (e.g., tuberculosis, osteomyelitis, leprosy, Hodgkin's disease, and carcinoma).

● Sudan Black B (SBB) Stain

The Sudan Black B (SBB) stain aids in differentiation of the immature cells of acute leukemias, especially acute myeloblastic leukemia. The SBB stains a variety of fats and lipids that are present in myeloid leukemias but are not present in the lymphoid leukemias.

Reference Values

Positive Reactions

Granulocytic cells (neutrophils and eosinophils)
Myeloblasts
Promyelocytes
Neutrophilic myelocytes
Metamyelocytes, bands, and segmented neutrophils
Eosinophils at all stages
Monocytes and precursors

Variable Reactions

Basophils

Negative Reactions (Sudanophobia)

Lymphocytes and lymphocytic precursors
Megakaryocytes and thrombocytes (platelets)
Erythrocytes
Erythroblasts may display a few granules that represent mitochondrial phospholipid components.

Procedure

1. Obtain bone marrow aspirate.
2. Prepare slide, stain with SBB, and scan microscopically. Use normal smear control.

Clinical Implications

1. Positive staining of primitive (blast) cells indicates myelogenous origin of cells. SBB is positive in acute myelocytic leukemia (AML).
2. SBB is negative in acute lymphocytic leukemia, monocytic leukemia, plasma cell leukemia, and megakaryocytic leukemia.
3. SBB is weak to negative in acute monocytic leukemia.

Interfering Factors

There are cases of acute leukemia in which the cytochemical stains are not useful and fail to reveal the differentiating features of any specific cell line.

Interventions

Pretest Patient Care

1. Explain test purposes and procedures. If bone marrow aspiration is done, see pages 58–61 for special care.
2. Follow guidelines in Chapter 1 for safe, effective, informed *pretest* care.

Posttest Patient Care

1. Review test results; report and record findings. Modify the nursing care plan as needed.
2. Counsel the patient regarding abnormal findings; explain the need for possible follow-up testing and treatment. Monitor for leukemia, amyloid disease, anemia, and infection.
3. Follow guidelines in Chapter 1 for safe, effective, informed *posttest* care.

Periodic Acid–Schiff (PAS) Stain

The periodic acid–Schiff (PAS) stain aids in the diagnosis of acute lymphoblastic leukemia (ALL). Early myeloid precursors and erythrocyte precursors are negative. As granulocytes mature, they increase in PAS positivity, whereas mature RBCs stay negative. The PAS stain cannot be used to distinguish between ALL and AML or between benign and malignant lymphocytic disorders.

Normal Findings

Lymphoblasts: stain (positive)
Myeloblasts: do not stain (negative)

Procedure

1. Obtain bone marrow aspirate.
2. Prepare slide, stain with PAS, and scan microscopically.

Clinical Implications

1. Positive reaction
   a. Blasts in ALL in childhood often have coarse clumps or masses of PAS-positive material within their scent cytoplasm. The staining pattern is usually heterogeneous, with some cells containing PAS-positive clumps and others virtually unstained.
   b. Acute monocytic leukemia
   c. Hairy cell leukemia
   d. Sézary's syndrome
   e. Conspicuous PAS positivity in the erythroid precursors is strongly suggestive of erythroleukemia (M_6).
2. Weakly positive
   a. In acute granulocytic leukemia, the blasts display either a negative or weakly positive, finely granular pattern.
   b. In some cases of thalassemia and in anemias with blocked or deficient iron, the RBC precursors also contain PAS-positive material.
   c. Hodgkin's lymphoma
   d. Infectious mononucleosis
3. Negative stain
   a. Lymphoblasts of Burkitt's lymphoma
   b. Megaloblastic leukemia

Interventions

Pretest Patient Care

1. Explain test purposes and procedures.
2. Follow guidelines in Chapter 1 for safe, effective, informed *pretest* care.

Posttest Patient Care

1. Review test results; report and record findings. Modify the nursing care plan as needed. Counsel the patient regarding abnormal findings; explain the need for possible follow-up testing and treatment.
2. Follow guidelines in Chapter 1 for safe, effective, informed *posttest* care.

● Terminal Deoxynucleotidyl Transferase (TDT) Stain

The thymus is the primary site of terminal deoxynucleotidyl transferase (TDT)-positive cells, and TDT is found in the nucleus of the more primitive T cells. A thymus-related population of TDT-positive cells resides in the bone marrow (normally a minor population, 0% to 2%). TDT is increased in >90% of cases of ALL of childhood. A minor (5% to 10%) population of patients with acute nonlymphoblastic leukemia has TDT-positive blasts. TDT-positive blasts are prominent in some cases of chronic myelogenous leukemia (CML), relating to the development of an acute blast phase. TDT has been reported to assist in establishing the diagnosis of ALL. TDT-positive cases of blast-phase CML correlate with a positive response to chemotherapy (vincristine and prednisone).

Normal Findings

Negative in nonlymphoblastic leukemia
Negative in peripheral blood
0% to 2% positive in bone marrow

Procedure

1. Obtain a 5-mL EDTA-anticoagulated peripheral blood sample or a 2-mL EDTA-anticoagulated bone marrow aspirate. Label the specimen with the patient's name, date and time of collection, and test(s) ordered.
2. Dry slides (store at room temperature for up to 5 days), process, and stain and then examine under the microscope for positive cells.

Clinical Implications

1. TDT is positive in ALL, lymphoblastic lymphoma, and CML (blast crisis).
2. TDT is negative in patients in remission and in those with CML or chronic lymphatic leukemia.

Interventions

Pretest Patient Care

1. Explain test purposes and procedures.
2. Follow guidelines in Chapter 1 for safe, effective, informed *pretest* care.

Posttest Patient Care

1. Review test results; report and record findings. Modify the nursing care plan as needed. Counsel the patient regarding abnormal findings; explain the need for possible follow-up testing and treatment.
2. Follow guidelines in Chapter 1 for safe, effective, informed *posttest* care.

● Leukocyte Alkaline Phosphatase (LAP) Stain

Neutrophils are the only leukocytes to contain various amounts of alkaline phosphatase.

The leukocyte alkaline phosphatase (LAP) stain is used as an aid to distinguish chronic granulocytic leukemia from a leukemoid reaction. A leukemoid reaction is a high WBC count that may look like leukemia but is not. In remission of CML, the LAP may return to normal. In the blast phase of CML, the LAP may be elevated.

Normal Findings

40 to 100 LAP units

NOTE *Normal values vary greatly; check with your reference laboratory.*

Procedure

1. Obtain specimen by capillary puncture, venous whole blood (EDTA), green-topped tube. Label the specimen with the patient's name, date and time of collection, and test(s) ordered.
2. Prepare smear and air-dry; stain with LAP.
3. Make a count of 100 granulocytes and score (from 0 to 4+) as to the degree of LAP units.

Clinical Implications

1. *Decreased* values (0 to 15 LAP units)
   a. CML
   b. Paroxysmal nocturnal hemoglobinuria (PNH)
   c. Idiopathic thrombocytopenic purpura
   d. Hereditary hypophosphatasia
   e. Progressive muscular dystrophy
   f. Marked eosinophilia
   g. Nephrotic syndrome
   h. Siderocytic anemia
2. *Increased* values
   a. Leukemoid reactions, all kinds of neutrophilia with elevated WBC count
   b. Polycythemia vera
   c. Thrombocytopenia (essential)
   d. Down syndrome (trisomy 21)
   e. Multiple myeloma
   f. Hodgkin's disease
   g. Hairy cell leukemia
   h. Aplastic leukemia, acute and chronic lymphatic leukemia, chronic granulocytic leukemia
   i. Myelofibrosis, myeloid metaplasia
3. Normal levels of LAP
   a. Secondary polycythemia
   b. Hemolytic anemia
   c. Infectious mononucleosis
   d. Iron-deficiency anemia
   e. Viral hepatitis
4. Serial LAP tests can be a useful adjunct in evaluating the activity of Hodgkin's disease and the response to therapy.

Interfering Factors

1. Any physiologic stress, such as third-trimester pregnancy, labor, or severe exercise, causes an *increased* LAP score.
2. Steroid therapy *increases* LAP score.
3. CML with infection *increases* LAP score.

Interventions

Pretest Patient Care

1. Explain test purposes and procedures.
2. Follow guidelines in Chapter 1 for safe, effective, informed *pretest* care.

Posttest Patient Care

1. Review test results; report and record findings. Modify the nursing care plan as needed.
2. Counsel the patient regarding abnormal findings; explain the need for possible follow-up testing and treatment. Monitor for blood diseases.
3. Follow guidelines in Chapter 1 for safe, effective, informed *posttest* care.

● Tartrate-Resistant Acid Phosphatase (TRAP) Stain

The malignant mononuclear cells of leukemic reticuloendotheliosis (hairy cell leukemia) are resistant to inhibition by tartaric acid. There is evidence that the reaction is not entirely specific because tartrate-resistant acid phosphatase (TRAP) reactions have been reported in prolymphocytic leukemia and malignant lymphoma and in some cases of infectious mononucleosis.

Normal Findings

No TRAP activity

Procedure

1. Obtain venous blood sample (5 mL) or bone marrow smear. Label the specimen with the patient's name, date and time of collection, and test(s) ordered.
2. Incubate blood smear with TRAP, counterstain, and examine microscopically.

Clinical Implications

1. TRAP is present in the leukemic cells of most patients with hairy cell leukemia; 5% of patients with otherwise typical hairy cell leukemia lack the enzyme.
2. TRAP occasionally occurs in malignant cells of patients with lymphoproliferative disorders other than hairy cell leukemia.
3. Histiocytes have weakly positive reactions.

Interventions

Pretest Patient Care

1. Explain test purposes and procedures. Assess for history of signs and symptoms of leukemia.
2. Follow guidelines in Chapter 1 for safe, effective, informed *pretest* care.

Posttest Patient Care

1. Review test results; report and record findings. Modify the nursing care plan as needed. Counsel the patient regarding abnormal findings; explain the need for possible follow-up testing and treatment.
2. Follow guidelines in Chapter 1 for safe, effective, informed *posttest* care.

TESTS FOR RED BLOOD CELLS

Many tests look at the RBCs: their number and size, amount of Hb, rate of production, and percent composition of the blood. The RBC count, Hct, and Hb are closely related but different ways to look at the adequacy of erythrocyte production. The same conditions cause an increase (or decrease) in each of these indicators.

• Red Blood Cell (RBC) Count (Erythrocyte Count)

The main function of the RBC (erythrocyte) is to carry oxygen from the lungs to the body tissues and to transfer carbon dioxide from the tissues to the lungs. This process is achieved by means of the Hb in the RBCs, which combines easily with oxygen and carbon dioxide and gives arterial blood a bright red appearance. To enable use of the maximal amount of Hb, the RBC is shaped like a biconcave disk—this affords more surface area for the Hb to combine with oxygen. The cell also is able to change its shape when necessary to allow for passage through the smaller capillaries.

The RBC count, an important measurement in the evaluation of anemia or polycythemia, determines the total number of erythrocytes in a microliter (cubic millimeter) of blood.

Normal Findings

See Table 2.4.

Procedure

1. Obtain 5 mL of whole blood in a lavender-topped tube (with EDTA). Label the specimen with the patient's name, date and time of collection, and test(s) ordered. Place the specimen in a biohazard bag.
2. Automated electronic devices are generally used to determine the number of RBCs.
3. Note patient age and time of day on the laboratory slip.

Clinical Implications

1. *Decreased RBC values* occur in:
   a. Anemia, a condition in which there is a reduction in the number of circulating erythrocytes, the amount of Hb, or the volume of packed cells (Hct). Anemia is associated with cell destruction, blood loss, or dietary insufficiency of iron or of certain vitamins that are essential in the

TABLE 2.4 Normal Values for Red Blood Cells

Men	4.2–5.4 × 10^6/mm^3 or × 10^{12}/L (average, 4.8)
Women	3.6–5.0 × 10^6/mm^3 or × 10^{12}/L (average, 4.3)
Children	
Birth–2 wk	4.1–6.1 × 10^6/mm^3 or × 10^{12}/L
2–8 wk	4.0–6.0 × 10^6/mm^3 or × 10^{12}/L
2–6 mo	3.8–5.6 × 10^6/mm^3 or × 10^{12}/L
6 mo–1 yr	3.8–5.2 × 10^6/mm^3 or × 10^{12}/L
1–6 yr	3.9–5.3 × 10^6/mm^3 or × 10^{12}/L
6–16 yr	4.0–5.2 × 10^6/mm^3 or × 10^{12}/L
16–18 yr	4.2–5.4 × 10^6/mm^3 or × 10^{12}/L
>18 yr (males)	4.5–5.5 × 10^6/mm^3 or × 10^{12}/L
>18 yr (females)	4.0–5.0 × 10^6/mm^3 or × 10^{12}/L

production of RBCs. See Chart 2.1 (later in this chapter) for a classification of anemias based on their underlying mechanisms and the test for reticulocyte count for a discussion of the purpose and clinical implications of the reticulocyte count.

b. Disorders such as:
   (1) Hodgkin's disease and other lymphomas
   (2) Multiple myeloma, myeloproliferative disorders, leukemia
   (3) Acute and chronic hemorrhage
   (4) Lupus erythematosus
   (5) Addison's disease
   (6) Rheumatic fever
   (7) Subacute endocarditis, chronic infection

(This list is not meant to be all inclusive.)

2. *Erythrocytosis* (increased RBC count) occurs in:
   a. Primary erythrocytosis
      (1) Polycythemia vera (myeloproliferative disorder)
      (2) Erythremic erythrocytosis (increased RBC production in bone marrow)
   b. Secondary erythrocytosis
      (1) Renal disease
      (2) Extrarenal tumors
      (3) High altitude
      (4) Pulmonary disease
      (5) Cardiovascular disease
      (6) Alveolar hypoventilation
      (7) Hemoglobinopathy
      (8) Tobacco, carboxyhemoglobin
   c. Relative erythrocytosis (decrease in plasma volume)
      (1) Dehydration (vomiting, diarrhea)
      (2) Gaisböck's syndrome

CLINICAL ALERT

Refer to pages 94–95 for a discussion of the combined clinical implications of increased and decreased RBC count, Hct, and Hb values (polycythemia and anemia, respectively).

Interfering Factors

1. Posture: When a blood sample is obtained from a healthy person in a recumbent position, the RBC count is 5% lower. (If the patient is anemic, the count will be lower still.)
2. Dehydration: Hemoconcentration in dehydrated adults (caused by severe burns, untreated intestinal obstruction, severe persistent vomiting, or diuretic abuse) may obscure significant anemia.
3. Age: The normal RBC count of a newborn is higher than that of an adult, with a rapid drop to the lowest point in life at 2 to 4 months. The normal adult level is reached at age 14 years and is maintained until old age, when there is a gradual drop (see Table 2.4).
4. Falsely high counts may occur because of prolonged venous stasis during venipuncture.
5. Stress can cause a higher RBC count.
6. Altitude: The higher the altitude, the greater the increase in RBC count. Decreased oxygen content of the air stimulates the RBC count to rise (erythrocytosis).

7. Pregnancy: There is a relative decrease in RBC count when the body fluid increases in pregnancy, with the normal number of erythrocytes becoming more diluted.
8. There are many drugs that may cause decreased or increased RBC count. See Appendix E for drugs that affect test outcomes.
9. The EDTA blood sample tube must be at least three fourths filled or values will be invalid because of cell shrinkage caused by the anticoagulant.
10. The blood sample must not be clotted (even slightly) or the values will be invalid.

Interventions

Pretest Patient Care

1. Explain test purpose and procedure. Assess for signs/symptoms of fatigue, shortness of breath, weakness, tachycardia, and pallor of skin and mucous membranes.
2. Refer to standard *pretest* care for hemogram, CBC, and differential count.
3. Have the patient avoid extensive exercise, stress, and excitement before the test. These cause elevated counts of doubtful clinical value.
4. Avoid overhydration or dehydration, if possible—either causes invalid results. If patient is receiving IV fluids or therapy, note on requisition.
5. Note any medications the patient is taking.
6. Follow guidelines in Chapter 1 for safe, effective, informed *pretest* care.

Posttest Patient Care

1. Review test results; report and record findings. Modify the nursing care plan as needed.
2. Counsel the patient regarding abnormal findings; explain the need for possible follow-up testing and treatment. Monitor for anemia and erythrocytosis.
3. Refer to standard *posttest* care for hemogram, CBC, and differential count.
4. Follow guidelines in Chapter 1 for safe, effective, informed *posttest* care.
5. Possible treatments include stop the source of bleeding, administer IV fluids, administer whole blood or packed cell infusions, give supplemental iron, and promote proper nutrition. Administer oxygen as ordered.
6. Resume normal activities and diet.

● Hematocrit (Hct); Packed Cell Volume (PCV)

The word *hematocrit* means "to separate blood," which underscores the mechanism of the test because the plasma and blood cells are separated by centrifugation.

The Hct test is part of the CBC. This test indirectly measures the RBC mass. The results are expressed as the percentage by volume of packed RBCs in whole blood (packed cell volume [PCV]). It is an important measurement in the determination of anemia or polycythemia.

Normal Findings

Women: 36% to 48% or 0.36 to 0.48
Men: 42% to 52% or 0.42 to 0.52
Children:
0 to 2 weeks: 44% to 64% or 0.44 to 0.64
2 to 8 weeks: 39% to 59% or 0.39 to 0.59
2 to 6 months: 35% to 49% or 0.35 to 0.49
6 months to 1 year: 29% to 43% or 0.29 to 0.43
1 to 6 years: 30% to 40% or 0.30 to 0.40
6 to 16 years: 32% to 42% or 0.32 to 0.42
16 to 18 years: 34% to 44% or 0.34 to 0.44

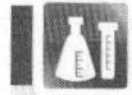
If blood is drawn from a capillary puncture and a microhematocrit is done, values are slightly higher.

CLINICAL ALERT

An Hct <20% (<0.20) can lead to cardiac failure and death; an Hct >60% (>0.60) is associated with spontaneous clotting of blood.

Procedure

1. Observe standard precautions. Obtain a 5-mL whole blood specimen in a lavender-topped tube (with EDTA). When doing a capillary puncture (finger puncture), the microcapillary tube is filled three fourths full with blood directly from the puncture site. These tubes are coated with an anticoagulative. Label the specimen with the patient's name, date and time of collection, and test(s) ordered.
2. Centrifuge the tubes in a microcentrifuge and measure the height of packed cells in the tube.
3. Record the measurement as a percentage of the total amount of blood in the capillary tube.
4. An Hct can be done on automated hematology instruments, in which case a 5-mL EDTA-anticoagulated venous blood sample is obtained.

Clinical Implications

1. *Decreased Hct values* are an indicator of anemia, a condition in which there is a reduction in the PCV. An Hct <30% (<0.30) means that the patient is moderately to severely anemic. Decreased values also occur in the following conditions:
   a. Leukemias, lymphomas, Hodgkin's disease, myeloproliferative disorders
   b. Adrenal insufficiency
   c. Chronic disease
   d. Acute and chronic blood loss
   e. Hemolytic reaction: This condition may be found in transfusion of incompatible blood or as a reaction to chemicals or drugs, infectious agents, or physical agents (e.g., severe burns, prosthetic heart valves).
2. The Hct may or may not be reliable immediately after even a moderate loss of blood or immediately after transfusion.
3. The Hct may be normal after acute hemorrhage. During the recovery phase, both the Hct and the RBC count drop markedly.
4. Usually, the Hct parallels the RBC count when the cells are of normal size. As the number of normal-sized erythrocytes increases, so does the Hct.
   a. However, for the patient with microcytic or macrocytic anemia, this relationship does not hold true.
   b. If a patient has iron-deficiency anemia with small RBCs, the Hct decreases because the microcytic cells pack to a smaller volume. The RBC count, however, may be normal or higher than normal.
5. *Increased Hct values* occur in:
   a. Erythrocytosis
   b. Polycythemia vera
   c. Shock, when hemoconcentration rises considerably

CLINICAL ALERT

Refer to pages 92–93 for a discussion of the combined clinical implications of increased and decreased Hct, Hb, and RBC values. The same underlying conditions cause an increase or decrease in each of these three tests of erythrocyte production.

Interfering Factors

1. People living at high altitudes have high Hct values as well as high Hb and RBC values.
2. Normally, the Hct slightly decreases in the physiologic hydremia of pregnancy.
3. The normal values for Hct vary with age and gender. The normal value for infants is higher because the newborn has many macrocytic red cells. Hct values in females are usually slightly lower than in males.
4. There is also a tendency toward lower Hct values in men and women older than 60 years of age, corresponding to lower RBC count values in this age group.
5. Severe dehydration from any cause falsely raises the Hct.

Interventions

Pretest Patient Care

1. Explain test purpose and procedure. Assess for signs/symptoms of fatigue, cool extremities, dyspnea, tachycardia, and pallor.
2. Refer to standard *pretest* care for hemogram, CBC, and differential count. Also, follow guidelines in Chapter 1 for safe, effective, informed *pretest* care.

Posttest Patient Care

1. Review test results; report and record findings. Modify the nursing care plan as needed.
2. Counsel the patient regarding abnormal findings; explain the need for possible follow-up testing and treatment. Monitor for anemia or polycythemia.
3. Possible treatments may include administration of whole blood products, iron supplements, and proper nutrition. Also, supplemental oxygen may be ordered.
4. Refer to standard *posttest* care for hemogram, CBC, and differential count. Also, follow guidelines in Chapter 1 for safe, effective, informed *posttest* care.

● Hemoglobin (Hb)

Hb, the main component of erythrocytes, serves as the vehicle for the transportation of oxygen and carbon dioxide. It is composed of amino acids that form a single protein called *globin*, and a compound called *heme*, which contains iron atoms and the red pigment porphyrin. It is the iron pigment that combines readily with oxygen and gives blood its characteristic red color. Each gram of Hb can carry 1.34 mL of oxygen per 100 mL of blood. The oxygen-combining capacity of the blood is directly proportional to the Hb concentration rather than to the RBC count because some RBCs contain more Hb than others. This is why Hb determinations are important in the evaluation of anemia.

The Hb determination is part of a CBC. It is used to screen for disease associated with anemia, to determine the severity of anemia, to monitor the response to treatment for anemia, and to evaluate polycythemia.

Hb also serves as an important buffer in the extracellular fluid. In tissue, the oxygen concentration is lower, and the carbon dioxide level and hydrogen ion concentration are higher. At a lower pH, more oxygen dissociates from Hb. The unoxygenated Hb binds to hydrogen ion, thereby raising the pH.

As carbon dioxide diffuses into the RBC, carbonic anhydrase converts carbon dioxide to bicarbonate and protons. As the protons are bound to Hb, the bicarbonate ions leave the cell. For every bicarbonate ion leaving the cell, a chloride ion enters. The efficiency of this buffer system depends on the ability of the lungs and kidneys to eliminate, respectively, carbon dioxide and bicarbonate. Refer to the discussion of ABGs in Chapter 14.

Normal Findings

Women: 12.0 to 16.0 g/dL or 120 to 160 g/L
Men: 14.0 to 17.4 g/dL or 140 to 174 g/L
Children:
- 0 to 2 weeks: 14.5 to 24.5 g/dL or 145 to 245 g/L
- 2 to 8 weeks: 12.5 to 20.5 g/dL or 125 to 205 g/L
- 2 to 6 months: 10.7 to 17.3 g/dL or 107 to 173 g/L
- 6 months to 1 year: 9.9 to 14.5 g/dL or 99 to 145 g/L
- 1 to 6 years: 9.5 to 14.1 g/dL or 95 to 141 g/L
- 6 to 16 years: 10.3 to 14.9 g/dL or 103 to 149 g/L
- 16 to 18 years: 11.1 to 15.7 g/dL or 111 to 157 g/L

CLINICAL ALERT

The critical Hb value is <5.0 g/dL (<50 g/L), a condition that leads to heart failure and death. A value >20 g/dL (>200 g/L) leads to clogging of the capillaries as a result of hemoconcentration.

Procedure

1. Obtain 5 mL of whole blood in a lavender-topped tube (with EDTA). Fill the Vacutainer tube at least three fourths full. Automated electronic devices are generally used to determine the Hb; however, a manual colorimetric procedure is also widely used. Label the specimen with the patient's name, date and time of collection, and test(s) ordered.
2. Do not allow the blood sample to clot, or the results will be invalid. Place the specimen in a biohazard bag.

Clinical Implications

1. *Decreased Hb levels* are found in anemia states (a condition in which there is a reduction of Hb, Hct, or RBC values). The Hb must be evaluated along with the RBC count and Hct.
   a. Iron deficiency, thalassemia, pernicious anemia, hemoglobinopathies
   b. Liver disease, hypothyroidism
   c. Hemorrhage (chronic or acute)
   d. Hemolytic anemia caused by:
      (1) Transfusions of incompatible blood
      (2) Reactions to chemicals or drugs
      (3) Reactions to infectious agents
      (4) Reactions to physical agents (e.g., severe burns, artificial heart valves)
      (5) Various systemic diseases, including but not limited to:
         (a) Hodgkin's disease
         (b) Leukemia
         (c) Lymphoma
         (d) SLE

(e) Carcinomatosis
(f) Sarcoidosis
(g) Renal cortical necrosis

2. *Increased Hb levels* are found in:
   a. Polycythemia vera
   b. Congestive heart failure
   c. Chronic obstructive pulmonary disease (COPD)
3. *Variation* in Hb levels
   a. Occurs after transfusions, hemorrhages, burns. (Hb and Hct are both high during and immediately after hemorrhage.)
   b. The Hb and Hct provide valuable information in an emergency situation if they are interpreted not in an isolated fashion but in conjunction with other pertinent laboratory data.
   c. Hb variants can cause variation in measured Hb:
      (1) Methemoglobin (Hb M)
      (2) Sickle cell hemoglobin (Hb S)
      (3) Fetal hemoglobin (Hb F)
      (4) Deoxyhemoglobin (HHb)

CLINICAL ALERT

See pages 92–93 for a discussion of the combined clinical implications of increased and decreased Hb, Hct, and RBC values. The same underlying conditions cause an increase or decrease in each of these three tests of erythrocyte production.

Clinical Implications of Polycythemia: Increased RBC Count, Hct, or Hb

Polycythemia is the term used to describe an abnormal increase in the number of RBCs. Although there are several tests to directly determine the RBC mass, these tests are expensive and somewhat cumbersome. For screening purposes, we rely on the Hct and Hb to evaluate polycythemia indirectly. Polycythemias are classified as follows:

1. *Relative* polycythemia: an increase in Hb, Hct, or RBC count caused by a decrease in the plasma volume (e.g., dehydration, spurious erythrocytosis from stress or smoking)
2. *Absolute* or *true* polycythemia
   a. Primary (e.g., polycythemia vera, erythemic erythrocytosis)
   b. Secondary
      (1) Appropriate (an appropriate bone marrow response to physiologic conditions)
         (a) Altitude
         (b) Cardiopulmonary disorder
         (c) Increased affinity for oxygen
      (2) Inappropriate (an overproduction of RBCs not necessary to deliver oxygen to the tissues)
         (a) Renal tumor or cyst
         (b) Hepatoma
         (c) Cerebellar hemangioblastoma

Clinical Implications of Anemia: Decreased RBC Count, Hct, or Hb

Anemia is the term used to describe a condition in which there is a reduction in the number of circulating RBCs, amount of Hb, or volume of packed cells (Hct). A pathophysiologic classification of anemias based on their underlying mechanisms follows. Anemias are further explained in Chart 2.1. Anemias are classified as follows:

1. *Hypoproliferative anemias* (inadequate production of RBCs)
    a. Marrow aplasias
    b. Myelophthisic anemia
    c. Anemia with blood dyscrasias
    d. Anemia of chronic disease
    e. Anemia with organ failure
2. *Maturation defect* anemias
    a. Cytoplasmic: hypochromic anemias
    b. Nuclear: megaloblastic anemias
    c. Combined: myelodysplastic syndromes
3. *Hyperproliferative* anemias (decreased Hb or Hct despite an increased production of RBCs)
    a. Hemorrhagic: acute blood loss
    b. Hemolytic: a premature, accelerated destruction of RBCs
        (1) Immune hemolysis
        (2) Primary membrane
        (3) Hemoglobinopathies
        (4) Toxic hemolysis (physical–chemical)
        (5) Traumatic or microangiopathic hemolysis
        (6) Hypersplenism
        (7) Enzymopathies
        (8) Parasitic infections
4. *Dilutional* anemias
    a. Pregnancy
    b. Splenomegaly

Interfering Factors

1. People living at high altitudes have increased Hb values as well as increased Hct and RBC count.
2. Excessive fluid intake causes a decreased Hb.
3. Normally, the Hb is higher in infants (before active erythropoiesis begins).
4. Hb is normally decreased in pregnancy as a result of increased plasma volume.
5. There are many drugs that may cause a decreased Hb. Drugs that may cause an increased Hb include gentamicin and methyldopa.
6. Extreme physical exercise causes increased Hb.

Interventions

Pretest Patient Care

1. Explain test purpose and procedure. Assess medication history.
2. Refer to standard *pretest* care for hemogram, CBC, and differential count. Also, follow guidelines in Chapter 1 for safe, effective, informed *pretest* care.

Posttest Patient Care

1. Review test results; report and record findings. Modify the nursing care plan as needed.
2. Counsel the patient regarding abnormal findings; explain the need for possible follow-up testing and treatment. Monitor for anemia or polycythemia.
3. Refer to standard *posttest* care for hemogram, CBC, and differential count. Also, follow guidelines in Chapter 1 for safe, effective, informed *posttest* care.

CHART 2.1 Anemias Characterized by Deficient Hemoglobin Synthesis

MICROCYTIC ANEMIAS (MCV 50–82 fL)

DISORDERS OF IRON METABOLISM

Iron-deficiency anemia: the most prevalent worldwide cause of anemia; the major causes are dietary inadequacy, malabsorption, increased iron loss, and increased iron requirements

Anemia of chronic disease, hereditary atransferrinemia

Congenital hypochromic-microcytic anemia with iron overload (Shahidi-Nathan-Diamond syndrome)

DISORDERS OF PORPHYRIN AND HEME SYNTHESIS

Acquired sideroblastic anemias

Idiopathic refractory sideroblastic anemia, complicating other diseases associated with drugs or toxins (ethanol, isoniazid, lead)

Hereditary sideroblastic anemias

X chromosome–linked, autosomal anemias

DISORDERS OF GLOBIN SYNTHESIS

Thalassemias, hemoglobinopathies, characterized by unstable Hb

Normocytic Normochromic Anemias (MCV 82–98 fL)

ANEMIA WITH APPROPRIATE BONE MARROW RESPONSE

Acute posthemorrhagic anemia

Hemolytic anemia (may be macrocytic when there is pronounced reticulocytosis)

ANEMIA WITH IMPAIRED MARROW RESPONSE

Marrow hypoplasia

Aplastic anemia, pure red cell aplasia

Marrow infiltration

Infiltration by malignant cells, myelofibrosis, inherited storage diseases

Decreased erythropoietin production

Kidney and liver disease, endocrine deficiencies, malnutrition, anemia of chronic disease

Macrocytic Anemias (MCV 100–150 fL)

COBALAMIN (B_{12}) DEFICIENCY

Decreased ingestion

Lack of animal products, strict vegetarianism

Impaired absorption

Intrinsic factor deficiency, pernicious anemia, gastrectomy (total or partial), destruction of gastric mucosa by caustics, anti-intrinsic factor antibody in gastric juice, abnormal intrinsic factor molecule, intrinsic intestinal disease, familial selective malabsorption (Imerslünd's syndrome), ileal resection, ileitis, sprue, celiac disease, infiltrative intestinal disease (e.g., lymphoma, scleroderma), drug-induced malabsorption

Competitive parasites

Fish tapeworm infestations (*Diphyllobothrium latum*); bacteria in diverticulum of bowel, blind loops

Increased requirements

Chronic pancreatic disease, pregnancy, neoplastic disease, hyperthyroidism

continues on pg. 95

CHART 2.1 continued

Impaired utilization
Enzyme deficiencies, abnormal serum cobalamin–binding protein, lack of transcobalamin II, nitrous oxide administration

FOLATE DEFICIENCY
Decreased ingestion
Lack of vegetables, alcoholism, infancy

Impaired absorption
Intestinal short circuits, steatorrhea, sprue, celiac disease, intrinsic intestinal disease, anticonvulsants, oral contraceptives, other drugs

Increased requirement
Pregnancy, infancy, hypothyroidism, hyperactive hematopoiesis, neoplastic disease, exfoliative skin disease

Impaired utilization
Folic acid antagonists: methotrexate, triamterene, trimethoprim, enzyme deficiencies

Increased loss
Hemodialysis

UNRESPONSIVE TO COBALAMIN OR FOLATE
Metabolic inhibitors
Purine synthesis: 6-mercaptopurine, 6-thioguanine, azathioprine

Pyrimidine synthesis: 6-azauridine

Thymidylate synthesis: methotrexate, 5-fluorouracil

Deoxyribonucleotide synthesis: hydroxyurea, cytarabine, severe iron deficiency

Inborn errors
Lesch-Nyhan syndrome, hereditary orotic aciduria, deficiency of formiminotransferase, methyltransferase, others

● Red Blood Cell Indices

The RBC indices define the size and Hb content of the RBC count and consist of the MCV, the MCHC, and the MCH.

The RBC indices are used in differentiating anemias. When they are used together with an examination of the erythrocytes on the stained smear, a clear picture of RBC morphology may be ascertained. On the basis of the RBC indices, the erythrocytes can be characterized as normal in every respect or as abnormal in volume or Hb content. In deficient states, the anemias can be classified by cell size as macrocytic, normocytic, or microcytic, or by cell size and color as microcytic hypochromic.

Procedure

1. These are calculated values.
2. Obtain 5 mL of whole blood in a lavender-topped tube (with EDTA) so that RBC count, Hb, and Hct determinations can be performed. Label the specimen with the patient's name, date and time of collection, and tests ordered.

Interventions

Pretest Patient Care for MCV, MCHC, and MCH

1. Explain the purpose and procedure for testing. Assess for possible causes of anemia. No fasting is required. Assess for signs/symptoms of fatigue, palpitations, dyspnea, angina, tachycardia, brittle hair and nails, and pallor.
2. Follow guidelines in Chapter 1 for safe, effective, informed *pretest* care.

Posttest Patient Care for MCV, MCHC, and MCH

1. Review test results; report and record findings. Modify the nursing care plan as needed.
2. Counsel the patient appropriately for proper diet, medication, related hormone and enzyme problems, and genetically linked disorders. Explain the need for possible follow-up testing and treatment.
3. Treatment includes iron-rich foods, control of chronic blood loss, or administration of iron.
4. Follow guidelines in Chapter 1 for safe, effective, informed *posttest* care.

● Mean Corpuscular Volume (MCV)

Individual cell size is the best index for classifying anemias. This index expresses the volume occupied by a single erythrocyte and is a measure in cubic micrometers (femtoliters [fL]) of the mean volume. The MCV indicates whether the RBC size appears normal (normocytic), smaller than normal ($<82\ \mu m^3$, microcytic), or larger than normal ($>100\ \mu m^3$, macrocytic).

Normal Findings

82 to 98 mm^3 or 82 to 98 fL (higher values in infants and newborns and for elderly patients)

Procedure

1. Calculate the MCV from the RBC count (the number of cells per cubic millimeter of blood) and the Hct (the proportion of the blood occupied by the RBCs).
2. Use the following formula:

$$\text{MCV (fL)} = \frac{\text{Hct (\%)} \times 10}{\text{RBC } (10^{12}/\text{L})}$$

Clinical Implications

The MCV results are the basis of the classification system used to evaluate an anemia. The categorizations shown in Chart 2.1 aid in orderly investigation.

Interfering Factors

1. Mixed (bimorphic) population of macrocytes and microcytes can result in a normal MCV. Examination of the blood film confirms this.
2. Increased reticulocytes can increase the MCV.
3. Marked leukocytosis increases the MCV.
4. Marked hyperglycemia increases the MCV.
5. Cold agglutinins increase the MCV.

Interventions

Pretest Patient Care

1. Explain test purposes and procedures.
2. Follow guidelines in Chapter 1 for safe, effective, informed *pretest* care.

Posttest Patient Care

1. Review test results; report and record findings. Modify the nursing care plan as needed. Counsel the patient regarding abnormal findings; explain the need for possible follow-up testing and treatment.
2. Follow guidelines in Chapter 1 for safe, effective, informed *posttest* care.

• Mean Corpuscular Hemoglobin Concentration (MCHC)

The MCHC measures the average concentration of Hb in the RBCs. The MCHC is most valuable in monitoring therapy for anemia because the two most accurate hematologic determinations (Hb and Hct) are used in its calculation.

Normal Findings

32 to 36 g/dL or 4.9 to 5.5 mmol/L

Procedure

1. The MCHC is a calculated value. It is an expression of the average concentration of Hb in the RBCs and, as such, represents the ratio of the weight of Hb to the volume of the erythrocyte.
2. Use the following formula:

$$\text{MCHC (g/dL)} = \frac{\text{Hb (g/dL)} \times 100}{\text{Hct (\%)}}$$

Clinical Implications

1. *Decreased MCHC values* signify that a unit volume of packed RBCs contains less Hb than normal. Hypochromic anemia (MCHC <30 g/dL) occurs in:
   a. Iron deficiency
   b. Microcytic anemias, chronic blood loss anemia
   c. Some thalassemias
2. Increased MCHC values (RBCs cannot accommodate >37 g/dL or 370 g/L Hb) occur in:
   a. Spherocytosis (hereditary)
   b. Newborns and infants

Interfering Factors

1. The MCHC may be falsely high in the presence of lipemia, cold agglutinins, or rouleaux and with high heparin concentrations.
2. The MCHC cannot be >37 g/dL (370 g/L) because the RBC count cannot accommodate >37 g/dL (370 g/L) Hb. (Check for errors in calculation or in Hb determination. MCHC can be used for laboratory quality control.)

Interventions

Pretest Patient Care

1. Explain test purposes and procedures.
2. Follow guidelines in Chapter 1 for safe, effective, informed *pretest* care.

Posttest Patient Care

1. Review test results; report and record findings. Modify the nursing care plan as needed. Counsel the patient regarding abnormal findings; explain the need for possible follow-up testing and treatment.
2. Follow guidelines in Chapter 1 for safe, effective, informed *posttest* care.

Mean Corpuscular Hemoglobin (MCH)

The MCH is a measure of the average weight of Hb per RBC. This index is of value in diagnosing severely anemic patients.

Normal Findings

26 to 34 pg/cell or 0.40 to 0.53 fmol/cell (normally higher in newborns and infants)

Procedure

The MCH is a calculated value. The average weight of Hb in the RBC is expressed as picograms of Hb per RBC. The formula is:

$$\frac{\text{MCH}}{\text{(pg/cell)}} = \frac{\text{Hb (g/dL)} \times 10}{\text{RBC } (10^{12}\text{/L})}$$

Clinical Implications

1. An increase of the MCH is associated with macrocytic anemia and in newborns.
2. A decrease of the MCH is associated with microcytic anemia.

Interfering Factors

1. Hyperlipidemia falsely elevates the MCH.
2. WBC count $>50{,}000/\text{mm}^3$ falsely raises the Hb value and therefore falsely elevates the MCH.
3. High heparin concentrations falsely elevate the MCH.
4. Cold agglutinins falsely elevate the MCH.

Interventions

Pretest Patient Care

1. Explain test purposes and procedures.
2. Follow guidelines in Chapter 1 for safe, effective, informed *pretest* care.

Posttest Patient Care

1. Review test results; report and record findings. Modify the nursing care plan as needed. Counsel the patient regarding abnormal findings; explain the need for possible follow-up testing and treatment.
2. Follow guidelines in Chapter 1 for safe, effective, informed *posttest* care.

Red Cell Size Distribution Width (RDW)

This automated method of measurement is helpful in the investigation of some hematologic disorders and in monitoring response to therapy. The RDW is essentially an indication of the degree of anisocytosis (abnormal variation in size of RBCs). Normal RBCs have a slight degree of variation.

Normal Findings

11.5 to 14.5 coefficient of variation (CV) of red cell size

Procedure

1. The CV of RDW is determined and calculated by the analyzer.
2. Use the CV of RDW with caution and not as a replacement for other diagnostic tests.
3. Use the following calculation:

$$\text{RDW (CV\%)} = \frac{\text{Standard deviation of RBC size} \times 100}{\text{MCV}}$$

Clinical Implications

1. The RDW can be helpful in distinguishing uncomplicated heterozygous thalassemia (low MCV, normal RDW) from iron-deficiency anemia (low MCV, high RDW).
2. The RDW can be helpful in distinguishing anemia of chronic disease (low-normal MCV, normal RDW) from early iron-deficiency anemia (low-normal MCV, elevated RDW).
3. *Increased* RDW occurs in:
   a. Iron deficiency
   b. Vitamin B_{12} (VB_{12}) or folate deficiency (pernicious anemia)
   c. Abnormal Hb: S, S-C, or H
   d. S-β-thalassemia (homogeneous)
   e. Immune hemolytic anemia
   f. Marked reticulocytosis
   g. Fragmentation of RBCs
4. Normal RDW—normal in anemias with homogeneous red cell size
   a. Chronic disease
   b. Acute blood loss
   c. Aplastic anemia
   d. Hereditary spherocytosis
   e. Hb E disease
   f. Sickle cell disease
5. There is no known cause of a decreased RDW.

Interfering Factors

1. This test is not helpful for persons who do not have anemia.
2. Alcoholism elevates RDW.
3. Cold agglutinins

Interventions

Pretest Patient Care

1. Explain the purpose and procedure for testing. Assess for possible causes of anemia. No fasting is required.
2. Follow guidelines in Chapter 1 for safe, effective, informed *pretest* care.

Posttest Patient Care

1. Review test results; report and record findings; monitor appropriately for response to therapy. Modify the nursing care plan as needed.
2. Counsel the patient regarding abnormal findings and proper diet, medication, related hormone and enzyme problems, and genetically linked disorders. Explain the need for possible follow-up testing and treatment.
3. Follow guidelines in Chapter 1 for safe, effective, informed *posttest* care.

● Stained Red Cell Examination (Film; Stained Erythrocyte Examination)

The stained film examination determines variations and abnormalities in erythrocyte size, shape, structure, Hb content, and staining properties. It is useful in diagnosing blood disorders such as anemia, thalassemia, and other hemoglobinopathies. This examination also serves as a guide to therapy and as an indicator of harmful effects of chemotherapy and radiation therapy. The leukocytes are also examined at this time.

Normal Findings

Size: normocytic (normal size, 7 to 8 μm)
Color: normochromic (normal)
Shape: normocyte (biconcave disk)
Structure: normocytes or erythrocytes (anucleated cells)

Procedure

1. Collect 5 mL of whole blood in a lavender-topped tube (with EDTA). Label the specimen with the patient's name, date and time of collection, and test(s) ordered. Stain a thin smear with Wright's stain and study under a microscope to determine size, shape, and other characteristics of the RBCs.
2. Be aware that a capillary smear may also be used and may be preferred for detection of some abnormalities.

Clinical Implications

Variations in staining, color, shape, and RBC inclusions are indicative of RBC abnormalities (Table 2.5).

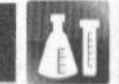

CLINICAL ALERT

Marked abnormalities in size and shape of RBCs without a known cause are an indication for more complete blood studies.

Interventions

Pretest Patient Care

1. Explain the purpose and procedure for testing. Assess for possible causes of anemia. No fasting is required.
2. Follow guidelines in Chapter 1 for safe, effective, informed *pretest* care.

Posttest Patient Care

1. Review test results; report and record findings. Modify the nursing care plan as needed. Counsel the patient regarding abnormal findings; explain the need for possible follow-up testing and treatment.
2. Follow guidelines in Chapter 1 for safe, effective, informed *posttest* care.

• Reticulocyte Count

A *reticulocyte*—a young, immature, nonnucleated RBC—contains reticular material (RNA) that stains gray-blue. Reticulum is present in newly released blood cells for 1 to 2 days before the cell reaches its full mature state. Normally, a small number of these cells are found in circulating blood. For the reticulocyte count to be meaningful, it must be viewed in relation to the total number of erythrocytes (absolute reticulocyte count = % reticulocytes × erythrocyte count).

The reticulocyte count is used to differentiate anemias caused by bone marrow failure from those caused by hemorrhage or hemolysis (destruction of RBCs), to check the effectiveness of treatment in pernicious anemia and folate and iron deficiency, to assess the recovery of bone marrow function in aplastic anemia, and to determine the effects of radioactive substances on exposed workers.

TABLE 2.5 Peripheral Red Blood Cell Abnormalities

Abnormality	Description	Associated Diseases
Anisocytosis (diameter)	Abnormal variation in size (normal diameter = 6–8 μm)	Any severe anemia (e.g., iron-deficiency, hemolytic hypersplenism)
Microcytes	Small cells, <6 μm (MCV < 80 fL)	Iron-deficiency and iron-loading (sideroblastic) anemia, thalassemia, lead poisoning, vitamin B_6 deficiency
Macrocytes	Large cells, >8 μm (MCV >100 fL)	Megaloblastic anemia, alcoholism, liver disease, hemolytic anemia (reticulocytes), hemolytic disease of newborn, myeloma, leukemia, myelophthisic anemia, metastatic carcinoma, hypothyroidism
Megalocytes	Large (>9 μm) oval cells	Megaloblastic anemia, pernicious anemia, cancer chemotherapy
Hypochromia	Pale cells with decreased concentration of hemoglobin (MCHC <30 g/dL)	Severe iron-deficiency and iron-loading (sideroblastic) anemia, thalassemia, lead poisoning, transferrin deficiency
Poikilocytes	Abnormal variation in shape	Any severe anemia (e.g., megaloblastic, iron-deficiency, myeloproliferative syndrome, hemolytic); certain shapes are diagnostically helpful (see entries below for Spherocytes through Teardrop cells)
Spherocytes	Spherical cells without pale centers; often small (i.e., microspherocytosis)	Hereditary spherocytosis, Coombs'-positive hemolytic anemia; small numbers are seen in any hemolytic anemia and after transfusion of stored blood
Elliptocytes	Oval cells—elongated	Hereditary elliptocytosis (>25% on smear), iron deficiency
Stomatocytosis	Red cells with slitlike (instead of circular) areas of central pallor	Congenital stomatocytosis, Rh-null disease, alcoholism, liver disease, artifact
Sickle cells	Crescent-shaped cells	Sickle cell disease (Hb S)
Target cells	Cells with a dark center and periphery and a clear ring in between	Liver disease, thalassemia, iron-deficiency anemia, hemoglobinopathies, (S, C, S-C, S-thalassemia), artifact
Schistocytes (helmet cells)	Irregularly contracted cells (severe poikilocytosis), fragmented cells	Vasculitis, artificial heart valve, disseminated intravascular coagulation, thrombocytopenia purpura and other microangiopathic anemias, toxins (lead, phenylhydrazine, snake bite), severe burns, renal graft rejection, and march hemoglobinuria
Burr cells (echinocytes)	Burrlike cells, spinous processes	Usually artifactual, uremia, stomach cancer, pyruvate kinase deficiency

table continues on pg. 102 >

TABLE 2.5 continued

Abnormality	Description	Associated Diseases
Acanthocytes	Small cells with thorny projections	Abetalipoproteinemia (hereditary acanthocytosis or Bassen-Kornzweig disease), postsplenectomy, hemolytic anemia, alcoholic cirrhosis, hepatitis of newborns, malabsorption states
Teardrop cells (dacryocytes)	Cells shaped like teardrops	Myeloproliferative syndrome, myelophthisic anemia (neoplastic, granulomatous, or fibrotic marrow infiltration), thalassemia, pernicious anemia, tuberculosis
Nucleated red cells	Erythrocytes with nuclei still present, normoblastic or megaloblastic	Hemolytic anemias, leukemias, myeloproliferative syndrome, polycythemia vera, myelophthisic anemia (neoplastic, granulomatous, or fibrotic marrow infiltration), multiple myeloma, extramedullary hematopoiesis, megaloblastic anemias, any severe anemia
Howell-Jolly bodies	Spherical purple bodies (Wright's) within or on erythrocytes, nuclear debris	Hyposplenism, postsplenectomy pernicious anemia, thalassemia, sickle cell anemia, other hemolytic anemias
Heinz inclusion bodies	Small round inclusions of denatured Hb seen under phase microscopy or with supravital staining (not seen with Wright's stain)	Congenital hemolytic anemias (e.g., glucose-6-phosphate dehydrogenase deficiency), hemolytic anemia secondary to drugs (dapsone, phenacetin), thalassemia (Hb H), hemoglobinopathies (Hb Zurich, Koln, Ube, I, etc.)
Pappenheimer bodies (siderocytes)	Siderotic granules, staining blue with Wright or Prussian blue stain	Iron-loading anemias (e.g., sideroblastic anemia), hyposplenism, lead poisoning, iron overload (hemochromatosis)
Cabot's rings	Purple, fine, ringlike, intraerythrocytic structure	Pernicious anemia, lead poisoning, severe hemolytic anemia
Basophilic stippling	Punctate stippling when Wright stained	Hemolytic anemia, punctate stippling seen in lead poisoning (mitochondrial RNA and iron), thalassemia, megaloblastic anemia, alcoholism
Rouleaux	Aggregated erythrocytes regularly stacked on one another—"rows of coins"	Multiple myeloma, Waldenström's macroglobulinemia, cord blood, pregnancy, hypergammaglobulinemia, hyperfibrinogenemia
Polychromatophilia (called reticulocytes when stained with supravital stain)	RBCs containing RNA, staining a pinkish blue color; stains supravitally as reticular network with new methylene blue	Hemolytic anemia, blood loss, uremia, after treatment of iron-deficiency or megaloblastic anemia

Hb, hemoglobin; MCHC, mean corpuscular hemoglobin concentration; MCV, mean corpuscular volume; RBCs, red blood cells.

Normal Findings

Adults: 0.5% to 1.5% of total erythrocytes (women may be slightly higher)
Newborns: 3% to 6% of total erythrocytes (drops to adult levels in 1 to 2 months)
Absolute count: 25 to 85 $\times$ 10^3/mm^3 or $\times$ 10^9 cells/L
Reticulocyte index (RI): 1% corrected reticulocyte count (CRC)
Hct correction for anemia: RI = reticulocyte count $\times$ (patient's Hct/45 $\times$ 1/1.85)

Procedure

1. Obtain 5 mL of whole blood in a lavender-topped tube (with EDTA). Label the specimen with the patient's name, date and time of collection, and test(s) ordered. Place the specimen in a biohazard bag.
2. Mix the blood sample with a supravital stain such as brilliant cresyl blue. Allow the stain to react with the blood, prepare a smear with this mixture, and scan under a microscope. Count and calculate the reticulocytes.

Retic % = Total retics / (1000 RBCs $\times$ 100)

3. Use the following formula:

RI (CRC) = reticulocyte count $\times$ (Patient's Hct / 45) $\times$ (1/1.85)

45 = normal Hct; 1.85 = number of days for reticulocyte to mature

Clinical Implications

1. Increased reticulocyte count (reticulocytosis) means that increased RBC production is occurring as the bone marrow replaces cells lost or prematurely destroyed. Identification of reticulocytosis may lead to the recognition of an otherwise occult disease, such as hidden chronic hemorrhage or unrecognized hemolysis (e.g., sickle cell anemia, thalassemia).
   Increased levels are observed in the following:
   a. Hemolytic anemia
      (1) Immune hemolytic anemia
      (2) Primary RBC membrane problems
      (3) Hemoglobinopathic and sickle cell disease
      (4) RBC enzyme deficits
      (5) Malaria
   b. After hemorrhage (3 to 4 days)
   c. After treatment of anemias
      (1) An increased reticulocyte count may be used as an index of the effectiveness of treatment.
      (2) After adequate doses of iron in iron-deficiency anemia, the rise in reticulocytes may exceed 20%.
      (3) There is a proportional increase when pernicious anemia is treated by transfusion or VB_{12} therapy.
2. *Decreased reticulocyte count* means that bone marrow is not producing enough erythrocytes; this occurs in:
   a. Untreated iron-deficiency anemia
   b. Aplastic anemia (a persistent deficiency of reticulocytes suggests a poor prognosis)
   c. Untreated pernicious anemia
   d. Anemia of chronic disease
   e. Radiation therapy
   f. Endocrine problems
   g. Tumor in marrow (bone marrow failure)
   h. Myelodysplastic syndromes
   i. Alcoholism

3. RI implications
   a. <2% indicates hypoproliferative component to anemia
   b. >2% to 3% indicates increased RBC production

Interventions

Pretest Patient Care

1. Explain test purpose and procedure. Pretest and posttest care are the same as for the hemogram. Follow guidelines in Chapter 1 for safe, effective, informed *pretest* care.
2. Note medications. Some drugs cause aplastic anemia.

Posttest Patient Care

1. Review test results; report and record findings. Modify the nursing care plan as needed. Counsel the patient regarding abnormal findings; explain the need for possible follow-up testing and treatment. Monitor for anemias.
2. Follow guidelines in Chapter 1 for safe, effective, informed *posttest* care.

● Sedimentation Rate (Sed Rate); Erythrocyte Sedimentation Rate (ESR)

Sedimentation occurs when the erythrocytes clump or aggregate together in a column-like manner (rouleaux formation). These changes are related to alterations in the plasma proteins. Normally, erythrocytes settle slowly because normal RBCs do not form rouleaux.

The erythrocyte sedimentation rate (ESR) is the rate at which erythrocytes settle out of anticoagulated blood in 1 hour. This test is based on the fact that inflammatory and necrotic processes cause an alteration in blood proteins, resulting in aggregation of RBCs, which makes them heavier and more likely to fall rapidly when placed in a special vertical test tube—the faster the settling of cells, the higher the ESR. The ESR should not be used to screen asymptomatic patients for disease. It is most useful for diagnosis of temporal arteritis, rheumatoid arthritis, and polymyalgia rheumatica. The sedimentation rate is not diagnostic of any particular disease but rather is an indication that a disease process is ongoing and must be investigated. It is also useful in monitoring the progression of inflammatory diseases; if the patient is being treated with steroids, the ESR will decrease with clinical improvement.

Normal Findings by Westergren's Method

Men: 0 to 15 mm/hr (over age 50 years: 0 to 20 mm/hr)
Women: 0 to 20 mm/hr (over age 50 years: 0 to 30 mm/hr)
Newborn: 0 to 2 mm/hr
Children: 0 to 10 mm/hr

Procedure

1. Obtain 5 mL of whole blood in a lavender-topped tube (with EDTA) or 3.8% sodium citrate. Label the specimen with the patient's name, date and time of collection, and test(s) ordered. Place the specimen in a biohazard bag.
2. Suction the specimen into a graduated sedimentation tube and allow to settle for exactly 1 hour. The amount of settling is the patient's ESR.

Clinical Implications

1. *Increased ESR* is found in:
   a. All collagen diseases, SLE
   b. Infections, pneumonia, syphilis, tuberculosis
   c. Inflammatory diseases (e.g., acute pelvic inflammatory disease)

   d. Carcinoma, lymphoma, neoplasms
   e. Acute heavy metal poisoning
   f. Cell or tissue destruction, myocardial infarction
   g. Toxemia, pregnancy (third month to 3 weeks postpartum)
   h. Waldenström's macroglobulinemia, increased serum globulins
   i. Nephritis, nephrosis
   j. Subacute bacterial endocarditis
   k. Anemia—acute or chronic disease
   l. Rheumatoid arthritis, gout, arthritis, polymyalgia rheumatica
   m. Hypothyroidism and hyperthyroidism
2. *Normal* ESR (no increase) is found in:
   a. Polycythemia vera, erythrocytosis
   b. Sickle cell anemia, Hb C disease
   c. Congestive heart failure
   d. Hypofibrinogenemia (from any cause)
   e. Pyruvate kinase (PK) deficiency
   f. Hereditary spherocytosis
   g. Anemia
      (1) ESR is normal in iron-deficiency anemia.
      (2) ESR is abnormal in anemia of chronic disease alone or in combination with iron-deficiency anemia and can be used to differentiate these.
   h. Uncomplicated viral disease and infectious mononucleosis—normal
   i. Active renal failure with heart failure—normal
   j. Acute allergy—normal
   k. Peptic ulcer—normal

CLINICAL ALERT

Extreme elevation of the ESR is found with malignant lymphocarcinoma of colon or breast, myeloma, and rheumatoid arthritis.

Interfering Factors

1. Allowing the blood sample to stand longer than 24 hours before the test is started causes the ESR to decrease.
2. In refrigerated blood, the ESR is increased. Refrigerated blood should be allowed to return to room temperature before the test is performed.
3. Factors leading to an increased ESR include:
   a. The presence of fibrinogen, globulins, C-reactive protein, high cholesterol
   b. Pregnancy after 12 weeks until about the fourth postpartum week
   c. Young children
   d. Menstruation
   e. Certain drugs (e.g., heparin, oral contraceptives; see Appendix E)
   f. Anemia (low Hct)
   g. Macrocytosis
4. The ESR may be very high (up to 60 mm/hr) in apparently healthy women ages 70 to 89 years.
5. Factors leading to reduced ESR include:
   a. High blood sugar, high albumin level, high phospholipids
   b. Decreased fibrinogen level in the blood in newborns, hypofibrinogenemia
   c. Certain drugs (e.g., steroids, high-dose aspirin; see Appendix E)

d. High Hb and RBC count—polycythemia
e. High WBC count
f. Abnormal RBCs (e.g., sickle cells, spherocytes, microcytosis)

Interventions

Pretest Patient Care

1. Explain test purpose and procedure. Assess for signs/symptoms of fever, chills, and acute infection. Obtain appropriate medication history. Fasting is not necessary, but a fatty meal can cause plasma alterations.
2. Possible treatments include preventing cross-infection and decreasing activity levels.
3. Follow guidelines in Chapter 1 for safe, effective, informed *pretest* care.

Posttest Patient Care

1. Have patient resume normal activities and diet.
2. Review test results; report and record findings. Modify the nursing care plan as needed. Counsel the patient regarding abnormal findings; explain the need for possible follow-up testing and treatment. Monitor for rheumatic disorders and inflammatory conditions.
3. Follow guidelines in Chapter 1 for safe, effective, informed *posttest* care.

TESTS FOR PORPHYRIA

Porphyrins are chemical intermediates in the synthesis of Hb, myoglobin, and other respiratory pigments called *cytochromes*. They also form part of the peroxidase and catalase enzymes, which contribute to the efficiency of internal respiration. Iron is chelated within porphyrins to form heme. Heme is then incorporated into proteins to become biologically functional hemoproteins.

Tests of blood, urine, and stool are done to diagnose porphyria, an abnormal accumulation of porphyrins in body fluids. Porphyrias are a group of diseases caused by a deficit in the enzymes involved in porphyrin metabolism and abnormalities in the production of the metalloporphyrin heme. These tests are indicated in persons who have unexplained neurologic manifestations, unexplained abdominal pain, cutaneous blisters, or the presence of a relevant family history. Test results may identify clinical conditions associated with abnormal heme production, including anemia and porphyria (abnormal accumulation of the porphyrins) associated with enzyme disorders that may be genetic (hereditary) or acquired (e.g., lead poisoning, alcohol). Accumulation of porphyrins occurs in blood plasma, serum, erythrocytes, urine, and feces. A discussion of erythrocyte totals and fractionation of erythrocytes and plasma follows. For details of urine, serum, and stool testing for porphyrias, see Chapters 3, 6, and 4, respectively.

● Erythropoietic Porphyrins; Free Erythrocyte Protoporphyrin (FEP)

Normally, there is a small amount of excess porphyrin at the completion of heme synthesis. This excess is cell free erythrocyte protoporphyrin (FEP). The amount of FEP in the erythrocyte is elevated when the iron supply is diminished.

This test is useful in screening for RBC disorders such as iron deficiency and lead exposure, especially in children 6 months to 5 years of age. This is the test of choice to diagnose erythropoietic protoporphyria. This test should not be used for screening for lead poisoning in children.

Normal Findings

<100 µg/dL of packed RBCs

NOTE *This depends on the method. Check with your laboratory.*

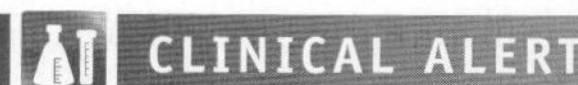

Critical Value

FEP >300 μg/dL or >3000 μg/L

Procedure

1. Obtain a 5-mL sample of anticoagulated (EDTA or heparin may be used) venous blood. Label the specimen with the patient's name, date and time of collection, and test(s) ordered. Place the specimen in a biohazard bag.
2. Protect the blood sample from light.
3. Wash the cells and then test for porphyrins.
4. Be aware that the Hct must be known for test interpretation.

Clinical Implications

1. *Increased* FEP is associated with:
   a. Iron-deficiency anemias (elevated before anemia)
   b. Lead poisoning (chronic)
   c. Halogenated solvents and many drugs (see Appendix E)
   d. Anemia of chronic disease
   e. Acquired idiopathic sideroblastic anemia (most cases)
   f. Erythropoietic protoporphyria
2. FEP is *normal* in:
   a. Thalassemia minor (and therefore can be used to differentiate this from iron deficiency and other disorders of globin synthesis)
   b. Pyridoxine-responsive anemia
   c. Certain forms of sideroblastic anemia due to proximal block to protoporphyrin

Interventions

Pretest Patient Care

1. Explain test purpose and sampling procedure.
2. Note on laboratory slip or computer any medications the patient is taking that cause intermittent porphyria. Discontinue such medications before testing (after checking with the healthcare provider).
3. Follow guidelines in Chapter 1 for safe, effective, informed *pretest* care.

Posttest Patient Care

1. Resume normal activities and diet.
2. Review test results; report and record findings. Modify the nursing care plan as needed. Counsel the patient regarding abnormal findings; explain the need for possible follow-up testing and treatment. Monitor for porphyria or lead poisoning.
3. Follow guidelines in Chapter 1 for safe, effective, informed *posttest* care.

● Porphyrins; Fractionation of Erythrocytes and of Plasma

The primary porphyrins of erythrocytes are protoporphyrin, uroporphyrin, and coproporphyrin.

Fractionation of erythrocytes is used to differentiate congenital erythropoietic coproporphyria from erythropoietic protoporphyria and to confirm a diagnosis of protoporphyria. This test establishes a specific type of porphyria by naming the specific porphyrin in plasma. In persons with renal failure, plasma fractionation can help to determine whether the porphyria is caused by a deficiency of uroporphyrinogenic decarboxylase or by failure of the renal system to excrete porphyrinogens.

Normal Findings

The value is reported in micrograms per deciliter (μg/dL). Check with your laboratory for reference values.

1. Erythrocyte porphyrins
   a. Protoporphyrin: 16 to 60 μg/dL packed cells or 0.3 to 1.7 μmol/L
   b. Uroporphyrin: <2 μg/dL or <24 nmol/L
   c. Hepatocarboxylic: <1 μg/dL or <10 μg/L
   d. Hexacarboxylic: <1 μg/dL or <10 μg/L
   e. Pentacarboxylic: <1 μg/dL or <10 μg/L
   f. Coproporphyrin: <1 μg/dL or <15 μg/L
2. Plasma porphyrins: Total porphyrins should not exceed 1.0 μg/dL or 12 nmol/L.

Procedure

1. Draw a 5-mL sample of anticoagulated (EDTA or heparin can be used) blood. Label the specimen with the patient's name, date and time of collection, and test(s) ordered. Place the specimen in a biohazard bag.
2. Protect the specimen from light.

Clinical Implications

1. *Increased erythrocyte porphyrins* are associated with primary porphyrias:
   a. Congenital erythropoietic protoporphyria
   b. Protoporphyria (autosomal-dominant deficiency of heme synthetase)
   c. Hereditary porphobilinogen synthase deficiency
   d. Intoxication porphyria
2. *Increased plasma porphyrins* are associated with:
   a. Congenital erythropoietic protoporphyria
   b. Coproporphyria
   c. Porphyria cutanea tarda
   d. Variegate porphyria
   e. Chronic renal failure porphyria

Interventions

Pretest Patient Care

1. Advise patient of test purpose and procedure.
2. Note on the requisition any drugs the patient is taking.
3. Before testing, discontinue drugs that are known to cause intermittent porphyria (after checking with the healthcare provider).
4. Follow guidelines in Chapter 1 for safe, effective, informed *pretest* care.

Posttest Patient Care

1. Resume medications.
2. Review test results; report and record findings. Modify the nursing care plan as needed. Counsel the patient regarding abnormal findings; explain the need for possible follow-up testing and treatment. Monitor for porphyria or lead poisoning.
3. Caution persons diagnosed with porphyria (with cutaneous manifestations) to avoid sun exposure.

4. Advise persons diagnosed with porphyria (with neurologic symptoms) that attacks can be precipitated by infections, various phases of the menstrual cycle, fasting states, and certain drugs. A listing of drugs (not all inclusive) that may precipitate acute attacks follows:
   a. Barbiturates
   b. Chlordiazepoxide
   c. Chloroquine
   d. Chlorpropamide
   e. Dichloralphenazone
   f. Ergot preparations
   g. Estrogens
   h. Ethanol
   i. Glutethimide
   j. Griseofulvin
   k. Hydantoins
   l. Imipramine
   m. Meprobamate
   n. Methsuximide
   o. Methyldopa
   p. Sulfonamides
5. Follow guidelines in Chapter 1 for safe, effective, informed *posttest* care.

CLINICAL ALERT

1. A blood test for uroporphyrinogen I synthase (also known as erythrocyte porphobilinogen deaminase) can be done to identify persons at risk for acute intermittent porphyria, to detect latent-phase intermittent porphyria, and to confirm the diagnosis during an acute episode.
2. The normal value is 5.3–9.2 nmol/L in women; 3.4–8.5 nmol/L in men. A value of <3.5 nmol/L is diagnostic of acute intermittent porphyria.

TESTS FOR HEMOLYTIC ANEMIA

Several RBC enzyme and fragility tests can be done to screen, detect, and confirm the cause of chronic hemolytic anemia. Many persons with hemolytic anemia have no clinical signs or symptoms. Abnormal test outcomes are associated with inherited deficiencies, abnormal Hb, and exposure to chemicals and drugs. Definitive test results indicate some type of injury to the RBC, oxidative activity that interferes with normal Hb function, or increased RBC fragility.

● Pyruvate Kinase (PK)

PK deficiency is a genetic disorder characterized by a lowered concentration of adenosine triphosphate in the RBC and consequential membrane defect. The result is a nonspherocytic, chronic hemolytic anemia. PK deficiency is the most common and most important form of hemolytic anemia resulting from a deficiency of glycolytic enzymes in the RBC.

Normal Findings

2.8 to 8.8 U/g Hb or 46.7 to 146.7 nkat/g Hb
To convert to U/mL of packed RBCs: U/g Hb × 0.34 = U/mL packed RBCs
Normal values vary greatly; check with your reference laboratory.

Procedure

1. Obtain 5 mL of whole blood in a green–topped tube (with EDTA or heparin anticoagulant). Label the specimen with the patient's name, date and time of collection, and test(s) ordered.
2. Refrigerate immediately.

Clinical Implications

PK is *decreased* in:

1. Congenital PK deficiency: recessive, nonspherocytic hemolytic anemia. Patients tolerate anemia well because of increased 2,3-diphosphoglycerate (2,3-DPG).
2. Acquired PK deficiency caused by (level returns to normal after treating underlying disorder):
   a. Myelodysplastic disorders
   b. Acute leukemias
   c. Anemias

Interfering Factors

In congenital PK deficiency, intravascular hemolysis increases during pregnancy or following use of oral contraceptives.

Interventions

Pretest Patient Care

1. Explain test purpose and procedure. There should be no exercising before tests.
2. Withhold transfusion until after blood samples are drawn (especially with osmotic fragility).
3. Follow guidelines in Chapter 1 for safe, effective, informed *pretest* care.

Posttest Patient Care

1. Review test results; report and record findings. Modify the nursing care plan as needed. Counsel the patient regarding abnormal findings; explain the need for possible follow-up testing and treatment. Monitor for hemolytic anemia, hypoxia, or polycythemia.
2. Splenectomy is indicated when anemia is severe enough to require transfusions.
3. Follow guidelines in Chapter 1 for safe, effective, informed *posttest* care.

CLINICAL ALERT

Many prescribed drugs interfere with the normal functioning of Hb in susceptible persons, especially sulfonamides, antipyretics, analgesics, large doses of vitamin K, and nitrofurans. Any increase in PK level should be brought to the immediate attention of the healthcare provider.

• Erythrocyte Fragility (Osmotic Fragility and Autohemolysis)

Spherocytes of any origin (including conditions other than hereditary spherocytosis) are more susceptible than normal RBCs to hemolysis in dilute (hypotonic) saline and show increased osmotic fragility. Generally, fully expanded cells (spheroidal cells or spherocytes) have increased osmotic fragility, whereas cells with higher surface area-to-volume ratios (e.g., thin cells, hypochromic cells, tart cells) have decreased osmotic fragility.

In hereditary spherocytosis, the osmotic fragility test may be normal initially. Therefore, the test is incubated at 37°C for 24 hours, at which time the test is positive for hereditary spherocytosis.

Normal Findings

Immediate test:
Hemolysis begins at 0.5% NaCl.
Hemolysis completes at 0.3% NaCl.
24-hour incubation:
Hemolysis begins at 0.7% NaCl.
Hemolysis completes at 0.4% NaCl.

Procedure

1. Obtain a 7-mL venous blood sample using a green top tube (heparin) or lavender-topped tube (EDTA). Label the specimen with the patient's name, date and time of collection, and test(s) ordered. Place the specimen in a biohazard bag.
2. Expose erythrocytes to varying dilutions of sodium chloride. Read hemolysis on a spectrophotometer (optical density measurement). Perform studies and measure both before and after 24-hour incubation of the RBCs.

Clinical Implications

1. *Increased* osmotic fragility is found in:
   a. Hemolytic anemia (acquired immune)
   b. Hereditary spherocytosis (stomatocytosis)
   c. Hemolytic disease of the newborn
   d. Malaria
   e. Severe PK deficiency
2. *Decreased* osmotic fragility occurs in:
   a. Iron-deficiency anemia (macrocytic hypochromic)
   b. Thalassemias
   c. Asplenia (postsplenectomy)
   d. Liver disease (obstructive jaundice)
   e. Reticulocytosis
   f. Hemoglobinopathies, especially Hb C, Hb S

Interventions

Pretest Patient Care

1. Explain test purpose and procedure. There should be no exercising before tests.
2. Withhold transfusion until after blood samples are drawn (especially with osmotic fragility).
3. Follow guidelines in Chapter 1 for safe, effective, informed *pretest* care.

Posttest Patient Care

1. Follow guidelines in Chapter 1 for safe, effective, informed *posttest* care.
2. Be aware that the usual treatment for hereditary spherocytosis is splenectomy, which removes the agent of RBC destruction and prevents complications such as aplastic anemia.

● Glucose-6-Phosphate Dehydrogenase (G6PD)

Glucose-6-phosphate dehydrogenase (G6PD) deficiency is a sex-linked disorder. The major variants occur in specific ethnic groups. In a large group of African American men, the incidence of type A G6PD deficiency was found to be 11%. Approximately 20% of African American women are heterozygous. With some variants, there is chronic lifelong hemolysis, but more commonly, the condition is asymptomatic and results only in susceptibility to acute hemolytic episodes, which may be triggered by certain drugs, ingestion of fava beans, or viral or bacterial infection. G6PD hemolysis is associated with formation of Heinz bodies in peripheral RBCs.

The other two most common types are Mediterranean, which is common in Iraqis, Kurds, Sephardic Jews, and Lebanese and less common in Greeks, Italians, Turks, and North Africans, and the MAHIDOL variant, which is common in Southeast Asians (22% of males).

Normal Findings

G6PD screen: G6PD detected
Adults: 8.6 to 18.6 U/g Hb or 0.14 to 0.31 nkat/g Hb
Children: 6.4 to 15.6 U/g Hb or 0.11 to 0.26 nkat/g Hb
Newborns: have values up to 50% higher than adults
If done as a screening test, G6PD activity is reported as within normal limits. Different laboratories have different ways of reporting.
To convert U/g Hb to U/mL of RBCs: U/g Hb × 0.34 = U/mL of RBCs

Procedure

1. Obtain 5 mL of whole blood in two lavender-topped tubes (with EDTA or heparin anticoagulant). Label the specimen with the patient's name, date and time of collection, and test(s) ordered.
2. Perform a G6PD screen and then place on ice in a biohazard bag.
3. Do not centrifuge.
4. Refrigerate.

Clinical Implications

1. G6PD is *decreased* in:
    a. G6PD deficiency (causes hemolytic episodes after exposure to certain drugs and fava beans)
    b. Congenital nonspherocytic anemia
    c. Nonimmunologic hemolytic disease of the newborn (Asian and Mediterranean)
2. G6PD is *increased* in:
    a. Untreated megaloblastic anemia (pernicious anemia)
    b. Thrombocytopenia purpura
    c. Hyperthyroidism
    d. Viral hepatitis

Interfering Factors

1. Marked reticulocytosis may give a falsely high G6PD.
2. G6PD may be falsely normal for 6 to 8 weeks after a hemolytic episode, especially in African Americans with the type A variant. Retest after the patient recovers from the episode of anemia.

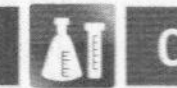

CLINICAL ALERT

In G6PD-Mediterranean, G6PD levels are grossly deficient in all RBCs. Patients with this variant commonly experience hemolysis induced by diabetic acidosis, infections, and oxidant drugs and potentially fatal hemolytic crises after ingestion of fava beans.

Interventions

Pretest Patient Care

1. Explain test purpose and procedure. There should be no exercising before tests.
2. Withhold transfusion until after blood samples are drawn (especially with osmotic fragility).
3. Follow guidelines in Chapter 1 for safe, effective, informed *pretest* care.

Posttest Patient Care

1. Follow guidelines in Chapter 1 for safe, effective, informed *posttest* care.
2. Possible treatments include providing the patient with a list of drugs that can precipitate hemolysis and teaching the patient to read labels and not to take over-the-counter drugs with aspirin.
3. There are certain drugs and chemicals that should be avoided by persons with G6PD deficiency.

● Heinz Bodies; Heinz Stain; Glutathione Instability

Heinz bodies are insoluble intracellular inclusions of Hb attached to the RBC membrane. Heinz bodies are uncommon except with G6PD deficiency immediately after hemolysis and in patients with unstable Hb variants.

Oxidative denaturation of the Hb molecule leads to Heinz body formation and is probably the mechanism for the precipitation of unstable Hb. Heinz bodies are usually removed by the spleen; after splenectomy, they increase in the peripheral blood and may appear in >50% of RBCs.

Normal Findings

Not seen in normal patients

Procedure

1. Obtain a 5-mL venous blood sample using either a green-topped (sodium heparin) tube or a lavender-topped (EDTA) tube. Label the specimen with the patient's name, date and time of collection, and test(s) ordered. Place the specimen in a biohazard bag.
2. Mix cells with a supravital stain and examine microscopically. They stain as pale blue bodies, as opposed to the dark purple RNA in reticulocytes.

Clinical Implications

1. Increased Heinz bodies are found in:
   a. G6PD deficiency, especially after hemolysis
   b. Congenital Heinz body hemolytic anemia
   c. Unstable Hb variants (e.g., Hb Zurich, Hb Philly)
   d. Homozygous β-thalassemia
2. Heinz bodies are found in blood of normal persons who have been poisoned by certain drugs used in treatment protocols (e.g., chlorates, phenylhydrazine, primaquine).
3. Heinz bodies are present in some newborns or in splenectomized patients.

Interfering Factors

See Appendix E for drugs that affect test outcomes.

Interventions

Pretest Patient Care

1. Explain test purposes and procedures.
2. Follow guidelines in Chapter 1 for safe, effective, informed *pretest* care.

Posttest Patient Care

1. Review test results; report and record findings. Modify the nursing care plan as needed. Counsel the patient regarding abnormal findings; explain the need for possible follow-up testing and treatment.
2. Follow guidelines in Chapter 1 for safe, effective, informed *posttest* care.

● 2,3-Diphosphoglycerate (2,3-DPG)

2,3-DPG assists in transporting oxygen in RBCs. 2,3-DPG increases in response to hypoxia or anemia and decreases in acidosis. Levels are lower in newborns and even lower in premature newborns.

Normal Findings

Adults: 10.4 to 14.2 μmol/g Hb or 3.6 to 4.8 μmol/mL RBCs
Check with your reference laboratory.

Procedure

1. Obtain a venous blood sample of at least 3 mL, anticoagulated with heparin. Label the specimen with the patient's name, date and time of collection, and test(s) ordered.
2. Place on ice immediately (2,3-DPG is stable for only 2 hours) and transport to the laboratory as soon as possible in a biohazard bag.

Clinical Implications

1. *Increased* 2,3-DPG occurs in:
   a. Emphysema, cystic fibrosis with pulmonary involvement (conditions of hypoxia)
   b. Cyanotic heart disease
   c. Pulmonary vascular disease
   d. Sickle cell anemia, iron-deficiency anemia
   e. PK deficiency
   f. Hyperthyroidism
   g. Chronic renal failure
   h. Cirrhosis
2. *Decreased* 2,3-DPG occurs in:
   a. Polycythemia vera
   b. Respiratory distress syndrome
   c. 2,3-DPG deficiency
   d. Hexokinase deficiency

Interfering Factors

1. High altitude *increases* 2,3-DPG.
2. Exercise *increases* 2,3-DPG.

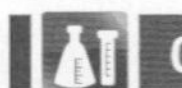

CLINICAL ALERT

If blood with decreased 2,3-DPG is used for transfusion, the Hb may not release O_2 when needed.

Interventions

Pretest Patient Care for Tests for Hemolytic Anemia

1. Explain test purpose and procedure. There should be no exercising before tests.
2. Withhold transfusion until after blood samples are drawn (especially with osmotic fragility).
3. Follow guidelines in Chapter 1 for safe, effective, informed *pretest* care.

Posttest Patient Care for Tests for Hemolytic Anemia

1. Review test results; report and record findings. Modify the nursing care plan as needed. Counsel the patient regarding abnormal findings; explain the need for possible follow-up testing and treatment. Monitor for hemolytic anemia, hypoxia, or polycythemia.
2. Follow guidelines in Chapter 1 for safe, effective, informed *posttest* care.

TESTS FOR ANEMIA

● Vitamin B_{12} (VB_{12})

VB_{12}, also known as the *antipernicious anemia factor*, is necessary for the production of RBCs. It is obtained only from ingestion of animal protein and requires an intrinsic factor for absorption. Both VB_{12} and folic acid depend on a normally functioning intestinal mucosa for their absorption and are important for the production of RBCs. Levels of VB_{12} and folate are usually tested in conjunction with one another because the diagnosis of macrocytic anemia requires measurement of both.

This determination is used in the differential diagnosis of anemia and conditions marked by high turnover of myeloid cells, as in the leukemias. When binding capacity is measured, it is the unsaturated fraction that is determined. The measurement of unsaturated VB_{12}–binding capacity (UBBC) is valuable in distinguishing between untreated polycythemia vera and other conditions in which there is an elevated Hct.

Normal Findings

Adults: 280 to 1500 pg/mL or 206 to 1107 pmol/L
Elderly (60 to 90 yr): 110 to 770 pg/mL (81 to 568 pmol/L)
Newborns: 160 to 1300 pg/mL or 118 to 959 pmol/L
UBBC: 600 to 1400 pg/mL or 443 to 1033 pmol/L

Procedure

1. Obtain a fasting venous blood sample of at least 5 mL, using a red-topped tube or serum separator tube (SST). Label the specimen with the patient's name, date and time of collection, and test(s) ordered.
2. Obtain the specimen before an injection of VB_{12} is administered and before a Schilling test is done.

Clinical Implications

1. *Decreased* VB_{12} (<100 pg/mL or <74 pmol/L) is associated with:
   a. Pernicious anemia (megaloblastic anemia)
   b. Malabsorption syndromes and inflammatory bowel disease
   c. Fish tapeworm infestation
   d. Primary hypothyroidism
   e. Loss of gastric mucosa, as in gastrectomy and resection
   f. Zollinger-Ellison syndrome
   g. Blind loop syndromes (bacterial overgrowth)
   h. Vegetarian diets (dietary insufficiency)
   i. Folic acid deficiency
   j. Iron deficiency may be present in some patients (e.g., gastrectomy)
2. *Increased* VB_{12} (>700 pg/mL or >517 pmol/L) is associated with:
   a. Chronic granulocytic leukemia, lymphatic and monocytic leukemia
   b. Chronic renal failure
   c. Liver disease (hepatitis, cirrhosis)
   d. Some cases of cancer, especially with liver metastasis
   e. Polycythemia vera

f. Congestive heart failure
g. Diabetes
h. Obesity
i. COPD
3. *Increased UBBC* is found in:
a. Sixty percent of cases of polycythemia vera. (This test is normal in secondary relative polycythemia, aiding in the differential diagnosis of these two states.)
b. Reactive leukocytosis (leukemoid reaction)
c. CML

Interfering Factors

The following result in increased VB_{12} values:

1. Pregnancy
2. Blood transfusion
3. Elderly persons
4. High vitamin C and A doses
5. Smoking
6. Drugs capable of interfering with VB_{12} absorption (see Appendix E)

Interventions

Pretest Patient Care

1. Explain test purpose and procedure.
2. Alert patient that overnight fasting from food is necessary. Water is permitted.
3. Withhold VB_{12} injection before the blood is drawn.
4. Follow guidelines in Chapter 1 for safe, effective, informed *pretest* care.

Posttest Patient Care

1. Resume normal activities and diet.
2. Review test results; report and record findings. Modify the nursing care plan as needed. Counsel the patient regarding abnormal findings; explain the need for possible follow-up testing and treatment. Monitor for anemia, leukemia, or polycythemia.
3. Follow guidelines in Chapter 1 for safe, effective, informed *posttest* care. See Appendix C for more information on vitamin testing.

CLINICAL ALERT

1. Persons who have recently received therapeutic or diagnostic doses of radionuclides will have unreliable results.
2. The Schilling test is used to confirm pernicious anemia and to determine whether VB_{12} deficiency is caused by malabsorption.
3. See Appendix C for more information on nutritional status of VB_{12}.

• Folic Acid (Folate)

Folic acid (pteroylmonoglutamate) is needed for normal RBC and WBC function and for the production of cellular genes. Folic acid is a more potent growth promoter than VB_{12}, although both depend on the normal functioning of intestinal mucosa for their absorption. Folic acid, like VB_{12}, is required for DNA production. Folic acid is formed by bacteria in the intestines; is stored in the liver; and is present in eggs, milk, leafy vegetables, yeast, liver, fruits, and other elements of a well-balanced diet.

This test is indicated for the differential diagnosis of megaloblastic anemia and in the investigation of folic acid deficiency, iron deficiency, and hypersegmental granulocytes. Measurement of both serum and RBC folate levels constitutes a reliable means of determining the existence of folate deficiency. The finding of low serum folate means that the patient's recent diet was subnormal in folate content, that the patient's recent absorption of folate was subnormal, or both. Low RBC folate can mean either that there is tissue folate depletion owing to folate deficiency requiring folate therapy or, alternatively, that the patient has primary VB_{12} deficiency that is blocking the ability of cells to take up folate. Serum levels are commonly high in patients with VB_{12} deficiency because this vitamin is needed to allow incorporation of folate into tissue cells. For thoroughness, the serum VB_{12} should also be determined because >50% of all patients with significant megaloblastic anemia have VB_{12} deficiency rather than folate deficiency.

Normal Findings

Serum:
Adults: 3 to 13 ng/mL or 6.8 to 29.5 nmol/L
Children: 5 to 21 ng/mL or 11.3 to 47.6 nmol/L
Infants: 14 to 51 ng/mL or 31.7 to 115.5 nmol/L
RBC folate:
Adults: 140 to 628 ng/mL or 317 to 1422 nmol/L
Children: >160 ng/mL or >362 nmol/L

Procedure

1. If a serum sample is ordered, obtain a fasting venous sample of 10 mL using a red-topped tube or SST. Protect the sample from light. Label the specimen with the patient's name, date and time of collection, and test(s) ordered.
2. If RBC folate is ordered, draw up to two 5-mL tubes of venous blood using a lavender-topped tube with EDTA anticoagulant. An Hct determination is also required. Patient should not have had a folic acid supplement (e.g., in a daily vitamin) for at least 3 to 5 days.

Clinical Implications

1. *Decreased* folic acid levels are associated with:
   a. Inadequate intake owing to alcoholism, chronic disease, malnutrition, diet devoid of fresh vegetables, or anorexia
   b. Malabsorption of folic acid (e.g., small bowel disease)
   c. Excessive use of folic acid by the body (e.g., pregnancy, hypothyroidism)
   d. Megaloblastic (macrocytic) anemia caused by VB_{12} deficiency
   e. Hemolytic anemia (sickle cell, phenocytosis, PNH)
   f. Liver disease associated with cirrhosis, alcoholism, hepatoma
   g. Adult celiac disease, sprue
   h. Vitamin B_6 deficiency
   i. Carcinomas (mainly metastatic), acute leukemia, myelofibrosis
   j. Crohn's disease, ulcerative colitis
   k. Infantile hyperthyroidism
   l. Intestinal resection, jejunal bypass procedure
   m. Drugs that are folic antagonists (interfere with nucleic acid synthesis)
      (1) Anticonvulsants (phenytoin)
      (2) Aminopterin and methotrexate
      (3) Antimalarials

    (4) Alcohol (ethanol)
    (5) Oral contraceptives
    (6) Heavy usage of antacids
2. *Increased* folic acid levels are associated with:
    a. Blind loop syndrome
    b. Vegetarian diet
    c. Pernicious anemia, VB_{12} deficiency
3. *Decreased* RBC folate occurs with:
    a. Untreated folate deficiency
    b. VB_{12} deficiency (60% of uncomplicated cases)

Interfering Factors

1. Drugs that are folic acid antagonists, among others (see Appendix E)
2. Hemolyzed specimens (false elevation)
3. Iron-deficiency anemia (false increase)

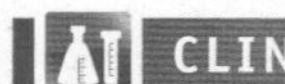

CLINICAL ALERT

Elderly persons and those with inadequate diets may develop folate-deficient megaloblastic anemia.

Interventions

Pretest Patient Care

1. Explain test purpose and procedure. Obtain pertinent medication history. Assess for sign/symptoms of anorexia, fainting, fatigue, headache, forgetfulness, pallor, palpitations, and weakness.
2. Alert patient that fasting from food for 8 hours before testing is required; water is permitted.
3. Draw blood before VB_{12} injection.
4. Do not administer radioisotopes for 24 hours before the specimen is drawn.
5. Follow guidelines in Chapter 1 for safe, effective, informed *pretest* care.

Posttest Patient Care

1. Resume normal activities and medications.
2. Review test results; report and record findings. Modify the nursing care plan as needed. Counsel the patient regarding abnormal findings; explain the need for possible follow-up testing and treatment. Monitor for anemia.
3. Possible treatments include administering folic acid supplements as ordered and teaching patients about a well-balanced diet.
4. Follow guidelines in Chapter 1 for safe, effective, informed *posttest* care. See Appendix C for more information on vitamin testing.

● Erythropoietin (Ep)

Erythropoietin (Ep) is a glycoprotein hormone that regulates erythropoiesis. The levels of Ep in anemia are primarily determined by the degree of anemia; Ep is inversely related to RBC volume and Hct.

Ep is used to investigate obscure anemias. This test is useful in differentiating primary from secondary polycythemia and in detecting the recurrence of Ep-producing tumors. It is also used as an indicator of need for Ep therapy in patients with renal failure (end-stage renal disease).

Normal Findings

5 to 36 mU/mL or 5 to 36 U/L

Procedure

1. Obtain a venous blood serum sample of 5 mL using a red-topped tube or SST. Label the specimen with the patient's name, date and time of collection, and test(s) ordered. Place the specimen in a biohazard bag.
2. Separate serum from cells as soon as possible and place in polypropylene tube (*not* clear plastic-polystyrene). Freeze.

Clinical Implications

1. Ep is *increased appropriately* in:
   a. Anemias with very low Hb (e.g., aplastic anemia, hemolytic anemia); hematologic cancers have very high levels
   b. Patients with any iron-deficiency anemia have moderately high levels
   c. Myelodysplasia, chemotherapy, AIDS
   d. Secondary polycythemia vera caused by tissue hypoxia (e.g., high altitude, COPD)
   e. Pregnancy (very high values)
2. Ep is *increased inappropriately* in Ep-producing tumors such as the following:
   a. Renal cysts, renal transplant rejection
   b. Renal adenocarcinoma
   c. Pheochromocytomas
   d. Cerebellar hemangioblastomas
   e. Polycystic kidney disease
   f. Occasionally, adrenal, ovarian, testicular, breast, and hepatic carcinoma
3. Ep is *decreased appropriately* in:
   a. Rheumatoid arthritis
   b. Multiple myeloma
   c. Cancer
4. Ep is *decreased inappropriately* in:
   a. Polycythemia vera (primary)
   b. After bone marrow transplantation (weeks 3 and 4)
   c. AIDS before initiating therapy
   d. Autonomic neuropathy
   e. Renal failure and adult nephrotic syndrome

Interfering Factors

1. Ep is *increased* in:
   a. Pregnancy
   b. Use of anabolic steroids
   c. Administration of thyroid-stimulating hormone, ACTH, epinephrine
   d. Growth hormone (see Appendix E)
2. Ep is *decreased* in:
   a. Transfusions
   b. Use of some prescribed drugs (see Appendix E)
   c. Drugs that increase renal blood flow (e.g., enalapril)
   d. High plasma viscosity

Interventions

Pretest Patient Care

1. Explain test purpose and procedure.
2. Draw blood at the same time for serial determinations: Circadian rhythm is lowest in the morning and 40% higher in late evening.

3. Alert patient that fasting is not necessary, but a morning specimen is needed.
4. Note use of any drugs.
5. Follow guidelines in Chapter 1 for safe, effective, informed *pretest* care.

Posttest Patient Care

1. Resume normal activities and medications.
2. Review test results; report and record findings. Modify the nursing care plan as needed. Counsel the patient regarding abnormal findings; explain the need for possible follow-up testing and treatment. Monitor for anemia.
3. Follow guidelines in Chapter 1 for safe, effective, informed *posttest* care. See Appendix C for more information on vitamin testing.

IRON TESTS

● Iron (Fe), Total Iron-Binding Capacity (TIBC), and Transferrin Tests

Iron is necessary for the production of Hb. Iron is contained in several components. Transferrin (also called siderophilin), a transport protein largely synthesized by the liver, regulates iron absorption. High levels of transferrin relate to the ability of the body to deal with infections. Total iron-binding capacity (TIBC) correlates with serum transferrin, but the relation is not linear. A serum iron test without a TIBC and transferrin determination has very limited value except in cases of iron poisoning. Transferrin saturation is a better index of iron saturation; it is evaluated as follows:

$$\text{Transferrin saturation \%} = \frac{(\text{Serum iron} \times 100)}{\text{TIBC}}$$

The combined results of transferrin, iron, and TIBC tests are helpful in the differential diagnosis of anemia, in assessment of iron-deficiency anemia, and in the evaluation of thalassemia, sideroblastic anemia, and hemochromatosis (Table 2.6).

Normal Findings

Iron
Adult men: 70 to 175 µg/dL or 12.5 to 31.3 µmol/L
Adult women: 50 to 150 µg/dL or 8.9 to 26.8 µmol/L
Children: 50 to 120 µg/dL or 9.0 to 21.5 µmol/L
Newborns: 100 to 250 µg/dL or 17.9 to 44.8 µmol/L
Total iron-binding capacity
Men: 250 to 450 µg/dL or 44.8 to 76.1 µmol/L
Women: 250 to 450 µg/dL or 44.8 to 76.1 µmol/L
Transferrin
Adults: 250 to 425 mg/dL or 2.5 to 4.2 g/L
Children: 203 to 360 mg/dL or 2.0 to 3.6 g/L
Newborns: 130 to 275 mg/dL or 1.3 to 2.7 g/L
Transferrin (iron) saturation
Men: 10% to 50%
Women: 15% to 50%

CLINICAL ALERT

1. Critical iron values: intoxicated child, 350–500 μg/dL or 63–90 μmol/L; fatally poisoned child, >800–1000 μg/dL or >145–180 μmol/L
2. Symptoms of iron poisoning include abdominal pain, vomiting, bloody diarrhea, cyanosis, and convulsions.

Procedure

1. Obtain a venous blood sample of 10 mL using a red-topped tube. Label the specimen with the patient's name, date and time of collection, and test(s) ordered.
2. Place the specimen in a biohazard bag. Serum is needed for these tests.

Clinical Implications

1. *Increased transferrin* is observed in:
    a. Iron-deficiency anemia (uncomplicated)
    b. Pregnancy
    c. Estrogen therapy
2. *Decreased transferrin* is found in:
    a. Microcytic anemia of chronic disease
    b. Protein deficiency or loss from burns or malnutrition
    c. Chronic infection
    d. Acute liver disease
    e. Renal disease (nephrosis)
    f. Genetic deficiency, hereditary atransferrinemia
    g. Iron-overload states (hemochromatosis)
3. *Decreased iron* occurs in:
    a. Iron-deficiency anemia
    b. Chronic blood loss
    c. Chronic diseases (e.g., lupus, rheumatoid arthritis, chronic infections)
    d. Third-trimester pregnancy and progesterone birth control pills
    e. Remission of pernicious anemia
    f. Inadequate absorption of iron
    g. Hemolytic anemia (PNH)
4. *Increased iron* occurs in:
    a. Hemolytic anemias, especially thalassemia, pernicious anemia in relapse (not hemolytic anemias)
    b. Acute iron poisoning (children)
    c. Iron-overload syndromes
    d. Hemochromatosis, iron overload
    e. Transfusions (multiple), intramuscular iron, inappropriate iron therapy
    f. Acute hepatitis, liver damage
    g. Vitamin B_6 deficiency
    h. Lead poisoning
    i. Acute leukemia
    j. Nephritis
5. *Increased TIBC* is found in:
    a. Iron deficiency
    b. Pregnancy (late)

   c. Acute and chronic blood loss
   d. Acute hepatitis
6. *Decreased TIBC* is observed in:
   a. Hypoproteinemia (malnutrition and burns)
   b. Hemochromatosis
   c. Non–iron-deficiency anemia (infection and chronic disease)
   d. Cirrhosis of liver
   e. Nephrosis and other renal diseases
   f. Thalassemia
   g. Hyperthyroidism
7. The iron saturation index is *increased* in:
   a. Hemochromatosis
   b. Increased iron intake
   c. Thalassemia
   d. Hemosiderosis
   e. Acute liver disease
8. The iron saturation index is *decreased* in:
   a. Iron-deficiency anemias
   b. Malignancy (standard and small intestine)
   c. Anemia of infection and chronic disease
   d. Iron neoplasms

Interfering Factors

1. Many drugs affect test outcomes (see Appendix E).
2. Drugs that may cause increased iron include ethanol, estrogens, and oral contraceptives.
3. Drugs that may cause decreased iron include some antibiotics, aspirin, and testosterone.
4. Hemolysis of the blood sample interferes with testing.
5. Iron contamination of glassware used in testing can give high values.
6. Menstruation causes decreased iron; iron is elevated in the premenstrual period.
7. There is a diurnal variation in iron: normal values in the morning, lower in midafternoon, very low in the evening.
8. Serum iron and TIBC may be normal in iron-deficiency anemia if the Hb is >9.0 g/dL (or >90 g/L).

Interventions

Pretest Patient Care

1. Explain test purpose and procedure.
2. Draw fasting blood in the morning, when levels are higher.
3. Draw iron sample before iron therapy is initiated or blood is transfused.
4. If the patient has received a transfusion, delay iron testing for 4 days.
5. Avoid any iron-chelating drug (e.g., deferoxamine [Desferal]).
6. Avoid sleep deprivation and extreme stress, which cause lower iron levels.
7. Note on laboratory slip or computer screen whether the patient is taking oral contraceptives or estrogen therapy or is pregnant.
8. Follow guidelines in Chapter 1 for safe, effective, informed *pretest* care.

Posttest Patient Care

1. Resume normal activities.
2. Review test results; report and record findings. Modify the nursing care plan as needed. Counsel the patient regarding abnormal findings; explain the need for possible follow-up testing and treatment. The combination of low serum iron, high TIBC, and high transferrin levels indicates iron deficiency.

Diagnosis of iron deficiency may lead further to detection of adenocarcinoma of the gastrointestinal tract, a point that cannot be overemphasized. A significant minority of patients with megaloblastic anemias (20% to 40%) have coexisting iron deficiency. Megaloblastic anemia can interfere with the interpretation of iron studies; repeat iron studies 1 to 3 months after folate or VB_{12} replacement.

3. Follow guidelines in Chapter 1 for safe, effective, informed *posttest* care.

● Ferritin

Ferritin, a complex of ferric (Fe^{2+}) hydroxide and a protein, apoferritin, originates in the reticuloendothelial system. Ferritin reflects the body iron stores and is the most reliable indicator of total-body iron status. A bone marrow examination is the only better test. Bone marrow aspiration may be necessary in some cases, such as low-normal ferritin and low serum iron in the anemia of chronic disease.

The ferritin test is more specific and more sensitive than iron concentration or TIBC for diagnosing iron deficiency. Ferritin decreases before anemia and other changes occur (see Table 2.6).

Normal Findings

Men: 18 to 270 ng/mL or 18 to 270 μg/L
With anemia of chronic disease: <100 ng/mL or <100 μg/L
In absence of inflammation: <20 ng/mL or <20 μg/L
Women: 18 to 160 ng/mL or 18 to 160 μg/L
With anemia of chronic disease: <20 ng/mL or <20 μg/L
In absence of inflammation: <10 ng/mL or <10 μg/L
Children: 7 to 140 ng/mL or 7 to 140 μg/L
Newborns: 25 to 200 ng/mL or 25 to 200 μg/L
1 month: 50 to 200 ng/mL or 50 to 200 μg/L
2 to 5 months: 50 to 200 ng/mL or 50 to 200 μg/L
Serum TfR–ferritin index: 1.5 in absence of anemia of chronic disease, 0.8 with anemia of chronic disease

NOTE *TfR is the transferrin receptor.*

TABLE 2.6 Ferritin, Iron, and Iron Saturation Changes in Anemias

Anemia	Ferritin	Iron	Iron Saturation
Hemorrhage, acute	N	D	D
Hemorrhage, chronic	D	D	D
Iron-deficiency	D	D	D
Aplastic	D	I	I
Megaloblastic	I	D	D
Hemolytic	I	I	I
Sideroblastic	I	I	I
Thalassemia major	I	I	I
Thalassemia minor	I	N/I	N/I
Bone marrow neoplasia	N/I	I	I
Uremia, nephrosis, or nephrotic syndrome	N/I	D/I	D
Liver disease	N/I	N/I	N/I
Chronic diseases	I	D	D

N, no change; D, decrease; I, increase.

CLINICAL ALERT

Critical Value

Iron deficiency: <10 ng/mL or <10 μg/L

Procedure

1. Obtain a venous sample of 6 mL using a red-topped tube or SST. Label the specimen with the patient's name, date and time of collection, and test(s) ordered.
2. Place the specimen in a biohazard bag.

Clinical Implications

1. *Decreased ferritin* (<10 ng/mL or <10 μg/L) usually indicates iron-deficiency anemia.
2. Increased ferritin (>400 ng/mL or >400 μg/L) occurs in iron excess and in the following:
   Iron overload from hemochromatosis or hemosiderosis
   Oral or parenteral iron administration
   Inflammatory diseases
   Acute or chronic liver disease involving alcoholism
   Acute myoblastic or lymphoblastic leukemia
   Other malignancies (Hodgkin's disease, breast carcinoma, malignant lymphoma)
   Hyperthyroidism
   Hemolytic anemia, megaloblastic anemia, thalassemia, sideroblastic anemia
   Renal cell carcinoma, end-stage renal disease

Interfering Factors

1. Recently administered radioactive medications cause spurious results.
2. Oral contraceptives and antithyroid therapy interfere with testing (see Appendix E).
3. Hemolyzed blood may cause high results.
4. Increases with age.
5. Higher in red-meat eaters than in vegetarians.
6. Ferritin is not of value to evaluate iron stores in persons with alcoholism who have liver disease.

Interventions

Pretest Patient Care

1. Explain test purpose and procedure. Fasting is not necessary. Assess for signs/symptoms of dyspnea; fatigue; listlessness; pallor; loss of consciousness; irritability; headache; tachycardia; brittle, spoon-shaped nails; and cracks at the corners of the mouth.
2. Radioactive medications may not be given for 3 to 4 days before testing.
3. Refrain from alcohol (higher levels of ferritin occur in alcoholism).
4. Follow guidelines in Chapter 1 for safe, effective, informed *pretest* care.

Posttest Patient Care

1. Resume normal activities.
2. Review test results; report and record findings. Modify the nursing care plan as needed. Counsel the patient regarding abnormal findings; explain the need for possible follow-up testing and treatment. Monitor for iron-deficiency anemia and ferritin increases. When iron and TIBC tests are used together with ferritin, they can better distinguish between iron-deficiency anemia and the anemia of chronic disease. Treatment may include VB_{12} and folic acid.
3. Follow guidelines in Chapter 1 for safe, effective, informed *posttest* care.

● Iron Stain (Stainable Iron in Bone Marrow; Prussian Blue Stain)

In the bone marrow, normoblasts containing iron granules (stainable) are known as *sideroblasts*. Erythrocytes (RBCs) that contain stainable iron are called *siderocytes*. Normally, about 33% of the normoblasts are sideroblasts. Other storage iron is readily identifiable in monophages in bone marrow particles on the marrow slides.

The bone marrow iron stain is the gold standard of iron deficiency: The presence of iron rules out iron deficiency. Marrow iron disappears before peripheral blood changes occur in iron-deficiency anemia. Only patients with decreased marrow iron are likely to benefit from iron therapy.

Normal Findings

Bone marrow: 33% sideroblasts present
Peripheral blood: no siderocytes present

Procedure

1. Make bone marrow slides (bone marrow biopsy material can be used), stain, and examine under the microscope for the presence of iron.
2. This test may also be done on peripheral blood for the detection of sideroblastic anemias.

Clinical Implications

1. Bone marrow iron is *decreased* in:
   a. Iron deficiency from all causes of chronic bleeding, hemorrhage, malignancy
   b. Polycythemia vera
   c. Pernicious anemia (early phase of therapy)
   d. Collagen diseases (e.g., rheumatoid arthritis, SLE)
   e. Infiltration of marrow by malignant lymphomas, carcinoma
   f. Chronic infection
   g. Myeloproliferative diseases
   h. Uremia
2. Bone marrow iron is *increased* in:
   a. Hemochromatosis (primary and secondary)
   b. Anemia, especially thalassemia major and minor, PNH, and other hemolytic anemias
   c. Megaloblastic anemia in relapse
   d. Chronic infections
   e. Chronic pancreatic insufficiency

Interfering Factors

Ingestion of iron dextran will bring values to normal despite other evidence of iron-deficiency anemia.

Interventions

Pretest Patient Care

1. See Pretest Patient Care for bone marrow aspiration (page 60).
2. Follow guidelines in Chapter 1 for safe, effective, informed *pretest* care.

Posttest Patient Care

1. See Posttest Patient Care for bone marrow aspiration (page 60).
2. Follow guidelines in Chapter 1 for safe, effective, informed *posttest* care.

TESTS FOR HEMOGLOBIN DISORDERS

Hemoglobin Electrophoresis

Normal and abnormal Hb can be detected by electrophoresis, which matches hemolyzed RBC material against standard bands for the various Hb types known. The most common forms of normal adult Hb are HbA_1, HbA_2, and Hb F. Of the various types of abnormal Hb (hemoglobinopathies), the best known are Hb S (responsible for sickle cell anemia) and Hb C (results in a mild hemolytic anemia). The most common abnormality is a significant increase in HbA_2, which is diagnostic of the thalassemias, especially β-thalassemia trait. More than 350 variants of Hb have been recognized and identified.

Normal Findings

HbA_1: 96.5% to 98.5% or 0.96 to 0.985 mass fraction
HbA_2: 1.5% to 3.5% or 0.015 to 0.035 mass fraction
Hb F: 0% to 1% or 0 to 0.01 mass fraction

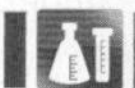
CLINICAL ALERT

The results may be questionable if a blood transfusion has been given in the months preceding testing.

Fetal Hemoglobin (Hemoglobin F; Alkali-Resistant Hemoglobin)

Hb F is a normal Hb manufactured in the RBCs of the fetus and infant; it makes up 50% to 90% of the Hb in the newborn. The remaining portion of the Hb in the newborn is made up of HbA_1 and HbA_2, the adult types.

Under normal conditions, the manufacture of Hb F is replaced by the manufacture of adult Hb types during the first year of life. But if Hb F persists and constitutes >5% of the Hb after 6 months of age, an abnormality should be expected.

Determination of Hb F is used to evaluate thalassemia (an inherited abnormality in the manufacture of Hb), hemolytic anemias, hereditary persistence of fetal Hb, and other hemoglobinopathies.

Normal Findings

Adults: 0% to 2% or 0 to 0.02 mass fraction Hb F
Newborns: 60% to 90% or 0.60 to 0.90 mass fraction Hb F
By 6 months of age: 2% or 0.02 mass fraction Hb F

Procedure

1. Use a 5-mL venous blood EDTA-anticoagulated sample for Hb electrophoresis.
2. A blood smear stain may also be done to identify cells containing Hb F (Kleihauer-Betke stain).

Clinical Implications

Increased Hb F is found in:

1. Thalassemias (major and minor)
2. Hereditary familial fetal hemoglobinemia (persistence of Hb F)
3. Hyperthyroidism
4. Sickle cell disease

5. Hb H disease
6. Anemia, as a compensatory mechanism (pernicious anemia, PNH, sideroblastic anemia)
7. Leakage of fetal blood into the maternal bloodstream
8. Aplastic anemia (acquired)
9. Juvenile myeloid leukemia with absence of Philadelphia chromosome
10. Myeloproliferative disorders, multiple myeloma, lymphoma

CLINICAL ALERT

In thalassemia minor, continued production of Hb F may occur on a minor scale (5%–10% or 0.05–0.10), and the patient usually lives. In thalassemia major, the values may reach 40%–90% or 0.40–0.90. This continued production of Hb F leads to severe anemia, and death usually ensues.

Interfering Factors

1. If analysis of the specimen is delayed for more than 2 to 3 hours, the level of Hb F may be falsely increased.
2. Infants small for gestational age or with chronic intrauterine anoxia have persistently elevated Hb F.
3. Hb F is increased during anticonvulsant drug therapy.

Interventions

Pretest Patient Care

1. Explain test purpose and procedure.
2. Ensure that the test is done before transfusion.
3. Follow guidelines in Chapter 1 for safe, effective, informed *pretest* care.

Posttest Patient Care

1. Review test results; report and record findings. Modify the nursing care plan as needed. Counsel the patient regarding abnormal findings; explain the need for possible follow-up testing and treatment. Monitor for thalassemia and anemia.
2. Follow guidelines in Chapter 1 for safe, effective, informed *posttest* care.

● Hemoglobin A_2 (HbA_2)

HbA_2 levels have special application to the diagnosis of β-thalassemia trait, which may be present even though the peripheral blood smear is normal. The microcytosis and other morphologic changes of β-thalassemia trait must be differentiated from iron deficiency. Low MCV may be present in most patients with β-thalassemia trait, but it does not differentiate iron-deficient patients.

This measurement is used in the investigation of hemolytic anemias for hemoglobinopathies, especially thalassemia and β-thalassemia.

Normal Findings

Adult: 1.5% to 3.5% or 0.015 to 0.035 mass fraction
Newborns: 0% to 1.8% or 0 to 0.018 mass fraction

Procedure

1. Draw a 5-mL venous sample of blood using a lavender-topped (EDTA) tube. Label the specimen with the patient's name, date and time of collection, and test(s) ordered.
2. Perform electrophoresis.

Clinical Implications

1. *Increased* HbA_2 occurs in:
   a. β-Thalassemia major (3% to 11%)
   b. Thalassemia minor (3.5% to 7.5%)
   c. Thalassemia intermedia (6% to 8%)
   d. Hb A/S (sickle cell trait) (15% to 45%)
   e. Hb S/S (sickle cell disease) (2% to 6%)
   f. S-β-thalassemia (3.0% to 8.5%)
   g. Megaloblastic anemia
   h. Hyperthyroidism
   i. VB_{12} or folate deficiency
2. *Decreased* HbA_2 occurs in:
   a. Untreated iron-deficiency anemia
   b. Sideroblastic anemia
   c. Hb H disease
   d. Erythroleukemia

Interfering Factors

1. Blood transfusions before electrophoresis will interfere with results.
2. High levels of Hb F usually are accompanied by low levels of A_2.
3. Hb C, Hb O and Hb E interfere with the electrophoric migration of A_2.
4. If a patient with β-thalassemia also has iron-deficiency anemia, the A_2 may be normal; therefore, retesting may be needed after iron therapy.

Interventions

Pretest Patient Care

1. Explain test purpose and procedure. Assess for signs/symptoms of anemia, abdominal enlargement, frequent infections, epistaxis, anorexia, small body, large head, and possible mental retardation.
2. Provide genetic counseling.
3. Follow guidelines in Chapter 1 for safe, effective, informed *pretest* care.

Posttest Patient Care

1. Review test results; report and record findings. Modify the nursing care plan as needed. Counsel the patient regarding abnormal findings; explain the need for possible follow-up testing and treatment.
2. Possible treatments include administering antibiotics as ordered, providing folic acid supplements, and administering blood transfusions as ordered.
3. Follow guidelines in Chapter 1 for safe, effective, informed *posttest* care.

• Hemoglobin S (Sickle Cell Test; Sickledex)

Sickle cell disease is a term for a group of hereditary blood disorders. Sickle cell anemia is caused by an abnormality of Hb, the red protein in RBCs that carries oxygen from the lungs to the tissues. People with sickle cell disease make an abnormal Hb, *hemoglobin S* (Hb S). The RBCs of a person with sickle cell disease do not last as long as normal RBCs. This result is chronic anemia. Also, these RBCs lose their normal disk shape. They become rigid and deformed and take on a sickle or crescent shape. These oddly shaped cells are not flexible enough to squeeze through small blood vessels. This may result in blood vessels being blocked. The areas of the body served by those blood vessels will then be deprived of their blood circulation, damaging tissues and organs. This homozygous state of Hb S disease is associated with considerable morbidity and mortality. The heterozygous state presents little mortality.

This blood measurement is routinely done as a screening test for sickle cell anemia or trait and to confirm these disorders. This test detects Hb S, an inherited, recessive gene. An examination is made of erythrocytes for the sickle-shaped forms characteristic of sickle cell anemia or trait. This is done by removing oxygen from the erythrocyte. In erythrocytes with normal Hb, the shape is retained, but erythrocytes containing Hb S assume a sickle shape. However, the distinction between sickle cell trait and sickle cell disease is done by electrophoresis, which identifies an Hb pattern. Screening in adult women and their partners is recommended during pre- and postnatal care and for newborns as early as 24 to 48 hours following birth.

Normal Findings

Adult: none present (i.e., negative)

Procedure

1. Obtain a venous blood sample of 5 mL in a lavender-topped tube with EDTA. Invert immediately 8 to 10 times to mix with the anticoagulant. Label the specimen with the patient's name, date and time of collection, and test(s) ordered. Place the specimen in a biohazard bag.
2. Perform the Sickledex test or Hb electrophoresis. Electrophoresis is more accurate and should be done in all positive Sickledex screens.

Clinical Implications

A *positive test* (Hb S present) means that great numbers of erythrocytes have assumed the typical sickle cell (crescent) shape. Positive tests are 99% accurate.

1. *Sickle cell trait*
   a. Definite confirmation of sickle cell trait by Hb electrophoresis reveals the following heterozygous (A/S) pattern: Hb S, 20% to 40%; HbA_1, 60% to 80%; and Hb F, small amount. This means that the patient has inherited a normal Hb gene from one parent and an Hb S gene from the other (heterozygous pattern). This patient does not have any clinical manifestations of the disease, but some of the children of this patient may inherit the disease if the patient's mate also has the recessive gene pattern.
   b. The diagnosis of sickle cell trait does not affect longevity and is not accompanied by signs and symptoms of sickle cell anemia. A/S occurs in 8.5% of African Americans.
   c. Sickle cell trait can lead to renal papillary necrosis, hematuria, increased risk for pulmonary embolus, and anterior segment ischemia.
2. *Sickle cell anemia* (Hb S disease)
   a. Definite confirmation of sickle cell anemia by Hb electrophoresis reveals the following homozygous (S/S) pattern: Hb S, 80% to 100%; Hb F, most of the rest; HbA_1, 0% (absent).
   b. This means that an abnormal Hb S gene has been inherited from both parents (homozygous pattern). Such a patient has all the clinical manifestations of the disease.
3. Hb C—Harlem (rare)
4. Hb C—Georgetown
5. Hb S in combination with other disorders, such as β-thalassemia or Hb S-C

Interfering Factors

1. False-negative results occur in:
   a. Infants younger than 3 months of age (maximal amounts reached by 6 months)
   b. Coexisting thalassemias or iron deficiency
2. False-positive results occur up to 4 months after transfusion with RBCs having sickle cell trait.
3. Hb D and Hb G migrate to the same place as Hb F in electrophoresis.
4. The solubility test is unreliable in pernicious anemia and polycythemia.

CLINICAL ALERT

A positive Sickledex test must be confirmed by electrophoresis.

Assess for sickle cell crisis: pale lips, tongue, palms, or nail beds; lethargy; listlessness; pain; and increased temperature.

Interventions

Pretest Patient Care

1. Explain test purpose and procedure. Assess for signs/symptoms of aching bones, cardiomegaly, chest pain, fatigue, murmurs, dyspnea, pallor, joint swelling, and jaundice.
2. Provide genetic counseling.
3. Follow guidelines in Chapter 1 for safe, effective, informed *pretest* care.

Posttest Patient Care

1. Review test results; report and record findings. Modify the nursing care plan as needed. Counsel the patient regarding abnormal findings; explain the need for possible follow-up testing and treatment.
2. A positive diagnosis of sickle cell disorder has genetic implications, including the need for genetic counseling.
3. A person with sickle cell disease should avoid situations in which hypoxia may occur, such as very strenuous exercise, traveling to high-altitude regions, or traveling in an unpressurized aircraft.
4. Because of the hypoxia created by general anesthetics and a state of shock, surgical and maternity patients with sickle cell disease need very close observation.
5. Possible treatments include administering vaccines (*Haemophilus influenzae* B) and analgesics as ordered.
6. Oral hydroxyurea (HU), an antineoplastic drug, was approved for the treatment of sickle cell anemia by the U.S. Food and Drug Administration in 1998. HU inhibits Hb S production and increases Hb F synthesis.
7. Follow guidelines in Chapter 1 for safe, effective, informed *posttest* care.

● Methemoglobin (Hemoglobin M)

Methemoglobin (Hb M) is formed when the iron in the heme portion of deoxygenated Hb is oxidized to a ferric form rather than a ferrous form. In the ferric form, oxygen and iron cannot combine. The formation of Hb M is a normal process and is kept within bounds by the reduction of Hb M to Hb. Hb M causes a shift to the left of the oxyhemoglobin dissociation curve. When a high concentration of Hb M is produced in the RBCs, it reduces their capacity to combine with oxygen—anoxia and cyanosis result.

This test is used to diagnose hereditary or acquired methemoglobinemia in patients with symptoms of anoxia or cyanosis and no evidence of cardiovascular or pulmonary disease. Hb M is an inherited disorder of the Hb that produces cyanosis.

Methemoglobinemia is most commonly encountered as an acquired state as a result of medications such as phenacetin, sulfonamides, or ingestion of nitrates.

Normal Findings

0.4% to 1.5% or 0.004 to 0.015 of total Hb

A value of >40% or >0.40 is a critical value.

CLINICAL ALERT

Critical Values

1. Hb M of 30% (or 0.30) results in headaches, cyanosis
2. Hb M of 70% (or 0.70) is usually fatal

Procedure

1. Obtain a 5-mL venous or arterial blood sample in a green-topped tube or lavender-topped tube anticoagulated with sodium fluoride. Label the specimen with the patient's name, date and time of collection, and test(s) ordered.
2. Place on ice immediately and transport to the laboratory in a biohazard bag. Hb M is very unstable and must be tested within 8 hours.

Clinical Implications

1. *Hereditary methemoglobinemia* (uncommon) is associated with:
   a. A hemoglobinopathy, Hb M (40% [or 0.40] of the total Hb)
   b. Deficiency of Hb M reductase (autosomal recessive)
   c. Glutathione deficiency (dominant mode of transmission)
2. *Acquired methemoglobinemia* is associated with:
   a. Black-water fever
   b. Paroxysmal hemoglobinuria
   c. Clostridial infection
3. Toxic effect of drugs or chemicals (most common cause)
   a. Analgesics, phenacetin
   b. Sulfonamide derivatives—sulfonamide S
   c. Nitrates and nitrites; nitroglycerin
   d. Antimalarials
   e. Isoniazid
   f. Quinones
   g. Potassium chloride
   h. Benzocaine, lidocaine
   i. Dapsone (most common drug causing methemoglobinemia)

Interfering Factors

1. Consumption of sausage, processed meats, or other foods rich in nitrites and nitrates
2. Absorption of silver nitrate used to treat extensive burns
3. Excessive intake of Bromo Seltzer is a common cause of methemoglobinemia. (The patient appears cyanotic but otherwise feels well.)
4. Smoking
5. Use of bismuth preparations for diarrhea (see Appendix E)

Interventions

Pretest Patient Care

1. Advise patient of purpose of test. Assess for history of Bromo Seltzer or toxic drugs or chemicals.
2. Follow guidelines in Chapter 1 for safe, effective, informed *pretest* care.

Posttest Patient Care

1. Review test results; report and record findings. Modify the nursing care plan as needed. Counsel the patient regarding abnormal findings; explain the need for possible follow-up testing and treatment. Explain the causes, signs, and symptoms of cyanosis and monitor for anoxia.
2. Treatment includes IV methylene blue and oral ascorbic acid.
3. Follow guidelines in Chapter 1 for safe, effective, informed *posttest* care.

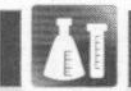

CLINICAL ALERT

Because Hb F is more easily converted to Hb M than to Hb A, infants are more susceptible than adults to methemoglobinemia, which may be caused by drinking well water containing nitrites. Bismuth preparations for diarrhea may also be reduced to nitrites by bowel action.

Sulfhemoglobin

Sulfhemoglobin is an abnormal Hb pigment produced by the combination of inorganic sulfides with Hb. Sulfhemoglobinemia manifests as a cyanosis. Sulfhemoglobinemia often accompanies drug-induced methemoglobinemia.

This test is indicated in persons with cyanosis. Sulfhemoglobinemia may occur in association with the administration of various drugs and toxins. The symptoms are few, but cyanosis is intense even though the concentration of sulfhemoglobin seldom exceeds 10%.

Normal Findings

None present or 0% to 1.0% or 0 to 0.01 of total Hb

Procedure

1. Draw a 5-mL venous blood sample using a lavender-topped (EDTA) tube. Label the specimen with the patient's name, date and time of collection, and test(s) ordered.
2. Place the specimen in a biohazard bag. Sulfhemoglobin is stable.

Clinical Implications

1. Sulfhemoglobin is observed in patients who take oxidant drugs such as phenacetin, Bromo Seltzer, sulfonamides, and acetanilid (see Appendix E).
2. Sulfhemoglobin is formed rarely without exposure to drugs or toxins, as in chronic constipation and purging.
3. Sulfhemoglobin can be due to exposure to trinitrotoluene or zinc ethylene bisdithiocarbamate (fungicide).

Interventions

Pretest Patient Care

1. Explain test purpose and procedure. Assess for exposure to drugs and toxins.
2. Follow guidelines in Chapter 1 for safe, effective, informed *pretest* care.

Posttest Patient Care

1. Review test results; report and record findings. Modify the nursing care plan as needed. Counsel the patient regarding abnormal findings; explain the need for possible follow-up testing and treatment. Explain the causes, signs, and symptoms of cyanosis and use of certain medications.

2. Sulfhemoglobin persists until the RBCs containing it are destroyed; therefore, the levels decline slowly over a period of weeks. There is no treatment.
3. Follow guidelines in Chapter 1 for safe, effective, informed *posttest* care.

● Carboxyhemoglobin; Carbon Monoxide (CO)

Carboxyhemoglobin is formed when Hb is exposed to carbon monoxide (CO). The affinity of Hb for CO is 240 times greater than for oxygen. CO poisoning causes anoxia because the carboxyhemoglobin formed does not permit Hb to combine with oxygen.

This test is done to detect CO poisoning. Because carboxyhemoglobin is not capable of transporting oxygen, hypoxia results, causing headache, nausea, vomiting, vertigo, collapse, or convulsions. Death may result from anoxia and irreversible tissue changes. Carboxyhemoglobin produces a cherry-red or violet color of the blood and skin, but this may not be present in chronic exposure. The most common causes of CO toxicity are automobile exhaust fumes, coal gas, water gas, and smoke inhalation from fires. Smoking is a minor cause.

Normal Findings

Nonsmokers: <2.0% of total Hb or <0.02 fraction of Hb saturation
Heavy smokers: 6.0% to 8.0% or 0.06 to 0.08 fraction of Hb saturation
Light smokers: 4.0% to 5.0% or 0.04 to 0.05 fraction of Hb saturation
Newborns: 10% to 12% or 0.10 to 0.12 fraction of Hb saturation

CLINICAL ALERT

1. With values of 10%–20% (0.10–0.20), the patient may be asymptomatic.
2. With 20%–30% (0.20–0.30), headache, nausea, vomiting, and loss of judgment occur.
3. With 30%–40% (0.30–0.40), tachycardia, hyperpnea, hypotension, and confusion occur.
4. With 50%–60% (0.50–0.60), there is loss of consciousness.
5. Values of >60% (>0.60) cause convulsions, respiratory arrest, and death.

Procedure

1. Obtain 5 mL of a venous blood sample using a green–topped tube (with EDTA). Label the specimen with the patient's name, date and time of collection, and test(s) ordered.
2. Keep the sample tightly capped and transport to the laboratory immediately in a biohazard bag.

Clinical Implications

1. Carboxyhemoglobin is *increased* in:
   a. CO poisoning from many sources, including smoking, exhaust fumes, fires
   b. Hemolytic disease
   c. Blood in intestines
   d. Newborns because of Hb F breakdown that yields endogenous CO
2. A direct correlation has been found between CO and symptoms of heart disease, angina, and myocardial infarction.

Interventions

Pretest Patient Care

1. Advise patient of purpose of test.
2. Draw blood sample before oxygen therapy has started.
3. Follow guidelines in Chapter 1 for safe, effective, informed *pretest* care.

Posttest Patient Care

1. Review test results; report and record findings. Modify the nursing care plan as needed. Counsel the patient regarding abnormal findings; explain the need for possible follow-up testing and treatment. Explain the causes of headache, dizziness, vomiting, convulsions, or coma.
2. Treatment consists of removal of the patient from the source of CO.
3. Initiate oxygen therapy either by supplemental oxygen at atmospheric pressure or by hyperbaric oxygen.
4. Possible treatments include administering high concentrations of O_2 under hyperbaric conditions as ordered.
5. Follow guidelines in Chapter 1 for safe, effective, informed *posttest* care.

• Myoglobin (Mb)

Myoglobin (Mb) is the oxygen-binding protein of striated muscle. It resembles Hb but is unable to release oxygen except at extremely low tension. Injury to skeletal muscle results in release of Mb. It is not specific to myocardial muscle. Mb is not tightly bound to protein and is rapidly excreted in the urine.

The Mb test is used as an early marker of muscle damage in myocardial infarction and to detect injury to or necrosis of skeletal muscle. Serum Mb is found earlier than creatine kinase (CK) enzymes in acute myocardial infarction.

Normal Findings

5 to 70 ng/mL or 5 to 70 μg/L

Procedure

1. Draw a venous blood sample of at least 5 mL (red-topped tube or SST); use serum. Lipemic or grossly hemolyzed specimens are not acceptable. Label the specimen with the patient's name, date and time of collection, and test(s) ordered.
2. Two or three samples taken 1 to 2 hours apart give optimal results in detecting myocardial infarction.

Clinical Implications

1. *Increased Mb values* are associated with:
   a. Myocardial infarction (elevates 1 to 3 hours after pain onset, earlier than CK). The amount of Mb correlates with size of infarct.
   b. Angina without infarction
   c. Other muscle injury (trauma, exercise, open heart surgery, intramuscular injections)
   d. Polymyositis and progressive muscular dystrophy
   e. Myositis
   f. Rhabdomyolysis
   g. Inflammatory myopathy (e.g., SLE)
   h. Toxin exposure: narcotics, Malayan sea snake toxin
   i. Malignant hyperthermia
   j. Renal failure
   k. Electric shock
   l. Tonic-clonic seizures
2. *Decreased Mb values* are found in:
   a. Circulating antibodies to Mb (many patients with polymyositis)
   b. Rheumatoid arthritis
   c. Myasthenia gravis

Interfering Factors

1. See Appendix E for drugs that affect test outcomes.
2. Cocaine use elevates Mb.
3. Decreased elimination due to kidney insufficiency causes increase of serum levels.

Interventions

Pretest Patient Care

1. Advise patient of test purpose.
2. Have patient avoid radioisotopes until after blood is drawn.
3. Avoid vigorous exercise before the test because it may elevate Mb.
4. Follow guidelines in Chapter 1 for safe, effective, informed *pretest* care.

Posttest Patient Care

1. Resume normal activities.
2. Review test results; report and record findings. Modify the nursing care plan as needed. Counsel the patient regarding abnormal findings; explain the need for possible follow-up testing and treatment. Monitor for myocardial infarction, muscle inflammation, and metabolic stress.
3. Follow guidelines in Chapter 1 for safe, effective, informed *posttest* care.

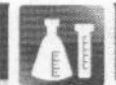

CLINICAL ALERT

Mb is the earliest biologic marker of myocardial necrosis. It appears in the peripheral blood 2–3 hr after pain onset and reaches peak levels at 6–9 hr. Mb is a sensitive indicator of acute myocardial infarction but is not specific for cardiac muscle.

● Haptoglobin (Hp)

Haptoglobin (Hp) is a transport glycoprotein synthesized solely in the liver. It is a carrier for free Hb in plasma; its primary physiologic function is the preservation of iron. Hp binds Hb and carries it to the reticuloendothelial system.

A decrease in Hp (with normal liver function) is most likely to occur with increased consumption of Hp due to intravascular hemolysis. The concentration of Hp is inversely related to the degree of hemolysis and to the duration of the hemolytic episode.

Normal Findings

Newborns: 5 to 48 mg/dL or 50 to 480 mg/L (may be absent at birth)
Children: reach adult levels by 1 year
Adults: 40 to 200 mg/dL or 0.4 to 2.0 g/L

Procedure

1. Obtain a venous blood sample of at least 2 mL (red-topped tube or SST). Label the specimen with the patient's name, date and time of collection, and test(s) ordered. Place the specimen in a biohazard bag.
2. Measure the serum for Hp by a radial immunodiffusion method. A single determination is of limited value.

Clinical Implications

1. *Hp is decreased in acquired disorders* such as:
   a. Intravascular hemolysis from any cause
   b. Autoimmune hemolytic anemia

   c. Other hemoglobinemias caused by intravascular hemorrhages, especially artificial heart valves, and acute bacterial endocarditis
   d. Transfusion reactions
   e. Erythroblastosis fetalis
   f. Malarial infestation
   g. PNH
   h. Hematoma, tissue hemorrhage
   i. Thrombotic thrombocytopenic purpura
   j. Drug-induced hemolytic anemia (methyldopa)
   k. Acute or chronic liver disease
2. *Hp is decreased in some inherited disorders* such as:
   a. Sickle cell disease
   b. G6PD and PK deficiency
   c. Hereditary spherocytosis
   d. Thalassemia and megaloblastic anemias
   e. Congenital absence is observed in 1% of African American and Asian populations
3. *Hp is increased* in:
   a. Infection and inflammation (acute or chronic)
   b. Neoplasias, lymphomas (advanced)
   c. Biliary obstruction
   d. Acute rheumatic disease and other collagen diseases
   e. Tissue destruction

Interfering Factors

1. Estrogen and oral contraceptives lower Hp.
2. Steroid therapy raises Hp.
3. Androgens increase Hp.
4. Regular strenuous exercise lowers Hp.

CLINICAL ALERT

Normal Hp results measured during inflammatory episodes or during steroid treatment do not rule out hemolysis.

Interventions

Pretest Patient Care

1. Advise patient of test purpose.
2. Avoid use of oral contraceptives and androgens before blood is drawn. (Check with the healthcare provider.)
3. Avoid exercise before test.
4. Follow guidelines in Chapter 1 for safe, effective, informed *pretest* care.

Posttest Patient Care

1. Resume normal activities and medications.
2. Review test results; report and record findings. Modify the nursing care plan as needed. Counsel the patient regarding abnormal findings; explain the need for possible follow-up testing and treatment. Monitor for abnormal bleeding.
3. Follow guidelines in Chapter 1 for safe, effective, informed *posttest* care.

Bart's Hemoglobin

Bart's Hb is an unstable Hb with high oxygen affinity. When there is complete absence of production of the chain of Hb and deletion of all four globin genes, the disorder is known as *Bart's hydrops fetalis*. Both parents of the affected infant have heterozygous thalassemia; they are almost all Southeast Asians. Affected infants are either stillborn or die shortly after birth.

This test determines the percentage of the abnormal Bart's Hb in cord blood and identifies α-thalassemia hemoglobinopathies.

Normal Findings

Adults: none
Children: none
Newborns: <0.5% or <0.005 mass fraction of total Hb

Procedure

1. Obtain a sample of cord blood and perform Hb electrophoresis.
2. Venous blood anticoagulated with EDTA or heparin can be used.

Clinical Implications

Increased levels are associated with:

1. Homozygous α-thalassemia (hydrops fetalis syndrome, which causes stillbirth)
2. Hb H disease
3. α-Thalassemia minor

Interventions

Pretest Patient Care

1. Explain test purpose and procedure to parents.
2. Obstetric complications may lead to significant morbidity and mortality for the mothers of these infants.
3. Provide genetic counseling in a sensitive manner.
4. Follow guidelines in Chapter 1 for safe, effective, informed *pretest* care.

Posttest Patient Care

1. Review test results and counsel the patient's parents or legal guardians regarding abnormal findings; explain the need for possible follow-up testing and treatment.
2. Follow guidelines in Chapter 1 for safe, effective, informed *posttest* care.

Paroxysmal Nocturnal Hemoglobinuria (PNH) Test; Acid Hemolysis Test; Ham's Test

PNH was first described by a patient who noted hemoglobinuria after sleep. In many patients, the hemolysis is irregular or occult. PNH is a hemolytic anemia in which there is also production of defective platelets and granulocytes. The diagnostic feature of PNH is an increased sensitivity of the erythrocytes to complement-mediated lysis. Although patients with PNH can present with hemoglobinuria or a hemolytic anemia, they may also present with iron deficiency (because of urinary loss of blood), bleeding secondary to thrombocytopenia, thrombosis, renal abnormalities, or neurologic abnormalities.

These tests are carried out to make a definitive diagnosis of PNH. The basis of these tests is that the cells peculiar to PNH have membrane defects, making them extra sensitive to complement in the plasma. Cells from patients with PNH undergo marked hemolysis after 15 minutes in the laboratory test. The tests are performed for patients who have hemoglobinuria, bone marrow aplasia (hypoplasia), or undiagnosed hemolytic anemia; they may be useful in the evaluation of patients with unexplained thrombosis or acute leukemia.

Normal Findings

Negative or <1% hemolysis

Procedure

1. Obtain a venous blood sample of 5 mL anticoagulated with EDTA. Label the specimen with the patient's name, date and time of collection, and test(s) ordered. Place the specimen in a biohazard bag.
2. Mix the patient's RBCs with normal serum and also with the patient's own serum, acidify, incubate at 37°C, and examine for hemolysis. Normally, there should be no lysis of the RBCs in this test (also called *Ham's test*).
3. Be aware that a separate test called the *sugar water test* or *sucrose hemolysis test* may also be done at this time.

Clinical Implications

A *positive test* (hemolysis) is found in:

1. PNH: a positive test (10% to 50% lysis) is needed for diagnosis. The sucrose hemolysis test is also positive in PNH.
2. Hereditary erythroblastic multinuclearity associated with a positive acidified serum test (HEMPAS): The sucrose hemolysis test is negative.

Interfering Factors

1. False-positive results may be obtained with the following:
   a. Blood containing large numbers of spherocytes (hereditary or acquired)
   b. Dyserythropoietic anemia
   c. Specimen >8 hours old, specimen hemolyzed
   d. Aplastic anemia
   e. Leukemia and myeloproliferative syndromes
2. These conditions can be distinguished from PNH by the fact that hemolysis occurs in both acidified serum and complement. In PNH, hemolysis occurs only in complement (complement dependent).

Interventions

Pretest Patient Care

1. Explain test purpose.
2. Follow guidelines in Chapter 1 for safe, effective, informed *pretest* care.

Posttest Patient Care

1. Review test results; report and record findings. Modify the nursing care plan as needed. Counsel the patient regarding abnormal findings; explain the need for possible follow-up testing and treatment. Monitor for anemia.
2. Follow guidelines in Chapter 1 for safe, effective, informed *posttest* care.

TESTS OF HEMOSTASIS AND COAGULATION

The prime function of the coagulation mechanism is to protect the integrity of the blood vessels while maintaining the fluid state of blood. Serious medical problems or even death may occur with the inability to stem the loss of blood or with the inability for a normal clot to form.

Hemostasis and coagulation tests are generally done for patients with bleeding disorders, vascular injury or trauma, or coagulopathies. Reflex vasoconstriction is the normal response to vascular insult once the first-line defenses (skin and tissue) are breached. In larger vessels, vasoconstriction may be the primary mechanism for hemostasis. With smaller vessels, vasoconstriction reduces the size of the area that must be occluded by the hemostatic plug. Part of this cascade of sequential clotting events relates to the fact that platelets adhere to the injured and exposed subendothelial tissues. This phenomenon initiates the complex clotting mechanism whereby thrombin and fibrin are formed and deposited to aid in intravascular clotting (Table 2.7).

The entire mechanism of coagulation and fibrinolysis (removal of fibrin clot) is one of balance. It may best be understood by referring to Figures 2.2 (page 150) and 2.3 (page 153). Abnormal bleeding does not always indicate coagulopathy in much the same way that lack of bleeding does not necessarily indicate absence of a bleeding disorder.

The most common causes of hemorrhage are thrombocytopenia (platelet deficiency) and other acquired coagulation disorders, including liver disease, uremia, disseminated intravascular coagulation (DIC), and anticoagulant administration. Together, they account for most hemorrhagic problems. Hemophilia and other inherited factor deficiencies are seen less frequently. Bleeding tendencies are associated with delays in clot formation or premature clot lysis. Thrombosis is associated with inappropriate clot activation or localization of the blood coagulation process. Finally, clotting disorders are divided into two classes: those caused by impaired coagulation and those caused by hypercoagulability.

TABLE 2.7 The Complex Chain of Coagulation Reactions

A balance normally exists between the factors that stimulate formation of thrombin and forces acting to delay thrombin formation. This balance maintains circulating blood as a fluid. When injury occurs or blood is removed from a vessel, this balance is upset, and coagulation occurs. Blood clotting involves four progressive stages. The Roman numerals assigned to the coagulation factors identify their order of discovery rather than their involvement in the stages of clot formation.

Stage	Components of Stages
Stage I (3–5 min)	
Phase I—platelet activity; platelets serve as a source of thromboplastin.	90% of all coagulation disorders are caused by defects in phase I.
Phase II—thromboplastin; factor III, an enzyme thought to be liberated by damaged cells, is formed by five different factors plus calcium.	Calcium Factor V Factor VIII Factor IX Factor X Factor XI } are involved in the formation of tissue thromboplastin (intrinsic prothrombin activation)
Stage II (8–15 s)	
Prothrombin factor II is converted to thrombin in the presence of calcium.	Factor II Factor X Factor VII Factor V } are involved in the conversion of fibrinogen to fibrin
Stage III (1 s)	
Thrombin interacts with fibrinogen (factor I) to form the framework of the clot.	At the end of stage III, factor XIII functions in the stabilization of the clot.
Stage IV	
Fibrinolytic system (antagonistic check-and-balance to the clotting mechanism) is activated.	Removal of fibrin clot through fibrinolysis. Plasminogen is converted to plasmin, which breaks clot into fibrin split products.

Hypercoagulability States

Two general forms of hypercoagulability exist: hyperreactivity of the platelet system, which results in arterial thrombosis, and accelerated activity of the clotting system, which results in venous thrombosis. Hypercoagulability refers to an unnatural tendency toward thrombosis. The thrombus is the actual insoluble mass (fibrin or platelets) present in the bloodstream or chambers of the heart.

Conditions and classifications associated with hypercoagulability include the following:

Platelet Abnormalities. These conditions are associated with arteriosclerosis, diabetes mellitus, increased blood lipids or cholesterol levels, increased platelet levels, and smoking. Arterial thrombosis may be related to blood flow disturbances, vessel wall changes, and increased platelet sensitivity to factors causing platelet adherence and aggregation.

Clotting System Abnormalities. These are associated with congestive heart failure, immobility, artificial surfaces (e.g., artificial heart valves), damaged vasculature, use of oral contraceptives or estrogen, pregnancy and the postpartum state, and the postsurgical state. Other influences include malignancy, myeloproliferative (bone marrow) disorders, obesity, lupus disorders, and genetic predisposition.

Venous Thrombosis. This can be related to stasis of blood flow, to coagulation alterations, or to increases in procoagulation factors or decreases in anticoagulation factors (Table 2.8).

Disorders of Hemostasis

Congenital Vascular Abnormalities (Vessel Wall Structure Defects). Defects of the actual blood vessel are poorly defined and difficult to test. Hereditary telangiectasia is the most commonly recognized vascular abnormality. Laboratory studies are normal, so the diagnosis must be made from clinical signs and symptoms. Patients frequently report epistaxis and symptoms of anemia. Another abnormality is congenital hemangiomas (Kasabach-Merritt syndrome).

Acquired Abnormalities of the Vessel Wall Structure. Causes include Henoch-Schönlein purpura as an allergic response to infection or drugs, diabetes mellitus, rickettsial diseases, septicemia, and amyloidosis present with some degree of vascular abnormalities. Purpura can also be associated with steroid therapy and easy bruising in females (infectious purpura), or it can be a result of drug use.

Hereditary Connective Tissue Disorders. These include Ehlers-Danlos syndrome (hyperplastic skin and hyperflexible joints) and pseudoxanthoma elasticum (rare connective tissue disorder).

Acquired Connective Tissue Defects. These can be caused by scurvy (vitamin C deficiency) or senile purpura.

Qualitative Platelet Abnormalities. These disorders can be divided into subclasses:

1. *Thrombocytopenia* (platelet count $<150 \times 10^3/mm^3$) is caused by decreased production of platelets, increased use or destruction of platelets, or hypersplenism. Contributing factors include bone marrow disease, autoimmune diseases, DIC, bacterial or viral infection, chemotherapy, radiation therapy, multiple transfusions, and certain drugs (e.g., NSAIDs, thiazides, estrogens).
2. *Thrombocytosis* (elevated platelet count) is caused by hemorrhage, iron-deficiency anemia, inflammation, or splenectomy.
3. *Thrombocythemia* (platelet count $>1000 \times 10^3/mm^3$ or $>1000 \times 10^9/L$) is caused by granulocytic leukemia, polycythemia vera, or myeloid metaplasia.

Quantitative Platelet Abnormalities. These are associated with Glanzmann's thrombasthenia, a hereditary autosomal-recessive disorder that can produce severe bleeding, especially with trauma and surgical procedures. Platelet factor 3 differences associated with aggregation, adhesion, or release defects may be manifested in storage pool disease, May-Hegglin anomaly, Bernard-Soulier syndrome (autosomal recessive coagulopathy), and Wiskott-Aldrich syndrome. Dialysis and use of drugs such as aspirin, other anti-inflammatory agents, dipyridamole, and prostaglandin E also can be tied to platelet abnormalities.

TABLE 2.8 Proteins Involved in Blood Coagulation

Protein[a]	Synonym	Plasma Concentration (mg/dL)	Function
Fibrinogen	Factor I	200–400	Is converted to fibrin along with platelets to form clot
Factor II	Prothrombin (prethrombin)	10–15	Is converted to thrombin (IIa), which splits fibrinogen into fibrin
Factor V	Proaccelerin; labile factor	0.5–1.0	Supports Xa activation of II to IIa
Factor VII	Stable factor; proconvertin	0.2	Activates X
Factor VIII:C	Antihemophilic factor (AHF); platelet; cofactor I	1.0–2.0	Supports IXa activation of X
Factor IX	Christmas factor; plasma thromboplastin component (PTC)	0.3–0.4	Activates X
Factor X	Stuart-Prower factor (AVTD prothrombin III)	0.6–0.8	Activates II
Factor XI	Plasma thromboplastin antecedent (antihemophilic factor C)	0.4	Activates XII and prekallikrein
Factor XII	Hageman factor	2.9	Activates XI and prekallikrein
Factor XIII	Fibrin-stabilizing factor; Laki-Lorand factor	2.5	Cross-links fibrin and other proteins
von Willebrand's factor	Factor VIII–related antigen VIII:VWD	1.0	Stabilizes VIII, mediates platelet adhesion
Prekallikrein	Fletcher factor	5.0	Activates XII and prekallikrein, cleaves HMWK
High-molecular-weight kininogen (HMWK)	Fitzgerald factor	4.7–12.2	Supports reciprocal activation of XII, XI, and prekallikrein
Fibronectin	Cold insoluble globulin	20–40	Mediates cell adhesion
Major antithrombin	Antithrombin III	20–40	Inhibits IIa, Xa, XIa, XIIa, and kallikrein
Protein C		0.5	Complexed with protein S, inactivates V and VIII
Plasminogen		20	Forms plasmin, which lyses the fibrin clot and inhibits other factors
α_2-Antiplasmin		9.6–13.5	Inhibits plasmin
α_1-Antitrypsin		245–335	Weak inhibitor of thrombin, potent inhibitor of XIa
Tissue plasminogen			Activates plasminogen
Plasminogen activator inhibitor I			Inactivates tissue plasminogen activator (tPA)
Plasminogen activator inhibitor II			Inactivates urokinase

[a]The clotting factors of the blood are proteins; they are present in the blood plasma in an inactive form called *zymogens*.

Congenital Coagulation Abnormalities. These include hemophilia A and B (deficiencies of factors VIII and IX, respectively), rare autosomal recessive traits (hemophilia C), and autosomal dominant traits (e.g., von Willebrand's disease).

Acquired Coagulation Abnormalities. These are associated with several disease states and are much more common than inherited deficiencies.

1. Circulatory anticoagulant activity may be evident in the presence of antifactor VIII, rheumatoid arthritis, immediate postpartum period, SLE, or multiple myeloma.
2. Vitamin D deficiency may be caused by oral anticoagulants, biliary obstruction and malabsorption syndrome, or intestinal sterilization by antibiotic therapy. Newborns are prone to vitamin D deficiency.
3. DIC causes continuous production of thrombin, which, in turn, consumes the other clotting factors and results in uncontrolled bleeding.
4. Primary fibrinolysis is the situation whereby isolated activation of the fibrinolytic mechanism occurs without prior coagulation activity, as in streptokinase therapy, severe liver disease, prostate cancer, or, more rarely, electroshock.
5. Most coagulation factors are manufactured in the liver. Consequently, in liver disease, the extent of coagulation abnormalities is directly proportional to the severity of the liver disease.

CLINICAL ALERT

An increased platelet count predisposes the patient to arterial thrombosis. Paradoxically, a substantially elevated platelet count can also cause easy bleeding after dental surgery, gastrointestinal bleeding, and epistaxis. When the platelet count is substantially decreased, bleeding can occur in the nose, gastrointestinal tract, skin, and gums.

Tests for Disseminated Intravascular Coagulation (DIC)

DIC is an acquired hemorrhagic syndrome characterized by uncontrolled formation and deposition of fibrin thrombi. Continuous generation of thrombin causes depletion (consumption) of the coagulation factors and results in uncontrolled bleeding. Also, fibrinolysis is activated in DIC. This further adds to the hemostasis defect caused by the consumption of clotting factors. The many coagulation test abnormalities found in acute DIC include the following:

1. Prolonged
   a. PT
   b. PTT or activated partial thromboplastin time (aPTT)
   c. Bleeding time
   d. Thrombin time (TT)
2. Decreased
   a. Fibrinogen
   b. Platelet count
   c. Clotting factors II, V, VIII, and X
   d. Antithrombin III (AT-III)
3. Increased
   a. Fibrinolysin test
   b. Fibrinopeptide A
4. Positive
   a. Fibrin split products
   b. D-Dimer

In chronic DIC, the results are variable, especially the PT, PTT, TT, and fibrinogen, making the diagnosis much more difficult. No single test or group of tests is diagnostic, and diagnosis usually depends on a combination of findings. Normal levels do not rule out DIC, and a repeat profile should be done a few hours later to look for changes in platelet count and fibrinogen.

Causes of DIC include septicemia, malignancies and cancer, obstetric emergencies, cirrhosis of the liver, sickle cell disease, trauma or crushing injuries, malaria, incompatible blood transfusion, cold hemoglobinuria or PNH, connective tissue diseases, snake bites, and brown recluse spider bites.

Paradoxically, the treatment of uncontrolled bleeding in DIC is heparin administration. The heparin blocks thrombin formation, which blocks consumption of the other clotting factors and allows hemostasis to occur.

Laboratory Investigation of Hemostasis

Usually, a blood sample of at least 20 mL is obtained by the two-tube technique. In the first tube, a 5-mL blood sample is obtained and discarded. Then, 15 to 20 mL of blood is drawn into Vacutainer tubes with sodium citrate as the anticoagulant. A butterfly needle may be used to prevent backflow or to make sampling easier in the case of a difficult draw. Coagulation studies (*coagulation profiles, coag panels, coagulograms*) are used for screening or as diagnostic tools for evaluation of symptoms such as easy or spontaneous bruising, petechiae, prolonged bleeding (e.g., from cuts), abnormal nosebleeds, heavy menstrual flow, family history of coagulopathies, or gastrointestinal bleeding (Table 2.9).

Many of the more common screening tests are automated and easily done. Platelet counts are included in the automated CBC. PT and PTT can be done on photo-optical instruments that sense the change in optical density when a clot forms. Tests for fibrinogen are on instruments that detect fibrin strands. Many patients can undergo testing at the same time with the help of automation. Some of the more specialized tests still must be done manually or using semiautomated methods.

1. These five primary screening tests are initially performed to diagnose suspected coagulation disorders:
   a. Platelet count, size, and shape
   b. Bleeding time—reflects data about the ability of platelets to function normally and the ability of the capillaries to constrict their walls
   c. PTT—determines the overall ability of the blood to clot
   d. PT—measures the function of second-stage clotting factors
   e. Fibrinogen level
2. Factor assays are definitive coagulation studies of a specific clotting factor (e.g., factor VIII for hemophilia). These are done if the screening test indicates a problem with a specific factor or factors.
3. Fibrinolysis is used to address problems of the fibrinolytic system and includes the following studies:
   a. Euglobulin clot lysis—identifies increased plasminogen activator activity. (Plasmin is *not* usually present in the blood plasma.)
   b. Factor XIII (fibrin-stabilizing factor)
   c. Fibrin split products (e.g., protamine sulfate test)
4. The investigation of hypercoagulable status (thrombotic tendency, thromboembolic disorders) covers both primary causes (deficiencies of AT-III, protein C, protein S, and factor XII; fibrinolytic mechanisms) and secondary causes (acquired platelet disorders and acquired diseases of coagulation and fibrinolytic impairment) and includes the following tests:
   a. PT
   b. PTT
   c. Fibrinogen test
   d. Antiplatelet factors (e.g., prostacyclin)
   e. Anticoagulant factors (e.g., AT-III, protein C, protein S, lupus anticoagulant)
   f. Fibrinolysis tests (e.g., fibrin degradation products [FDPs], euglobulin lysis time, fibrin monomers)
   g. TT

TABLE 2.9 Laboratory Tests to Measure Hemostasis[a]

Name of Test	Vascular Function	Platelet Function	Stage I	Stage II	Stage III	Stage IV
Bleeding time	X	X				
Platelet count		X				
Platelet adhesiveness		X				
Platelet aggregation		X				
Aspirin tolerance	X					
Platelet factor III assay		X				
Activated clotting	X	X	X	X		
Activated recalcification time			X	X		
Activated partial thromboplastin			X	X		
Prothrombin time			X			
Stypven[b] time				X		
Circulating anticoagulant factor			X	X	X	
Factor assay			X	X	X	
Thrombin time				X	X	X
Reptilase time				X		
Fibrinogen assay					X	
Factor XIII assay			X			
Euglobulin lysis time						X
Thrombin time—diluted				X	X	
Plasminogen assay						X
Protamine sulfate (ethanol gelation)					X	X
D-Dimer					X	
Fibrin monomer						X
Fibrinopeptide A					X	
Latex agglutination for fibrin split products						X

[a]These tests measure all facets of hemostasis: vascular function, platelets, and clotting factors.

[b]Activates factor X.

NOTE *The lupus inhibitor (lupus anticoagulant) is an antibody (against the phospholipid used in the PT and PTT tests) that is responsible for inhibition of the PT, PTT, Russell viper venom time (dRVVT), and kaolin clotting time (kCT). To demonstrate its presence, 1 mL of the patient's plasma is mixed with 1 mL of normal plasma, and a PTT test of the mixture is done. When an inhibitor of any sort is present, the PTT will not return to normal range. An inhibitor of the lupus type can be shown by correcting the PTT through use of platelets as a phospholipid source or by demonstrating a characteristic pattern in the PTT that results from sequential dilution of the phospholipid reagent. Lupus anticoagulants may be associated with false-positive Venereal Disease Research Laboratory (VDRL) test reports and with another antiphospholipid—the anticardiolipin antibody (β_2-glycoprotein I).*

CLINICAL ALERT

Conditions associated with the presence of the lupus anticoagulant include:

1. SLE (one fifth of patients)
2. Multiple myeloma
3. Other autoimmune diseases (rheumatoid arthritis, Raynaud's syndrome)
4. Spontaneous abortions (associated with presence of anticardiolipin autoantibody) and postpartum complications
5. Lupus anticoagulant is more often associated with thromboembolism than with bleeding problems.
6. Most lupus anticoagulant antibodies are directed against prothrombin or β_2-glycoprotein I.

CLINICAL ALERT

1. All patients with hemorrhagic or thrombotic tendencies, or undergoing coagulation studies, should be observed closely for possible bleeding emergencies. A comprehensive history and physical examination should be done.
2. Blood samples for coagulation studies should be drawn last if other blood studies are indicated.

PROCEDURAL ALERT

When a blood sample is obtained for PT, PTT, and TT, sodium citrate is used as the anticoagulant in the sampling tubes.

Patient Assessment for Bleeding Tendency

1. Examine all skin for bruising.
2. Record petechiae associated with use of blood pressure cuffs or tourniquets.
3. Note bleeding from the nose or gums with no apparent cause.
4. Estimate blood quantity in vomitus, expectorated mucus, urine, stools, and menstrual flow.
5. Note prolonged bleeding from injection sites.
6. Watch for symptoms, especially changes in levels of consciousness or neurologic checks that may signal an intracranial bleed.
7. Determine whether the patient is taking anticoagulants or aspirin.

Bleeding Time (Ivy Method; Template Bleeding Time)

Bleeding time measures the primary phase of hemostasis: the interaction of the platelet with the blood vessel wall and the formation of a hemostatic plug. Bleeding time is the best single screening test for platelet function disorders and is one of the primary screening tests for coagulation disorders.

This test is of value in detecting vascular abnormalities and platelet abnormalities or deficiencies. It is not recommended for routine presurgical workup.

A small stab wound is made in either the earlobe or the forearm; the bleeding time (the amount of time it takes to form a clot) is recorded. The duration of bleeding from a punctured capillary depends on the quantity and quality of platelets and the ability of the blood vessel wall to constrict.

The principal use of this test today is in the diagnosis of von Willebrand's disease, an inherited defective molecule of factor VIII and a type of pseudohemophilia. It has been established that aspirin may cause abnormal bleeding in some normal persons, but the bleeding time test has not proved consistently valuable in identifying such persons.

Normal Findings

3 to 10 minutes in most laboratories
Duke method (earlobe): 5 minutes (not recommended—not very reproducible with a wide range of normal values)
Ivy method (forearm with template): 25 to 90 minutes
Mielke's method (Surgicut):
Adults: 1 to 7 minutes
Teens: 3.0 to 8 minutes
Children: 2.5 to 13 minutes

CLINICAL ALERT

1. The critical value for bleeding time is >15 min.
2. If the puncture site is still bleeding after 15 min, discontinue the test and apply pressure to the site. Document and report the results to the healthcare provider.
3. Patients on heparin or Lovenox have a risk of heparin-induced thrombocytopenia with thrombosis syndrome (HITTS). Tests to diagnosis HITTS include IgG immune-mediated decrease and platelet count decrease. Stop heparin immediately when platelet count falls by 50%.

Procedure (Ivy Method)

1. Cleanse the area three finger-widths below the antecubital space with alcohol and allow to dry.
2. Place a blood pressure cuff on the arm above the elbow and inflate to 40 mm Hg.
3. Select a cleansed area of the forearm without superficial veins. Stretch the skin laterally and tautly between the thumb and forefinger.
4. Start a stopwatch. Use the edge of a 4- × 4-inch filter paper to blot the blood through capillary action by gently touching the drop every 30 seconds. Do not disturb the wound itself. Remove the blood pressure gauge when bleeding stops and a clot has formed. Apply a sterile dressing when the test is completed.
5. The end point (by the Ivy or the earlobe method) is reached when blood is no longer blotted from the forearm puncture. Report in minutes and half minutes (e.g., 5 minutes, 30 seconds).

Clinical Implications

1. Bleeding time is *prolonged* when the level of platelets is decreased or when platelets are qualitatively abnormal:
   a. Thrombocytopenia (platelet count <80 × 10^3/mm^3)
   b. Platelet dysfunction syndromes
   c. Decrease or abnormality in plasma factors (e.g., von Willebrand's factor, fibrinogen)
   d. Abnormalities in the walls of the small blood vessels, vascular disease
   e. Advanced renal failure
   f. Severe liver disease
   g. Leukemia, other myeloproliferative diseases
   h. Scurvy
   i. DIC disease (owing to the presence of FDPs)
2. In von Willebrand's disease, bleeding time can be variable; it will definitely be prolonged if aspirin is taken before testing (aspirin tolerance test).
3. A single prolonged bleeding time does not prove the existence of hemorrhagic disease. Because a larger vessel can be punctured, the puncture should be repeated on an alternate body site, and the two values obtained should be averaged.
4. Bleeding time is normal in the presence of coagulation disorders other than platelet dysfunction, vascular disease, or von Willebrand's disease.
5. Aspirin therapy (antiplatelet function therapy): when thrombus formation is thought to be mediated by platelet activation, the patient frequently is given agents to interrupt normal platelet function, which may be monitored by bleeding times or platelet aggregation studies. Aspirin is the most commonly used inhibitor; it inhibits platelet adhesion or "stickiness."

Interfering Factors

1. Normal values for bleeding time vary when the puncture site is not of uniform depth and width.
2. Touching the puncture site during this test will break off fibrin particles and prolong the bleeding time.
3. Excessive alcohol consumption (as in alcoholic patients) may cause increased bleeding time.
4. Prolonged bleeding time can reflect ingestion of 10 g of aspirin as long as 5 days before the test.
5. Other drugs that may cause increased bleeding times include dextran, streptokinase-streptodornase (fibrinolytic agents), mithramycin, and pantothenyl alcohol (see Appendix E).
6. Extreme hot or cold conditions can alter the results.
7. Edema of patient's hands or cyanotic hands will invalidate the test.

Interventions

Pretest Patient Care

1. Explain test purpose and procedure. (See Patient Assessment for Bleeding Tendency on page 145.)
2. Instruct patient to abstain from aspirin and aspirin-like drugs for at least 7 days before the test.
3. Advise the patient to abstain from alcohol before the test.
4. Inform the patient that scar tissue may form at the puncture site (keloid formation).
5. If the patient has an infectious skin disease, postpone the test.
6. Follow guidelines in Chapter 1 for safe, effective, informed *pretest* care.

Posttest Patient Care

1. Review test results; report and record findings. Modify the nursing care plan as needed. Counsel the patient regarding abnormal findings; explain the need for possible follow-up testing and treatment. Monitor for prolonged bleeding. (See Patient Assessment for Bleeding Tendency on page 145.)
2. Follow guidelines in Chapter 1 for safe, effective, informed *posttest* care.

CLINICAL ALERT

Critical Values

1. A decrease in platelets to $<20 \times 10^3/mm^3$ or $<20 \times 10^9/L$ is associated with a tendency for spontaneous bleeding, prolonged bleeding time, petechiae, and ecchymosis.
2. Platelet counts $>50 \times 10^3/mm^3$ or $>50 \times 10^9/L$ are not generally associated with spontaneous bleeding.

Platelet Count; Mean Platelet Volume (MPV)

Platelets (thrombocytes) are the smallest of the formed elements in the blood. These cells are nonnucleated, round or oval, flattened, disk-shaped structures. Platelet activity is necessary for blood clotting, vascular integrity and vasoconstriction, and the adhesion and aggregation activity that occurs during the formation of platelet plugs that occlude (plug) breaks in small vessels. Thrombocyte development takes place primarily in the bone marrow. The life span of a platelet is about 7.5 days. Normally, two thirds of all the body platelets are found in the circulating blood and one third in the spleen.

The platelet count is of value for assessing bleeding disorders that occur with thrombocytopenia, uremia, liver disease, or malignancies and for monitoring the course of disease associated with bone marrow failure. This test is indicated when the estimated platelet count (on a blood smear) appears abnormal. It is also part of a coagulation profile or workup.

The MPV is sometimes ordered in conjunction with a platelet count. The MPV indicates the uniformity of size of the platelet population. It is used for the differential diagnosis of thrombocytopenia.

Normal Findings

Platelet count:
Adults: 140 to 400 $\times 10^3/mm^3$ or 140 to 400 $\times 10^9/L$
Children: 150 to 450 $\times 10^3/mm^3$ or 150 to 450 $\times 10^9/L$

Mean platelet volume:
Adults: 7.4 to 10.4 μm^3 or fL
Children: 7.4 to 10.4 μm^3 or fL

Procedure

1. Obtain a 7-mL venous whole blood sample in a lavender-topped tube (with EDTA). Label the specimen with the patient's name, date and time of collection, and test(s) ordered.
2. Count the platelets by phase microscopy or by an automated counting instrument. The MPV is also calculated by many instruments at the time of the platelet count.
3. Make a blood smear and note the size, shape, and clumping of the platelets.
4. Place the specimen in a biohazard bag.

Clinical Implications

1. *Abnormally increased numbers* of platelets (thrombocythemia, thrombocytosis) occur in:
   a. Essential thrombocythemia
   b. Chronic myelogenous and granulocytic leukemia, myeloproliferative diseases
   c. Polycythemia vera and primary thrombocytosis
   d. Splenectomy
   e. Iron-deficiency anemia

   f. Asphyxiation
   g. Rheumatoid arthritis and other collagen diseases, SLE
   h. Rapid blood regeneration caused by acute blood loss, hemolytic anemia
   i. Acute infections, inflammatory diseases
   j. Hodgkin's disease, lymphomas, malignancies
   k. Chronic pancreatitis, tuberculosis, inflammatory bowel disease
   l. Renal failure
   m. Recovery from bone marrow suppression (thrombocytopenia)
2. *Abnormally decreased numbers* of platelets (thrombocytopenia) occur in:
   a. Idiopathic thrombocytopenic purpura, neonatal purpura
   b. Pernicious, aplastic, and hemolytic anemias
   c. Massive blood transfusion (dilution effect)
   d. Viral, bacterial, and rickettsial infections
   e. Congestive heart failure, congenital heart disease
   f. Thrombopoietin deficiency
   g. During cancer chemotherapy and radiation, exposure to dichlorodiphenyl-trichloroethane (DDT) and other chemicals
   h. HIV infection
   i. Lesions involving the bone marrow (e.g., leukemias, carcinomas, myelofibrosis)
   j. DIC and thrombotic thrombocytopenic purpura
   k. Inherited syndromes such as Bernard-Soulier syndrome (autosomal recessive coagulopathy), May-Hegglin anomaly, Wiskott-Aldrich syndrome, Fanconi's syndrome
   l. Toxemia of pregnancy, eclampsia
   m. Alcohol toxicity, ethanol abuse
   n. Hypersplenism
   o. Renal insufficiency
   p. Antiplatelet antibodies
3. *Increased MPV* is observed in:
   a. Idiopathic thrombocytopenic purpura (autoimmune)
   b. Thrombocytopenia caused by sepsis
   c. Prosthetic heart valve
   d. Massive hemorrhage
   e. Myeloproliferative disorders
   f. Acute and CML
   g. Splenectomy
   h. Vasculitis
   i. Megaloblastic anemia
4. *Decreased MPV* occurs in Wiskott-Aldrich syndrome.

CLINICAL ALERT

1. In 50% of patients who exhibit unexpected platelet increases, a malignancy is found.
2. In patients with an extremely elevated platelet count (>1000 × 10^3/mm^3 or >1000 × 109/L) as a result of a myeloproliferative disorder, assess for bleeding caused by abnormal platelet function.

NOTE *Many drugs have toxic effects. The dosage does not have to be high to be toxic. Toxic thrombocytopenia depends on the inability of the body to metabolize and secrete the toxic substance.*

Interfering Factors

1. Platelet counts normally increase at high altitudes; after strenuous exercise, trauma, or excitement; and in winter.
2. Platelet counts normally decrease before menstruation and during pregnancy.
3. Clumping of platelets may cause falsely lowered results.
4. Oral contraceptives cause a slight increase.
5. See Appendix E for drugs that affect test outcomes.

Interventions

Pretest Patient Care

1. Explain test purpose and procedure.
2. Avoid strenuous exercise before blood is drawn.
3. Note what medications and what treatments the patient is receiving.
4. Follow guidelines in Chapter 1 for safe, effective, informed *pretest* care.

Posttest Patient Care

1. Review test results; report and record findings. Modify the nursing care plan as needed. Counsel the patient regarding abnormal findings; explain the need for possible follow-up testing and treatment. Observe for signs and symptoms of gastrointestinal bleeding, hemolysis, hematuria, petechiae, vaginal bleeding, epistaxis, and bleeding from the gums. When hemorrhage is apparent, use emergency measures to control bleeding and notify the attending healthcare provider.
2. Use platelet transfusions if the platelet count is $<20 \times 10^3/mm^3$ ($<20 \times 10^9/L$) or if there is a specific bleeding lesion. One unit of platelet concentrate raises the count by $15 \times 10^3/mm^3$ ($15 \times 10^9/L$).
3. Follow guidelines in Chapter 1 for safe, effective, informed *posttest* care.

● Platelet Aggregation

Platelet aggregation is used to evaluate congenital qualitative functional disorders of adhesion, release, or aggregation. It is rarely used to evaluate acquired bleeding disorders. In vivo, the clotting process follows two pathways: blood coagulation cascade and platelet activation (Fig. 2.2).

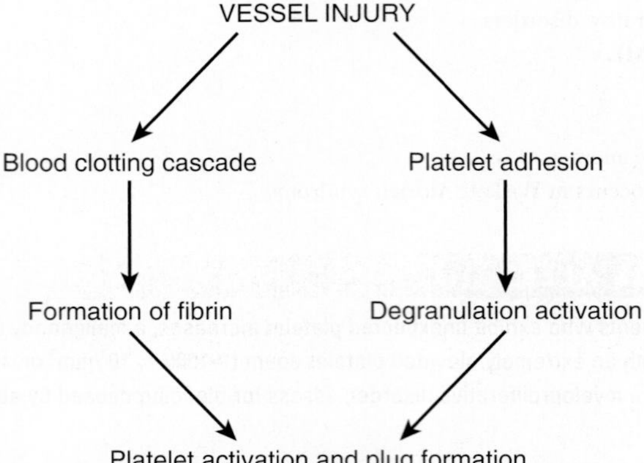

FIGURE 2.2. In vivo, the clotting process follows two pathways: blood coagulation cascade and platelet activation. (Source: Karon BS, Jaben E: Platelet function: Laboratory methods for evaluating effectiveness of anti-platelet therapy. Clin Lab News, 37(4):8–10, 2011)

Normal Findings

Full platelet aggregation in response to the following:
Adenosine diphosphate
Collagen
Epinephrine
Thrombin
Ristocetin

Procedure

1. Obtain a 5-mL venous blood sample (anticoagulated in a tube containing sodium citrate). Label the specimen with the patient's name, date and time of collection, and test(s) ordered.
2. Place the sample in a biohazard bag. The sample is kept at room temperature (never refrigerate) and must be run within 30 minutes after the blood is drawn.
3. Increase the transmission of light through a sample of platelet-rich plasma when platelets aggregate. This increase in light transmission can be used as an index to the aggregation in response to various agonists.

Clinical Implications

1. Decreased platelet aggregation occurs in congenital diseases:
   a. Bernard-Soulier syndrome (autosomal recessive coagulopathy)
   b. Glanzmann's thrombasthenia (abnormality of platelets, resulting in inability for platelets to bridge with other platelets)
   c. Storage pool diseases (e.g., Chédiak-Higashi syndrome, gray platelet disease)
   d. Cyclo-oxygenase deficiency
   e. Wiskott-Aldrich syndrome (X-linked recessive disease, resulting in a low platelet count)
   f. Albinism
   g. β-Thalassemia major
   h. May-Hegglin anomaly (abnormally large platelets)
   i. Various connective tissue disorders (e.g., Marfan's syndrome)
   j. von Willebrand's disease
2. Decreased platelet aggregation also occurs in acquired disorders:
   a. Uremia
   b. Antiplatelet antibodies
   c. Cardiopulmonary bypass
   d. Myeloproliferative disorders
   e. Dysproteinemias (macroglobulinemia)
   f. Idiopathic thrombocytopenic purpura
   g. Polycythemia vera
   h. Use of drugs and aspirin, some antibiotics, anti-inflammatory drugs, psychotropic drugs, and others (see Appendix E)
   i. DIC
3. *Increased* aggregation occurs in primary and secondary Raynaud's syndrome.

Interfering Factors

1. Platelet count $<100,000/mm^3$
2. Patient cannot be taking drugs that interfere with aggregation (see Appendix E).
3. Lipemia will interfere with testing.

Interventions

Pretest Patient Care

1. Explain test purpose and procedure.
2. Ten days before test, drugs that inhibit platelet aggregation are contraindicated. These include aspirin, antihistamines, steroids, cocaine, anti-inflammatories, theophylline, and antibiotics.
3. On the day of the test, avoid caffeine.
4. Avoid warfarin (Coumadin) for 2 weeks and heparin therapy for 1 week before testing.
5. Follow guidelines in Chapter 1 for safe, effective, informed *pretest* care.

Posttest Patient Care

1. Review test results; report and record findings. Modify the nursing care plan as needed. Counsel the patient regarding abnormal findings; explain the need for possible follow-up testing and treatment.
2. Resume medications and normal diet.
3. Possible treatments include applying pressure to venipuncture site and assessing for bleeding; hematoma may occur.
4. Follow guidelines in Chapter 1 for safe, effective, informed *posttest* care.

● Thrombin Time (TT); Thrombin Clotting Time (TCT)

Stage III fibrinogen defects can be detected by the TT test. It can detect DIC and hypofibrinogenemia and may also be used for monitoring streptokinase therapy. The test actually measures the time needed for plasma to clot when thrombin is added. Normally, a clot forms rapidly; if it does not, a stage III deficiency is present (Fig. 2.3). A TT test is often included as part of a panel for coagulation defects.

Normal Findings

7.0 to 12.0 seconds (varies widely by laboratory)
Check with your laboratory for values.

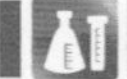

CLINICAL ALERT

TT is severely prolonged in the presence of afibrinogenemia (<80 mg/dL or <0.8 g/L of fibrinogen).

Critical Value
>60 seconds

Procedure

1. Use the procedure for two-tube specimen collection to anticoagulate a 7-mL venous blood sample with sodium citrate and put on ice. Take care not to contaminate the specimen with heparin from IV apparatus or other sources. Label the specimen with the patient's name, date and time of collection, and test(s) ordered.
2. Ensure that the specimen is tested within 2 hours, or it must be frozen for later testing.

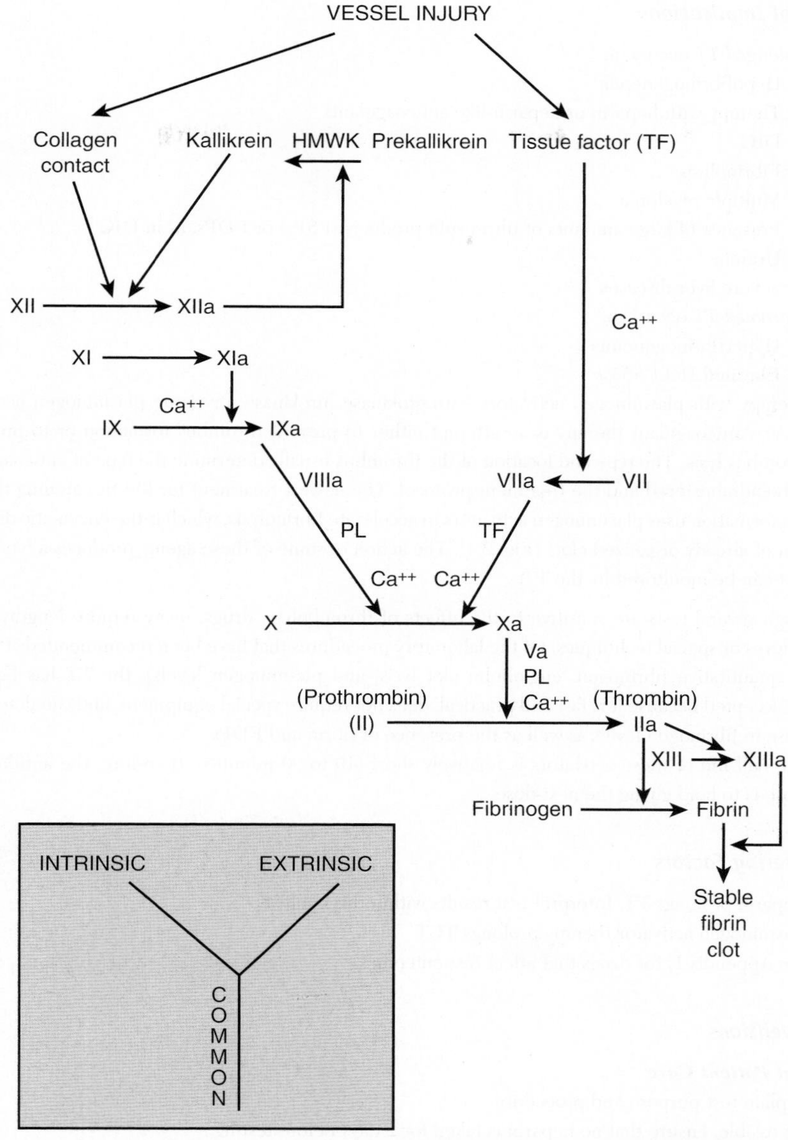

FIGURE 2.3. Intrinsic, extrinsic, and common pathways of coagulation. Vessel injury initiates intrinsic pathway through contact activation by exposed collagen. Extrinsic pathway is initiated by endothelial release of tissue factor (i.e., tissue thromboplastin). Extrinsic and intrinsic pathways each initiate common pathway to create stable fibrin clot. HMWK, high-molecular-weight kininogen; PL, platelet membrane phospholipid. (Lotspeich-Steininger CA, et al: Clinical Hematology. Philadelphia, JB Lippincott, 1992)

Clinical Implications

1. *Prolonged TT* occurs in:
   a. Hypofibrinogenemia
   b. Therapy with heparin or heparin-like anticoagulants
   c. DIC
   d. Fibrinolysis
   e. Multiple myeloma
   f. Presence of large amounts of fibrin split products (FSPs) or FDPs, as in DIC
   g. Uremia
   h. Severe liver diseases
2. *Shortened TT* occurs in:
   a. Hyperfibrinogenemia
   b. Elevated Hct (>55%)
3. Therapy with plasminogen activators—streptokinase, urokinase, or tissue plasminogen activator (tPA). Anticoagulant therapy is an attempt either to prevent thrombus formation or to promote thrombus lysis. The type and location of the thrombus usually determine the type of anticoagulant to be administered and the treatment protocol. The newest treatment for life-threatening thrombus formation uses plasminogen activators to accelerate fibrinolysis, which is the enzymatic dissolution of already organized clots (Fig. 2.4). The action of some of these agents produces a lytic state that can be monitored by the TT.

Although several tests are sensitive to the effects of thrombolytic drugs, many require lengthy assay procedures or special techniques. Of the laboratory procedures that have been recommended (PT, TT, aPTT, quantitative fibrinogen, euglobulin clot lysis, and plasminogen levels), the TT has become widely accepted because it is fast and practical, does not require special equipment, and can detect the decrease in fibrinogen levels as well as the presence of fibrin and FDPs.

The half-life of these activators is relatively short (10 to 90 minutes); therefore, the antidote for overdose is to hold giving the next dose.

Interfering Factors

1. Heparin prolongs TT. Interpret test results within this context.
2. Plasminogen activator therapy prolongs TCT.
3. See Appendix E for drugs that affect test outcomes.

Interventions

Pretest Patient Care

1. Explain test purpose and procedure.
2. If possible, ensure that no heparin is taken for 2 days before testing.
3. Follow guidelines in Chapter 1 for safe, effective, informed *pretest* care.

Posttest Patient Care

1. Resume normal activities and medications as ordered.
2. Review test results; report and record findings. Modify the nursing care plan as needed. Counsel the patient regarding abnormal findings; explain the need for possible follow-up testing and treatment. Check for excess bleeding. If plasminogen activator is being monitored, see Posttest Patient Care for aPTT.
3. Follow guidelines in Chapter 1 for safe, effective, informed *posttest* care.

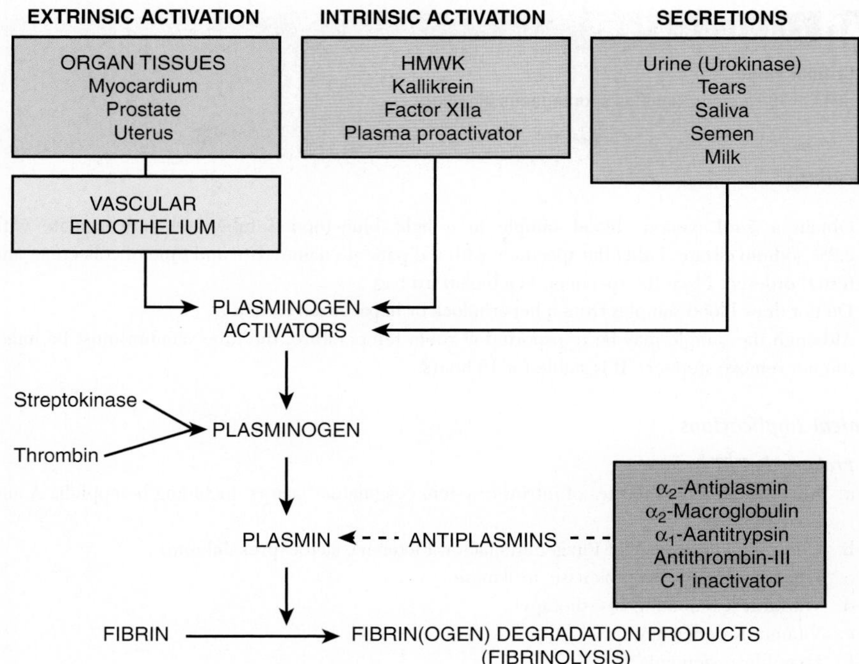

Fibrinolytic system may be activated by plasminogen activators from extrinsic sources such as vascular endothelium or by intrinsic sources such as factor XIIa and others as shown. These plasminogen activators convert plasminogen to plasmin. Thrombin also activates plasminogen; streptokinase, administered therapeutically in thrombotic disorders, acts in the same way. Plasmin promotes fibrinolysis. Antiplasmins control (inhibit and neutralize) excess plasmin, thus preventing excessive and premature fibrinolysis.

FIGURE 2.4. Stage four activation of the fibrinolytic system. HMWK, high-molecular-weight kininogen.

• Partial Thromboplastin Time (PTT); Activated Partial Thromboplastin Time (aPTT)

The PTT, a one-stage clotting test, screens for coagulation disorders. Specifically, it can detect deficiencies of the intrinsic thromboplastin system and also reveal defects in the extrinsic coagulation mechanism pathway.

NOTE *The PTT and aPTT test for the same functions. aPTT is a more sensitive version of PTT that is used to monitor heparin therapy.*

The aPTT is used to detect deficiencies in the intrinsic coagulation system, to detect incubating anticoagulants, and to monitor heparin therapy. It is part of a coagulation panel workup.

Normal Findings

aPTT: 21.0 to 35.0 seconds

Check with your laboratory for therapeutic range values during heparin therapy (2 to 2.5 times normal).

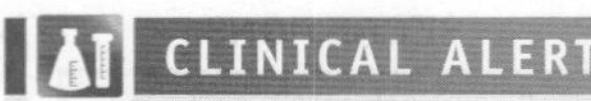

Critical Value

aPTT >70 seconds signifies spontaneous bleeding.

Procedure

1. Obtain a 5-mL venous blood sample in a light blue–topped tube and anticoagulate with 3.2% sodium citrate. Label the specimen with the patient's name, date and time of collection, and test(s) ordered. Place the specimen in a biohazard bag.
2. Do not draw blood samples from a heparin lock or heparinized catheter.
3. Although the sample may be transported at room temperature, the tube vacuum must be intact (do not remove stopper). It is stable for 12 hours.

Clinical Implications

1. *Prolonged aPTT* occurs in:
   a. All congenital deficiencies of intrinsic system coagulation factors, including hemophilia A and hemophilia B
   b. Congenital deficiency of Fitzgerald's factor, Fletcher's factor (prekallikrein)
   c. Heparin therapy, streptokinase, urokinase
   d. Warfarin (Coumadin)-like therapy
   e. Vitamin K deficiency
   f. Hypofibrinogenemia
   g. Liver disease
   h. DIC (chronic or acute)
   i. Fibrin degradation products (FDPs)
2. When aPTT is performed in conjunction with PT, a further clarification of coagulation defects is possible. For example, a normal PT with an abnormal aPTT means that the defect lies within the first stage of the clotting cascade (factor VIII, IX, X, XI, or XII). The pattern of a normal PTT with an abnormal PT suggests a possible factor VII deficiency. If both PT and aPTT are prolonged, a deficiency of factor I, II, V, or X is suggested. Used together, aPTT and PT will detect approximately 95% of coagulation defects.
3. *Shortened aPTT* occurs in:
   a. Extensive cancer, except when the liver is involved
   b. Immediately after acute hemorrhage
   c. Very early stages of DIC
4. *Circulating anticoagulants* (inhibitors) usually occur as inhibitors of a specific factor (e.g., factor VIII). These are most commonly seen in the development of anti–factor VIII or anti–factor IX in 5% to 10% of hemophiliac patients. Anticoagulants that develop in the treated hemophiliac are detected through prolonged aPTT. Circulating anticoagulants are also associated with other conditions:
   a. After many plasma transfusions
   b. Drug reactions
   c. Tuberculosis
   d. Chronic glomerulonephritis
   e. SLE
   f. Rheumatoid arthritis
5. *Heparin therapy*: In deep vein thrombosis or acute myocardial infarction, the usual protocol requires injection of heparin (monitored by the aPTT), followed by long-term therapy with oral anticoagulants (monitored by the PT, aPTT, or both).

a. In the blood, heparin combines with an α-globulin (heparin cofactor) to form a potent antithrombin. It is a direct anticoagulant.
b. IV heparin injection produces an immediate anticoagulant effect; it is chosen when rapid anticoagulant effects are desired.
c. Because the half-life of heparin is 3 hours, the aPTT is measured 3 hours after heparin administration, or 1 hour before the next dose.
d. Therapeutic aPTT levels are ordinarily maintained at 2 to 2.5 times the normal values.
e. To evaluate heparin effects, blood is tested:
   (1) For baseline values before therapy is initiated
   (2) One hour before the next dose is due (when a 4-hour administration cycle is ordered)
   (3) According to the patient's status (e.g., bleeding)

NOTE *Mixing equal parts of patient plasma and normal plasma corrects the aPTT if it is caused by a coagulation factor defect but does not correct the aPTT to normal if it is caused by a circulating inhibitor. A more sensitive test is the Russell viper venom test, which demonstrates the presence of the lupus anticoagulant. This test is unaffected by inhibitors of factor VIII or deficiencies of factors VIII, IX, or XI, or is affected by deficiencies of factors II, V, or X and by the use of sodium, warfarin, or heparin. Because lupus-type anticoagulants vary greatly in their reactivity in various test systems, it is recommended that this test be done in conjunction with the aPTT and the anticardiolipin antibody assay. The reference range is 33.5 to 41.5 seconds.*

NOTE *Not all individuals respond ideally or predictably to heparin. Anaphylaxis and erythematous reactions may occur. There is no shortcut to adequate and safe anticoagulation.*

Interfering Factors

1. See Appendix E for drugs that affect test outcomes.
2. Hemolyzed plasma shortens aPTT in normal patients but not in abnormal (heparinized) patients.
3. Very increased or decreased Hct
4. Incorrect ratio of blood to citrate ("short" fill of blood in collection tube)

Interventions

Pretest Patient Care

1. Explain test purpose, procedure, benefits, and risks.
2. Follow guidelines in Chapter 1 for safe, effective, informed, *pretest* care.
3. Draw blood sample 1 hour before next dose of heparin. The heparin dose given relates to the aPTT result.

Posttest Patient Care

1. Review test results; report and record findings. Modify the nursing care plan as needed. Counsel the patient regarding abnormal findings; explain the need for possible follow-up testing and treatment. Protamine sulfate is the antidote for heparin overdose or for reversal of heparin anticoagulation therapy.
2. Follow guidelines in Chapter 1 for safe, effective, informed *posttest* care.
3. Watch for signs of spontaneous bleeding; notify the healthcare provider immediately and treat accordingly.
4. Alert the patient to watch for bleeding gums, hematuria, oozing from wounds, and excessive bruising.

5. Instruct the patient to use an electric shaver instead of a blade and to exercise caution in all activities.
6. Avoid use of aspirin or ASA-like drugs (unless specifically prescribed) because they contribute to bleeding tendencies.
7. Long-term use of heparin can cause development of osteoporosis with fractures.
8. Thrombocytopenia can also develop with high-dose heparin therapy, along with progressive thromboembolic syndrome. This platelet abnormality quickly reverses when heparin is discontinued.

Activated Clotting Time (ACT)

The activated clotting time (ACT) test evaluates coagulation status. The ACT responds linearly to heparin level changes and responds to wider ranges of heparin concentrations than does the aPTT. The ACT, however, assays overall coagulation activity. Therefore, prolonged values may not be exclusively the result of heparin.

The ACT can be a bedside procedure and requires only 0.4 mL of blood. Heparin infusion or reversal with protamine can then be titrated almost immediately according to the ACT results. ACT also is routinely used during dialysis, coronary artery bypass procedures, arteriograms, and percutaneous transluminal coronary arteriography. This test is hard to standardize, and no controls are available; therefore, it is used with caution mainly in cardiac surgery. The results are backed up by the aPTT.

Normal Findings

ACT: 70 to 120 seconds
Therapeutic range: 180 to 240 seconds (two times normal range)

Prothrombin Time (Pro Time; PT)

Prothrombin is a protein produced by the liver for clotting of blood. Prothrombin production depends on adequate vitamin K intake and absorption. During the clotting process, prothrombin is converted to thrombin. The prothrombin content of the blood is reduced in patients with liver disease.

The PT is one of the four most important screening tests used in diagnostic coagulation studies. It directly measures a potential defect in stage II of the clotting mechanism (extrinsic coagulation system) through analysis of the clotting ability of five plasma coagulation factors (prothrombin, fibrinogen, factor V, factor VII, and factor X). In addition to screening for deficiency of prothrombin, the PT is used to evaluate dysfibrinogenemia, the heparin effect and coumarin effect, liver failure, and vitamin K deficiency.

Normal Findings

PT: 11.0 to 13.0 seconds (can vary by laboratory)
Therapeutic levels are at a P/C ratio of 2.0 to 2.5. Recommended therapeutic ranges are shown in Table 2.10.
P/C ratio (prothrombin time ratio): the observed patient PT divided by the laboratory PT mean normal value
INR (International Normalized Ratio): a comparative rating of PT ratios (representing the observed PT ratio adjusted by the International Reference Thromboplastin)
Normal: 0.8 to 1.2
Patients on anticoagulants: 2.0 to 3.0 (<2.0 may indicate inadequate protection from clotting and if >4.0 may indicate blood is clotting too slowly)

TABLE 2.10 Therapeutic Context

	INR	Target
Preoperative oral anticoagulant started 2 weeks before surgery		
Non–hip surgery	1.5–2.5	2.0
Hip surgery	2.0–3.0	2.5
Primary and secondary prevention of deep vein thrombosis	2.0–3.0	2.5
Prevention of systemic embolism in patients with atrial fibrillation	2.0–3.0	2.5
Recurrent systemic embolism	3.0–4.5	3.5
Prevention of recurrent deep vein thrombosis (two or more episodes)	2.5–4.0	3.0
Cardiac stents	3.0–4.5	3.5
Prevention of arterial thrombosis, including patients with mechanical heart valves	2.5–3.5	3.0

INR, International Normalized Ratio.

ISI (International Sensitivity Index): a comparative rating of thromboplastin (supplied by the manufacturer of the reagent, generally between 1.0 and 2.0) with an international World Health Organization standard.

INR = $[\text{PTpatient}/\text{MNPT}]^{\text{ISI}}$
PT = prothrombin time
MNPT = mean of the normal range of prothrombin time

NOTE *Recent studies have shown that at-home (weekly self-testing) testing did result in patients spending more time in the therapeutic range; however, there was no benefit in major clinical outcomes as compared to clinic testing (Matchar et al., 2010).*

CLINICAL ALERT

1. Critical value: If P/C is >2.5 or >30.0 s, notify the healthcare provider (for patients on anticoagulant).
2. If PT is excessively prolonged (>30 s), vitamin K may be ordered.
3. Critical value: >20 s (for nonanticoagulated persons)
4. Baseline PT levels should be determined before anticoagulant administration.
5. Critical value: INR >3.6; notify the healthcare provider (for patients on anticoagulants)

Procedure

1. Draw a 5-mL venous whole blood sample (by the two-tube technique) into a tube containing a calcium-binding anticoagulant (sodium citrate). The ratio of sodium citrate to blood is critical.
2. Use blue-topped vacuum tubes that keep prothrombin levels stable at room temperature for 12 hours if left capped (vacuum intact). Label the specimen with the patient's name, date and time of collection, and test(s) ordered. Place the specimen in a biohazard bag.

Oral Anticoagulant Therapy

Oral anticoagulant drugs (e.g., warfarin, dicumarol) are commonly prescribed to treat blood clots. These are indirect anticoagulants (compared with heparin, which is a direct anticoagulant). However, if necessary, heparin is the anticoagulant of choice for initiating treatment because it acts rapidly and also partially lyses the clot.

1. These drugs act through the liver to delay coagulation by interfering with the action of the vitamin K–related factors (II, VII, IX, and X), which promote clotting.
2. Oral anticoagulants delay vitamin K formation and cause the PT to increase as a result of decreased factors II, VII, IX, and X.
3. The usual procedure is to run a PT test every day when beginning therapy. The anticoagulant dose is adjusted until the therapeutic range is reached. Then, weekly to monthly PT testing continues for the duration of therapy.
4. Coumadin takes 48 to 72 hours to cause a measurable change in the PT (3 to 4 days of drug therapy).

Drug Therapy and PT Protocols

1. Patients with cardiac problems are usually maintained at a PT level 2 to 2.5 times the normal (baseline) values.
2. Use of the INR values allows more sensitive control. A reasonable INR target for virtually all thromboembolic problems is 2.0 to 3.0. See Table 2.10 for more specific guidelines.
3. For treatment of blood clots, the PT is maintained within 2 to 2.5 times the normal range. If the PT drops below this range, treatment may be ineffective, and old clots may expand or new clots may form. Conversely, if the PT rises above 30 seconds, bleeding or hemorrhage may occur.

Clinical Implications

1. Conditions that cause *increased PT* include:
   a. Deficiency of factors II (prothrombin), V, VII, or X
   b. Vitamin K deficiency, newborns of mother with vitamin K deficiency
   c. Hemorrhagic disease of the newborn
   d. Liver disease (e.g., alcoholic hepatitis), liver damage
   e. Current anticoagulant therapy with warfarin (Coumadin)
   f. Biliary obstruction
   g. Poor fat absorption (e.g., sprue, celiac disease, chronic diarrhea)
   h. Current anticoagulant therapy with heparin
   i. DIC
   j. Zollinger-Ellison syndrome
   k. Hypofibrinogenemia (factor I deficiency), dysfibrinogenemia
   l. Circulating anticoagulants, lupus anticoagulant
   m. Premature newborns
2. Conditions that *do not affect the PT* include:
   Polycythemia vera
   Tannin disease
   Christmas disease (factor IX deficiency)
   Hemophilia A (factor VIII deficiency)
   von Willebrand's disease
   Platelet disorders (idiopathic thrombocytopenic purpura)

Interfering Factors

1. Diet: Ingestion of excessive green, leafy vegetables increases the body's absorption of vitamin K, which promotes blood clotting.
2. Alcoholism or excessive alcohol ingestion prolongs PT levels.
3. Diarrhea and vomiting decrease PT because of dehydration.
4. Quality of venipuncture: PT can be shortened if technique is traumatic and tissue thromboplastin is introduced to the sample and if collection tube is not filled properly.
5. Influence of prescribed medications: antibiotics, aspirin, cimetidine, isoniazid, phenothiazines, cephalosporins, cholestyramines, phenylbutazone, metronidazole, oral hypoglycemics, phenytoin
6. Prolonged storage of plasma at 4°C activates factor VII and shortens PT.

Interventions

Pretest Patient Care

1. Explain the purpose, procedure, and need for frequent testing. Emphasize the need for regular monitoring through frequent blood testing if long-term therapy is prescribed. *Do not refer to anticoagulants as "blood thinners."* One explanation might be, "Your blood will be tested periodically to determine the pro time, which is an indication of how the blood clots." The anticoagulant dose will be adjusted according to PT results.
2. Caution against self-medication. Ascertain what drugs the patient has been taking. Many drugs, including over-the-counter medications, alter the effects of anticoagulants and the PT value. Aspirin, acetaminophen, and laxative products should be avoided unless specifically ordered by the healthcare provider.
3. Instruct the patient never to start or discontinue any drug without the doctor's permission. This will affect PT values and may also interfere with the healing process.
4. Counsel regarding diet. Excessive amounts of green, leafy vegetables (e.g., spinach, broccoli) will increase vitamin K levels and could interfere with anticoagulant metabolism. Caution against using razor blades; electric shavers should be used.
5. These guidelines also apply to posttest patient care.

Posttest Patient Care

1. Review test results; report and record findings. Modify the nursing care plan as needed. Counsel the patient regarding abnormal findings; explain the need for possible follow-up testing and treatment.
2. Avoid intramuscular injections during anticoagulant therapy because hematomas may form at the injection site. As the PT increases to upper limits (>30 seconds), assess carefully for bleeding from different areas; this may require neurologic assessment (if cranial bleeding is suspected), lung assessment and auscultation, gastrointestinal and genitourinary assessments, or other assessments as appropriate. Instruct the patient to observe for bleeding from gums, blood in the urine, or other unusual bleeding. Advise that care should be exercised in all activities to avoid accidental injury.
3. Alert patients who are being monitored by PT for long-term anticoagulant therapy that they should not take any other drugs unless they have been specifically prescribed.
4. When unexpected adjustments in anticoagulant doses are required to maintain a stable PT, or when there are erratic changes in PT levels, a drug interaction should be suspected and further investigation should take place.
5. Make changes in exercise intensity gradually or not at all. Active sports and contact sports should be avoided because of the potential for injury.
6. Follow guidelines in Chapter 1 for safe, effective, informed *posttest* care.

Coagulant Factors (Factor Assay)

Assay of specific factors of coagulation is done in the investigation of inherited and acquired bleeding disorders. For example, tests of factor VIII–related antigen are used in the differential diagnosis of classic hemophilia and von Willebrand's disease in cases in which there is no family history of bleeding and bleeding times are borderline or abnormal. A test for ristocetin cofactor is done to help diagnose von Willebrand's disease by determining the degree or rate of platelet aggregation that is taking place.

Normal Findings

Factor II—prothrombin: 80% to 120% of normal
Factor V—labile factor: 50% to 150% of normal
Factor VII—stable factor: 65% to 140% of normal or 65 to 135 AU
Factor VIII—antihemophilic factor: 55% to 145% of normal or 55 to 145 AU
Factor IX—Christmas factor: 60% to 140% of normal or 60 to 140 AU
Factor X: 45% to 155% of normal or 45 to 155 AU
Factor XI: 65% to 135% of normal or 65 to 135 AU
Factor XII—Hageman factor: 50% to 150% of normal or 50 to 150 AU
Ristocetin (von Willebrand's factor): 45% to 140% of normal or 45 to 140 AU
Factor VIII antigen: 100 μg/L or 50% to 150% of normal or 50 to 150 AU
Factor VIII–related antigen: 45% to 185% of normal or 45 to 185 AU
Fletcher's factor (prekallikrein): 80% to 120% of normal or 0.80 to 1.20

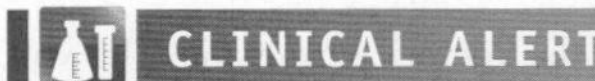

Critical Value
For any coagulation factor: <10% of normal

Procedure

1. Draw a 5-mL venous blood sample by the two-tube method and add to a collection tube containing sodium citrate as the anticoagulant. Label the specimen with the patient's name, date and time of collection, and test(s) ordered.
2. Cap samples, put on ice, and send to the laboratory as soon as possible.

Clinical Implications

1. *Inherited deficiencies*:
   Any of the specific factors—I, II, V, VII, VIII, IX, X, XI, XII, and XIII—may be deficient on a familial basis.
   Factor VII is decreased in hypoproconvertinemia (autosomal recessive).
   Factor VIII is decreased in classic hemophilia A and von Willebrand's disease (inherited autosomally).
   Factor IX is decreased in Christmas disease or hemophilia B (sex-linked recessive).
   Factor XI is decreased in hemophilia C (autosomal dominant, occurring predominantly in Jews).
2. *Acquired disorders*:
   a. Factor II is decreased in:
      (1) Liver disease
      (2) Vitamin K deficiency
      (3) Oral anticoagulants (last factor to decrease after starting warfarin therapy)
      (4) Normal newborns
      (5) Circulating inhibitors or lupus-like anticoagulants

b. Factor V is decreased in:
   (1) Liver disease
   (2) Factor V inhibitors
   (3) Myeloproliferative disorders
   (4) DIC and fibrinolysis
   (5) Normal newborns (mildly decreased)
c. Factor VII is decreased in:
   (1) Liver disease
   (2) Treatment with coumarin-type drugs (first factor to decrease)
   (3) Normal newborns
   (4) Kwashiorkor
d. Factor VIII is increased in:
   (1) Late normal pregnancy
   (2) Thromboembolic conditions
   (3) Liver disease
   (4) Postoperative period
   (5) Rebound activity after sudden cessation of a coumarin-type drug
   (6) Normal newborns
e. Factor VIII is decreased in:
   (1) Presence of factor VIII inhibitors (anticoagulants capable of specifically neutralizing a coagulation factor and thereby disrupting hemostasis), associated with hemophilia A and immunologic reactions, and postpartum
   (2) von Willebrand's disease
   (3) DIC, fibrinolysis
   (4) Myeloproliferative disorders
f. Factor IX is decreased in:
   (1) Uncompensated cirrhosis, liver disease
   (2) Nephrotic syndrome
   (3) Development of circulating anticoagulants against factor IX (rare)
   (4) Normal newborns
   (5) Dicumarol and related anticoagulant drugs
   (6) DIC
   (7) Vitamin K deficiency
g. Factor X is decreased in:
   (1) Vitamin K deficiency
   (2) Liver disease
   (3) Oral anticoagulants
   (4) Amyloidosis
   (5) DIC
   (6) Normal newborns
h. Factor XI is decreased in:
   (1) Liver disease
   (2) Intestinal malabsorption (vitamin K)
   (3) Occasional development of circulatory anticoagulants against factor IX
   (4) DIC
   (5) Newborns (do not reach adult levels for up to 6 months)
i. Factor XII is decreased in:
   (1) Nephrotic syndrome
   (2) Liver disease

(3) Chronic granulocytic leukemia
(4) Normal newborns

j. Factor XIII is decreased in:
(1) Postoperative patients
(2) Liver disease
(3) Persistent increased fibrinogen levels
(4) Obstetric complications with hypofibrinogenemia
(5) Acute myelogenous leukemia
(6) Circulating anticoagulants
(7) DIC

Interventions

Pretest Patient Care

1. Explain test purpose and procedure.
2. Follow guidelines in Chapter 1 for safe, effective, informed *pretest* care.

Posttest Patient Care

1. Review test results; report and record findings. Modify the nursing care plan as needed. Counsel the patient regarding abnormal findings; explain the need for possible follow-up testing and treatment.
2. Follow guidelines in Chapter 1 for safe, effective, informed *posttest* care.

● Plasminogen (Plasmin; Fibrinolysin)

Plasminogen is a glycoprotein, synthesized in the liver, present in plasma. Under normal circumstances, plasminogen is a part of any clot because of the tendency of fibrin to absorb plasminogen from the plasma. When plasminogen activators perform their function, plasmin is formed within the clot; this gradually dissolves the clot while leaving time for tissue repair. Free plasmin also is released to the plasma; however, antiplasmins there immediately destroy any plasmin released from the clot (see Fig. 2.3).

This test is done to determine plasminogen activity in persons with thrombosis or DIC. When pathologic coagulation processes are involved, excessive free plasmin is released to the plasma. In these situations, the available antiplasmin is depleted, and plasmin begins destroying components other than fibrin, including fibrinogen, factors V and VIII, and other factors. Plasmin acts more quickly to destroy fibrinogen because of fibrinogen's instability.

For therapeutic destruction of thrombi, urokinase, a trypsin-like protease purified from urine, may be administered to a patient to activate plasminogen to plasmin and induce fibrinolysis. Streptokinase is another therapeutic agent used for the same purpose.

Normal Findings

Plasminogen activity:
Males: 76% to 124% of normal for plasma or 0.76 to 1.24 fraction of normal
Females: 65% to 153% of normal for plasma or 0.65 to 1.53 fraction of normal
Infants: 27% to 59% of normal for plasma or 0.27 to 0.59 fraction of normal

Procedure

1. Add a 5-mL venous blood sample to a light blue–topped collection tube containing sodium citrate. Use the two-tube method. Label the specimen with the patient's name, date and time of collection, and test(s) ordered. Place the specimen in a biohazard bag.

2. Put the sample on ice and transport to the laboratory immediately.
3. The test must be started within 30 minutes after the blood is drawn.

Clinical Implications

1. *Decreased* plasminogen activity occurs in:
   a. Some familial or isolated cases of idiopathic deep vein thrombosis
   b. DIC and systemic fibrinolysis
   c. Liver disease and cirrhosis
   d. Neonatal hyaline membrane disease
   e. Therapy with plasminogen activators
2. Decreased levels of plasminogen or abnormally functioning plasminogen can lead to venous and arterial clotting (thrombosis).
3. *Increased* plasminogen activity occurs in:
   a. Pregnancy (third trimester)
   b. Regular vigorous physical exercise

Interfering Factors

See Appendix E for drugs that affect test outcomes.

Interventions

Pretest Patient Care

1. Explain test purpose and procedure.
2. Follow guidelines in Chapter 1 for safe, effective, informed *pretest* care.

Posttest Patient Care

1. Review test results; report and record findings. Modify the nursing care plan as needed. Counsel the patient regarding abnormal findings; explain the need for possible follow-up testing and treatment. Monitor for thrombotic tendency.
2. Follow guidelines in Chapter 1 for safe, effective, informed *posttest* care.

● Fibrinolysis (Euglobulin Lysis Time; Diluted Whole Blood Clot Lysis)

Primary fibrinolysis, without any sign of intravascular coagulation, is extremely rare. Secondary fibrinolysis is usually seen and follows or occurs simultaneously with intravascular coagulation. This secondary fibrinolysis is a protective mechanism against generalized clotting.

This test is done to evaluate fibrinolytic activity. Shortened time indicates excessive fibrinolytic activity. Lysis is marked and rapid with primary fibrinolysis but can be minimal in secondary fibrinolysis. The diluted whole blood is used to monitor urokinase and streptokinase therapy.

Normal Findings

Euglobulin lysis—no lysis of plasma clot at 37°C in 60 to 120 minutes. The clot is observed for 24 hours.
Diluted whole blood clot lysis: no lysis of clot in 120 minutes at 37°C.

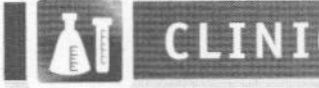

CLINICAL ALERT

A lysis time of <1 hr signifies that abnormal fibrinolysis is occurring.

Procedure

1. Collect a 5-mL venous blood sample in a tube containing sodium citrate using the two-tube method. Label the specimen with the patient's name, date and time of collection, and test(s) ordered. Place the specimen in a biohazard bag.
2. Put the sample on ice and transport to the laboratory immediately or start at bedside.
3. The test must be started within 90 minutes after the blood is centrifuged.

NOTE *To avoid release of plasminogen activator, do not massage vein, pump fist, or leave tourniquet on for a prolonged period of time.*

Clinical Implications

1. *Increased* fibrinolysis time occurs in the following conditions:
   a. Primary fibrinolysis
   b. Within 48 hours after surgery
   c. Cancer of prostate or pancreas
   d. Circulatory collapse, shock
   e. During lung and cardiac surgery
   f. Obstetric complications (e.g., antepartum hemorrhage, amniotic embolism, septic abortion, death of fetus, hydatidiform mole)
   g. Long-term DIC (may be normal if plasminogen is depleted)
   h. Liver disease
   i. Administration of plasminogen activators (tPA, streptokinase, urokinase)
2. Heparin does not interfere with the euglobulin lysis test.

Interfering Factors

1. Increased fibrinolysis occurs with moderate exercise and increasing age.
2. Decreased fibrinolysis occurs in arterial blood, compared with venous blood. This difference is greater in arteriosclerosis (especially in young persons).
3. Decreased fibrinolysis occurs in postmenopausal women and in normal newborns.
4. FDPs interfere with fibrinolysis.
5. Normal results can occur if fibrinolysis is far advanced (plasminogen depleted).
6. Fibrinolysis is increased by very low fibrinogen levels (<80 mg/dL or <0.8 g/L) and decreased by high fibrinogen levels.
7. Increased fibrinolysis can be caused by traumatic venipuncture or a tourniquet that is too tight.
8. See Appendix E for drugs that affect test outcomes.

Interventions

Pretest Patient Care

1. Advise the patient of test purpose and procedure; no exercise before test.
2. Follow guidelines in Chapter 1 for safe, effective, informed *pretest* care.

Posttest Patient Care

1. Review test results; report and record findings. Modify the nursing care plan as needed. Counsel the patient regarding abnormal findings; explain the need for possible follow-up testing and treatment. Monitor for fibrinolytic crisis.
2. Follow guidelines in Chapter 1 for safe, effective, informed *posttest* care.

● Fibrin Split Products (FSPs); Fibrin Degradation Products (FDPs)

When fibrin is split by plasmin, positive tests for fibrin degradation (split) products, identified by the letters X, Y, D, and E, are produced. These products have an anticoagulant action and inhibit clotting when they are present in excess in the circulation. Increased levels of FDPs may occur with a variety of pathologic processes in which clot formation and lysis occur.

This test is done to establish the diagnosis of DIC and other thromboembolic disorders.

Normal Findings

Negative at 1:4 dilution or <10 μg/mL (<10 mg/L)

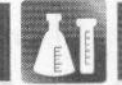

CLINICAL ALERT

Patients with very high levels of FSP/FDP have blood that does not clot or clots poorly.

Critical Value

>40 μg/mL (>40 mg/L)

Procedure

1. Place a venous blood sample of at least 4.5 mL in a tube containing thrombin and an inhibitor of fibrinolysis (reptilase, aprotinin, and calcium). Label the specimen with the patient's name, date and time of collection, and test(s) ordered. Place the specimen in a biohazard bag.
2. The blood should be completely clotted before the test is started because the end products (X, Y, D, and E) are due to degradation of fibrinogen and fibrin.

Clinical Implications

Increased FSP and FDP are associated with DIC and are seen in:

1. Primary fibrinolysis
2. Venous thrombosis
3. Thoracic and cardiac surgery or renal transplantation
4. Acute myocardial infarction
5. Pulmonary embolism
6. Carcinoma
7. Liver disease

Interfering Factors

1. Because all of the laboratory methods are sensitive to fibrinogen as well as FDP, it is essential that no unclotted fibrinogen be left in the serum preparation. False-positive reactions can result if any fibrinogen is present.
2. False-positive results occur with heparin therapy.
3. The presence of rheumatoid factor (rheumatoid arthritis) may cause falsely high FSP and FDP values.
4. See Appendix E for drugs that affect test outcomes.

Interventions

Pretest Patient Care

1. Explain test purpose and procedure.
2. Follow guidelines in Chapter 1 for safe, effective, informed *pretest* care.

Posttest Patient Care

1. Review test results; report and record findings. Modify the nursing care plan as needed. Counsel the patient regarding abnormal findings; explain the need for possible follow-up testing and treatment. Monitor for DIC and thrombosis.
2. Follow guidelines in Chapter 1 for safe, effective, informed *posttest* care.

D-Dimer

D-Dimers are produced as a degradation product of fibrin clots resulting from the action of three enzymes: (1) thrombin, due to activation of the coagulation cascade that converts fibrinogen into fibrin clots; (2) activated factor XIII, which cross-links fibrin clots; and (3) plasmin. The presence of D-dimer confirms that both thrombin generation and plasmin generation have occurred.

This test is used in the diagnosis of DIC, venous thromboembolism (VTE), and excluding the diagnosis of acute pulmonary embolism. The D-dimer test is more specific for DIC than are tests for FSPs. The test verifies in vivo fibrinolysis because D-dimers are produced only by the action of plasmin on cross-linked fibrin, not by the action of plasmin on unclotted fibrinogen.

Normal Findings

Quantitative
<250 μg/L or <1.37 nmol/L D-Dimer Units (DDU)
0 to 0.6 mg/L fibrinogen equivalent units (FEU)
Qualitative: no D-dimer fragments present

Procedure

A venous blood sample of 5 mL is collected into a light blue–topped tube containing 3.2% sodium citrate and aprotinin. Label the specimen with the patient's name, date and time of collection, and test(s) ordered. Place the specimen in a biohazard bag and return it to the laboratory immediately.

Clinical Implications

1. *Increased* D-dimer values are associated with:
   a. DIC (secondary fibrinolysis)
   b. Arterial or venous thrombosis (deep vein thrombosis)
   c. Renal or liver failure
   d. Pulmonary embolism
   e. Late in pregnancy, preeclampsia
   f. Myocardial infarction
   g. Malignancy, inflammation, and severe infection
2. D-Dimer values are increased with tPA anticoagulant therapy.

NOTE *D-Dimer analysis of spinal fluid can rapidly and accurately differentiate cases of subarachnoid hemorrhage (SAH) from a traumatic tap. Positive in SAH.*

Interfering Factors

1. False-positive tests are obtained with high titers of rheumatoid factor.
2. False-positive D-dimer levels increase as the tumor marker CA-125 for ovarian cancer increases.
3. The D-dimer test will be positive in all patients after surgery or trauma.
4. False-positive results found in estrogen therapy, normal pregnancy.

Interventions

Pretest Patient Care

1. Explain test purpose and procedure.
2. Follow guidelines in Chapter 1 for safe, effective, informed *pretest* care.

Posttest Patient Care

1. Review test results; report and record findings. Modify the nursing care plan as needed. Counsel the patient regarding abnormal findings; explain the need for possible follow-up testing and treatment. Monitor for DIC and thrombosis.
2. Follow guidelines in Chapter 1 for safe, effective, informed *posttest* care.

● Fibrinopeptide A (FPA)

Fibrinopeptides A (FPA) and B are formed by the action of thrombin on fibrinogen; therefore, the presence of FPA indicates that thrombin has acted on fibrinogen.

The measurement is the most sensitive assay done to determine thrombin action. FPA reflects the amount of active intravascular blood clotting; this occurs in subclinical DIC, which is common in patients with leukemia of various types and may be associated with tumor progression. FPA elevations can occur without intravascular thrombosis, decreasing the value of a positive test.

Normal Findings

Male: 0.4 to 2.6 mg/mL
Female: 0.7 to 3.1 mg/mL

Procedure

1. Collect a venous blood sample of 5 mL in special Vacutainer tube containing aprotinin EDTA and thrombin to prevent activation in vitro. Use a two-tube method of draining blood.
2. Draw the specimen in a prechilled tube and place immediately on ice.
3. Label the specimen with the patient's name, date and time of collection, and test(s) ordered. Place the specimen in a biohazard bag. Clean venipuncture and gentle handling of specimen are required. The specimen must be transported to the lab within 30 minutes.

Clinical Implications

1. *Increased* FPA occurs in:
   a. DIC
   b. Leukemia of various types
   c. Venous thrombosis and pulmonary embolus
   d. Myocardial infarction
   e. Postoperative patients
   f. Patients with widespread solid tumors, malignancies

2. *Decreased* FPA occurs in:
   a. Clinical remission of leukemia achieved with chemotherapy
   b. Therapeutic heparinization

Interfering Factors

1. A traumatic venous puncture may result in falsely increased levels.
2. The biologic half-life (stable for 2 hours or more) imposes limitations on the interpretation of a negative FPA test.

> **CLINICAL ALERT**
>
> DIC occurs commonly in association with death of tumor cells in acute promyelocytic leukemia. For this reason, heparin is used prophylactically and in association with the initiation of chemotherapy for promyelocytic leukemia. DIC occurs less commonly during the treatment of acute myelomonocytic leukemia and acute lymphocytic leukemia. Evidence of DIC should be sought in every patient with leukemia before initiation of treatment.

Interventions

Pretest Patient Care

1. Explain test purpose and procedure.
2. Avoid prolonged use of tourniquet.
3. Follow guidelines in Chapter 1 for safe, effective, informed *pretest* care.

Posttest Patient Care

1. Review test results; report and record findings. Modify the nursing care plan as needed. Counsel the patient regarding abnormal findings; explain the need for possible follow-up testing and treatment. Monitor for DIC and thrombosis.
2. Follow guidelines in Chapter 1 for safe, effective, informed *posttest* care.
3. Resume normal activities.

● Prothrombin Fragment (F1 + 2)

The prothrombin F1 + 2 fragment is liberated from the prothrombin molecule when it is activated by factor Xa to form thrombin. Thrombin may be rapidly inactivated by AT-III. The F1 + 2 fragment, however, has a half-life of about 1.5 hours, making it a useful marker for activated coagulation.

Prothrombin F1 + 2 is used to detect activation of the coagulation system before actual thrombosis occurs. It is used to identify patients with low-grade intravascular coagulation (DIC) and to judge the effectiveness of oral anticoagulant therapy. F1 + 2 levels may assist in the study of the hypercoagulable states and in the assessment of thrombotic risk.

Normal Findings

7.4 to 102.9 μg/L or 0.2 to 2.78 nmol/L
Levels rise slightly with age older than 45 years.

Procedure

1. Draw a 5-mL sample of venous blood into a blue-topped (sodium citrate anticoagulant) Vacutainer. Label the specimen with the patient's name, date and time of collection, and test(s) ordered.
2. Use the two-tube technique. (Some methods may use lithium heparin.)

Clinical Implications

Increased prothrombin F1 + 2 is found in the following:

1. DIC (early)
2. Congenital deficiencies of AT-III
3. Congenital deficiencies of protein S and protein C
4. Leukemias
5. Severe liver disease
6. Post–myocardial infarction

NOTE *Failure to achieve a reduction in prothrombin F1 + 2 levels during oral anticoagulant therapy, despite an adequately prolonged PT, suggests inadequate anticoagulation.*

Interfering Factors

1. Levels will be high in the immediate postoperative period.
2. Decreased with oral anticoagulants (warfarin)
3. Decreased in patients treated with AT-III

Interventions

Pretest Patient Care

1. Explain test purpose and procedure.
2. Avoid prolonged use of tourniquet.
3. Follow guidelines in Chapter 1 for safe, effective, informed *pretest* care.

Posttest Patient Care

1. Review test results; report and record findings. Modify the nursing care plan as needed. Counsel the patient regarding abnormal findings; explain the need for possible follow-up testing and treatment. Monitor for DIC and thrombosis.
2. Follow guidelines in Chapter 1 for safe, effective, informed *posttest* care.
3. Resume normal activities.

● Fibrin Monomers (Protamine Sulfate Test; Fibrin Split Products)

A positive test result reflects the presence of fibrin monomers, indicative of thrombin activity and consistent with a diagnosis of intravascular coagulation. A negative result does not mean that intravascular coagulation is not present. A positive result may also be seen in some cases of severe liver disease and in inflammatory disorders caused by accumulation of products of coagulation in the circulation.

The detection of fibrin monomers and early-stage FSPs in plasma is useful in the diagnosis of DIC. Heparin therapy does not interfere with this test.

Normal Findings

Negative; no fibrin monomer present

Procedure

1. Obtain a 5-mL venous blood sample anticoagulated with sodium citrate (blue-topped tube). The two-tube technique is used.
2. Label the specimen with the patient's name, date and time of collection, and test(s) ordered.
3. Place the specimen on ice and transport to the laboratory. The test must be performed within 1 hour after collection.

Clinical Implications

1. A positive test is indicative of DIC.
2. Patients with deep vein thrombosis occasionally have positive results.
3. The test may be positive in severe liver disease or metastatic cancer.

Interfering Factors

False-positive results may occur in the following situations:

1. Traumatic venipuncture
2. During or immediately before menstruation
3. During streptokinase therapy (thrombolytic therapy)

Interventions

Pretest Patient Care

1. Explain test purpose and procedure. If possible, drain blood before heparin therapy is started.
2. Avoid prolonged use of tourniquet.
3. Follow guidelines in Chapter 1 for safe, effective, informed *pretest* care.

Posttest Patient Care

1. Review test results; report and record findings. Modify the nursing care plan as needed. Counsel the patient regarding abnormal findings; explain the need for possible follow-up testing and treatment. Monitor for DIC and thrombosis.
2. Follow guidelines in Chapter 1 for safe, effective, informed *posttest* care.
3. Resume normal activities.

• Fibrinogen

Fibrinogen is a complex protein (polypeptide) that, with enzyme action, is converted to fibrin. The fibrin, along with platelets, forms the network for the common blood clot. Although it is of primary importance as a coagulation protein, fibrinogen is also an acute-phase protein reactant. It is increased in diseases involving tissue damage or inflammation.

This test is done to investigate abnormal PT, aPTT, and TT and to screen for DIC and fibrin-fibrinogenolysis. It is part of a coagulation panel.

Normal Findings

200 to 400 mg/dL or 2.0 to 4.0 g/L

1. Values of <50 mg/dL or <0.5 g/L can result in hemorrhage after traumatic surgery.
2. Values of >700 mg/dL or >7.0 g/L constitute a significant risk for both coronary artery and cerebrovascular disease.

CLINICAL ALERT

<100 mg/dL or 1.0 g/L—possible critical value, notify the healthcare provider

Procedure

1. Obtain a 5-mL venous plasma blood sample using the two-tube technique with a collection tube containing sodium citrate (light blue–topped tube). Label the specimen with the patient's name, date and time of collection, and test(s) ordered.
2. Place the specimen in a biohazard bag.

Clinical Implications

1. *Increased* fibrinogen values occur in:
   a. Inflammation and infections (rheumatoid arthritis, pneumonia, tuberculosis, streptomycin)
   b. Acute myocardial infarction
   c. Nephrotic syndrome
   d. Cancer, multiple myeloma, Hodgkin's disease
   e. Pregnancy, eclampsia
   f. Various cerebral accidents and diseases
2. *Decreased* fibrinogen values occur in:
   a. Liver disease
   b. DIC (secondary fibrinolysis)
   c. Cancer
   d. Primary fibrinolysis
   e. Hereditary and congenital hypofibrinogenemia
   f. Dysfibrinogenemia

Interfering Factors

1. High levels of heparin interfere with test results.
2. High levels of FSP and FDP cause low fibrinogen values.
3. Oral contraceptives cause high fibrinogen values.
4. Elevated AT-III may cause decreased fibrinogen.
5. See Appendix E for other drugs that affect test outcomes.

Interventions

Pretest Patient Care

1. Explain test purpose and procedure.
2. Have the patient avoid aggressive muscular exercise before the test.
3. Follow guidelines in Chapter 1 for safe, effective, informed *pretest* care.

Posttest Patient Care

1. Review test results; report and record findings. Modify the nursing care plan as needed. Counsel the patient regarding abnormal findings; explain the need for possible follow-up testing and treatment. Monitor for DIC and response to treatment. If fibrinogen is low, cryoprecipitate is the preferred product for therapeutic replacement.
2. Follow guidelines in Chapter 1 for safe, effective, informed *posttest* care.

● Protein C (PC Antigen)

Protein C, a vitamin K–dependent protein that prevents thrombosis, is produced in the liver and circulates in the plasma. It functions as an anticoagulant by inactivating factors V and VIII. Protein C is also a profibrinolytic agent (i.e., it enhances fibrinolysis). The protein C mechanism therefore functions to prevent extension of intravascular thrombi. This test is used for evaluation of patients suspected of having congenital protein C deficiency. Resistance to protein C is caused by an inherited defect in the factor V gene (factor V Leiden) and causes significant risk for thrombosis. It is the underlying defect in up to 60% of patients with unexplained thrombosis and is the most common cause of pathologic thrombosis. If functional protein C is abnormal, a protein C resistance test should be performed.

This test evaluates patients with severe thrombosis and those with an increased risk for or predisposition to thrombosis. Patients with partial protein C or partial protein S deficiency (heterozygotes) may experience venous thrombotic episodes, usually in early adult years. There may be deep vein thromboses, episodes of thrombophlebitis or pulmonary emboli (or both), and manifestations of a hypercoagulable state. Patients who are heterozygous may have type I protein C deficiency, with decreased protein C antigen, or type II deficiency, with normal protein C antigen levels but decreased functional activity.

NOTE *The protein S level should always be determined when a protein C test is ordered.*

NOTE *Protein C resistance (factor V Leiden) should be tested in all patients with abnormal protein C activity.*

Normal Findings

Qualitative: 70% to 150% or 0.70 to 1.50 of increased functional activity
Quantitative: 60% to 125% or 0.60 to 1.25 of normal PC antigen

Procedure

1. Anticoagulate a 5-mL venous plasma blood sample with sodium citrate (light blue–topped tube). The two-tube method is used. Label the specimen with the patient's name, date and time of collection, and test(s) ordered.
2. Cap the specimen and place on ice.

Clinical Implications

1. *Decreased* protein C is associated with:
   a. Severe thrombotic complications in the neonatal period (neonatal purpura fulminans)
   b. Increased risk for venous thrombotic episodes
   c. Warfarin (Coumadin)-induced skin necroses (pathognomonic for protein C deficiency)
   d. DIC, especially when it occurs with cancer (presumably owing to consumption by cofactor thrombin–thrombomodulin catalyst activities)
   e. Thrombophlebitis and pulmonary embolism, especially in early adult years
   f. Other acquired causes of protein C deficiency include:
      (1) Liver disease
      (2) Acute respiratory distress syndrome
      (3) L-Asparaginase therapy
      (4) Malignancies
      (5) Vitamin K deficiency
2. A deficiency of protein C may also be congenital (35% to 58%).

CLINICAL ALERT

Homozygous protein C–deficient patients have absent or almost-absent protein C antigen and usually succumb in infancy with clinical presentation of purpura fulminans neonatalis, including lower extremity skin ecchymoses, anemia, fever, and shock.

Interfering Factors

1. Decreased protein C is found in the postoperative state.
2. Pregnancy or use of oral contraceptives decreases protein C.
3. A transient drop in protein C occurs with a high loading dose of warfarin (Coumadin).
4. Protein C decreases with age.
5. High doses of heparin decrease protein C.
6. Lipemic serum may interfere with the assay.

Interventions

Pretest Patient Care

1. Explain test purpose and procedure. Patient should be fasting.
2. Follow guidelines in Chapter 1 for safe, effective, informed *pretest* care.

Posttest Patient Care

1. Review test results; report and record findings. Modify the nursing care plan as needed. Counsel the patient regarding abnormal findings; explain the need for possible follow-up testing and treatment. Monitor for thrombosis. In the case of a protein C deficiency, educate the patient concerning the symptoms and implications of the disease. The risk factors include obesity, oral contraceptives, varicose veins, infection, trauma, surgery, pregnancy, immobility, and congestive heart failure.
2. Follow guidelines in Chapter 1 for safe, effective, informed *posttest* care.

● Protein S

Both protein S and protein C are dependent on vitamin K for their production and function. A deficiency of either one is associated with a tendency toward thrombosis. Protein S serves as a cofactor to enhance the anticoagulant effects of activated protein C. Slightly more than half of protein S is complexed with C4-binding protein and is inactive. Activated protein C in the presence of protein S rapidly inactivates factors V and VIII.

This test is done to differentiate acquired from congenital protein S deficiency. Congenital deficiency of protein S is associated with a high risk for thromboembolism. Acquired deficiency of protein S can be seen in various autoimmune disorders and inflammatory states owing to elevation of C4-binding protein. This protein forms an inactive complex with protein S. C4-binding protein levels should be determined in all patients who demonstrate a reduced level of protein S.

Normal Findings

Males: 60% to 130% or 0.60 to 1.30 of normal activity
Females: 50% to 120% or 0.50 to 1.20 of normal activity
Newborns: 15% to 50% or 0.15 to 0.50 of normal activity

Procedure

1. Anticoagulate a 5-mL venous blood sample with sodium citrate (blue-topped tube). The two-tube method is used. Label the specimen with the patient's name, date and time of collection, and test(s) ordered.
2. Keep the specimen capped and on ice. Place in a biohazard bag and take to the laboratory immediately.

Clinical Implications

1. *Decreased* values are associated with protein S deficiency. Familial protein S deficiency is associated with recurrent thrombosis. Abnormal plasma distribution of protein S occurs in functional

protein S deficiency. In type I, free protein S is decreased, although the level of total protein may be normal; in type II, total protein is markedly reduced.

2. Hypercoagulable-state acquired protein S deficiency is found in:
   a. Diabetic nephropathy
   b. Chronic renal failure caused by hypertension
   c. Cerebral venous thrombosis
   d. Coumarin-induced skin necrosis
   e. DIC
   f. Thrombotic thrombocytopenia purpura
   g. Acute inflammation

Interfering Factors

The following factors cause decreased protein S:

1. Heparin therapy or specimen contaminated with heparin
2. Patient on unstable warfarin (Coumadin should be discontinued for 30 days for a true protein S determination)
3. Pregnancy
4. Contraceptives (oral)
5. First month of life
6. l-Asparaginase therapy

NOTE *This test is not useful in diagnosing DIC.*

Interventions

Pretest Patient Care

1. Explain test purpose and procedure.
2. Follow guidelines in Chapter 1 for safe, effective, informed *pretest* care.

Posttest Patient Care

1. Review test results; report and record findings. Modify the nursing care plan as needed. Counsel the patient regarding abnormal findings; explain the need for possible follow-up testing and treatment. Monitor for thrombotic tendency.
2. Follow guidelines in Chapter 1 for safe, effective, informed *posttest* care.

● Antithrombin III (AT-III; Heparin Cofactor Activity)

AT-III inhibits the activity of activated factors XII, XI, IX, and X as well as factor II. AT-III is the main physiologic inhibitor of activated factor X, on which it appears to exert its most critical effect. AT-III is a "heparin cofactor." Heparin interacts with AT-III and thrombin, increasing the rate of thrombin neutralization (inhibition) but decreasing the total quantity of thrombin inhibited.

This test detects a decreased level of antithrombin that is indicative of thrombotic tendency. Only the test of functional activity gives a direct clue to thrombotic tendency. In some families, several members may have a combination of recurrent thromboembolism and reduced plasma antithrombin (30% to 60%). A significant number of patients with mesenteric venous thrombosis have AT-III deficiency. It has been recommended that patients with such thrombotic disease be screened for AT-III levels to identify those patients who may benefit from coumarin anticoagulant prophylaxis rather than heparin therapy.

Normal Findings

Functional Assay

Infants (1 to 30 days): 26% to 61% or 0.26 to 0.61 (premature); 44% to 76% or 0.44 to 0.76 (full-term)
Adults and infants older than 6 months: 80% to 120% or 0.80 to 1.20

Immunologic assay

Adults and infants older than 6 months: 17 to 30 mg/dL or 170 to 300 mg/L

Procedure

1. Anticoagulate a venous blood sample (5 mL) with sodium citrate. Mix gently.
2. Use the two-tube method. Label the specimen with the patient's name, date and time of collection, and test(s) ordered.
3. Place the sample on ice and transport to the laboratory immediately.

Clinical Implications

1. *Increased* AT-III values are associated with:
   a. Acute hepatitis
   b. Renal transplantation
   c. Inflammation, patients with increased ESR
   d. Menstruation
   e. Use of warfarin (Coumadin) anticoagulant
   f. Hyperglobulinemia
2. *Decreased* AT-III values are associated with:
   a. Congenital deficiency (hereditary)
   b. Liver transplantation and partial liver removal, cirrhosis, nephrotic syndrome, liver failure
   c. DIC, fibrinolytic disorders (not diagnostically useful)
   d. Acute myocardial infarction
   e. Active thrombotic disease (deep vein thrombosis), thrombophlebitis
   f. Carcinoma, trauma, severe inflammations
   g. Pulmonary embolism
   h. Heparin failure (low levels of AT-III exhibit heparin resistance)
   i. Protein-wasting diseases

Interfering Factors

1. Antithrombin decreases after 3 days of heparin therapy.
2. Use of oral contraceptives interferes with the test (decreased values).
3. Results are unreliable in the last trimester of pregnancy and in the early postpartum period.
4. Decreased after surgery, prolonged bed rest.
5. Decreased in L-asparaginase therapy.

Interventions

Pretest Patient Care

1. Explain test purpose and procedure.
2. Follow guidelines in Chapter 1 for safe, effective, informed *pretest* care.

Posttest Patient Care

1. Review test results; report and record findings. Modify the nursing care plan as needed. Counsel the patient regarding abnormal findings; explain the need for possible follow-up testing and treatment. Monitor for thrombotic tendency.

2. If patient has decreased levels of AT-III, coumarin anticoagulant would be used as a prophylaxis.
3. Follow guidelines in Chapter 1 for safe, effective, informed *posttest* care.

BIBLIOGRAPHY

Baglin TP: Heparin induced thrombocytopenia thrombosis (HIT/T) syndrome: Diagnosis and treatment. J Clin Pathol 54(4):272–274, 2001

Black JM, Hawks JH: Medical-Surgical Nursing: Clinical Management for Positive Outcomes, 8th ed. Philadelphia, Saunders Elsevier, 2009

Centers for Disease Control and Prevention: Get Screened to Know Your Sickle Cell Status. Available at: https://www.cdc.gov/ncbddd/sicklecell/documents/factsheet_scicklecell_status.pdf

D'Orazio P: Blood Gas and pH Analysis and Related Measurements: Approved Guideline, vol. 29, no. 8, 2nd ed. Wayne, PA, Clinical and Laboratory Standards Institute, 2009

Freeman J, Rodgers BA: Lupus: A Patient Care Guide for Nurses and Other Health Professionals, 3rd ed. Bethesda, MD, National Institutes of Health, National Institute of Arthritis and Musculoskeletal and Skin Diseases, 2006

Goldman L, Schafer AI: Goldman's Cecil Medicine, 24th ed. Philadelphia, Saunders Elsevier, 2011

Goroll AH, Mulley GA: Primary Care Medicine: Office Evaluation and Management of the Adult Patient, 7th ed. Philadelphia, Lippincott Williams & Wilkins, 2014

Greer JP, Foerster J, Rodgers GM, et al: Wintrobe's Clinical Hematology, 13th ed. Philadelphia, Lippincott Williams & Wilkins, 2013

Grossman S: Porth's Pathophysiology: Concepts of Altered Health States, 9th ed. Philadelphia, Lippincott Williams & Wilkins, 2014

Handin RI, Lux SE, Stossel TP: Blood: Principles and Practice of Hematology, 2nd ed. Philadelphia, Lippincott Williams & Wilkins, 2002

Haymond S: Oxygen saturation: A guide to laboratory assessment. Clin Lab News 10–12, 2006

Jacobs DS, DeMott WR, Oxley DK: Laboratory Test Handbook, 5th ed. Hudson, OH, Lexi-Comps Clinical Reference Library, 2001

Kjeldsberg CR, Perkins SL: Practical Diagnosis of Hematologic Disorders, 5th ed. Chicago, ASCP Press, 2010

Leavelle DE (ed): Mayo Medical Laboratories Interpretative Handbook. Rochester, MN, Mayo Clinic Laboratories, 2017

Matchar DB, Jacobson A, Dolor R, et al: Effect of home testing of international normalized ratio on clinical events. N Engl J Med 363:1608–1620, 2010

McPherson RA, Pincus MR: Henry's Clinical Diagnosis and Management by Laboratory Methods, 23rd ed. Philadelphia, Elsevier, 2016

Rodak BF, Carr JH: Clinical Hematology Atlas, 4th ed. St Louis, MO, Elsevier Saunders, 2013

Stamatoyannopoulos G, Majerus PW, Perlmutter RM, et al: The Molecular Basis of Blood Diseases, 3rd ed. Philadelphia, WB Saunders, 2001

Stedman's Medical Dictionary for the Health Professions and Nursing. Philadelphia, Lippincott Williams & Wilkins, 2012

Torn M, Cannegieter SC, Bollen WL, et al: Optimal level of oral anticoagulant therapy for the prevention of arterial thrombosis in patients with mechanical heart valve prostheses, atrial fibrillation, or myocardial infarction: A prospective study of 4202 patients. Arch Intern Med 169(13):1203–1209, 2009

Turgeon ML: Clinical Hematology: Theory and Procedures, 5th ed. Philadelphia, Lippincott Williams & Wilkins, 2011

Williamson MA, Snyder LM: Wallach's Interpretation of Diagnostic Tests, 10th ed. Philadelphia, Lippincott Williams & Wilkins, 2014

Wu AHB: Tietz Clinical Guide to Laboratory Tests, 4th ed. Philadelphia, Elsevier, 2006

Urine Studies

3

OVERVIEW OF URINE STUDIES

Urine Formation

Urine is continuously formed by the kidneys. It is an ultrafiltrate of plasma from which glucose, amino acids, water, and other substances essential to body metabolism have been reabsorbed. A complex physiologic process converts approximately 170,000 mL of filtered plasma to the average daily urine output of 1200 mL.

Urine formation takes place in the kidneys, two fist-sized organs located outside the peritoneal cavity on each side of the spine, at about the level of the last thoracic and first two lumbar vertebrae. The kidneys, together with the skin and the respiratory system, are the chief excretory organs of the body. Each kidney is a highly discriminatory organ that maintains the internal environment of the body by selective secretion or reabsorption of various substances according to specific body needs.

The main functional unit of the kidney is the nephron. There are about 1 to 1.5 million nephrons per kidney, each composed of two main parts: a glomerulus, which is essentially a filtering system, and a tubule, through which the filtered liquid passes. Each glomerulus consists of a capillary network surrounded by a membrane called *Bowman's capsule*, which continues on to form the beginning of the renal tubule. The kidney's ability to clear waste products selectively from the blood while maintaining the essential water and electrolyte balances in the body is controlled in the nephron by renal blood flow, glomerular filtration, and tubular reabsorption and secretion.

Blood is supplied to the kidney by the renal artery and enters the nephron through the afferent arteriole. It flows through the glomerulus and into the efferent arteriole. The varying size of these arterioles creates the hydrostatic pressure difference necessary for glomerular filtration and serves to maintain glomerular capillary pressure and consistent renal blood flow within the glomerulus. (The smaller size of the efferent arteriole produces an increase in the glomerular capillary pressure, which aids in urine formation.)

As the filtrate passes along the tubule, more solutes are added by excretion from the capillary blood and secretions from the tubular epithelial cells. Essential solutes and water pass back into the blood through the mechanism of tubular reabsorption. Finally, urine concentration and dilution occur in the renal medulla. The kidney has the remarkable ability to dilute or concentrate urine, according to the needs of the individual, and to regulate sodium excretion. Blood chemistry, blood pressure, fluid balance, and nutrient intake, together with the general state of health, are key elements in this entire metabolic process.

Urine Constituents

In general, urine consists of urea and other organic and inorganic chemicals dissolved in water. Considerable variations in the concentrations of these substances can occur as a result of the influence of factors such as dietary intake, physical activity, body metabolism, endocrine function, and even body position. Urea, a metabolic waste product produced in the liver from the breakdown of protein and amino acids, accounts for almost half of the total dissolved solids in urine. Other organic substances include primarily creatinine and uric acid. The major inorganic solid dissolved in urine is chloride, followed by sodium and potassium. Small or trace amounts of many additional inorganic chemicals are also present in urine. The concentrations of these inorganic compounds are greatly influenced by dietary intake, making it difficult to establish normal levels. Other substances found in urine include hormones, vitamins, and medications. Although they are not a part of the original plasma filtrate, the urine may also contain formed elements such as cells, casts, crystals, mucus, and bacteria. Increased amounts of these formed elements are often indicative of disease.

Types of Urine Specimens

During the course of 24 hours, the composition and concentration of urine changes continuously. Urine concentration varies according to water intake and pretest activities. To obtain a specimen that is truly representative of a patient's metabolic state, it is often necessary to regulate certain aspects of specimen collection, such as time of collection, length of collection period, patient's dietary and medicinal intake, and method of collection. It is important to instruct patients when special collection procedures must be followed. For additional guidelines, see Appendix A: Standard Precautions for Prevention and Control of Infection and Appendix B: Guidelines for Specimen Transport and Storage.

URINE TESTING

Urinalysis (UA) is one of the most frequently ordered tests. The results of UA are used to diagnose, treat, and provide follow-up for a variety of conditions, especially urinary tract infections (UTIs). In general, UA is obtained for symptoms of irritation, burning, pain, change in frequency of urination, or change in appearance of the urine.

UA is an essential procedure for patients undergoing hospital admission or physical examination. It is a useful indicator of a healthy or diseased state and has remained an integral part of the patient examination. Two unique characteristics of urine specimens can account for this continued popularity:

1. Urine specimens are readily available and easy to collect.
2. Urine contains information about many of the body's major metabolic functions, and this information can be obtained by simple laboratory tests.

These characteristics fit in well with the current trends toward preventive medicine and lower medical costs. By offering an inexpensive way to test large numbers of people, not only for renal disease but also for the asymptomatic beginnings of conditions such as diabetes mellitus and liver disease, the UA can be a valuable metabolic screening procedure. Urine tests can even be used to detect prostate and breast cancer markers.

Should it be necessary to determine whether a particular fluid is actually urine, the specimen can be tested for its urea and creatinine content. Both of these substances are present in much higher concentrations in urine than in other body fluids (Chart 3.1).

Laboratory Testing for Routine Urinalysis

Laboratory facilities allow for a wide range of urine tests. In a laboratory routine UA, first the physical characteristics of the urine are noted and recorded. Second, a series of chemical tests is run. A chemically impregnated dipstick can be used for many of these tests. Standardized results can be obtained by processing the urine-touched dipstick through special automated instruments. Third, the urine sediment is examined under the microscope to identify its components.

CHART 3.1 Overview of the Urinary System and Related Tests

Organs and Function

The kidneys, ureters, bladder, and urethra compose the urinary system. Kidneys must be able to excrete dietary and waste products (not eliminated by other organs) through the urine. Urine is formed within the functional unit of the kidneys, the nephron, which consists of glomeruli and tubules.

Functions of Kidney Glomerulus

Formation of filtrate

Filtration

Functions of Kidney Tubule

Secretion of waste products

Reabsorption of waste products needed by the body

Reabsorption of water, sodium chloride, bicarbonates, potassium, and calcium, among others

Functions of Kidney: Pelvis, Ureters, and Bladder

Excretion and storage of formed urine

Main urine constituents: water, urea, uric acid, creatinine, sodium, potassium, chloride, calcium, magnesium, phosphates, sulfates, and ammonia

Examples of Selective Filtration, Reabsorption, and Excretion by the Urinary System

Constituent	Filtered (g/24 hr)	Reabsorbed (g/24 hr)	Excreted (g/24 hr)
Sodium	540	537	3.3
Chloride	630	625	5.3
Bicarbonate	300	300	0.3
Potassium	28	24	3.9
Glucose	140	140	0.0
Urea	53	28	25
Creatinine	1.4	0.0	1.4
Uric acid	8.5	7.7	0.8

Dipstick Testing

Some types of tablet, tape, and dipstick tests are available for UA outside the laboratory setting. They can be used and read directly by patients and healthcare providers.

Similar in appearance to pieces of blotter paper on a plastic strip, dipsticks actually function as miniature laboratories. Chemically impregnated reagent strips provide quick determinations of pH, protein, glucose, ketones (acetone or acetoacetic acid), bilirubin, hemoglobin (blood), nitrite, leukocyte esterase, urobilinogen, and specific gravity. The dipstick is impregnated with chemicals that react with specific substances in the urine to produce color-coded visual results. The depth of color produced relates to the concentration of the substance in the urine. Color controls provided with the dipstick are compared against the actual color produced by the urine sample. The reaction times of the impregnated chemicals are standardized for each category of dipstick; it is vital that color changes be matched to the control chart at the correct elapsed time after each stick is dipped into the urine specimen. Instructions that accompany each type of dipstick outline the procedure. When more than one type of test is incorporated on a single stick (e.g., pH, protein, and glucose), the chemical reagents for each test are separated by a water-impermeable barrier made of plastic so that results do not become altered (Table 3.1). Figure 3.1 is an example of a form used to record dipstick testing results.

TABLE 3.1 Urine Testing by Dipstick/Reagent Strip

	Possible Reaction Interference		
Measurement	**False Positive**	**False Negative**	**Correlations with Other Tests**
pH	None	Runover from the protein pad may lower pH level	Nitrite Leukocytes Microscopic examination
Protein	Highly alkaline urine, ammonium compounds (antiseptics), detergents	High salt concentration	Blood Nitrite Leukocytes Microscopic examination
Glucose	Peroxide, oxidizing detergents	Ascorbic acid, 5-hydroxyindoleacetic acid, homogentisic acid, aspirin, levodopa, ketones, high specific gravity with low pH	Ketones
Ketones	Levodopa, phenylketones	None	Glucose
Blood	Oxidizing agents, vegetable and bacterial peroxidases	Ascorbic acid, nitrite, protein, pH <5.0, high specific gravity, captopril	Protein Microscopic examination
Bilirubin	Lodine, pigmented urine, indican	Ascorbic acid, nitrite	Urobilinogen
Urobilinogen	Ehrlich-reactive compounds (Multistix), medication color	Nitrite, formalin	Bilirubin
Nitrite	Pigmented urine on automated readers	Ascorbic acid, high specific gravity	Protein Leukocytes Microscopic examination
Leukocytes	Oxidizing detergents	Glucose, protein, high specific gravity, oxalic acid, gentamycin, tetracycline, cephalexin, cephalothin	Protein Nitrite Microscopic examination
Specific gravity	Protein	Alkaline urine	None

In addition to dipsticks, reagent strips, tablets, and treated slides for special determinations such as bacteria, phenylketonuria (PKU), mucopolysaccharides, salicylate, and cystinuria are available for UA.

NOTE *Tablets are becoming obsolete but are still used for certain tests, such as glucose and reducing agents.*

Procedure

1. Use a fresh urine sample within 1 hour of collection or a sample that has been refrigerated; if refrigerated, bring to room temperature and mix specimen.
2. Read or review directions for use of the reagent. Periodically check for changes in procedure.

□UA CHEMSTRIP SCREEN

Color ______________________ Clarity ______________________

Specific Gravity	□1.000	□1.005	□1.010	□1.015	□1.020	□1.025	□1.030	1.005–1.030
pH	□5	□6	□7	□8	□9			5–8
Leukocyte	□negative		□trace		□1+*	□2+*		Negative
Nitrite	□negative		□positive					Negative
Protein	□negative		□trace	□1+	□2+	□3+		Negative
Glucose	□normal		□50**	□100	□250	□500	□1000	Normal
Ketone	□negative		□1+	□2+	□3+			Negative
Urobilinogen	□normal		□01	□04	□08	□012		Normal
Bilirubin	□negative		□1+	□2+	□3+			Negative
Blood	□negative		□trace	□1+(about 50 #)	□2+(about 250)			Negative

□MICROSCOPIC URINALYSIS (performed by technologists, MD or NP only)

WBC ________ /hpf (<5/hpf) Bacteria ________ Negative

RBC ________ /hpf (<5/hpf) Casts ________ /lpf Type ________

Epi ________ /lpf Crystals ________

*arbitrary units based on the sensitivity of the reagent strip (see manufacturer's insert)

**mg/dL

#intact red blood cells/microliter

FIGURE 3.1. Urinalysis Chemstrip screen.

3. Dip a reagent strip into well-mixed urine and then remove it, blot, and compare each reagent area on the dipstick with the corresponding color control chart within the established time frame. Correlate color comparisons as closely as possible using good lighting.

Interfering Factors

1. If the dipstick is kept in the urine sample too long, the impregnated chemicals in the strip might be dissolved and could produce inaccurate readings and values.
2. If the reagent chemicals on the impregnated pad become mixed, the readings will be inaccurate. To avoid this, blot off excess urine after withdrawing the dipstick from the sample.

CLINICAL ALERT

1. Precise timing is essential. If the test is not timed correctly, color changes may produce invalid or false results.
2. When not in use, the container of dipsticks should be kept tightly closed and stored in a cool, dry environment. If the reagents absorb moisture from the air before they are used, they will not produce accurate results. A desiccant comes with the reagents and should be kept in the container.
3. Quality control protocols must be followed:
   a. The expiration date must be honored even if there is no detectable deterioration of strips.
   b. Bottles must be discarded 6 months after opening, regardless of expiration date.
   c. Known positive and negative (abnormal and normal) controls must be run for each new bottle of reagent strips when it is opened and whenever there is a question of deterioration.

COLLECTION OF URINE SPECIMENS

Standard urine specimens for UA can be collected any time, whereas first morning, fasting, and timed specimens require collection at specific times of day. Patient preparation and education needs vary according to the type of specimen required (Table 3.2) and the patient's ability to cooperate with specimen collection. Clear instructions and assessment of the patient's understanding of the process are key to a successful outcome. Assess the patient's usual urination patterns and encourage fluid intake (unless contraindicated). Provide verbal and written directions for self-collection of specimens. Assess for presence of interfering factors: Failure to follow collection instructions, inadequate fluid intake, certain medications, and patient use of illegal drugs may affect test results. Certain foods, or any type of food consumption in some instances, may also affect test results.

● Single, Random Urine Specimen

This is the most commonly requested specimen. Because the composition of urine changes over the course of the day, the time of day when the specimen is collected may influence the findings. The first voided morning specimen is particularly valuable because it is usually more concentrated and therefore more likely to reveal abnormalities as well as the presence of formed substances. It is also relatively free of dietary influences and of changes caused by physical activity because the specimen is collected after a period of fasting and rest.

Procedure

1. Instruct the patient to void directly into a clean, dry container or bedpan. Transfer the specimen directly into an appropriate container. Disposable containers are recommended. Women should always have a clean-catch specimen if a microscopic examination is ordered (see Chapter 7).
2. Collect specimens from infants and young children into a disposable collection apparatus consisting of a plastic bag with an adhesive backing around the opening that can be fastened to the perineal area or around the penis to permit voiding directly into the bag. The specimen bag is carefully removed, and the urine is transferred to an appropriate specimen container.
3. Cover all specimens tightly; label properly with the patient's name, date and time of collection, and test(s) ordered; and send immediately to the laboratory. Place the label on the cup, not on the lid.
4. Obtain a clean specimen using the same procedure as for bacteriologic examination (see Chapter 7) if a urine specimen is likely to be contaminated with drainage, vaginal discharge, or menstrual blood.
5. If a urine specimen is obtained from an indwelling catheter, it may be necessary to clamp off the catheter for about 15 to 30 minutes before obtaining the sample. Clean the specimen port in the tubing with antiseptic before aspirating the urine sample with a needle and syringe or a Luer-Lok syringe.
6. Observe standard precautions when handling urine specimens (see Appendix A).
7. If the specimen cannot be delivered to the laboratory or tested within 1 hour, it should be refrigerated or have an appropriate preservative added.

Interfering Factors

1. Feces, discharges, vaginal secretions, and menstrual blood will contaminate the urine specimen. A clean voided specimen must be obtained.
2. If the specimen is not refrigerated within 1 hour of collection, the following changes in composition may occur:
   a. Increased pH from the breakdown of urea to ammonia by urease-producing bacteria
   b. Decreased glucose from glycolysis and bacterial utilization
   c. Decreased ketones because of volatilization

TABLE 3.2 Collection of Urine by Type of Specimen[a]

Type of Specimen	Characteristics
First morning specimen	Most concentrated Free of dietary influences Bladder-incubated Formed elements may disintegrate if pH is high and/or specific gravity is low Best for nitrate, protein, pregnancy tests, microscopic examination, routine screening
Random specimen	Most common Most convenient Collected any time Good for chemical screening, routine screening, microscopic examination
Clean-catch (midstream)	Minimizes bacterial counts Used for random collection and bacterial culture
Second (double-voided) specimen	The first morning specimen is discarded; the second specimen is collected and tested Used for diabetic monitoring Reflects blood glucose/usually fasting; less concentrated urine Formed elements remain intact Accurately reflects components
Postprandial	Used for glucose determination, diabetic monitoring Collected 2 hr after a meal
Timed	Requires collection at certain time Total specimen must be collected
Timed 2-hr volume	Used for urobilinogen determination All urine saved for 2-hr period
Timed 24-hr volume	Necessary for accurate quantitative results Chemical testing All urine saved for 24-hr period
Catheter specimen	Used for bacterial culture Clamp catheter 15–30 min before collection Cleanse sample port with alcohol Insert needle into sample port; after aspirating sample, transfer to specimen container ALERT: Unclamp catheter
Suprapubic aspiration	Sterile bladder urine Used for bacterial culture cytology

[a]Place urine specimens in a biohazard bag.

d. Decreased bilirubin from exposure to light
e. Decreased urobilinogen as a result of its oxidation to urobilin
f. Increased nitrite from bacterial reduction of nitrate
g. Increased bacteria from bacterial reproduction
h. Increased turbidity caused by bacterial growth and possible precipitation of amorphous material
i. Disintegration of red blood cells (RBCs) and casts, particularly in dilute alkaline urine
j. Changes in color caused by oxidation or reduction of metabolites

● Long-Term, Timed Urine Specimen (2-Hour, 24-Hour)

Some diseases or conditions require a second morning specimen or a 2-hour or 24-hour urine specimen to evaluate kidney function accurately (see Table 3.2). Substances excreted by the kidney are not excreted at the same rate or in the same amounts during different periods of the day and night; therefore, a random urine specimen might not give an accurate picture of the processes taking place over a 24-hour period. For measurement of total urine protein, creatinine, electrolytes, and so forth, more accurate information is obtained from a long-term specimen. All urine voided in a 24-hour period is collected into a suitable receptacle; depending on the intended test, a preservative is added, the collection is kept refrigerated, or both (Table 3.3).

Procedure

1. Ask the patient to void at the beginning of a 24-hour timed urine specimen collection (or any other timed specimen collection). *Discard* this first specimen and note the time.
2. Mark the time the test begins and the time the collection should end on the container. As a reminder, it may be helpful to post a sign above the toilet (e.g., "24-Hour Collection in Progress"), with the beginning and ending times noted.
3. Collect all urine voided over the next 24 hours into a large container (usually glass or polyethylene) and label it with the patient's name, the time frame for collection, the test ordered, and other pertinent information. It is not necessary to measure the volume of individual voidings, unless specifically ordered.
4. Ask the patient to void 24 hours after the first voiding to conclude the collection. Add urine from this last voiding to the specimen in the container.
5. Storage
   a. Keep nonrefrigerated samples in a specified area or in the patient's bathroom.
   b. Refrigerate the collection bottle immediately after the patient has voided or place it into an iced container if refrigeration is necessary.

NOTE *Because the patient may not always be able to void on request, the last specimen should be obtained as closely as possible to the stated end-time of the test.*

Special Considerations

1. In a healthcare facility, responsibility for the collection of urine specimens should be specifically assigned.
2. When instructing a patient about 24-hour urine collections, make certain the patient understands that the bladder must be emptied just before the 24-hour collection starts and that this preliminary specimen must be discarded; then, all urine voided until the ending time is saved.
3. Do not predate and pretime requisitions for serial collections. It is difficult for some patients to void at specific times. Instead, mark the actual times of collection on containers.
4. Documentation of the exact times at which the specimens are obtained is crucial to many urine tests.
5. Instruct the patient to urinate as near to the end of the collection period as possible.
6. When a preservative is added to the collection container (e.g., HCl preservative in 24-hour urine collection for vanillylmandelic acid [VMA]), the patient must take precautions against splashing or spilling the contents and receiving an acid burn. Provide instructions regarding spillage before the test begins.
7. The preservative used is determined by the urine substance to be tested for. The laboratory usually provides the container and the proper preservative when the test is ordered. If in doubt, verify this with the laboratory personnel.

TABLE 3.3 24-Hour Collection: Standards for Timed Urine Specimen Collection

Test Element and Purpose	Preservative	Specimen Handling and Storage
Acid mucopolysaccharides (inherited enzyme deficiency in infants with mental retardation or failure to thrive)	20 mL of toluene (add at start of collection)	Refrigerate during collection; include patient's age
Aldosterone (cause of hypertension)	1 g of boric acid per 100 mL of urine	Refrigerate
Amino acids, quantitative (aminoaciduria, screen for inborn errors of metabolism and genetic abnormalities)	None	Refrigerate during collection
Aminolevulinic acid (porphyria and lead poisoning)	25 mL of 50% acetic acid; for children $<$5 yr, use 15 mL of 50% acetic acid	Refrigerate or ice; protect from light
Amylase (differentiates acute pancreatitis from other abdominal diseases)	None	Refrigerate during collection
Arsenic (arsenic poisoning—occupational exposure)	20 mL of 6N HNO_3 in a metal-free container	Refrigerate during collection
Cadmium (toxic levels, including occupational exposure)	20 mL of 6N HNO_3 in a metal-free container	Refrigerate during collection
Calcium, quantitative Sulkowitch (hypercalciuria as in hyperparathyroidism, hyperthyroidism, vitamin D toxicity, Paget's disease, osteolytic diseases, and renal tubular acidosis)	30 mL of 6N HCl	Refrigerate during collection
Catecholamine fractions, urinary free catecholamines (measure adrenomedullary function to diagnose pheochromocytoma)	25 mL of 50% acetic acid; for children $<$5 yr, use 15 mL of 50% acetic acid	Refrigerate or freeze, pH 1–3
Chloride (electrolyte imbalance, dehydration, metabolic alkalosis)	None	Refrigerate during collection
Chromium (toxic levels, including occupational exposure)	20 mL of 6N HNO_3 in a metal-free container	Refrigerate
Citrate/citric acid (renal disease)	10 g of boric acid	Refrigerate
Copper (Wilson's disease)	20 mL of 6N HNO_3 in a metal-free container	Refrigerate during collection
Cortisol, free (hydrocortisone levels in adrenal hormone function)	30 mL of 6N HCl	Refrigerate during collection
Creatinine (to evaluate disorders of kidney function)	None	Refrigerate during collection
Creatinine clearance (measures kidney function, primarily glomerular filtration)	None	Refrigerate during collection
Cyclic adenosine monophosphate	None	Refrigerate during collection; freeze a portion after collection
Cystine, quantitative (to diagnose cystinuria, inherited disease characterized by bladder calculi)	20 mL of toluene	Refrigerate during collection, pH 2–3; if not acidified, freeze
Δ-Aminolevulinic acid (porphyria and lead poisoning)	30 mL of 33% glacial acetic acid	Protect from light; refrigerate during collection

table continues on pg. 189 >

TABLE 3.3, continued

Test Element and Purpose	Preservative	Specimen Handling and Storage
Electrolytes, sodium, potassium (electrolyte imbalance)	None, or 1.0 g of boric acid	Refrigerate
Estriol, estradiol (menstrual and fertility problems, male feminization characteristics, estrogen-producing tumors, and pregnancy)	1.0 g of boric acid	Refrigerate during collection
Estrogens, total, nonpregnancy or third trimester (estrogen levels for menstrual and fertility problems, pregnancy and estrogen-producing tumors)	1.0 g of boric acid	Refrigerate during collection
Follicle-stimulating/luteinizing hormone (gonadotropic hormones, follicle-stimulating hormone and luteinizing hormone to determine cause of gonadal deficiency)	1.0 g of boric acid or none	Store frozen
Glucose (glucosuria to screen, confirm, or monitor diabetes mellitus, rapid intestinal absorption)	1.0 g of boric acid or NaF	Store in dark bottle
Histamine (chronic myelogenous leukemia, carcinoids, polycythemia vera)	None	Refrigerate; freeze portion after collection
Homogentisic acid	None	Freeze portion after collection
Homovanillic acid (to diagnose neuroblastoma, pheochromocytoma, ganglioblastoma)	15 mL of 50% acetic acid <5 yr, 25 mL of 50% acetic acid >5 yr, to maintain pH 2.0–4.0	Refrigerate during collection
17-Hydroxycorticosteroids (adrenal function by measuring urine excretion of steroids to diagnose endocrine disturbances of the adrenal androgens, Cushing's, Addison's, and so forth)	1.0 g of boric acid	Refrigerate, pH 5–7; freeze portion after collection
5-Hydroxyindoleacetic acid, serotonin (carcinoid tumors)	15 mL of 50% acetic acid <5 yr, 25 mL of 50% acetic acid >5 yr, to maintain pH 2.0–4.0	Refrigerate during collection; freeze portion after collection
Hydroxyproline, free (measures the free hydroxyproline [<10% normally]; rapid growth and increased collagen turnover)	10 mL of 6N HCl per liter of urine, maintain pH <3	Refrigerate during collection; store frozen
Hydroxyproline, total 24-hr collection (bone collagen reabsorption and the degree of bone destruction from bone tumors)	10 mL of 6N HCl per liter of urine, maintain pH <3	Refrigerate during collection; use gelatin-free and low-collagen diet
Immunofixation electrophoresis (measures immune status and competence by identifying monoclonal and particle protein band immunoglobulins)	None	Refrigerate
κ and γ chains quantitative, also in serum (monoclonal gammopathies, myeloma tumor burden)	None	Refrigerate

table continues on pg. 190 >

TABLE 3.3, continued

Test Element and Purpose	Preservative	Specimen Handling and Storage
17-Ketogenic steroids (Porter-Silber and Cushing's syndrome, adrenogenital syndrome)	1.0 g of boric acid	Do not refrigerate
17-Ketosteroid, fractions (adrenal and gonadal abnormalities)	1.0 g of boric acid	Do not refrigerate
Lead (lead poisoning and chelation therapy)	20 mL of 6N HNO_3 in a metal-free container	Refrigerate
Lipase (acute pancreatitis and to differentiate pancreatitis from other abdominal disorders)	None	Refrigerate
Lysozyme, muramidase (to differentiate acute myelogenous or monocytic leukemia from acute lymphatic leukemia)	None	Refrigerate
Magnesium (magnesium metabolism, electrolyte status, and nephrolithiasis)	20 mL of 6N HCl in a metal-free container	Refrigerate
Manganese (toxicity, parenteral nutrition)	None	Refrigerate during collection
Mercury (toxicity, industrial and dental overexposure; inorganic mercury)	20 mL of 6N HNO_3 in a metal-free container	Refrigerate; pH 2 with nitric acid
Metanephrine, total (assays of catecholamines and vanillylmandelic acid; frequently to diagnose pheochromocytoma)	30 mL of 6N HCl	pH 1–3
Metanephrine, fractions (to diagnose and monitor pheochromocytoma and ganglioneuroblastoma)	30 mL of 6N HCl, final pH <3	Refrigerate; no caffeine before or during testing
Metanephrine, total (pheochromocytoma, children with neuroblastoma, ganglioneuroma)	25 mL of 50% acetic acid; for children <5 yr, use 15 mL of 50% acetic acid, or 30 mL of 6N HCl	Refrigerate; no caffeine before or during testing
MHPG (3-methoxy-4-hydroxyphenylglycol) (to classify bipolar manic depression for drug therapy)	None	Refrigerate, ship frozen
Microalbumin, 24-hr (diabetic nephropathy)	None	Refrigerate
Osmolality, 24-hr (diabetes insipidus, primary polydipsia)	None	Refrigerate
Oxalate (nephrolithiasis and inflammatory bowel diseases)	20 mL of 6N HCl	Refrigerate, pH 2–3
Phosphorous, 24-hr (renal losses; hyperparathyroidism and hypoparathyroidism)	Acid-washed, detergent-free container	Refrigerate during collection; acidify after collection
Porphobilinogens	None	Refrigerate during collection; freeze a portion; protect from light
Porphyrins, quantitative (to diagnose porphyrias and lead poisoning)	5 g of sodium carbonate (do not use sodium bicarbonate)	Refrigerate; protect specimen from light

table continues on pg. 191 >

TABLE 3.3, continued

Test Element and Purpose	Preservative	Specimen Handling and Storage
Porphyrins (to diagnose porphyrias and lead poisoning)	None (preservative is added on receipt in laboratory)	Refrigerate; protect specimen from light
Potassium, 24-hr (electrolyte imbalance, renal and adrenal disorders)	None	Refrigerate during collection
Pregnanediol, 24-hr (measures ovarian and placental function)	Boric acid	Refrigerate during collection
Pregnanetriol (adrenogenital syndrome)	25 mL of 50% acetic acid; for children <5 yr, use 15 mL of 50% acetic acid	Refrigerate during collection; pH 4–4.5 after receipt in laboratory
Protein electrophoresis, 24-hr	None	Refrigerate
Protein, total (proteinuria, differential diagnosis of renal disease)	None	Refrigerate during collection
Selenium (nutritional deficiency, industrial exposure)	None	Refrigerate; transport entire specimen to laboratory
Sodium, 24-hr (electrolyte imbalance, acute renal failure, oliguria and hyponatremia, sodium excreted for diagnosis of renal and adrenal imbalances)	None	Refrigerate during collection
Substance abuse screen (specific drugs and alcohol involved in substance abuse)	None	Refrigerate or freeze
Thallium (thallium toxicity, occupational exposure)	None	Refrigerate
Thiocyanate (short-term nitroprusside therapy, cyanide poisoning)	None	Refrigerate during collection
Total protein (renal disease)	None	Refrigerate during collection
Urea nitrogen, 24-hr (kidney function, hyperalimentation)	10 g of boric acid	Refrigerate
Uric acid, 24-hr (uric acid metabolism in gout and renal calculus formation)	None	Refrigerate during collection
Urobilinogen (liver function and liver cell damage)	5 g of sodium carbonate and 100 mL of petroleum ether (do not use sodium bicarbonate)	Refrigerate during collection; protect specimen from light; check with laboratory
Vanillylmandelic acid, quantitative (adrenomedullary pheochromocytoma, hypertension)	15 mL of 50% acetic acid <5 yr, 25 mL of 50% acetic acid >5 yr	Refrigerate, pH 1–3; protect from light
Zinc (industrial exposure, toxicity, nutritional, acrodermatitis enteropathica)	20 mL of 6N HNO_3 in a metal-free container	Refrigerate

Interfering Factors

1. Failure of patient or attending personnel to follow the procedure is the most common source of error.
   a. The patient should be given both verbal and written instructions. If the patient is unable to comprehend these directions, a significant other should be instructed in the process.
   b. If required, the proper preservative must be used.
2. Instruct the patient to use toilet paper *after* transferring the urine to the 24-hour collection container. Toilet paper placed in the specimen decreases the actual amount of urine available and contaminates the specimen.
3. The presence of feces contaminates the specimen. Patients should void first and transfer the urine to the collection receptacle before defecating.
4. If heavy menstrual flow or other discharges or secretions are present, the test may have to be postponed, or an indwelling catheter may need to be inserted to keep the specimen free of contamination. In some cases, thorough cleansing of the perineal or urethral area before voiding may be sufficient. If in doubt, communicate with laboratory personnel and the healthcare provider who ordered the test.

Interventions

Pretest Patient Care

Most 24-hour urine specimen collections start in the early morning at about 7:00 a.m. (0700). Instruct the patient to do the following:

1. Empty the bladder completely on awakening and then discard that urine specimen. Record the time the voided specimen is discarded and the time the test is begun.
2. Save all urine voided during the next 24 hours, including the first specimen voided the next morning.
3. Add the urine voided the next morning (as close to the ending time as possible) to the collection container. The 24-hour test is then terminated, and the ending time is recorded.
4. Use a urinal, wide-mouth container, special toilet device, or bedpan to catch urine. It is probably easier for women to void into another wide-mouth receptacle first and then to transfer the entire specimen *carefully* to the collection bottle.
5. It is most important that *all* urine be saved in the 24-hour container. Ideally, the container should be refrigerated or placed on ice.
6. Test results are calculated on the basis of a 24-hour output. Unless *all* urine is saved, results will not be accurate. Moreover, these tests are usually expensive, complicated, and necessary for the evaluation and treatment of the patient's condition.
7. If the laboratory requests an aliquot, record total amount, mix well, and aliquot the requested amount.
8. Always check with your laboratory as to the preservative needed; different laboratories may have different requirements.
9. Follow guidelines in Chapter 1 for safe, effective, informed *pretest* care.

Posttest Patient Care

1. Review test results; report and record findings. Modify the nursing care plan as needed.
2. Follow guidelines in Chapter 1 for safe, effective, informed *posttest* care.

ROUTINE URINALYSIS (UA) AND RELATED TESTS

The process of UA determines the following properties of urine: color, odor, turbidity, specific gravity, pH, glucose, ketones, blood, protein, bilirubin, urobilinogen, nitrite, leukocyte esterase, and other abnormal constituents revealed by microscopic examination of the urine sediment. A 10-mL urine specimen is usually sufficient for conducting these tests (Table 3.4).

Figure 3.2 shows sample reports of routine UA and culture sensitivity.

TABLE 3.4 Normal Values in Urinalysis

General Characteristics and Measurements	Chemical Determinations	Microscopic Examination of Sediment
Color: pale yellow to amber	Glucose: negative	Casts negative: occasional hyaline casts
Appearance: clear to slightly hazy	Ketones: negative	Red blood cells: negative or rare
Specific gravity: 1.005–1.025 with a normal fluid intake	Blood: negative	Crystals: negative (none)
pH: 4.5–8.0; average person has a pH of about 5–6	Protein: negative	White blood cells: negative or rare
Volume: 600–2500 mL/24 hr; average 1200 mL/24 hr	Bilirubin: negative	Epithelial cells: few; hyaline casts 0–1/lpf
	Urobilinogen: 0.5–4.0 mg/d	
	Nitrite for bacteria: negative	
	Leukocyte esterase: negative	

lpf, low-power field.

Urine Volume

Urine volume measurements are part of the assessment for fluid balance and kidney function. The normal volume of urine voided by the average adult in a 24-hour period ranges from 600 to 2500 mL; the typical amount is about 1200 mL. The amount voided over any period is directly related to the individual's fluid intake, the temperature and climate, and the amount of perspiration that occurs. Children void smaller quantities than adults, but the total volume voided is greater in proportion to their body size.

The volume of urine produced at night is <700 mL, making the day-to-night ratio approximately 2:1 to 4:1.

Urine volume depends on the amount of water excreted by the kidneys. Water is a major body constituent; therefore, the amount excreted is usually determined by the body's state of hydration. Factors that influence urine volume include fluid intake, fluid loss from nonrenal sources, variations in the secretion of antidiuretic hormone (ADH), and the necessity to excrete increased amount of solutes such as glucose or salts. *Polyuria* is marked increase of urine production. *Oliguria* is decreased urinary output. The extreme form of this process is *anuria*, a total lack of urine production.

Normal Findings

Children: 500 to 1400 mL/24 hours or 500 to 1400 mL/day
Adults: 800 to 2500 mL/24 hours or 800 to 2500 mL/day

Procedure

1. Collect a 24-hour urine specimen and keep it refrigerated or on ice.
2. Record the exact collection starting time and collection ending time on the specimen container and in the patient's healthcare record. Discard first voided urine and include the last voided urine.
3. Transfer the specimen container to the laboratory refrigerator when the collection is completed. Complete the proper forms and document accordingly.

An 82-year-old female resident displayed the following signs and symptoms related to a urinary tract infection: high fever (101.0°F) for 24 hours; lethargy past 2 days; cloudy, foul-smelling urine; and dysuria. Urinalysis, microscopic exam, and culture sensitivity were ordered.

A. URINALYSIS

Interpretation of test results for routine urinalysis and urine culture with interventions.

Urinalysis Report:

Macroscopic Analysis	Normal	Date: 06/16/10 Time: 2130
Color	Pale yellow-amber	Yellow
Clarity	Clear to slightly hazy	Cloudy*
Urine chemistries		
Specific gravity	1.005–1.030	1.0–2.0*
Glucose	Negative	Negative
Ketones	Negative	Negative
pH	5.0–8.0	8.5 High
Protein	Negative	30*
Blood	Negative	Small*
Bilirubin	Negative	Negative
Urobilinogen	0.2–1.0 EU/dL	0.2
Nitrite	Negative	Pos*
Leukocyte ester	Negative	Small
Microscopic examination		
BACT/hpf	None	4+*
WBC/hpf	0–2	50–100
RBC/hpf	0–2	2–5*
SQ EPITH/lpf	0–2	10–20*
Casts/lpf	None	Present*
Hyaline/lpf	Occasional	2–5*
Triple Phos	None	Few* (occurs in alkaline, neutral, or slightly acid urine)

* = abnormal, HPF = high-powered field, LPF = low-powered field, NEG = negative, BACT = bacteria, WBC = white blood cells, RBC = red blood cells, SPEC = specific (as in specific gravity), POS = positive, TRC = trace, ABN = abnormal, EU = Ehrlich units, MIC = minimum inhibitory concentration (the lowest concentration of the antibiotic that inhibits the organism's growth), S = sensitive or susceptible, R = resistant, TMP-SMX = trimethoprim sulfamethoxazole

FIGURE 3.2. Sample reports of routine urinalysis **(A)** and culture sensitivity **(B)**.

4. Ascertain volume by measuring the entire urine amount in a graduated and appropriately calibrated pitcher or other receptacle. The total volume is recorded as urine volume in milliliters (cubic centimeters) per 24 hours.

Clinical Implications

1. *Polyuria* (increased urine output) with elevated blood urea nitrogen (BUN) and creatinine levels
   a. Diabetic ketoacidosis
   b. Partial obstruction of urinary tract
   c. Some types of tubular necrosis

B. Urine Culture Antibiotic Drug Sensitivity and Organism Susceptibility
Collected: 06/16/10—Time 2130
Received: 06/17/10—Time 1006

Final Report—6/19/10 of antibiotic drug sensitivity and organism susceptibility
>100,000 colonies/mL *Streptococcus agalactiae,* Group B hemolytic
>100,000 colonies/mL *Escherichia coli*
Susceptibility Testing—*E. coli*
S = sensitivity or susceptibility; R = resistant; TMP-SMX = trimethoprim sulfamethoxazole

	Interpretation of Organism Susceptibility to Antibiotic	Minimum Inhibitory Concentration (MIC) (the lowest concentration of antibiotic that inhibits the organism's growth)
Ampicillin	S	2
Piperacillin	S	<8
Ampicill/Sulbac	S	≤8/4
Cefazolin	S	<8
Gentamicin	S	≤1
Tobramycin	S	≤1
Tetracycline	S	2
Ciprofloxacin	S	≤1
Levofloxacin	S	<2
Nitrofurantoin	S	<32
TMP-SMX Bactrim	S	≤5/9.5

Results of the tests were abnormal outcomes and the following interventions started on 06/19/10 with Bactrim DS (double strength) BID × 7 days; then Bactrim SS (single strength) every day until further orders; force fluids as appropriate. Repeat urinalysis and culture and sensitivity in 2 weeks. The rationale for Bactrim as drug of choice was because of both sensitivity and MIC.

FIGURE 3.2. Continued

2. *Polyuria* with normal BUN and creatinine
   a. Diabetes mellitus and diabetes insipidus
   b. Neurotic states (compulsive water drinking)
   c. Certain tumors of brain and spinal cord
3. *Oliguria* (50 to 400 mL in adults, or <15 to 20 mL/kg in children per 24 hours)
   a. Renal causes
      (1) Renal ischemia
      (2) Renal disease due to toxic agents
      (3) Glomerulonephritis
   b. Dehydration caused by prolonged vomiting, diarrhea, excessive diaphoresis, or burns
   c. Obstruction (mechanical) of some area of the urinary tract or system
   d. Cardiac insufficiency
4. *Anuria* (<50 mL in 24 hours)
   a. Complete urinary tract obstruction
   b. Acute cortical necrosis
   c. Glomerulonephritis (acute, necrotizing)
   d. Acute tubular necrosis
   e. Hemolytic transfusion reaction

Interfering Factors

1. Polyuria
   a. Intravenous glucose or saline
   b. Pharmacologic agents such as thiazides and other diuretics
   c. Coffee, alcohol, tea, caffeine
2. Oliguria
   a. Water deprivation, dehydration
   b. Excessive salt intake

Interventions

Pretest Patient Care

1. Explain purpose of test, procedure for urine collection, and interfering factors.
2. Advise patient to avoid excessive fluid intake and to eliminate caffeine and alcohol. Determine the patient's usual liquid intake and request that intake not be increased beyond this daily amount during testing.
3. Advise the patient to void salty foods and added salt in the diet.
4. Obtain healthcare provider's approval to withhold diuretics for 3 days before specimen collection, if possible
5. Follow guidelines in Chapter 1 for safe, effective, informed *pretest* care.

Posttest Patient Care

1. Patient may resume normal diet, fluid intake, and medications, unless specifically ordered otherwise.
2. Review test results; report and record findings. Modify the nursing care plan as needed. Counsel the patient regarding abnormal findings.
3. Follow guidelines in Chapter 1 for safe, effective, informed *posttest* care.

● Urine Specific Gravity (SG)

Specific gravity (SG) is a measurement of the kidneys' ability to concentrate urine. The test compares the density of urine against the density of distilled water, which has an SG of 1.000. Because urine is a solution of minerals, salts, and compounds dissolved in water, the SG is a measure of the density of the dissolved chemicals in the specimen. As a measurement of specimen density, SG is influenced by both the number of particles present and the size of the particles. Osmolality is a more exact measurement and may be needed in certain circumstances.

The range of urine SG depends on the state of hydration and varies with urine volume and the load of solids to be excreted under standardized conditions; when fluid intake is restricted or increased, SG measures the concentrating and diluting functions of the kidney. Loss of these functions is an indication of renal dysfunction.

Normal Findings

Normal hydration and volume: 1.005 to 1.030 (usually between 1.010 and 1.025)
Concentrated urine: ≥1.025
Dilute urine: 1.001 to 1.010
Infant <2 years old: 1.001 to 1.006

NOTE *Specific gravity should be corrected for protein (increases SG 0.001 per 0.4 g/dL) and glucose (increases SG 0.004 per 10 g/L).*

Procedure

There are three methods of determining SG:

1. A multiple-test *dipstick* has a separate reagent area for SG. An indicator changes color in relation to ionic concentration, and this result is translated into a value for SG.
2. A *refractometer,* or total solids meter, is used to determine the specimen's refractive index, or the ratio of the velocity of light in air to the velocity of light in the test solution. A drop of urine is placed on a clear glass plate of the refractometer, and another plate is pressed on top of the urine sample. The path of light is deviated when it enters the solution, and the degree of deviation (refraction) is directly proportional to the density of the solution.
3. A *urinometer* (hydrometer) is the least accurate method. It consists of a bulb-shaped instrument that contains a scale calibrated in SG readings. Urine (10 to 20 mL) is transferred into a small test tube–like cylinder, and the urinometer is floated in the urine. The SG is read off the urinometer at the meniscus level of the urine. This method is becoming obsolete owing to the ease of dipstick testing.

Specimen collection:

1. For regular UA testing, about 20 mL of a random sample is needed (UA including SG).
2. When a special evaluation of SG is ordered separately from the UA, the patient should fast for 12 hours before specimen collection.

Clinical Implications

1. *Normal SG:* SG values usually vary inversely with the amount of urine excreted (decreased urine volume = increased SG). However, this relationship is not valid in certain conditions, including:
   a. Diabetes—increased urine volume, increased SG
   b. Hypertension—normal volume, decreased SG
   c. Early chronic renal disease—increased volume, decreased SG
2. *Hyposthenuria* (low SG, 1.001 to 1.010) occurs in the following conditions:
   a. Diabetes insipidus (low SG with large urine volume). It is caused by absence or decrease of ADH, a hormone that triggers kidney absorption of water. Without ADH, the kidneys produce excessive amounts of urine that are not reabsorbed (sometimes 15 to 20 L/day).
   b. Glomerulonephritis and pyelonephritis. SG can be low in glomerulonephritis, with decreased urine volume. Tubular damage affects the kidneys' ability to concentrate urine.
   c. Severe renal damage with disturbance of both concentrating and diluting abilities of urine. The SG is low (1.010) and fixed (varying little from specimen to specimen); this is termed *isosthenuria*.
3. *Hypersthenuria* (increased SG, 1.025 to 1.035) occurs in the following conditions:
   a. Diabetes mellitus
   b. Nephrosis
   c. Excessive water loss (due to dehydration, fever, vomiting, diarrhea)
   d. Increased secretion of ADH and diuretic effects related to the stress of a surgical procedure
   e. Congestive heart failure
   f. Toxemia of pregnancy

Interfering Factors

1. Radiopaque x-ray contrast media, minerals, and dextran may cause falsely high SG readings on the refractometer. The reagent dipstick method is not affected by high-molecular-weight substances. SG >1.040 suggests radiopaque contrast material is in the urine.
2. Temperature of urine specimens affects SG; cold specimens produce falsely high values using the hydrometer.

3. Highly buffered alkaline urine may also cause low readings (with dipsticks only).
4. Elevated readings may occur in the presence of moderate amounts of protein (100 to 750 mg/dL) or with patients receiving intravenous albumin.
5. Detergent residue (on specimen containers) can produce elevated SG results.
6. Diuretics and antibiotics cause high readings.
7. See Appendix E for drugs that affect test outcomes.

Intervention

Pretest Patient Care

1. Explain purpose of test, procedure for urine collection, and interfering factors.
2. Follow guidelines in Chapter 1 for safe, effective, informed *pretest* care.

Posttest Patient Care

1. Review test results; report and record findings. Modify the nursing care plan as needed. Counsel the patient regarding abnormal findings. Monitor appropriately for conditions associated with altered SG.
2. Follow guidelines in Chapter 1 for safe, effective, informed *posttest* care.

● Urine Osmolality

Osmolality, a more exact measurement of urine concentration than SG, depends on the number of particles of solute in a unit of solution. More information concerning renal function can be obtained if serum and urine osmolality tests are run at the same time. The normal ratio between urine and serum osmolality is 3:1. A high urine-to-serum ratio is seen with concentrated urine. With poor concentrating ability, the ratio is low.

Whenever a precise measurement is indicated to evaluate the concentrating and diluting ability of the kidney, this test is done. Urine osmolality during water restriction is an accurate test of decreased kidney function. It is also used to monitor the course of renal disease; to monitor fluid and electrolyte therapy; to establish the differential diagnosis of hypernatremia, hyponatremia, and polyuria; and to evaluate the renal response to ADH.

Normal Findings

24-hour specimen: 300 to 900 mOsm/kg of H_2O
Random specimen: 50 to 1200 mOsm/kg of H_2O
Urine-to-serum ratio: 1:1 to 3:1

Procedure

1. Inform the patient whether the test will be a done using a random specimen or 24-hour urine specimen.
2. For the 24-hour test, follow procedure for Long Term, Timed Urine Specimen (2-Hour, 24-Hour).
3. Simultaneous determination of serum osmolality may be done. A high urine-to-serum ratio is seen with concentrated urine.

Clinical Implications

1. Osmolality is *increased* in:
   a. Prerenal azotemia
   b. Congestive heart failure
   c. Addison's disease
   d. Syndrome of inappropriate antidiuretic hormone secretion (SIADH)
   e. Dehydration
   f. Amyloidosis
   g. Hyponatremia

2. Osmolality is *decreased* in:
   a. Acute renal failure
   b. Diabetes insipidus
   c. Hypokalemia
   d. Hypernatremia
   e. Primary polydipsia
   f. Hypercalcemia
   g. Compulsive water drinking (causing increased fluid intake)
3. Urine-to-serum ratio is:
   a. *Increased* in prerenal azotemia
   b. *Decreased* in acute tubular necrosis

Interfering Factors

1. Intravenous sodium administration
2. Intravenous dextrose and water administration

Interventions

Pretest Patient Care

1. Explain purpose of test, procedure for urine collection, and interfering factors.
2. To increase sensitivity of the osmolality test, a fasting urine specimen may be collected, which requires a high-protein diet for 3 days before the test. On the day before the test, no liquids should be taken with the evening meal, and no food or liquids should be taken after the evening meal until collection. Check with your laboratory if the patient has diabetes.
3. Follow guidelines in Chapter 1 for safe, effective, informed *pretest* care.

Posttest Patient Care

1. Provide patient with food and fluids as soon as the last urine sample is obtained.
2. Review test results; report and record findings. Modify the nursing care plan as needed. Counsel the patient regarding abnormal findings. Monitor appropriately.
3. Follow guidelines in Chapter 1 for safe, effective, *posttest* care.

● Urine Appearance

The first observation made about a urine specimen is usually its appearance, which generally refers to the clarity of the specimen.

Cloudy urine signals a possible abnormal constituent, such as white blood cells (WBCs), RBCs, or bacteria. Cloudy urine may also be due to normal urinary components within the bladder, which can be caused by a change in urine pH. Alkaline urine may appear cloudy because of phosphates; acid urine may appear cloudy because of urates.

Normal Findings

Fresh urine is clear to slightly hazy.

Procedure

1. Observe the clarity of a fresh urine sample by visually examining a well-mixed specimen in front of a light source.
2. Use common terms to report appearance, including the following: clear, hazy, slightly cloudy, cloudy, turbid, and milky.
3. Document results. The degree of turbidity should correspond to the amount of material observed under the microscope.

Clinical Implications

1. Pathologic urines are often turbid or cloudy; however, normal urine can also appear cloudy.
2. Urine turbidity may result from UTIs.
3. Urine may be cloudy because of the presence of RBCs, WBCs, epithelial cells, or bacteria.

Interfering Factors

1. After ingestion of food, urates, carbonates, or phosphates may produce cloudiness in normal urine on standing.
2. Semen or vaginal discharges mixed with urine are common causes of turbidity.
3. Fecal contamination causes turbidity.
4. Extraneous contamination (e.g., talcum powder, vaginal creams, radiographic contrast media) can cause turbidity.
5. "Greasy" cloudiness may be caused by large amounts of fat.
6. Often, normal urine develops a haze or turbidity after refrigeration or standing at room temperature because of precipitation of crystals of calcium oxalate or uric acid.

● Urine Color

The yellow color of urine is caused by the presence of the pigment urochrome, a product of metabolism that under normal conditions is produced at a constant rate. The actual amount of urochrome produced depends on the body's metabolic state, with increased amounts being produced in thyroid conditions and fasting states.

Urine specimens may vary in color from pale yellow to dark amber. Variations in the yellow color are related to the body's state of hydration. The darker amber color may be directly related to the urine concentration or SG.

Normal Findings

The normal color of urine is pale yellow to amber.

Straw-colored (almost colorless) urine is normal and indicates a low SG, usually <1.010. (The exception may be a patient with an elevated blood glucose concentration, whose urine is very pale yellow but has a high SG.)

Amber-colored urine is normal and indicates a high SG and a small output of urine.

Procedure

Observe and record the color of freshly voided urine.

Clinical Implications

1. *Straw-colored* (almost colorless) urine
   a. Large fluid intake
   b. Chronic interstitial nephritis
   c. Untreated diabetes mellitus
   d. Diabetes insipidus
   e. Alcohol and caffeine ingestion
   f. Diuretic therapy
   g. Nervousness
2. *Amber* (orange-colored) urine
   a. Concentrated urine caused by fever, sweating, reduced fluid intake, or first morning specimen
   b. Bilirubin present (produces yellow foam when shaken)
   c. Carrots or vitamin A ingestion (large amounts)
   d. Certain urinary tract medications (e.g., phenazopyridine [Pyridium], nitrofurantoin)
3. *Brownish yellow or greenish yellow* urine may indicate bilirubin in the urine that has been oxidized to biliverdin (produces greenish foam when shaken).

4. *Green* urine
   a. Pseudomonal infection
   b. Indican
   c. Chlorophyll
5. *Pink to red* urine
   a. RBCs
   b. Hemoglobin, methemoglobin, oxyhemoglobin
   c. Myoglobin
   d. Porphyrins
6. *Brown-black* urine
   a. RBCs oxidized to methemoglobin
   b. Methemoglobin
   c. Homogentisic acid (alkaptonuria)
   d. Melanin or melanogen
   e. Phenol poisoning
7. *Smoky* urine may be caused by RBCs.
8. *Milky* urine is associated with fat, cystinuria, large amounts of WBCs, or phosphates.

Interfering Factors

1. Normal urine color darkens on standing because of the oxidation of urobilinogen to urobilin. This decomposition process starts about 30 minutes after voiding.
2. Some foods cause changes in urine color:
   a. Beets turn the urine *red*.
   b. Rhubarb can cause *brown* urine.
3. Many drugs alter the color of urine:
   a. Cascara and senna laxatives in the presence of acid urine turn the urine *reddish brown*; in the presence of alkaline urine, they turn the urine *red*.
   b. *Bright-yellow* color in alkaline urine may be a result of riboflavin or phenazopyridine.
   c. Urine that *darkens* on standing may indicate antiparkinsonian agents such as levodopa (Sinemet).
   d. *Black* urine may be caused by cascara, chloroquine, iron salts (ferrous sulfate, ferrous fumarate, ferrous gluconate), metronidazole, nitrofurantoin, quinine, or senna.
   e. *Blue* urine may be caused by triamterene.
   f. *Blue-green* urine may be caused by amitriptyline, methylene blue, or mitoxantrone.
   g. *Orange* urine may be caused by heparin, phenazopyridine, rifampin, sulfasalazine, or warfarin.
   h. *Red-pink* urine may be caused by chlorzoxazone, daunorubicin, doxorubicin, heparin, ibuprofen, methyldopa, phenytoin, rifampin, or senna.
   i. *Pink to brown* urine may be caused by laxatives.
   j. *Brown* urine may be caused by chloroquine, furazolidone, or primaquine.
   k. *Green* urine may be caused by indomethacin.

CLINICAL ALERT

1. If the urine is a red color, do not assume drug causation. Check the urine for hemoglobin. Question the patient regarding hematuria and recent activity, injury, or infection. Sometimes, vigorous exercise can bring on hematuria.
2. Red urine that is negative for occult blood is an indication that porphyria may be present. Report at once and document test results.
3. Other grossly abnormal colors (e.g., black, brown) should be documented and reported.

Interventions

Pretest Patient Care

1. Explain purpose of test, procedure for urine collection, and interfering factors.
2. Assess color of urine; instruct patient to monitor and to report abnormal urine colors.

Posttest Patient Care

1. Interpret abnormal urine colors; report and record findings. Modify the nursing care plan as needed.
2. Counsel the patient regarding abnormal findings. Explain possible need for follow-up testing.

Urine Odor

Normal, freshly voided urine has a faint odor owing to the presence of volatile acids. It is not generally offensive. Although not part of the routine UA, abnormal odors should be noted.

Normal Findings

Fresh urine from most healthy persons has a characteristic odor.

Procedure

Smell the urine and record perceptions.

Clinical Implications

1. The urine of patients with diabetes mellitus may have a fruity (acetone) odor because of ketosis.
2. UTIs result in foul-smelling urine because of the presence of bacteria, which split urea to form ammonia.
3. The urine of infants with an inherited disorder of amino acid metabolism known as *maple syrup urine disease* smells like maple syrup or burnt sugar.
4. Cystinuria and homocystinuria result in a sulfurous odor.
5. Oasthouse urine (Smith-Strang) disease, methionine malabsorption syndrome, causes an odor associated with the smell of a brewery (yeasts, hops).
6. In PKU, a musty, mousy smell may be evident.
7. Tyrosinemia is characterized by a cabbage-like or fishy urine odor.
8. Butyric/hexanoic acidemia produces a urine odor resembling that of sweaty feet.

Interfering Factors

1. Some foods, such as asparagus, produce characteristic urine odors.
2. Bacterial activity produces ammonia from the decomposition of urea, with its characteristic pungent odor.

Urine pH

The symbol *pH* expresses the urine as a dilute acid or base solution and measures the free hydrogen ion (H^+) concentration in the urine; 7.0 is the point of neutrality on the pH scale. The lower the pH, the greater the acidity; the higher the pH, the greater the alkalinity. The pH is an indicator of the renal tubules' ability to maintain normal hydrogen ion concentration in the plasma and extracellular fluid. The kidneys maintain normal acid–base balance primarily through reabsorption of sodium and tubular secretion of hydrogen and ammonium ions. Secretion of an acid or alkaline urine by the kidneys is one of the most important mechanisms the body has for maintaining a constant body pH.

Urine becomes increasingly acidic as the amount of sodium and excess acid retained by the body increases. Alkaline urine, usually containing bicarbonate–carbonic acid buffer, is normally excreted when there is an excess of base or alkali in the body.

The importance of urinary pH lies primarily in determining the existence of systemic acid–base disorders of metabolic or respiratory origin and in the management of urinary conditions that require the urine to be maintained at a specific pH.

Control of Urine pH

Control of urinary pH is important in the management of several diseases, including bacteriuria, renal calculi, and drug therapy in which streptomycin or methenamine mandelate is being administered.

1. *Renal calculi*
   a. Renal stone formation partially depends on the pH of urine. Patients being treated for renal calculi are frequently given diets or medication to change the pH of the urine so that kidney stones will not form.
   b. Calcium phosphate, calcium carbonate, and magnesium phosphate stones develop in alkaline urine. In such instances, the urine must be kept acidic (see No. 4 "Diet" below).
   c. Uric acid, cystine, and calcium oxalate stones precipitate in acid urines. Therefore, as part of treatment, the urine should be kept alkaline (see No. 4 "Diet" below).
2. *Drug treatment*
   a. Streptomycin, neomycin, and kanamycin are effective for treating genitourinary tract infections, provided the urine is alkaline.
   b. During sulfa therapy, alkaline urine should help prevent formation of sulfonamide crystals.
   c. Urine should also be kept persistently alkaline in the presence of salicylate intoxication (to enhance excretion) and during blood transfusions.
3. *Clinical conditions*
   a. The urine should be kept acidic during treatment of UTI or persistent bacteriuria and during management of urinary calculi that develop in alkaline urine.
   b. An accurate measurement of urinary pH can be made only on a freshly voided specimen. If the urine must be kept for any length of time before analysis, it must be refrigerated.
   c. Highly concentrated urine, such as that formed in hot, dry environments, is strongly acidic and may produce irritation.
   d. During sleep, decreased pulmonary ventilation causes respiratory acidosis; as a result, urine becomes more acidic.
   e. Chlorothiazide diuretic administration causes acid urine to be excreted.
   f. Bacteria from a UTI or from bacterial contamination of the specimen produce alkaline urine. Urea is converted to ammonia.
4. *Diet*
   a. A vegetarian diet that emphasizes citrus fruits and most vegetables, particularly legumes, helps keep the urine alkaline. Alkaline urine after meals is a normal response to the secretion of hydrochloric acid in gastric juice.
   b. A diet high in meat and protein keeps the urine acidic.

Normal Findings

The pH of normal urine can vary widely, from 4.6 to 8.0.
The average pH value is about 6.0 (acidic).

Procedure

1. Use reagent strips for a dipstick measurement. They produce a spectrum of color changes from orange to green-blue to identify pH ranges from 5.0 to 9.0.
2. Dip the reagent strip into a freshly voided urine specimen and compare the color change with the standardized color chart on the bottle that correlates color results with pH values.
3. Maintenance of the urine at a consistent pH requires frequent urine pH testing.

Clinical Implications

To be useful, the urine pH measurement must be used in conjunction with other diagnostic information. For example, in renal tubular necrosis, the kidney is not able to excrete urine that is strongly acidic. Therefore, if the urine pH is 5.0, renal tubular necrosis is eliminated as a possible diagnosis.

1. *Acidic urine* (pH <7.0) occurs in:
   a. Metabolic acidosis, diabetic ketosis, diarrhea, starvation, uremia
   b. UTIs caused by *Escherichia coli*
   c. Respiratory acidosis (carbon dioxide retention)
   d. Renal tuberculosis
   e. Pyrexia
2. *Alkaline urine* (pH >7.0) occurs in:
   a. UTIs caused by urea-splitting bacteria (*Proteus* and *Pseudomonas*)
   b. Renal tubular acidosis, chronic renal failure
   c. Metabolic acidosis (vomiting)
   d. Respiratory alkalosis involving hyperventilation ("blowing off" carbon dioxide)
   e. Potassium depletion

CLINICAL ALERT

The pH of urine never reaches 9, either in normal or abnormal conditions. Therefore, a pH finding of 9 indicates that a fresh specimen should be obtained to ensure the validity of the UA.

Interfering Factors

1. With prolonged lapse of time since voiding, the pH of a urine specimen becomes alkaline because bacteria split urea and produce ammonia. Note: A urine pH of >9.0 is indicative of prolonged standing.
2. Ammonium chloride and mandelic acid may produce acid urines.
3. Runover between the pH testing area and the highly acidic protein area on the dipsticks may cause alkaline urine to give an acidic reading.
4. Sodium bicarbonate, potassium citrate, and acetazolamide may produce alkaline urine.
5. Urine becomes alkaline after eating because of excretion of stomach acid.
6. The pH tends to be low following overnight fasting and high following ingestion of a meal.

Interventions

Pretest Patient Care

1. Explain purpose of test, procedure for urine collection, and interfering factors.
2. Follow guidelines in Chapter 1 for safe, effective, informed *pretest* care.

Posttest Patient Care

1. Review test results; report and record findings. Modify the nursing care plan as needed. Monitor patient appropriately (see Control of Urine pH).
2. Follow guidelines in Chapter 1 for safe, effective, informed *posttest* care.

• Urine Blood or Hemoglobin (Hb)

The presence of free hemoglobin (Hb) in the urine is referred to as *hemoglobinuria.* Hemoglobinuria can be related to conditions outside the urinary tract and occurs when there is such extensive or rapid destruction (intravascular hemolysis) of circulating erythrocytes that the reticuloendothelial system cannot metabolize or store the excess free Hb. The Hb is then filtered through the glomerulus. Hemoglobinuria may also occur as a result of lysis of RBCs in the urinary tract.

When intact RBCs are present in the urine, the term *hematuria* is used. Hematuria is most closely related to disorders of the renal or genitourinary systems in which bleeding is the result of trauma or damage to these organs or systems.

This test detects RBCs, Hb, and myoglobin in urine. Blood in urine is *always* an indicator of damage to the kidney or urinary tract.

The use of both a urine dipstick measurement and microscopic examination of urine provides a complete clinical evaluation of hemoglobinuria and hematuria. Some forms of dipsticks contain a lysing reagent that reacts with occult blood and detects intact as well as lysed RBCs.

When urine sediment is positive for occult blood but no RBCs are seen microscopically, *myoglobinuria* can be suspected. Myoglobinuria is caused by excretion of myoglobin, a muscle protein, into the urine as a result of (1) traumatic muscle injury, such as may occur in automobile accidents, football injuries, or electric shock; (2) a muscle disorder, such as an arterial occlusion to a muscle or muscular dystrophy; (3) certain kinds of poisoning, such as carbon monoxide or fish poisoning; or (4) malignant hyperthermia related to administration of certain anesthetic agents. Myoglobin can be distinguished from free Hb in the urine by chemical tests.

Normal Findings

Negative (<0.03 mg free Hb/dL or <10 Ercs/μL)
Ercs = erythrocytes

Procedure

1. Collect a fresh random urine specimen.
   a. *Hemoglobinuria* (Hb in urine)
      (1) Dip reagent stick into the urine; the color change on the dipstick correlates with a standardized color chart specifically used with that particular type of dipstick.
      (2) The color chart indicates color gradients for negative, moderate, and large amounts of Hb.
   b. *Hematuria* (RBCs in urine)
      (1) This dipstick method allows detection of intact RBCs when the number is >10 cells/mL of urine. The color change appears stippled on the dipstick.
      (2) The degree of hematuria can be estimated by the intensity of the speckled pattern.
2. Centrifuge the urine sample and examine the sediment microscopically (see Microscopic Examination of Urine Sediment) to verify the presence of RBCs.
   a. Hemoglobinuria is suspected when no RBCs are seen or the number seen does not correspond to the degree of color on the dipstick.
   b. Myoglobinemia may be suspected if the urine is cherry-red, no RBCs are seen, and blood serum enzymes for muscle destruction are elevated.

Clinical Implications

1. *Hematuria* is found in:
   a. Acute UTI (cystitis)
   b. Lupus nephritis
   c. Urinary tract or renal tumors
   d. Urinary calculi (intermittent hematuria)
   e. Malignant hypertension
   f. Glomerulonephritis (acute or chronic)
   g. Pyelonephritis
   h. Trauma to kidneys

i. Polycystic kidney disease
j. Leukemia
k. Thrombocytopenia
l. Strenuous exercise
m. Benign familial or recurrent hematuria (asymptomatic hematuria without proteinuria; other clinical and laboratory data are normal)
n. Heavy smokers

2. *Hemoglobinuria* is found in:
   a. Extensive burns
   b. Transfusion reactions (incompatible blood products)
   c. Febrile intoxication
   d. Certain chemical agents and alkaloids (poisonous mushrooms, snake venom)
   e. Malaria
   f. Bleeding resulting from operative procedures on the prostate (can be difficult to control, especially in the presence of malignancies)
   g. Hemolytic disorders such as sickle cell anemia, thalassemia, and glucose-6-phosphate dehydrogenase deficiency
   h. Paroxysmal hemoglobinuria (large quantities of hemoglobin appear in urine at irregular intervals)
   i. Kidney infarction
   j. Hemolysis occurring while the urine is in the urinary tract (RBC lysis from hypotonic urine or alkaline urine)
   k. Fava bean (broad bean) sensitivity (causes severe hemolytic anemia)
   l. Disseminated intravascular coagulation (DIC)
   m. Strenuous exercise

CLINICAL ALERT

One of the early indicators of possible renal or urinary tract disease is the appearance of blood in the urine. This does not mean that blood will be present in every voided specimen, but in most cases of renal or urinary tract disease, occult blood will appear in the urine with a reasonable degree of frequency. Any positive test for blood should be rechecked on a new urine specimen. If blood still appears, the patient should be further evaluated.

Interfering Factors

1. Drugs causing a positive result for blood or hemoglobin include:
   a. Drugs toxic to the kidneys (e.g., bacitracin, amphotericin)
   b. Drugs that alter blood clotting (warfarin [Coumadin])
   c. Drugs that cause hemolysis of RBCs (aspirin)
   d. Drugs that may give a false-positive result (e.g., bromides, copper, iodides, oxidizing agents)
2. High doses of ascorbic acid or vitamin C may cause a false-negative result.
3. High SG or elevated protein reduces sensitivity.
4. Myoglobin produces a false-positive result.
5. Hypochlorites or bleach used to clean urine containers causes false-positive results.
6. Menstrual blood may contaminate the specimen and alter results.
7. Prostatic infections may cause false-positive results.
8. See Appendix E for a complete list of drugs that affect test outcomes.

Interventions

Pretest Patient Care

1. Explain purpose of test, procedure for urine collection, and interfering factors.
2. Follow guidelines in Chapter 1 for safe, effective, informed *pretest* care.

Posttest Patient Care

1. Review test results; report and record findings. Modify the nursing care plan as needed. Explain possible need for follow-up testing.
2. Follow guidelines in Chapter 1 for safe, effective, informed *posttest* care.

● Urine Protein (Albumin), Qualitative and 24-Hour

Increased amounts of protein in the urine can be an important indicator of renal disease. It may be the first sign of a serious problem and may appear before any other clinical symptoms. However, there are other physiologic conditions (e.g., exercise, fever) that can lead to increased protein excretion in urine. Also, there are some renal disorders in which proteinuria is absent.

In a healthy renal and urinary tract system, the urine contains no protein or only trace amounts. These consist of albumin (one third of normal urine protein is albumin) and globulins from the plasma. Because albumin is filtered more readily than the globulins, it is usually abundant in pathologic conditions. Therefore, the term *albuminuria* is often used synonymously with *proteinuria*.

Normally, the glomeruli prevent passage of protein from the blood to the glomerular filtrate. Therefore, the presence of protein in the urine is the *single most important indication* of renal disease. If more than a trace amount of protein is found persistently in the urine, a quantitative 24-hour evaluation of protein excretion is necessary.

Postural proteinuria results from the excretion of protein by some patients when they stand or move about. This type of proteinuria is intermittent and disappears when the patient lies down. Postural proteinuria occurs in 3% to 15% of healthy young adults. It is also known as *orthostatic proteinuria*.

Normal Findings

Qualitative
Negative
24-Hour Urine
Adult male: 10 to 140 mg/L or 1 to 14 mg/dL
Adult female: 30 to 100 mg/L or 3 to 10 mg/dL
Child: <10 years old: 10 to 100 mg/L or 1 to 10 mg/dL

Procedure

Qualitative Protein Collection

1. Collect a random urine sample in a clean container and test it as soon as possible.
2. Use a protein reagent dipstick and compare the test result color with the color comparison chart provided on the reagent strip bottle. Protein can also be detected by turbidimetric methods using sulfosalicylic acid.
3. Test a new second specimen and investigate any interfering factors if one of these methods produces positive results. A 24-hour urine test may then be ordered for a quantitative measurement of protein.

24-Hour Urine Protein Collection

1. Label a 24-hour urine container with the name of the patient, the test, and the date and time the test is started.
2. Refrigerate the specimen as it is being collected.

3. See general instructions for 24-hour urine collection listed (see Long-Term, Timed Urine Specimen [2-Hour, 24-Hour]).
4. Record the exact starting and ending times for the 24-hour collection on the specimen container and on the patient's record. (The usual starting and ending times are 0700 to 0700.)

Orthostatic Proteinuria Collection

1. The patient is instructed to void at bedtime and to discard this urine.
2. The next morning, a urine specimen is collected immediately after the patient awakens and before the patient has been in an upright position for longer than 1 minute. This may involve the use of a bedpan or urinal.
3. A second specimen is collected after the patient has been standing or walking for at least 2 hours.
4. With orthostatic (postural) proteinuria, the first specimen contains no protein, but the second one is positive for protein.
5. The urine looks microscopically normal; no RBCs or WBCs are apparent. Orthostatic proteinuria is considered a benign condition and slowly disappears with time. Progressive renal impairment usually does not occur.

Clinical Implications

1. Proteinuria occurs by two main mechanisms: damage to the glomeruli or a defect in the reabsorption process that occurs in the tubules.
   a. *Glomerular damage*
      (1) Glomerulonephritis, acute and chronic
      (2) Systemic lupus erythematosus (SLE)
      (3) Malignant hypertension
      (4) Amyloidosis
      (5) Diabetes mellitus
      (6) Nephrotic syndrome
      (7) Polycystic kidney disease
   b. *Diminished tubular reabsorption*
      (1) Renal tubular disease
      (2) Pyelonephritis, acute and chronic
      (3) Cystinosis
      (4) Wilson's disease
      (5) Fanconi's syndrome (defect of proximal tubular function)
      (6) Interstitial nephritis
2. In pathologic states, the level of proteinuria is rarely constant, so not every sample of urine is abnormal in patients with renal disease, and the concentration of protein in the urine is not necessarily indicative of the severity of renal disease.
3. Proteinuria may result from glomerular blood flow changes without the presence of a structural abnormality, as in congestive heart failure.
4. Proteinuria may be caused by increased serum protein levels.
   a. Multiple myeloma (Bence Jones protein)
   b. Waldenström's macroglobulinemia
   c. Malignant lymphoma
5. Proteinuria can occur in other nonrenal disease ("functional proteinuria").
   a. Acute infection, septicemia
   b. Trauma, stress
   c. Leukemia, hematologic disorders
   d. Toxemia, preeclampsia of pregnancy
   e. Hyperthyroidism

f. Vascular disease (hypertension), cardiac disease
g. Renal transplant rejection
h. Central nervous system lesions
i. Poisoning from turpentine, phosphorus, mercury, gold, lead, phenol, opiates, or other drugs
j. Hereditary, sickle cell, oxalosis

6. Large numbers of leukocytes accompanying proteinuria usually indicate infection at some level in the urinary tract. Large numbers of both leukocytes and erythrocytes indicate a noninfectious inflammatory disease of the glomerulus. Proteinuria associated with pyelonephritis may have as many RBCs as WBCs.
7. Proteinuria does not always accompany renal disease.
8. Proteinuria is often associated with the finding of casts on sediment examination because protein is necessary for cast formation.

CLINICAL ALERT

1. Proteinuria of >2000 mg/24 hr in an adult or ≥40 mg/24 hr in a child usually indicates a glomerular cause.
2. Proteinuria of >3500 mg/24 hr points to a nephrotic syndrome.

Interfering Factors for Qualitative Protein Test

1. Because of renal vasoconstriction, the presence of a functional, mild, and transitory proteinuria is associated with:
   a. Strenuous exercise leading to urine protein values of up to 300 mg/24 hours
   b. Severe emotional stress, seizures
   c. Cold baths, exposure to very cold temperatures
2. Increased protein in urine occurs in these benign states:
   a. Fever and dehydration (salt depletion)
   b. Non–immunoglobulin E food allergies
   c. Salicylate therapy
   d. In the premenstrual period and immediately after delivery
3. False or accidental proteinuria may occur because of a mixture of pus and RBCs in the urinary tract related to infections, menstrual or vaginal discharge, mucus, or semen.
4. False-positive results can occur from incorrect use and interpretation of the color reagent strip test.
5. Alkaline, highly buffered urine can produce false-positive results on the dipstick test.
6. Very dilute urine may give a falsely low protein value.
7. Certain drugs may cause false-positive or false-negative urine protein tests (see Appendix E).
8. Radiographic contrast agents may produce false-positive results with turbidimetric measurements.

Interventions

Pretest Patient Care

1. Explain purpose of test, procedure for 24-hour urine collection, and interfering factors. Emphasize the importance of compliance with the procedure.
2. Allow food and fluids, but advise the patient that fluids should not be forced because very dilute urine can produce false-negative values.
3. Follow guidelines in Chapter 1 for safe, effective, informed *pretest* care.

Posttest Patient Care

1. Review test results; report and record findings. Modify the nursing care plan as needed. Explain possible need for follow-up testing (e.g., urine differential/electrophoresis) and treatment (to prevent progression to renal failure).
2. Follow guidelines in Chapter 1 for safe, effective, informed *posttest* care.
3. See Chapter 8 for protein electrophoresis.

● Microalbuminuria/Albumin (24-Hour Urine)

Microalbuminuria is an increase in urinary albumin that is below the detectable range of the standard protein dipstick test. It is not a different chemical form of albumin. Microalbuminuria occurs long before clinical proteinuria becomes evident.

This test allows for the routine detection of low concentrations of albumin in the urine. This test has become a standard for the screening, monitoring, and detection of deteriorating renal function in diabetic patients. Studies have shown that diabetic patients who progress to renal failure first excrete microscopic amounts of albumin and that, at this stage, intervening treatment can reverse the proteinuria and thus prevent progression to renal failure. This test is also used to monitor compliance with blood pressure control, glucose control, and protein restriction.

Normal Findings

<30 mg/24 hours (<30 mg/day) or <20 mg/L (10-hour collection)

Procedure

1. 24-hour: same as for total urine protein
2. 10-hour: overnight collection
   a. Last voiding before sleep (10:00 p.m. or 2200)
   b. Collect all urine at first morning voiding (8:00 a.m. or 0800)

   These results approximate 24-hour collection.

Clinical Implications

Increased microalbuminuria is associated with:

1. Diabetes with early diabetic nephropathy
2. Hypertension—heart disease
3. Generalized vascular disease
4. Preeclampsia

Interfering Factors

1. Strenuous exercise
2. Hematuria
3. High-protein diet or high salt levels

Interventions

Pretest Patient Care

The *pretest* care is the same as for 24-hour protein.

Posttest Patient Care

1. Albumin excretion of >30 mg/24 hours or >20 mg/L/10 hours indicates an abnormal excretion.
   a. Patient management should be reviewed.
   b. Patient compliance can be checked by glycosylated hemoglobin to determine further control.

2. Patients with borderline results should be assessed on more than one occasion before the significance of a given urine measurement is finally judged.
3. The *posttest* care is the same as for 24-hour total protein.

● Urine β_2-Microglobulin

β_2-Microglobulin, an amino acid peptide component of the lymphatic human lymphocyte antibody (HLA) major histocompatibility complex, is found on the outside of the plasma membrane. It is structurally related to the immunoglobulins.

This test measures β_2-microglobulin, which is nonspecifically increased in inflammatory conditions and in patients with malignancies (e.g., lymphoma, active chronic lymphatic leukemia, or multiple myeloma). It may be used to differentiate glomerular from tubular dysfunction. In glomerular disease, β_2-microglobulin is increased in serum and decreased in urine, whereas in tubular disorders, it is decreased in serum and increased in urine. In aminoglycoside toxicity, β_2-microglobulin levels become abnormal before creatinine levels begin to show abnormal values. Serum is also used to evaluate the prognosis of multiple myeloma.

Normal Findings

Urine 24-hour specimen: <1 mg/24 hours or <1 mg/day
Blood serum specimen: <2.7 μg/mL or <2.7 mg/L

Procedure

1. Collect a 24-hour urine specimen or a serum sample (~5 mL).
2. Keep the pH neutral or alkaline (pH >6.0).
3. Freeze specimen if not analyzed immediately. Not stable at room temperature.

Clinical Implications

1. Increased urine β_2-microglobulin occurs in:
   a. Renal tubular disorders (>50 mg/24 hours or >50 mg/day)
   b. Heavy metal poisoning (mercury, cadmium)
   c. Drug toxicity (aminoglycosides, cyclosporine)
   d. Fanconi's syndrome
   e. Wilson's disease
   f. Pyelonephritis
   g. Renal allograft rejection
   h. Lymphoid malignancies associated with B-lymphocyte lineage
   i. AIDS (can be used as a predictor of the progression to AIDS)
2. Increased serum β_2-microglobulin occurs in:
   a. Multiple myeloma
   b. Amyloidosis
   c. Viral infection

Interfering Factors

1. Acid urine
2. Certain antibiotics (e.g., gentamicin, tobramycin)
3. Recent nuclear medicine scan
4. Increased synthesis in certain diseases (e.g., Crohn's disease, hepatitis, sarcoidosis) decreases the usefulness of the blood serum test.
5. Random specimens are not recommended.

Interventions

Pretest Patient Care

1. Explain purpose of test, procedure for 24-hour urine collection, and interfering factors.
2. See instructions for 24-hour urine collection (see Long-Term, Timed Urine Specimen [2-Hour, 24-Hour]).
3. Follow guidelines in Chapter 1 for safe, effective, informed *pretest* care.

Posttest Patient Care

1. Review test results; report and record findings. Modify the nursing care plan as needed. Monitor appropriately.
2. Follow guidelines in Chapter 1 for safe, effective, informed *posttest* care.

Urine Glucose (Sugar)

Glucose is present in glomerular filtrate and is reabsorbed by the proximal convoluted tubule. If the blood glucose level exceeds the reabsorption capacity of the tubules, glucose will appear in the urine. Tubular reabsorption of glucose is by active transport in response to the body's need to maintain an adequate concentration of glucose. The blood level at which tubular reabsorption stops is termed the *renal threshold*, which for glucose is between 160 and 180 mg/dL (9 to 10 mmol/L).

Types of Glucose Tests

1. *Reduction tests* (Clinitest)
   a. These are based on reduction of cupric ions by glucose. When the compounds are added to urine, a heat reaction takes place. This results in precipitation and a change in the color of the urine if glucose is present.
   b. These tests are nonspecific for glucose because the reaction can also be caused by other reducing substances in the urine, including:
      (1) Creatinine, uric acid, ascorbic acid
      (2) Other sugars such as galactose, lactose, fructose, pentose, and maltose
   c. These tests have a lower sensitivity than enzyme tests.
2. *Enzyme tests* (Clinistix, Diastix, Tes-Tape)
   a. These tests are based on interaction between glucose oxidase (an enzyme) and glucose. When dipped into urine, the enzyme-impregnated strip changes color according to the amount of glucose in the urine. The manufacturer's color chart provides a basis for comparison of colors between the sample and the manufacturer's control.
   b. These tests are specific for glucose only.

Normal Findings

Random specimen: negative
24-hour specimen: 1 to 15 mg/dL (60 to 830 μmol/L) or <0.5 g/24 hours (<2.8 mmol/day)

Procedure

1. Use a freshly voided specimen.
2. Follow directions on the test container exactly. Timing must be exact; the color reaction must be compared with the closest matching control color on the manufacturer's color chart to ascertain accurate results.
3. Record the results on the patient's record.
4. Refrigerate or ice the entire urine sample during collection if a 24-hour urine specimen is also ordered. See Table 3.3 on pages 188–191 for proper preservative.

CLINICAL ALERT

1. Urine glucose >1000 mg/dL (>55 mmol/L) (4+) is a critical value.
2. Determine exactly what drugs the patient is taking and whether the metabolites of these drugs can affect the urine glucose results. Frequent updating in regard to the effects of drugs on blood glucose levels is necessary in light of the many new drugs introduced and prescribed.
3. Test results may be reported as "plus" (+) or as percentages. Percentages are more accurate.
4. When screening for galactose (galactosuria) in infants, the reduction test must be used. The enzyme test does not react with galactose.
5. Newborns should always be tested by both methods (reduction and enzymatic).

Clinical Implications

1. *Increased glucose* occurs in:
   a. Diabetes mellitus
   b. Endocrine disorders (thyrotoxicosis, Cushing's syndrome, acromegaly)
   c. Liver and pancreatic disease
   d. Central nervous system disorders (brain injury, stroke)
   e. Impaired tubular reabsorption
      (1) Fanconi's syndrome
      (2) Advanced renal tubular disease
   f. Pregnancy with possible latent diabetes (gestational diabetes)
2. *Increase of other sugars* (react only with reduction tests, not dipstick tests)
   a. Lactose—pregnancy, lactation, lactose intolerance
   b. Galactose—hereditary galactosuria (severe enzyme deficiency in infants; must be treated promptly)
   c. Xylose—excessive ingestion of fruit
   d. Fructose—hereditary fructose intolerance, hepatic disorders
   e. Pentose—certain drug therapies and rare hereditary conditions

CLINICAL ALERT

Urine glucose >1000 mg/dL (>55 mmol/L)—test blood glucose, notify healthcare provider, and begin appropriate treatment.

Interfering Factors

1. Interfering factors for reduction test (false-positive results)
   a. Presence of non–sugar-reducing substances such as ascorbic acid, homogentisic acid, creatinine
   b. Tyrosine
   c. Nalidixic acid, cephalosporins, probenecid, and penicillin
   d. Large amounts of urine protein (slows reaction)
2. Interfering factors for dipstick enzyme tests
   a. Ascorbic acid (in large amounts) may cause a false-negative result.
   b. Large amount of ketones may cause a false-negative result.
   c. Peroxide or strong oxidizing agents may cause a false-positive result.
3. Stress, excitement, myocardial infarction, testing after a heavy meal, and testing soon after the administration of intravenous glucose may all cause false-positive results, most frequently trace reactions.

4. Contamination of the urine sample with bleach or hydrogen peroxide may invalidate results.
5. False-negative results may occur if urine is left to sit at room temperature for an extended period, owing to the rapid glycolysis of glucose.
6. High SG depresses color development; low SG intensifies it. See Appendix E for other drugs that affect test outcomes.

Interventions

Pretest Patient Care

1. Explain purpose of test, procedure for urine collection, the double-voiding technique, and interfering factors.
   a. Discard the first voided morning specimen and then void 30 to 45 minutes later for the test specimen. This second specimen reflects the immediate state of glucosuria more accurately because the first morning specimen consists of urine that has been present in the bladder for several hours.
   b. Advise the patient not to drink liquids between the first and second voiding so as not to dilute the glucose present in the specimen.
   c. A urine glucose test combined with a blood glucose test gives a more complete assessment of diabetes.
2. Instruct the patient about the 24-hour urine collection procedure when applicable (see Long-Term, Timed Urine Specimen [2-Hour, 24-Hour]).
3. Follow guidelines in Chapter 1 for safe, effective, informed *pretest* care.

Posttest Patient Care

1. Review test results; report and record findings. Modify the nursing care plan as needed. Counsel the patient regarding abnormal findings.
2. Follow guidelines in Chapter 1 for safe, effective, informed *posttest* care.

● Urine Ketones (Acetone; Ketone Bodies)

Ketones, which result from the metabolism of fatty acid and fat, consist mainly of three substances: acetone, β-hydroxybutyric acid, and acetoacetic acid. The last two substances readily convert to acetone, in essence making acetone the main substance being tested. However, some testing products measure only acetoacetic acid.

In healthy persons, ketones are formed in the liver and are completely metabolized so that only negligible amounts appear in the urine. However, when carbohydrate metabolism is altered, an excessive amount of ketones is formed (acidosis) because fat becomes the predominant body fuel instead of carbohydrates. When the metabolic pathways of carbohydrates are disturbed, carbon fragments from fat and protein are diverted to form abnormal amounts of ketone bodies. Increased ketones in the blood lead to electrolyte imbalance, dehydration, and, if not corrected, acidosis and eventual coma.

The excess presence of ketones in the urine (ketonuria) is associated with diabetes or altered carbohydrate metabolism. Some diets that are low in carbohydrates and high in fat and protein also produce ketones in the urine. Testing for urine ketones in patients with diabetes may provide the clue to early diagnosis of ketoacidosis and diabetic coma.

Indications for ketone testing include:

1. *General*: Screening for ketonuria is frequently done in hospitalized patients, presurgical patients, pregnant women, children, and persons with diabetes.
2. *Glycosuria* (diabetes)
   a. Testing for ketones is indicated in any patient showing elevated urine and blood sugars.
   b. When treatment is being switched from insulin to oral hypoglycemic agents, the development of ketonuria within 24 hours after withdrawal of insulin usually indicates a poor response to the oral hypoglycemic agents.

c. The urine of diabetic patients treated with oral hypoglycemic agents should be tested regularly for glucose and ketones because oral hypoglycemic agents, unlike insulin, do not control diabetes when acute complications such as infection develop.
d. Ketone testing is done to differentiate between diabetic coma (positive ketones) and insulin shock (negative ketones).

3. *Acidosis*
   a. Ketone testing is used to judge the severity of acidosis and to monitor the response to treatment.
   b. Urine ketone measurement frequently provides a more reliable indicator of acidosis than blood testing. It is especially useful in emergency situations.
   c. Ketones appear in the urine before there is any significant increase of ketones in the blood.
4. *Pregnancy*: During pregnancy, the early detection of ketones is essential because ketoacidosis is a prominent factor that contributes to intrauterine death.

Normal Findings

Urine: negative (<0.3 mg/dL or <0.05 mmol/L)
Serum or plasma:
Acetone: <2.0 mg/dL or <0.34 mmol/L
Acetoacetate: <1 mg/dL or <0.1 mmol/L
β-Hydroxybutyric acid: 0.21 to 2.81 mg/dL or 20 to 270 μmol/L

NOTE *β-Hydroxybutyrate is a useful indicator for monitoring insulin therapy in patients with diabetic ketoacidosis.*

Procedure

1. Dip the ketone reagent strip in fresh urine, tap off excess urine, time the reaction accurately, and then compare the strip with the control color chart on the container.
2. Follow the manufacturer's directions exactly if procedure differs from the technique just described.
3. Do not use dipsticks to test for ketones in blood. Special testing products are designed for blood.

Clinical Implications

1. Ketosis and ketonuria may occur whenever increased amounts of fat are metabolized, carbohydrate intake is restricted, or the diet is rich in fats. This state can occur in the following situations:
   a. Metabolic conditions
      (1) Diabetes mellitus (diabetic acidosis)
      (2) Renal glycosuria
      (3) Glycogen storage disease (von Gierke's disease)
   b. Dietary conditions
      (1) Starvation, fasting
      (2) High-fat diets
      (3) Prolonged vomiting, diarrhea
      (4) Anorexia
      (5) Low-carbohydrate diet
      (6) Eclampsia
   c. Increased metabolic states caused by:
      (1) Hyperthyroidism
      (2) Fever
      (3) Pregnancy or lactation

2. In nondiabetic persons, ketonuria occurs frequently during acute illness, severe stress, or strenuous exercise. Approximately 15% of hospitalized patients have ketones in their urine even though they do not have diabetes.
3. Children are particularly prone to developing ketonuria and ketosis.
4. Ketonuria occurs after anesthesia (ether or chloroform).

CLINICAL ALERT

Ketonuria signals a need for caution, rather than crisis intervention, in either a diabetic or a nondiabetic patient. However, this condition should not be taken lightly.

1. In the diabetic patient, ketone bodies in the urine suggest that the diabetes is not adequately controlled and that adjustments of either the medication or the diet should be made promptly.
2. In the nondiabetic patient, ketone bodies indicate a reduced carbohydrate metabolism and excessive fat metabolism.
3. Positive urine ketones in a child younger than 2 yr of age is a critical alert.

Interfering Factors

1. Drugs that may cause a false-positive result include:
   a. Levodopa
   b. Phenothiazines
   c. Ether
   d. Insulin
   e. Isopropyl alcohol
   f. Metformin
   g. Penicillamine
   h. Phenazopyridine (Pyridium)
   i. Captopril
2. False-negative results occur if urine stands too long, owing to loss of ketones into the air.
3. See Appendix E for other drugs that affect test outcomes.

Interventions

Pretest Patient Care

1. Explain purpose of test, procedure for urine collection, and interfering factors.
2. Follow guidelines in Chapter 1 for safe, effective, informed *pretest* care.

Posttest Patient Care

1. Review test results; report and record findings. Modify the nursing care plan as needed. Monitor appropriately.
2. Follow guidelines in Chapter 1 for safe, effective, informed *posttest* care.

● Urine Nitrite (Bacteria)

This test is a rapid, indirect method for detecting bacteria in the urine. Significant UTI may be present in a patient who does not experience any symptoms. Common gram-negative organisms contain enzymes that reduce the nitrate in the urine to nitrite.

Healthcare providers frequently request the urine nitrite test to screen high-risk patients: pregnant women, school-age children (especially females), diabetic patients, elderly patients, and patients with a history of recurrent infections.

The majority of UTIs are believed to start in the bladder as a result of extreme contamination; if left untreated, they can progress to the kidneys. Pyelonephritis is a frequent complication of untreated cystitis and can lead to renal damage. Detection of bacteria using the nitrite test and subsequent antibiotic therapy can prevent these serious complications. The nitrite test can also be used to evaluate the success of antibiotic therapy.

Normal Findings

Negative for bacteria

Procedure

1. Obtain a first morning specimen because urine that has been in the bladder for several hours is more likely to yield a positive nitrite test than a random urine sample that may have been in the bladder for only a short time. A clean-catch (midstream) urine specimen is needed to minimize bacterial contamination from adjacent anatomical areas.
2. Follow the exact testing procedure according to prescribed guidelines for reliable test results. Any shade of pink is positive for nitrite-producing bacteria.
3. Compare the reacted reagent area on the dipstick with a white background to aid in the detection of a faint pink hue that might otherwise be missed.
4. Perform a microscopic examination to verify results, if at all possible.

Clinical Implications

1. Under the light microscope, the presence of >20 bacteria per high-power field (hpf) may indicate a UTI. Untreated bacteriuria can lead to serious kidney disease.
2. The presence of a few bacteria suggests a UTI that cannot be confirmed or excluded until more definitive studies, such as culture and sensitivity tests, are performed. Again, this finding merits serious consideration for treatment.
3. A positive nitrite test is a reliable indicator of significant bacteriuria and is a cue for performing urine culture.
4. A negative result should *not* be interpreted as indicating absence of bacteriuria, for the following reasons:
   a. If an overnight urine sample is not used, there may not have been enough time for the nitrate to convert to nitrite in the bladder.
   b. Some UTIs are caused by organisms that do not convert nitrate to nitrite (e.g., staphylococci, streptococci).
   c. Sufficient dietary nitrate may not be present for the nitrate-to-nitrite reaction to occur.

Interfering Factors

1. Azo dye metabolites and bilirubin can produce false-positive results.
2. Ascorbic acid can produce false-negative results.
3. False-positive results can be obtained if the urine sits too long at room temperature, allowing contaminant bacteria to multiply.
4. High SG will reduce the sensitivity.

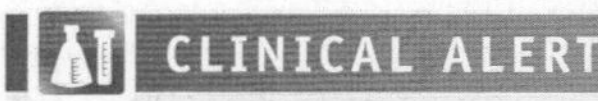

A negative urine nitrite test should not be interpreted as indicating the absence of bacteria.

Interventions

Pretest Patient Care

1. Explain purpose of test, procedure for clean-catch (midstream) urine collection, and interfering factors.
2. Follow guidelines in Chapter 1 for safe, effective, informed *pretest* care.

Posttest Patient Care

1. Interpret test outcomes and monitor appropriately.
2. Follow guidelines in Chapter 1 for safe, effective, informed *posttest* care.

● Urine Leukocyte Esterase

Usually, the presence of leukocytes (WBCs) in the urine indicates a UTI. The leukocyte esterase test detects esterase released by the leukocytes into the urine. Elevation of leukocyte esterase, a bacteria-related enzyme, is consistent with infection. This is a standardized means for the detection of WBCs.

Microscopic examination and chemical testing are used to determine the presence of leukocytes in the urine. The chemical test is done with a leukocyte esterase dipstick. This test can also detect intact leukocytes, lysed leukocytes, and WBC casts.

Normal Findings

Negative

Procedures

1. Collect a fresh, random urine specimen with a clean-catch or midstream technique.
2. Follow directions for dipstick use exactly. Timing is critical for accurate results.
3. Note that a positive result causes a purple color on the dipstick. The test is not designed to measure the amount of leukocytes.

Clinical Implications

1. Positive results are clinically significant and indicate:
    a. Cystitis (UTI)
    b. Acute pyelonephritis
    c. Acute Bright's disease
    d. Bladder tumor
    e. SLE
    f. Tuberculosis infection
2. Urine with positive results from the dipstick should be examined microscopically for WBCs and bacteria.

Interfering Factors

1. False-positive results
    a. Vaginal discharge, parasites, histocytes
    b. Drug therapies (e.g., ampicillin, kanamycin)
    c. Salicylate toxicity
    d. Strenuous exercise
2. False-negative results
    a. Large amounts of glucose or protein
    b. High SG
    c. Certain drugs (e.g., tetracycline)

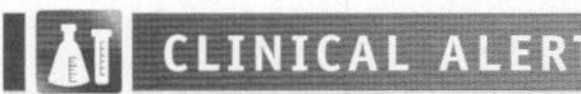

A urine sample that tests positive for both nitrite and leukocyte esterase should be cultured for pathogenic bacteria.

Interventions

Pretest Patient Care

1. Explain purpose of test, procedure for urine collection, and interfering factors.
2. Follow guidelines in Chapter 1 for safe, effective, informed *pretest* care.

Posttest Patient Care

1. Review test results; report and record findings. Modify the nursing care plan as needed. Monitor appropriately.
2. Follow guidelines in Chapter 1 for safe, effective, informed *posttest* care.

● Urine Bilirubin

Bilirubin is formed in the reticuloendothelial cells of the spleen and bone marrow as a result of the breakdown of hemoglobin; it is then transported to the liver. Urinary bilirubin levels are increased to significant levels in the presence of any disease process that increases the amount of conjugated bilirubin in the bloodstream (see Chapter 6). Elevated amounts appear when the normal degradation cycle is disrupted by obstruction of the bile duct or when the integrity of the liver is damaged.

Urine bilirubin aids in the diagnosis and monitoring of treatment for hepatitis and liver damage. Urine bilirubin is an early sign of hepatocellular disease or intrahepatic or extrahepatic biliary obstruction. It should be a part of every UA because bilirubin often appears in the urine before other signs of liver dysfunction (e.g., jaundice, weakness) become apparent. Not only does the detection of urinary bilirubin provide an early indication of liver disease but also its presence or absence can be used in determining the cause of clinical jaundice.

Normal Findings

Negative (0 to 0.02 mg/dL or 0 to 0.34 μmol/L)

Procedure

1. Examine the urine within 1 hour of collection because urine bilirubin is unstable, especially when exposed to light. If the urine is yellow-green to brown, shake the urine. If a yellow-green foam develops, bilirubin is probably present. Bilirubin alters the surface tension and allows foam to form. The yellow color is the bilirubin.
2. Chemical strip testing
   a. Dip a chemically reactive dipstick into the urine sample according to the manufacturer's directions.
   b. Close comparison of color changes on the dipstick with control colors on the color chart is an absolute necessity. Failure to make a close approximation of color may result in failure to recognize urine bilirubin. Good lighting is required.
   c. Interpret results as "negative" to "3+" or as "small," "moderate," or "large" amounts of bilirubin.
3. When it is crucial to detect even very small amounts of bilirubin in the urine, as in the earliest phase of viral hepatitis, Ictotest tablets are preferred for testing because they are more sensitive to urine bilirubin. When elevated amounts of urine bilirubin are present, a blue to purple color forms on the absorptive mat. The intensity of the color and the rapidity of its development are directly proportional to the amount of bilirubin in the urine.

Clinical Implications

1. Even trace amounts of bilirubin are abnormal and warrant further investigation. Normally, there is no detectable bilirubin in the urine.
2. Increased bilirubin occurs in:
   a. Hepatitis and liver diseases caused by infections or exposure to toxic agents (cirrhosis)
   b. Obstructive biliary tract disease
   c. Liver or biliary tract tumors
   d. Septicemia
   e. Hyperthyroidism

NOTE *Urine bilirubin is negative in hemolytic disease.*

Interfering Factors

1. Drugs may cause false-positive or false-negative results (see Appendix E).
2. Bilirubin rapidly decomposes when exposed to light; therefore, urine should be tested immediately.
3. High concentrations of ascorbic acid or nitrate cause decreased sensitivity.

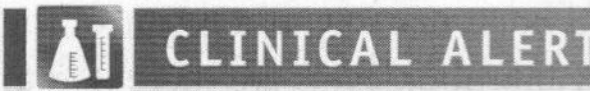

CLINICAL ALERT

Pyridium-like drugs or urochromes may give the urine an amber or reddish color and can mask the bilirubin reaction.

Interventions

Pretest Patient Care

1. Explain purpose of test, procedure for urine collection, and interfering factors.
2. Follow guidelines in Chapter 1 for safe, effective, informed *pretest* care.

Posttest Patient Care

1. Review test results; report and record findings. Modify the nursing care plan as needed. Monitor appropriately for liver disease.
2. Follow guidelines in Chapter 1 for safe, effective, informed *posttest* care.

● Urine Urobilinogen, Random and Timed

Bilirubin, which is formed from the degradation of hemoglobin, is transformed through the action of bacterial enzymes into *urobilinogen* after it enters the intestines. Some of the urobilinogen formed in the intestine is excreted as part of the feces, where it is oxidized to urobilin; another portion is absorbed into the portal bloodstream and carried to the liver, where it is metabolized and excreted in the bile. Traces of urobilinogen in the blood that escape removal by the liver are carried to the kidneys and excreted in the urine. This is the basis of the urine urobilinogen test. Unlike bilirubin, urobilinogen is *colorless*.

Urine urobilinogen is one of the most sensitive tests available to determine impaired liver function. Urinary urobilinogen is increased by any condition that causes an increase in the production of bilirubin and by any disease that prevents the liver from normally removing the reabsorbed urobilinogen from the portal circulation. An increased urobilinogen level is one of the earliest signs of liver disease and hemolytic disorders.

Although it cannot be determined by reagent strip, the absence of urobilinogen is also diagnostically significant and represents an obstruction of the bile duct.

Normal Findings

Random specimen: 0.1 to 1 Ehrlich U/dL or <1 mg/dL
2-hour specimen: 0.1 to 1.0 Ehrlich U/2 hours or <1 mg/2 hours
24-hour specimen: 0.5 to 4.0 Ehrlich U/24 hours or 0.5 to 4.0 mg/day

Procedure

1. Follow instructions for collecting a timed 24-hour, 2-hour, or random specimen. Check with the laboratory for specific protocols.
2. Perform the 2-hour timed collection from 1:00 p.m. to 3:00 p.m. (1300 to 1500) or from 2:00 p.m. to 4:00 p.m. (1400 to 1600) for best results because peak excretion occurs during this time. No preservatives are necessary. Record the total amount of urine voided. Protect the collection receptacle from light. Test immediately after specimen collection is completed.

Clinical Implications

1. Urine urobilinogen is *increased* when there is:
   a. Increased destruction of RBCs
      (1) Hemolytic anemias
      (2) Pernicious anemia (megaloblastic)
      (3) Malaria
   b. Hemorrhage into tissues
      (1) Pulmonary infarction
      (2) Excessive bruising
   c. Hepatic damage
      (1) Biliary disease
      (2) Cirrhosis (viral and chemical)
      (3) Acute hepatitis
   d. Cholangitis
2. Urine urobilinogen is *decreased* or absent when normal amounts of bilirubin are not excreted into the intestinal tract. This usually indicates partial or complete obstruction of the bile ducts. The stool is pale in color. Decreased urinary urobilinogen is associated with:
   a. Cholelithiasis
   b. Severe inflammation of the biliary ducts
   c. Cancer of the head of the pancreas
3. During antibiotic therapy, suppression of normal gut flora may prevent the breakdown of bilirubin to urobilinogen; therefore, urine levels will be decreased or absent.
4. More comprehensive information is obtained when the tests for urobilinogen and bilirubin are correlated (see Table 3.5 for comparisons).

CLINICAL ALERT

Urine urobilinogen rapidly decomposes at room temperature or when exposed to light.

Interfering Factors

1. Drugs that may affect urobilinogen levels include those that cause cholestasis and those that reduce the bacterial flora in the gastrointestinal tract. Review and update medication list; consult pharmacist if necessary.
2. Peak excretion is known to occur from noon to 4:00 p.m. (1600). The amount of urobilinogen in the urine is subject to diurnal variation.

TABLE 3.5 Comparison of Urine Urobilinogen and Urine Bilirubin Values

Test	In Health	In Hemolytic Disease	In Hepatic Disease	In Biliary Obstruction
Urine urobilinogen	Normal	Increased	Increased	Low or absent
Urine bilirubin	Negative	Negative	Positive or negative	Positive

3. Strongly alkaline urine shows a higher urobilinogen level, and strongly acidic urine shows a lower urobilinogen level.
4. Drugs that may cause *increased* urobilinogen include drugs that cause hemolysis. Review and update medication list; consult pharmacist if necessary.
5. If the urine is highly colored, the strip will be difficult to read.

Interventions

Pretest Patient Care

1. Explain purpose of test, procedure for urine collection, and interfering factors.
2. Follow guidelines in Chapter 1 for safe, effective, informed *pretest* care.

Posttest Patient Care

1. Review test results; report and record findings. Modify the nursing care plan as needed. Monitor appropriately for anemia and gastrointestinal disorders. Explain the need for follow-up testing.
2. Follow guidelines in Chapter 1 for safe, effective, informed *posttest* care.

MICROSCOPIC EXAMINATION OF URINE SEDIMENT

In healthy persons, the urine contains small numbers of cells and other formed elements from the entire genitourinary tract: casts and epithelial cells from the nephron; epithelial cells from the kidney, pelvis, ureters, bladder, and urethra; mucous threads and spermatozoa from the prostate; and possibly RBCs or WBCs and an occasional cast. In renal parenchymal disease, the urine usually contains increased numbers of cells and casts discharged from an organ that is otherwise accessible only by biopsy or surgery (Table 3.6 and Table 3.7). Urinary sediment provides information useful for both diagnosis and prognosis. It provides a direct sampling of urinary tract morphology.

The urinary sediment is obtained by pouring 1 mL of fresh, well-mixed urine into a conical tube and centrifuging the sample at a specific speed for 10 minutes. The supernatant is poured off, and 1 mL of the sediment is resuspended. A small drop is placed on a slide, cover-slipped, and examined microscopically.

The urine sediment can be broken down into cellular elements (RBCs, WBCs, and epithelial cells), casts, crystals, and bacteria. These may originate anywhere in the urinary tract. When casts do occur in the urine, they may indicate tubular or glomerular disorders.

Casts are the only elements found in urinary sediment that are unique to the kidneys. They are formed primarily within the lumen of the distal convoluted tubule and collecting duct, providing a microscopic view of conditions within the nephron. Their shapes are representative of the tubular lumen.

TABLE 3.6 Microscopic Examination of Urine Sediment

Urine Sediment Component	Clinical Significance
Bacteria	Urinary tract infection
Casts	Tubular or glomerular disorders
Broad casts	Formation occurs in collecting tubules; serious kidney disorder, extreme stasis of flow
Epithelial (renal) casts	Tubular degeneration
Fatty casts	Nephrotic syndrome
Granular	Renal parenchymal disease
Waxy	Stasis of flow
Hyaline casts	Chronic renal failure, chronic renal disease, congestive heart failure; stress or exercise
Red blood cell casts	Acute glomerulonephritis
White blood cell casts	Pyelonephritis, acute interstitial nephritis
Epithelial cells	Damage to various parts of urinary tract
Renal cells	Tubular damage
Squamous cells	Normal or contamination
Erythrocytes	Most renal disorders, menstruation; strenuous exercise
Fat bodies (oval)	Nephrotic syndrome
Leukocytes	Most renal disorders; urinary tract infection; pyelonephritis

Cast width is significant in determining the site of origin and may indicate the extent of renal damage. The width of the cast indicates the diameter of the tubule responsible for its formation. Cast width is described as *narrow* (as wide as 1 to 2 RBCs), *medium-broad* (3 to 4 RBCs), or *broad* (5 RBCs). The broad casts form in the collecting tubule and may be of any composition. Their presence usually indicates a marked reduction in the functional capacity of the nephron and suggests severe renal damage or end-stage renal disease.

The major constituent of casts is Tamm-Horsfall protein, a glycoprotein excreted by the renal tubular cells. It is found in normal and abnormal urine and is not detected by the urine dipstick method.

Procedure for Microscopic Urine Examination

1. Collect a random urine specimen. Transport the specimen to the laboratory as soon as possible.
2. Urinary sediment is microscopically examined under both the low-power field (lpf) and the high-power field (hpf). Low power is used to find and count casts; RBCs, WBCs, and bacteria show up and are counted under high power. Amounts present are defined in the following terms: few, moderate, packed, and packed solid; or 1+, 2+, 3+, and 4+. Crystals and other elements are also noted.
3. Microscopic results should be correlated with the physical and chemical findings to ensure the accuracy of the report (Table 3.8).

CLINICAL ALERT

Microscopic examination of urine sediment can provide the following information:

1. Evidence of renal disease as opposed to infection of the lower urinary tract
2. Type and status of a renal lesion or disease

TABLE 3.7 Interpreting Urine Laboratory Findings

Disease	Cause	Laboratory Findings	Signs	Chemical Findings	Microscopic Findings
Acute glomerulonephritis	Anti–basement membrane antibodies associated with strep infection, variety of infectious agents, toxins, allergens Inflammation of the glomeruli by which they become abnormally permeable and leak plasma proteins and blood into the renal tubules	Rapid appearance of hematuria, proteinuria, and casts Varying degree of hypertension, renal insufficiency, and edema Frequently seen in children and young adults	Gross hematuria, turbid, smoky	Protein <1.0 g/dL Blood positive	Increased RBCs, WBCs, renal tubular epithelial Casts: RBCs, granular, waxy, broad
Chronic glomerulonephritis	Represents end-stage result of persistent glomerular damage with continuing and irreversible loss of renal function Progresses to end-stage renal disease	Symptoms include edema, hypertension, anemia, metabolic acidosis, oliguria progressing to anuria	Hematuria	Protein >2.5 g/dL Blood, small amount SG low and fixed	Increased RBCs, WBCs, renal epithelial Casts: granular, waxy, broad
Nephrotic syndrome	Glomeruli whose basement membrane has become highly permeable to plasma proteins of large molecular weight and lipids, allowing them to pass in the tubules	Massive protein, edema, high levels of serum lipids, and low levels of serum albumin	Cloudy	Protein >3.5 g/dL Blood, small amount	Increased RBCs, oval fat bodies, free fat, renal epithelial Casts: fatty, waxy, renal
Acute tubular necrosis	Destruction of renal tubular epithelial cells Usually following a hypotensive event (shock), toxic element, or drugs and heavy metals	Oliguria and complete renal failure	Slightly cloudy	Protein <1.0 g/dL Blood positive SG low	Increased RBCs, WBCs, renal epithelial Casts: renal, granular, waxy, broad
Cystitis (lower urinary tract)	Infection of the bladder most commonly caused by bacteria; *Escherichia coli* most common (85%)	Frequent and painful urination	Cloudy, foul smelling	Protein <0.5 g/dL Blood, small amount	Increased WBCs, bacteria, RBCs, transitional epithelial

Urethritis (urethra in males)				Nitrite positive (usually) Leukocyte esterase positive (usually)	
Acute pyelonephritis (upper urinary tract)	An infection of the kidney or renal pelvis Caused by infectious organism that has traveled through the urinary tract and invaded the kidney tissue	More frequently in women with repeated urinary tract infections	Turbid, foul smelling	Protein <1.0 g/dL Blood positive Nitrite positive (usually) Leukocyte esterase positive (usually)	Increased WBCs (clumps), bacteria, renal epithelial Casts: WBCs, granular, renal, occasionally waxy
Chronic pyelonephritis	Permanent scarring of the renal tissue	Polyuria and nocturia develop as tubular function is lost With disease progression, there is hypertension and altered renal and glomerular flow	Cloudy	Protein <2.5 g/dL Nitrite positive (usually) Leukocyte esterase positive (usually) SG low	Increased WBCs Casts: granular, waxy, broad
Acute interstitial nephritis	Inflammation of the renal interstitium caused by drug toxicity or an allergic reaction	Fever, eosinophilia Skin rash	Cloudy	Protein <1 g/dL Blood positive Leukocyte esterase positive (usually)	Increased WBCs, RBCs, eosinophils, epithelial Increased casts: granular, renal hyaline

RBC, red blood cell; SG, specific gravity; WBC, white blood cell.

Adapted from Finnegan K: Routine urinalysis. In Lehmann CA (ed): Saunders Manual of Clinical Laboratory Science. Philadelphia, WB Saunders, 1998.

TABLE 3.8 Common Correlations in Urinalysis

Microscopic Elements	Physical Examination	Dipstick Measurement[a]
Red blood cells	Turbidity, red to brown color	Blood
White blood cells	Turbidity	Protein Nitrite Leukocytes
Epithelial cast cells	Turbidity	Protein
Bacteria	Turbidity, odor	pH Nitrite Leukocytes
Crystals	Turbidity, odor	pH

[a]Positive result.

Interventions

Pretest Patient Care

1. Explain purpose of test, procedure for random urine sample collection, and interfering factors.
2. Follow guidelines in Chapter 1 for safe, effective, informed *pretest* care.

Posttest Patient Care

1. Review test results; report and record findings. Modify the nursing care plan as needed. Monitor appropriately. Counsel the patient regarding abnormal findings.
2. Follow guidelines in Chapter 1 for safe, effective, informed *posttest* care.

● Urine Red Blood Cells and Red Blood Cell Casts

In healthy persons, erythrocytes (RBCs) occasionally appear in the urine. However, *persistent* findings of even small numbers of RBCs should be thoroughly investigated because these cells come from the kidney and may signal serious renal disease. They are usually diagnostic of glomerular disease. The presence of increased red cells in the urine is referred to as *hematuria*.

Normal Findings

RBCs: 0 to 3/hpf (high-power field, 40× objective)
RBC casts: 0/lpf (low-power field, 20× objective)

Procedure

1. Observe the Procedure for Microscopic Urine Examination on pages 223 through 224 of this chapter.
2. Urinary sediment is microscopically examined under high power for cells and under low power for casts.

Clinical Implications

1. *RBC casts* indicate hemorrhage in the nephron.
   a. RBC casts are found in three forms:
      (1) Intact RBCs
      (2) Degenerating cells within a protein matrix
      (3) Homogeneous blood casts ("hemoglobin casts")

b. RBC casts indicate acute inflammatory or vascular disorders in the glomerulus and are found in:
   (1) Glomerulonephritis (acute and chronic)
   (2) Renal infarction
   (3) Lupus nephritis
   (4) Goodpasture's syndrome
   (5) Severe pyelonephritis
   (6) Congestive heart failure
   (7) Renal vein thrombosis
   (8) Acute bacterial endocarditis
   (9) Malignant hypertension
   (10) Periarteritis nodosa

c. RBCs *should be present* if RBC casts are in the sediment.

2. *RBCs*

a. The finding of more than 1 or 2 RBCs/hpf is abnormal and can indicate:
   (1) Renal or systemic disease (glomerulonephritis)
   (2) Trauma to the kidney (vascular injury)

b. Increased numbers of RBCs occur in:
   (1) Pyelonephritis
   (2) SLE
   (3) Renal stones
   (4) Cystitis (acute or chronic)
   (5) Prostatitis
   (6) Tuberculosis (renal)
   (7) Genitourinary tract malignancies
   (8) Hemophilia, coagulation disorders
   (9) Malaria
   (10) Polyarteritis nodosa
   (11) Malignant hypertension
   (12) Acute febrile episodes

c. Greater numbers of RBCs than WBCs indicate bleeding into the urinary tract, as may occur with:
   (1) Trauma
   (2) Tumors of rectum, colon, pelvis
   (3) Aspirin overdose or other toxic drugs
   (4) Anticoagulant therapy overdose
   (5) Thrombocytopenia

CLINICAL ALERT

1. In health, RBCs are occasionally found in the urine. However, persistent findings of even small numbers of RBCs should be thoroughly investigated, the first step being to request a fresh urine specimen for repeat testing.
2. Rule out the possible presence of menstrual blood, vaginal bleeding, or trauma to the perineal area in a female patient.

Interfering Factors

1. Increased numbers of RBCs may be found after a traumatic catheterization and after passage of urinary tract or kidney stones.
2. Alkaline urine hemolyzes RBCs and dissolves casts ("ghosts").

3. Some drugs can cause increased numbers of RBCs in the urine (see Appendix E).
4. RBC casts and RBCs may appear after very strenuous physical activity or participation in contact sports.
5. Heavy smokers show small numbers of RBCs in the urine.
6. Yeast or oil droplets may be mistaken for RBCs.

Interventions

Refer to the Pretest Patient Care and Posttest Patient Care guidelines for Microscopic Examination of Urine Sediment on page 224.

● Urine White Blood Cells and White Blood Cell Casts

Leukocytes (WBCs) may originate from anywhere in the genitourinary tract. They are also capable of ameboid migration through the tissues to sites of infection or inflammation. An increase in urinary WBCs is called *pyuria* and indicates the presence of an infection or inflammation in the genitourinary system. However, WBC casts always come from the kidney tubules.

Normal Findings

WBCs: 0 to 4/hpf
Normal: Women may have slightly more WBCs.
WBC casts: 0/lpf

Procedure

1. Observe the Procedure for Microscopic Urine Examination on pages 223 through 224 of this chapter.
2. Urinary sediment is microscopically examined under high power for cells and under low power for casts.

Clinical Implications

1. *White blood cells*
   a. Large numbers of WBCs (>30/hpf) usually indicate acute bacterial infection within the urinary tract.
   b. Increased WBCs (pyuria) are seen in:
      (1) All renal disease
      (2) Urinary tract disease (e.g., cystitis, prostatitis, urethritis)
      (3) Appendicitis, pancreatitis
      (4) Strenuous exercise
      (5) Chronic pyelonephritis
      (6) Bladder tumors
      (7) Tuberculosis
      (8) SLE
      (9) Interstitial nephritis
      (10) Glomerulonephritis
   c. In bladder infections, WBCs tend to be associated with bacteria, epithelial cells, and relatively few RBCs.
   d. Large numbers of lymphocytes and plasma cells in the presence of a kidney transplant may indicate early tissue rejection (acute renal allograft rejection).
   e. Eosinophils are associated with tubulointerstitial disease and hypersensitivity to penicillin.
   f. WBC clumps suggest renal origin of WBCs and should be reported when present.

2. *WBC casts*
   a. WBC casts indicate renal parenchymal infection and may occur in:
      (1) Pyelonephritis
      (2) Acute glomerulonephritis
      (3) Interstitial nephritis
      (4) Lupus nephritis
   b. It can be very difficult to differentiate between WBC casts and epithelial cell casts.

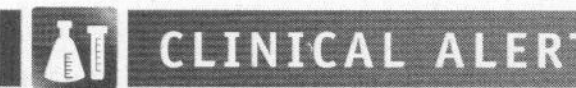

A urine culture (see Chapter 7) should be done if elevated urine WBCs are found.

Interfering Factors

Vaginal discharge can contaminate a specimen with WBCs. A clean-catch urine specimen or a catheterized urine specimen should be obtained to rule out contamination as the cause for WBCs in the urine.

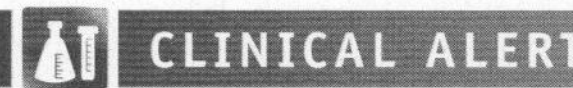

Pyelonephritis may remain completely asymptomatic even though renal tissue is being progressively destroyed. Therefore, careful examination (using low power) of urinary sediment for leukocyte casts is vital.

Interventions

Refer to the Pretest Patient Care and Posttest Patient Care guidelines for Microscopic Examination of Urine Sediment on page 224.

● Urine Epithelial Cells and Epithelial Casts

Renal epithelial cell casts are formed from cast-off tubule cells that slowly degenerate, first into coarse and then into fine granular material. Epithelial casts are the rarest.

Urine epithelial cells are of three kinds:

1. *Renal tubule epithelial cells* are round and slightly larger than WBCs. Each cell contains a single large nucleus. These are the types of epithelial cells associated with renal disease. However, the presence of an occasional renal epithelial cell is not unusual because the renal tubules are continually sloughing old cells. In cases of acute tubular necrosis, renal tubular epithelial cells containing large nonlipid vacuoles may be seen. These are referred to as *bubble cells*. When lipids cross the glomerular membrane, the renal epithelial cells absorb the lipids and become highly refractive. These are called *oval fat bodies*. Both of these findings are significant and should be reported.
2. *Bladder epithelial cells* are larger than renal epithelial cells. They range from round to pear-shaped to columnar. Also known as "transitional" epithelial cells, they line the urinary tract from the renal pelvis to the proximal two thirds of the urethra.
3. *Squamous epithelial cells* are large, flat cells with irregular borders; a single small nucleus; and abundant cytoplasm. Most of these cells are urethral and vaginal in origin and do not have much diagnostic importance.

Normal Findings

Renal tubule epithelial cells: 0 to 3/hpf
Squamous epithelial cells are common in normal urine sample.
Renal tubule epithelial casts: 0 (not seen)

Procedure

Observe the Procedure for Microscopic Urine Examination on pages 223 through 224 of this chapter.

Clinical Implications

1. Epithelial cell casts are found when they are also present in the urine after exposure to toxic agents or viruses.
2. Renal tubular epithelial cells are found in:
   a. Acute tubular necrosis
   b. Acute glomerulonephritis (secondary effects)
   c. Pyelonephritis
   d. Salicylate overdose (toxic reaction)
   e. Impending allograft rejection
   f. Viral infections (e.g., cytomegalovirus)
   g. Poisoning from heavy metals or other toxins

Interventions

Refer to the Pretest Patient Care and Posttest Patient Care guidelines for Microscopic Examination of Urine Sediment on page 224.

● Urine Hyaline Casts

Hyaline casts are clear, colorless casts that are formed when a renal protein within the tubules (Tamm-Horsfall protein) precipitates and gels. Tamm-Horsfall protein is excreted at a fairly constant rate by the tubule cells and provides immunologic protection from infection. Hyaline casts can be seen in physiologic states such as strenuous exercise and even in the mildest renal disease. They are not associated with any one particular disorder.

Normal Findings

Occasional, 0 to 2/lpf (low-power field, 10× objective)

Procedure

1. Observe the Procedure for Microscopic Urine Examination on pages 223 through 224 of this chapter.
2. Examine urinary sediment microscopically for casts under low power.
3. Examine casts when the light intensity is reduced because they are colorless and transparent.
4. Note that wrinkling and convoluting of the cast occurs as it ages.

Clinical Implications

1. Hyaline casts indicate possible damage to the glomerular capillary membrane. These casts appear in:
   a. Glomerulonephritis, pyelonephritis
   b. Malignant hypertension
   c. Chronic renal disease

    d. Congestive heart failure
    e. Diabetic nephropathy
2. Hyaline casts may be a temporary phenomenon in the presence of:
    a. Fever (dehydration)
    b. Postural orthostatic lordotic strain
    c. Emotional stress
    d. Strenuous exercise
    e. Heat exposure
3. Nephrotic syndrome may be suspected when large numbers of hyaline casts appear in the urine together with significant proteinuria, fine granular casts, fatty casts, oval bodies, or fat droplets.
4. In cylindroiduria, large numbers of hyaline casts may be present, but protein in the urine is absent. Cylindroids are hyaline casts that have been formed at the junction of the ascending loop of Henle and therefore have tapered ends.

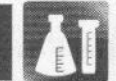

CLINICAL ALERT

Casts may not be found even when proteinuria is significant if the urine is dilute (1.010 SG) or alkaline. In these cases, the casts are dissolved as soon as they are formed.

Interfering Factors

Delays between specimen collection and testing may result in disintegration of casts.

Interventions

Refer to the Pretest Patient Care and Posttest Patient Care guidelines for Microscopic Examination of Urine Sediment on page 224.

● Urine Granular Casts

Granular casts appear homogeneous, coarsely granular, colorless, and very dense. They then further degenerate into finely granular casts. It is not necessary to distinguish the different granular casts. Granular casts may result from degradation of cellular casts, or they may represent direct aggregation of serum proteins into a matrix of Tamm-Horsfall microprotein.

Normal Findings

Occasional, 0 to 2/lpf (low-power field, 10× objective)

Procedure

1. Observe the Procedure for Microscopic Urine Examination on pages 223 through 224 of this chapter.
2. Examine urinary sediment microscopically under low power.

Clinical Implications

1. Granular casts are found in:
    a. Acute tubular necrosis
    b. Advanced glomerulonephritis

c. Pyelonephritis
d. Malignant nephrosclerosis

2. Granular casts are found with hyaline casts after strenuous exercise or severe stress.

Interventions

Refer to the Pretest Patient Care and Posttest Patient Care guidelines for Microscopic Examination of Urine Sediment on page 224.

● Urine Waxy Casts or Broad Casts (Renal Failure Casts) and Fatty Casts

Casts are formed in the collecting tubules under conditions of extreme renal stasis. Waxy casts form from the degeneration of granular casts.

Broad, waxy casts are 2 to 6 times the width of ordinary casts and appear waxy and granular. Casts may vary in size as disease distorts the tubular structure (they get wider because they are a mold of the tubules). Also, as urine flow from the tubules becomes compromised, casts are more likely to form. The finding of broad, waxy casts suggests a serious prognosis—hence, the term *renal failure casts*.

Fatty casts are formed from the attachment of fat droplets and degenerating oval fat bodies to a protein matrix. Fatty casts are highly refractile and contain yellow-brown fat droplets, or oval fat bodies.

Normal Findings

Negative (not seen)

Procedure

1. Observe the Procedure for Microscopic Urine Examination on pages 223 through 224 of this chapter.
2. Examine urine sediment microscopically under low power.

Clinical Implications

1. Broad and waxy casts occur in:
   a. Severe renal failure
   b. Tubular inflammation and degeneration (nephrotic syndrome)
   c. Localized nephron obstruction (extreme stasis of urine flow)
   d. Malignant hypertension
   e. Renal amyloidosis
   f. Diabetic nephropathy
   g. Renal allograft rejection
2. Fatty casts are found in:
   a. Disorders causing lipiduria, such as nephrotic syndrome and lipoid nephrosis
   b. Chronic glomerulonephritis
   c. Kimmelstiel-Wilson syndrome
   d. Systemic lupus erythematosus (SLE)
   e. Toxic renal poisoning

CLINICAL ALERT

The presence of broad, waxy casts signals serious renal disease.

Interfering Factors

Recent exposure to radiographic contrast may result in precipitation of crystals.

Interventions

Refer to the Pretest Patient Care and Posttest Patient Care guidelines for Microscopic Examination of Urine Sediment on page 224.

● Urine Crystals

A variety of crystals may appear in the urine. They can be identified by their specific appearance and solubility characteristics. Crystals in the urine may present no symptoms, or they may be associated with the formation of urinary tract calculi and give rise to clinical manifestations associated with partial or complete obstruction of urine flow.

The type and quantity of crystalline precipitate varies with the pH of the urine. Amorphous crystalline material has no significance and forms as normal urine cools.

Normal Findings

Negative for crystals

Procedure

1. Observe the Procedure for Microscopic Urine Examination on pages 223 through 224 of this chapter. Crystal identification should be done on freshly voided specimens.
2. Examine the urinary sediment microscopically under high power.
3. The pH of the urine is an important aid to identification of crystals and must be noted.
4. The problems associated with the identification of abnormal crystals can be resolved by a check on the medications the patient is receiving, saving considerable time and energy.

Clinical Implications

Table 3.9 describes the meaning of urine crystal findings.

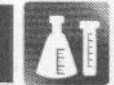 CLINICAL ALERT

Specific drugs (most commonly, ampicillin and sulfonamides) can cause increased levels of their own crystals, which could be a sign of improper hydration.

Interfering Factors

1. Refrigerated urine will precipitate out many crystals because the solubility properties of the compound are altered.
2. Urine left standing at room temperature will also cause precipitation of crystals or the dissolving of the crystals.
3. Radiographic dye can cause crystals in improperly hydrated patients. These resemble uric acid crystals and can be suspected in specimens that have an abnormally high SG (>1.030).

Interventions

Refer to the Pretest Patient Care and Posttest Patient Care guidelines for Microscopic Examination of Urine Sediment on page 224.

TABLE 3.9 Urine Crystals

Type of Crystal	Color	Shape	Clinical Implications
Acid Urine			
Amorphous urates	Pink to brick red	Granules	Normal
Uric acid	Yellow-brown	Polymorphous—whetstones, rosettes or prisms, rhombohedral prisms, hexagonal plate	Normal; increased purine metabolism, gout, Lesch-Nyhan syndrome
Sodium urate	Colorless to yellow	Fan of slender prisms	No clinical significance
Cystine (rare)	Colorless, highly refractile	Flat hexagonal plates with well-defined edges, singly or in clusters	Cystinuria; cystinosis—cystine stones in kidney, crystals also in spleen and eyes
Cholesterol (rare)	Colorless	"Broken window panes" with notched corners	Nephritis, nephrotic syndrome, chyluria
Leucine (rare)	Yellow or brown, highly refractile	Spheroids with striations; pure form hexagonal	Protein breakdown, severe liver disease, Fanconi's syndrome
Tyrosine (rare)	Colorless or yellow	Fine, silky needles in sheaves or rosettes	Protein breakdown, severe liver disease, oasthouse urine disease, tyrosinosis
Bilirubin	Reddish brown	Cubes, rhombic plates, amorphous needles	Elevated bilirubin
Acid, Neutral, or Slightly Alkaline Urine			
Calcium oxalate	Colorless	Octahedral dumbbells, often small—use high power	Normal; large amounts in fresh urine may indicate severe chronic renal disease, liver disease, ethylene glycol poisoning, diabetes mellitus, large doses of vitamin C
Hippuric acid (rare)	Colorless	Rhombic plates, four-sided prisms	No significance
Alkaline, Neutral, or Slightly Acid Urine			
Triple phosphate	Colorless	"Coffin lids," 3- to 6-sided prism; occasionally fern-leaf	Urine stasis and chronic cystitis, chronic pyelitis and enlarged prostate
Alkaline Urine			
Calcium carbonate	Colorless	Needles, spheres, dumbbells	Normal
Ammonium biurate	Yellow, opaque brown	"Thorn apple" spheres, dumbbells, sheaves of needles	Normal
Calcium phosphate	Colorless	Prisms, plates, needles	Normal
Amorphous phosphates	White	Granules	Normal

URINE CHEMISTRY

● Urine Pregnancy Test; Human Chorionic Gonadotropin (hCG) Test

From the earliest stage of development, the placenta produces hormones, either on its own or in conjunction with the fetus. The very young placental trophoblast produces appreciable amounts of the hormone human chorionic gonadotropin (hCG), which is excreted in the urine. This hormone is not found in the urine of men or of healthy, young, nonpregnant women.

Increased urinary hCG levels form the basis of the tests for pregnancy; hCG is present in blood and urine whenever there is living chorionic/placental tissue. hCG is made up of α- and β-subunits. The β-subunit is the most sensitive and specific test for early pregnancy. hCG can be detected in the urine of pregnant women 26 to 36 days after the first day of the last menstrual period (i.e., 5 to 7 days after conception). Pregnancy tests should return to negative 3 to 4 days after delivery.

Normal Findings

Positive: Pregnancy exists.
Negative: Pregnancy does not exist.

NOTE *Over-the-counter (home) pregnancy kits can typically detect hCG in the urine soon after the first missed menstrual period.*

Procedure

1. Collect an early morning urine specimen. The first morning specimen generally contains the greatest concentration of hCG. A random specimen may be used, but the SG must be >1.005.
2. Do not use grossly bloody specimens. If necessary, a catheterized specimen should be used.

Clinical Implications

1. A *positive* result usually indicates pregnancy.
2. *Positive* results also occur in:
   a. Choriocarcinoma
   b. Hydatidiform mole
   c. Testicular and trophoblastic tumors in males
   d. Chorioepithelioma
   e. Chorioadenoma destruens
   f. About 65% of ectopic pregnancies
3. *Negative or decreased* results occur in:
   a. Fetal demise
   b. Abortion, threatened abortion (test remains positive for 1 week after procedure)

Interfering Factors

1. False-negative test results and falsely low levels of hCG may be caused by dilute urine (low SG) or by using a specimen obtained too early in pregnancy.
2. False-positive tests are associated with
   a. Proteinuria
   b. Hematuria
   c. The presence of excess pituitary gonadotropin
   d. Certain drugs (e.g., chlorpromazine, phenothiazines, methadone)

Urine Estrogen, Total and Fractions (Estradiol [E_2] and Estriol [E_3]), 24-Hour Urine, and Total Estrogen—Blood

Measurements of *estradiol* (E_2), *estriol* (E_3), and total estrogen, together with the gonadotropin (follicle-stimulating hormone [FSH]) level (see Chapter 6), are useful in evaluating menstrual and fertility problems, male feminization characteristics, estrogen-producing tumors, and pregnancy.

- E_2 is the most active of the endogenous estrogens. The test evaluates female menstrual and fertility problems. In men, E_2 is useful for evaluating estrogen-producing tumors.
- E_3 is the prominent urinary estrogen in pregnancy. E_3 levels in both plasma and urine rise as pregnancy advances; significant amounts are produced in the third trimester. Serial measurements reflect the integrity of the fetal-placental complex. E_3 is not considered useful for detection of fetal distress. *Total estrogens* evaluate ovarian estrogen-producing tumors in premenarchal or postmenopausal females. Total estrogens may be helpful to establish time of ovulation and the optimum time for conception.

Normal Findings

Normal values vary widely between women and men and in the presence of pregnancy; the menopausal state; or the follicular, ovulatory, or luteal stage of the menstrual cycle.

Urine Estradiol (E_2)

Men: 0 to 6 μg/24 hours or 0 to 22 nmol/day
Women: follicular phase, 0 to 3 μg/24 hours or 0 to 11 nmol/day
Ovulatory peak, 4 to 14 μg/24 hours or 15 to 51 nmol/day
Luteal phase, 4 to 10 μg/24 hours or 15 to 37 nmol/day
Postmenopausal, 0 to 4 μg/24 hours or 0 to 15 nmol/day

Urine Estriol (E_3) (wide range of normal)

Men: 1 to 11 μg/24 hours or 4 to 40 nmol/day
Women: follicular phase, 0 to 14 μg/24 hours or 0 to 51 nmol/day
Ovulatory phase, 13 to 54 μg/24 hours or 48 to 198 nmol/day
Luteal phase, 8 to 60 μg/24 hours or 29 to 220 nmol/day
Postmenopausal, 0 to 11 μg/24 hours or 0 to 40 nmol/day
Pregnancy: 1st trimester, 0 to 800 μg/24 hours or 0 to 2900 nmol/day
2nd trimester, 800 to 12,000 μg/24 hours or 2900 to 44,000 nmol/day
3rd trimester, 5000 to 50,000 μg/24 hours or 18,000 to 180,000 nmol/day

Urine Total Estrogens

Men: 15 to 40 μg/24 hours or 55 to 147 nmol/day
Women: Menstruating, 15 to 80 μg/24 hours or 55 to 294 nmol/day
Postmenopausal, <20 μg/24 hours or <73 nmol/day
Pregnancy: 1st trimester, 0 to 800 μg/24 hours or 0 to 2900 nmol/day
2nd trimester, 800 to 5000 μg/24 hours or 2900 to 18,350 nmol/day
3rd trimester, 5000 to 50,000 μg/24 hours or 2900 to 183,000 nmol/day

Blood Total Estrogens

Men: 20 to 80 pg/mL or 20 to 80 ng/L
Women: Menstruating, 60 to 400 pg/mL or 60 to 400 ng/L
Postmenopausal, <130 pg/mL or <130 ng/L
Prepuberty, <25 pg/mL or <25 ng/L
Puberty, 30 to 280 pg/mL or 30 to 280 ng/mL

NOTE *Total serum estrogen does not measure estriol (E_3) and should not be used in pregnancy or to assess fetal well-being.*

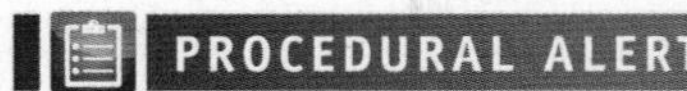

PROCEDURAL ALERT

Normal values are guidelines and must be interpreted in conjunction with clinical findings.

Procedure

1. Obtain a venous blood sample if needed for total estrogen.
2. Collect a 24-hour urine specimen and use boric acid preservative for all estrogen tests. Keep the container refrigerated or on ice during collection.
3. Follow general collection procedures for a 24-hour urine specimen (see Long-Term, Timed Urine Specimen [2-Hour, 24-Hour]).
4. Record the age and sex of the patient.
5. Ensure that the number of gestation weeks is communicated if patient is pregnant.
6. Document the number of days into the menstrual cycle for the nonpregnant woman.

CLINICAL ALERT

Estradiol may be used for monitoring persons on Pergonal (menotropins; i.e., combination of FSH and luteinizing hormone used to promote ovarian follicular growth). Serial measurements of E_2 during ovulation induction enable the healthcare provider to minimize high E_2 levels caused by ovarian overstimulation and thereby decrease side effects.

Clinical Implications

1. *Increased urine E_2* is found in the following conditions:
   a. Feminization in children (testicular feminization syndrome)
   b. Estrogen-producing tumors
   c. Precocious puberty related to adrenal tumors
   d. Hepatic cirrhosis
   e. Hyperthyroidism
   f. In women, E_2 increases during menstruation, before ovulation, and during the 23rd to 41st weeks of pregnancy.
2. *Decreased urine E_2* occurs in:
   a. Primary and secondary hypogonadism
   b. Kallmann's syndrome
   c. Hypofunction or dysfunction of the pituitary or adrenal glands
   d. Menopause
3. *Increased urine E_3* occurs in pregnancy; there is a sharp rise when delivery is imminent.
4. *Decreased urine E_3* is found in:
   a. Cases of placental insufficiency or fetal distress (abrupt drop of >40% on 2 consecutive days). Serial monitoring of E_3 for 4 consecutive days is recommended to evaluate fetal distress.

   b. Congenital heart disease
   c. Down's syndrome
5. Blood and urine total estrogens are *increased* in:
   a. Malignant neoplasm of adrenal gland
   b. Malignant neoplasm of ovary
   c. Benign neoplasm of ovary
   d. Granulosa cell tumor of ovary
   e. Lutein cell tumor of ovary
   f. Theca cell tumor of ovary
   g. Testicular tumors
6. Blood and urine total estrogens are *decreased* in:
   a. Ovarian hypofunction (ovarian agenesis, primary ovarian malfunction)
   b. Intrauterine death
   c. Preeclampsia
   d. Hypopituitarism
   e. Hypofunction of adrenal cortex
   f. Menopause
   g. Anorexia nervosa

Interfering Factors

1. Total estrogens
   a. Oral contraceptives
   b. Estrogen therapy
   c. Progesterone therapy
   d. Pregnancy and after administration of acetazolamide during pregnancy
2. E_2
   a. Radioactive pharmaceuticals
   b. Oral contraceptives
3. E_3
   a. Glucose and protein interfere with outcome.
   b. Day-to-day physiologic variation can be as much as 30%; therefore, single determinations are of limited use.
   c. Renal disease—in which case a serum assay would be more accurate

Interventions

Pretest Patient Care

1. Explain purpose of test, procedure for urine collection, and interfering factors.
2. Emphasize the importance of compliance with the procedure. The patient must be able to adjust daily activities to accommodate urine collection protocols.
3. Do not administer radioisotopes for 48 hours before specimen collection.
4. Obtain healthcare provider's approval to discontinue all medications for 48 hours before specimen collection. Drugs deemed necessary must be documented and communicated.
5. Follow guidelines in Chapter 1 for safe, effective, informed *pretest* care.

Posttest Patient Care

1. Patient may resume medications and normal activity.
2. Review test results; report and record findings. Modify the nursing care plan as needed. Counsel patient regarding abnormal findings. Monitor appropriately.
3. Follow guidelines in Chapter 1 for safe, effective, informed *posttest* care.

TIMED URINE TESTS

Timed urine tests, with collection times ranging from 2 to 24 hours, provide important information about the substances that are excreted in urine over time.

● Urine Chloride (Cl), Quantitative (24-Hour)

Normally, the urinary chloride excretion approximates the dietary intake. The amount of chloride excreted in the urine in a 24-hour period is an indication of the state of the electrolyte balance. Chloride is most often associated with sodium balance and fluid change.

The urine chloride measurement may be used to diagnose dehydration or as a guide in adjusting fluid and electrolyte balance in postoperative patients. It also serves as a means of monitoring the effects of reduced-salt diets, which are of great therapeutic importance in patients with cardiovascular disease, hypertension, liver disease, and kidney ailments.

Urine chloride is often ordered along with sodium and potassium as a 24-hour urine test. The urinary anion gap $[(Na + K) - (Cl + HCO_3)]$ is useful for initial evaluation of hyperchloremic metabolic acidosis. It is also used to determine whether a case of metabolic alkalosis is salt responsive.

Normal Findings

Adult: 140 to 250 mEq/24 hours or 140 to 250 mmol/day
Child <6 years old: 15 to 40 mEq/24 hours or 15 to 40 mmol/day
Child 10 to 14 years old: 64 to 176 mEq/24 hours or 64 to 176 mmol/day
Children's values are much lower than adult values.
Values vary greatly with salt intake and perspiration.
Different laboratories may have different values. Test results are interpreted in relation to salt intake and output.

Procedure

1. Collect a 24-hour urine specimen.
2. Record the exact starting and ending times on the specimen container and in the patient's health-care record.
3. The complete specimen should be sent to the laboratory for refrigeration until it can be analyzed.

CLINICAL ALERT

Because the electrolytes and water balance are so closely related, evaluate the patient's state of hydration by checking daily weight, by recording accurate intake and output, and by observing and recording skin turgor, the appearance of the tongue and mucous membranes, and the appearance of the urine sample.

Clinical Implications

1. *Decreased* urine chloride occurs in:
   a. Chloride-depleted patients (<10 mEq/L or <10 mmol/L); these patients have low serum chloride and are chloride responsive.
      (1) SIADH secretion
      (2) Vomiting, diarrhea, excessive sweating
      (3) Gastric suction

(4) Addison's disease
(5) Metabolic alkalosis
(6) Massive diuresis from any cause
(7) Villous tumors of the colon

b. Chloride is decreased by endogenous or exogenous corticosteroids (>20 mEq/L or >20 mmol/L); this condition is not responsive to chloride administration. Diagnosis of a chloride-resistant metabolic alkalosis helps identify a corticotropin (adrenocorticotropic hormone [ACTH]) or aldosterone-producing neoplasm, such as:
(1) Cushing's syndrome
(2) Conn's syndrome
(3) Mineralocorticoid therapy
(4) Postoperative chloride retention

2. *Increased* urine chloride occurs in:
a. Increased salt intake
b. Adrenocortical insufficiency
c. Potassium depletion
d. Bartter's syndrome
e. Salt-losing nephritis

Interfering Factors

1. Decreased chloride is associated with:
a. Carbenicillin therapy
b. Reduced dietary intake of chloride
c. Ingestion of large amounts of licorice
d. Alkali ingestion
e. Dehydration

2. Increased chloride is associated with:
a. Ammonium chloride administration
b. Excessive infusion of normal saline
c. Ingestion of sulfides, cyanides, halogens, bromides, and sulfhydryl compounds

Interventions

Pretest Patient Care

1. Explain purpose of test, procedure for 24-hour urine collection, and interfering factors.
2. Follow guidelines in Chapter 1 for safe, effective, informed *pretest* care.

Posttest Patient Care

1. Review test results; report and record findings. Modify the nursing care plan as needed. Monitor appropriately for fluid imbalances.
2. Follow guidelines in Chapter 1 for safe, effective, informed *posttest* care.

● Urine Sodium (Na), Quantitative (24-Hour)

Sodium is a primary regulator for retaining or excreting water and maintaining acid–base balance. The body has a strong tendency to maintain a total base content; on a relative scale, only small shifts are found even under pathologic conditions. As the predominant base substance in the blood, sodium helps to regulate acid–base balance because of its ability to combine with chloride and bicarbonate. Sodium also promotes the normal balance of electrolytes in the intracellular and extracellular fluids by acting in conjunction with potassium under the effect of aldosterone. This hormone promotes the 1:1 exchange of sodium for potassium or the hydrogen ion.

This test measures one aspect of electrolyte balance by determining the amount of sodium excreted in a 24-hour period. It is done for diagnosis of renal, adrenal, water, and acid–base imbalances.

Normal Findings

Adult: 40 to 220 mEq/24 hours or 40 to 220 mmol/day
Child: 41 to 115 mEq/24 hours or 41 to 115 mmol/day
Values are diet dependent.

Procedure

1. Properly label a 24-hour urine container with the patient's name, date and time of collection, and test(s) ordered.
2. The urine container must be refrigerated or kept on ice.
3. Follow general instructions for 24-hour urine collections (see Long-Term, Timed Urine Specimen [2-Hour, 24-Hour]).
4. Record exact starting and ending times on the specimen container and in the patient's healthcare record.
5. Transfer the specimen to the laboratory for proper storage when the test is completed.

Clinical Implications

1. *Increased* urine sodium occurs in:
   a. Adrenal failure (Addison's disease) (primary and secondary)
   b. Salt-losing nephritis
   c. Renal tubular acidosis
   d. SIADH
   e. Diabetic acidosis
   f. Aldosterone defect (AIDS-related hypoadrenalism)
   g. Tubulointerstitial disease
   h. Bartter's syndrome
2. *Decreased* urine sodium occurs in:
   a. Excessive sweating, diarrhea
   b. Congestive heart failure
   c. Adrenocortical hyperfunction
   d. Nephrotic syndromes with acute oliguria
   e. Prerenal azotemia
   f. Cushing's disease
   g. Primary aldosteronism

Interfering Factors

1. Increased sodium levels are associated with caffeine intake, diuretic therapy, dehydration, dopamine, postmenstrual diuresis, increased sodium intake, and vomiting (see Appendix E).
2. Decreased sodium levels are associated with intake of corticosteroids and propranolol, low sodium intake, premenstrual water retention, overhydration, and stress diuresis (see Appendix E).

Interventions

Pretest Patient Care

1. Explain purpose of test, procedure for urine collection (including the need to refrigerate or place specimen on ice), and interfering factors. Written instructions can be helpful.
2. Encourage food and fluids.
3. Follow guidelines in Chapter 1 for safe, effective, informed *pretest* care.

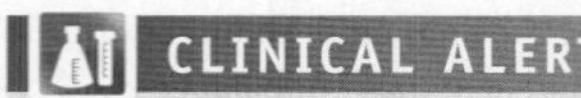

Because electrolytes and water balance are so closely related, determine the patient's state of hydration by checking and recording daily weights, accurate intake and output of fluids, and observations about skin turgor, the appearance of the tongue and mucous membranes, and the appearance of the urine.

Posttest Patient Care

1. Review test results; report and record findings. Modify the nursing care plan as needed. Monitor as necessary for fluid and electrolyte state.
2. Follow guidelines in Chapter 1 for safe, effective, informed *posttest* care.

• Urine Potassium (K), Quantitative (24-Hour) and Random

Potassium (K) acts as a part of the body's buffer system and serves a vital function in the body's overall electrolyte balance. Because the kidneys cannot completely conserve potassium, this balance is regulated by the excretion of potassium through the urine. It takes the kidney 1 to 3 weeks to conserve potassium effectively.

This test provides insight into electrolyte balance by measuring the amount of potassium excreted in 24 hours. This measurement is useful in the study of renal and adrenal disorders and water and acid–base imbalances. An evaluation of urinary potassium can be helpful in determining the origin of abnormal potassium levels. Urine potassium values of <20 mEq/L (or <20 mmol/L) are associated with nonrenal conditions, whereas values of >20 mEq/L (or >20 mmol/L) are associated with renal causes.

Normal Findings

Adult: 25 to 125 mEq/24 hours or 25 to 125 mmol/day
Child: 10 to 60 mEq/24 hours or 10 to 60 mmol/day
Values are diet dependent.
The transtubular potassium gradient (TTKG) is an index that reflects potassium conservation by the kidneys.
TTKG = urine K/plasma K ÷ urine osmolality/plasma osmolality
Normal TTKG = 8 to 9 is seen in a normal diet.
TTKG >10 is seen with high potassium intake and more excretion by the kidneys.
TTKG <3 is seen with low potassium intake and less excretion by the kidneys.
TTKG <7 is seen with hyperkalemia and may indicate mineralocorticoid deficiency.

Procedure

1. Label a 24-hour urine container properly with the patient's name, date and time of collection, and test(s) ordered.
2. Refrigerate the urine container or keep it on ice during the collection.
3. Follow general instructions for 24-hour urine collection (see Long-Term, Timed Urine Specimen [2-Hour, 24-Hour]).
4. Record exact starting and ending times on the container and in the patient's healthcare record.
5. Transfer the specimen to the laboratory for proper storage.
6. A random urine potassium determination may be done.

Clinical Implications

1. *Increased* urine potassium occurs in:
   a. Primary renal diseases
   b. Diabetic and renal tubule acidosis
   c. Albright-type renal disease
   d. Starvation (onset)

   e. Primary and secondary aldosteronism
   f. Cushing's syndrome
   g. Onset of metabolic alkalosis
   h. Fanconi's syndrome
   i. Bartter's syndrome
2. *Decreased* urine potassium occurs in:
   a. Addison's disease
   b. Severe renal disease (e.g., pyelonephritis, glomerulonephritis)
   c. In patients with potassium deficiency, regardless of the cause, the urine pH tends to decrease. This occurs because hydrogen ions are released in exchange for sodium ions, given that both potassium and hydrogen are excreted by the same mechanism.

Interfering Factors

1. *Increased* urinary potassium is associated with:
   a. Acetazolamide and other diuretics
   b. Cortisone
   c. Ethylenediaminetetraacetic acid (EDTA) anticoagulant
   d. Penicillin, carbenicillin
   e. Thiazides
   f. Licorice
   g. Sulfates (see Appendix E)
2. *Decreased* urinary potassium is associated with:
   a. Amiloride
   b. Diazoxide
   c. Intravenous glucose infusion (see Appendix E)

CLINICAL ALERT

In the presence of excessive vomiting or gastric suctioning, the resulting alkalosis maintains urinary potassium excretion at levels inappropriately high for the degree of actual potassium depletion that occurs.

Interventions

Pretest Patient Care

1. Explain purpose of test, procedure for 24-hour urine collection (including the need to refrigerate or place the specimen on ice), and interfering factors. Written instructions can be helpful.
2. Encourage food and fluids.
3. Follow guidelines in Chapter 1 for safe, effective, informed *pretest* care.

CLINICAL ALERT

1. Because electrolytes and water balance are so closely related, determine the patient's state of hydration by checking and recording daily weights, accurate intake and output of fluids, and observations about skin turgor, the appearance of the tongue and mucous membranes, and the appearance of the urine.
2. Observe for signs of muscle weakness, tremors, changes in electrocardiographic tracings, and dysrhythmias. The degree of hypokalemia or hyperkalemia at which these symptoms occur varies with each person.

Posttest Patient Care

1. Review test results; report and record findings. Modify the nursing care plan as needed. Monitor appropriately for signs and symptoms of electrolyte imbalances and kidney disorders.
2. Follow guidelines in Chapter 1 for safe, effective, informed *posttest* care.

● Urine Uric Acid, Quantitative (24-Hour)

Uric acid is formed from the metabolic breakdown of nucleic acids composed of purines. Excessive uric acid relates to excessive dietary intake of purines or to endogenous uric acid production in certain disorders. Normally, one third of the uric acid formed is degraded by bacteria in the intestines.

This test evaluates uric acid metabolism in gout and renal calculus formation. Evaluation of excess uric acid excretion is important to aid in evaluating stone formation and nephrolithiasis. It also reflects the effects of treatment with uricosuric agents by measuring the total amount of uric acid excreted within a 24-hour period.

Normal Findings

With normal diet: 250 to 750 mg/24 hours or 1.48 to 4.43 mmol/day
With purine-free diet: <400 mg/24 hours or <2.48 mmol/day
With high-purine diet: <1000 mg/24 hours or <5.90 mmol/day

Procedure

1. Properly label a 24-hour urine container to which the appropriate preservative has been added. Label with the patient's name, date and time of collection, and test(s) ordered.
2. Follow general instructions for 24-hour urine collection (see Long-Term, Timed Urine Specimen [2-Hour, 24-Hour]).
3. Record exact starting and ending times on the specimen container and in the patient's healthcare record.
4. When collection is completed, send the specimen to the laboratory.

Clinical Implications

1. *Increased* urine uric acid (uricosuria) occurs in:
   a. Nephrolithiasis (primary gout)
   b. Chronic myelogenous leukemia (secondary nephrolithiasis)
   c. Polycythemia vera
   d. Lesch-Nyhan syndrome
   e. Wilson's disease
   f. Viral hepatitis
   g. Sickle cell anemia
   h. High uric acid concentration in urine with low urine pH may produce uric acid stones in the urinary tract. (These patients do not have gout.)
2. *Decreased* urine uric acid is found in:
   a. Chronic kidney disease
   b. Xanthinuria
   c. Folic acid deficiency
   d. Lead toxicity

Interfering Factors

1. Many drugs increase uric acid levels, including:
   a. Salicylates (aspirin) and other nonsteroidal anti-inflammatory drugs (NSAIDs)
   b. Diuretics
   c. Vitamin C (ascorbic acid)

   d. Warfarin
   e. Cytotoxic drugs used to treat lymphoma and leukemia (see Appendix E)
2. Other factors increasing uric acid urine levels include:
   a. X-ray contrast media
   b. Strenuous exercise
   c. Diet high in purines (e.g., kidney, sweetbreads) (see Chapter 6)
3. Allopurinol decreases uric acid levels (see Appendix E)

Interventions

Pretest Patient Care

1. Explain purpose of test, procedure for 24-hour urine collection (including the need to refrigerate or place the specimen on ice), and interfering factors. Written instructions can be helpful.
2. Encourage food and fluids. In some situations, a diet high or low in purines may be ordered during and before specimen collection.
3. Follow guidelines in Chapter 1 for safe, effective, informed *pretest* care.

Posttest Patient Care

1. Patient may resume normal diet.
2. Review test results; report and record findings. Modify the nursing care plan as needed. Counsel the patient regarding abnormal findings; explain the prescribed treatment and possible need for further testing.
3. Follow guidelines in Chapter 1 for safe, effective, informed *posttest* care.

• Urine Calcium (Ca), Quantitative (24-Hour)

Calcium (Ca) homeostasis is maintained by the parathyroid hormone. The bulk of calcium excreted is eliminated in the stool. However, a small quantity of calcium is normally excreted in the urine. This amount varies with the quantity of dietary calcium ingested. Increased calcium in urine results from an increase in intestinal calcium absorption, a lack of renal tubule reabsorption of calcium, resorption or loss of calcium from bone, or a combination of these mechanisms. Values in both healthy and sick persons have a wide range.

The urine calcium test is used for evaluation of calcium intake and/or the rate of intestinal absorption, bone resorption, and renal loss. Urine calcium is high in 30% to 80% of cases of primary hyperparathyroidism but does not reliably diagnose this disease.

Normal Findings

Normal diet: 100 to 300 mg/24 hours or 2.50 to 7.50 mmol/day
Low-calcium diet: 50 to 150 mg/24 hours or 1.25 to 3.75 mmol/day
Rate of calcium excretion can be expressed as the ratio of calcium/creatinine (Ca/Cr).
Ca (mg/dL)/Cr (mg/dL): <0.14 or Ca (mmol/L)/Cr (mmol/L) <0.40
Ca (mg/dL)/Cr (mg/dL): >0.20 or Ca (mmol/L)/Cr (mmol/L) >0.57 are consistent with hypercalciuria.

Procedure

1. Properly label a 24-hour urine container with the patient's name, date and time of collection, and test(s) ordered.
2. Procure an acid-washed bottle. See Table 3.3 regarding 24-hour urine collection data.
3. Follow general instructions for 24-hour urine collection (see Long-Term, Timed Urine Specimen [2-Hour, 24-Hour]). Refrigerate during collection.
4. Record exact starting and ending times of the collection on the specimen container and in the patient's healthcare record.

5. Send the specimen to the laboratory when collection is completed.
6. Perform a random (Sulkowitch) test in an emergency. Follow directions for random urine collection.

Clinical Implications

1. *Increased* urine calcium (hypercalciuria: >350 mg/24 hours or >8.75 mmol/day) is found in:
   a. Hyperparathyroidism (30% to 80% of cases)
   b. Sarcoidosis
   c. Primary cancers of breast and bladder
   d. Osteolytic bone metastases (carcinoma, sarcoma)
   e. Multiple myeloma
   f. Paget's disease
   g. Renal tubular acidosis
   h. Fanconi's syndrome
   i. Vitamin D intoxication
   j. Idiopathic hypercalciuria
   k. Osteoporosis (especially after immobilization)
   l. Osteitis deformans
   m. Thyrotoxicosis
2. Increased urinary calcium almost always accompanies increased blood calcium levels.
3. Calcium excretion levels greater than calcium intake levels are always excessive; urine excretion values >400 to 500 mg/24 hours (>10 to 12.5 mmol/d) are reliably abnormal.
4. Increased calcium excretion occurs whenever calcium is mobilized from the bone, as in metastatic cancer or prolonged skeletal immobilization.
5. When calcium is excreted in increasing amounts, the situation creates the potential for nephrolithiasis or nephrocalcinosis, especially with high protein intake.
6. *Decreased* urine calcium is found in:
   a. Hypoparathyroidism
   b. Familial hypocalciuric hypercalcemia
   c. Vitamin D deficiency
   d. Preeclampsia
   e. Acute nephrosis, nephritis, renal failure
   f. Renal osteodystrophy
   g. Vitamin D–resistant rickets
   h. Metastatic carcinoma of prostate
   i. Malabsorption syndrome—celiac disease (sprue), steatorrhea
7. Urine calcium decreases late in normal pregnancy.

Interfering Factors

1. Falsely elevated levels may be caused by:
   a. Some drugs (e.g., calcitonin; vitamins A, K, and C; and corticosteroids) (see Appendix E)
   b. Urine procured immediately after meals in which high calcium intake has occurred (e.g., milk)
   c. Increased exposure to sunlight
   d. Immobilization (especially in children)
2. Falsely decreased levels may be found with:
   a. Increased ingestion of phosphate, bicarbonate, antacids
   b. Alkaline urine
   c. Thiazide diuretics (can be used to lower calcium levels therapeutically)
   d. Oral contraceptives, estrogens
   e. Lithium (see Appendix E)

Interventions

Pretest Patient Care

1. Explain purpose of test, procedure for urine collection, and interfering factors. Written instructions can be helpful.
2. Encourage food and fluids.
3. If the urine calcium test is done because of a metabolic disorder, the patient should eat a low-calcium diet, and calcium medications should be restricted for 1 to 3 days before specimen collection.
4. For a patient with a history of renal stone formation, urinary calcium results will be more meaningful if the patient's usual diet is followed for 3 days before specimen collection. Do *not* stop medications.
5. Follow guidelines in Chapter 1 for safe, effective, informed *pretest* care.

Posttest Patient Care

1. Review test results; report and record findings. Modify the nursing care plan as needed. Counsel the patient regarding abnormal findings. Monitor accordingly for calcium imbalances.
2. Follow guidelines in Chapter 1 for safe, effective, informed *posttest* care.

CLINICAL ALERT

1. Observe patients with very low urine calcium levels for signs and symptoms of tetany (muscle spasms, twitching, hyperirritable nervous system).
2. The first sign of calcium imbalance may be pathologic fracture that can be related to calcium excess.
3. The Sulkowitch test (random urine sample) can be used in an emergency, especially when hypercalcemia is suspected because hypercalcemia is life-threatening.

● Urine Magnesium (Mg), Quantitative (24-Hour)

Magnesium (Mg) excretion controls serum magnesium balance. Mg also helps regulate calcium absorption and bone and teeth integrity. Urinary magnesium excretion is diet dependent. With normal dietary intake of 200 to 500 mg/day, urine excretion is normally 75 to 150 mg/24 hours (3 to 6 mmol/day). The remainder of the dietary intake is excreted in the stool.

This test evaluates magnesium metabolism, investigates electrolyte status, and is a component of a workup for nephrolithiasis. It is useful for assessing the cause of abnormal serum magnesium. The magnesium load test is used to identify magnesium deficiency in individuals with normal renal function.

Normal Findings

75 to 150 mg/24 hours or 6.0 to 10.0 mEq/24 hours or 3.00 to 5.00 mmol/day
Values are diet dependent.

Magnesium Load Test
>18 nmol Mg/24 hours
<18 nmol Mg/24 hours indicates Mg deficiency

Procedure

1. Collect a 24-hour urine specimen in a metal-free and acid-rinsed container. The pH must be <2.
2. Record exact starting and ending times.

3. See Long-Term, Timed Urine Specimen (2-Hour, 24-Hour) for 24-hour urine collection guidelines.
4. In the magnesium load test, the patient is given 30 mmol of $MgSO_4$ in 1.0 L of normal saline via IV over an 8-hour period. Urine is collected for 24 hours beginning with the start of the IV.

Clinical Implications

1. *Increased* urine magnesium is associated with:
   a. Increased blood alcohol
   b. Bartter's syndrome
   c. Chronic glomerulonephritis
2. *Decreased* urine magnesium is associated with:
   a. Malabsorption
   b. Long-term chronic alcoholism
   c. Long-term parenteral therapy
   d. Magnesium deficiency
   e. Chronic renal disease
   f. Hypoparathyroidism
   g. Hypercalciuria
   h. Decreased renal function (e.g., Addison's disease)

Interfering Factors

1. Increased magnesium levels are associated with:
   a. Corticosteroids
   b. Cisplatin therapy
   c. Thiazide diuretics
   d. Amphotericin (see Appendix E)
   e. Blood in urine
2. Decreased magnesium levels: Many drugs affect test outcomes (see Appendix E).

Interventions

Pretest Patient Care

1. Explain purpose of test, procedure for urine collection, and interfering factors.
2. Instruct that the specimen will be unacceptable if it comes in contact with any type of metal.
3. Follow guidelines in Chapter 1 for safe, effective, informed *pretest* care.

Posttest Patient Care

1. Review test results; report and record findings. Modify the nursing care plan as needed. Monitor appropriately for abnormal magnesium excretion.
2. Follow guidelines in Chapter 1 for safe, effective, informed *posttest* care.

● Urine Oxalate, Quantitative (24-Hour)

Oxalate is an end product of metabolism. Normal oxalate is derived from dietary oxalic acid (10%) and from the metabolism of ascorbic acid (35% to 50%) and glycine (40%). Patients who form calcium oxalate kidney stones appear to absorb and excrete a higher proportion of dietary oxalate in the urine.

The 24-hour urine collection for oxalate is indicated in patients with surgical loss of distal small intestine, especially those with Crohn's disease. The incidence of nephrolithiasis in patients who have inflammatory bowel disease is 2.6% to 10%. Hyperoxaluria is regularly present after jejunoileal bypass for morbid obesity; such patients may develop nephrolithiasis.

Oxaluria is also a characteristic of ethylene glycol intoxication. In addition, vitamin C increases oxalate excretion and in some people may be a risk factor for calcium oxalate nephrolithiasis. Such ingestion can usually be determined through the patient's history. If oxalate excretion becomes normal after reduction of vitamin C intake, additional therapy to prevent stones may not be required.

Normal Findings

Men: <55 mg/24 hours or <611 μmol/day
Women: <50 mg/24 hours or <555 μmol/day

Procedure

1. Collect and refrigerate or place on ice a 24-hour urine specimen according to protocols. Do not acidify.
2. See Long-Term, Timed Urine Specimen (2-Hour, 24-Hour) for directions for a 24-hour urine collection.

Clinical Implications

1. *Increased* urine oxalate is associated with:
    a. Ethylene glycol poisoning (>150 mg/24 hours or >1700 μmol/day)
    b. Primary hyperoxaluria, a rare genetic disorder (100 to 600 mg/24 hours or 1100 to 6700 μmol/day [nephrocalcinosis])
    c. Pancreatic disorders (diabetes, steatorrhea)
    d. Cirrhosis, biliary diversion
    e. Vitamin B_6 (pyridoxine) deficiency
    f. Sarcoidosis
    g. Crohn's disease (inflammatory bowel disease)
    h. Celiac disease (sprue)
    i. Jejunoileal bypass for treatment of morbid obesity
2. *Decreased* urine oxalate occurs in renal failure.

Interfering Factors

1. Foods containing oxalates, such as rhubarb, strawberries, beans, beets, spinach, tomatoes, gelatin, chocolate, cocoa, and tea, cause increased levels.
2. Ethylene glycol and methoxyflurane cause increased levels (see Appendix E).
3. Calcium causes decreased levels (see Appendix E).
4. Ascorbic acid (vitamin C) increases levels.

Interventions

Pretest Patient Care

1. Explain purpose of test, procedure for urine collection, and interfering factors.
2. Advise the patient continue normal fluid intake and to avoid foods that promote oxalate excretion before the test. A written list of such foods is helpful.
3. Vitamin C should not be taken within 24 hours before the beginning of the test or during the test.
4. The patient should be ambulatory and preferably at home.
5. Follow guidelines in Chapter 1 for safe, effective, informed *pretest* care.

Posttest Patient Care

1. Patient may resume normal diet.
2. Review test results; report and record findings. Modify the nursing care plan as needed. Counsel the patient regarding abnormal findings
3. Follow guidelines in Chapter 1 for safe, effective, informed *posttest* care.

Urine Pregnanediol (24-Hour)

Pregnanediol levels in women with normal menstrual cycles are constant during the follicular phase. Levels increase sharply during the luteal phase. During pregnancy, levels gradually increase, falling sharply before the onset of labor and delivery.

This test measures ovarian and placental function. Specifically, it measures a part of the hormone progesterone and its principal excreted metabolite, pregnanediol. Progesterone exerts its main effect on the endometrium by causing the endometrium to enter the secretory phase and to become ready for the implantation of the blastocyte should fertilization take place.

Pregnanediol excretion is elevated in pregnancy and decreased in luteal deficiency or placental failure.

NOTE *A serum progesterone test is more informative than a urine pregnanediol test and is used as an index of progesterone production.*

Normal Findings

This test is difficult to standardize; it varies with age, sex, and length of existing pregnancy.
Child: <0.1 mg/24 hours or <0.312 μmol/day
Men: 0 to 1.9 mg/24 hours or 0 to 5.9 μmol/day
Women: follicular phase, 0 to 2.6 mg/24 hours or 0 to 8.1 μmol/day
Luteal, 2.6 to 10.6 mg/24 hours or 8.1 to 33.1 μmol/day
Pregnancy: 1st trimester, 10 to 35 mg/24 hours or 31 to 109 μmol/day
2nd trimester, 35 to 70 mg/24 hours or 109 to 218 μmol/day
3rd trimester, 70 to 100 mg/24 hours or 218 to 312 μmol/day

Procedure

1. Properly label a 24-hour urine container with the patient's name, date and time of collection, and test(s) ordered.
2. Refrigerate the specimen or use a boric acid preservative. Check laboratory policy. Protect the specimen from light.
3. Follow general instructions for 24-hour urine collection (see Long-Term, Timed Urine Specimen [2-Hour, 24-Hour]).
4. Record exact starting and ending times on the specimen container and in the patient's healthcare record.
5. Send the completed specimen to the laboratory.

Clinical Implications

1. *Increased* urine pregnanediol is associated with:
   a. Luteal cysts of ovary
   b. Arrhenoblastoma of the ovary
   c. Congenital hyperplasia of adrenal gland
   d. Granulosa theca cell tumor of ovary
2. *Decreased* urine pregnanediol is associated with:
   a. Amenorrhea (ovarian hypofunction)
   b. Threatened abortion (if <5.0 mg/24 hours or <15.6 μmol/day, abortion is imminent)
   c. Fetal death, intrauterine death, placental insufficiency
   d. Toxemia, eclampsia
   e. Ovarian failure
   f. Chronic nephritis in pregnancy

Interfering Factors

Decreased values occur with estrogen or progesterone therapy and with the use of oral contraceptives.

Interventions

Pretest Patient Care

1. Explain purpose of test, procedure for 24-hour urine collection, and interfering factors. Written instructions can be helpful.
2. Allow food and fluids.
3. Follow guidelines in Chapter 1 for safe, effective, informed *pretest* care.

Posttest Patient Care

1. Review test results; report and record findings. Modify the nursing care plan as needed. Counsel the patient regarding abnormal findings.
2. Follow guidelines in Chapter 1 for safe, effective, informed *posttest* care.

● Urine Pregnanetriol (24-Hour)

Pregnanetriol is a ketogenic steroid reflecting one segment of adrenocortical activity. Pregnanetriol should not be confused with pregnanediol despite the similarity of name. This 24-hour urine test is done to diagnose congenital adrenal hyperplasia, adrenogenital syndrome, owing to a defect in 21-hydroxylation. The diagnosis of adrenogenital syndrome is indicated in:

1. Adult women who show signs and symptoms of excessive androgen production with or without hypertension
2. Craving for salt
3. Sexual precocity in boys
4. Infants who exhibit signs of failure to thrive
5. Presence of external genitalia in females (pseudohermaphroditism). In males, differentiation must be made between a virilizing tumor of the adrenal gland, neurogenic and constitutional types of sexual precocity, and interstitial cell tumor of the testes.

Normal Findings

Adult female: 0 to 1.4 mg/24 hours or 0 to 4.4 μmol/day
Adult male: 0.02 to 0.7 mg/24 hours or 0.3 to 2.2 μmol/day
Child (<9 years old): <0.3 mg/24 hours or <0.9 μmol/day
Child (10 to 16 years old): 0.1 to 0.6 mg/24 hours or 0.3 to 1.9 μmol/day

NOTE *Above reference values are based on use of boric acid as the preservative.*

Procedure

1. Properly label a 24-hour urine container with the patient's name, date and time of collection, and test(s) ordered.
2. Refrigerate the specimen if necessary; some laboratories may require a boric acid preservative in the collection receptacle.
3. Follow general instructions for 24-hour urine collection (see Long-Term, Timed Urine Specimen [2-Hour, 24-Hour]).
4. Record exact starting and ending times on the specimen container and in the patient's healthcare record.
5. Send the completed specimen to the laboratory.

Clinical Implications

1. *Elevated* urine pregnanetriol occurs in:
   a. Congenital adrenocortical hyperplasia
   b. Stein-Leventhal syndrome
   c. Ovarian and adrenal tumors

2. *Decreased* urine pregnanetriol occurs in:
   a. Hydroxylase deficiency (rare)
   b. Ovarian failure

Interventions

Pretest Patient Care

1. Explain purpose of test, procedure for 24-hour urine collection, and interfering factors. Written instructions can be helpful.
2. Allow food and fluids.
3. Avoid muscular exercise before and during specimen collection.
4. Follow guidelines in Chapter 1 for safe, effective, informed *pretest* care.

Posttest Patient Care

1. Review test results; report and record findings. Modify the nursing care plan as needed. Counsel patient regarding abnormal findings.
2. Follow guidelines in Chapter 1 for safe, effective, informed *posttest* care.

● Urine 5-Hydroxyindoleacetic Acid (5-HIAA) (24-Hour)

Serotonin is a vasoconstricting hormone normally produced by the argentaffin cells of the gastrointestinal tract. The principal function of the cells is to regulate smooth muscle contraction and peristalsis. 5-Hydroxyindoleacetic acid (5-HIAA) is the major urinary metabolite of serotonin. 5-HIAA assays are more useful than the parent hormone serotonin.

This urine test is conducted to diagnose the presence of a functioning carcinoid tumor, which can be shown by significant elevations of 5-HIAA. Excess amounts of 5-HIAA are produced by most carcinoid tumors. Carcinoid tumors produce symptoms of flushing, hepatomegaly, diarrhea, bronchospasm, and heart disease.

Normal Findings

Qualitative: negative
Quantitative: 2 to 7 mg/24 hours or 11 to 37 μmol/day

Procedure

1. Tell the patient to not eat any bananas, pineapple, tomatoes, eggplants, plums, or avocados for 48 hours before or during the 24-hour test because these foods contain serotonin.
2. Properly label (patient's name, date and time of collection, and test ordered) a 24-hour urine container that contains a preservative.
3. Discontinue the following drugs 48 hours before sample collection with healthcare provider approval: acetaminophen, salicylates, phenacetin, naproxen, imipramine, and monoamine oxidase inhibitors.
4. Follow general directions for 24-hour urine collection (see Long-Term, Timed Urine Specimen [2-Hour, 24-Hour]).
5. Record exact starting and ending times of the collection on the specimen container and in the patient's healthcare record.
6. Send the completed specimen to the laboratory.

Clinical Implications

1. Levels >25 mg/24 hours or >131 μmol/day indicate large carcinoid tumors, especially when metastatic:
   a. Ileal tumors
   b. Pancreatic tumors
   c. Duodenal tumors
   d. Biliary tumors

2. *Increased* urine 5-HIAA is found in:
   a. Ovarian carcinoid tumor
   b. Nontropical sprue
   c. Bronchial adenoma (carcinoid type)
   d. Malabsorption
   e. Celiac disease
   f. Whipple's disease
   g. Oat cell cancer of the respiratory system
3. *Decreased* urine 5-HIAA is found in:
   a. Depressive illness
   b. Small intestine resection
   c. PKU
   d. Hartnup's disease
   e. Mastocytosis

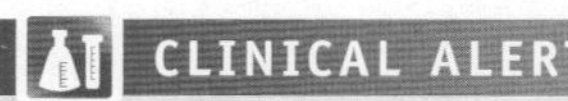

CLINICAL ALERT

A serum serotonin assay may detect some carcinoids missed by the urine 5-HIAA assay.

Interfering Factors

1. False-positive results occur with:
   a. Ingestion of banana, pineapple, plum, tomato, eggplant, chocolate, walnuts, and avocado because of their serotonin content
   b. Many drugs (see Appendix E)
   c. After surgery (surgical stress)
2. False-negative results can be caused by specific drugs that depress 5-HIAA production.

Interventions

Pretest Patient Care

1. Explain purpose of test, procedure for 24-hour urine collection, and interfering factors. Written instructions can be helpful.
2. Encourage food and fluids. Foods high in serotonin content must not be eaten for 48 hours before or during the test.
3. Obtain healthcare provider's approval to discontinue medications for 72 hours before or during specimen collection, if possible, especially aforementioned drugs and including over-the-counter drugs.
4. Follow guidelines in Chapter 1 for safe, effective, informed *pretest* care.

Posttest Patient Care

1. Patient may resume normal diet and medications.
2. Review test results; report and record findings. Modify the nursing care plan as needed. Counsel patient regarding abnormal findings.
3. Follow guidelines in Chapter 1 for safe, effective, informed *pretest* care.

• Urine Vanillylmandelic Acid (VMA); Catecholamines (24-Hour)

The principal substances formed by the adrenal medulla and excreted in urine are epinephrine, norepinephrine, metanephrine, and normetanephrine. These substances contain a catechol nucleus together with an amine group and therefore are referred to as *catecholamines*. Most of these hormones are changed into metabolites, the principal one being 3-methoxy-4-hydroxymandelic acid, known as VMA.

VMA is the primary urinary metabolite of the catecholamine group. It has a urine concentration 10 to 100 times greater than the concentrations of the other amines. It is also fairly simple to detect; methods used for catecholamine determination are much more complex.

This 24-hour urine test of adrenomedullary function is done primarily when pheochromocytoma, a tumor of the chromaffin cells of the adrenal medulla, is suspected in a patient with hypertension.

The assay for pheochromocytoma is most valuable when a urine specimen is collected during a hypertensive episode. Because a 24-hour urine collection represents a longer sampling time than a symptom-directed serum sample, the 24-hour urine test may detect a pheochromocytoma missed by a single blood level determination.

Normal Findings

Adults
VMA: up to 9 mg/24 hours or up to 45 μmol/day
Catecholamines (total): <100 μg/day or <591 nmol/day
Epinephrine: 0 to 20 μg/24 hours or 0 to 109 nmol/day
Metanephrine: 74 to 297 μg/24 hours or 375 to 1506 nmol/day
Norepinephrine: 15 to 80 μg/24 hours or 89 to 473 nmol/day
Normetanephrine: 105 to 354 μg/24 hours or 573 to 1933 nmol/day
Dopamine: 65 to 400 μg/24 hours or 420 to 2612 nmol/day
Children's levels are different from those of adults. Check with your laboratory for values in children.

NOTE *Different laboratories report values in different units—this should be kept in mind when analyzing results.*

Procedure

1. Properly label (patient's name, date and time of collection, and test[s] ordered) a 24-hour container with acid preservative (20 mL of HCl, 6 mol/L) and refrigerate the container or keep it on ice. Stable up to 14 days.
2. Follow general instructions for 24-hour urine collection (see Long-Term, Timed Urine Specimen [2-Hour, 24-Hour]).
3. Record exact starting and ending times of the collection on the specimen container and in the patient's healthcare record.
4. Send the specimen to the laboratory.

Clinical Implications

1. *Increased urine VMA* occurs as follows:
   a. High levels in pheochromocytoma
   b. Slight to moderate elevations in:
      (1) Neuroblastoma
      (2) Ganglioneuroma
      (3) Ganglioblastoma
      (4) Carcinoid tumor (some cases)
2. *Increased urine catecholamines* are found in:
   a. Pheochromocytoma
      (1) Norepinephrine, >170 mg/24 hours or >170 mg/day
      (2) Epinephrine, >35 mg/24 hours or >35 mg/day

   b. Neuroblastomas
   c. Ganglioneuromas
   d. Myocardial infarction (acute)
   e. Hypothyroidism
   f. Diabetic acidosis
   g. Long-term manic-depressive states
3. *Decreased urine catecholamines* are found in:
   a. Diabetic neuropathy
   b. Parkinson's disease

Interfering Factors

1. Increased urine VMA and catecholamines are caused by:
   a. Hypoglycemia—for this reason, the test should *not* be scheduled while the patient is NPO (nothing by mouth).
   b. Many foods, such as the following:
      (1) Caffeine-containing products (e.g., tea, coffee, cocoa, carbonated drinks)
      (2) Vanilla
      (3) Fruit, especially bananas
      (4) Licorice
   c. Many drugs cause increased VMA levels, especially reserpine, α-methyldopa, levodopa, monoamine oxidase inhibitors, sinus and cough medicines, bronchodilators, and appetite suppressants.
   d. Exercise, stress, smoking, and pain cause physiologic increases of catecholamines.
   e. Heavy alcohol intake increases catecholamine levels.
2. Falsely decreased levels of VMA and catecholamines are caused by:
   a. Alkaline urine
   b. Uremia (causes toxicity and impaired excretion of VMA)
   c. Radiographic contrast agents—for this reason, an intravenous pyelogram should not be scheduled before a VMA test.
   d. Certain drugs (see Appendix E)

Interventions

Pretest Patient Care

1. Explain purpose of test, procedure for 24-hour urine collection, and interfering factors. Written instructions can be helpful, especially regarding restricted foods.
2. Explain diet and drug restrictions. Diet restrictions vary among laboratories, but coffee, tea, bananas, cocoa products, vanilla products, and aspirin are always excluded for 3 days (2 days before and 1 day during specimen collection).
3. Many laboratories require that all medications be discontinued for 1 week before specimen collection. Obtain healthcare provider's approval.
4. Encourage adequate rest, food, and fluids.
5. Stress, strenuous exercise, and smoking should be avoided during the test.
6. Follow guidelines in Chapter 1 for safe, effective, informed *pretest* care.

Posttest Patient Care

1. Patient may resume normal diet, medications, and activity.
2. Review test results; report and record findings. Modify the nursing care plan as needed. Counsel patient regarding abnormal findings.
3. Follow guidelines in Chapter 1 for safe, effective, informed *posttest* care.

Urine Porphyrins and Porphobilinogens (24-Hour and Random); Δ-Aminolevulinic Acid (ALA, Δ-ALA)

Porphyrins are cyclic compounds formed from Δ-aminolevulinic acid (Δ-ALA), which plays a role in the formation of hemoglobin and other hemoproteins that function as carriers of oxygen in the blood and tissues. In health, insignificant amounts of porphyrin are excreted in the urine. However, in certain conditions, such as porphyria (disturbance in metabolism of porphyrin), liver disease, and lead poisoning, increased levels of porphyrins and Δ-ALA are found in the urine. Disorders in porphyrin metabolism also result in increased amounts of porphobilinogen in urine. The most common signs and symptoms of acute intermittent porphyria are abdominal pain, photosensitivity, sensory neuropathy, or psychosis. Patients with the porphyrias may pass urine that is pink, port wine, or burgundy colored.

When urine is tested for the presence of porphyrins, porphobilinogen, or ALA, it is also given the black-light screening test (Wood's light test). Porphyrins are fluorescent when exposed to black or ultraviolet light. See Chapter 2 for other tests for porphyria.

This test is used to diagnose porphyrias and lead poisoning in children. The following is a summary of laboratory findings for various porphyrias.

- *Congenital Erythropoietic Porphyria.* Elevations of urine uroporphyrin and coproporphyrin occur, with the former exceeding the latter. Lesser amounts of hepta-, hexa-, and pentacarboxyporphyrins are secreted. ALA and porphobilinogen levels are normal.
- *Acute Intermittent Porphyria.* Porphobilinogen and Δ-ALA are elevated in acute attacks, and small increases of urine uroporphyrin and coproporphyrin may be found. During periods of latency, the values are normal.
- *Porphyria Cutanea Tarda.* In this more common form of porphyria, increased uroporphyrins, uroporphyrinogen, and heptacarboxyporphyrins are seen.
- *Protoporphyria.* Mild disease, which mainly has the clinical symptoms of solar urticaria and solar eczema (from exposure to sunshine); increased fecal protoporphyrin.
- *Hereditary Coproporphyria.* Urine coproporphyrin and porphobilinogen are markedly increased during acute attacks; increases of urine uroporphyrin may also be found.
- *Variegate Porphyria.* In acute attacks, results are similar to those seen in acute intermittent porphyria. Porphobilinogen and Δ-ALA usually return to normal between attacks. Urine coproporphyrin exceeds uroporphyrin excretion during acute attacks.
- *Chemical Porphyrias* ("Intoxication porphyria"). Porphyrinogenic chemicals include certain halogenated hydrocarbons, which cause increased uroporphyrin levels in the urine. Also increased are ALA, coproporphyrin, and porphobilinogen.
- *Lead Poisoning.* Δ-ALA levels exceed those of porphobilinogen, which may remain normal. In children, ALA secretion in urine is more sensitive than blood lead levels.

Normal Findings

Porphyrins

Total and fractions: see Table 3.10

Porphobilinogens

Random specimen: 0 to 2.0 mg/L or negative or 0 to 8.8 μmol/L
24-hour specimen: 0 to 1.5 mg/24 hours or 0 to 6.6 mg/day

Δ-ALA

Random specimen: 0 to 4.5 mg/L or 0 to 34 μmol/L
24-hour specimen: 1.5 to 7.5 mg/24 hours or 11.4 to 57.2 μmol/day

TABLE 3.10 Specimen Values

	Male		Female	
Porphyrins[a]	(mg/24 hr)	(nmol/d)	(mg/24 hr)	(nmol/d)
Random and 24-hr specimens:	Negative		Negative	
Uroporphyrin	8–44	10–53	4–22	10–26
Coproporphyrin	10–109	15–167	3–56	5–86
Heptacarboxyporphyrin	0–12	0–15	0–9	0–11
Pentacarboxyporphyrin	0–4	0–6	0–3	0–4
Hexacarboxyporphyrin	0–5	0–7	0–5	0–5

[a]Total porphyrins: 20–121 mg/L or 24–146 nmol/L.

Procedure

1. Properly label a 24-hour clean-catch urine container with the patient's name, date and time of collection, and test(s) ordered.
2. Provide refrigeration or icing. The specimen must be kept protected from exposure to light. Check with your laboratory regarding the need for preservatives (e.g., 5 g of Na_2CO_3).
3. Follow general instructions for 24-hour urine collection (see Long-Term, Timed Urine Specimen [2-Hour, 24-Hour]).
4. Record exact starting and ending times on the specimen container and in the patient's healthcare record.
5. Send the specimen to the laboratory.
6. Obtain midmorning or midafternoon specimens for random tests because it is more likely that the patient will excrete porphyrins at those times. Transport the specimen to the laboratory immediately. Protect the specimen from light.
7. Observe and record the urine color. If porphyrins are present, the urine may appear amber-red or burgundy in color, or it may vary from pale pink to almost black. Some patients excrete urine of normal color that turns dark after standing in the light.

Clinical Implications

1. *Increased urine porphobilinogen* occurs in:
   a. Porphyria (acute intermittent type)
   b. Variegate porphyria
   c. Hereditary coproporphyria
2. *Increased fractionated porphyrins* occur in:
   a. Acute intermittent porphyria
   b. Congenital erythropoietic porphyria
   c. Hereditary porphyria
   d. Variegate porphyria
   e. Chemical porphyria caused by heavy metal poisoning or carbon tetrachloride
   f. Lead poisoning
   g. Viral hepatitis
   h. Cirrhosis (alcoholism)
   i. Newborn of mother with porphyria
   j. Congenital hepatic porphyria
3. *Increased urine Δ-ALA* can occur in:
   a. Acute intermittent porphyria (acute phase)
   b. Variegate porphyria (during crisis)
   c. Hereditary coproporphyria

d. Lead poisoning does *not* increase urine Δ-ALA until serum lead levels reach >40 μg/dL; urine Δ-ALA may remain elevated for several months after control of lead exposure.
e. Congenital hepatic porphyria
f. Slight increase in pregnancy, diabetic acidosis

4. *Decreased urine Δ-ALA* is found in alcoholic liver disease.

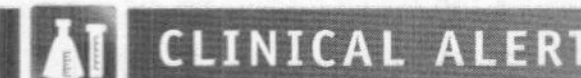

CLINICAL ALERT

Porphobilinogen is not increased in lead poisoning.

Interfering Factors

1. Oral contraceptives and diazepam can cause acute porphyria attacks in susceptible patients.
2. Alcohol ingestion interferes with the test.
3. Many other drugs, especially phenazopyridine, procaine, sulfamethoxazole, and the tetracyclines, interfere with the test (see Appendix E).

Interventions

Pretest Patient Care

1. Explain purpose of test, procedure for 24-hour urine collection, and interfering factors. Written instructions can be helpful.
2. Allow food and fluids but advise the patient to avoid alcohol and excessive fluid intake during the 24-hour collection.
3. Obtain healthcare provider's approval to discontinue all medications for 2 to 4 weeks before specimen collection, if possible, so that results will be accurate.
4. Follow guidelines in Chapter 1 for safe, effective, informed *pretest* care.

Posttest Patient Care

1. Patient may resume normal activities and medications.
2. Review test results; report and record findings. Modify the nursing care plan as needed. Counsel patient regarding abnormal findings.
3. Follow guidelines in Chapter 1 for safe, effective, informed *posttest* care.

CLINICAL ALERT

This test should not be ordered for patients receiving Donnatal (phenobarbital, hyoscyamine sulfate, atropine sulfate and scopolamine hydrobromide) or other barbiturate preparations. However, if intermittent porphyria is suspected, the patient should take those medications according to prescribed protocols because these drugs may provoke an attack of porphyria.

• Urine Amylase Excretion and Clearance (Random, Timed Urine, and Blood)

Amylase is an enzyme that changes starch to sugar. It is produced in the salivary glands, pancreas, liver, and fallopian tubes and is normally excreted in small amounts in the urine. If the pancreas or salivary glands are inflamed, much more of the enzyme enters the blood, and consequently, more amylase is excreted in the urine.

This test of blood and urine indicates pancreatic function and is done to differentiate acute pancreatitis from other causes of abdominal pain, epigastric discomfort, or nausea and vomiting.

In patients with acute pancreatitis, the urine often shows a prolonged elevation of amylase, compared with a short-lived peak in the blood. Moreover, urine amylase may be elevated when blood amylase is within normal range, and, conversely, the blood amylase may be elevated when the urine amylase is within normal range. The advantage of the amylase-creatinine clearance test is that it can be done on a single random urine specimen and a single serum sample instead of having to wait for a 2- or 24-hour urine collection. The ratio is increased in certain conditions other than acute pancreatitis, such as diabetic acidosis and renal insufficiency. Although the usefulness of this test in pancreatic disease has been questioned, it can be helpful to screen for macroamylasemia.

Normal Findings

Amylase/Creatinine Clearance Ratio

1% to 4% or 0.01 to 0.04 clearance fraction. This is a ratio calculated as follows:

$$\frac{\text{Urine amylase}}{\text{Serum amylase}} \times \frac{\text{Serum creatinine}}{\text{Urine creatinine}} \times 100$$

Urine Amylase

2-hour specimen: 2 to 34 U or 16 to 283 nkat/hour
24-hour specimen: 24 to 408 U or 400 to 6800 nkat/day
Values vary according to laboratory methods used. Check with your lab.

NOTE *kat = katal, which is a measure of enzyme activity.*

Procedure

For the amylase clearance test, a venous blood sample of 4 mL must be collected at the same time the random urine specimen is obtained.

1. Order a random, 2-hour, or 24-hour timed urine specimen. A 2-hour specimen is usually collected.
2. Refrigerate the urine specimen. Amylase is unstable in acidic urine. The pH must be adjusted to pH >7.0.
3. Follow general instructions for the appropriate urine collection.
4. Record exact starting and ending times on the specimen container and on the healthcare record. This is very important for calculation of results.
5. Send the specimen to the laboratory.

Clinical Implications

1. Amylase/creatinine clearance is *increased* in:
   a. Pancreatitis, pancreatic cancer
   b. Diabetic ketoacidosis (some patients)
   c. Toxemia of pregnancy, hyperemesis of pregnancy
   d. Renal insufficiency
2. Amylase/creatinine clearance is *decreased* in macroamylasemia.
3. Urine amylase is *increased* in:
   a. Pancreatitis
   b. Parotitis
   c. Intestinal obstruction
   d. Diabetic ketoacidosis
   e. Strangulated bowel
   f. Pancreatic cyst
   g. Peritonitis
   h. Biliary tract disease
   i. Some lung and ovarian tumors

4. Urine amylase is *decreased* in:
   a. Pancreatic insufficiency
   b. Advanced cystic fibrosis
   c. Severe liver disease
   d. Renal failure
   e. Macroamylasemia

Interfering Factors

1. Acid pH decreases urine amylase.
2. Some drugs produce increased amylase and possible pancreatitis.

Interventions

Pretest Patient Care

1. Explain purpose of test, procedure for urine collection, and interfering factors. Written instructions can be helpful.
2. Encourage fluids if they are not restricted.
3. Follow guidelines in Chapter 1 for safe, effective, informed *pretest* care.

Posttest Patient Care

1. Review test results; report and record findings. Modify the nursing care plan as needed. Monitor appropriately.
2. Follow guidelines in Chapter 1 for safe, effective, informed *posttest* care.

CLINICAL ALERT

Follow-up calcium levels should be checked in fulminating pancreatitis because extremely low calcium levels can occur.

Phenylketonuria (PKU); Urine Phenylalanine (Random Urine and Blood)

Routine blood and urine tests are done on newborns to detect PKU, an autosomal-recessive inherited disease that can lead to mental retardation and brain damage if untreated. This disease is characterized by a lack of the enzyme that converts phenylalanine, an amino acid, to tyrosine, which is necessary for normal metabolic function. Because dietary phenylalanine is not converted to tyrosine, phenylalanine, phenylpyruvic acid, and other metabolites accumulate in blood and urine. Tyrosine and the derivative catecholamines are deficient, which results in mental retardation. Both sexes are affected equally, with most cases occurring in persons of northern European ancestry.

This test is used for newborns to detect the metabolic disorder hyperphenylalaninemia. If untreated, this disorder can lead to mental retardation. Dietary restrictions of phenylalanine have shown good results.

Normal Findings

Blood: <2 mg/dL (2 to 5 days after birth) or <121 μmol/L
Urine: negative dipstick (detects phenylalanine in range of 5 to 10 mg/dL or 302 to 605 μmol/L)
24-hour urine:
    Newborns: 1.2 to 1.7 mg/24 hours (10 days to 7 weeks after birth) or 7.2 to 10.3 μmol/day
    Adults: <16.5 mg/24 hours or <100 μmol/day
    Children (3 to 12 years old): 4.0 to 17.5 mg/24 hours or 24 to 106 μmol/day

Procedure

The established standard is that all newborn infants should be tested for PKU and congenital hypothyroidism before discharge.

1. The blood test must be performed at least 3 days after birth or after the child has ingested protein (milk) for at least 24 to 48 hours.
2. Urine testing is usually done at the 4- or 6-week checkup if a blood test was not done.
3. PKU studies should be done on all infants who weigh ≥5 pounds (≥2.3 kg) before they leave the hospital.
4. Sick or premature infants should be tested within 7 days after birth regardless of protein intake, weight, or antibiotic therapy.

Collecting the Blood Sample

1. Cleanse the skin with an antiseptic and pierce the infant's heel with a sterile disposable lancet.
2. Support the infant, if bleeding is slow, so that the blood flows by means of gravity while spotting the blood with filter paper.
3. Fill the circles on the filter paper completely. This can best be done by placing one side of the filter paper against the infant's heel and watching for the blood to appear on the other side of the paper until it completely fills the circle.
4. Do not touch blood circles until they are completely dry. Keep in cool, dry area.
5. Transport samples to testing site within 12 to 24 hours.
6. Confirm all positive filter paper tests with a quantitative blood or urine test.

Collecting the Urine Sample in Nursery or at Home

1. Dip the reagent strip into a fresh sample of urine or press it against a wet diaper (phenylalanines and phenylpyruvic acid may not appear in urine until the infant is 2 to 3 weeks of age).
2. After exactly 30 seconds, compare the strip with a color chart according to manufacturer's directions.
3. Salicylates and phenothiazine may cause abnormal color reactions.
4. All positive tests must be confirmed with a quantitative chemical test.

Collecting the 24-Hour Urine Sample

1. Properly label a 24-hour clean-catch urine container with the patient's name, date and time of collection, and test(s) ordered.
2. Provide refrigeration or icing. Check with your laboratory regarding the need for preservatives (e.g., 10 mL of 6 mol/L HCl).
3. Follow general instructions for 24-hour urine collection (see Long-Term, Timed Urine Specimen [2-Hour, 24-Hour]).
4. Record exact starting and ending times on the specimen container and in the patient's healthcare record.
5. Send the specimen to the laboratory.

Clinical Implications

Increased phenylalanine is found in:

1. Hyperphenylalaninemia. In a positive test for PKU, the blood phenylalanine is >15 mg/dL or >907 μmol/L. Blood tyrosine is <5 mg/dL or <276 μmol/L; it is never increased in PKU.
2. Obesity
3. In low-birth-weight or premature infants, transient hyperphenylalaninemia, along with transient hypertyrosinemia, may occur.

Interfering Factors

1. Premature infants, those weighing <5 pounds (<2.3 kg), may have elevated phenylalanine and tyrosine levels without having the genetic disease. This is a result of delayed development of appropriate enzyme activity in the liver (liver immaturity).

2. Antibiotics interfere with the blood assay.
3. Cord blood cannot be used for analysis.
4. Two days of protein feeding must be done before blood is taken.

Interventions

Pretest Patient Care

Explain purpose of test, procedure for specimen collection, and interfering factors to the caregiver.

Posttest Patient Care

Interpret test outcomes and counsel regarding diet if results are positive.

● D-Xylose Absorption (Timed Urine and Blood)

The D-xylose test is a diagnostic measure for evaluating malabsorptive conditions and intestinal absorption of D-xylose, a pentose not normally present in the blood in significant amounts. It is passively absorbed in the proximal small bowel, passes unchanged in the liver, and is excreted by the kidneys.

This test directly measures intestinal absorption. When D-xylose (which is not metabolized by the body) is administered orally, blood and urine levels are checked for absorption rates. Absorption is normal in pancreatic insufficiency but is impaired in intestinal malabsorption. It is a reliable index of the functional integrity of the jejunum in pediatric patients.

Normal Findings

Blood

1-hour absorption of 5-g dose—infant: >15 mg/dL or >1.0 mmol/L
1-hour absorption of 5-g dose—child: >20 mg/dL or >1.3 mmol/L
2-hour absorption of 5-g dose—adult: >20 mg/dL or >1.3 mmol/L
2-hour absorption of 25-g dose—adult: >25 mg/dL or >1.6 mmol/L

Urine Xylose 5-Hour Reference Range for 25-g Dose

Child: 16% to 33% of 5-g dose
Adult: >16% of 5-g dose or >4.0 g of maximum (0.5 g/kg to a maximum of 25 g)
Adult, 65 years of age and older: >14% of dose or >3.5 g of maximum

Procedure

1. Have the patient refrain from foods containing pentose for 24 hours before test.
2. Do not allow food or liquids by mouth for at least 8 hours before the start of the test. Pediatric patients should fast only 4 hours.
3. Have the patient void at the beginning of the test. Discard this urine.
4. Administer the oral dose of D-xylose after it has been dissolved in 100 mL of water. Adult dosage is 25 g; for children younger than 12 years of age, a 5-g oral dose is recommended. For adults, additional water up to 250 mL should be taken at this time and another 250 mL in 1 hour. Record times on the patient's healthcare record. Give no further fluids (except water) or food until the test is completed.
5. Draw a 3-mL sample of venous blood within 60 to 120 minutes later.
6. Have the patient rest quietly in one place until the test is completed.
7. Have the patient void 5 hours from the start of the test. Save all urine voided during the test.

CLINICAL ALERT

Nausea, vomiting, and diarrhea may result from ingestion of the D-xylose. If vomiting occurs, the test is invalid and must be repeated. A 5-g dose is more tolerated but is less sensitive.

Clinical Implications

1. Urine D-xylose is *decreased* in:
   a. Intestinal malabsorption
   b. Impaired renal function
   c. Small bowel ischemia
   d. Whipple's disease
   e. Viral gastroenteritis (vomiting)
   f. Bacterial overgrowth in small intestine
2. The D-xylose test is *normal* in the following conditions:
   a. Malabsorption due to pancreatic insufficiency
   b. Postgastrectomy
   c. Malnutrition

Interfering Factors

1. Many drugs and antibiotics (see Appendix E)
2. Nonfasting state, treatment with hyperalimentation
3. Foods rich in pentose (fruits and preserves)
4. Vomiting of the xylose test meal (25-g dose may cause gastrointestinal distress)
5. Impaired renal function—use serum test only
6. In adults, the serum test has little value—use 5-hour urine test.

Interventions

Pretest Patient Care

1. Explain purpose of test, procedure for urine collection, and interfering factors. The entire 5-hour specimen must be collected.
2. The patient must fast at least 8 hours before the start of the test; children younger than 9 years of age should fast for only 4 hours.
3. Water may be taken at any time.
4. Weigh the patient to determine the proper dose of D-xylose.
5. The patient must discontinue contraindicated medications for 1 week before specimen collection. Obtain healthcare provider's approval.
6. Follow guidelines in Chapter 1 for safe, effective, informed *pretest* care.

Posttest Patient Care

1. Patient may resume normal food, fluids, and activities.
2. Follow guidelines in Chapter 1 for safe, effective, informed *posttest* care.

● Urine Creatinine; Blood (Serum) Creatinine, Creatinine Clearance (CrCl) (Timed Urine and Blood), Estimated Glomerular Filtration Rate (eGFR)

Creatinine is a substance that, in health, is easily excreted by the kidney. It is the byproduct of muscle energy metabolism and is produced at a constant rate according to the muscle mass of the individual. Endogenous creatinine production is constant as long as the muscle mass remains constant. Because all creatinine filtered by the kidneys in a given time interval is excreted into the urine, creatinine levels are equivalent to the glomerular filtration rate (GFR). Disorders of kidney function prevent maximum excretion of creatinine. The creatinine clearance test is part of most batteries of quantitative urine tests. Creatinine clearance is measured together with other urinary components in order to interpret the overall excretion rate of the various urinary components.

The creatinine clearance test is a specific measurement of kidney function, primarily glomerular filtration. It measures the rate at which the kidneys clear creatinine from the blood. In a broad sense, clearance of a substance may be defined as the imaginary volume (in milliliters) of plasma from which the substance would have to be completely extracted in order for the kidney to excrete that amount in 1 minute. In addition to estimating the GFR, this test is used to evaluate renal function in patients.

Because the excretion of creatinine in a given person is relatively constant, the 24-hour urine creatinine level is used as a check on the completeness of a 24-hour urine collection. It is of no help in the evaluation of renal function unless it is done as part of a creatinine clearance test.

Normal Findings

Urine creatinine, men: 14 to 26 mg/kg/24 hours or 124 to 230 μmol/kg/day
Urine creatinine, women: 11 to 20 mg/kg/24 hours or 97 to 177 μmol/kg/day
Blood (serum) creatinine: 0.6 to 1.2 mg/dL or 71 to 106 μmol/L for males (Table 3.11)
0.4 to 1.0 mg/dL or 36 to 90 μmol/L for females

NOTE *The National Kidney Disease Education Program (NKDEP) recommends that clinical laboratories report an estimated glomerular filtration rate when reporting serum creatinine.*

The following equations can be used to estimate the glomerular filtration rate (eGFR) when the method used to measure serum creatinine has not been calibrated to be traceable to isotope dilution mass spectrometry (IDMS).

When S_{cr} is in mg/dL (conventional units):

$$\text{eGFR (mL/min/1.73 m}^2) = 186 \times (S_{cr})^{-1.154} \times (\text{Age})^{-0.203} \times (0.742 \text{ if female}) \times (1.210 \text{ if African American})$$

When S_{cr} is in μmol/L (SI units):

$$\text{eGFR (mL/min/1.73 m}^2) = 186 \times (S_{cr}/88.4)^{-1.154} \times (\text{Age})^{-0.203} \times (0.742 \text{ if female}) \times (1.210 \text{ if African American})$$

Example:
Creatinine = 1.82 mg/dL
63-year-old African American female
eGFR = 36 mL/min/1.73 m^2

The following equations can be used to estimate the GFR when the method used to measure serum creatinine has been calibrated to be traceable to IDMS.

When S_{cr} is in mg/dL (conventional units):

$$\text{eGFR (mL/min/1.73 m}^2) = 175 \times (S_{cr})^{-1.154} \times (\text{Age})^{-0.203} \times (0.742 \text{ if female}) \times (1.210 \text{ if African American})$$

TABLE 3.11 Mean Creatinine Clearance (mL/min/1.73 m^2)[a]

Age (yr)	Men	Women
20–30	90–140 or 0.8–1.3 mL/sec/m^2	72–110 or 0.69–1.06 mL/sec/m^2
30–40	59–137 or 0.5–1.3 mL/sec/m^2	71–121 or 0.68–1.17 mL/sec/m^2

[a]Values slowly increase to adult levels and then slowly decrease each decade thereafter (the decrease per decade is approximately 6.5 mL/min/1.73 m^2 or 0.06 mL/sec/m^2).

When S_{cr} is in μmol/L (SI units):

$$\text{eGFR (mL/min/1.73 m}^2) = 175 \times (S_{cr}/88.4)^{-1.154} \times (\text{Age})^{-0.203} \times (0.742 \text{ if female}) \times (1.210 \text{ if African American})$$

Procedure

1. Properly label a 12-hour or 24-hour urine container with the patient's name, date and time of collection, and test(s) ordered.
2. Refrigerate or ice the specimen.
3. Follow general instructions for 24-hour urine collection (see Long-Term, Timed Urine Specimen [2-Hour, 24-Hour]).
4. Record exact starting and ending times on the specimen container and in the patient's healthcare record.
5. Send the entire specimen to the laboratory.
6. For serum creatinine, obtain a 5-mL venous blood sample in a red-topped or serum separator tube.
7. Record the patient's height and weight on the container and in the patient's healthcare record. Creatinine clearance values are based on the body surface area, and these values are needed to calculate the surface area.
8. Ensure that the patient is adequately hydrated throughout the test to provide proper urine flow.

Clinical Implications

1. *Decreased* creatinine clearance is found in any condition that decreases renal blood flow:
   a. Impaired kidney function, intrinsic renal disease, glomerulonephritis, pyelonephritis, nephrotic syndrome, acute tubular dysfunction, amyloidosis, interstitial nephritis
   b. Shock, dehydration
   c. Hemorrhage
   d. Chronic obstructive lung disease
   e. Congestive heart failure
2. *Increased* creatinine clearance is found in:
   a. State of high cardiac output
   b. Pregnancy
   c. Burns
   d. Carbon monoxide poisoning
3. *Increased* urine creatinine is found in:
   a. Acromegaly
   b. Gigantism
   c. Diabetes mellitus
   d. Hypothyroidism
4. *Decreased* urine creatinine is found in:
   a. Hyperthyroidism
   b. Anemia
   c. Muscular dystrophy
   d. Polymyositis, neurogenic atrophy
   e. Inflammatory muscle disease
   f. Advanced renal disease, renal stenosis
   g. Leukemia

Interfering Factors

1. Exercise may increase creatinine clearance and urine creatinine.
2. Pregnancy substantially increases creatinine clearance.
3. Many drugs decrease creatinine clearance (see Appendix E).
4. The creatinine clearance overestimates the GFR when there is severe renal impairment. The serum creatinine is more indicative of the GFR in this situation.

5. A diet high in meat may elevate the urine creatinine concentration.
6. Proteinuria and advanced renal failure make creatinine clearance an unreliable method for determining GFR.

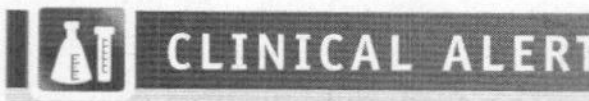

Determination of urine creatinine is of little value for evaluating renal function unless it is done as part of a creatinine clearance test.

Interventions

Pretest Patient Care

1. Explain purpose of test, procedure for urine collection, and interfering factors. Written instructions can be helpful.
2. Encourage fluids for good hydration. Large urine volumes ensure optimal test results. Advise patient to avoid tea and coffee (diuretics).
3. Allow food but advise patient to avoid eating large amounts of meat. Check with healthcare provider.
4. Avoid vigorous exercise during the test.
5. Obtain healthcare provider's approval to discontinue medications affecting the results before specimen collection, especially ACTH, cortisone, or thyroxine.
6. Follow guidelines in Chapter 1 for safe, effective, informed *pretest* care.

Posttest Patient Care

1. Patient may resume normal food, fluids, and activity.
2. Review test results; report and record findings. Modify the nursing care plan as needed. Monitor appropriately.
3. Follow guidelines in Chapter 1 for safe, effective, informed *posttest* care.

• Urine Cystine (Random and 24-Hour)

Cystinuria is a condition characterized by increased amounts of the amino acid cystine in the urine. The presence of increased urinary cystine is caused not by a defect in the metabolism of cystine but rather by the inability of the renal tubules to reabsorb cystine filtered by the glomeruli. The tubules fail to reabsorb not only cystine but also lysine, ornithine, and arginine; this rules out the possibility of an error in metabolism, even though the condition is inherited.

These urine tests are useful for the differential diagnosis of cystinuria, an inherited disease characterized by bladder calculi (cystine has low solubility). Patients with cystine stones face recurrent urolithiasis and repeated urinary infections.

Normal Findings

Random specimen: negative
24-hour specimen, adult: <38 mg/24 hours or <316 μmol/day
24-hour specimen, child: 5 to 31 mg/24 hours or 42 to 258 μmol/day
Values are age dependent; that is, they decrease throughout life.

Procedure

1. Obtain a random 20-mL urine specimen for a qualitative screening test. Label the specimen with the patient's name, date and time of collection, and test(s) ordered.
2. When collecting a 24-hour urine specimen, the container needs a preservative (toluene). Follow general procedures for a 24-hour urine specimen (see Long-Term, Timed Urine Specimen [2-Hour, 24-Hour]).

Clinical Implications

1. Urine cystine is *increased* in cystinuria (up to 20 times normal).
2. Urine cystine is *decreased* in burn patients.

CLINICAL ALERT

1. Cystinosis, a different entity from cystinuria, is not detected by cystine studies. Most patients with infantile nephropathic cystinosis have neurologic defects that become apparent in infancy. Failure to thrive and renal dysfunction are evidence of this disease.
2. Patients with cystinosis have a defect in renal tubular reabsorption that develops into Fanconi's syndrome, which leads to a generalized aminoaciduria. Cystine is elevated in the urine in the same proportion as all amino acids; the concentration is not high enough to form cystine stones. Plasma cystine is normal, but cystine is elevated in kidneys, eyes, spleen, and bone marrow; for purposes of diagnosis, it is usually measured in WBCs.

Interventions

Pretest Patient Care

1. Explain purpose of test, procedure for timed urine collection, and interfering factors.
2. Follow guidelines in Chapter 1 for safe, effective, informed *pretest* care.

Posttest Patient Care

1. Review test results; report and record findings. Modify the nursing care plan as needed. Counsel patient regarding abnormal findings.
2. Follow guidelines in Chapter 1 for safe, effective, informed *posttest* care.

● Urine Hydroxyproline (Timed Urine and Blood)

Hydroxyproline is an amino acid found only in collagen. It increases during periods of rapid growth, in bone diseases, and in some endocrine disorders. Urine hydroxyproline is almost entirely peptide bound, and only 10% is in the free form.

Total hydroxyproline is considered to be a marker for bone resorption because 50% of human collagen resides in bone. This test indicates the presence of reabsorption of bone collagen in various disorders and evaluates the degree of destruction from primary or secondary bone tumors. Free hydroxyproline is used as an aid to diagnose hydroxyprolinemia, a rare genetic disorder characterized by mental retardation and thrombocytopenia.

NOTE *During periods of rapid growth in early childhood and in puberty, total hydroxyproline is greatly increased.*

Normal Findings

Urine

Total hydroxyproline (24-hour): 15 to 45 mg/24 hours or 115 to 345 μmol/day
Adult females: 0.4 to 2.9 mg/2-hour specimen or 3 to 22 μmol/2 hours
Adult males: 0.4 to 5.0 mg/2-hour specimen or 3 to 38 μmol/2 hours
Children <5 years old: 100 to 400 μg/mg creatinine or 86 to 345 mmol/day
Children 5 to 12 years: 100 to 150 μg/mg creatinine or 86 to 129 mmol/day

Blood (Plasma)—Free Hydroxyproline

Newborn: 0.52 ± 0.52 mg/dL or 40 ± 40 µmol/L
Child (male): <0.66 mg/dL or <50 µmol/L
Child (female): <0.58 mg/dL or <44 µmol/L
Adult (male): <0.55 mg/dL or <42 µmol/L
Adult (female): <0.45 mg/dL or <34 µmol/L

Procedure

1. Obtain a 2-hour specimen after the patient has fasted overnight (preferred method). Label with the patient's name, date and time of collection, and test(s) ordered.
2. Notify the laboratory of the patient's age and sex.
3. If ordered, collect a 24-hour urine specimen. No preservative is required; however, to maintain proper pH, 25 mL of HCl, 6 mol/L is added. Specimen must be refrigerated or placed on ice.
4. Follow 24-hour urine collection procedures. The laboratory will record the total 24-hour volume.
5. Note that the preferred method of testing in the first few months of life is blood sampling (free hydroxyproline only for genetic screening).

Clinical Implications

1. *Free hydroxyproline is increased* in:
   a. Hydroxyprolinemia, a hereditary autosomal recessive condition (very rare)
   b. Familial iminoglycinuria, also inherited and rare
2. *Total hydroxyproline is increased* in:
   a. Hyperparathyroidism, hyperthyroidism
   b. Paget's disease—measures the severity and the response to treatment
   c. Marfan's syndrome, acromegaly
   d. Osteoporosis
   e. Myeloma
   f. Severe burns
3. *Total hydroxyproline is decreased* in:
   a. Hypopituitarism
   b. Hypothyroidism
   c. Hypoparathyroidism

Interfering Factors

1. Gelatin or collagen may affect test results (false-positive test); therefore, patient should avoid ingestion of meat. For best results, the patient should be on a nonprotein diet.
2. Bed rest increases values.
3. Pregnancy increases values.
4. Hydroxyproline excretion is highest at night due to diurnal variation.

Interventions

Pretest Patient Care

1. Explain purpose of test, procedure for timed urine collection, and interfering factors. Fasting and special fluid requirements before testing are often required for a 24-hour timed procedure. Check with laboratory.
2. Avoid gelatin- or collagen-containing foods for several days before the test.
3. Follow guidelines in Chapter 1 for safe, effective, informed *pretest* care.

Posttest Patient Care

1. Patient may resume normal diet and activity.
2. Review test results; report and record findings. Modify the nursing care plan as needed. Counsel patient regarding abnormal findings.
3. Follow guidelines in Chapter 1 for safe, effective, informed *posttest* care.

● Urine Lysozyme (Random, 24-Hour Urine, and Blood)

Lysozyme (muramidase) in blood or urine is a bacteriolytic enzyme that comes from degradation of granulocytes and monocytes but not lymphocytes. It is increased in leukemia owing to degradation of granulocytic or monocytic cells.

This blood and urine test differentiates acute myelogenous or monocytic leukemia from acute lymphatic leukemia. It is useful to monitor the response to treatment of acute myelogenous and active monocytic leukemia.

Normal Findings

Blood plasma: 0.4 to 1.3 mg/dL or 4 to 13 mg/L
Urine, 24-hour specimen: 0 to 3 mg/24 hours or 0 to 3 mg/day

NOTE *If collection time is less than or greater than 24 hours, value should be reported as mg/L.*

Reference values are not established for random urine specimens.

Procedure

1. Collect a 5-mL EDTA-anticoagulated blood sample or urine specimen.
2. Follow general instructions for 24-hour urine collections. *Transport the sample to the laboratory immediately after collection.*

Clinical Implications

1. *Lysozyme levels are increased* in:
   a. Acute myelogenous leukemia (granulocytic)
   b. Acute monocytic leukemia
   c. Malignant histiocytosis
2. *Lysozyme levels may be increased* in:
   a. Renal disorders and transplant rejection
   b. Tuberculosis
   c. Sarcoidosis (sarcoid lymph nodes)
   d. Crohn's disease
   e. Polycythemia vera
3. *Lysozyme levels are normal* in acute lymphatic leukemia.
4. *Lysozyme levels are decreased* in neutropenia with hypoplasia of bone marrow.

Interventions

Pretest Patient Care

1. Explain purpose of test, procedure for urine or blood collection, and interfering factors.
2. Follow guidelines in Chapter 1 for safe, effective, informed *pretest* care.

Posttest Patient Care

1. Review test results; report and record findings. Modify the nursing care plan as needed Counsel patient regarding abnormal findings.
2. Follow guidelines in Chapter 1 for safe, effective, informed *posttest* care.

● Urine Amino Acids, Total and Fractions (Random, 24-Hour Urine, and Blood)

Many abnormalities in amino acid transport or metabolism can be detected by physiologic fluid analysis (urine, plasma, or cerebrospinal fluid). Free amino acids are found in urine and in acid filtrates of protein-containing fluids. Urine is used for initial screening of inborn metabolic errors. Both transport errors and metabolic errors can be detected by changes in observed amino acid patterns. In many cases, metabolic errors are detected when amino acid or metabolite exceeds its renal threshold.

This test is useful for the diagnosis and monitoring of inborn errors of metabolism and transport in cases of suspected genetic abnormalities in patients with mental retardation, reduced growth, or other unexplained symptoms. More than 50 aminoacidopathies are now recognized.

Normal Findings

Urine and blood amino acid values are age dependent.

Procedure

1. Obtain a fasting blood specimen.
2. Collect a random 24-hour timed urine specimen. Keep the specimen refrigerated or on ice.

Clinical Implications

1. *Total plasma amino acids are increased* in:
   a. Specific aminoacidopathies (Table 3.12)
   b. Secondary causes
      (1) Diabetes with ketosis
      (2) Malabsorption
      (3) Hereditary fructose intolerance
      (4) Conditions with severe brain damage
      (5) Reye's syndrome
      (6) Acute and chronic renal failure
      (7) Eclampsia
2. *Total plasma amino acids are decreased* in:
   a. Adrenocortical hyperfunction
   b. Huntington's chorea
   c. *Phlebotomus* fever
   d. Nephritic syndrome
   e. Rheumatoid arthritis
   f. Hartnup's disease
3. *Total urine amino acids are increased* in specific aminoacidurias (see Table 3.12).
4. *Absence of amino acids* occurs as listed in Table 3.13.
5. *Renal transport aminoacidurias*
6. *Secondary aminoacidurias* occur in the following:
   a. Viral hepatitis
   b. Multiple myeloma
   c. Hyperparathyroidism
   d. Rickets (vitamin D resistant)

TABLE 3.12 Aminoacidurias

Aminoacidurias	Amino Acids Increased in Urine and Blood	Presence of Abnormal Enzymes
Phenylketonuria	Phenylketonuria	Phenylamine hydroxylase
Tyrosinosis	Tyrosine	p-Hydroxyphenyl-pyruvic acid oxidase
Histidinemia	Histidine	Histidase
Maple syrup urine disease	Valine, leucine, and isoleucine	Branched chain ketoacid decarboxylase
Hypervalinemia	Valine	Probably valine transaminase
Hyperglycinemia	Glycine (lysine on high-protein diet)	Increased glycine and propionic acid
Hyperprolinemia		
Type I	Proline	Proline oxidase,
Type II		pyrroline-5-carboxylate dehydrogenase
Hydroxyprolinemia	Hydroxyproline	Hydroxyproline oxidase
Homocystinuria	Methionine, homocystine	Cystathionine synthetase
Hyperlysinemia	Lysine	Lysine-α-ketoglutarate reductase
Citrullinemia	Citrulline	Argininosuccinic acid synthetase
Alkaptonuria	Homogentisic acid (2,5-dihydroxyphenylacetic acid); no abnormal amino acid	Homogentisic acid oxidase
Oasthouse urine disease	Methionine, phenylalanine, valine, leucine, isoleucine, and tyrosine, and also α-hydroxybutyric acid in urine	Possibly methionine malabsorption syndrome

e. Osteomalacia
f. Hereditary fructose intolerance
g. Galactosemia
h. Liver disease or necrosis
i. Renal failure, renal disease
j. Cystinosis
k. Muscular dystrophy (progressive)

TABLE 3.13 Absence of Amino Acids

Disease	Amino Acids in Urine	Presence of Abnormal Enzyme
Argininosuccinic aciduria	Argininosuccinic acid (also citrulline)	Argininosuccinase
Cystathioninuria	Cystathionine	Cystathionines
Homocystinuria	Homocystine	Cystathionine synthetase
Hypophosphatasia	Phosphoethanolamine	Serum alkaline phosphate

Interfering Factors

1. Amino acid concentration displays a marked circadian rhythm—30% variation, highest in midafternoon and lowest in morning.
2. Hyperalimentation and intravenous therapy affect outcome.
3. Drugs such as amphetamines, norepinephrine, levodopa, and all antibiotics affect results.
4. Age is a significant factor, especially in newborns and infants.
5. Pregnancy decreases values.

Interventions

Pretest Patient Care

1. Genetic counseling is recommended before specimen collection.
2. Explain purpose of test, procedure for urine collection (including the need for refrigeration), and interfering factors. Written instructions can be helpful.
3. Allow food and moderate amounts of fluids (do not overhydrate).
4. It may be necessary to consume proteins or carbohydrates for a challenge load to produce certain amino acid metabolites.
5. Follow guidelines in Chapter 1 for safe, effective, informed *pretest* care.

Posttest Patient Care

1. Review test results; report and record findings. Modify the nursing care plan as needed. Counsel patient regarding abnormal findings. Genetic counseling may be necessary.
2. Follow guidelines in Chapter 1 for safe, effective, informed *posttest* care.

BIBLIOGRAPHY

Goroll AH, Mully AG: Primary Care Medicine: Office Evaluation and Management of the Adult Patient, 7th ed. Philadelphia, Lippincott Williams & Wilkins, 2014

Mundt L, Shanahan K: Graff's Textbook of Urinalysis and Body Fluids, 3rd ed. Philadelphia, Lippincott Williams & Wilkins, 2015

Myers GL, Miller WR, Coresh J, et al: Recommendations for improving serum creatinine measurements: A report from the laboratory working group of the National Kidney Disease Education Program. Clin Chem 52:5–18, 2006

Strasinger SK, Dilorenzo M: Urinalysis and Body Fluids, 6th ed. Philadelphia, FA Davis, 2014

van Kuilenburg ABP, van Lenthe H, Löffler M, van Gennip AH: Analysis of pyrimidine synthesis "de novo" intermediates in urine and dried urine filter-paper strips with HPLC-electrospray tandem mass spectrometry. Clin Chem 50(11):2117–2124, 2004

Williamson MA, Snyder LM: Wallach's Interpretation of Diagnostic Tests, 10th ed. Philadelphia, Lippincott Williams & Wilkins, 2014

Wu AHB: Tietz Clinical Guide to Laboratory Tests, 4th ed. Philadelphia, Saunders Elsevier, 2006

Young DS: Effects of Drugs on Clinical Laboratory Tests, 5th ed. Washington, DC, AACC Press, 2000

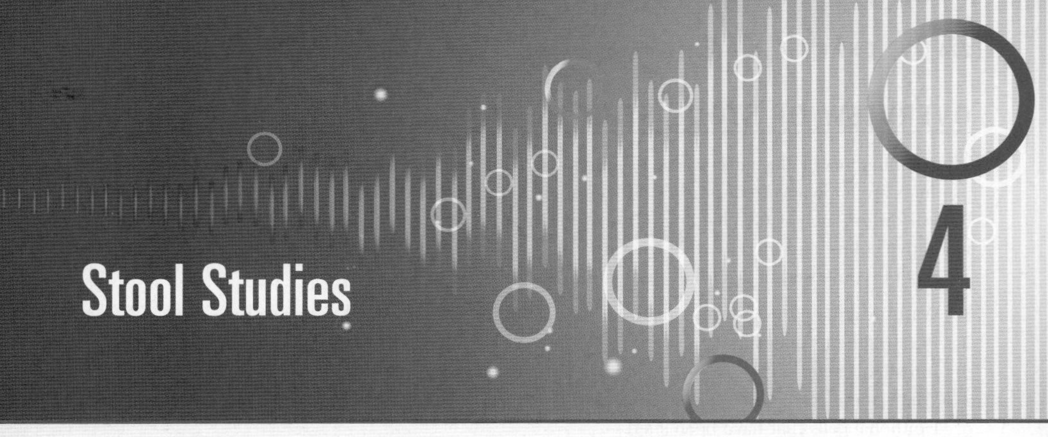

Stool Studies

4

OVERVIEW OF STOOL STUDIES

The elimination of digestive waste products from the body is essential to health. Excreted waste products are known as *stool* or *feces*. Stool examination is often done for evaluation of gastrointestinal (GI) disorders such as GI bleeding, GI obstruction, obstructive jaundice, parasitic disease, dysentery, ulcerative colitis, and increased fat excretion.

Stool is composed of the following materials:

1. Waste residue of indigestible material (e.g., cellulose) from food eaten during the previous 4 days
2. Bile (pigments and salts)
3. Intestinal secretions
4. Water and electrolytes
5. Epithelial cells that have been shed
6. Bacteria
7. Inorganic material, mainly calcium and phosphates
8. Undigested or unabsorbed food (normally present in very small quantities)

The output of feces depends on a complex series of absorptive, secretory, and fermentative processes. Normal function of the colon involves three physiologic processes: (1) absorption of fluid and electrolytes, (2) contractions that churn and expose the contents to the GI tract mucosa and transport the contents to the rectum, and (3) defecation.

The small intestine is approximately 23 feet (7 m) long, and the large intestine is 4 to 5 feet (1.2 to 1.5 m) long. The small intestine degrades ingested fats, proteins, and carbohydrates to absorbable units and then absorbs them. Pancreatic, gastric, and biliary secretions exert their effects on the GI contents to prepare this material for active mucosal transport. Other active substances absorbed in the small intestine include fat-soluble vitamins, iron, and calcium. Vitamin B_{12}, after combining with intrinsic factors, is absorbed in the ileum. The small intestine also absorbs as much as 9.5 L of water and electrolytes for return to the bloodstream. Small intestine contents (i.e., chyme, which contains fragments of proteins, droplets of fat, salt, and water) begin to enter the rectum as soon as 2 to 3 hours after a meal, but the process is not complete until 6 to 9 hours after eating.

The large intestine performs less complex functions than the small intestine. The proximal, or right, colon absorbs most of the water remaining after the GI contents have passed through the small intestine. Colonic absorption of water, sodium, and chloride is a passive process. Fecal water excretion is only about 100 mL/day. The colon mainly moves the luminal contents by seemingly random contractions of circular smooth muscle. Increased propulsive activity (i.e., peristalsis) occurs after eating. Peristaltic waves are caused by the gastrocolic and duodenocolic reflexes, which are initiated after meals and stimulated by the emptying of the stomach into the duodenum. The muscles of the colon are innervated by the autonomic nervous system. In addition, the parasympathetic nervous system stimulates movement, and the sympathetic system inhibits movement. Massive peristalsis (progressive waves of muscular contractions pushing the contents ahead) usually occurs several times a day. Resultant distention of the rectum initiates the urge to defecate. In persons with normal motility and a mixed dietary intake, normal colon transit time is 24 to 48 hours.

STOOL ANALYSIS

Stool analysis determines the various properties of the stool for diagnostic purposes. Some of the more frequently ordered tests on feces include tests for leukocytes, blood, fat, ova, parasites, and pathogens (Table 4.1). (See Chapter 7 for stool culture.) Stool is also examined by *chromatographic* analysis for the presence of gallstones. The recovery of a gallstone (precipitated by cholesterol or bile pigments) from feces provides the only proof that a common bile duct stone

TABLE 4.1 Stool Testing for Infections

Source of Stool Infection	Clinical Signs or Symptoms	Laboratory Test (Sequence or Follow-up)
Community Acquired from intermediate hosts, such as: Home—domestic pets, contaminated water Occupational Fishers—from snails and worms Meat cutters—from contaminated animals Healthcare workers—from patients Farm workers—from animals (cows, pigs), garden, flies, mosquitoes, fleas, other insects Recreational—backpacking, poor sanitation Travel—Third World—contaminated water supply Contact with fair animals Hookworm infection—not fecal or oral; passed via direct penetration of skin by larva in contaminated soil or in animal droppings	Diarrhea, bloody, purulent Steatorrhea Cramping, bloating, belching Small bowel obstruction, weight loss Generalized skin rash Huge swelling of legs, arms, or scrotum Huge lymphatic swelling Fever, chills, night sweats	Screen stool for ova and parasites Microscopic exam of stool for ova and parasites Stool culture for *Clostridium difficile* (some patients may require more than one assay) Eosinophilia in blood sample Exam for worms in stool or around anus Fecal smear for leukocytes and yeast
Nosocomial Acquired from institutions such as hospitals or nursing homes	Diarrhea Medication history of antibiotic use	Eosinophilia in blood sample Exam for worms in stool or around anus Microscopic exam of stool for ova and parasites Stool culture for *C. difficile* Fecal smear for leukocytes and yeast
Personal Contact with an infected host when patient is compromised (weakened immune system; i.e., HIV) or debilitated (such as a frail child or elderly patient)	Testing may occur following contact with infected host but before symptoms appear.	Screen stool for ova and parasites Microscopic exam of stool for ova and parasites Stool culture for *C. difficile* Toxin stool assay Acid-fast bacilli (AFB) in stool for tuberculosis Microsporidium

has been dislodged and excreted. Stool analysis also screens for colon cancer and asymptomatic ulcerations or other masses of the GI tract and evaluates GI diseases in the presence of diarrhea or constipation. Stool analysis is done in immunocompromised persons for parasitic diseases. Fat analysis is used as the gold standard to diagnose malabsorption syndrome. The Centers for Disease Control and Prevention recommend that stool samples submitted for enteric pathogen testing should also be tested for Shiga toxin (produced by *Escherichia coli* O157:H7 and other strains of *E. coli*).

Patients and healthcare personnel may dislike collecting and examining stool samples; however, this natural aversion must be overcome in light of the value of a stool examination for diagnosing disturbances and diseases of the GI tract, the liver, and the pancreas.

STOOL SPECIMEN COLLECTION AND TRANSPORT PROCEDURES

● Collection and Transport Procedures for All Types of Stool Collection

Procedure

1. Observe standard precautions (see Appendix A) when procuring and handling specimens to avoid infectious pathogens (e.g., hepatitis A, *Salmonella*, and *Shigella*).
2. Collect stool sample in a dry, clean, urine-free container that has a properly fitting cover. If unsure of how to collect the specimen, contact the laboratory before collection is begun.
3. The fresh specimen should not be contaminated with urine or other bodily secretions such as menstrual blood. Stool can be collected from the diaper of an infant or incontinent adult. Samples can be collected from temporary ostomy bags.
4. Accurately label all stool specimens with the patient's name, date, and tests ordered on the specimen. Keep the outside of the container free from contamination and immediately send the sealed container to the laboratory.
5. Place the specimen in a biohazard bag.
6. Post signs in bathrooms that say "DO NOT DISCARD STOOL" or "SAVE STOOL" to serve as reminders that stool sample collection is in progress.

Interfering Factors

1. Stool specimens from patients receiving tetracyclines, antidiarrheal medications, barium, bismuth, oil, iron, or magnesium may not yield accurate results.
2. Bismuth found in paper towels and toilet tissue interferes with accurate results.
3. Do not collect or retrieve stool from the toilet bowl or use a specimen that has been contaminated with urine, water, or toilet bowl cleaner. A clean, dry bedpan may be the best receptacle for defecation.
4. Inaccurate test results may result if the sample is *not representative* of the entire stool evacuation.
5. Lifestyle, personal habits, travel, home and work environments, and bathroom accessibility are some of the factors that may interfere with proper sample procurement.
6. Prompt transport of the specimen is necessary for accurate results. Trophozoites (protozoa in the early growth stage) in liquid stool disintegrate rapidly after defecation; therefore, the specimen needs to be examined 30 minutes from start of collection of specimen, not 30 minutes from end of collection. Semi-formed stool should be examined within 60 minutes after defecation. No trophozoites are seen in formed stool.

Interventions

Pretest Patient Care

1. Explain purpose of test, procedure for stool collection, and interfering factors using a culturally competent and culturally sensitive approach. Because the specimen cannot be obtained on demand, it is important to provide detailed instructions before the test so that the specimen is collected when the opportunity presents itself. Provide written instructions if necessary.
2. Provide proper containers and other collection supplies. Instruct the patient to defecate in a large-mouthed plastic container, bag, or clean bedpan. Provide for and respect the patient's privacy.
3. Instruct the patient *not to urinate* into the collecting container or bedpan.
4. Do not place toilet paper in the container or bedpan because it interferes with testing.
5. If the patient has diarrhea, a large plastic bag attached by adhesive tape to the toilet seat may be helpful in the collection process. After defecation, the bag can be placed into a container.
6. Specimens for most tests can be produced by a warm saline enema or Fleet Phospho-Soda enema.
7. Tests for both ova and parasites and cultures for enteric pathogens may be ordered together. In this case, the specimen should be divided into two samples, with one portion refrigerated for culture testing and one portion kept at room temperature for ova and parasite testing. Commercial collection kits are available that require the stool to be divided and placed into separate vials for better recovery of ova and parasites and enteric pathogens. (See Chapter 7, Microbiologic Studies.)
8. Follow guidelines in Chapter 1 for safe, effective, informed *pretest* care.

Posttest Patient Care

1. Provide patient privacy and the opportunity to cleanse perineal area and hands. Assist as necessary.
2. Review test results; report and record findings. Modify the nursing care plan as needed.
3. Follow guidelines in Chapter 1 for safe, effective, informed *posttest* care.

CLINICAL ALERT

1. Any stool collected may harbor highly infective pathogens. Observe standard precautions and proper handling techniques at all times.
2. Instruct patients in proper handwashing techniques after each use of the bathroom.

● Collection and Transport of Random Specimens

1. Observe the Collection and Transport Procedures for All Types of Stool Collection on pages 276 through 277 of this chapter.
2. Collect the entire stool sample and transfer it to a clean container using a clean tongue blade or similar object. A sample 2.5-cm (1-inch) long or 64.7 mg (1 oz) of liquid stool may be sufficient for some tests.
3. For best results, cover specimens and deliver to the laboratory immediately after collection. Depending on the examination to be performed, the specimen should be either refrigerated or kept warm. Contact the laboratory for detailed instructions concerning the temperature of stool specimen before collection is begun to avoid delay once the specimen is obtained.

● Collection and Transport of Specimens for Ova and Parasites

1. Observe the Collection and Transport Procedures for All Types of Stool Collection on pages 276 through 277 of this chapter.
2. Warm stools are best for detection of ova and parasites. Do *not* refrigerate specimens for ova and parasites.

3. Special vials that contain 10% formalin and polyvinyl alcohol (PVA) fixative may be used for collecting stool samples to test for ova and parasites.
4. Because of the life cycle of parasites, three separate random stool specimens for analysis are recommended.

Collection and Transport of Specimens for Enteric Pathogens

1. Observe the Collection and Transport Procedures for All Types of Stool Collection on pages 276 through 277 of this chapter.
2. Some coliform bacilli produce antibiotic substances that destroy enteric pathogens. Refrigerate the specimen immediately to prevent this from happening in the sample.
3. Samples that are diarrheal rather than formed stool are usually still adequate to give accurate results.
4. A freshly passed stool is the specimen of choice.
5. Collect stool specimens before antibiotic therapy is initiated and as early in the course of the disease as possible.
6. If mucus or blood is present, it should be included with the specimen because pathogens are more likely to be found in these substances. If only a small amount of stool is available, a walnut-sized specimen is usually adequate.
7. Keep the outside of the collection container free from contamination and immediately send the sealed container to the laboratory.
8. For best preservation and transport of specimens suspected of containing pathogens, a Cary-Blair solution (which contains sodium thioglycolate, disodium phosphate, sodium chloride, agar, and distilled water) vial with indicator should be used.

Collection and Transport of 24-, 48-, 72-, and 96-Hour Stool Specimens

This method is used to test for fat, porphyrins, urobilinogen, nitrogen, and electrolytes.

Procedure for Submitting Individual Specimens

1. Observe the Collection and Transport Procedures for All Types of Stool Collection on pages 276 through 277 of this chapter.
2. Collect all stool specimens for 1 to 3 days. The entire stool should be collected. Some procedures may require 4 days.
3. Label specimens with day of test (e.g., *Day 1, Day 2, Day 3, Day 4*), time of day collected, patient's name, and test(s) ordered. It is important to disclose the number of days collected because this information is needed for calculations.
4. Submit individual specimens to the laboratory as soon as they are collected.

Procedure for Submitting Total Specimens

1. Observe the Collection and Transport Procedures for All Types of Stool Collection on pages 276 through 277 of this chapter.
2. Obtain a 1-gallon container from the laboratory (a 1-gallon paint tin or covered plastic pail is preferred).
3. Save all stool and place in the container. Keep refrigerated or in a container with canned ice and replace ice as needed.
4. Label the specimen with the patient's name, dates and times of collections, duration of collection time, and test(s) ordered.
5. Transfer the properly labeled container to the laboratory at the end of the collection period.

STOOL STUDIES

● Stool Consistency, Shape, Form, Amount, and Odor

Inspection of the feces is an important diagnostic tool. The quantity, form, consistency, and color of the stool should be noted. Normally, stool reflects the shape and caliber of the colonic lumen as well as the colonic motility. The normal consistency is somewhat plastic and neither fluid, mushy, nor hard. Consistency can also be described as formed, soft, mushy, frothy, or watery. When diarrhea is present, the stool is watery. Large amounts of mushy, frothy, foul-smelling stool are characteristic of steatorrhea (excess fat in the feces). Constipation is associated with hard, spherical masses of stool.

Feces have a characteristic odor that varies with diet and the pH of the stool. The odor of normal stool is caused by indole (produced in intestine by breakdown of tryptophan) and skatole (formed from decomposition of protein) formed by bacterial fermentation and putrefaction.

Normal Findings

1. 100 to 200 g/24 hours or 100 to 200 g/day
2. Characteristic odor present; plastic, soft, formed; soft and bulky on a high-fiber diet; small and dry on a high-protein diet; seeds and small amounts of vegetable fiber present (as opposed to muscle fiber) (Table 4.2)

Procedure

Collect a random, fresh stool specimen following the procedure for Collection and Transport of Random Specimens. Observe standard precautions.

Clinical Implications

1. Stool consistency alterations
   a. Diarrhea due to the following:
      (1) Infection—*Salmonella*, *Shigella*, *Yersinia*, HIV enteropathy, *Campylobacter*
      (2) Inflammatory disorder—Crohn's disease, ulcerative colitis
      (3) Steatorrhea—celiac disease
      (4) Carbohydrate malabsorption—lactose or sucrose deficiency
      (5) Endocrine abnormalities—diabetes mellitus, hyperthyroidism or hypothyroidism, adrenal insufficiency
      (6) Hormone-producing tumors—Zollinger-Ellison syndrome (pancreatic gastrin-secreting tumor leading to increased acid activity in the stomach), gastrinoma, medullary thyroid carcinoma, villous adenoma
      (7) Colon carcinoma
      (8) Infiltration of lesions due to lymphoma, scleroderma of bowel
      (9) Drugs, antibiotics, cardiac medications, chemotherapy
      (10) Osmotically active dietary items—sorbitol, psyllium fiber, caffeine, ethanol
      (11) GI surgery—gastrectomy, stomach stapling, intestinal resection
      (12) Factitious—self-induced laxative abuse associated with psychiatric disorders
   b. "Pasty" stool associated with high-fat content can be caused by the following:
      (1) Common bile duct obstruction
      (2) Celiac disease
      (3) Cystic fibrosis—greasy "butter" stool appearance due to pancreatic involvement
   c. Bulky or frothy stool is usually due to steatorrhea and celiac disease.

TABLE 4.2 Normal Values in Stool Analysis

Macroscopic Examination	Normal Value
Amount	100–200 g/24 hr (100–200 g/d)
Color	Brown
Odor	Varies with pH of stool and depends on bacterial fermentation and putrefaction
Consistency	Plastic; not unusual to see fiber, vegetable skins, and seeds; soft and bulky in high-vegetable diet; small and dry in high-meat diet
Size and shape	Formed
Gross blood	None
Mucus	None
Pus	None
Parasites	None
Microscopic Examination	**Normal Value**
Fat	Colorless, neutral fat (18%) and fatty acid crystals and soaps
Undigested food, meat fibers, starch, trypsin	None to small amount
Eggs and segments of parasites	None
Bacteria and viruses	None
Yeasts	None
Leukocytes	None
Chemical Examination	**Normal Values**
Water	Up to 75% (0.75)
pH	Neutral to weakly alkaline (pH 7.0–7.5)
Occult blood	Negative
Urobilinogen	50–300 mg/24 hr (50–300 mg/d)
Porphyrins	Coproporphyrins: 400–1200 μg/24 hr (611–1832 nmol/d) Uroporphyrins: 10–40 μg/24 hr (12–48 nmol/d)
Nitrogen	<2.5 g/24 hr (<178 mmol/d)
Apt test for swallowed blood	Negative in adults; positive in newborns
Trypsin	20–95 U/g
Osmolality, used with stool	200–250 mOsm
Sodium	5.8–9.8 mEq/24 hr (5.8–9.8 mmol/d)
Chloride	2.5–3.9 mEq/24 hr (2.5–3.9 mmol/d)
Potassium	15.7–20.7 mEq/24 hr (15.7–20.7 mmol/d)
Lipids (fatty acids)	0–6 g/24 hr (0–21 mmol/d)
Carbohydrates (as reducing substances)	<0.25 g/dL (<2.5 g/L)

Note: Normal values for electrolytes vary greatly; check with your reference laboratory.

2. Stool size or shape alterations indicate altered motility or colon wall abnormalities.
   a. A narrow, ribbon-like stool suggests the possibility of spastic bowel, rectal narrowing or stricture, decreased elasticity, or a partial obstruction.
   b. Excessively hard stools are usually due to increased fluid absorption because of prolonged contact of luminal contents with colon mucosa during delayed transmit time through the colon.
   c. A large-circumference stool indicates dilation of the viscus.

   d. Small, round, hard stools (i.e., scybala) accompany habitual, moderate constipation.
   e. Severe fecal retention can produce huge, firm, impacted stool masses with a small amount of liquid stool as overflow. These must be removed manually, occasionally under light anesthesia.
3. Fecal odor should be assessed whenever a stool specimen is collected.
   a. A foul odor is caused by dehydration of undigested protein and is produced by excessive carbohydrate ingestion.
   b. A sickly sweet odor is produced by volatile fatty acids and undigested lactose.
4. Mucus in stool occurs in constipation, malignancy, and colitis.

Interventions

Pretest Patient Care

1. Explain purpose of test and procedure for stool collection. Instruct the patient to refrigerate the specimen. Provide clean, dry, leakproof collection container.
2. Advise the patient to avoid barium procedures and laxatives for 1 week before stool specimen collection.
3. Follow guidelines in Chapter 1 for safe, effective, informed *pretest* care.

Assessment of Diarrhea and Constipation

1. When performing a workup for the differential diagnosis of diarrhea or constipation, a patient history is most important. The following factors should be charted:
   a. An estimate of volume and frequency of fecal output
   b. Stool consistency and presence of blood, pus, mucus, oiliness, or bad odor in specimen; evaluate through direct observation when possible
   c. Decrease or increase in frequency of defecation
   d. Sensations of rectal fullness with incomplete stool evacuation
   e. Painful defecation
2. Assess dietary habits and food allergies.
3. Assess emotional state of patient—psychological stress may be major cause of altered bowel habits.
4. Assess for signs of laxative abuse.

Posttest Patient Care

1. Review test results; report and record findings. Modify the nursing care plan as needed. Counsel the patient regarding abnormal findings. If patient has watery diarrhea, note history of contact with affected family members, travel to a developing country, vacation or resort travel to areas at high risk for travelers' diarrhea, community and municipal water supply, or contact with farm animals. Explain that additional testing (e.g., colonoscopy) may be necessary.
2. Follow guidelines in Chapter 1 for safe, effective, informed *posttest* care.

● Stool Color

The brown color of normal stool is probably due to stercobilin (end product of heme catabolism), a bile pigment derivative, which results from the action of reducing bacteria in bilirubin and other undetermined factors.

The first indication of GI disturbances is often a change in the normal brown color of the feces. A change in color can provide information about pathologic conditions, organic dysfunction, or intake of drugs. Color abnormalities may aid the healthcare provider in selection of appropriate diagnostic chemical and microbiologic stool tests.

Normal Findings

Brown

Procedure

Collect a random, fresh stool specimen following the procedure for Collection and Transport of Random Specimens. Observe standard precautions.

Clinical Implications

The color of feces changes in some disease states as follows:

1. Yellow, yellow-green, or green: severe diarrhea
2. Black, with a tarry consistency: usually the result of bleeding in the upper GI tract (>100 mL blood)
3. Maroon, red, or pink: possibly the result of bleeding of the lower GI tract from tumors, hemorrhoids, fissures, or an inflammatory process
4. Clay colored (tan, gray, or white): biliary obstruction
5. Pale, with a greasy consistency: pancreatic deficiency causing malabsorption of fat

CLINICAL ALERT

Grossly visible blood always indicates an abnormal state.

1. Blood streaked on the outer surface of stool usually indicates hemorrhoids or anal abnormalities.
2. Blood present in stool can also be caused by abnormalities higher in the colon. If transit time is sufficiently rapid, blood from the stomach or duodenum can appear as bright red, dark red, or maroon in stool.

Interfering Factors

1. Stool darkens on standing.
2. The color of stool is influenced by dietary intake, food dyes, and drugs (see Appendix E).
   a. Yellow-rhubarb, yellow to yellow-green color occurs in the stool of breast-fed infants who lack normal intestinal flora.
   b. Pale yellow, white, or gray stools can be due to barium intake.
   c. Green color occurs with diets high in chlorophyll-rich green vegetables such as spinach or with some drugs (see Appendix E). An increase in biliverdin, green pigment formed during hemoglobin breakdown, may also contribute to green color.
   d. Black color may be due to foods such as cherries, a high proportion of dietary meat, artificially colored foods such as black jelly beans, or drugs and supplements such as charcoal, bismuth, or iron.
   e. Light-colored stool with little odor may be due to diets high in milk and low in meat.
   f. Clay-like color may be due to a diet with excessive fat intake or to barium intake.
   g. Red color may be due to a diet high in beets or tomatoes, red food coloring, or peridium compounds.
   h. Certain color changes may result from specific drugs (see Appendix E).

CLINICAL ALERT

A complete dietary and drug history will help to differentiate significant abnormalities from interfering factors.

Interventions

Pretest Patient Care

1. Explain purpose of test, procedure for stool collection, and interfering factors. Ask the patient to notify the healthcare provider about stool color changes.

2. Record dietary and drug history.
3. Advise the patient to avoid barium procedures and laxatives and for 1 week before specimen collection.
4. Follow guidelines in Chapter 1 for safe, effective, informed *pretest* care.

Posttest Patient Care

1. Report and record abnormal appearance and colors of stool. Modify the nursing care plan as needed. Counsel the patient regarding the meaning of color changes and explain the need for further testing (e.g., GI studies).
2. Follow guidelines in Chapter 1 for safe, effective, informed *posttest* care.

● Blood in Stool; Occult Blood

The most frequently performed fecal analysis is chemical screening for the detection of occult (i.e., hidden) blood. Bleeding in the upper GI tract may produce a black, tarry stool. Bleeding in the lower GI tract may result in an overtly bloody stool. However, no visible signs of bleeding may be present with smaller amounts of blood found in early stages of GI diseases; thus, the chemical detection of occult blood is necessary to identify and treat disease early in its course. Occult blood testing is also controversial owing to many false-positive and false-negative results. If the patient preparation and collection of specimen are followed explicitly, the results are more accurate.

An average, healthy person passes up to 2.0 mL of blood per 150 g of stool into the GI tract daily. Passage of >2.0 mL of blood in the stool in 24 hours is pathologically significant. Detection of occult blood in the stool is very useful in detecting early disease of the GI tract. This test demonstrates the presence of blood produced by upper GI bleeding, as in the presence of gastric ulcer; it also screens for colonic carcinomas while they are still in the localized stages. With proper medical follow-up, an 87% 5-year relative survival rate has been demonstrated for treatment of stage I colon cancer.

NOTE *Recent studies have demonstrated that fecal DNA testing may be more sensitive for detecting invasive cancers than fecal occult blood testing (FOBT). Another study looked at single digital FOBT (office based, screening) versus six-sample FOBT (home collected) and concluded that single digital FOBT is a poor screening tool. The fecal immunochemical test (FIT) also detects occult blood in the stool. The FIT is an antibody test that detects ungraded human hemoglobin. A positive FIT is more specific for bleeding in the lower GI tract.*

Normal Findings

Negative for blood

Procedure

1. Collect a random, fresh stool specimen following the procedure for Collection and Transport of Random Specimens. Observe standard precautions. Tests for detecting fecal blood use the pseudoperoxidase activity of hemoglobin reacting with hydrogen peroxide to oxidize a colorless compound to a colored one (usually blue). Hemoccult II (Beckman Coulter) is a widely used commercial test with a low percentage of false-positive results. This test system uses guaiac-impregnated filter paper as the chromogen that produces the blue color in a positive reaction.
2. Apply a thin smear of stool inside the indicated circle using a wood applicator stick and allow it to dry. If stool is bloody, the collector may be at risk for hepatitis B, hepatitis C, or HIV infection.
3. Protect the Hemoccult slide from light, heat, and humidity. Do not refrigerate.
4. Do not allow the delay between smearing the stool and testing to exceed 14 days. Do not refrigerate sample before testing.

Clinical Implications

1. Stool that appears dark red to tarry black indicates a loss of 50 to 75 mL of blood from the upper GI tract. Smaller quantities of blood in the GI tract can produce similar-appearing stools or appear as bright red blood.
2. A stool sample should be considered grossly bloody *only* after a chemical testing for presence of blood. This will eliminate the possibility that abnormal coloring caused by diet or drugs may be mistaken for bleeding in the GI tract.
3. Positive test for occult blood may be caused by the following conditions:
   a. Carcinoma of colon
   b. Ulcerative colitis and other inflammatory lesions
   c. Adenoma
   d. Diaphragmatic hernia
   e. Gastric carcinoma
   f. Rectal carcinoma
   g. Peptic ulcer
   h. Gastritis
   i. Vasculitis
   j. Amyloidosis
   k. Kaposi's sarcoma (tumors caused by human herpesvirus 8 [HHV8] presenting with cutaneous lesions)

CLINICAL ALERT

1. To be accurate, the test employed must be repeated 3–6 times on different stool samples; some bowel lesions may bleed intermittently.
2. The patient's diet should be free of red/rare meat and fruit and vegetable sources of peroxidase activity (e.g., turnips, parsnips, horseradish, radishes, mushrooms, cauliflower, broccoli, cantaloupe, apples, bananas). Only after following this regimen can a positive series of tests be considered an indication for further patient evaluation and testing.

Interfering Factors

1. Drugs such as salicylates (aspirin), steroids, indomethacin, nonsteroidal anti-inflammatory drugs (NSAIDs), anticoagulants, colchicine, and antimetabolites are associated with increased GI blood loss in average, healthy persons and with more pronounced bleeding when disease is present. GI bleeding can also follow parenteral administration of the aforementioned drugs and should be avoided 7 days before testing.
2. Drugs that may cause false-positive results for occult blood testing include the following:
   a. Boric acid
   b. Bromides
   c. Colchicine
   d. Iodine, povidone-iodine (Betadine)
   e. Other drugs (see Appendix E)
3. Foods that may cause false-positive results for occult blood testing include the following:
   a. Meats, including processed meats and liver, that contain hemoglobin, myoglobin, and certain enzymes and can give false-positive test results for up to 4 days after consumption
   b. Vegetables and fruits with peroxidase activity (e.g., turnips, parsnips, radishes, horseradish, mushrooms, broccoli, cauliflower, apples, bananas, cantaloupe)

4. Substances that cause false-negative results for occult blood testing include the following:
   a. Ascorbic acid (vitamin C) in excess of 250 mg/day
   b. Vitamin C–enriched foods and juices
   c. Iron supplements that contain vitamin C in excess of 250 mg
   d. Other drugs (see Appendix E)
5. Other factors affecting test results include the following:
   a. Bleeding hemorrhoids may produce erroneous results; take samples from center of stool to avoid this error.
   b. Collection of specimen during menstrual period
   c. Hematuria (i.e., blood in urine)
   d. Some long-distance runners have positive outcomes for occult blood.
   e. Toilet bowl cleansers may interfere with the chemical reaction of the test; remove bowl cleaners and flush twice before proceeding with test.

Interventions

Pretest Patient Care

1. Explain purpose of test, procedure for stool collection, and interfering factors, as well as the need to follow appropriate stool collection protocols for using a special kit for fecal occult blood or a plastic container with a lid.
2. Recommend that the patient consume a high-residue diet, starting 72 hours before and continuing throughout the collection period. Roughage in diet can increase test accuracy by helping to uncover silent lesions that bleed intermittently. The diet may include the following:
   a. Meats: only small amounts of chicken, turkey, and tuna
   b. Vegetables: generous amounts of both raw and cooked vegetables, including lettuce, corn, spinach, carrots, and celery; avoid vegetables with high peroxidase activity (see 3b, Interfering Factors)
   c. Fruits: plenty of fruits, especially prunes
   d. Cereals: bran and bran-containing cereals
   e. Moderate amounts of peanuts and popcorn daily. If any of the foods listed earlier are known to cause discomfort, the patient should consult the healthcare provider.
3. Advise the patient to avoid barium enemas for 72 hours before and during stool specimen collection.
4. Follow guidelines in Chapter 1 for safe, effective, informed *pretest* care.

PROCEDURAL ALERT

Instruct patients to observe the following procedures:

- Do not collect samples during or until 3 d after menstrual period or while the patient has bleeding hemorrhoids or blood in the urine.
- Do not consume the following medications, vitamins, and foods: For 7 d before and during the test period, avoid aspirin or other NSAIDs; for 72 hr before and during the test period, avoid vitamin C in excess of 250 mg/24 hr (250 mg/d) (from all sources, dietary and supplementary), red meat (e.g., beef, lamb), including processed meats and liver, and raw fruits and vegetables (see items listed in 3b, Interfering Factors).
- Remove toilet bowl cleaners from toilet tank and flush twice before proceeding to defecate.
- Collect samples from three consecutive bowel movements or three bowel movements closely spaced in time and spread a small stool sample (about 1 mL) on each of the three slides or card provided.
- Protect card or slides from heat, light, and volatile chemicals (e.g., iodine, bleach). Keep cover flap of slides closed when not in use.

Posttest Patient Care

1. Patient may resume normal diet after testing is complete.
2. Review occult blood test results; report and record findings. Modify the nursing care plan as needed. Counsel the patient regarding abnormal findings and monitor as necessary. Explain that further testing (e.g., barium enema, defecography) and follow-up may be required.
3. Follow guidelines in Chapter 1 for safe, effective, informed *posttest* care.

CLINICAL ALERT

Blood in the stool is abnormal and should be reported and recorded.

● Apt Test for Swallowed Blood

Dr. Leonard Apt developed the test for identifying the swallowed blood syndrome. The swallowed blood syndrome refers to bloody stools usually passed on the second or third day of life. The blood may be swallowed during delivery or may be from a fissure of the mother's nipple in breast-fed infants. This condition must be differentiated from GI hemorrhage of the newborn. The test is based on the fact that the infant's blood contains largely fetal hemoglobin (HbF), which is alkali resistant. This blood can be differentiated from the mother's blood using laboratory methods.

The Apt test is used to differentiate swallowed blood syndrome from infant GI hemorrhage or blood from the mother. The test can be done on stool or vomitus. Test result will indicate whether blood present in newborn stool or vomitus is of maternal or fetal origin.

Normal Findings

Qualitative: The specimen is dissolved and treated with 1% NaOH (5:1 ratio) for alkali denaturation. If blood is of fetal origin, the solution remains pink. If the blood is of maternal origin, the mixture will turn a yellowish brown. HbF is more resistant to alkali denaturation than adult hemoglobin.

Procedure

1. Collect a random, fresh specimen from a newborn infant. Observe standard precautions. Label the specimen with the patient's name, date and time of collection, and test(s) ordered.
2. The following are acceptable specimens:
   a. Blood-stained diaper
   b. Grossly bloody stool
   c. Bloody vomitus or gastric aspiration
3. Place specimen or specimens in a biohazard bag and deliver to the laboratory as soon as possible. Refrigerate the specimen or specimens if there is any delay.

Clinical Implications

1. HbF, which is pink in color, is present in gastric hemorrhage of the newborn.
2. Adult hemoglobin, which is brownish in color, is present in swallowed blood syndrome in the infant.

Interfering Factors

1. The test is invalid with black, tarry stools because the blood has already been converted to hematin (stimulates the synthesis of globin).
2. The test is invalid if there is insufficient blood present; grossly visible blood must be present in the specimen.
3. Vomitus with pH <3.9 produces an invalid test result.
4. The presence of maternal thalassemia major produces a false-positive test result because of increased maternal hemoglobin F.

Interventions

Pretest Patient Care

1. Explain purpose of test, procedure for stool collection, and interfering factors to the parent(s) or guardian(s).
2. Follow guidelines in Chapter 1 for safe, effective, informed *pretest* care.

Posttest Patient Care

1. Review test results; report and record findings. Modify the nursing care plan as needed. Counsel the parent(s) or guardian(s) regarding abnormal findings; explain the need for further testing and possible treatment for infant GI hemorrhage.
2. Follow guidelines in Chapter 1 for safe, effective, informed *posttest* care.

● Mucus in Stool

The mucosa of the colon secretes mucus in response to parasympathetic stimulation. Recognizable mucus in a stool specimen is abnormal and should be reported and recorded.

Normal Findings

Qualitative: negative for mucus

Procedure

Collect a random, fresh stool specimen following the procedure for Collection and Transport of Random Specimens. Observe standard precautions. Observe and report findings of mucus.

Clinical Implications

1. Translucent gelatinous mucus clinging to the surface of formed stool occurs in the following conditions:
    a. Spastic constipation
    b. Mucous colitis
    c. Emotionally affected patients
    d. Excessive straining to defecate
2. Bloody mucus clinging to the feces suggests the following conditions:
    a. Neoplasm
    b. Inflammation of the rectal canal
3. In villous adenoma of the colon, copious quantities of mucus may be passed (up to 3 to 4 L in 24 hours).
4. Mucus and diarrhea with white and red blood cells is associated with the following conditions:
    a. Ulcerative colitis (*Shigella*)
    b. Bacillary dysentery (*Salmonella*)
    c. Ulcerating cancer of colon
    d. Acute diverticulitis
    e. Intestinal tuberculosis
    f. Regional enteritis
    g. Amebiasis (infection caused by an amoeba, *Entamoeba histolytica*)

Interventions

Pretest Patient Care

1. Explain purpose of test and procedure for stool collection.
2. Advise the patient to avoid barium procedures and laxatives for 1 week before stool specimen collection.
3. Follow guidelines in Chapter 1 for safe, effective, informed *pretest* care.

Posttest Patient Care

1. Report and record presence, type, and amount of mucus. Modify the nursing care plan as needed.
2. Counsel the patient appropriately. Monitor bowel habits. Explain that further testing and follow-up monitoring may be necessary.
3. Follow guidelines in Chapter 1 for safe, effective, informed *posttest* care.

● Stool pH

Stool pH is diet dependent and is based on bacterial fermentation in the small intestine. Carbohydrate fermentation changes the pH to acid; protein breakdown changes the pH to alkaline.

Stool pH testing is done to evaluate carbohydrate and fat malabsorption and assess disaccharidase deficiency. Breast-fed infants have slightly acid stool; bottle-fed infants have slightly alkaline stools.

Normal Findings

1. Neutral to slightly acid or alkaline: pH 7.0 to 7.5 depending on diet
2. Newborns: pH 5.0 to 7.5 (In bottle-fed newborns, the pH will be slightly alkaline, whereas in breast-fed newborns, the pH will be slightly acidic.)

Procedure

1. Collect a random, fresh stool specimen following the procedure for Collection and Transport of Random Specimens. Observe standard precautions.
2. Refrigerate specimen.

Clinical Implications

1. Increased pH (alkaline)
   a. Secretory diarrhea without food intake
   b. Colitis
   c. Villous adenoma
   d. Antibiotic use (impaired colonic fermentation)
2. Decreased pH (acid)
   a. Carbohydrate malabsorption
   b. Fat malabsorption
   c. Disaccharidase deficiency (intestinal)

Interfering Factors

1. Barium procedures and laxatives affect test outcomes. They should be avoided for 1 week before stool sample collection.
2. Specimens contaminated with urine will invalidate the test.

Interventions

Pretest Patient Care

1. Explain purpose of test, procedure for stool collection, and interfering factors.
2. Advise the patient to avoid barium procedures and laxatives for 1 week before stool specimen collection.
3. Follow guidelines in Chapter 1 for safe, effective, informed *pretest* care.

Posttest Patient Care

1. Review test results; report and record findings. Modify the nursing care plan as needed. If abnormal pH is found, assess dietary patterns and antibiotic use. Counsel the patient regarding abnormal findings; explain the need for possible further testing.

2. Monitor as appropriate for malabsorption syndrome.
3. Order a stool reducing substance test if disaccharidase deficiency is suspected (see Stool Reducing Substances Test).
4. Follow guidelines in Chapter 1 for safe, effective, informed *posttest* care.

● Stool Reducing Substances Test

Normally, sugars are rapidly absorbed in the upper small intestine. However, if this is not the case, they remain in the intestine and cause osmotic diarrhea due to osmotic pressure of the unabsorbed sugar in the intestine, drawing fluid and electrolytes into the gut. The unabsorbed sugars are measured as reducing substances. Reducing substances that can be detected in the stool include glucose, fructose, lactose, galactose, and pentose. Carbohydrate malabsorption is a major cause of watery diarrhea and electrolyte imbalance seen in patients with the short bowel syndrome. Idiopathic lactase deficiency is common in people of African and Asian descent.

The finding of elevated levels of reducing substances in the stool is abnormal and suggests carbohydrate malabsorption. A presumptive diagnosis of disaccharide intolerance can be made with an elevated reducing substance level along with an acid (i.e., low) pH.

Normal Findings

1. Normal: <0.25 g/dL or <13.9 mmol/L reducing substances in stool
2. Questionable: 0.25 to 0.50 g/dL or 13.9 to 27.8 mmol/L reducing substances in stool

Abnormal

>0.5 g/dL (or >27.8 mmol/L) reducing substances in stool

Procedure

Collect a random, fresh stool specimen following the procedure for Collection and Transport of Random Specimens. Observe standard precautions and immediately deliver specimen to the laboratory.

Clinical Implications

Elevated reducing substances in stool are found in the following conditions:

1. Disaccharidase deficiency (intestinal)
2. Short bowel syndrome (as a result of the surgical removal of the small intestine, there is a malabsorptive disorder)
3. Idiopathic lactase deficiency, primary alactasia (enzyme deficiency leading to lactose intolerance)
4. Carbohydrate malabsorption abnormalities due to:
   a. Celiac disease (celiac sprue)
   b. Viral gastroenteritis

Interfering Factors

1. Bacterial fermentation of sugars may give falsely low results if the stool is not tested immediately.
2. Newborns may normally have elevated results.
3. Some drugs may cause malabsorption (e.g., neomycin, kanamycin, methotrexate).

Interventions

Pretest Patient Care

1. Explain purpose of test procedure for stool collection and interfering factors.
2. Follow guidelines in Chapter 1 for safe, effective, informed *pretest* care.

Posttest Patient Care

1. Review test results; report and record findings. Modify the nursing care plan as needed.
2. Counsel the patient regarding abnormal findings; explain the need for further testing (lactose intolerance) and treatment (dietary therapy).
3. Follow guidelines in Chapter 1 for safe, effective, informed *posttest* care.

● Leukocytes in Stool

Microscopic examination of the stool for the presence of leukocytes (white blood cells) is performed as a preliminary procedure in determining the cause of diarrhea. Leukocytes are normally not present in stool and are a response to infection or inflammation.

The presence or absence of fecal leukocytes can provide diagnostic information before the isolation of a bacterial pathogen. Neutrophils (>3 neutrophils per high-power field) are seen in the stool in conditions that affect the intestinal wall (e.g., ulcerative colitis, invasive bacterial pathogen infection). Viruses and parasites usually do not cause neutrophils in the stool. The greater the number of leukocytes, the greater the likelihood that an invasive pathogen is present.

Normal Findings

Negative for leukocytes

Procedure

Collect a random stool specimen following the procedure for Collection and Transport of Random Specimens. Observe standard precautions. Mucus or a liquid stool specimen can be used. A fresh specimen is preferred, or it may be preserved in PVA.

Clinical Implications

1. Large amounts of leukocytes (primarily neutrophils) accompany the following conditions:
   a. Chronic ulcerative colitis
   b. Bacillary dysentery
   c. Localized abscesses
   d. Fistulas of the sigmoid rectum or anus
   e. Shigellosis
   f. Salmonellosis
   g. *Yersinia* infection
   h. Invasive *E. coli* diarrhea
   i. *Campylobacter* infection
2. Primarily mononuclear leukocytes appear in typhoid. A few leukocytes are sometimes seen in amebiasis.
3. Absence of leukocytes is associated with the following conditions:
   a. Cholera
   b. Nonspecific diarrhea (e.g., drug or food induced)
   c. Viral diarrhea
   d. Amebic colitis (many red blood cells)
   e. Noninvasive *E. coli* diarrhea
   f. Toxigenic bacteria (e.g., *Staphylococcus*, *Clostridium*)
   g. Parasites (e.g., *Giardia*, *Entamoeba*)

Interfering Factors

Testing for fecal leukocytes cannot be performed on formalin-preserved specimens.

Interventions

Pretest Patient Care

1. Explain purpose of test, procedure for stool collection, and interfering factors.
2. Advise the patient to avoid barium procedures and laxatives for 1 week before stool specimen collection.
3. Do not start antibiotic therapy until after collection.
4. Follow guidelines in Chapter 1 for safe, effective, informed *pretest* care.

Posttest Patient Care

1. Review test results; report and record findings. Modify the nursing care plan as needed. Monitor for diarrhea. Counsel the patient regarding abnormal findings; explain the need for follow-up tests (stool culture) and treatment (e.g., antibiotics).
2. Follow guidelines in Chapter 1 for safe, effective, informed *posttest* care.

● Fat in Stool; Fecal Fat Stain

Fecal fat is the gold standard test for diagnosing steatorrhea (malabsorption). The three major causes of steatorrhea, which is a pathologic increase in fecal fat, are impairment of intestinal absorption, deficiency of pancreatic digestive enzymes, and deficiency of bile.

Specimens from patients suspected of having steatorrhea can be screened microscopically for the presence of excess fecal fat. This procedure can also be used to monitor patients undergoing treatment for malabsorption disorders. In general, there is good correlation between the qualitative and quantitative fecal fat procedures. Lipids included in the microscopic examination of feces are neutral fats (triglycerides), fatty acid salts (soaps), fatty acids, and cholesterol. The presence of these lipids can be observed microscopically by staining with Sudan III, Sudan IV, or oil red O dye. The staining procedure consists of two parts: the neutral fat stain and the split fat stain for fatty acids.

Normal Findings

1. Qualitative
   a. Neutral fat: <60 fat globules per high-power field
   b. Fatty acids: <100 fat globules per high-power field
2. Quantitative
   a. Adult: 2 to 7 g/24 hours or 2 to 7 g/day and <20% of total solids
   b. Child: <2.0 g/24 hours or <2.0 g/day
   c. Infant: <1.0 g/24 hours or <1.0 g/day and breast-fed 10% to 40% of total solids; bottle-fed 30% to 50% of total solids
   d. Coefficient of fat absorption (%) = (fat ingested − fat excreted)/fat ingested × 100

Procedure

1. Collect a 48- to 96-hour specimen following the procedure for Collection and Transport of 24-, 48-, 72-, and 96-Hour Stool Specimens for the quantitative test. Observe standard precautions. A random specimen can be used for the qualitative test. Label each individual stool specimen with the patient's name, date and time of collection, and test(s) ordered. Also indicate the length (actual time frame) of the collection period. The specimen should be sent immediately to the laboratory.
2. Follow the procedure for the collection of 24-, 48-, or 72-hour specimens.

Clinical Implications

1. Increases in fecal fat and fatty acids are associated with malabsorption syndrome caused by the following conditions:
   a. Celiac disease
   b. Crohn's disease

   c. Whipple's disease (systemic infectious disease caused by *Tropheryma whipplei*)
   d. Cystic fibrosis
   e. Regional enteritis
   f. Atrophy of malnutrition
2. Increases in fecal fat and fatty acids are also found in the following conditions:
   a. Enteritis and pancreatic diseases in which there is a lack of lipase (e.g., chronic pancreatitis)
   b. Surgical removal of a section of the intestine
3. Fecal fat test does not provide a diagnostic explanation for the presence of steatorrhea. It is not useful for differentiating among pancreatic diseases.
   a. D-Xylose absorption test may be ordered for the differential diagnosis of malabsorption.

Interfering Factors

1. Increased neutral fat may occur under the following nondisease conditions:
   a. Use of rectal suppositories and/or oily creams applied to the perineum
   b. Ingestion of castor oil, mineral oil
   c. Ingestion of dietetic low-calorie mayonnaise, oily salad dressings
   d. Ingestion of high-fiber diet (>100 g/24 hours or >100 g/day)
   e. Use of psyllium-based stool softeners (e.g., Metamucil)
2. Use of barium and bismuth interferes with test results.
3. Urine contaminates the specimen.
4. A random stool specimen is not an acceptable sample for the quantitative fat test.

Interventions

Pretest Patient Care

1. Explain purpose of test, procedure for stool collection, and interfering factors.
2. For a 72- to 96-hour stool collection, ensure the patient has a diet containing 100 to 150 g of fat, 100 g of protein, and 180 g of carbohydrate for 6 days before and during the test.
3. Advise the patient to avoid laxatives for 3 days before stool specimen collection.
4. Follow the procedure for the collection of 72-hour stool specimens.
5. Follow guidelines in Chapter 1 for safe, effective, informed *pretest* care.

Posttest Patient Care

1. Patient may resume normal diet after testing is complete.
2. Report and record appearance, color, and odor of all stools in persons suspected of having steatorrhea. The typical stool in patients with this condition is foamy, greasy, soft, pasty, and foul smelling. Modify the nursing care plan as needed.
3. Counsel the patient regarding abnormal findings; explain the possible need for further testing (e.g., colonoscopy) and treatment (e.g., elimination of certain foods from the diet).
4. Follow guidelines in Chapter 1 for safe, effective, informed *posttest* care.

● Urobilinogen in Stool

Increased destruction of red blood cells, as in hemolytic anemia, increases the amount of urobilinogen excreted. Liver disease, in general, reduces the flow of bilirubin to the intestine and thereby decreases the fecal excretion of urobilinogen. In addition, complete obstruction of the bile duct reduces urobilinogen to very low levels.

This test investigates hemolytic diseases and hepatic obstructive conditions. Determination of stool urobilinogen is an estimation of the total excretion of bile pigments, which are the breakdown products of hemoglobin.

Normal Findings

1. 50 to 300 mg/24 hours or 100 to 400 Ehrlich units/100 g
2. Newborns to 6 months: negative

Procedure

1. Collect a 48-hour specimen following the procedure for Collection and Transport of 24-, 48-, 72-, and 96-Hour Stool Specimens. Observe standard precautions.
2. Protect the specimen from light. Send to the laboratory as soon as possible.

Clinical Implications

1. *Increased values* are associated with hemolytic anemias.
2. *Decreased values* are associated with the following conditions:
   a. Complete biliary obstruction (clay-colored feces result)
   b. Severe liver disease (e.g., infectious hepatitis)
   c. Oral antibiotic therapy that alters intestinal bacterial flora
   d. Aplastic anemia, which results in decreased hemoglobin turnover

Interfering Factors

See Appendix E for drugs that affect test outcomes.

Interventions

Pretest Patient Care

1. Explain purpose of test, procedure for stool collection, and interfering factors.
2. Ensure that the patient does not receive oral antibiotic therapy for 1 week before test.
3. Advise the patient to avoid barium procedures and laxatives for 1 week before stool specimen collection.
4. Follow guidelines in Chapter 1 for safe, effective, informed *pretest* care.

Posttest Patient Care

1. Review test results; report and record findings. Modify the nursing care plan as needed. Counsel the patient regarding abnormal findings; explain the need for further testing. Monitor patient for liver disease, biliary obstruction, and diarrhea.
2. Follow guidelines in Chapter 1 for safe, effective, informed *posttest* care.

● Trypsin in Stool: Fecal Chymotrypsin

Trypsin is a proteolytic enzyme formed in the small intestine. In older children and adults, trypsin is destroyed by bacteria in the GI tract. Inadequate trypsin secretion can lead to malabsorption and abdominal discomfort. Chymotrypsin, an intestinal proteolytic enzyme secreted by the pancreas, can be used to assess pancreatic function. Fecal chymotrypsin is a more reliable measurement of pancreatic function than trypsin.

PROCEDURAL ALERT

This test is not reliable in older children and adults.

Normal Findings

Trypsin, 20 to 950 U/g or 20 to 950 µg/g stool
Chymotrypsin, 74 to 1200 µg/g or 74 to 1200 mg/kg stool

Procedure

1. Collect random stools specimens following the procedure for Collection and Transport of Random Specimens. Three separate, fresh stools are usually collected. Observe standard precautions.
2. Ensure that the specimen is taken to the laboratory and tested within 2 hours.
3. Give a cathartic (laxative) before obtaining a specimen from older children (saline or Fleet only).

Clinical Implications

Decreased amounts of trypsin occur in the following conditions:

1. Pancreatic deficiency syndromes (0 to 33 U/g or 0 to 33 μg/g stool)
2. Cystic fibrosis (sweat chloride test is diagnostic) (<20 U/g or <20 μg/g stool)

Interfering Factors

1. No trypsin activity is detectable in constipated stools owing to prolonged exposure to intestinal bacteria, which inactivates trypsin.
2. Barium and laxatives used <1 week before test affect results.
3. In adults and older children, the test is unreliable owing to trypsin inactivation by intestinal flora.
4. Bacterial proteases may produce positive reactions when no trypsin is present.

Interventions

Pretest Patient Care

1. Explain purpose of test, procedure for stool collection, and interfering factors.
2. Advise the patient to avoid barium procedures and laxatives for 1 week before stool collection.
3. Follow guidelines in Chapter 1 for safe, effective, informed *pretest* care.

Posttest Patient Care

1. Review test results; report and record findings. Modify the nursing care plan as needed. Counsel the patient regarding abnormal findings; explain the possible need for follow-up testing (e.g., sweat testing) and treatment (enzymes).
2. Follow guidelines in Chapter 1 for safe, effective, informed *posttest* care.

CLINICAL ALERT

1. Diagnosis of pancreatic insufficiency should not be made until three specimens exhibit no trypsin activity.
2. Bacterial protease may produce positive reactions when no trypsin is present; therefore, both positive and negative reactions should be carefully interpreted.

Stool Electrolytes: Sodium, Chloride, Potassium, and Osmolality

Normal colon function involves absorption of fluid and electrolytes.

Stool electrolyte tests are used to assess electrolyte imbalance in patients with diarrhea. Stool electrolytes must be evaluated along with the serum and urine electrolytes as well as clinical findings in the patient. Stool osmolality is used in conjunction with blood serum osmolality to calculate the osmotic gap and to diagnose intestinal disaccharide deficiency.

Normal Findings

1. Sodium: 5.8 to 9.8 mEq/24 hours or 5.8 to 9.8 mmol/day
2. Chloride: 2.5 to 3.9 mEq/24 hours or 2.5 to 3.9 mmol/day

3. Potassium: 15.7 to 20.7 mEq/24 hours or 15.7 to 20.7 mmol/day
4. Osmolality: 275 to 295 mOsm/kg
5. Osmotic gap: >50 mOsm/kg (secretory diarrhea); >50 mOsm/kg (osmotic diarrhea). Note: Osmotic gap = measured osmolality − (2 [stool Na + stool K]).

Normal values vary greatly; check with your reference laboratory.

Procedure

1. Collect a random or 24-hour liquid stool specimen following the procedures given earlier in this chapter. Observe standard precautions.
2. Keep the specimen covered and refrigerated.

Clinical Implications

1. Electrolyte abnormalities occur in the following conditions:
   a. Idiopathic proctocolitis: *increased* sodium (Na) and chloride (Cl); *normal* potassium (K)
   b. Ileostomy: *increased* sodium (Na) and chloride (Cl), *low* potassium (K)
   c. Cholera: *increased* sodium (Na) and chloride (Cl)
2. Chloride is greatly increased in stool in the following conditions:
   a. Congenital chloride diarrhea
   b. Acquired chloride diarrhea or secondary chloride diarrhea
   c. Idiopathic proctocolitis
   d. Cholera
3. Stool osmolality 500 mg/dL per day is suspicious for factitious disorders (e.g., laxative abuse). Higher levels indicate high amounts of reducing substances in the stool. The osmotic gap is increased in osmotic diarrhea caused by the following:
   a. Saline laxatives
   b. Sodium or magnesium citrate
   c. Carbohydrates (lactulose or sorbitol candy)
4. Osmotic gap >50 mOsm/kg (osmotic diarrhea)
   a. Lactose intolerance
   b. Malabsorption
   c. Poorly absorbed sugars (e.g., sorbitol, mannitol)
   d. Magnesium-containing laxatives
5. Osmotic gap <50 mOsm/kg (secretory diarrhea)
   a. Acute (e.g., cholera)
   b. Chronic (e.g., celiac disease or sprue, collagenous colitis, hyperthyroidism)

Interfering Factors

1. Formed stools invalidate the results. Stools *must* be liquid for electrolyte tests.
2. The stool cannot be contaminated with urine.
3. Surreptitious addition of water to the stool specimen considerably lowers the osmolality. Stool osmolality must be <240 mOsm/kg (or <240 mmol/kg H_2O) to calculate the osmotic gap.
4. See Appendix E for drugs that cause increased values.

Interventions

Pretest Patient Care

1. Explain purpose of test, procedure for stool collection, and interfering factors.
2. Advise the patient to avoid barium procedures and laxatives for 1 week before stool specimen collection.
3. Follow guidelines in Chapter 1 for safe, effective, informed *pretest* care.

Posttest Patient Care

1. Review test results; report and record findings. Modify the nursing care plan as needed. Counsel the patient regarding abnormal findings; explain the need for further testing and treatment. Monitor diarrhea episodes and record findings. Assess the patient for electrolyte imbalances.
2. Follow guidelines in Chapter 1 for safe, effective, informed *posttest* care.

BIBLIOGRAPHY

Centers for Disease Control and Prevention: Diagnostic Procedures: Stool Specimens. Available at: http://www.dpd.cdc.gov/dpdx/HTML/DiagnosticProcedures.htm

Centers for Disease Control and Prevention: *E. coli*. Available at: http://www.cdc.gov/ecoli/index.html

Centers for Disease Control and Prevention: Multistate Outbreak of Shiga Toxin-producing *Escherichia coli* O145 Infections (Final Update), 2012. Available at: http://www.cdc.gov/ecoli/2012/O145-06-12/index.html

Collins JF, Lieberman DA, Durbin TE, et al: Accuracy of screening for fecal occult blood on a single stool sample obtained by digital rectal examination: A comparison with recommended sampling practice. Ann Intern Med 142:81–85, 2005

Goldman L, Schafer AI: Goldman's Cecil Medicine, 24th ed. Philadelphia, Saunders Elsevier, 2012

Imperiale TF, Ransohoff DF, Itzkowitz SH, et al: Fecal DNA versus fecal occult blood for colorectal-cancer screening in an average-risk population. N Engl J Med 351(26):2704–2714, 2004

Leavelle DE (ed): Mayo Medical Laboratories Interpretive Handbook. Rochester, MN, Mayo Medical Laboratories, 2001

Levin B, Lieberman DA, McFarland B, et al; American Cancer Society Colorectal Cancer Advisory Group; US Multi-Society Task Force; American College of Radiology Colon Cancer Committee: Screening and surveillance for the early detection of colorectal cancer and adenomatous polyps, 2008: A joint guideline from the American Cancer Society, the US Multi-Society Task Force on Colorectal Cancer, and the American College of Radiology. CA Cancer J Clin 58(3):130–160, 2008

McPherson RA, Pincus MR: Henry's Clinical Diagnosis and Management by Laboratory Methods, 22nd ed. Philadelphia, Saunders Elsevier, 2011

Mylonakis E, Ryan ET, Calderwood SB: Clostridium difficile–associated diarrhea. Arch Intern Med 161:525–533, 2001

National Cancer Institute. Statistical Summaries. Surveillance, Epidemiology, and End Results Program database. Available at: https://seer.cancer.gov/statistics/summaries/html

Smith RA, Brooks D, Cokkinides V, et al: Cancer screening in the United States, 2013: A review of current American Cancer Society guidelines, current issues in cancer screening, and new guidance on cervical cancer screening and lung cancer screening. CA Cancer J Clin 63:87–105, 2013

Smith RA, Cokkinides V, Eyre HJ: American Cancer Society guidelines for the early detection of cancer. CA Cancer J Clin 55:31–44, 2005

Strasinger S, DiLorenzo MS: Urinalysis and Body Fluids, 5th ed. Philadelphia, FA Davis, 2008

Williamson MA, Snyder LM: Wallach's Interpretation of Laboratory Tests, 9th ed. Philadelphia, Lippincott Williams & Wilkins, 2011

Wu AHB: Tietz Clinical Guide to Laboratory Tests, 4th ed. Philadelphia, Saunders Elsevier, 2006

Young DS: Effects of Drugs on Clinical Laboratory Tests, 5th ed. Washington, DC, AACC Press, 2000

Young DS, Friedman RB: Effects of Disease on Clinical Laboratory Tests, 4th ed. Washington, DC, AACC Press, 2001

Cerebrospinal Fluid Studies

5

OVERVIEW OF CEREBROSPINAL FLUID (CSF)

Description, Formation, and Composition of CSF

Cerebrospinal fluid (CSF) is a clear, colorless fluid formed within the cavities (i.e., ventricles) of the brain. The choroid plexus produces about 70% of the CSF by ultrafiltration and secretion. The ependymal lining of the ventricles and cerebral subarachnoid space produce the remainder of the CSF total volume. About 500 mL of CSF is formed per day, although only 90 to 150 mL is present in the system at any one time. Reabsorption of CSF occurs at the arachnoid villi.

CSF circulates slowly from the ventricular system into the space surrounding the brain and spinal cord and serves as a hydraulic shock absorber, diffusing external forces to the skull that might otherwise cause severe injury. The CSF also helps to regulate intracranial pressure (ICP), supply nutrients to the nervous tissues, and remove waste products. The chemical composition of CSF does not resemble an ultrafiltrate of plasma. Certain chemicals in the CSF are regulated by specific transport systems (e.g., K^+, Ca^{2+}, Mg^{2+}), whereas other substances (e.g., glucose, urea, creatinine) diffuse freely. Proteins enter the CSF by passive diffusion at a rate dependent on the plasma-to-CSF concentration gradient. The term *blood–brain barrier* is used to represent the control and filtration of blood plasma components (e.g., restriction of protein diffusion from blood into brain tissue) to the CSF and then to the brain capillaries. The ratio of increased albumin in CSF to blood serum is always caused by blood–brain barrier dysfunction because albumin is found extensively in blood. A decreased CSF flow rate is due to decreased production or restriction or blockage of flow.

Most CSF constituents are present in the same or lower concentrations as in the blood plasma, except for chloride concentrations, which are usually higher (Table 5.1). Disease, however, can cause elements ordinarily restrained by the blood–brain barrier to enter the spinal fluid. Erythrocytes and leukocytes can enter the CSF from the rupture of blood vessels or from meningeal reaction to irritation. Bilirubin can be found in the spinal fluid after intracranial hemorrhage. In such cases, the arachnoid granulations and the nerve root sheaths will reabsorb the bloody fluid. Normal CSF pressure will consequently be maintained by the reabsorption of CSF in amounts equal to its production. Blockage causes an increase in the amount of CSF, resulting in hydrocephalus in infants or increased ICP in adults. Of the many factors that regulate the level of CSF pressure, venous pressure is the most important because the reabsorbed fluid ultimately drains into the venous system.

Despite the continuous production (~0.3 mL/min) and reabsorption of CSF and the exchange of substances between the CSF and the blood plasma, considerable pooling occurs in the lumbar sac. The lumbar sac, located at L4–L5, is the usual site used for puncture to obtain CSF specimens because damage to the nervous system is less likely to occur in this area. In infants, the spinal cord is situated more caudally than in adults (L3–L4 until 9 months of age, when the cord ascends to L1–L2); therefore, a low lumbar puncture should be made in these patients.

Explanation of Tests

CSF, obtained by lumbar intrathecal puncture, is the main diagnostic tool for neurologic disorders. A lumbar intrathecal puncture is done for the following reasons:

1. To examine the spinal fluid for diagnosis of four major disease categories:
   a. Meningitis
   b. Subarachnoid hemorrhage
   c. Central nervous system (CNS) malignancy (meningeal carcinoma, tumor metastasis)
   d. Autoimmune disease and multiple sclerosis (MS)
2. To determine level of CSF pressure, to document impaired CSF flow, or to lower pressure by removing volume of fluid
3. To identify disease-related immunoglobulin patterns (IgG, IgA, and IgM referenced to albumin) in neurotuberculosis, neuroborreliosis, or opportunistic infections

TABLE 5.1 Normal CSF Values

	Normal Values	
Volume	Adult: 90–150 mL; child: 60–100 mL	
Appearance	Clear, colorless	
Pressure	Adult: 90–180 mm H_2O; child: 10–100 mm H_2O	
Total cell count	Essentially free cells	
	Normal Values	
Microscopic Examination of Cells	**Adults**	**Newborn (0–14 d)**
WBCs	0–5 cells	0–30 cells
Differential		
Lymphocytes	40%–80% (0.40–0.80)	5%–35% (0.05–0.35)
Monocytes	15%–45% (0.15–0.45)	50%–90% (0.50–0.90)
Polys (neutrophils)	0%–6% (0–0.06)	0%–8% (0–0.08)
RBCs (has limited diagnostic value)		
Specific gravity	1.006–1.008	
	Normal Values	
Clinical Tests	**Adults**	**Newborn (0–14 d)**
Glucose	40–70 mg/dL (2.2–3.9 mmol/L)	60–80 mg/dL (3.3–4.4 mmol/L)
Protein		
Lumbar	Adults: 15–45 mg/dL (150–450 mg/L) Elderly (>60 yr): 15–60 mg/dL (150–600 mg/L)	Neonates: 15–100 mg/dL (150–1000 mg/L)
Cisternal	15–25 mg/dL (150–250 mg/L)	
Ventricular	5–15 mg/dL (50–150 mg/L)	
Lactic acid (lactate)	10–24 mg/dL (1.11–2.66 mmol/L)	
Glutamine	5–20 mg/dL (0.34–1.37 mmol/L)	
Albumin	10–35 mg/dL (1.52–5.32 mmol/L)	
Urea nitrogen	6–16 mg/dL (2.14–5.71 mmol/L)	
Creatinine	0.5–1.2 mg/dL (44–106 mmol/L)	
Uric acid	0.5–4.5 mg/dL (29.7–268 mmol/L)	
Bilirubin	0 (none)	
Phosphorus	1.2–2.0 mg/dL (387–646 mmol/L)	
Ammonia	10–35 mg/dL (5.87–20.5 mmol/L)	
Lactate dehydrogenase (LDH) (10% of serum level)	Adult: 0–40 U/L (0–0.67 mkat/L)	
	Normal Values	
Electrolytes and pH	**Adults**	**Newborn (0–14 d)**
pH		
Lumbar	7.28–7.32	
Cisternal	7.32–7.34	
Chloride	115–130 mEq/L (mmol/L)	
Sodium	135–160 mEq/L (mmol/L)	
Potassium	2.6–3.0 mEq/L (mmol/L)	
CO_2 content	20–25 mEq/L (mmol/L)	

table continues on pg. 300 >

TABLE 5.1, continued

Electrolytes and pH	Normal Values: Adults	Newborn (0–14 d)
PCO_2	44–50 mm Hg (5.8–6.6 kPa)	
PO_2	40–44 mm Hg (5.3–5.8 kPa)	
Calcium	2.0–2.8 mEq/L (mmol/L)	1.0–1.4 mEq/L (mmol/L)
Magnesium	2.4–3.0 mEq/L (mmol/L)	1.2–1.5 mEq/L (mmol/L)
Osmolality	280–300 mOsm/kg (280–300 mmol/kg)	
Serology and Microbiology	**Normal Values**	
VDRL	Negative	
Bacteria	None present	
Viruses	None present	
Antibody index	>1.5 indicates chronic inflammatory process <0.4 probably not acute inflammatory process	

CSF, cerebrospinal fluid; RBCs, red blood cells; VDRL, Venereal Disease Research Laboratory; WBCs, white blood cells.
Be sure to include patient's age because it is needed to evaluate borderline values.

4. To introduce anesthetics, drugs, or contrast media used for radiographic studies and nuclear scans into the spinal cord
5. To confirm the identity of pathogens involved in acute inflammatory or chronic inflammatory disorders (e.g., MS and blood–brain barrier dysfunction)
6. To identify extent of brain infarction or stroke
7. To formulate antibody index (AI) of the IgG class for polyspecific immune response in the CNS. Examples: measles, rubella, and zoster (MRZ) antibodies to viruses in MS; herpes simplex virus (HSV) antibodies in MS; toxoplasma antibodies in MS; and autoantibodies to double-stranded DNA (ds-DNA)
8. To identify brain-derived proteins, such as neuron-specific enolase present after brain trauma

See Figure 5.1 for an example of a CSF analysis report.

CLINICAL ALERT

The MRZ reaction occurs in MS, lupus erythematosus, Sjögren's syndrome, and Wegener's granulomatosis.

Certain observations are made each time lumbar puncture is performed:

1. CSF pressure is measured.
2. General appearance, consistency, and tendency of the CSF to clot are noted.
3. CSF cell count is performed to distinguish types of cells present; this must be done within 2 hours of obtaining the CSF sample.
4. CSF protein and glucose concentrations are determined.
5. Other clinical serologic and bacteriologic tests are done when the patient's condition warrants (e.g., culture for aerobes and anaerobes or tuberculosis).
6. Tumor markers may be present in CSF; these tests are useful as supplements to CSF cytology analysis (Table 5.2).

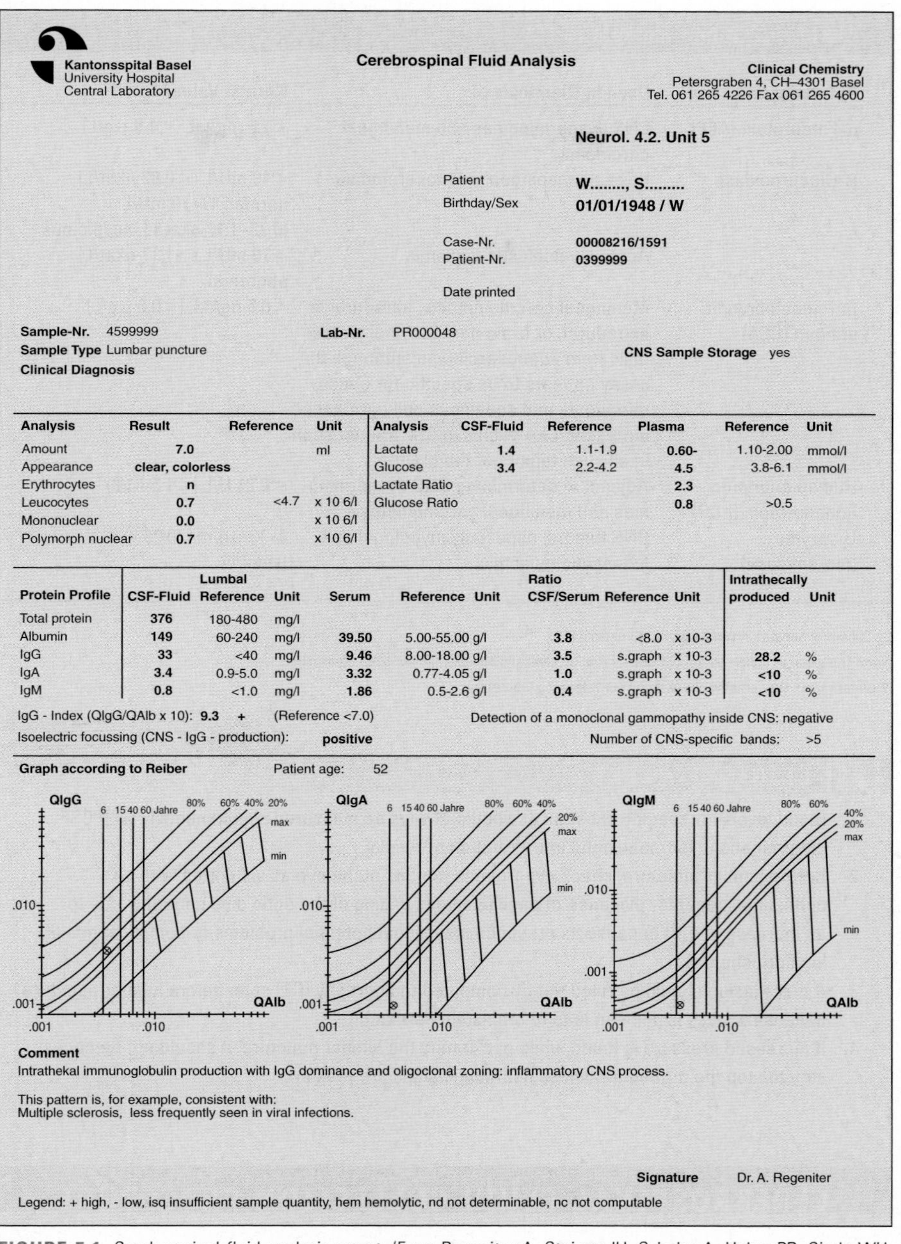

Kantonsspital Basel
University Hospital
Central Laboratory

Cerebrospinal Fluid Analysis

Clinical Chemistry
Petersgraben 4, CH–4301 Basel
Tel. 061 265 4226 Fax 061 265 4600

Neurol. 4.2. Unit 5

Patient **W........, S........**
Birthday/Sex **01/01/1948 / W**

Case-Nr. **00008216/1591**
Patient-Nr. **0399999**

Date printed

Sample-Nr. 4599999 **Lab-Nr.** PR000048
Sample Type Lumbar puncture **CNS Sample Storage** yes
Clinical Diagnosis

Analysis	Result	Reference	Unit
Amount	**7.0**		ml
Appearance	**clear, colorless**		
Erythrocytes	**n**		
Leucocytes	**0.7**	<4.7	x 10 6/l
Mononuclear	**0.0**		x 10 6/l
Polymorph nuclear	**0.7**		x 10 6/l

Analysis	CSF-Fluid	Reference	Plasma	Reference	Unit
Lactate	**1.4**	1.1-1.9	**0.60-**	1.10-2.00	mmol/l
Glucose	**3.4**	2.2-4.2	**4.5**	3.8-6.1	mmol/l
Lactate Ratio			**2.3**		
Glucose Ratio			**0.8**	>0.5	

	Lumbal						Ratio			Intrathecally	
Protein Profile	**CSF-Fluid**	**Reference**	**Unit**	**Serum**	**Reference**	**Unit**	**CSF/Serum**	**Reference**	**Unit**	**produced**	**Unit**
Total protein	**376**	180-480	mg/l								
Albumin	**149**	60-240	mg/l	**39.50**	5.00-55.00	g/l	**3.8**	<8.0	x 10-3		
IgG	**33**	<40	mg/l	**9.46**	8.00-18.00	g/l	**3.5**	s.graph	x 10-3	**28.2**	%
IgA	**3.4**	0.9-5.0	mg/l	**3.32**	0.77-4.05	g/l	**1.0**	s.graph	x 10-3	**<10**	%
IgM	**0.8**	<1.0	mg/l	**1.86**	0.5-2.6	g/l	**0.4**	s.graph	x 10-3	**<10**	%

IgG - Index (QlgG/QAlb x 10): **9.3 +** (Reference <7.0) Detection of a monoclonal gammopathy inside CNS: negative
Isoelectric focussing (CNS - IgG - production): **positive** Number of CNS-specific bands: >5

Graph according to Reiber Patient age: 52

Comment
Intrathekal immunoglobulin production with IgG dominance and oligoclonal zoning: inflammatory CNS process.

This pattern is, for example, consistent with:
Multiple sclerosis, less frequently seen in viral infections.

Signature Dr. A. Regeniter

Legend: + high, - low, isq insufficient sample quantity, hem hemolytic, nd not determinable, nc not computable

FIGURE 5.1. Cerebrospinal fluid analysis report. (From Regeniter A, Steiger JU, Scholer A, Huber PR, Siede WH: Windows to the ward: Graphically oriented report forms. Presentation of complex, interrelated laboratory data for electrophoresis/immunofixation, cerebrospinal fluid, and urinary protein profiles. Clin Chem 49:1, 41–50, 2003, Fig. 2; Reprinted with permission of AACC.)

TABLE 5.2 Tumor Markers in CSF

Determination	Used in Diagnosis of	Normal Values[a]
α-Fetoprotein (AFP)	CNS dysgerminomas and meningeal carcinomas	<1.5 mg/mL (<1.5 μg/L)
β-Glucuronidase	Possible meningeal adenocarcinoma	<49 mU/L (<0.82 nkat/L) normal; 47–70 mU/L (0.78–1.17 nkat/L), suspicious
	Acute myeloblastic leukemia	>70 mU/L (>1.17 nkat/L) abnormal
Carcinoembryonic antigen (CEA)	Meningeal carcinomatosis; intradural or extradural, or brain parenchymal metastasis from adenocarcinoma; although the assay appears to be specific for adenocarcinoma and squamous cell carcinoma, increased CEA values in CSF are not seen in all such tumors of the brain	<0.6 ng/mL (<0.6 μg/L)
Human chorionic gonadotropin (hCG)	Adjunct in determining CNS dysgerminomas and meningeal carcinomatosis	<0.21 U/L (<1.5 IU/L)
Lysozyme (muramidase)	CNS tumors, especially myoclonal and monocytic leukemia	4–13 μg/mL (0.28–0.91 μmol/L)

CNS, central nervous system; CSF, cerebrospinal fluid.

Note: The value of tumor markers in CSF for routine clinical diagnosis has not been established.

[a]Normal values vary greatly; check with your reference laboratory.

CLINICAL ALERT

1. Blood levels for specific substances should always be measured simultaneously with CSF determinations for meaningful interpretation of results.
2. Before lumbar puncture, check eyegrounds (fundus of the eye as visualized with an ophthalmoscope) for evidence of papilledema (swelling of the optic disc generally due to an increase in ICP) because its presence may signal potential problems or complications of lumbar puncture.
3. A mass lesion should be ruled out by computed tomography (CT) scan before lumbar puncture because a mass lesion can lead to brainstem herniation.
4. If increased pressure is found while performing the lumbar puncture, it should not be necessary to stop the procedure unless neurologic signs are present.

CEREBROSPINAL FLUID COLLECTION PROCEDURE

● Lumbar Puncture (Spinal Tap)

Procedure

1. Place the patient in a side-lying position with the head flexed onto the chest and knees drawn up to, but not compressing, the abdomen to "bow" the back. This position helps to increase the space between the lower lumbar vertebrae so that the spinal needle can be inserted more easily between

the spinal processes. However, a sitting position with the head flexed to the chest can be used. The patient is helped to relax and instructed to breathe slowly and deeply with his or her mouth open.

2. Select the puncture site, usually between L4 and L5 or lower. There is a small bony landmark at the L5–S1 interspace that helps to locate the puncture site. The site is thoroughly cleansed with an antiseptic solution, and the surrounding area is draped with sterile towels in such a way that the drapes do not obscure important landmarks (Fig. 5.2).
3. Inject a local anesthetic slowly into the dermis around the intended puncture site.
4. Insert a spinal needle with stylet into the midline between the spines of the lumbar space and slowly advance until it enters the subarachnoid space. The patient may feel the entry as a "pop" of the needle through the dura mater. Once this happens, the patient can be helped to straighten his or her legs slowly to relieve abdominal compression.
5. Remove the stylet with the needle remaining in the subarachnoid space and attach a pressure manometer to the needle to record the opening CSF pressure.
6. Remove a specimen consisting of up to 20 mL of CSF. Take up to four samples of 2 to 3 mL each, place in separate sterile screw-top tubes, and label with the patient's name, date and time of collection, and test(s) ordered. Label the tubes sequentially: Tube 1 is used for chemistry and serology; tube 2 is used for microbiology studies; tube 3 is used for hematology cell counts; and tube 4 is used for special studies such as cryptococcal antigens, syphilis testing (Venereal Disease Research Laboratory [VDRL]), protein electrophoresis, and other immunologic studies. A closing pressure reading may be taken before the needle is withdrawn. In cases of increased ICP, no more than 2 mL is withdrawn because of the risk that the brainstem may shift.

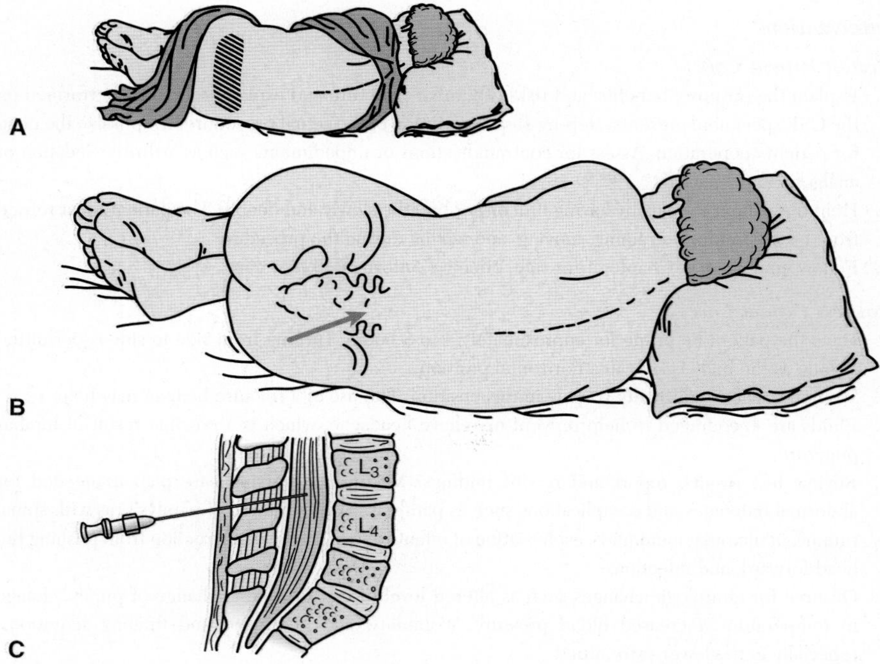

FIGURE 5.2. Spinal tap technique. The patient lies on one side with knees flexed and back arched to separate the lumbar vertebrae. The patient is surgically draped, and an area overlying the lumbar spine is disinfected **(A)**. The space between lumbar vertebrae L4 and L5 is palpated with a sterile gloved forefinger **(B)**, and the spinal needle is carefully directed between the spinous processes, through the infraspinous ligaments, and into the spinal canal **(C)**.

7. Apply a small sterile dressing to the puncture site.
8. The correctly labeled specimens of CSF must be immediately delivered to the laboratory, where they should be given to laboratory personnel with specific instructions regarding the testing. CSF samples should never be placed in the refrigerator because refrigeration alters the results of bacteriologic and fungal studies. Analysis should be started immediately. If viral studies are to be performed, a portion of the specimen should be frozen.
9. Record procedure start and completion times, patient's status, CSF appearance, and CSF pressure readings.

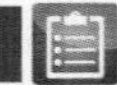

PROCEDURAL ALERT

1. If the opening pressure is >200 mm H_2O in a relaxed patient, no more than 2 mL of CSF should be withdrawn.
2. If the initial pressure is normal, Queckenstedt's test may be done. (This test is not done if a CNS tumor is suspected.) In this test, pressure is placed on both jugular veins to occlude them temporarily and to produce an acute rise in CSF pressure. Normally, pressure rapidly returns to average levels after jugular vein occlusion is removed. Total or partial spinal fluid blockage is diagnosed if the lumbar pressure fails to rise when both jugular veins are compressed or if the pressure requires >20 seconds to fall after compression is released.

Interventions

Pretest Patient Care

1. Explain the purpose, benefits, and risks of lumbar puncture and explain tests to be performed on the CSF specimen; present a step-by-step description of the actual procedure. Emphasize the need for patient cooperation. Assess for contraindications or impediments such as arthritis. Sedation or analgesia may be used.
2. Help the patient to relax by having him or her breathe slowly and deeply. The patient must refrain from breath holding, straining, moving, and talking during the procedure.
3. Follow guidelines in Chapter 1 for safe, effective, informed *pretest* care.

Posttest Patient Care

1. Have the patient lie prone for approximately 4 to 8 hours. Turning from side to side is permitted as long as the body is kept in a horizontal position.
2. Women may have difficulty voiding in this position. The use of a fracture bedpan may help.
3. Fluids are encouraged to help prevent or relieve headache, which is a possible result of lumbar puncture.
4. Review test results; report and record findings. Modify the nursing care plan as needed for abnormal outcomes and complications such as paralysis (or progression of paralysis, as with spinal tumor), hematoma, meningitis, asphyxiation of infants due to tracheal obstruction from pushing the head forward, and infection.
5. Observe for neurologic changes such as altered level of consciousness, change of pupils, change in temperature, increased blood pressure, irritability, and numbness and tingling sensations, especially in the lower extremities.
6. If headache occurs, administer analgesics as ordered and encourage a longer period of prone bed rest. If severe headache persists, an epidural blood patch may need to be done, in which a small amount of the patient's own blood is introduced into the epidural space at the same level that the canal was previously entered.

7. Check the puncture site for leakage.
8. Document the procedure completion and any problems encountered or complaints voiced by the patient.
9. Follow guidelines in Chapter 1 for safe, effective, informed *posttest* care.

CLINICAL ALERT

1. Extreme caution should be used when performing lumbar puncture in the following cases:
   a. If ICP is elevated, especially in the presence of papilledema or split cranial sutures. However, with some cases of increased ICP, such as with a coma, intracranial bleeding, or suspected meningitis, the need to establish a diagnosis is absolutely essential and outweighs the risks of the procedure.
   b. If ICP is from a suspected mass lesion. To reduce the risk for brain herniation, a less invasive procedure such as a CT scan or magnetic resonance imaging (MRI) should be done.
2. Contraindications to lumbar puncture include the following conditions:
   a. Suspected epidural infection
   b. Infection or severe dermatologic disease in the lumbar area, which may be introduced into the spinal canal
   c. Severe psychiatric or neurotic problems
   d. Chronic back pain
   e. Anatomic malformations, scarring in puncture site areas, or previous spinal surgery at the site
3. If there is CSF leakage at the puncture site, notify the healthcare provider immediately and document findings.
4. Follow standard precautions (see Appendix A) when handling CSF specimens.

CEREBROSPINAL FLUID TESTS

● CSF Pressure

The CSF pressure is directly related to pressure in the jugular and vertebral veins that connect with the intracranial dural sinuses and the spinal dura. In conditions such as congestive heart failure or obstruction of the superior vena cava, CSF pressure is increased, whereas in circulatory collapse, CSF pressure is decreased.

Pressure measurement is done to detect impairment of CSF flow or to lower the CSF pressure by removing a small volume of CSF fluid. Provided that initial pressure is not elevated and there is no marked fall in the pressure as fluid is removed, 10 to 20 mL of CSF may be removed without danger to the patient. Elevation of the opening CSF pressure may be the only abnormality found in patients with cryptococcal meningitis and pseudotumor cerebri. Repeated lumbar punctures are performed for ICP elevation in cryptococcal meningitis to decrease the CSF pressure.

Normal Findings

Adult: 90 to 180 mm H_2O (or 9 to 18 cm H_2O) in the lateral recumbent position. (This value is position dependent and will change with a horizontal or sitting position.)
Child (<8 years of age): 80 to 100 mm H_2O (or 8 to 10 cm H_2O)

Procedure

1. A lumbar puncture is performed (see Lumbar Puncture [Spinal Tap]).
2. Measure the CSF pressure before any fluid is withdrawn.
3. Take up to four samples of 2 to 3 mL each, place in separate sterile screw-top tubes, and label with the patient's name, date and time of collection, and test(s) ordered. Label the tubes sequentially: Tube 1 is used for chemistry and serology, tube 2 is used for microbiology studies, tube 3 is used for hematology cell counts, and tube 4 is used for special studies.

Clinical Implications

1. Increases in CSF pressure can be a significant finding in the following conditions:
   a. Intracranial tumors; abscess; lesions
   b. Meningitis (bacterial, fungal, viral, or syphilitic)
   c. Hypo-osmolality as a result of hemodialysis
   d. Congestive heart failure
   e. Superior vena cava syndrome
   f. Subarachnoid hemorrhage
   g. Cerebral edema
   h. Thrombosis of venous sinuses
   i. Conditions inhibiting CSF absorption
2. Decreases in pressure can be a significant finding in the following conditions:
   a. Circulatory collapse
   b. Severe dehydration
   c. Hyperosmolality
   d. Leakage of spinal fluid
   e. Spinal-subarachnoid block
3. Significant variations between opening and closing CSF pressure can be found in the following conditions:
   a. Tumors or spinal blockage above the puncture site when there is a large pressure drop (no further fluid should be withdrawn)
   b. Hydrocephalus when there is a small pressure drop that is indicative of a large CSF pool

Interfering Factors

1. Slight elevations of CSF pressure may occur in an anxious patient who holds his or her breath or tenses his or her muscles.
2. If the patient's knees are flexed too firmly against the abdomen, venous compression will cause an elevation in CSF pressure. This can occur in patients of normal weight and in those who are obese.

Interventions

Pretest Patient Care

1. Follow pretest patient care for lumbar puncture (see Lumbar Puncture [Spinal Tap]).
2. Follow guidelines in Chapter 1 for safe, effective, informed *pretest* care.

Posttest Patient Care

1. Review abnormal pressure levels; report and record findings. Modify the nursing care plan as needed to prevent complications.
2. Follow posttest patient care for lumbar puncture (see Lumbar Puncture [Spinal Tap]).
3. Follow guidelines in Chapter 1 for safe, effective, informed *posttest* care.

● CSF Color and Appearance

Normal CSF is clear, with the appearance and viscosity of water. Abnormal CSF may appear hazy, cloudy, smoky, or bloody. Clotting of CSF is abnormal and indicates increased protein or fibrinogen levels.

The initial appearance of CSF can provide various types of diagnostic information. Inflammatory diseases, hemorrhage, tumors, and trauma produce elevated cell counts and corresponding changes in appearance.

Normal Findings

Clear and colorless

Procedure

1. A lumbar puncture is performed (see Lumbar Puncture [Spinal Tap]).
2. Compare the CSF with a test tube of distilled water held against a white background. If there is no turbidity, newsprint can be read through normal CSF in the tube.

Clinical Implications

1. Abnormal appearance (Table 5.3)—causes and indications:
   a. Blood in CSF can be due to hemorrhage or result from trauma from the lumbar puncture. If blood in CSF is caused by subarachnoid or cerebral hemorrhage, the blood is evenly mixed in all three tubes. Table 5.4 describes differentiation of bloody spinal tap from cerebral hemorrhage. Clear CSF fluid does not rule out intracranial hemorrhage.
   b. Turbidity is graded from 1+ (slightly cloudy) to 4+ (very cloudy) and may be caused by the following conditions:
      (1) Leukocytes (pleocytosis [i.e., an increase in the number of cells—in this case, white blood cells (WBCs)—which is referred to as *leukocytosis*])
      (2) Erythrocytes
      (3) Microorganisms such as fungi and amebae
      (4) Protein
      (5) Aspirated epidural fat (pale pink to dark yellow)
      (6) Contrast media
   c. Xanthochromia (pale pink to dark yellow) can be caused by the following conditions:
      (1) Oxyhemoglobin from lysed red blood cells (RBCs) present in CSF before lumbar puncture

TABLE 5.3 Color Changes in CSF Suggestive of Disease States

Appearance	Condition
Opalescent, slightly yellow, with delicate clot	Tuberculous meningitis
Opalescent to purulent, slightly yellow, with coarse clot	Acute pyogenic meningitis
Slightly yellow; may be clear or opalescent, with delicate clot	Acute anterior poliomyelitis
Bloody, purulent, may be turbid	Primary amebic meningoencephalitis
Generally clear, but may be xanthochromic	Tumor of brain or cord
Xanthochromic	Toxoplasmosis
Viscous	Metastatic colon cancer, severe meningeal infection, cryptococcus, injury

TABLE 5.4 Differentiation of Bloody CSF Caused by Subarachnoid Hemorrhage versus Traumatic Lumbar Puncture

CSF Findings	Subarachnoid Hemorrhage	Traumatic Lumbar Puncture[a]
CSF pressure	Often increased	Normal
Blood in tubes for collecting CSF	Mixture with blood is uniform in all tubes	Tubes 1 and 2 more bloody than tube 3 or 4
CSF clotting	Does not clot	Often clots
Xanthochromia	Present if >8–12 hr since cerebral hemorrhage	Absent unless patient is jaundiced
Immediate repeat of lumbar puncture at higher level	CSF same as initial puncture	CSF clear (if atraumatic)

CSF, cerebrospinal fluid.

[a]CSF with red blood cells >6000 per mm³ appears grossly bloody.

(2) Methemoglobin (iron in the heme group of the hemoglobin molecule is in the Fe^{3+}, not the Fe^{2+}, state)
(3) Bilirubin (>6 mg/dL or >103 μmol/L) (breakdown product of normal heme catabolism)
(4) Increased protein (>150 mg/dL or >1500 mg/L)
(5) Melanin (meningeal melanocarcinoma)
(6) Carotene (systemic carotenemia)
(7) Prior bleeding within 2 to 36 hours (e.g., traumatic puncture >72 hours before)

d. Yellow color (bilirubin, >10 mg/dL or >171 μmol/L) due to a prior hemorrhage (10 hours to 4 weeks before)

CLINICAL ALERT

1. Spinal fluid should be cultured for bacteria, fungi, and tuberculosis. In children, *Haemophilus influenzae* type B is the most common cause of bacterial meningitis; in adults, the most common bacterial pathogens for meningitis are meningococci and pneumococci.
2. Spinal fluid with any degree of cloudiness should be treated with extreme care because this could be an indication of contagious disease.

Interfering Factors

1. CSF can look xanthochromic (yellow discoloration) from contamination with methylate used to disinfect the skin.
2. If the blood in the specimen is due to a traumatic spinal tap (which occurs in 10% to 30% of cases), the CSF in the third tube should be clearer than that in tube 1 or 2; a traumatic tap makes interpretation of results very difficult to impossible.

Interventions

Pretest Patient Care

1. Observations of color and appearance of CSF are always noted.
2. Follow pretest patient care for lumbar puncture (see Lumbar Puncture [Spinal Tap]).
3. Follow guidelines in Chapter 1 for safe, effective, informed *pretest* care.

Posttest Patient Care

1. Recognize abnormal color and presence of turbidity and monitor patient appropriately.
2. Follow posttest patient care for lumbar puncture (see Lumbar Puncture [Spinal Tap]).
3. Follow guidelines in Chapter 1 for safe, effective, informed *posttest* care.

● CSF Microscopic Examination of Cells; Total Cell Count; Differential Cell Count

Normal CSF contains a small number of lymphocytes and monocytes in a ratio of approximately 70:30 in adults. A higher proportion of monocytes is present in young children. An increase in the number of WBCs in CSF is termed *pleocytosis*. Disease processes may lead to abrupt increases or decreases in numbers of cells.

CSF is examined for the presence of RBCs and WBCs. The cells are counted and identified by cell type; the percentage of cell type is compared with the total number of WBCs or RBCs present. In general, inflammatory disease, hemorrhage, neoplasms, and trauma cause an elevated WBC count.

Normal Findings

Normal CSF is essentially free of cells (Tables 5.5 and 5.6).
Adult: 0 to 5 WBCs/μL or 0 to 5 × 10^6 WBCs/L
Newborn: 0 to 30 WBCs/μL or 0 to 30 × 10^6 WBCs/L
Child: 0 to 15 WBCs/μL or 0 to 15 × 10^6 WBCs/L

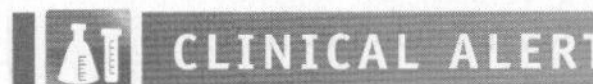

CLINICAL ALERT

Critical Values
>20 segmented neutrophils

Procedure

1. A lumbar puncture is performed (see Lumbar Puncture [Spinal Tap]).
2. Typically, approximately 20 mL of CSF is obtained and subsequently divided into four separate sterile screw-top tubes.
3. One of the tubes is used for counting the cells present in the CSF sample. The cells are counted by a manual counting chamber or by electronic means. A CSF smear is made, and various types of cells present are counted to determine differentiation of cells.

Clinical Implications

1. The total CSF cell count (includes neutrophils, lymphocytes, mixed cells, and cells after hemorrhage) is the most sensitive index of acute inflammation of the CNS.

TABLE 5.5 Cell Counts

Differential	Adults	Newborn (0–14 d)
Lymphocytes	40%–80% (0.40–0.80)	5%–35% (0.05–0.35)
Monocytes	15%–45% (0.15–0.45)	50%–90% (0.50–0.90)
Polys (neutrophils)	0%–6% (0–0.06)	0%–8% (0–0.08)

TABLE 5.6 Major Cells Seen in Microscopic Examination of CSF

Cell Types	Occurrence	Findings
Blast forms	Acute leukemia	Lymphoblasts or myeloblasts
Ependymal and choroidal cells	Trauma (diagnostic procedures)	Clusters with distinct nuclei and distinct cell walls
Lymphocytes	Normal Viral, tubercular, and fungal meningitis Multiple sclerosis	All stages of development possible
Macrophages	Viral and tubercular meningitis RBCs in spinal fluid Contrast media	May contain phagocytized RBCs (appearing as empty vacuoles or ghost cells) and hemosiderin granules
Malignant cells	Metastatic carcinomas	Clusters with fusing of cell borders and nuclei
Monocytes	Chronic bacterial meningitis Viral, tubercular, and fungal meningitis Multiple sclerosis	Mixed with lymphocytes and neutrophils
Neutrophils	Bacterial meningitis Early cases of viral, tubercular, and fungal meningitis	Granules may be less prominent than in blood
Pia arachnoid mesothelial (PAM) cells	Normal, mixed reactions, including lymphocytes, neutrophils, monocytes, and plasma cells	Resemble young monocytes with a round, not indented, nucleus
Plasma cells	Multiple sclerosis Tuberculosis Meningitis Sarcoidosis	Transitional and classic forms seen

RBCs, red blood cells.

2. WBC counts >500 WBCs/μL or >500 × 10^6 WBCs/L usually arise from a purulent infection and are predominantly granulocytes (i.e., neutrophils). Neutrophilic reaction classically suggests meningitis caused by a pyogenic organism, in which case the WBC count can exceed 1000 WBCs/μL or 1000 × 10^6 WBCs/L and even reach 20,000 WBCs/μL or 20,000 × 10^6 WBCs/L.
   a. Increases in neutrophils are associated with the following conditions:
      (1) Bacterial meningitis (Table 5.7)
      (2) Early viral meningitis
      (3) Early tubercular meningitis
      (4) Fungal mycotic meningitis
      (5) Amebic encephalomyelitis
      (6) Early stages of cerebral abscess
   b. Noninfectious causes of neutrophilia include the following:
      (1) Reaction to CNS hemorrhage
      (2) Injection of foreign materials into the subarachnoid space (e.g., x-ray contrast medium, anticancer drugs)

TABLE 5.7 Abnormal CSF Findings in Types of Meningitis

	Bacterial	Viral	Tubercular	Fungal
Total WBCs	Increased	Increased	Increased	Increased
Differential	Neutrophils present	Lymphocytes present	Lymphocytes and monocytes present	Lymphocytes and monocytes present
Protein	Marked increase	Moderate increase	Moderate to marked increase; clots occur with protein >150 mg/dL (>1500 mg/L)	Moderate to marked increase
Glucose	Markedly decreased	Normal	Decreased	Normal to decreased
Lactate	Increased	Normal	Increased	Increased
LDH fractions	Lactate dehydrogenase isoenzymes 4 and 5 increased	Lactate dehydrogenase isoenzymes 1, 2, and 3 increased	Lactate dehydrogenase isoenzymes 1, 2, and 3 increased	—
Limulus amebocyte Lysate: indicator of endotoxin produced by gram-negative bacteria (not affected by antibiotic therapy)	Positive	—	Pellicle formation when protein >150 mg/dL (>1500 mg/L)	Positive India ink with neoformans

LDH, lactate dehydrogenase; WBCs, white blood cells.

(3) CSF infarct

(4) Metastatic tumor in contact with CSF

(5) Reaction to repeated lumbar puncture

3. WBC counts of 300 to 500/μL or 300 to 500 × 10^6/L with preponderantly lymphocytes are indicative of the following conditions:
   a. Viral meningitis
   b. Syphilis of CNS (i.e., meningoencephalitis)
   c. Tuberculous meningitis
   d. Parasitic infestation of the CNS
   e. Bacterial meningitis due to unusual organisms (e.g., *Listeria* species)
   f. MS (reactive lymph present)
   g. Encephalopathy caused by drug abuse
   h. Guillain-Barré syndrome (15%)
   i. Acute disseminated encephalomyelitis
   j. Sarcoidosis of meninges
   k. Human T-lymphotropic virus type III (HTLV III)

   l. Aseptic meningitis due to peptic focus adjacent to meninges
   m. Fungal meningitis
   n. Polyneuritis
4. WBC counts with ≥40% monocytes occur in the following conditions:
   a. Chronic bacterial meningitis
   b. Toxoplasmosis and amebic meningitis
   c. MS
   d. Rupture of brain abscess
5. Malignant cells (lymphocytes or histiocytes) may be present with primary and metastatic brain tumors, especially when there is meningeal extension.
6. Increased numbers of plasma cells occur in the following conditions:
   a. Acute viral infections
   b. MS
   c. Sarcoidosis
   d. Syphilitic meningoencephalitis
   e. SSPE
   f. Tuberculous meningitis
   g. Parasitic infestations of CSF
   h. Guillain-Barré syndrome
   i. Lymphocytic reactions
7. Plasma cells are responsible for an increase in IgG and altered patterns in immunoelectrophoresis.
8. Macrophages are present in tuberculous or viral meningitis and in reactions to erythrocytes, foreign substances, or lipids in the CSF.
9. Ependymal (neuronal support cell) and plexus cells may be present after surgical procedures or trauma to the CNS (not clinically significant).
10. Blast cells appear in CSF when acute leukemia is present (lymphoblasts or myeloblasts).
11. Eosinophils are present in the following conditions:
   a. Parasitic infections
   b. Fungal infections
   c. Rickettsial infections (Rocky Mountain spotted fever)
   d. Idiopathic hypereosinophilic syndrome
   e. Reaction to foreign materials in CSF (e.g., drugs, shunts)
   f. Sarcoidosis

CLINICAL ALERT

Neutrophilic reaction classically suggests meningitis caused by a pyogenic organism.

Interfering Factors

1. Patient position or movement, such as that caused by crying, gasping, or coughing, may cause changes in CSF pressure.
2. Delay in time from collection to testing may affect results.

Interventions

Pretest Patient Care

1. Follow pretest patient care for lumbar puncture (see Lumbar Puncture [Spinal Tap]).
2. Follow guidelines in Chapter 1 for safe, effective, informed *pretest* care.

Posttest Patient Care

1. Review abnormal cell counts; report and record findings. Modify the nursing care plan as needed for infection and malignancy.
2. Follow posttest patient care for lumbar puncture (see Lumbar Puncture [Spinal Tap]).
3. Follow guidelines in Chapter 1 for safe, effective, informed *posttest* care.

● CSF Glucose

The CSF glucose level varies with the blood glucose levels. It is usually about 60% of the blood glucose level. A blood glucose specimen should be obtained at least 60 minutes before lumbar puncture for comparisons. Any changes in blood sugar are reflected in the CSF approximately 1 hour later because of the lag in CSF glucose equilibrium time.

This measurement is helpful in determining impaired transport of glucose from plasma to CSF, increased use of glucose in the CNS, and glucose use by leukocytes and microorganisms. The finding of a markedly decreased CSF glucose level accompanied by an increased WBC count with a large percentage of neutrophils is indicative of bacterial meningitis.

Normal Findings

Adult: 40 to 70 mg/dL or 2.2 to 3.9 mmol/L
Child: 60 to 80 mg/dL or 3.3 to 4.4 mmol/L
CSF-to-plasma glucose ratio: <0.5
CSF glucose level: 60% to 70% of blood glucose levels

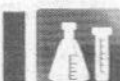 **CLINICAL ALERT**

The critical value for CSF glucose level is <20 mg/dL (<1.1 mmol/L); below this level, damage to the CNS will occur.

Procedure

1. A lumbar puncture is performed (see Lumbar Puncture [Spinal Tap]).
2. Place 1 mL of CSF in a sterile screw-top tube. The glucose test should be done on tube 1 when three tubes of CSF are taken. Accurate evaluation of CSF glucose requires a plasma glucose measurement. A blood glucose level ideally should be drawn 1 hour before the lumbar puncture.

Clinical Implications

1. Decreased CSF glucose levels are associated with the following conditions:
   a. Acute bacterial meningitis
   b. Tuberculous, fungal, and amebic meningitis
   c. Systemic hypoglycemia
   d. Subarachnoid hemorrhage
2. CSF glucose levels are uncommonly decreased in the following conditions:
   a. Malignant tumor with meningeal involvement
   b. Acute syphilitic meningitis
   c. Nonbacterial meningoencephalitis
3. Increased CSF glucose levels are associated with the following conditions:
   a. Diabetic hyperglycemia
   b. Increased serum glucose
   c. Epidemic encephalitis

CLINICAL ALERT

1. **Decreased glucose levels reflect abnormal activity due to infectious microorganisms metabolizing glucose.**
2. **The findings of a markedly decreased CSF glucose and an increased WBC count with a high percentage of neutrophils are indicative of bacterial meningitis.**

Interfering Factors

1. Falsely decreased levels may be due to cellular and bacterial metabolism if the test is not performed immediately after specimen collection.
2. A traumatic tap may produce misleading results owing to glucose present in blood.
3. See Appendix E for drugs that affect test outcomes.

Interventions

Pretest Patient Care

1. Follow pretest patient care for lumbar puncture (see Lumbar Puncture [Spinal Tap]).
2. Explain the need for a blood specimen test for glucose to compare with CSF glucose.
3. Follow guidelines in Chapter 1 for safe, effective, informed *pretest* care.

Posttest Patient Care

1. Review abnormal CSF glucose levels; report and record findings. Modify the nursing care plan as needed to prevent complications. Correlate with the presence of meningitis, cancer, hemorrhage, and diabetes.
2. Follow posttest patient care for lumbar puncture (see Lumbar Puncture [Spinal Tap]).
3. Follow guidelines in Chapter 1 for safe, effective, informed *posttest* care.

● CSF Glutamine

Glutamine, an amino acid, is synthesized in brain tissue from ammonia and α-ketoglutarate. Production of glutamine, the most prominent amino acid in CSF, provides a mechanism for removing the ammonia, a toxic metabolic waste product, from the CNS.

The determination of CSF glutamine level provides an indirect test for the presence of excess ammonia in the CSF. As the concentration of ammonia in the CSF increases, the supply of α-ketoglutarate becomes depleted; consequently, glutamine can no longer be produced to remove the toxic ammonia, and coma ensues. A CSF glutamine test is therefore frequently requested for patients with coma of unknown origin.

Normal Findings

8.6 ± 0.50 mg/dL or 0.60 ± 0.03 mmol/L or 590 ± 34 μmol/L (A CSF glutamine value >35 mg/dL [>2.4 mmol/L] usually results in loss of consciousness.)

Procedure

1. A lumbar puncture is performed (see Lumbar Puncture [Spinal Tap]).
2. Use 1 mL of CSF for the glutamine test in a sterile screw-top tube.
3. Centrifuge the samples if cells are present.

Clinical Implications

Increased CSF glutamine levels are associated with the following conditions:

1. Hepatic encephalopathy (glutamine values >35 mg/dL or >2.4 mmol/L are diagnostic)
2. Reye's syndrome (typically affects the brain and liver of children after a viral infection)

3. Encephalopathy secondary to hypercapnia or sepsis
4. Bacterial meningitis

Interventions

Pretest Patient Care

1. Follow pretest patient care for lumbar puncture (see Lumbar Puncture [Spinal Tap]).
2. Follow guidelines in Chapter 1 for safe, effective, informed *pretest* care.

Posttest Patient Care

1. Review abnormal glutamine levels; report and record findings. Modify the nursing care plan as needed to prevent complications. Correlate with clinical symptoms.
2. Follow posttest patient care for lumbar puncture (see Lumbar Puncture [Spinal Tap]).
3. Follow guidelines in Chapter 1 for safe, effective, informed *posttest* care.

● CSF Lactic Acid, L-Lactate

The source of CSF lactic acid (L-lactate) is CNS anaerobic metabolism. Lactic acid in CSF varies independently with the level of lactic acid in the blood. Destruction of tissue within the CNS because of oxygen deprivation causes the production of increased CSF lactic acid levels. Thus, elevated CSF lactic acid levels can result from any condition that decreases the flow of oxygen to brain tissues.

The CSF lactic acid test is used to differentiate between bacterial and nonbacterial meningitis. Elevated CSF lactate levels are not limited to meningitis and can result from any condition that decreases the flow of oxygen to the brain. CSF lactate levels are frequently used to monitor severe head injuries.

Normal Findings

Adult: 10 to 22 mg/dL or 1.1 to 2.4 mmol/L
Newborn: 10 to 60 mg/dL or 1.1 to 6.7 mmol/L

Procedure

1. A lumbar puncture is performed (see Lumbar Puncture [Spinal Tap]).
2. Collect 0.5 mL of CSF in a sterile screw-top tube.

Clinical Implications

Increased CSF lactic acid levels are associated with the following conditions:

1. Bacterial meningitis (>38 mg/dL or >4.2 mmol/L)
2. Brain abscess or tumor
3. Cerebral ischemia
4. Cerebral trauma
5. Seizures
6. Stroke
7. Increased ICP

NOTE *Generally, in viral meningitis, the CSF lactic acid will be <38 mg/dL or <4.2 mmol/L.*

Interfering Factors

Traumatic tap causes elevated levels: RBCs contain large amounts of lactate. Hemolyzed or xanthochromic specimens will give falsely elevated results.

Interventions

Pretest Patient Care

1. Follow pretest patient care for lumbar puncture (see Lumbar Puncture [Spinal Tap]).
2. Follow guidelines in Chapter 1 for safe, effective, informed *pretest* care.

Posttest Patient Care

1. Review test outcomes; report and record findings. Modify the nursing care plan as needed to detect CNS disease and prevent complications.
2. Follow posttest patient care for lumbar puncture (see Lumbar Puncture [Spinal Tap]).
3. Follow guidelines in Chapter 1 for safe, effective, informed *posttest* care.

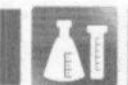

CLINICAL ALERT

Increases in CSF lactic acid levels must be interpreted in light of the clinical findings and in conjunction with glucose levels, protein levels, and cell counts in the CSF. Equivocal results in some instances of aseptic meningitis may lead to erroneous diagnosis of a bacterial etiology. Increased lactate in CSF following head injury suggests poor prognosis.

CSF Lactate Dehydrogenase (LD/LDH); CSF Lactate Dehydrogenase (LDH) Isoenzymes

Although many different enzymes have been measured in CSF, only lactate dehydrogenase (LDH) appears useful clinically. Sources of LDH in normal CSF include diffusion across the blood–CSF barrier, diffusion across the brain–CSF barrier, and LDH activity in cellular elements of the CSF, such as leukocytes, bacteria, and tumor cells. Because brain tissue is rich in LDH, damaged CNS tissue can cause increased levels of LDH in the CSF.

High levels of LDH occur in about 90% of cases of bacterial meningitis and in only 10% of cases of viral meningitis. When high levels of LDH do occur in viral meningitis, the condition is usually associated with encephalitis and a poor prognosis. Tests of LDH isoenzymes (LDH exists in four enzyme classes; two are cytochrome c–dependent enzymes and two are NAD[P]-dependent enzymes) have been used to improve the specificity of LDH measurements and are useful for making the differential diagnosis of viral versus bacterial meningitis (see Chapter 6 for a complete description of isoenzymes). Elevated LDH levels following resuscitation predict a poor outcome in patients with hypoxic brain injury.

Normal Findings

Adults: <40 U/L or approximately 10% of serum levels (total LD activity)
Neonates: <70 U/L

NOTE *Depending on the upper limit or cutoff value, sensitivity and specificity can vary between 70% and 85%.*

Procedure

1. A lumbar puncture is performed (see Lumbar Puncture [Spinal Tap]).
2. Obtain 1 mL of CSF for the LDH test in a sterile screw-top tube.
3. Take the sample to the laboratory as quickly as possible.

Clinical Implications

1. Increased CSF LDH levels are associated with the following conditions:
   a. Bacterial meningitis (90% of cases)
   b. Viral meningitis (10% of cases)
   c. Massive cerebrovascular accident
   d. Leukemia or lymphoma with meningeal infiltration
   e. Metastatic carcinoma of the CNS
2. The presence of CSF LDH isoenzymes 1, 2, and 3 reflects a CNS lymphocytic reaction, suggesting viral meningitis.
3. The CSF LDH isoenzyme pattern reflects a granulocytic (neutrophilic) reaction with LDH isoenzymes 4 and 5, suggesting bacterial meningitis.
4. High levels of CSF LDH isoenzymes 1 and 2 suggest extensive CNS damage and a poor prognosis (i.e., they are indicative of destruction of brain tissue).
5. CSF LDH isoenzymes 3 and 4 suggest lymphatic leukemia or lymphoma.

Interfering Factors

For the LDH test to be valid, CSF must not be contaminated with blood. A traumatic lumbar tap will make results difficult to interpret.

Interventions

Pretest Patient Care

1. Follow pretest patient care for lumbar puncture (see Lumbar Puncture [Spinal Tap]).
2. Follow guidelines in Chapter 1 for safe, effective, informed *pretest* care.

Posttest Patient Care

1. Review abnormal LDH test patterns; report and record findings. Modify the nursing care plan as needed to appropriately detect and prevent complications.
2. Follow posttest patient care for lumbar puncture (see Lumbar Puncture [Spinal Tap]).
3. Follow guidelines in Chapter 1 for safe, effective, informed *posttest* care.

● CSF Total Protein

The CSF normally contains very little protein because the protein in the blood plasma does not cross the blood–brain barrier easily. Protein concentration normally increases caudally from the ventricles to the cisterns and finally to the lumbar sac.

The CSF protein is a nonspecific but reliable indication of CNS pathology such as meningitis, brain abscess, MS, and other degenerative processes causing neoplastic disease. Elevated CSF protein levels may be caused by increased permeability of the blood–brain barrier, decreased resorption of the arachnoid villi, mechanical obstruction of the CSF flow, or increased intrathecal immunologic synthesis.

Normal Findings

Results vary by method used; check with the laboratory for reference values.
Total Protein
Adults: 15 to 45 mg/dL or 150 to 450 mg/L (lumbar)
Adults: 15 to 25 mg/dL or 150 to 250 mg/L (cisternal)
Adults: 5 to 15 mg/dL or 50 to 150 mg/L (ventricular)
Neonates: 15 to 100 mg/dL or 150 to 1000 mg/L (lumbar)
Elderly patients (>60 years of age): 15 to 60 mg/dL or 150 to 600 mg/L (lumbar)

CLINICAL ALERT

Critical Values

Low: none

High: >45 mg/mL or >450 mg/L in the adult

Procedure

1. A lumbar puncture is performed (see Lumbar Puncture [Spinal Tap]).
2. Obtain 1 mL of CSF for protein analysis in a sterile screw-top tube.
3. Measure serum protein levels concurrently to interpret CSF protein values.

Clinical Implications

1. Increased CSF protein occurs in the following situations:
   a. Traumatic tap with normal CSF pressure: CSF initially streaked with blood, clearing in subsequent tubes
   b. Increased permeability of blood–CSF barrier ("influx syndrome"): CSF protein 100 to 500 mg/dL (1000 to 5000 mg/L)
      (1) Infectious conditions
         i. Bacterial meningitis: Gram stain usually positive; culture may be negative if antibiotics have been administered
         ii. Tuberculosis: CSF protein 50 to 300 mg/dL (500 to 3000 mg/L); mixed cellular reaction typical
         iii. Fungal meningitis: CSF protein 50 to 300 mg/dL (500 to 3000 mg/L); special stains helpful
         iv. Viral meningitis: CSF protein usually <200 mg/dL (<2000 mg/L)
      (2) Noninfectious conditions
         i. Subarachnoid hemorrhage: xanthochromia 2 to 4 hours after onset
         ii. Intracerebral hemorrhage: CSF protein 20 to 200 mg/dL (200 to 2000 mg/L); marked fall in pressure after removing small amounts of CSF; xanthochromia
         iii. Cerebral thrombosis: slightly increased CSF protein in 40% of cases (usually, <100 mg/dL or <1000 mg/L)
         iv. Endocrine disorders, diabetic neuropathy, myxedema, hyperadrenalism, hypoparathyroidism: CSF protein 50 to 150 mg/dL (500 to 1500 mg/L) in about 50% of cases
         v. Metabolic disorders, uremia, hypercalcemia, hypercapnia, dehydration: CSF protein slightly elevated (usually, <100 mg/dL or <1000 mg/L)
         vi. Drug toxicity, ethanol, phenytoin, phenothiazines: CSF protein slightly elevated in about 40% of cases (usually, <200 mg/dL or <2000 mg/L)
   c. Obstruction to circulation of CSF occurs in the following circumstances:
      (1) Mechanical obstruction (e.g., tumor, abscess), herniated disk: rapid fall in pressure (yellow CSF, contains excess protein)
      (2) Loculated effusion of CSF: repeated taps may show a progressive increase in CSF protein; diagnosis by myelography
   d. Increased CSF IgG synthesis occurs in the following conditions:
      (1) MS: CSF protein level slightly increased
      (2) Subacute sclerosing panencephalitis (SSPE): increased CSF protein
      (3) Neurosyphilis: CSF protein normal or slightly increased (usually, <100 mg/dL or <1000 mg/L)

e. Increased CSF IgG synthesis and increased permeability of blood–CSF barrier occur in the following conditions:
   (1) Guillain-Barré syndrome: CSF protein usually 100 to 400 mg/dL (1000 to 4000 mg/L)
   (2) Systemic autoimmune diseases: CSF protein usually <400 mg/dL (or <4000 mg/L)
   (3) Chronic inflammatory demyelinating polyradiculopathy
f. Decreased CSF protein occurs in the following conditions:
   (1) Leakage of CSF due to trauma
   (2) Removal of a large volume of CSF
   (3) Intracranial hypertension
   (4) Hyperthyroidism
   (5) Young children between 6 months and 2 years of age

CLINICAL ALERT

More than 1000 mg/dL (>10,000 mg/L) of protein in CSF suggests subarachnoid block. In a complete spinal block, the lower the tumor location, the higher the CSF protein value.

Interfering Factors

1. Hemolyzed or xanthochromic drugs may falsely depress results.
2. Traumatic tap will invalidate the protein results.
3. See Appendix E for drugs that affect test outcomes.

Interventions

Pretest Patient Care

1. Follow pretest patient care for lumbar puncture (see Lumbar Puncture [Spinal Tap]).
2. Follow guidelines in Chapter 1 for safe, effective, informed *pretest* care.

Posttest Patient Care

1. Review abnormal CSF protein levels; report and record findings. Modify the nursing care plan as needed to prevent and detect complications for both infectious and noninfectious conditions.
2. Follow posttest patient care for lumbar puncture (see Lumbar Puncture [Spinal Tap]).
3. Follow guidelines in Chapter 1 for safe, effective, informed *posttest* care.

● CSF Albumin and Immunoglobulin G (IgG)

Albumin composes most (50% to 75%) of the proteins in CSF. The albumin and IgG that are present in normal CSF are derived from the serum. Increased levels of either or both are indicative of damage to the blood–CNS barrier.

The combined measurement of albumin and IgG is used to evaluate the integrity and permeability of the blood–CSF barrier and to measure the synthesis of IgG within the CNS. The IgG index is the most sensitive method to determine local CNS synthesis of IgG and to detect increased permeability of the blood–CNS barrier.

$$\text{CSF IgG Index} = \frac{\text{CSF IgG} \times \text{serum albumin}}{\text{CSF albumin} \times \text{serum IgG}}$$

The IgG index method is superior to the IgG-to-albumin ratio or measurement of IgG only.

Normal Findings

Albumin: 10 to 35 mg/dL or 1.5 to 5.3 μmol/L
IgG: <4.0 mg/dL or <40 mg/L
CSF serum albumin index: <9.0

$$\text{CSF serum albumin index} = \frac{\text{CSF albumin}}{\text{Serum albumin}}$$

CSF IgG index: <0.60
CSF IgG index = (CSF IgG × serum albumin)/(Serum IgG × CSF albumin)
CSF-to-serum IgG ratio: <0.003

$$\text{CSF-to-serum IgG ration} = \frac{\text{CSF IgG}}{\text{Serum IgG}}$$

Procedure

1. A lumbar puncture is performed (see Lumbar Puncture [Spinal Tap]).
2. Obtain 0.5 mL of CSF in a sterile screw-top tube.
3. Freeze the sample if the determination is not done immediately.

Clinical Implications

1. Increased CSF albumin occurs in most of the same conditions as increased total protein, especially:
   a. Lesions of the choroid plexus
   b. Blockage of CSF flow
   c. Bacterial meningitis
   d. Guillain-Barré syndrome
   e. Many infectious diseases, such as typhoid fever, tularemia, diphtheria, and septicemia
   f. Malignant neoplasms of the CNS
2. CSF serum albumin index
   a. An index of <9.0 is consistent with an intact blood–brain barrier.
   b. An index between 9 and 14 is considered slight impairment to the barrier.
   c. An index from 15 to 30 is considered moderate impairment of the barrier.
   d. An index >30 is severe impairment.
3. Increased CSF IgG index occurs in the following conditions:
   a. MS
   b. Subacute sclerosing leukoencephalitis
   c. Neurosyphilis
   d. Chronic phases of CNS infections (SSPE)

Interfering Factors

A traumatic tap will invalidate the results.

Interventions

Pretest Patient Care

1. Follow pretest patient care for lumbar puncture (see Lumbar Puncture [Spinal Tap]).
2. Follow guidelines in Chapter 1 for safe, effective, informed *pretest* care.

Posttest Patient Care

1. Review test results; report and record findings. Modify the nursing care plan as needed to prevent and detect complications.
2. Follow posttest patient care for lumbar puncture (see Lumbar Puncture [Spinal Tap]).
3. Follow guidelines in Chapter 1 for safe, effective, informed *posttest* care.

● CSF Protein Electrophoresis; Oligoclonal Bands; Multiple Sclerosis Panel

Agarose gel electrophoresis of concentrated CSF is used to detect oligoclonal bands, defined as two or more discrete bands in the γ region that are absent or of less intensity than in the concurrently tested patient's serum.

Fractionation (i.e., electrophoresis) of CSF is used to evaluate bacterial and viral infections and tumors of the CNS. However, the most important application of CSF protein electrophoresis is the detection and diagnosis of MS. Abnormalities of CSF in MS include an increase in total protein, primarily from IgG, which is the main component of the γ-globulin fraction. Abnormal immunoglobulins migrate as discrete, sharp bands, called *oligoclonal bands*. This is the pattern observed in MS: a pattern of discrete bands within the γ-globulin portion of the electrophoretic pattern. However, oligoclonal bands are found in the CSF of patients with other types of nervous system disorders of the immune system, including HIV.

Electrophoresis is also the method of choice to determine whether a fluid is actually CSF. Identification can be made based on the appearance of an extra band of transferrin (referred to as *TAV*), which occurs in CSF and not in serum.

Normal Findings

Globulins
Oligoclonal banding: none present
α_1-Globulin: 2% to 7% (0.02 to 0.07)
α_2-Globulin: 4% to 12% (0.04 to 0.12)
β-Globulin: 8% to 18% (0.08 to 0.18)
γ-Globulin: 3% to 12% (0.03 to 0.12)
Prealbumin: 2% to 7%; (0.02 to 0.07)
Albumin: 56% to 76% (0.56 to 0.76)
IgA: 0.10 mg/dL or 1.0 mg/L
IgD: 3.0 U/mL or 3.0 kU/L
IgG: 5.0 mg/dL or 50 mg/L
IgG synthesis rate: 0.0 to 8.0 mg/24 hours (average is 3.0) or 0.0 to 8.0 mg/day
IgG-to-albumin ratio: 0.09 to 0.25
IgM: 0.017 mg/dL or 0.17 mg/L

Procedure

1. A lumbar puncture is performed (see Lumbar Puncture [Spinal Tap]).
2. Obtain 3 mL of CSF for this test in a sterile screw-top tube. The sample must be frozen if the test is not performed immediately.
3. Apply a sample of the concentrate to a thin-layer agarose gel. Subject the agarose gel to electrophoresis. CSF is concentrated approximately 80-fold by selective permeability. Serum electrophoresis must be done concurrently for interpretation of the bands.

Clinical Implications

1. Increases in CSF IgG or in the IgG-to-albumin index occur in the following conditions:
   a. MS
   b. SSPE
   c. Tumors of the brain and meninges
   d. Chronic CNS infections
   e. Some patients with meningitis, Guillain-Barré syndrome, lupus erythematosus involving the CNS, and other neurologic conditions

2. Increases in the CSF albumin index occur in the following conditions:
   a. Obstruction of CSF circulation
   b. Damage to the CNS blood–brain barrier
   c. Diabetes mellitus
   d. Systemic lupus erythematosus of the CNS
   e. Guillain-Barré syndrome
   f. Polyneuropathy
   g. Cervical spondylosis
3. Increased CSF γ-globulin and the presence of oligoclonal bands occur in the following conditions:
   a. MS
   b. Neurosyphilis
   c. SSPE
   d. Cerebral infarction
   e. Viral and bacterial meningitis
   f. Progressive rubella panencephalitis
   g. Cryptococcal meningitis
   h. Idiopathic polyneuritis
   i. Burkitt's lymphoma
   j. HIV-1 (AIDS)
   k. Guillain-Barré syndrome
4. Increased CSF synthesis of IgG occurs in the following conditions:
   a. MS (90% of definite cases)
   b. Inflammatory neurologic diseases
   c. Postpolio syndrome

CLINICAL ALERT

1. A serum electrophoresis must be done at the same time as the CSF electrophoresis. An abnormal result is the finding of two or more bands in the CSF that are *not* present in the serum specimen (Fig. 5.3).
2. Oligoclonal bands are not specific for multiple sclerosis; however, the sensitivity is 83% to 94%. (0.83 to 0.94).
3. Diagnostic differentiation between MS and CSF autoimmune disease relies on further testing (e.g., antinuclear antibodies [ANAs] in blood [see Chapter 8]).

Interfering Factors

1. A traumatic tap invalidates the results.
2. Recent myelography affects the results.

Interventions

Pretest Patient Care

1. Follow pretest patient care for lumbar puncture (see Lumbar Puncture [Spinal Tap]).
2. Follow guidelines in Chapter 1 for safe, effective, informed *pretest* care.

Posttest Patient Care

1. Review test results; report and record findings. Modify the nursing care plan as needed to prevent and detect complications for MS and other CNS disorders.
2. Follow posttest patient care for lumbar puncture (see Lumbar Puncture [Spinal Tap]).
3. Follow guidelines in Chapter 1 for safe, effective, informed *posttest* care.

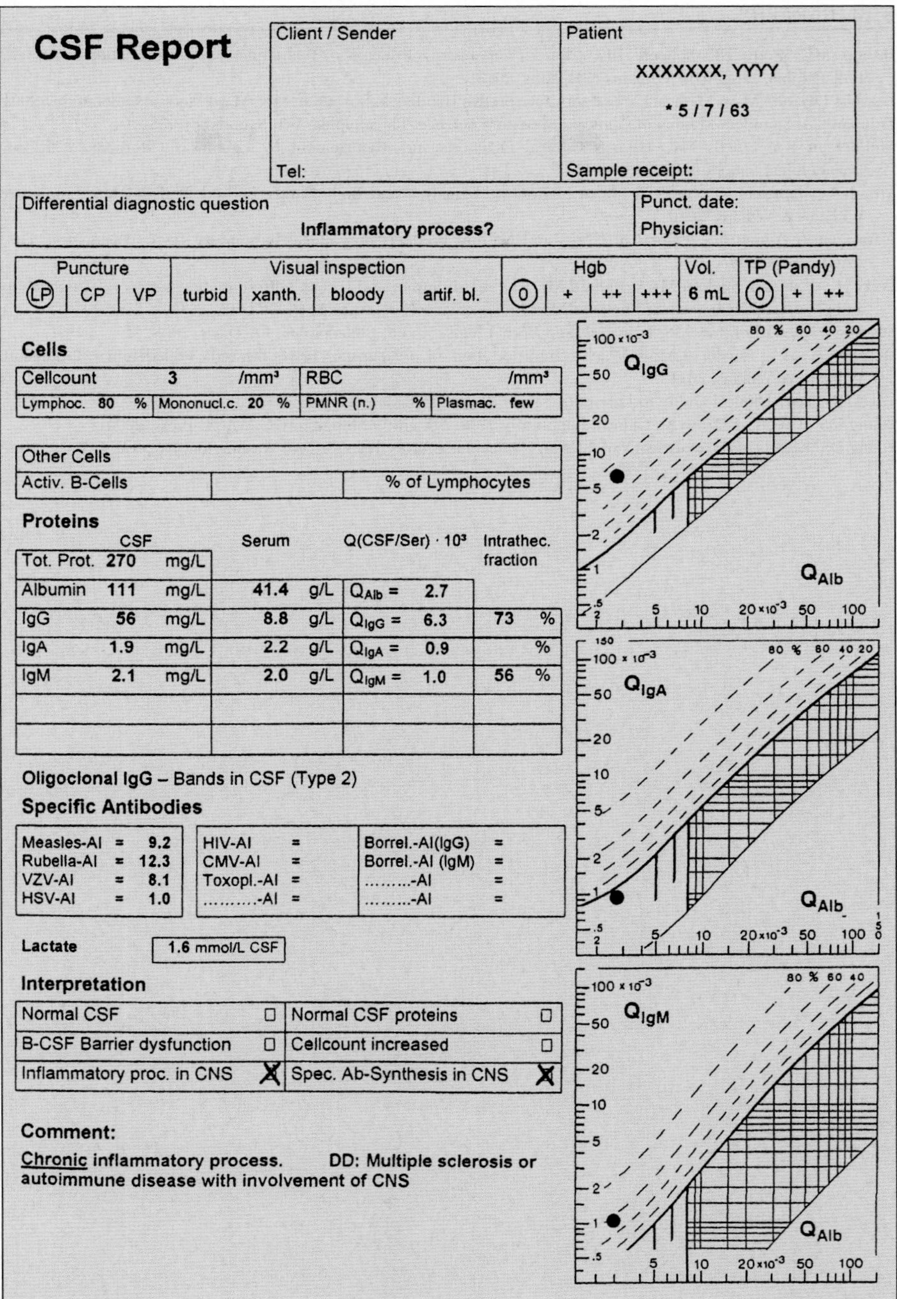

CSF Report

Client / Sender	Patient
	XXXXXXX, YYYY
	* 5 / 7 / 63
Tel:	Sample receipt:

Differential diagnostic question	Punct. date:
Inflammatory process?	Physician:

Puncture			Visual inspection				Hgb				Vol.	TP (Pandy)		
(LP)	CP	VP	turbid	xanth.	bloody	artif. bl.	(0)	+	++	+++	6 mL	(0)	+	++

Cells

Cellcount	3 /mm³	RBC	/mm³
Lymphoc. 80 %	Mononucl.c. 20 %	PMNR (n.) %	Plasmac. few

Other Cells		
Activ. B-Cells		% of Lymphocytes

Proteins

	CSF	Serum	Q(CSF/Ser) · 10³	Intrathec. fraction
Tot. Prot.	270 mg/L			
Albumin	111 mg/L	41.4 g/L	Q_{Alb} = 2.7	
IgG	56 mg/L	8.8 g/L	Q_{IgG} = 6.3	73 %
IgA	1.9 mg/L	2.2 g/L	Q_{IgA} = 0.9	%
IgM	2.1 mg/L	2.0 g/L	Q_{IgM} = 1.0	56 %

Oligoclonal IgG – Bands in CSF (Type 2)

Specific Antibodies

Measles-AI = 9.2	HIV-AI =	Borrel.-AI(IgG) =
Rubella-AI = 12.3	CMV-AI =	Borrel.-AI (IgM) =
VZV-AI = 8.1	Toxopl.-AI =	.........-AI =
HSV-AI = 1.0	..........-AI =	.........-AI =

Lactate 1.6 mmol/L CSF

Interpretation

Normal CSF	☐	Normal CSF proteins	☐
B-CSF Barrier dysfunction	☐	Cellcount increased	☐
Inflammatory proc. in CNS	X	Spec. Ab-Synthesis in CNS	X

Comment:

Chronic inflammatory process. DD: Multiple sclerosis or autoimmune disease with involvement of CNS

FIGURE 5.3. Cerebrospinal fluid report—patient with multiple sclerosis. (Reprinted from Reiber H, Peter JB: Cerebrospinal fluid analysis: Disease-related data patterns and evaluation programs. J Neurol Sci 184:101–122, 2001.)

BIBLIOGRAPHY

Bishop ML, Fody EP, Schoeff LE: Clinical Chemistry—Principles, Techniques, and Correlations, 7th ed. Philadelphia, Lippincott Williams & Wilkins, 2013

Leavelle DE (ed): Mayo Medical Laboratories Interpretive Handbook. Rochester, MN, Mayo Medical Laboratories, 2001

Lehman CA: Saunders Manual of Clinical Laboratory Science. Philadelphia, WB Saunders, 1998

McPherson RA, Pincus MR: Henry's Clinical Diagnosis and Management by Laboratory Methods, 22nd ed. Philadelphia, Saunders Elsevier, 2011

Mundt L, Shanahan K: Graff's Textbook of Routine Urinalysis and Body Fluids, 2nd ed. Philadelphia, Lippincott Williams & Wilkins, 2010

Narayanan S, Young DS: Effects of Herbs and Natural Products on Clinical Laboratory Tests. Washington, DC, AACC Press, 2007

Perry JJ, Alyahya B, Sivilotti MLA, Bullard MJ, Emond M, Sutherland J, et al: Differentiation between traumatic tap and aneurysmal subarachnoid hemorrhage: Prospective cohort study. BMJ 350:h568, 2015

Strasinger SK, DiLorenzo MS: Urinalysis and Body Fluids, 5th ed. Philadelphia, FA Davis, 2008

Williamson MA, Snyder LM: Wallach's Interpretation of Diagnostic Tests, 9th ed. Philadelphia, Lippincott Williams & Wilkins, 2011

Wu AHB: Tietz Clinical Guide to Laboratory Tests, 4th ed. Philadelphia, Saunders Elsevier, 2006

Young DS: Effects of Drugs on Clinical Laboratory Tests, 5th ed. Washington, DC, AACC Press, 2000

Young DS: Effects of Preanalytical Variables on Clinical Laboratory Tests, 3rd ed. Washington, DC, AACC Press, 2007

Chemistry Studies

6

OVERVIEW OF CHEMISTRY STUDIES

Blood chemistry testing identifies many chemical blood constituents. It is often necessary to measure several blood chemicals to establish a pattern of abnormalities. A wide range of tests can be grouped under the headings of enzymes, electrolytes, blood sugars, lipids, hormones, proteins, vitamins, minerals, and drug investigation. Other tests have no common denominator. Selected tests serve as screening devices to identify target organ damage. When collecting specimens for chemistry studies, refer to Standard Precautions for Prevention and Control of Infection in Appendix A, Guidelines for Specimen Transport and Storage in Appendix B, and Effects of Drugs on Laboratory Tests in Appendix E.

General Biochemical Profiles

Profiles are a group of select tests that screen for certain conditions. Some of the more common profiles or panels are listed in Table 6.1.

Use of the Autoanalyzer

Sophisticated automated instrumentation makes it possible to conduct a wide variety of chemical tests on a single sample of blood and to report results in a timely manner. Numerical results may be reported with low, high, panic (or critical values), toxic, or D (i.e., fails Delta check) comments along with normal reference range. Computerized interfaces allow direct transmission of results

TABLE 6.1 Common Screening Profiles

Group Headings	Tests Suggested
Cardiac markers (MI)	Troponin, myoglobin
Electrolyte panel	Na, K, Cl, CO_2
Kidney functions, disease	BUN, phosphorus, LDH, creatinine, creatinine clearance, total protein, A/G ratio, albumin, calcium, glucose, CO_2
Lipids (coronary risk)	Cholesterol, triglycerides, HDL, LDL
Liver function, disease	Total bilirubin, alkaline phosphatase, GGT, total protein, A/G ratio, albumin, AST, LDH, viral hepatitis panel, PT
Thyroid function	Free T_4, TSH
Basic metabolic screen	Cl, Na, K, CO_2, glucose, BUN, creatinine

A/G ratio, albumin-to-globulin ratio; AST, aspartate aminotransferase; BUN, blood urea nitrogen; GGT, γ-glutamyl transpeptidase; HDL, high-density lipoprotein; LDH, lactate dehydrogenase; LDL, low-density lipoprotein; MI, myocardial infarction; PT, prothrombin time; T_4, thyroxine; TSH, thyroid-stimulating hormone.

Adapted from Expert panel on detection, evaluation and treatment of high blood cholesterol in adults. Executive summary of NCEP-ATP III. JAMA 285:2486–2497, 2001

between laboratory and clinical settings. Not only does this method of record keeping provide a baseline for future comparisons, but it can also allow unsuspected diseases to be uncovered and can lead to early diagnosis when symptoms are vague or absent. Chemistry tests may be grouped into lipid, basic metabolic, comprehensive metabolic, hepatic, or electrolyte panels. A list of standard panels appears in Table 6.2.

NOTE *Normal or reference values (intervals) for any chemistry determination vary with the method or assay used. For example, differences in substrates or temperature at which the assay is run will alter the normal range. Thus, normal ranges vary from laboratory to laboratory.*

DIABETES TESTING, BLOOD GLUCOSE, BLOOD SUGAR, AND RELATED TESTS

● Fasting Blood Glucose (FBG); Fasting Blood Sugar (FBS); Fasting Plasma Glucose (FPG); Casual Random Plasma Glucose (PG)

Glucose is formed from carbohydrate digestion and conversion of glycogen to glucose by the liver. The two hormones that directly regulate blood glucose are glucagon and insulin. Glucagon accelerates glycogen breakdown in the liver and causes the blood glucose level to rise. Insulin increases cell membrane permeability to glucose, transports glucose into cells (for metabolism), stimulates glycogen formation, and reduces blood glucose levels. Driving insulin into the cells requires insulin and insulin receptors. For example, after a meal, the pancreas releases insulin for glucose metabolism, provided there are enough insulin receptors. Insulin binds to these receptors on the surface of target cells such as are found in fat and muscle. This opens the channels so that glucose can pass into cells, where it can be converted into energy. As cellular glucose metabolism occurs, blood glucose levels fall. Adrenocorticotropic hormone (ACTH), adrenocorticosteroids, epinephrine, and thyroxine also play key roles in glucose metabolism.

TABLE 6.2 Standard Panels

Panel Tests	Specimen Collection
Arthritis Panel (ARTH PN) Uric acid, ESR, ANA (antinuclear antibody screen), rheumatoid factor	Two 7-mL red-topped tubes and 1 lavender-topped tube
Basic Metabolic Panel (BC MET) Creatinine, CO_2, chloride, glucose, potassium, sodium, BUN, calcium	1-mL unhemolyzed serum (red-topped tube or SST tube)
Comprehensive Metabolic Panel (CM MET) Albumin, alkaline phosphatase, ALT, AST, total bilirubin, calcium, CO_2, chloride, creatinine, glucose, potassium, sodium, total protein, BUN	1-mL unhemolyzed serum (red-topped tube or SST tube)
Electrolytes (LYTES) CO_2, chloride, potassium, sodium	1-mL unhemolyzed serum (red-topped tube or SST tube)
Hepatic Function Panel (HEPFUN) ALT, albumin, alkaline phosphatase, AST, direct bilirubin and total bilirubin, total protein	1-mL unhemolyzed serum (red-topped tube or SST tube)
Acute Hepatitis Panel (ACUTE HEP) Hepatitis A Ab-IgM, hepatitis B core Ab-IgM, hepatitis B surface antigen–IgM, hepatitis C Ab	7-mL red-topped tube
Lipid Panel (LIPID PN) Cholesterol, HDL, triglycerides (LDL and CHOL/HDL ratio included, as calculated values)	2-mL serum (red-topped tube or SST tube)
Obstetric Panel (OB PN) Type and Rh, antibody screen, RPR, rubella Ab-IgG, hepatitis B surface antigen	One 7-mL red-topped tube, one lavender-topped tube, and SST tube
Prenatal Screen (PRESCP) Type and Rh, antibody screening and studies if indicated, RPR for syphilis, rubella Ab-IgG, hepatitis B surface antigen	One lavender-topped tube, one 7-mL red- topped tube, and SST tube

Ab, antibodies; Ab-IgG, antibodies for immunoglobulin G; Ab-IgM, antibodies for immunoglobulin M; ALT, alanine aminotransferase; AST, aspartate aminotransferase; BUN, blood urea nitrogen; CHOL, cholesterol; ESR, erythrocyte sedimentation rate; HDL, high-density lipoprotein; LDL, low-density lipoprotein; RPR, rapid plasma reagin; SST, serum separator tube.

There are four categories of diabetes:

1. Type 1 (formerly known as insulin-dependent diabetes mellitus or juvenile-onset diabetes mellitus), due to destruction of pancreatic β cells which leads to deficiency in insulin, accounts for about 5% to 10% of individuals diagnosed with diabetes.
2. Type 2 (formerly known as non–insulin-dependent diabetes mellitus or adult-onset diabetes mellitus), a progressive form of insulin deficiency concomitant with insulin resistance, accounts for 90% to 95% of individuals diagnosed with diabetes.
3. Due to other causes (e.g., genetic defects [see Chapter 11 for genetic causes]), disease of the pancreas, drug- or chemical-induced, and so forth.
4. Gestational (i.e., diagnosed during pregnancy)

The American Diabetes Association (ADA) uses the term *prediabetes*, also known as impaired glucose tolerance or impaired fasting glucose. Individuals with prediabetes demonstrate higher levels of blood plasma glucose (PG) (100 to 125 mg/dL or 5.6 to 6.9 mmol/L) than normal subjects (<100 mg/dL or <5.6 mmol/L) and, if left untreated, go on to develop type 2 diabetes within 10 years.

Diagnosing latent autoimmune diabetes in adults (LADA) early in the course of the disease process is critical because of the high risk for developing insulin dependency. It has been found that most patients with LADA have at least two of the following: age of onset <50 years, body mass index (BMI) <25 kg/m^2, personal history of autoimmune disease, acute symptoms before diagnosis, or family history of autoimmune disease.

Fasting blood glucose is a vital component of diabetes management. The term *random/casual* is defined as any time of day without regard to time since the last meal. *Fasting* is defined as no caloric intake for at least 8 hours. Abnormal glucose metabolism may be caused by inability of pancreatic islet β cells to produce insulin, reduced numbers of insulin receptors, faulty intestinal glucose absorption, inability of the liver to metabolize glycogen, or altered levels of hormones (e.g., ACTH) that play a role in glucose metabolism.

In most cases, significantly elevated fasting plasma glucose (FPG) levels (i.e., >140 mg/dL or >7.77 mmol/L; hyperglycemia) are, in themselves, usually diagnostic of diabetes. However, mild, borderline cases may present with normal fasting glucose values. If diabetes is suspected, a glucose tolerance test (GTT) can confirm the diagnosis. Occasionally, other diseases may produce elevated PG levels; therefore, a comprehensive history, physical examination, and workup should be done before a definitive diagnosis of diabetes is established.

CLINICAL ALERT

1. The National Institutes of Health (NIH) guidelines endorse diabetic testing of all adults ≥45 yr of age every 3 yr. The ADA recommends the following guidelines for testing:
   - Should be *considered* if patient is >45 yr of age
   - *Strongly recommended* if patient is >45 yr of age and overweight
   - *Considered* if patient is <45 yr of age and overweight with another risk factor
2. Diabetes mellitus, a group of metabolic disorders, is characterized by hyperglycemia and abnormal protein, fat, and carbohydrate metabolism due to defects in insulin secretions—that is, inadequate and deficient insulin action (insulin resistance) on target organs.
3. Criteria for diagnosing diabetes
   a. Symptoms of diabetes plus random/casual PG concentration of ≥200 mg/dL (≥11.1 mmol/L). Random/casual is defined as any time of day without regard to time since last meal. The classic symptoms of diabetes include polyuria, polydipsia, and unexplained weight loss, *or*
   b. FPG ≥126 mg/dL (≥7.0 mmol/L) on at least two occasions (fasting is defined as no caloric intake for at least 8 hr), *or*
   c. Two-hour PG ≥200 mg/dL (≥11.1 mmol/L) during an oral glucose tolerance test (OGTT). The test should be performed as described by the World Health Organization (WHO), using a glucose load containing the equivalent of 75 g of anhydrous glucose dissolved in water, *or*
   d. Hemoglobin A_{1c} ≥6.5% (48 mmol/mol). Method used for testing should be NGSP certified and standardized to Diabetes Control and Complications Trial (DCCT) assay.
      1) In the absence of unequivocal hyperglycemia with acute metabolic decompensation, these criteria should be confirmed by repeat testing of b through d on a different day. OGTT is not recommended for routine clinical use.

Source: American Diabetes Association: Standards of medical care in diabetes: Prevention/delay of type 2 diabetes. Diabetes Care 30:S4–S41, 2007, and Sacks DB, Arnold M, Bakris GL, et al: Guidelines and recommendations for laboratory analysis in the diagnosis and management of diabetes mellitus. Diabetes Care 34:e61–e99, 2011.

Normal Findings

FPG, adults: ≤100 mg/dL or ≤5.6 mmol/L
Fasting, children (2 to 18 years): 60 to 100 mg/dL or 3.3 to 5.6 mmol/L
Fasting, young children (0 to 2 years): 60 to 110 mg/dL or 3.3 to 6.1 mmol/L
Fasting, premature infants: 40 to 65 mg/dL or 2.2 to 3.6 mmol/L

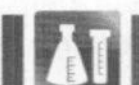

CLINICAL ALERT

Critical values for fasting blood glucose (FBG): <40 mg/dL (<2.22 mmol/L) may cause brain damage (women and children), <50 mg/dL (<2.77 mmol/L) (men); >400 mg/dL (>22.2 mmol/L) may cause coma.

Procedure

1. Draw a 5-mL venous blood sample from a fasting person or a random PG (FPG) (any time of day). In known cases of diabetes, blood drawing should precede administration of insulin or oral hypoglycemic agent. Observe standard precautions. Serum is acceptable if separated from red cells within an hour. A gray-topped tube, which contains sodium fluoride, is acceptable for 24 hours without separation.
2. Self-monitoring of blood glucose by the person (or healthcare provider) with diabetes can be done by finger-stick blood drop sampling several times per day if necessary. Several devices are commercially available for this procedure; they are relatively easy to use and have been established as a major component in satisfactory diabetes control. Calibration of monitoring devices should be done on a regular basis.
3. Noninvasive methods using skin pads to check blood glucose level are being developed for self-monitoring that eliminate the dreaded finger-prick test; for example, a GlucoWatch (Cygnus, Redwood City, CA), worn on the wrist and powered by an AAA battery.

NOTE *When whole blood glucose values are not equivalent to plasma values, plasma values are about 10% to 15% higher than whole blood values. However, most glucose meters convert the whole blood values to plasma equivalent values.*

Patient Checklist for Self-Monitoring of Blood Glucose Testing

This list is a general outline. Each brand of meter has its own instructions. Read the instructions on each new meter carefully to get accurate results. Know whether the monitor and strips give whole blood or plasma equivalent results (Fig. 6.1).

1. General instructions
   a. Make sure hands are clean, dry, and warm.
   b. Prick finger with the lancet.
   c. Squeeze out a drop of capillary blood.
   d. Apply SECOND drop of blood onto the test strip or sensor.
   e. Wait for the test strip or sensor to develop.
   f. Compare the test strip to the chart or insert it into the meter.
   g. Safely dispose of the lancet in an approved sharps container.
   h. Record blood glucose results with date and time.
2. If type 1 diabetes mellitus is present, also monitor urine for ketones or blood β-hydroxybutyrate for possible dangerous complications such as diabetic ketoacidosis (e.g., during stress or acute illness).
3. Test more often on days when illness occurs, when blood glucose is too high, when meal or exercise plans change, when traveling, or if it is thought that the blood glucose is low.

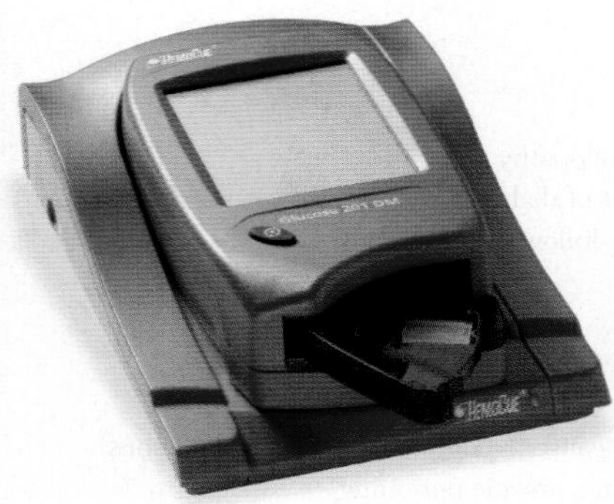

FIGURE 6.1. Portable blood glucose analyzer. (Reprinted with permission from HemoCue AB, Angelholm, Sweden.)

4. If concerned about getting accurate results, consult with the diabetes educator or contact the manufacturer to ensure proper use of the monitor.
5. Several blood glucose meters currently available are approved by the U.S. Food and Drug Administration (FDA), the agency that approves medical devices, for what is called "alternate site testing."
6. Alternate sites (other than fingertips) include forearm, bicep area, palm of hand, between fingers, and sometimes the calf.
7. Tips for using alternate sites
   a. Rub the site to be used to check blood glucose vigorously before pricking skin. This increases blood flow to the site.
   b. Use one type of monitor; do not alternate between different monitors. This will help to obtain consistent results.
   c. Consistently use the same alternate site. For example, always use forearms. This will also help to obtain consistent results.

CLINICAL ALERT

A recent warning was published by the FDA, alerting users of portable glucose monitors to be cognizant of the units of measurement displayed; that is, mg/dL or mmol/L. Reporting a glucose value without reporting the unit of measurement could result in an adverse event.

Clinical Implications

1. *Elevated blood glucose (hyperglycemia)* occurs in the following conditions:
   a. Diabetes mellitus: a fasting glucose ≥126 mg/dL (>7.0 mmol/L) or a 2-hour postprandial load PG ≥200 mg/dL (>11.1 mmol/L) during an oral GTT.
   b. Other conditions that produce elevated PG glucose levels include the following:
      (1) Cushing's disease (increased glucocorticoids cause elevated blood sugar levels)
      (2) Acute emotional or physical stress situations (e.g., myocardial infarction [MI], cerebrovascular accident, convulsions)
      (3) Pheochromocytoma, acromegaly, gigantism
      (4) Pituitary adenoma (increased secretion of growth hormone causes elevated blood glucose levels)
      (5) Hemochromatosis
      (6) Pancreatitis (acute and chronic), neoplasms of pancreas

(7) Glucagonoma
(8) Advanced liver disease
(9) Chronic renal disease
(10) Vitamin B deficiency: Wernicke's encephalopathy
(11) Pregnancy (may signal potential for onset of diabetes later in life)

2. *Decreased blood PG (hypoglycemia)* occurs in the following conditions:
   a. Pancreatic islet cell carcinoma (insulinomas)
   b. Extrapancreatic stomach tumors (carcinoma)
   c. Addison's disease (adrenal insufficiency), carcinoma of adrenal gland
   d. Hypopituitarism, hypothyroidism, ACTH deficiency
   e. Starvation, malabsorption (starvation does not cause hypoglycemia in normal persons)
   f. Liver damage (alcoholism, chloroform poisoning, arsenic poisoning)
   g. Premature infant; infant delivered to a mother with diabetes
   h. Enzyme-deficiency diseases (e.g., galactosemia, inherited maple syrup urine disease, von Gierke's syndrome)
   i. Insulin overdose (accidental or deliberate)
   j. Reactive hypoglycemia, including alimentary hyperinsulinism, prediabetes, endocrine deficiency
   k. Postprandial hypoglycemia may occur after gastrointestinal (GI) surgery and is described with hereditary fructose intolerance, galactosemia, and leucine sensitivity.
3. According to the ADA criteria, there are four definitive tests for diabetes:
   a. Symptoms of diabetes plus a random/casual PG ≥200 mg/dL (>11.1 mmol/L), or
   b. An FPG ≥126 mg/dL (>6.99 mmol/L; in the absence of unequivocal hyperglycemia, criteria b to d should be confirmed by repeat testing), or
   c. An OGTT with a 2-hour postload (75-g glucose load) level ≥200 mg/dL (>11.1 mmol/L; in the absence of unequivocal hyperglycemia, criteria b to d should be confirmed by repeat testing), or
   d. Hemoglobin A_{1c} (HbA_{1c}) ≥6.5% (in the absence of unequivocal hyperglycemia, criteria b to d should be confirmed by repeat testing)
4. The classification of diabetes diagnosis reflects a shift to the etiology or pathology of the disease from a classification based on pharmacologic treatment.
5. Impaired fasting glucose (IFG) or impaired glucose tolerance (IGT) is referred to as *prediabetes*.

Interfering Factors

1. *Elevated glucose*
   a. Steroids, diuretics, other drugs (see Appendix E)
   b. Pregnancy (a slight blood glucose elevation normally occurs)
   c. Surgical procedures, anesthesia, and hospitalization in intensive care unit (ICU)
   d. Obesity or sedentary lifestyle
   e. Parenteral glucose administration (e.g., from total parenteral nutrition)
   f. Intravenous (IV) glucose (recent or current)
   g. Heavy smoking
   h. The dawn phenomenon occurs in both non–insulin-dependent and insulin-dependent diabetes mellitus. There is an increase in blood glucose, typically between 4:00 a.m. and 8:00 a.m., due to counter-regulatory hormones, including growth hormone, cortisol, and glucagon.
2. *Decreased glucose*
   a. Hematocrit >55%
   b. Intense exercise
   c. Toxic doses of aspirin, salicylates, and acetaminophen
   d. Other drugs (see Appendix E), including ethanol, quinine, and haloperidol

Interventions

Pretest Patient Care

1. Explain test purpose (to detect hyperglycemia) and blood-drawing procedure. Note time.
2. Tell patient that the test requires at least an overnight fast; water is permitted. Instruct the patient to defer insulin or oral hypoglycemics until after blood is drawn, unless specifically instructed to do otherwise.
3. Note the last time the patient ate in the record and on the laboratory requisition.
4. Follow guidelines in Chapter 1 for safe, effective, informed *pretest* care.

Posttest Patient Care

1. Tell the patient that he or she may eat and drink after fasting blood is drawn. Note time.
2. Review test results; report and record findings. Modify the nursing care plan as needed. Monitor appropriately for hyperglycemia and hypoglycemia. Counsel regarding necessary lifestyle changes (e.g., diet, exercise, glycemic control, medication). Target blood glucose levels: before meals or upon waking, 80 to 120 mg/dL (4.4 to 6.6 mmol/L); and at bedtime, 100 to 140 mg/dL (5.5 to 7.7 mmol/L).

   Pharmacologic intervention may include pioglitazone (targets insulin resistance) plus glimepiride (increases amount of insulin) to improve glycemic control in type 2 diabetes.
3. Treatment regimens
   a. Initial medical treatment includes use of metformin. The addition of other glucose-lowering medications may be necessary.
   b. When target goals are not achieved and glucose and A_{1c} remain elevated, early (basal) insulin therapy may be indicated.
   c. In hospitalized patients (ICU, surgery, critical illnesses), strict glycemic controls, interventions (blood checking at least four times daily and sliding scale insulin administration), and aggressive insulin therapy are indicated.
   d. Glucose may be monitored by three methods: (1) intermittent laboratory analysis, (2) bedside monitor, and (3) continuous glucose monitoring. The continuous glucose monitor system has been used to safely lower blood sugar in children with type 1 diabetes. In this instance, a tiny glucose-sensing device is inserted under the skin of the abdomen. This sensor and computer (attached to a belt) measure and record blood glucose every 10 seconds for 3 days.
4. Give the patient the following checklist:
   a. Take special care of feet.
   b. Use a lubricant or unscented hand cream on dry, scaly skin.
   c. Look for calluses on soles. Rub them gently with a pumice stone.
   d. Make sure new shoes fit properly; wear freshly washed socks or stockings.
   e. Never go barefoot.
   f. Avoid using hot water bottles, tubs of hot water, or heating pads on the feet.
   g. Trim toenails straight across.
   h. Make sure doctor inspects feet as part of every visit.
   i. Use a team approach to help make decisions about care. The team may include a doctor, nurse diabetes educator, dietitian, pharmacist, ophthalmologist or optometrist, exercise physiologist, podiatrist, psychologist, and the family.
   j. Follow the most healthful lifestyle possible, focusing on diet, exercise, and weight management.
5. Persons with glucose levels >200 mg/dL (>11.1 mmol/L) should be placed on a strict intake and output program.
6. In-home test kits are available for patients to evaluate whether they have lost protective sensation in a foot, which would put them at high risk for lower extremity amputation. The lower extremity amputation prevention (LEAP) monofilament test includes a 10-g reusable monofilament that is touched to eight sites on each foot for 1 to 2 seconds. A diagram of each foot with the sites marked is included in the kit for recording whether sensation was felt at each site. The results can then be reviewed by the healthcare provider and further evaluation undertaken if indicated.
7. Follow guidelines in Chapter 1 for safe, effective, informed *posttest* care.

CLINICAL ALERT

1. If a person with known or suspected diabetes experiences headaches, irritability, dizziness, weakness, fainting, or impaired cognition, a blood glucose test or finger stick test must be done before giving insulin. Similar symptoms may be present for both hypoglycemia and hyperglycemia. If a blood glucose level cannot be obtained and one is uncertain regarding the situation, glucose may be given in the form of orange juice, sugar-containing soda, or candy (e.g., hard candy, jelly beans). Make certain the person is sufficiently conscious to manage eating or swallowing. In the acute care setting, IV glucose may be given in the event of severe hypoglycemia. A glucose gel is also commercially available and may be rubbed on the inside of the mouth by another person if the person with diabetes is unable to swallow or to respond properly. Instruct persons prone to hypoglycemia to carry sugar-type items on their person and to wear a necklace or bracelet that identifies the person as diabetic.
2. Frequent blood glucose monitoring, including self-monitoring, allows better control and management of diabetes than urine glucose monitoring.
3. When blood glucose values are >300 mg/dL (>16.6 mmol/L), urine output increases, as does the risk for dehydration.
4. Diabetes is a "disease of the moment": Persons living with diabetes are continually affected by fluctuations in blood glucose levels and must learn to manage and adapt their lifestyle within this framework. For some, adaptation is relatively straightforward; for others, especially those identified as being "brittle," lifestyle changes and management are more complicated, and these patients require constant vigilance, attention, encouragement, and support.
5. Each person with diabetes may experience certain symptoms in his or her own unique way and in a unique pattern.

CLINICAL ALERT

1. Infants with tremor, convulsion, or respiratory distress should have STAT glucose done, particularly in the presence of maternal diabetes or with hemolytic disease of the newborn.
2. Newborns who are too small or too large for gestational age should have their glucose level measured in the first day of life.
3. Diseases related to neonatal hypoglycemia
   a. Glycogen storage diseases
   b. Galactosemia
   c. Hereditary fructose intolerance
   d. Ketogenic hypoglycemia of infancy
   e. Carnitine deficiency (Reye's syndrome)

• Hemoglobin A_{1c} (HbA_{1c}); Glycohemoglobin (G-Hb); Glycated Hemoglobin (GhB); Diabetic Control Index; Glycated Serum Protein (GSP)

Glycohemoglobin (G-Hb) is a normal, minor type of hemoglobin. Glycosylated hemoglobin is formed at a rate proportional to the average glucose concentration by a slow, nonenzymatic process within the red blood cells (RBCs) during their 120-day circulating life span. G-Hb is blood glucose bound to hemoglobin. In the presence of hyperglycemia, an increase in G-Hb causes an increase in HbA_{1c} (formed as a result of irreversible attachment of glucose to an amino acid in the β chain of the adult hemoglobin molecule). If the glucose concentration increases because of insulin deficiency, then glycosylation is irreversible.

Glycosylated hemoglobin values reflect average blood sugar levels for the 2- to 3-month period before the test. This test provides information for evaluating diabetic treatment modalities (every 3 months), is useful in determining treatment for juvenile-onset diabetes with acute ketoacidosis, and tracks control of blood glucose in milder cases of diabetes. It can be a valuable adjunct in determining which therapeutic choices and directions (e.g., oral antihypoglycemic agents, insulin, β-cell transplantation) will be most effective. A blood sample can be drawn at any time. The measurement is of particular value for specific groups of patients: diabetic children; diabetic patients in whom the renal threshold for glucose is abnormal; unstable type 1 diabetic patients (taking insulin) in whom blood sugar levels vary markedly from day to day; type 2 diabetic patients who become pregnant; and persons who, before their scheduled appointments, change their usual habits, dietary or otherwise, so that their metabolic control appears better than it actually is.

Normal Findings

Results are expressed as percentage of total hemoglobin. Values vary slightly by method and laboratory.

G-Hb: 4.0% to 7.0% or 0.04 to 0.07
HbA_{1c}: 5.0% to 7.0% (100 to 170 mg/dL or 5.5 to 9.3 mmol/L)
Plasma blood glucose (mg/dL) = (HbA_{1c} × 35.6) − 77.3
Plasma blood glucose (mmol/L) = (HbA_{1c} × 1.98) − 4.29

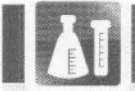

CLINICAL ALERT

Critical Value

1. G-Hb: >10.1% (>0.101)
2. HbA_{1c}: >8.1% (>0.08) corresponds to an estimated average glucose >186 mg/dL (>10.3 mmol/L)

Procedure

1. Obtain a 5-mL venous blood sample with ethylenediaminetetraacetic acid (EDTA) purple-topped anticoagulant additive. Serum may not be used.
2. Observe standard precautions. Label the specimen with the patient's name, date and time of collection, and test(s) ordered. Place the specimen in a biohazard bag.

Clinical Implications

1. Values are frequently increased in persons with poorly controlled or newly diagnosed diabetes.
2. With optimal control, the HbA_{1c} moves toward normal levels.
3. A diabetic patient who recently comes under good control may still show higher concentrations of glycosylated hemoglobin. This level declines gradually over several months as nearly normal glycosylated hemoglobin replaces older RBCs with higher concentrations.
4. Increases in glycosylated hemoglobin occur in the following nondiabetic conditions:
   a. Iron-deficiency anemia
   b. Splenectomy
   c. Alcohol toxicity
   d. Lead toxicity

5. Decreases in HbA_{1c} occur in the following nondiabetic conditions:
   a. Hemolytic anemia
   b. Chronic blood loss
   c. Pregnancy
   d. Chronic renal failure

Interfering Factors (varies by method)

1. Presence of HbF and H causes falsely elevated values.
2. Presence of HbS, C, E, D, G, and Lepore (autosomal recessive mutation resulting in a hemoglobinopathy) causes falsely decreased values.

Interventions

Pretest Patient Care

1. Explain test purpose and blood-drawing procedure. Observe standard precautions. Fasting is not required.
2. Note that this test is *not* meant for short-term diabetes mellitus management; instead, it assesses the efficacy of long-term management modalities over several weeks or months. It is not useful more often than 4 to 6 weeks.
3. Follow guidelines in Chapter 1 for safe, effective, informed *pretest* care.

Posttest Patient Care

1. Review test outcome, with target HbA_{1c} of <5.7%, and counsel patient appropriately for management of diabetes with oral hypoglycemics and insulin. If test results are not consistent with clinical findings, check the patient for HbF, which elevates HbA_{1c} results.
2. Follow guidelines in Chapter 1 regarding safe, effective, informed *posttest* care.

CLINICAL ALERT

A number of different tests can determine glycosylated hemoglobin levels. The most specific of these measures is HbA_{1c}. There are different expected values for each test. Keep in mind that HbA_1 is always 2%–4% higher than HbA_{1c}. When reviewing results, be certain of the specific test used.

• Gestational Diabetes Mellitus (GDM)

Glucose intolerance *during* pregnancy (gestational diabetes mellitus [GDM]) is associated with an increase in perinatal morbidity and mortality, especially in women who are aged >25 years, overweight, or hypertensive. In addition, more than one half of all pregnant patients with an abnormal GTT do not have any of the same risk factors. It is therefore recommended by the ADA that all pregnant women be screened for GDM as follows: Women with presence of risk factors should be screened at the first prenatal visit, and women with no known prior diabetes should be screened at 24 to 28 weeks.

A diabetes risk assessment should be done at the first prenatal visit. Screening for very-high-risk pregnancies should be done as soon as possible. At this stage, screening can be done using standard criteria. An OGTT is done to detect GDM and screen nonsymptomatic pregnant women. During pregnancy, abnormal carbohydrate metabolism is evaluated by screening all pregnant women at the first prenatal visit and then again at 24 to 28 weeks.

Two approaches may be followed for GDM screening at 24 to 28 weeks:

1. Two-step approach:
   A. Perform initial screening by measuring plasma or serum glucose 1 hour after a 50-g load of 140 mg/dL identifies 80% of women with GDM, whereas the sensitivity is further increased to 90% by a threshold of 130 mg/dL.
   B. Perform a diagnostic 100-g OGTT on a separate day in women who exceed the chosen threshold on 50-g screening.
2. One-step approach (may be preferred in clinics with high prevalence of GDM): Perform a diagnostic 100-g OGTT in all women to be tested at 24 to 28 weeks. The 100-g OGTT should be performed in the morning after an overnight fast of at least 8 hours.

Reference Values

To make a diagnosis of GDM, at least two of the following PG values must be found:

- FPG >95 mg/dL (>5.3 mmol/L)
- 1-hour >180 mg/dL (>10.0 mmol/L)
- 2-hour >155 mg/dL (>8.6 mmol/L)
- 3-hour >140 mg/dL (>7.8 mmol/L)

Procedure

1. Draw a 5-mL venous blood sample (sodium fluoride) after an 8- to 14-hour fast, at least 3 days of unrestricted diet and activity, and after glucose load.
2. Observe standard precautions. Label the specimen with the patient's name, date and time of collection, and test(s) ordered. Place the specimen in a biohazard bag.

Clinical Implications

1. A positive result in a pregnant woman means she is at much greater risk (seven times) for having GDM.
2. GDM is any degree of glucose intolerance with onset during pregnancy or first recognized during pregnancy.

Interventions

Pretest Patient Care

1. Explain test purpose (to evaluate abnormal carbohydrate metabolism and predict diabetes in later life) and procedure. No fasting is usually required. Obtain pertinent history of diabetes and record any signs or symptoms of diabetes.
2. Instruct the woman about obtaining a urine sample for glucose testing to check before drinking the glucose load. Positive urine glucose should be checked with the healthcare provider before glucose load. Those with glycosuria >250 mg/dL (>13.8 mmol/L) must have a blood glucose test before GDM testing.
3. Give the patient the appropriate glucose beverage (150 mL dissolved in water or Trutol or Orange DEX).
4. Explain to the patient that no eating, drinking, smoking, or gum chewing is allowed during the test. The patient should not leave the office. She may void if necessary.
5. After 1 hour, draw one NaF or EDTA tube (5-mL venous blood) using standard venipuncture technique.

Posttest Patient Care

1. Normal activities, eating, and drinking may be resumed.
2. Review test results; report and record findings. Modify the nursing care plan as needed. Explain to the patient what to expect for a normal outcome.
3. Six to 12 weeks after delivery, the patient should be retested and reclassified. In most cases, glucose will return to normal.

Glucose Tolerance Test (GTT); Oral Glucose Tolerance Test (OGTT)

In a healthy individual, the insulin response to a large oral glucose dose is almost immediate. It peaks in 30 to 60 minutes and returns to normal levels within 3 hours when sufficient insulin is present to metabolize the glucose ingested at the beginning of the test. The test should be performed according to WHO guidelines using glucose load containing the equivalent of 75 g of anhydrous glucose dissolved in water or other solution.

If fasting and postload glucose test results are borderline, the GTT can support or rule out a diagnosis of diabetes mellitus; it can also be a part of a workup for unexplained hypertriglyceridemia, neuropathy, impotence, renal diseases, or retinopathy. This test may be ordered when there is sugar in the urine or when the fasting blood sugar level is significantly elevated. The GTT/OGTT should *not* be used as a screening test in nonpregnant adults or children.

Indications for Test

The GTT/OGTT is done on certain patients, with the following indications (few indications still meet wide acceptance):

1. Family history of diabetes
2. Obesity
3. Unexplained episodes of hypoglycemia
4. History of recurrent infections (boils and abscesses)
5. In women, history of delivery of large infants, stillbirths, neonatal death, premature labor, and spontaneous abortions
6. Transitory glycosuria or hyperglycemia during pregnancy, surgery, trauma, stress, MI, and ACTH administration

Normal Findings

FPG
Adults: 100 mg/dL or 5.6 mmol/L
120-Minute (2-Hour GTT Test) 2-Hour PG after 75-g Glucose Load
Adults: ≤200 mg/dL or ≤11.1 mmol/L
Adults: 140 to 199 mg/dL (7.8 to 11.0 mmol/L), IGT

Procedure

This is a timed test for glucose tolerance. A 2-hour PG test is done after glucose load to detect diabetes in individuals other than pregnant women.

1. Have the patient eat a diet with >150 g of carbohydrates for 3 days before the test.
2. Ensure that the following drugs are discontinued 3 days before the test because they may influence test results:
   a. Hormones, oral contraceptives, steroids
   b. Salicylates, anti-inflammatory drugs
   c. Diuretic agents
   d. Hypoglycemic agents
   e. Antihypertensive drugs
   f. Anticonvulsants (see Appendix E)
3. Insulin and oral hypoglycemic agents should be withheld until the test is completed.
4. Record the patient's weight.
   a. Pediatric doses of glucose are based on body weight, calculated as 1.75 g/kg not to exceed a total of 75 g.
   b. Nonpregnant adults: 75 g of glucose

5. A 5-mL sample of venous blood is drawn. Serum or gray-topped tubes are used. The patient should fast 12 to 16 hours before testing. After the blood is drawn, the patient drinks all of a specially formulated glucose solution within a 5-minute time frame.
6. Blood samples are obtained at fasting and 2 hours after glucose ingestion.
7. Tolerance tests can also be performed for pentose, lactose, galactose, and D-xylose.
8. The GTT is not indicated in these situations:
   a. Persistent fasting hyperglycemia >140 mg/dL or >7.8 mmol/L
   b. Persistent fasting normal PG
   c. Patients with overt diabetes mellitus
   d. Persistent 2-hour PG >200 mg/dL or >11.1 mmol/L
9. Test has limited value in diagnosis of diabetes mellitus in children and is rarely indicated for that purpose.

PROCEDURAL ALERT

1. GTT is contraindicated in patients with a recent history of surgery, MI, or labor and delivery—these conditions can produce invalid values.
2. The GTT should be postponed if the patient becomes ill, even with common illnesses such as the flu or a severe cold.
3. Record and report any reactions during the test. Weakness, faintness, and sweating may occur between the second and third hours of the test. If this occurs, a blood sample for a glucose level should be drawn immediately and the GTT aborted.
4. Should the patient vomit the glucose solution, the test is declared invalid; it can be repeated in 3 d (~72 hr).

Clinical Implications

1. The presence of abnormal GTT values (decreased tolerance to glucose) is based on the International Classification for Diabetes Mellitus and the following glucose intolerance categories:
   a. At least two GTT values must be abnormal for a diagnosis of diabetes mellitus to be validated.
   b. In cases of overt diabetes, no insulin is secreted; abnormally high glucose levels persist throughout the test.
   c. Glucose values that fall above normal values but below the diagnostic criteria for diabetes or IGT should be considered nondiagnostic.
2. See Table 6.3 for an interpretation of glucose tolerance levels.
3. Decreased glucose tolerance occurs with high glucose values in the following conditions:
   a. Diabetes mellitus
   b. Postgastrectomy
   c. Hyperthyroidism
   d. Excess glucose ingestion
   e. Hyperlipidemia types III, IV, and V
   f. Hemochromatosis
   g. Cushing's disease (steroid effect)
   h. Central nervous system (CNS) lesions
   i. Pheochromocytoma
4. Decreased glucose tolerance with hypoglycemia can be found in persons with von Gierke's disease, severe liver damage, or increased epinephrine levels.

TABLE 6.3 Glucose Tolerance Test Levels

	Conventional Units (mg/dL)	SI Units (mmol/L)
Fasting adult	140	7.8
Adult diabetes mellitus 1-hr glucose	>200	>11.1
and 2-hr glucose	>200	>11.1
Fasting adult	140	7.8
Adult impaired glucose tolerance 1-hr glucose	>200	>11.1
and 2-hr glucose	>140–200	>7.8–11.1
Juvenile diabetes mellitus (fasting glucose)	>140	>7.8
and 1-hr glucose	>200	>11.1
and 2-hr glucose	>200	>11.1
Impaired glucose tolerance in children (fasting glucose)	—	—
and 2-hr glucose	>140	>7.8

5. Increased glucose tolerance with flat curve (i.e., glucose does not increase but may decrease to hypoglycemic levels) occurs in the following conditions:
   a. Pancreatic islet cell hyperplasia or tumor
   b. Poor intestinal absorption caused by diseases such as sprue, celiac disease, or Whipple's disease
   c. Hypoparathyroidism
   d. Addison's disease
   e. Liver disease
   f. Hypopituitarism, hypothyroidism

Interfering Factors

1. Smoking increases glucose levels.
2. Altered diets (e.g., weight reduction) before testing can diminish carbohydrate tolerance and suggest "false diabetes."
3. Glucose levels normally tend to increase with aging.
4. Prolonged oral contraceptive use causes significantly higher glucose levels in the second hour or in later blood specimens.
5. Infectious diseases, illnesses, and operative procedures affect glucose tolerance. Two weeks of recovery should be allowed before performing the test.
6. Certain drugs impair glucose tolerance levels (this list is not all inclusive; see Appendix E for other drugs):

   If possible, these drugs should be discontinued for at least 3 days before testing. Check with the healthcare provider for specific orders.

   a. Insulin
   b. Oral hypoglycemics
   c. Large doses of salicylates, anti-inflammatory drugs
   d. Thiazide diuretics
   e. Oral contraceptives
   f. Corticosteroids
   g. Estrogens
   h. Heparin

i. Nicotinic acid
j. Phenothiazines
k. Lithium
l. Metyrapone (Metopirone)

7. Prolonged bed rest influences GTT results. If possible, the patient should be ambulatory. A GTT in a hospitalized patient has limited value.

Interventions

Pretest Patient Care

1. Explain test purpose and procedure. A written reminder may be helpful.
   a. A diet high in carbohydrates (150 g) should be eaten for 3 days preceding the test. Instruct the patient to abstain from alcohol.
   b. The patient should fast for at least 12 hours but not more than 16 hours before the test. Only water may be ingested during fasting time and test time. Use of tobacco products is not permitted during testing.
   c. Patients should rest or walk quietly during the test period. They may feel weak, faint, or nauseated during the test. Vigorous exercise alters glucose values and should be avoided during testing.
2. Collect blood specimens at the prescribed times and record exact times collected. Urine glucose testing is no longer recommended.
3. Follow guidelines in Chapter 1 for safe, effective, informed *pretest* care.

Posttest Patient Care

1. Have the patient resume normal diet and activities at the end of the test. Encourage eating complex carbohydrates and protein if permitted.
2. Administer prescribed insulin or oral hypoglycemics when the test is done. Arrange for the patient to eat within a short time (30 minutes) after these medications are taken.
3. Review test results; report and record findings. Modify the nursing care plan as needed. Counsel the patient appropriately. Patients newly diagnosed with diabetes will need diet, medication, and lifestyle modification instructions.
4. Follow guidelines in Chapter 1 for safe, effective, informed *posttest* care.

CLINICAL ALERT

1. If fasting glucose is >140 mg/dL (>7.8 mmol/L) on two separate occasions, or if the 2-hr postprandial blood glucose is >200 mg/dL (>11.1 mmol/L) on two separate occasions, GTT is not necessary for a diagnosis of diabetes mellitus to be established.
2. The GTT is of limited diagnostic value for children.

● Lactose Tolerance; Breath Hydrogen Test

Lactose intolerance often begins in infancy, with symptoms of diarrhea, vomiting, failure to thrive, and malabsorption. The patient becomes asymptomatic when lactose is removed from the diet. This syndrome is caused by a deficiency of sugar-splitting enzymes (lactase) in the intestinal tract.

This test is actually a GTT done to diagnose intestinal disaccharidase (lactase) deficiency. Glucose is measured, and it is the increase or lack of increase over the fasting specimen that is used for the interpretation. Breath samples reveal increased hydrogen levels, which are caused by lactose buildup in the intestinal tract. Colonic bacteria metabolize the lactose and produce hydrogen gas.

Normal Findings

Change in glucose from normal value >30 mg/dL or >1.7 mmol/L
Inconclusive: 20 to 30 mg/dL or 1.1 to 1.7 mmol/L
Abnormal: <20 mg/dL or <1.1 mmol/L
Hydrogen (breath):
Fasting: <5 ppm or $<5 \times 10^{-6}$
After lactose ingestion: <12 ppm or $<12 \times 10^{-6}$ increase from fasting level

Procedure

1. Follow instructions given for the GTT.
2. Draw a blood specimen from a fasting patient. The patient then drinks 50 g of lactose mixed with 200 mL of water (2 g of lactose/kg body weight).
3. Draw blood lactose samples at 0, 30-, 60-, and 90-minute intervals.
4. Take breath hydrogen samples at the same time intervals as the blood specimens. Contact your laboratory for collection procedures.

Clinical Implications

1. Lactose intolerance occurs as follows:
   a. A "flat" lactose tolerance finding (i.e., no rise in glucose) points to a deficiency of sugar-splitting enzymes, as in irritable bowel syndrome. This type of deficiency is more prevalent in American Indians, African Americans, Asians, and Jews.
   b. A monosaccharide tolerance test such as the glucose/galactose tolerance test should be done as a follow-up.
      (1) The patient ingests 25 g of both glucose and galactose.
      (2) A normal increase in glucose indicates a lactose deficiency.
   c. Secondary lactose deficiency found in:
      (1) Infectious enteritis
      (2) Bacterial overgrowth in intestines
      (3) Inflammatory bowel disease, Crohn's disease
      (4) *Giardia lamblia* infestation
      (5) Cystic fibrosis of pancreas
2. The breath hydrogen test is abnormal in the lactose deficiency test because:
   a. Malabsorption causes hydrogen (H_2) production through the process of fermentation of lactose in the colon.
   b. The H_2 formed is directly proportional to the amount of test dose lactose *not* digested by lactase.
3. In diabetes:
   a. Blood glucose values may show increases >20 mg/dL (>1.11 mmol/L) despite impaired lactose absorption.
   b. There may be an abnormal lactose tolerance curve due to faulty metabolism, not necessarily from lactose intolerance.

Interventions

Pretest Patient Care

1. Explain test purpose and procedure. The patient must fast for 8 to 12 hours before the test.
2. Do not allow the patient to eat dark bread, peas, beans, sugars, or high-fiber foods within 24 hours of the test.
3. Do not permit smoking during the test and for 8 hours before testing; no gum chewing.
4. Do not allow antibiotics to be taken for 2 weeks before the test unless specifically ordered.
5. Follow guidelines in Chapter 1 for safe, effective, informed *pretest* care.

Posttest Patient Care

1. Have the patient resume normal diet and activity.
2. Review test results; report and record findings. Modify the nursing care plan as needed. Counsel the patient appropriately. Patients with irritable bowel syndrome with gas, bloating, abdominal pain, constipation, and diarrhea have lactose deficiency. Restricting milk intake relieves symptoms.
3. Follow guidelines in Chapter 1 regarding safe, effective, informed *posttest* care.

● Related Tests That Influence Glucose Metabolism

C-PEPTIDE

C-peptide is formed during the conversion of proinsulin to insulin. Proinsulin is cleaved (holds α- and β-insulin chains together in the proinsulin molecule) into insulin and biologically inactive C-peptide. C-peptide assay provides distinction between exogenous and endogenous circulating insulin.

The main use of C-peptide is to evaluate hypoglycemia. C-peptide levels provide reliable indicators for pancreatic and secretory functions and insulin secretions. In a patient with type 1 diabetes mellitus, C-peptide measurements can be an index of insulin production and mark endogenous β-cell activity. C-peptide levels can also be used to confirm suspected surreptitious insulin injections (i.e., factitious hypoglycemia). Findings in these patients reveal that insulin levels are usually high, insulin antibodies may be high, but C-peptide levels are low or undetectable. This test also monitors the patient's recovery after excision of an insulinoma. Rising C-peptide levels suggest insulinoma tumor recurrence or metastases.

Normal Findings

Fasting: 0.51 to 2.72 ng/mL or 0.17 to 0.90 mmol/L
Values vary with laboratory.

Procedure

1. Draw a 1-mL venous blood sample from a fasting patient using a red-topped chilled tube. Serum is needed for test. Label the specimen with the patient's name, date and time of collection, and test(s) ordered. Date and time must be correct. Centrifuge blood for 30 minutes. Follow standard precautions.
2. Separate the blood at 4°C and freeze if it will not be tested until later.
3. A sample for glucose testing is usually drawn at the same time.
4. Label the specimen with the patient's name, date and time of collection, and test(s) ordered. Place specimen in a biohazard bag.

Clinical Implications

1. *Increased C-peptide* values occur in the following conditions:
   a. Endogenous hyperinsulinism (insulinemia)
   b. Oral hypoglycemic drug ingestion
   c. Pancreas or β-cell transplantation
   d. Insulin-secreting neoplasms (islet cell tumor)
   e. Type 2 diabetes mellitus (non–insulin-dependent)
2. *Decreased C-peptide* values occur in the following conditions:
   a. Factitious hypoglycemia (surreptitious insulin administration)
   b. Radical pancreatectomy
   c. Type 1 diabetes mellitus
3. C-peptide stimulation test can determine the following:
   a. Distinguish between type 1 and type 2 diabetes mellitus.
   b. Identify patients with diabetes whose C-peptide stimulation values are >1.8 ng/mL (>0.59 nmol/L) who can be managed without insulin treatment.

Interfering Factors

Increased C-Peptide

1. Renal failure
2. Ingestion of sulfonylurea

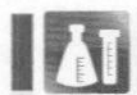

CLINICAL ALERT

To differentiate insulinoma from factitious hypoglycemia, an insulin–to–C-peptide ratio can be performed.

<1.0 ratio: increased endogenous insulin secretion

>1.0 ratio: exogenous insulin

Interventions

Pretest Patient Care

1. Explain the test purpose and blood-drawing procedure. Obtain history of signs and symptoms of hypoglycemia.
2. Ensure that the patient fasts, except for water, for 8 to 12 hours before blood is drawn.
3. If a radioisotope test is necessary, it should take place *after* blood is drawn for C-peptide levels.
4. If the C-peptide stimulation test is done, give IV glucagon after a baseline value blood sample is drawn.
5. Follow guidelines in Chapter 1 for safe, effective, informed *pretest* care.

Posttest Patient Care

1. Resume normal activities.
2. Review test results; report and record findings. Modify the nursing care plan as needed. Explain possible need for further testing. See Chapter 8 for anti-insulin antibody testing.
3. Follow guidelines in Chapter 1 for safe, effective, informed *posttest* care.

GLUCAGON

Glucagon is a peptide hormone that originates in the α cells of the pancreatic islets of Langerhans. This hormone promotes glucose production in the liver. Normally, glucagon is a counterbalance to insulin. Glucagon provides a sensitive, coordinated control mechanism for glucose production and storage. For example, low blood glucose levels cause glucagon to stimulate glucose release into the bloodstream, whereas elevated blood glucose levels reduce the amount of circulating glucagon to about 50% of that found in the fasting state. The kidneys also affect glucagon metabolism. Elevated fasting glucagon levels in the presence of renal failure return to normal levels following successful renal transplantation. Abnormally high glucagon levels drop toward normal once insulin therapy effectively controls diabetes. However, when compared with a healthy person, glucagon secretion in the person with diabetes does not decrease after eating carbohydrates. Moreover, in healthy persons, arginine infusion causes increased glucagon secretion.

This test measures glucagon production and metabolism. A glucagon deficiency reflects pancreatic tissue loss. Failure of glucagon levels to rise during arginine infusion confirms glucagon deficiency. Hyperglucagonemia (i.e., elevated glucagon levels) occurs in diabetes, acute pancreatitis, and situations in which catecholamine secretion is stimulated (e.g., pheochromocytoma, infection).

Normal Findings

Adults: 20 to 100 pg/mL or 20 to 100 ng/L
Children: 0 to 148 pg/mL or 0 to 148 ng/L
Newborns: 0 to 1750 pg/mL or 0 to 1750 ng/L
Normal ranges vary with different laboratories.

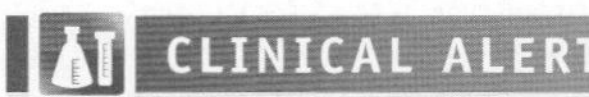

During a GTT in healthy persons, glucagon levels will decline significantly compared with baseline fasting levels because normal hyperglycemia takes place during the first hour of testing.

Procedure

1. Draw a 5-mL blood sample from a fasting person into a chilled EDTA Vacutainer tube containing aprotinin (Trasylol) proteinase inhibitor. Special handling is required because glucagon is very prone to enzymatic degradation. Tubes used to draw blood must be chilled before the sample is collected and placed on ice afterward, and plasma must be frozen as soon as possible after centrifuging.
2. Observe standard precautions. Label the specimen with the patient's name, date and time of collection, and test(s) ordered. Place the specimen in a biohazard bag.

Clinical Implications

1. *Increased glucagon levels* are associated with the following conditions:
   a. Acute pancreatitis (e.g., pancreatic α-cell tumor)
   b. Diabetes mellitus: Persons with severe diabetic ketoacidosis are reported to have fasting glucagon levels five times normal despite marked hyperglycemia.
   c. Glucagonoma (familial), which may be manifested by three different syndromes:
      (1) The first syndrome exhibits a characteristic skin rash, necrolytic migratory erythema, diabetes mellitus or IGT, weight loss, anemia, and venous thrombosis. This form usually shows elevated glucagon levels (>1000 pg/mL or >1000 ng/L) (diagnostic).
      (2) The second syndrome occurs with severe diabetes.
      (3) The third form is associated with multiple endocrine neoplasia syndrome and can show relatively lower glucagon levels as compared with the others.
   d. Chronic renal failure
   e. Hyperlipidemia
   f. Stress (trauma, burns, surgery)
   g. Uremia
   h. Hepatic cirrhosis
   i. Hyperosmolality
   j. Acute pancreatitis
   k. Hypoglycemia
2. *Reduced levels of glucagon* are associated with the following conditions:
   a. Loss of pancreatic tissue
      (1) Pancreatic neoplasms
      (2) Pancreatectomy
   b. Chronic pancreatitis
   c. Cystic fibrosis

NOTE *After glucose load, there is no suppression of glucagon in patients with glucagonoma.*

Interventions

Pretest Patient Care

1. Explain purpose of test and blood-drawing procedure. A minimum 8-hour fast (no calorie intake for at least 8 hours) is necessary before the test.
2. Promote relaxation in a low-stress environment; stress alters normal glucagon levels.
3. Do not administer radiopharmaceuticals within 1 week before the test.
4. Follow guidelines in Chapter 1 for safe, effective, informed *pretest* care.

Posttest Patient Care

1. Have the patient resume normal activities.
2. Review the test outcome and monitor for the three different syndromes of glucagonoma.
3. Follow guidelines in Chapter 1 for safe, effective, informed *posttest* care.

INSULIN

Insulin, a hormone produced by the pancreatic β cells of the islets of Langerhans, regulates carbohydrate metabolism together with contributions from the liver, adipose tissue, and other target cells. Insulin is responsible for maintaining blood glucose levels at a constant level within a defined range. The rate of insulin secretion is primarily regulated by the level of blood glucose perfusing the pancreas; however, it can also be affected by hormones, the autonomic nervous system, and nutritional status.

Insulin levels are valuable for establishing the presence of an insulinoma (i.e., tumor of the islets of Langerhans). This test is also used for investigating the causes of fasting hypoglycemic states and neoplasm differentiation. The insulin study can be done in conjunction with a GTT or FBG test or a FPG test.

Normal Findings

Immunoreactive
Adults: 0 to 35 μIU/mL or 0 to 243 pmol/L
Children: 0 to 10 μIU/mL or 0 to 69 pmol/L
Free
Adults: 0 to 17 μIU/mL or 0 to 118 pmol/L
Children (prepubertal): 0 to 13 μIU/mL or 0 to 90 pmol/L

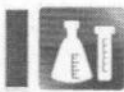

CLINICAL ALERT

Critical range: >35 μIU/mL or >243 pmol/L (fasting)

Procedure

1. Obtain a 5-mL blood sample (red-topped tube) from a fasting (8 hours) person; serum is preferred. Observe standard precautions. Heparinized blood may be used.
2. If done in conjunction with a GTT, draw the specimens before administering oral glucose, at ingestion, and 120 minutes after glucose ingestion (the same times as the GTT).

Clinical Implications

1. *Increased insulin values* are associated with the following conditions:
   a. Insulinoma (pancreatic islet tumor). Diagnosis is based on the following findings:
      (1) Hyperinsulinemia with hypoglycemia (glucose <30 mg/dL or <1.66 mmol/L)
      (2) Persistent hypoglycemia together with hyperinsulinemia (>20 μIU/mL or >139 pmol/L) after tolbutamide injection (rapid rise and rapid fall)
      (3) Failed C-peptide suppression with a PG level <30 mg/dL or <1.66 mmol/L and insulin/glucose ratio >0.3.
   b. Type 2 diabetes mellitus, untreated
   c. Acromegaly
   d. Cushing's syndrome
   e. Endogenous administration of insulin (factitious hypoglycemia)
   f. Obesity (most common cause)
   g. Pancreatic islet cell hyperplasia

2. *Decreased insulin values* are found in the following conditions:
   a. Type 1 diabetes mellitus, severe
   b. Hypopituitarism

Interfering Factors

1. Surreptitious insulin or oral hypoglycemic agent ingestion or injection causes elevated insulin levels (with low C-peptide values).
2. Oral contraceptives and other drugs cause falsely elevated values.
3. Recently administered radioisotopes affect test results.
4. In the second to third trimester of pregnancy, there is a relative insulin resistance with a progressive decrease of PG and immunoreactive insulin.

Interventions

Pretest Patient Care

1. Explain test purpose and procedure.
2. Ensure that the patient fasts from all food and fluid, except water, unless otherwise directed.
3. Insulin release from an insulinoma may be erratic and unpredictable; therefore, it may be necessary for the patient to fast for as long as 72 hours before the test.
4. Follow guidelines in Chapter 1 regarding safe, effective, informed *pretest* care.

Posttest Patient Care

1. Have patient resume normal activity and diet.
2. Review test results; report and record findings. Modify the nursing care plan as needed. Obese patients may have insulin resistance and unusually high fasting and postprandial (after eating) insulin levels. Explain possible need for further testing and treatment.
3. Follow guidelines in Chapter 1 regarding safe, effective, informed *posttest* care.

CLINICAL ALERT

A potentially fatal situation may exist if the insulinoma secretes unpredictably high levels of insulin. In this case, the blood glucose may drop to such dangerously low levels as to render the person comatose and unable to self-administer oral glucose forms. Patients and their families must learn how to deal with such an emergency and to be vigilant until the problem is treated.

END PRODUCTS OF METABOLISM AND OTHER TESTS

● Ammonia (NH_3)

Ammonia, an end product of protein metabolism, is formed by bacteria acting on intestinal proteins together with glutamine hydrolysis in the kidneys. The liver normally removes most of this ammonia through the portal vein circulation and converts the ammonia to urea. Because any appreciable level of ammonia in the blood affects the body's acid–base balance and brain function, its removal from the body is essential. The liver accomplishes this by synthesizing urea so that it can be excreted by the kidneys.

Blood ammonia levels are used to diagnose Reye's syndrome, to evaluate metabolism, and to determine the progress of severe liver disease and its response to treatment. Blood ammonia measurements are useful in monitoring patients on hyperalimentation therapy.

Normal Findings

When Measured as NH_3

Adults: 15 to 60 μg/dL or 11 to 35 μmol/L
10 days to 2 years: 70 to 135 μg/dL or 41 to 80 μmol/L
Birth to 10 days: 170 to 340 μg/dL or 100 to 200 μmol/L

When Measured as N

Adults: 15 to 45 μg/dL or 11 to 32 μmol/L
>1 month of age: 30 to 70 μg/dL or 21 to 50 μmol/L
Birth to 14 days: 80 to 130 μg/dL or 57 to 93 μmol/L

Values test somewhat higher in capillary blood samples. Values can vary with testing method used.

Procedure

1. Obtain a 5-mL venous plasma sample from a fasting patient. A green-topped (heparin) or purple-topped (EDTA) tube may be used. Observe standard precautions.
2. Place the sample in an iced container. The specimen must be centrifuged at 4°C. Promptly remove plasma from cells. Perform the test within 20 minutes or freeze plasma immediately.
3. Note all antibiotics the patient is receiving; these drugs lower ammonia levels.

Clinical Implications

Increased ammonia levels occur in the following conditions:

1. Reye's syndrome (a potentially fatal disease associated with aspirin use secondary to viral infections primarily in children)
2. Liver disease, cirrhosis
3. Hepatic coma (does not reflect degree of coma)
4. GI hemorrhage
5. Renal disease
6. HHH syndrome: hyperornithinemia, hyperammonemia, homocitrullinuria
7. Transient hyperammonemia of newborn
8. Certain inborn errors of metabolism of urea except for argininosuccinic aciduria
9. GI tract infection with distention and stasis
10. Total parenteral nutrition
11. Ureterosigmoidostomy

Interfering Factors

1. Ammonia levels vary with protein intake and many drugs.
2. Exercise may cause an increase in ammonia levels.
3. Ammonia levels may be increased by use of a tight tourniquet or by tightly clenching the fist while samples are drawn.
4. Ammonia levels can rise rapidly in the blood tubes.
5. Hemolyzed blood gives falsely elevated levels.

Interventions

Pretest Patient Care

1. Explain test purpose and procedure. Instruct the patient to fast (if possible) for 8 hours before the blood test. Water is permitted.
2. Do not allow the patient to smoke for several hours before the test (raises levels).
3. Follow guidelines in Chapter 1 regarding safe, effective, informed *pretest* care.

Posttest Patient Care

1. Review test results; report and record findings. Modify the nursing care plan as needed. Begin treatment.
2. In patients with impaired liver function demonstrated by elevated ammonia levels, the blood ammonia level can be lowered by reduced protein intake and by use of antibiotics to reduce intestinal bacteria counts.
3. Follow guidelines in Chapter 1 for safe, effective, informed *posttest* care.

CLINICAL ALERT

Ammonia should be measured in all cases of unexplained lethargy and vomiting, in encephalitis, or in any neonate with unexplained neurologic deterioration.

● Bilirubin

Bilirubin results from the breakdown of hemoglobin in the RBCs and is a byproduct of hemolysis (i.e., RBC destruction). It is produced by the reticuloendothelial system. Removed from the body by the liver, which excretes it into the bile, bilirubin gives the bile its major pigmentation. Usually, a small amount of bilirubin is found in the serum. A rise in serum bilirubin levels occurs when there is excessive destruction of RBCs or when the liver is unable to excrete the normal amounts of bilirubin produced.

There are two major forms of bilirubin in the body: conjugated bilirubin and unconjugated bilirubin, sometimes termed direct and indirect bilirubin, respectively. Unconjugated bilirubin circulates freely in the blood until it reaches the liver, where it is conjugated with glucuronide transferase and then excreted into the bile. An increase in unconjugated bilirubin is more frequently associated with increased destruction of RBCs (hemolysis) as well as in neonatal jaundice. An increase in free-flowing bilirubin is more likely seen in dysfunction or blockage of the liver. A routine examination measures only the total bilirubin. A normal level of total bilirubin rules out any significant impairment of the excretory function of the liver or excessive hemolysis of red cells. Only when total bilirubin levels are elevated will there be a call for differentiation of the bilirubin levels by conjugated and unconjugated types.

The measurement of bilirubin allows evaluation of liver function and hemolytic anemias. For infants younger than 15 days of age, a neonatal, or more specifically an unconjugated, bilirubin measurement may be necessary.

Normal Findings

Adults
Total: 0.3 to 1.0 mg/dL or 5 to 17 μmol/L
Conjugated (direct): 0.0 to 0.2 mg/dL or 0.0 to 3.4 μmol/L

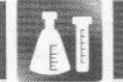

CLINICAL ALERT

Critical Value for Bilirubin in Adults
12 mg/dL or >200 μmol/L

Procedure

1. Obtain a 5-mL nonhemolyzed sample (red-topped tube) from a fasting patient. Observe standard precautions. Serum is used.
2. Protect the sample from ultraviolet light (sunlight).

3. Avoid air bubbles and unnecessary shaking of the sample during blood collection.
4. If the specimen cannot be examined immediately, store it away from light and in a refrigerator.

Clinical Implications

1. *Total bilirubin elevations accompanied by jaundice* may be due to hepatic, obstructive, or hemolytic causes.
   a. *Hepatocellular jaundice* results from injury or disease of the parenchymal cells of the liver and can be caused by the following conditions:
      (1) Viral hepatitis
      (2) Cirrhosis
      (3) Infectious mononucleosis
      (4) Reactions to certain drugs such as chlorpromazine (antipsychotic medication used to treat manic depression or schizophrenia)
   b. *Obstructive jaundice* is usually the result of obstruction of the common bile or hepatic ducts due to stones or neoplasms. The obstruction produces high conjugated bilirubin levels due to bile regurgitation.
   c. *Hemolytic jaundice* is due to overproduction of bilirubin resulting from hemolytic processes that produce high levels of unconjugated bilirubin. Hemolytic jaundice can be found in the following conditions:
      (1) After blood transfusions, especially those involving many units
      (2) Pernicious anemia
      (3) Sickle cell anemia
      (4) Transfusion reactions (ABO or Rh incompatibility)
      (5) Crigler-Najjar syndrome (a severe disease that results from a genetic deficiency of a hepatic enzyme needed for the conjugation of bilirubin)
      (6) Erythroblastosis fetalis (see Neonatal Bilirubin, Total and Fractionated ["Baby Bili"])
   d. Miscellaneous diseases
      (1) Dubin-Johnson syndrome (autosomal recessive disorder resulting in an increase in the serum levels of conjugated bilirubin)
      (2) Gilbert's disease (familial hyperbilirubinemia)
      (3) Nelson's disease (with acute liver failure)
      (4) Pulmonary embolism/infarct
      (5) Congestive heart failure
2. *Elevated indirect (unconjugated) bilirubin levels* occur in the following conditions:
   a. Neonatal jaundice
   b. Hemolytic anemias due to a large hematoma
   c. Trauma in the presence of a large hematoma
   d. Hemorrhagic pulmonary infarcts
   e. Crigler-Najjar syndrome (rare)
   f. Gilbert's disease (conjugated hyperbilirubinemia; rare)
3. *Elevated direct (conjugated) bilirubin levels* occur in the following conditions:
   a. Cancer of the head of the pancreas
   b. Choledocholithiasis
   c. Dubin-Johnson syndrome

Interfering Factors

1. A 1-hour exposure of the specimen to sunlight or high-intensity artificial light at room temperature will decrease the bilirubin content.
2. No contrast media should be administered 24 hours before measurement; a high-fat meal may also cause decreased bilirubin levels by interfering with the chemical reactions.

3. Air bubbles and shaking of the specimen may cause decreased bilirubin levels.
4. Certain foods (e.g., carrots, yams) and drugs (see Appendix E) increase the yellow hue in the serum and can falsely increase bilirubin levels when tests are done using certain methods (e.g., spectrophotometry).
5. Prolonged fasting and anorexia raises the bilirubin level.
6. Nicotinic acid increases unconjugated bilirubin.

Interventions

Pretest Patient Care

1. Explain test purpose and procedure and relation of results to jaundice.
2. Ensure that the patient is fasting, if possible.
3. Follow guidelines in Chapter 1 for safe, effective, informed *pretest* care.

NOTE *Excessive amounts of bilirubin eventually seep into the tissues, which assume a yellow hue as a result. This yellow color is a clinical sign of jaundice. In newborns, signs of jaundice may indicate hemolytic anemia or congenital icterus. Total bilirubin must be >2.5 mg/dL (>41.6 mmol/L) to detect jaundice in adults.*

Posttest Patient Care

1. Review test results; report and record findings. Modify the nursing care plan as needed.
2. Have the patient resume normal activities.
3. Follow guidelines in Chapter 1 for safe, effective, informed *posttest* care.

● Neonatal Bilirubin, Total and Fractionated ("Baby Bili")

In newborns, signs of jaundice may indicate hemolytic anemia or congenital icterus. If bilirubin levels reach a critical point in the infant, damage to the CNS may occur in a condition known as *kernicterus*. Therefore, in these infants, the level of bilirubin is the deciding factor in whether or not to perform an exchange transfusion.

Neonatal bilirubin is used to monitor erythroblastosis fetalis (hemolytic disease of the newborn), which usually causes jaundice in the first 2 days of life. All other causes of neonatal jaundice, including physiologic jaundice, hematoma or hemorrhage, liver disease, and biliary disease, should also be monitored. Normal, full-term neonates experience a normal, neonatal, physiologic, transient hyperbilirubinemia by the 3rd day of life, which rapidly falls by the 5th to 10th day of life.

Normal Findings

Newborns (0 to 7 days)
Interpretation of newborn bilirubin concentrations should be done using a nomogram comparing the age of the infant in hours to the bilirubin concentration. This nomogram provides the risk for a subsequent bilirubin result to be consistent with hyperbilirubinemia. See Figure 6.2.
Cord Blood Total
Full term: <2.5 mg/dL or <43 μmol/L
Premature: <2.9 mg/dL or <50 μmol/L

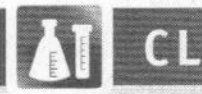
CLINICAL ALERT

Critical Value for Neonatal Bilirubin
>15 mg/dL or >256 μmol/L (mental retardation can occur)

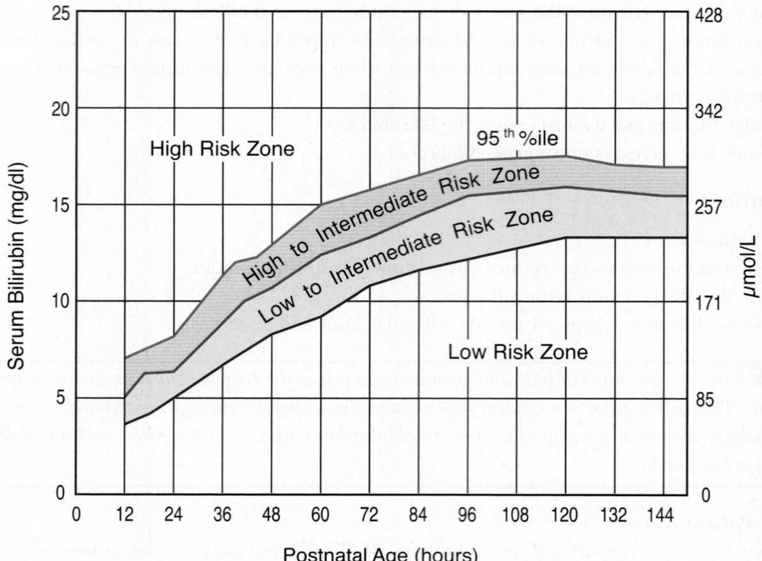

FIGURE 6.2. Nomogram for designation of risk in 2840 well newborns at 36 or more weeks' gestational age with birth weight of 2000 g or more, or at 35 or more weeks' gestational age and birth weight of 2500 g or more, based on the hour-specific serum bilirubin values. The serum bilirubin level was obtained before discharge, and the zone in which the value fell predicted the likelihood of a subsequent bilirubin level exceeding the 95th percentile (high-risk zone). (Used with permission from Bhutani VK, Johnson L, Sivieri EM: Predictive ability of a predischarge hour-specific serum bilirubin for subsequent significant hyperbilirubinemia in healthy term and near-term newborns. Pediatrics 103:6–14, 1999. Reprinted from American Academy of Pediatrics: Management of hyperbilirubinemia in the newborn infant 35 or more weeks of gestation. Pediatrics 114:297–316, 2004.)

See Table 6.4 for a comparison of premature and full-term infants.

NOTE *The American Academy of Pediatrics recommends that total bilirubin values for normal-term newborns be assessed for risk for developing hyperbilirubinemia using the Bhutani nomogram (Fig. 6.2).*

Procedure

1. Draw blood from heel of newborn using a capillary pipette and amber Microtainer tube; 0.5 mL of serum is needed. Cord blood may also be used.
2. Protect sample from light.

TABLE 6.4 Total Bilirubin Comparison

	Premature (mg/dL)	SI Units (μmol/L)	Full Term (mg/dL)	SI Units (μmol/L)
<24 hr	<8.0	<137	<6.0	<103
<48 hr	<12.0	<205	<10.0	<170
3–5 d	<15.0	<256	<12.0	<205
7 d	<15.0	<256	<10.0	<170

SI, International System of Units (Système International).

Clinical Implications

1. *Elevated total bilirubin* (neonatal) is associated with the following conditions:
   a. Erythroblastosis fetalis occurs as a result of blood group incompatibility between mother and fetus.
      (1) Rh (D) antibodies and other Rh factors
      (2) ABO antibodies
      (3) Other blood groups, including Kidd, Kell, and Duffy (see Chapter 8)
   b. Galactosemia
   c. Sepsis
   d. Infectious diseases (e.g., syphilis, toxoplasmosis, cytomegalovirus)
   e. RBC enzyme abnormalities
      (1) Glucose-6-phosphate dehydrogenase (G6PD) deficiency
      (2) Pyruvate kinase (PK) deficiency
      (3) Spherocytosis (autohemolytic anemia causing the RBCs to become sphere-shaped and not the typical biconcave shape)
   f. Subdural hematoma, hemangiomas
2. *Elevated unconjugated (indirect) neonatal bilirubin* is associated with the following conditions:
   a. Erythroblastosis fetalis
   b. Hypothyroidism
   c. Crigler-Najjar syndrome
   d. Obstructive jaundice
   e. Infants of diabetic mothers
3. *Elevated conjugated (direct) neonatal bilirubin* is associated with the following conditions:
   a. Biliary obstruction
   b. Neonatal hepatitis
   c. Sepsis

Interventions

Pretest Patient Care

1. Explain test purpose and procedure and its relation to jaundice to the mother.
2. See Chapter 1 guidelines for safe, informed, effective *pretest* care.

Posttest Patient Care

1. Review test results; report and record findings. Modify the nursing care plan as needed.
2. For slight elevations (i.e., <10.0 mg/dL or <170 μmol/L), phototherapy may be initiated.
3. Monitor neonatal bilirubin levels to determine indications for exchange transfusion. Tests should be done every 12 hours in jaundiced newborns. See Table 6.5 for exchange transfusion indications.

TABLE 6.5 Indications for Exchange Transfusion

Birth Weight (g)	Serum Bilirubin (mg/dL)	Serum Bilirubin (μmol/L)
<1000	10.0	170
1001–1250	13.0	222
1251–1500	15.0	256
1501–2000	17.0	291
2001–2500	18.0	309
>2500	20.0	>342

4. Transfuse at one step earlier in the presence of the following conditions:
   a. Coombs' test positive
   b. Serum protein <5 g/dL
   c. Metabolic acidosis (pH <7.25)
   d. Respiratory distress (with O_2 <50 mm Hg or 6.6 kPa)
   e. Certain clinical findings (e.g., hypothermia, CNS or other clinical deterioration, sepsis, hemolysis)

Other criteria for exchange transfusion are suddenness and rate of bilirubin increase and when such an increase occurs; for example, an increase of 3 mg/dL (51 µmol/L) in 12 hours, especially after bilirubin has already leveled off, must be followed by frequent serial determinations, especially if it occurs on the first or seventh day of life rather than on the third day. Be cognizant of a rate of bilirubin increase of >1 mg/dL (>17 µmol/L) during the first day of life. Serum bilirubin of 10 mg/dL (170 µmol/L) after 24 hours or 15 mg/dL (256 µmol/L) after 48 hours despite phototherapy usually indicates that serum bilirubin will reach 20 mg/dL (342 µmol/L).

Blood Urea Nitrogen (BUN, Urea Nitrogen)

Urea forms in the liver and, along with CO_2, constitutes the final product of protein metabolism. The amount of excreted urea varies directly with dietary protein intake, increased excretion in fever, diabetes, and increased adrenal gland activity.

The test for blood urea nitrogen (BUN), which measures the nitrogen portion of urea, is used as an index of glomerular function in the production and excretion of urea. Rapid protein catabolism and impairment of kidney function will result in an elevated BUN level. The rate at which the BUN level rises is influenced by the degree of tissue necrosis, protein catabolism, and the rate at which the kidneys excrete the urea nitrogen. A markedly increased BUN is conclusive evidence of severe impaired glomerular function. In chronic renal disease, the BUN level correlates better with symptoms of uremia than does the serum creatinine.

Normal Findings

Adults: 6 to 20 mg/dL or 2.1 to 7.1 mmol/L
Older adults (>60 years): 8 to 23 mg/dL or 2.9 to 8.2 mmol/L
Children: 5 to 18 mg/dL or 1.8 to 6.4 mmol/L

CLINICAL ALERT

Critical value for BUN is >100 mg/dL (>35 mmol/L).

Procedure

1. Obtain a 5-mL venous blood sample (red-topped tube). Serum is preferred.
2. Observe standard precautions.

Clinical Implications

1. *Increased BUN levels (azotemia)* occur in the following conditions:
   a. Impaired renal function caused by the following conditions:
      (1) Congestive heart failure
      (2) Salt and water depletion
      (3) Shock
      (4) Stress
      (5) Acute MI
   b. Chronic renal disease such as glomerulonephritis and pyelonephritis

c. Urinary tract obstruction
d. Hemorrhage into GI tract
e. Diabetes mellitus with ketoacidosis
f. Excessive protein intake or protein catabolism as occurs in burns or cancer
g. Anabolic steroid use

2. *Decreased BUN levels* are associated with the following conditions:
   a. Liver failure (severe liver disease), such as that resulting from hepatitis, drugs, or poisoning
   b. Acromegaly
   c. Malnutrition, low-protein diets
   d. Impaired absorption (celiac disease)
   e. Nephrotic syndrome (occasional)
   f. Syndrome of inappropriate antidiuretic hormone (SIADH)

Interfering Factors

1. A combination of a low-protein and high-carbohydrate diet can cause a decreased BUN level.
2. The BUN is normally lower in children and women because they have less muscle mass than adult men.
3. Decreased BUN values normally occur in late pregnancy because of increased plasma volume (physiologic hydremia).
4. Older persons may have an increased BUN when their kidneys are not able to concentrate urine adequately.
5. IV feedings only may result in overhydration and decreased BUN levels.
6. Many drugs may cause increased or decreased BUN levels.

Interventions

Pretest Patient Care

1. Explain test purpose and blood-drawing procedure. Assess dietary history.
2. Follow guidelines in Chapter 1 for safe, effective, informed *pretest* care.

Posttest Patient Care

1. Review test outcome and monitor as appropriate for impaired kidney function. Modify the nursing care plan as needed.
2. In patients with an elevated BUN level, fluid and electrolyte regulation may be impaired.
3. Follow guidelines in Chapter 1 for safe, effective, informed *posttest* care.

CLINICAL ALERT

If a patient is confused, disoriented, or has convulsions, the BUN level should be checked. If the level is high, it may help to explain these signs and symptoms.

● Albumin

Albumin (along with total protein) is a part of a diverse microenvironment. Its primary function is the maintenance of colloidal osmotic pressure (COP) in the vascular and extravascular spaces (e.g., urine, cerebrospinal fluid, amniotic fluid). Albumin is a source of nutrition and a part of a complex buffer system. It is a "negative" acute-phase reactant. It decreases in response to acute inflammatory infectious processes.

Albumin is used to evaluate nutritional status, albumin loss in acute illness, liver disease and renal disease with proteinuria, hemorrhage, burns, exudates or leaks in the GI tract, and other chronic diseases. Hypoalbuminuria is an independent risk factor for older adults for mortality—admission serum albumin in geriatric patients is a predictor of outcome.

Normal Findings

Using Bromcresol Green Dye
Children: 3.8 to 5.4 g/dL or 38 to 54 g/L
Adults: 3.5 to 5.2 g/dL or 35 to 52 g/L

Older than age 40 years and in persons living in subtropics and tropics (secondary to parasitic infections), level slowly declines.

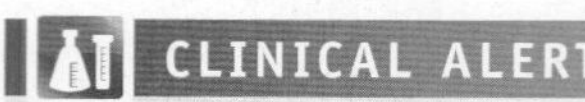

CLINICAL ALERT

Critical Range
<1.5 g/dL or 15 g/L

Procedure

1. Obtain 5 mL of serum in a light green tube. Fasting is not necessary.
2. Centrifuge within 30 minutes of blood draw. Label the specimen with the patient's name, date and time of collection, and test(s) ordered. Place specimen in a biohazard bag.
3. Observe standard procedures.
4. Urine specimens may also be collected (see Chapter 3).

Clinical Implications

1. Increased albumin is not associated with any naturally occurring condition. When albumin is increased, the only cause is decreased plasma water that increases the albumin proportionally: dehydration.
2. Decreased albumin is associated with the following conditions:
   a. Acute and chronic inflammation and infections
   b. Cirrhosis, liver disease, alcoholism
   c. Nephrotic syndrome, renal disease (increased loss in urine)
   d. Crohn's disease, colitis
   e. Congenital albuminemia
   f. Burns, severe skin disease
   g. Heart failure
   h. Starvation, malnutrition, malabsorption, anorexia (decreased synthesis)
   i. Thyroid diseases: Cushing's disease, thyrotoxicosis

Interfering Factors

Albumin is decreased in:

1. Pregnancy (last trimester, owing to increased plasma volume)
2. Oral birth control (estrogens) and other drugs (see Appendix E)
3. Prolonged bed rest
4. IV fluids, rapid hydration, overhydration

CLINICAL ALERT

Levels at 2.0–2.5 g/dL or 20–25 g/L may be the cause of edema.
Low levels occur with prolonged hospital stay.
Lipemic specimens with a high fat content interfere.

Interventions

Pretest Patient Care

1. Explain test purpose and specimen collection procedure. No fasting is required.
2. Follow guidelines in Chapter 1 for safe, effective, informed *pretest* care.

Posttest Patient Care

1. Review test results; report and record findings. Modify the nursing care plan as needed. Explain possible need for treatment (replacement therapy).
2. Low levels are associated with edema. Assess the patient for these signs and symptoms.
3. Follow guidelines in Chapter 1 for safe, effective, informed *posttest* care.
4. Further tests may be indicated:
   a. Total protein
   b. Protein electrophoresis
   c. 24-Hour urine protein

● Prealbumin (PAB)

The proteins most often used in nutrition assessment include albumin, prealbumin (PAB), C-reactive protein, and retinol-binding protein. When used in combination, they can very accurately reflect a subclinical deficit and assess response to restorative therapy.

For years, albumin was the widely accepted marker for malnutrition. However, mounting evidence points to PAB as the better choice. Because albumin has a half-life of 21 days, it is slow to respond to a patient's recent increase in nutrients and, therefore, is not a good indicator of recent changes in protein levels. In contrast, PAB responds more rapidly and gives a timelier picture of a change in dietary status. Because of its short half-life (2 days), PAB responds quickly to a decrease in nutritional intake and nutritional restoration. It reflects the current nutritional status within a patient's body, not the status from 3 weeks ago.

Normal Findings

19 to 38 mg/dL (190 to 380 mg/L) by nephelometry

Procedure

1. Collect a 7-mL blood serum sample in a red-topped tube. Observe standard precautions.
2. Label the specimen with the patient's name, date and time of collection, and test(s) ordered. Place the specimen in a biohazard bag for transport to the laboratory.

Clinical Implications

1. Hospital laboratories, in conjunction with dietitians, administration, pharmacists, nurses, physicians, and other healthcare providers, may develop a clinical pathway that includes running a PAB upon admission of each surgical, ICU, and medical patient.
2. Values of 0 to 5, 5 to 10, and 10 to 15 mg/dL (0 to 50, 50 to 100, and 100 to 150 mg/L) indicate severe, moderate, and mild protein depletion, respectively.

Interventions

Pretest Patient Care

1. Explain test purpose. PAB is useful in assessing nutritional status, especially in monitoring the response to nutritional support in the acutely ill patient.
2. Follow guidelines in Chapter 1 regarding safe, effective, informed, *pretest* care.

Posttest Patient Care

1. Review test outcomes and determine the need for possible follow-up testing. Hospital protocol may require patients to be retested twice a week until discharge if their PAB level is less than 18 mg/dL (<180 mg/L). Possible treatment includes replacement and restorative therapy. Modify the nursing care plan as needed.
2. Follow guidelines in Chapter 1 regarding safe, effective, informed *posttest* care.

● Cholinesterase, Serum (Pseudocholinesterase); Cholinesterase, Red Blood Cell (Acetylcholinesterase)

The cholinesterase of serum is referred to as *pseudocholinesterase* to distinguish it from the true cholinesterase of the RBC. Both of these enzymes act on acetylcholine and other cholinesters. Alkylphosphates are potent inhibitors of both serum and RBC cholinesterase.

Patients who are homozygous for the atypical gene that controls serum cholinesterase activity have low levels of cholinesterase that are not inhibited by dibucaine. Persons with normal serum cholinesterase activity show 70% to 90% inhibition by dibucaine (an amino amide). The red cell (true cholinesterase) enzyme is specific for the substrate acetylcholine.

These are two separate tests. The primary use of serum cholinesterase measurement (pseudocholinesterase) is to monitor the effect of muscle relaxants (e.g., succinylcholine), which are used in surgery. Patients for whom suxamethonium anesthesia is planned should be tested using the dibucaine inhibition test for the presence of atypical cholinesterase variants that are incapable of hydrolyzing this widely used muscle relaxant.

The RBC cholinesterase test is used when poisoning by pesticides such as parathion or malathion is suspected. Severe insecticide poisoning causes headaches, visual distortions, nausea, vomiting, pulmonary edema, confusion, convulsions, respiratory paralysis, and coma.

Normal Findings

Acetylcholinesterase: 7 ± 3.8 (SD) U/g Hb or 2 ± 0.2 mU/mol Hb
Serum cholinesterase: 4.9 to 11.9 U/mL or 4.9 to 11.9 kU/L
Dibucaine inhibition: 79% to 84% or 0.79 to 0.84
Fluoride inhibition: 58% to 64% or 0.58 to 0.64
RBC cholinesterase: 30 to 40 U/g Hb

Values vary with substrate and method. These are two different tests. Values are low at birth and for the first 6 months of life.

Procedures

1. For serum cholinesterase, obtain a 5-mL blood sample; 3 mL of serum is needed. This is stable for 1 week at 39°F to 77°F or 4°C to 25°C. Observe standard precautions.
2. For RBC cholinesterase, draw a blood sample using sodium heparin as an anticoagulant; do not use serum. Observe standard precautions. This is stable for 1 week at 39°F to 77°F or 4°C to 25°C.

Clinical Implications

1. *Decreased or no serum cholinesterase* occurs in the following conditions:
   a. Congenital inherited recessive disease. These patients are not able to hydrolyze drugs such as muscle relaxants used in surgery. These patients may have a prolonged period of apnea and may die if they are given succinylcholine.
   b. Poisoning from organic phosphate insecticides
   c. Liver diseases, hepatitis, cirrhosis with jaundice

    d. Conditions that may have decreased blood albumin, such as malnutrition, anemia, infections, skin diseases, and acute MI
    e. Congestive heart failure
2. *Decreased RBC cholinesterase levels* occur in the following conditions:
    a. Congenital inherited recessive disease
    b. Organic phosphate poisoning
    c. Paroxysmal nocturnal hemoglobinemia
    d. Megaloblastic anemia (returns to normal with therapy)
3. *Increased serum cholinesterase* is associated with:
    a. Type IV hyperlipidemia
    b. Nephrosis
    c. Obesity
    d. Diabetes
4. *Increased RBC cholinesterase* is associated with:
    a. Reticulocytosis (increase in immature RBCs or reticulocytes)
    b. Sickle cell anemia
    c. Hemolytic anemias
5. *Increased RBC cholinesterase* in amniotic fluid, along with elevated α-fetoprotein (AFP), is presumptive evidence of open neural tube defect (not normally present in amniotic fluid).

Interventions

Pretest Patient Care

1. Explain test purpose and procedure.
2. Draw blood for serum cholinesterase 2 days before surgery.
3. Be aware that blood should not be drawn in the recovery room; prior administration of surgical drugs and anesthesia invalidates the test results.
4. Follow guidelines in Chapter 1 for safe, effective, informed *pretest* care.

Posttest Patient Care

1. Review test results; report and record findings. Modify the nursing care plan as needed.
2. Consider patients exhibiting <70% inhibition to have an atypical cholinesterase variant and be aware that the administration of succinylcholine or similar type drugs may pose a risk.
3. Follow guidelines in Chapter 1 for safe, effective, informed *posttest* care.

CLINICAL ALERT

1. In industrial exposure, workers should not return to work until cholinesterase values rise to at least 75% of normal. RBC cholinesterase regenerates at the rate of 1% per day. Plasma cholinesterase regenerates at the rate of 25% in 7–10 d and returns to baseline in 4–6 wk.
2. Cholinesterase activity is completely and irreversibly inhibited by organophosphate pesticides.

● Creatinine and Estimated Glomerular Filtration Rate

Creatinine is a byproduct in the breakdown of muscle creatine phosphate resulting from energy metabolism. It is produced at a constant rate depending on the muscle mass of the person and is removed from the body by the kidneys. Production of creatinine is constant as long as muscle mass remains constant. A disorder of kidney function reduces excretion of creatinine, resulting in increased blood creatinine levels. Thus, creatinine levels give an approximation of the glomerular filtration rate (GFR).

An estimated GFR (eGFR) can be calculated using the Modification of Diet in Renal Disease (MDRD) study equation, which requires a serum creatinine result, gender, age, and race.

$$\text{eGFR (mL/min/1.73 m}^2) = 186 \times (S_{cr})^{-1.154} \times (\text{age})^{-0.203} \times (0.742 \text{ if female}) \times (1.210 \text{ if African American}) \text{ (conventional units)}$$

Many labs are reporting the eGFR with the creatinine result.

This test diagnoses impaired renal function. It is a more specific and sensitive indicator of kidney disease than BUN, although in chronic renal disease, both BUN and creatinine are ordered to evaluate renal problems because the BUN-to-creatinine ratio provides more information.

Normal Findings

Adult men: 0.9 to 1.3 mg/dL or 80 to 115 μmol/L
Adult women: 0.6 to 1.1 mg/dL or 53 to 97 μmol/L
Children (3 to 18 years): 0.5 to 1.0 mg/dL or 44 to 88 μmol/L
Young children (0 to 3 years): 0.3 to 0.7 mg/dL or 27 to 62 μmol/L
BUN-to-creatinine ratio: 10:1 to 20:1

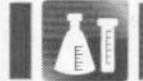

CLINICAL ALERT

Critical value is 10 mg/dL or 890 μmol/L in nondialysis patients.

Procedure

1. Obtain a 5-mL venous blood sample. Serum is preferred, but heparinized blood can be used. Label the specimen with the patient's name, date and time of collection, and test(s) ordered. Place the specimen in a biohazard bag.
2. Observe standard precautions.

Clinical Implications

1. *Increased blood creatinine levels* occur in the following conditions:
   a. Impaired renal function
   b. Chronic nephritis
   c. Obstruction of urinary tract
   d. Muscle disease
      (1) Gigantism
      (2) Acromegaly
      (3) Myasthenia gravis
      (4) Muscular dystrophy
      (5) Poliomyelitis
   e. Congestive heart failure
   f. Shock
   g. Dehydration
   h. Rhabdomyolysis (skeletal muscle tissue breakdown)
   i. Hyperthyroidism
2. *Decreased creatinine levels* occur in the following conditions:
   a. Small stature
   b. Decreased muscle mass
   c. Advanced and severe liver disease

   d. Inadequate dietary protein
   e. Pregnancy (0.4 to 0.6 mg/dL or 36 to 53 μmol/L is normal; >0.8 mg/dL or >71 μmol/L is abnormal and should be noted)
3. *Increased ratio* (>20:1) with normal creatinine occurs in the following conditions:
   a. Increased BUN (prerenal azotemia), heart failure, salt depletion, dehydration
   b. Catabolic states with tissue breakdown
   c. GI hemorrhage
   d. Impaired renal function plus excess protein intake, production, or tissue breakdown
4. *Increased ratio* (>20:1) with elevated creatinine occurs in the following conditions:
   a. Obstruction of urinary tract
   b. Prerenal azotemia with renal disease
5. *Decreased ratio* (<10:1) with decreased BUN occurs in the following conditions:
   a. Acute tubular necrosis
   b. Decreased urea synthesis as in severe liver disease or starvation
   c. Repeated dialysis
   d. SIADH
   e. Pregnancy
6. *Decreased ratio* (<10:1) with increased creatinine occurs in the following conditions:
   a. Phenacemide therapy (accelerates conversion of creatine to creatinine)
   b. Rhabdomyolysis (releases muscle creatinine)
   c. Muscular patients who develop renal failure

Interfering Factors

1. High levels of ascorbic acid and cephalosporin antibiotics can cause a falsely increased creatinine level; these agents also interfere with the BUN-to-creatinine ratio.
2. Drugs that influence kidney function plus other medications can cause a change in the blood creatinine level (see Appendix E).
3. A diet high in meat can cause increased creatinine levels.
4. Creatinine is falsely decreased by bilirubin, glucose, histidine, and quinidine compounds.
5. Ketoacidosis may increase serum creatinine substantially.

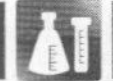 **CLINICAL ALERT**

Creatinine level should always be checked before administering nephrotoxic chemotherapeutics such as methotrexate, cisplatin, cyclophosphamide, mithramycin, and semustine.

Interventions

Pretest Patient Care

1. Explain test purpose and procedure.
2. Assess diet for meat and protein intake.
3. Follow guidelines in Chapter 1 for safe, effective, informed *pretest* care.

Posttest Patient Care

1. Review test results and monitor as appropriate for impaired renal function. Modify nursing care plan as needed.
2. Possible treatment includes hemodialysis and renal replacement therapy, including kidney transplant.
3. Follow guidelines in Chapter 1 for safe, effective, informed *posttest* care.

Cystatin C

Cystatin C is a low-molecular-weight protein inhibitor found in blood serum and is an indicator of glomerular filtration in kidney function.

This test is done to assess GFR. Cystatin C may be a more reliable indicator of renal function than creatinine. Cystatin C is independent of muscle mass and age and is not reabsorbed in the kidney. Measurements of cystatin C are not as common as creatinine measurements.

Normal Findings

Young adults: <0.70 mg/mL (<2.9 µmol/mL)
Older adults (>60 years): <0.85 mg/mL (<3.5 µmol/mL)

NOTE *Cystatin C can be used to estimate the GFR:*

$$\text{GFR (mL/min/1.73 m}^2) = -4.32 + 80.35/\text{cys C}$$

Source: Hoek FJ, Kemperman FAW, Krediet RT: A comparison between cystatin C, plasma creatinine and the Cockcroft and Gault formula for the estimation of glomerular filtration rate. Nephrol Dial Transplant 18:2024–2031, 2003.

Procedure

1. No fasting is required.
2. Obtain a 5-mL venous blood sample (heparin or EDTA).

Clinical Implications

Cystatin C levels abnormally increase in association with impaired renal function and loss of kidney homeostasis, as in acute renal failure, chronic renal failure, diabetic nephropathy, and infections.

Interventions

Pretest Patient Care

1. Explain purpose and sampling procedure for cystatin C.
2. Assess for signs of abnormal kidney function (hypertension, pain, edema, uremia, disorders of urination, and urine composition). Some conditions have no symptoms of nephrotic syndrome.
3. Follow Chapter 1 guidelines for safe, effective, informed *pretest* care.

Posttest Patient Care

1. Review outcomes and provide the patient with support and counseling.
2. Explain follow-up testing and possible treatment for kidney disease.
3. See Chapter 1 guidelines for safe, effective, informed *posttest* care.

Uric Acid

Uric acid is formed from the breakdown of nucleonic acids and is an end product of purine metabolism. Uric acid is transported by the plasma from the liver to the kidney, where it is filtered and where about 70% is excreted. The remainder of uric acid is excreted into the GI tract and degraded. A lack of the enzyme uricase allows this poorly soluble substance to accumulate in body fluids.

The basis for this test is that an overproduction of uric acids occurs when there is excessive cell breakdown and catabolism of nucleonic acids (as in gout), excessive production and destruction of cells (as in leukemia), or an inability to excrete the substance produced (as in renal failure). Measurement of uric acid is used most commonly in the evaluation of renal failure, gout, and leukemia. In hospitalized patients, renal failure is the most common cause of elevated uric acid levels, and gout is the least common cause.

Normal Findings

Men: 3.4 to 7.0 mg/dL or 202 to 416 μmol/L
Women: 2.4 to 6.0 mg/dL or 143 to 357 μmol/L
Children: 2.0 to 5.5 mg/dL or 119 to 327 μmol/L

Procedure

1. Obtain a 5-mL venous blood sample. Serum is preferred; heparinized blood is acceptable. Label the specimen with the patient's name, date and time of collection, and test(s) ordered. Place the specimen in a biohazard bag.
2. Observe standard precautions.

Clinical Implications

1. *Elevated uric acid levels (hyperuricemia)* occur in the following conditions:
   a. Gout (the amount of increase is not directly related to the severity of the disease)
   b. Renal diseases and renal failure, prerenal azotemia
   c. Alcoholism (ethanol consumption)
   d. Down syndrome
   e. Lead poisoning
   f. Leukemia, multiple myeloma, lymphoma
   g. Lesch-Nyhan syndrome (hereditary gout)
   h. Starvation, weight-loss diets
   i. Metabolic acidosis, diabetic ketoacidosis
   j. Toxemia of pregnancy (serial determination to follow therapy)
   k. Liver disease
   l. Hyperlipidemia, obesity
   m. Hypoparathyroidism, hypothyroidism
   n. Hemolytic anemia, sickle cell anemia
   o. Following excessive cell destruction, as in chemotherapy and radiation treatment (acute elevation sometimes follows treatment)
   p. Psoriasis
   q. Glycogen storage disease (G6PD deficiency)
2. *Decreased levels of uric acid* occur in the following conditions:
   a. Fanconi's syndrome (disease of the proximal renal tubules)
   b. Wilson's disease (autosomal recessive disorder resulting in the accumulation of copper in tissues)
   c. SIADH
   d. Some malignancies (e.g., Hodgkin's disease, multiple myeloma)
   e. Xanthinuria (deficiency of xanthine oxidase)

Interfering Factors

1. Stress and strenuous exercise will falsely elevate uric acid.
2. Many drugs cause increase or decrease of uric acid (see Appendix E).

3. Purine-rich diet (e.g., liver, kidney, sweetbreads) increases uric acid levels.
4. High levels of aspirin decrease uric acid levels.
5. Low purine intake, coffee, and tea decrease uric acid levels.

Interventions

Pretest Patient Care

1. Advise the patient of test purpose and blood-drawing procedure; fasting is preferred.
2. Promote relaxation; avoid strenuous exercise.
3. Follow guidelines in Chapter 1 for safe, effective, informed *pretest* care.

Posttest Patient Care

1. Have the patient resume normal activities.
2. Review test results and monitor appropriately for renal failure, gout, or leukemia. Uric acid level should fall in patients who are treated with uricosuric drugs such as allopurinol, probenecid, and sulfinpyrazone. Modify the nursing care plan as needed.
3. Follow guidelines in Chapter 1 for safe, effective, informed *posttest* care.

CLINICAL ALERT

1. Monitor uric acid levels during treatment of leukemia.
2. Acute, dangerous levels may occur following administration of cytotoxic drugs.

● Lead (Pb)

Lead is absorbed into the body through both the respiratory and GI tracts. It also moves transplacentally to the fetus. Absorption through these different routes varies and is affected by age, nutritional status, particle size, and chemical form of the lead. Absorption is inversely proportional to particle size; this factor makes lead-bearing dust important. Adults absorb 6% to 10% of dietary lead and retain very little of it; however, children from birth to 2 years of age have been shown to absorb 40% to 50% and to retain 20% to 25% of dietary lead. Spontaneous excretion of lead in urine by infants and young toddlers is normally about 1 μg/kg/24 hours, which may increase somewhat in cases of acute poisoning. Dietary intake of lead is <1 μg/kg of lead, which provides a margin of safety in the sense that a child goes into positive lead balance when intake exceeds 5 μg/kg of body weight. Early symptoms of lead poisoning include anorexia, apathy or irritability, fatigue, and anemia. Toxic effects include GI distress, joint pain, colic, headache, stupor, convulsions, and coma. Another, less sensitive test that may be used to evaluate lead intoxication is free erythrocyte protoporphyrin. However, a blood lead assay is the definitive test.

The blood lead assay is used to screen adults and children for lead poisoning (plumbism). In adults, high levels are caused mainly by industrial exposure to lead-based paints, gasoline, and ceramics. High-risk children usually are ages 3 to 12 years and live in or visit old or dilapidated housing with lead-based paint. A single paint chip can contain as much as 10,000 μg of lead.

Normal Findings

Blood

0 to 10 μg/dL or 0 to 0.48 μmol/L

24-hour urine: <80 μg/L or <0.39 μmol/L

Hair

Adult: <155 μg/g dry weight or <0.75 μmol/g dry weight

Child: <70 μg/g dry weight or <0.34 μmol/g dry weight

CLINICAL ALERT

Critical Values

1. <15 yr of age, >20 μg/dL or >0.97 μmol/L; ≥15 yr of age, >30 μg/dL or >1.45 μmol/L
2. Patients with blood lead concentrations >80 μg/dL or >3.86 μmol/L (panic value) should be hospitalized immediately and treated as a medical emergency.
3. A single lead determination cannot distinguish between chronic and acute exposure.

Procedure

1. Obtain a sample by finger stick using lead-free heparinized capillary tubes (capillary specimens are not considered diagnostic) or venous blood drawn in a 3-mL trace element–free tube. Label the specimen with the patient's name, date and time of collection, and test(s) ordered. Place the specimen in a lead-free biohazard bag or container.
2. Do not separate plasma from cells. Refrigerate the sample.
3. 24-Hour urine specimens can also be collected.
4. Hair may also be used.
5. Observe standard precautions.

Clinical Implications

Blood lead levels in adults

1. <10 μg/dL or <0.48 μmol/L: normal without occupational exposure
2. <20 μg/dL or <0.97 μmol/L: acceptable with occupational exposure
3. >40 μg/dL or >1.9 μmol/L: report to state occupational agency
4. >60 μg/dL or >2.9 μmol/L: remove from occupational exposure and begin chelation therapy

Table 6.6 lists the U.S. Centers for Disease Control and Prevention (CDC) classifications for levels of blood lead. Table 6.7 shows the effects of blood lead in children.

Interfering Factors

1. Failing to use lead-free Vacutainer tubes invalidates results.
2. An elevated level should be confirmed with a second specimen to ensure that the first specimen was not contaminated.

TABLE 6.6 U.S. Centers for Disease Control and Prevention Classifications of Blood Lead Levels

Class	Blood Lead[a]	Action
I	<10 μg/dL or 0.48 μmol/L	Not lead poisoned
IIA	10–14 μg/dL or 0.48–0.68 μmol/L	Rescreen frequently and consider prevention activities
IIB	15–19 μg/dL or 0.72–0.92 μmol/L	Institute nutritional and educational interventions
III	20–44 μg/dL or 0.97–2.1 μmol/L	Evaluate environment and consider chelation therapy
IV	45–69 μg/dL or 2.17–3.33 μmol/L	Institute environmental intervention and chelation therapy
V	>69 μg/dL or >3.33 μmol/L	Medical emergency

[a]Owing to possible contamination during collection, elevated levels should be confirmed with a second specimen before therapy is instituted.

TABLE 6.7 Effects of Increased Blood Lead Levels on Children

Blood Lead Level	Effects in Children
>10 μg/dL or >0.48 μmol/L	Reduced IQ, hearing, and growth
>20 μg/dL or >0.97 μmol/L	Impaired nerve function
>30 μg/dL or >1.45 μmol/L	Reduced vitamin D metabolism
>40 μg/dL or >1.93 μmol/L	Damage to blood-forming system
>50 μg/dL or >2.41 μmol/L	Severe stomach cramps
>60 μg/dL or >2.90 μmol/L	Severe anemia
>80 μg/dL or >3.86 μmol/L	Severe brain damage
>125 μg/dL or >6.04 μmol/L	Death

From the President's Task Force on Environmental Health Risks and Safety Risks to Children: Federal strategy to eliminate childhood lead poisoning, March 2002 (Online). Available at www.hud.gov/lea

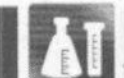

CLINICAL ALERT

1. Following chelation therapy, lead levels are assessed at varying intervals, and it is not unusual to see a slight increase due to lead leaching from bones.
2. Pregnant women with blood lead level (BLL) >10 μg/dL or >0.48 μmol/L are at risk for delivering a child with a BLL also >10 μg/dL or >0.48 μmol/L.

Interventions

Pretest Patient Care

1. Explain test purpose and procedure.
2. Explain the importance of follow-up if lead levels are elevated.
3. Follow guidelines in Chapter 1 for safe, effective, informed *pretest* care.

Posttest Patient Care

1. Have the patient resume normal activities.
2. Review test results, counsel, and monitor appropriately for elevated lead levels. Explain chelation therapy and possible need for further testing, such as iron deficiency and blood protoporphyrins. Modify the nursing care plan as needed.
   a. Parental compliance is necessary. Parent education about lead poisoning can be given face to face, by pamphlet distribution, or in both ways.
   b. The most important component of medical management is to facilitate reduction in the child's exposure to the environmental lead. In providing intervention for the child with an elevated blood lead level, the initial step is to obtain a detailed environmental history. The causes of childhood lead poisoning are multiple and must take into account potential environmental hazards as well as characteristics of the individual child. Once a child is found to have lead intoxication, all potential sources must be identified and removed from the child's environment.
   c. The recommended diet for a child with lead toxicity is simply a good diet with adequate protein and mineral intake and limitation of excess fat. It is no longer necessary to exclude canned foods and beverages when the cans are manufactured in the United States because the manufacture of cans with lead-soldered seams ended in the United States in 1991.
   d. Iron deficiency can enhance absorption and toxicity of lead and often coexists with overexposure to lead. All children with a blood lead concentration >20 μg/dL or >0.97 μmol/L whole blood should have appropriate testing for iron deficiency.

e. In class IV lead intoxication, chelation is necessary. Chelation therapy must be done in conjunction with eliminating the source of the lead poisoning. Chelation therapy, when promptly administered, can be life-saving and can reduce the period of morbidity associated with lead toxicity.
f. Additional follow-up tests may be ordered, including free erythrocyte protoporphyrin, erythrocyte protoporphyrin, or zinc protoporphyrin.

3. Follow guidelines in Chapter 1 for safe, effective, informed *posttest* care.

● Osteocalcin (Bone G1a Protein)

Osteocalcin, also referred to as *bone Gla protein*, is a protein produced by the osteoblasts and dentin and has a function in bone mineralization and calcium ion homeostasis. A small amount of osteocalcin, an integral part in bone formation, is released into the blood and therefore can serve as a marker for recent bone formation. Osteocalcin levels are influenced by age (rapid growth) and gender (males somewhat higher) and are increased during menopause. This test is used to screen for osteoporosis in postmenopausal women, assess risk for fractures, and determine eligibility for treatment for osteoporosis. The U.S. Preventive Task Force recommends screening for osteoporosis in women over the age of 65 years, and in women under age 65 years who have a risk of fracture that is equal to or greater than that of a 65-year-old white woman. Screening is not recommended for men. Osteocalcin is a specific marker for bone formation and is regulated by 1,25-dehydroxyvitamin D.

Normal Findings

Osteocalcin: 8.1 ± 4.6 μg/L or 1.4 ± 0.8 nmol/L
Carboxylated osteocalcin: 9.9 ± 0.5 μg/L or 1.7 ± 0.1 nmol/L
Undercarboxylated osteocalcin: 3.7 ± 1.0 μg/L or 0.6 ± 0.2 nmol/L
Normal Using RIA
Adult male: 3.0 to 13.0 ng/mL or 3.0 to 13.0 μg/L
Premenopausal female: 0.4 to 8.2 ng/mL or 0.4 to 8.2 μg/L
Postmenopausal female: 1.5 to 11.0 ng/mL or 1.5 to 11.0 μg/L

There is a diurnal variation, a peak during the night and a decrease in the morning.

Procedure

Collect a venous blood sample of serum on ice, separate within 1 hour, and immediately freeze. Avoid a freeze–thaw cycle.

Interfering Factors

1. Increased during bed rest and no increase in bone formation.
2. Increased with impaired renal function and no increase in bone formation.

Clinical Implications

1. Abnormally increased levels indicate increased bone formation in persons with hyperparathyroidism, fractures, and acromegaly.
2. Decreased levels are associated with hypoparathyroidism, a deficiency of growth hormone, and medications such as glucocorticoids, bisphosphonates, and calcitonin.

Interventions

Pretest Patient Care

1. Explain purpose and procedure of test. Record age and menopausal state. Tell the patient that the risk for osteoporosis increases steadily with age. Also, obtain pertinent personal and family history of osteoporotic fractures, history of falls, and so forth.
2. Follow Chapter 1 guideline for safe, effective, informed *pretest* care.

Posttest Patient Care

1. Review test outcomes, report and record findings, and counsel regarding further tests (e.g., dual-energy x-ray absorptiometry [DXA], bone density of the femoral neck, or quantitative ultrasound) and possible treatment (e.g., medical: alendronate, raloxifene). Sixteen percent of postmenopausal women will be found to have lumbar spine osteoporosis. Other blood test markers of bone resorption include pyridinolines, telopeptides, acid phosphatase, and urine tests of hydroxyproline and galactosyl hydroxylysine. These markers are known as *collagen crosslinks*. Modify the nursing care plan as needed.
2. See Chapter 1 for safe, effective, informed *posttest* care.

HORMONE TESTS

Androstenedione

Androstenedione is one of the major androgens produced by the ovaries in females and, to a lesser extent, in the adrenal gland in both genders. This hormone is converted to estrogens by hepatic enzymes. Levels rise sharply after puberty and peak at age 20 years.

This hormone measurement is helpful in the evaluation of conditions characterized by hirsutism (excessive hair growth in women) and virilization. In females, there is poor correlation of plasma levels with clinical severity.

Normal Findings

Newborns: 20 to 290 ng/dL or 0.7 to 10.1 mmol/L
Prepuberty: 8 to 50 ng/dL or 0.3 to 1.7 mmol/L
Women: 75 to 205 ng/dL or 2.6 to 7.2 mmol/L
Men: 85 to 275 ng/dL or 3.0 to 9.6 mmol/L
Postmenopausal women: $<$10 ng/dL or 0.35 mmol/L (abrupt decline at menopause)

Different laboratories may have variation in reference values.

Procedure

1. Obtain a 5-mL venous blood sample in the morning and place on ice. Serum or EDTA can be used. Observe standard precautions. Label the specimen with the patient's name, date and time of collection, and test(s) ordered. Place specimen in a biohazard bag.
2. In women, collect this specimen 1 week before or after the menstrual period. Record date of last menstrual period on the laboratory form.

Clinical Implications

1. *Increased androstenedione values* are associated with the following conditions:
   a. Polycystic ovary syndrome (Stein-Leventhal syndrome)
   b. Cushing's syndrome
   c. Atypical ovarian tumors
   d. Ectopic ACTH-producing tumor
   e. Late-onset congenital adrenal hyperplasia
   f. Ovarian stromal hyperplasia
   g. Osteoporosis in females
2. *Decreased androstenedione values* are found in the following conditions:
   a. Sickle cell anemia
   b. Adrenal and ovarian failure

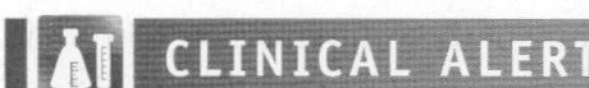

CLINICAL ALERT

>1000 ng/dL or >34.9 mmol/L (suggests virilizing tumor)

Interventions

Pretest Patient Care

1. Explain purpose of test and blood-drawing procedure. Obtain pertinent history of signs and symptoms (e.g., excessive hair growth and infertility).
2. Ensure that the patient is fasting and that blood is drawn at peak production (7:00 a.m. or 0700 hours). Lowest levels are at 4:00 p.m. or 1600 hours.
3. Collect specimen 1 week before menstrual period in women.
4. Follow guidelines in Chapter 1 for safe, effective, informed *pretest* care.

Posttest Patient Care

1. Have the patient resume normal activities.
2. Review test results; report and record findings. Modify the nursing care plan as needed. Counsel appropriately for ovarian and adrenal dysfunction.
3. Follow guidelines in Chapter 1 for safe, effective, informed *posttest* care.

● Aldosterone

Aldosterone is a mineralocorticoid hormone produced in the adrenal zona glomerulosa under complex control by the renin-angiotensin system. Its action is on the renal distal tubule, where it increases resorption of sodium and water at the expense of increased potassium excretion.

This test is useful in detecting primary or secondary aldosteronism (also called *hyperaldosteronism*). Patients with primary aldosteronism characteristically have hypertension, muscular pains and cramps, weakness, tetany, paralysis, and polyuria. This test is also used to evaluate causes of hypertension or low blood potassium levels and to check for adrenal tumors.

NOTE *A random aldosterone test is of no diagnostic value unless a plasma renin activity is performed at the same time.*

Normal Findings

In Upright Position
Adults: 7 to 30 ng/dL or 0.19 to 0.83 nmol/L
Adolescents: 4 to 48 ng/dL or 0.11 to 1.33 nmol/L
Children: 5 to 80 mg/dL or 0.14 to 2.22 nmol/L

In Supine Position
Adults: 3 to 16 ng/dL or 0.08 to 0.44 nmol/L
Adolescents: 2 to 22 ng/dL or 0.06 to 0.61 nmol/L
Children: 3 to 35 mg/dL or 0.08 to 0.97 nmol/L
Low-sodium diet: values 3 to 5 times higher

Procedure

1. Take plasma with the patient in an upright position for 2 hours and with normal salt intake.
2. Obtain a 5-mL venous blood specimen in a heparinized or EDTA Vacutainer tube. Serum, EDTA, or heparinized blood may be used. The cells must be separated from plasma immediately. Blood should be drawn with the patient sitting. Observe standard precautions. Label the specimen with the patient's name, date and time of collection, and test(s) ordered.

3. Specify patient position (upright or supine) and record the site and time of the venipuncture. Circadian rhythm exists in normal subjects, with levels of aldosterone peaking in the morning. Specify if the blood has been drawn from the adrenal vein (values are much higher: 200 to 800 ng/dL or 5.5 to 22.6 nmol/L).
4. A 24-hour urine specimen with boric acid preservative may also be ordered. Refrigerate immediately following collection.
5. Have the patient follow a normal sodium diet 2 to 4 weeks before the test.

Clinical Implications

1. *Elevated levels of aldosterone (primary aldosteronism)* occur in the following conditions:
   a. Aldosterone-producing adenoma (Conn's disease)
   b. Adrenocortical hyperplasia (pseudoprimary aldosteronism)
   c. Indeterminate hyperaldosteronism
   d. Glucocorticoid remediable hyperaldosteronism
2. *Secondary aldosteronism*, in which aldosterone output is elevated because of external stimuli or greater activity in the renin-angiotensin system, occurs in the following conditions:
   a. Renovascular hypertension
   b. Salt depletion
   c. Potassium loading
   d. Laxative abuse
   e. Cardiac failure
   f. Cirrhosis of liver with ascites
   g. Nephrotic syndrome
   h. Bartter's syndrome
   i. Diuretic abuse
   j. Hypovolemia and hemorrhage
   k. After 10 days of starvation
   l. Toxemia of pregnancy
3. *Decreased aldosterone levels* are found in the following conditions:
   a. Aldosterone deficiency
   b. Primary adrenal insufficiency (e.g., Addison's disease). Aldosterone is usually not affected in secondary adrenal insufficiency (hypopituitarism with decreased pituitary ACTH production) because the renin-angiotensin system is still intact.
   c. Syndrome of renin deficiency (very rare)
   d. Low aldosterone levels associated with hypertension are found in Turner's syndrome, diabetes mellitus, and alcohol intoxication.

Interfering Factors

1. Values are increased by upright posture.
2. Recently administered radioactive medications affect test outcomes.
3. Heparin therapy causes levels to fall. See Appendix E for drugs that increase or decrease levels.
4. Thermal stress, late pregnancy, and starvation cause levels to rise.
5. Aldosterone levels decrease with age.
6. Many drugs—diuretics, antihypertensives, progestogens, estrogens—and licorice should be terminated 2 to 4 weeks before test.

CLINICAL ALERT

1. The simultaneous measurement of aldosterone and renin is helpful in differentiating primary from secondary hyperaldosteronism. Renin levels are high in secondary aldosteronism and low in primary aldosteronism.
2. Potassium deficiencies should be corrected before testing for aldosterone.

Interventions

Pretest Patient Care

1. Explain test purpose and procedures. Assess for history of diuretic or laxative abuse. If 24-hour urine specimen is required, follow protocols in Chapter 3.
2. Discontinue diuretic agents, progestational agents, estrogens, and black licorice for 2 weeks before the test.
3. Ensure that the patient's diet for 2 weeks before the test is normal (other than the previously listed restrictions) and includes 3 g/day (135 mEq/L/day) of sodium. Check with your laboratory for special protocols.
4. Follow guidelines in Chapter 1 for safe, effective, informed *pretest* care.

Posttest Patient Care

1. Have the patient resume normal activities and diet.
2. Review test results and monitor appropriately for aldosteronism and aldosterone deficiency. Report and record findings. Modify the nursing care plan as needed.
3. Follow guidelines in Chapter 1 for safe, effective, informed *posttest* care.

● Antidiuretic Hormone (ADH); Arginine Vasopressin Hormone

Antidiuretic hormone (ADH) is secreted by the posterior pituitary gland. Its major physiologic function is regulation of body water. In the dehydrated (hyperosmolar) state, ADH release results in decreased urine excretion and conservation of water. ADH increases blood pressure.

When ADH activity is present, small volumes of concentrated urine are excreted. When ADH is absent, large amounts of diluted urine are produced. Higher secretion occurs at night, with erect posture, and with pain, stress, or exercise. Measurement of the level of ADH is useful in the differential diagnosis of polyuric and hyponatremic states. ADH testing aids in diagnosis of urine concentration disorders, especially diabetes insipidus, SIADH, psychogenic water intoxication, and syndromes of ectopic ADH production.

Normal Findings

<2.5 pg/mL or <2.3 pmol/L

Procedure

1. Draw venous blood samples, 5 mL, into prechilled tubes and put on ice. Plasma with EDTA anticoagulant is needed. Observe standard precautions. Label the specimen with the patient's name, date and time of collection, and test(s) ordered. Place the specimen in a biohazard bag.
2. Ensure that the patient is in a sitting position and calm during blood collection.

Clinical Implications

1. *Increased secretion of ADH* is associated with the following conditions:
   a. SIADH (with respect to plasma osmolality)
   b. Ectopic ADH production (systemic neoplasm)
   c. Nephrogenic diabetes insipidus
   d. Acute intermittent porphyria
   e. Guillain-Barré syndrome (acute polyneuropathy, ascending paralysis)
   f. Brain tumor, diseases, injury, neurosurgery
   g. Pulmonary diseases (tuberculosis)
2. *Decreased secretion of ADH* occurs in the following conditions:
   a. Central diabetes insipidus (hypothalamic or neurogenic)
   b. Psychogenic polydipsia (water intoxication)
   c. Nephrotic syndrome

Interfering Factors

1. Recently administered radioisotopes cause spurious results.
2. Many drugs affect results (e.g., thiazide diuretics, oral hypoglycemics, narcotics); see Appendix E.

Interventions

Pretest Patient Care

1. Explain test purpose and procedure.
2. Encourage relaxation before and during blood-drawing procedure.
3. Follow guidelines in Chapter 1 for safe, effective, informed *pretest* care.

Posttest Patient Care

1. Resume normal activities.
2. Review test results; report and record findings. Modify the nursing care plan as needed. Counsel appropriately for urine concentration disorders and polyuria.
3. Follow guidelines in Chapter 1 for safe, effective, informed *posttest* care.

CLINICAL ALERT

To distinguish SIADH from other conditions that cause dilutional hyponatremia, other tests must be done, such as plasma osmolality, plasma sodium, and water-loading tests.

Brain Natriuretic Peptide (BNP) and NT-proBNP

Brain natriuretic peptide—B-type natriuretic peptide (BNP) and the N-terminal portion of its precursor form (NT-proBNP)—includes hormones produced by the ventricles of the heart. Both BNP and NT-proBNP have been shown to increase in response to ventricular volume expansion (i.e., a decrease in left ventricular ejection fraction) and pressure overload. Although they are markers of ventricular dysfunction, BNP and NT-proBNP cannot clearly differentiate between ventricular systolic or ventricular diastolic dysfunction. However, these markers are useful in diagnosing and assessing the severity of congestive heart failure. These tests are particularly useful in the emergency department setting, where chest pain is a common presentation. Results for BNP and NT-proBNP are not interchangeable and cannot be compared. Chart 6.1 describes types of heart failures; Chart 6.2 offers a scale for grading them. Figure 6.3 illustrates the relationship of BNP to heart disease.

Normal Findings

BNP: <100 pg/mL or <100 ng/L; NT-proBNP: <400 pg/mL or <400 ng/L (values tend to increase with age and are higher in women than men)

Procedure

1. Obtain a plasma sample by venipuncture from a fasting patient. Use a lavender-topped (EDTA) tube. If a nonfasting sample is obtained, notify the laboratory. Label the specimen with the patient's name, date and time of collection, and test(s) ordered.
2. Prechill the tube at 4°C before drawing a sample. After drawing the sample, chill the tube in wet ice for 10 minutes. Place the specimen in a biohazard bag.

Clinical Implications

Increased BNP levels occur in:

1. Diastolic dysfunction
2. Decrease in left ventricular ejection fraction
3. Congestive heart failure

CHART 6.1 Heart Failure

Type of Heart Failure	Signs and Symptoms	Tests to Diagnose
Left heart failure (*congestive heart failure*) • Systolic heart failure (systolic ventricular dysfunction); inability of the heart to generate an adequate cardiac output to perfuse vital tissues • Diastolic heart failure (diastolic ventricular failure); pulmonary congestion despite a normal stroke volume **Right heart failure** An increase in left ventricular filling pressure that is reflected back in the pulmonary circulation **High-output failure** Inability of the heart to supply the body with blood-borne nutrients despite adequate blood volume and normal myocardial contractility	Shortness of breath at rest and exercise Persistent cough Weakness or fatigue Edema in feet, ankles, legs Weight gain	History/physical exam Electrocardiogram Echocardiography Chest x-ray Blood tests: brain natriuretic peptide, atrial natriuretic factor Pulmonary function tests Cardiac ultrasound Treadmill stress test Thallium stress test

Interfering Factors

See Appendix E for drugs that affect test outcomes.

Interventions

Pretest Patient Care

1. Explain test purpose and need to fast. Assess for signs and symptoms indicating need for testing (e.g., chronic fatigue, cough, heart palpitations, hypertension).
2. Withhold cardiovascular medications per healthcare provider's order (e.g., β and calcium antagonists, cardiac glycosides, diuretics, vasodilators) before drawing the specimen.
3. Follow guidelines in Chapter 1 for safe, effective, informed *pretest* care.

CHART 6.2 Grading Heart Diseases

Class I—no limitation of physical activity; no fatigue, shortness of breath, or heart palpitations with ordinary activities

Class II—slight limitation in physical activity; with fatigue, shortness of breath, or heart palpitations during ordinary activities

Class III—marked limitation of physical activity; with fatigue, shortness of breath, or heart palpitations with less-than-ordinary physical activity

Class IV—severe to complete limitation of physical activity with fatigue, shortness of breath, or heart palpitations with any exertion; symptoms occur even at rest

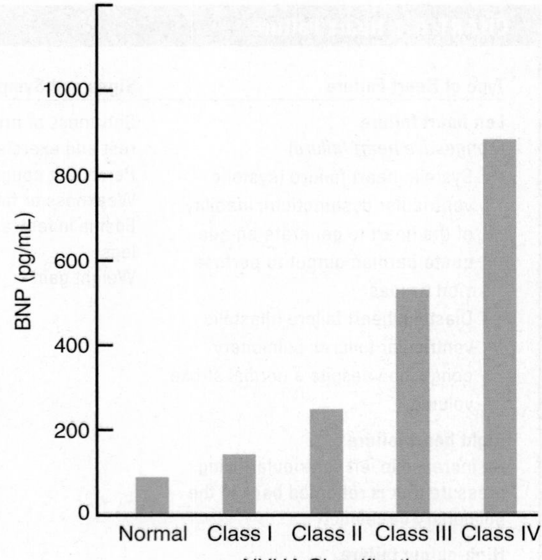

FIGURE 6.3. Relationship of brain natriuretic peptide (BNP) to heart disease (classification of the New York Heart Association [NYHA]). (Data from Maisel AS, Nowak RM, McCord J, et al: Rapid measurement of B-type natriuretic peptide in the emergency diagnosis of heart failure. N Engl J Med 347:161–167, 2002.)

Posttest Patient Care

1. Medications and usual diet may be restarted per healthcare provider's order.
2. Evaluate patient outcomes and monitor appropriately for congestive heart failure.
3. In collaboration with the healthcare provider, explain need for possible follow-up tests and medication therapy. Nesiritide (Natrecor), a synthetic B-type natriuretic peptide, is indicated for treatment of patients with acute decompensated congestive heart failure who are short of breath at rest or with minimal activity.
4. Follow guidelines in Chapter 1 for safe, effective, informed *posttest* care.

● Cortisol (Hydrocortisone)

Cortisol (hydrocortisone/compound F) is a glucocorticosteroid of the adrenal cortex and affects metabolism of proteins, carbohydrates, and lipids. Cortisol stimulates glucogenesis by the liver, inhibits the effect of insulin, and decreases the rate of glucose use by the cells. In health, the secretion rate of cortisol follows a diurnal pattern, being higher in the early morning (6:00 to 8:00 a.m.) and lower in the evening (4:00 to 6:00 p.m.). This variation is lost in patients with Cushing's syndrome and in persons under stress.

The cortisol test evaluates adrenal hormone function. Suppression and stimulation tests may also be done. Cortisol (dexamethasone) suppression test (DST) screens for Cushing's syndrome and identifies depressed persons who are likely to respond to antidepressants or electroshock therapy. It is based on the fact that ACTH production is suppressed in healthy persons after a low dose of dexamethasone but not in persons with Cushing's syndrome or in some depressed persons.

Eighty to 90% of cortisol is carried in the blood bound to corticosteroid-binding globulin (CBG), 5% to 7% bound loosely to albumin, and the remainder unbound.

Normal Findings

Cortisol

8:00 a.m.: 5 to 23 μg/dL or 138 to 635 nmol/L
4:00 p.m.: 3 to 16 μg/dL or 83 to 441 nmol/L

Midnight: <50% of 8:00 a.m. level
Newborns: 2 to 11 μg/dL or 55 to 304 nmol/L
Maternal (at birth): 51.2 to 57.4 μg/dL or 1413 to 1584 nmol/L
After the first week of life, cortisol levels attain adult values.

Suppression

8:00 a.m. or 0800 hours following administration of dexamethasone: <5 μg/dL (a.m. value) or <138 nmol/L

Stimulation

Baseline: at least 5 μg/dL or 138 nmol/L
After Cortrosyn (cosyntropin) administration: rise of at least 10 μg/dL or 276 nmol/L

Procedure

1. Obtain 5-mL venous blood samples at 8:00 a.m. (0800 hours) and at 4:00 p.m. (1600 hours). Serum is preferred. Heparin anticoagulant may be used. Label the specimen with the patient's name, date and time of collection, and test(s) ordered. Place the specimen in a biohazard bag.
2. Observe standard precautions.

Clinical Implications

1. *Decreased cortisol levels* are found in the following conditions:
   a. Adrenal hyperplasia
   b. Addison's disease (primary cortisol deficiency)
   c. Anterior pituitary hyposecretion (pituitary destruction)
   d. Hypothyroidism (hypopituitarism)
2. *Increased cortisol levels* are found in the following conditions:
   a. Hyperthyroidism
   b. Stress (trauma, surgery)
   c. Carcinoma (extreme elevation in the morning and no variation later in the day)
   d. Cushing's syndrome (high on rising but no variation later in the day)
   e. Overproduction of ACTH due to tumors (oat cell cancers)
   f. Adrenal adenoma
   g. Obesity

Interfering Factors

1. Pregnancy will cause an increased value.
2. There is no normal diurnal variation in patients under stress.
3. Drugs such as spironolactone and oral contraceptives will give falsely elevated values (see Appendix E).
4. Decreased levels occur in persons taking dexamethasone, prednisone, or prednisolone (steroids) (see Appendix E).
5. Random cortisol tests are useless and provide no pertinent information.

Interventions

Pretest Patient Care

1. Explain test purpose and blood-drawing procedure. Blood must be drawn at 8:00 a.m. (0800 hours) and 4:00 p.m. (1600 hours).
2. Encourage relaxation.
3. Ensure that no radioisotopes are administered within 1 day before the test.
4. Follow guidelines in Chapter 1 for safe, effective, informed *pretest* care.

Posttest Patient Care

1. Have patient resume normal activities.
2. Review test results; report and record findings. Modify the nursing care plan as needed. Counsel appropriately for adrenal dysfunction.
3. Follow guidelines in Chapter 1 for safe, effective, informed *posttest* care.

● Cortisol Suppression (Dexamethasone Suppression Test; DST)

See foregoing cortisol test for purpose and indications. The DST helps to differentiate causes of elevated cortisol. Cortisol level <15 μg/dL (<41.4 nmol/L) is an indication of adrenal cortisol insufficiency.

Normal Findings

<5 μg/dL or <138 nmol/L or <50% or 0.50 of baseline

Procedure

1. Obtain a 5-mL venous blood sample the day after administration of dexamethasone. Serum or heparinized plasma is acceptable. Observe standard precautions. Label the specimen with the patient's name, date and time of collection, and test(s) ordered. Place the specimen in a biohazard bag.
2. Administer dexamethasone tablets in the late evening or at bedtime. There is a low-dose and high-dose suppression test in which either 1.0 mg or 8.0 mg of dexamethasone is given, respectively, at 11:00 p.m. (2300 hours). The following morning at 8:00 a.m. (0800 hours), a blood sample is drawn to measure cortisol. (Some Cushing's disease patients have false-positive results with the low dose.)

Clinical Implications

1. Suppression occurs in persons with:
   a. Cushing's syndrome (>10 μg/dL or >276 nmol/L)
   b. Endogenous depression (50% of cases)
2. No suppression occurs in:
   a. Adrenal adenoma, carcinoma
   b. Ectopic ACTH-producing tumors

Interfering Factors

False suppression can occur in the following conditions:

1. Pregnancy
2. High doses of estrogens
3. Alcoholism
4. Uncontrolled diabetes
5. Trauma, high stress, fever, dehydration
6. Phenytoin (Dilantin) (see Appendix E for other drugs)

Interventions

Pretest Patient Care

1. Explain test purpose and procedure. Fasting is required for the 8:00 a.m. (0800 hours) test.
2. Discontinue all medications for 24 to 48 hours before the study. Especially important are spironolactone, estrogens, birth control pills, cortisol, tetracycline, stilbestrol, and phenytoin. Check with the healthcare provider.
3. Weigh the patient and record weight.
4. Have baseline blood cortisol drawn at 8:00 a.m. (0800 hours) and 4:00 p.m. (1600 hours). Give 1 mg dexamethasone at 11:00 p.m. (2300 hours) the same day. Draw blood at 8:00 a.m. (0800 hours) the next morning.

5. Ensure that no radioisotopes are administered within 1 week before test.
6. Follow guidelines in Chapter 1 regarding safe, effective, informed *pretest* care.

Posttest Patient Care

1. Have patient resume normal activities.
2. Review test results; report and record findings. Modify the nursing care plan as needed. Counsel appropriately for Cushing's syndrome or depression.
3. Follow guidelines in Chapter 1 for safe, effective, informed *posttest* care.

● Cortisone Stimulation (Cosyntropin, Cortrosyn Stimulation); Adrenocorticotropin Hormone (ACTH) Stimulation

This detects adrenal insufficiency after Cortrosyn administration. Cortrosyn is a synthetic subunit of ACTH that exhibits the full corticosteroid-stimulating effect of ACTH in healthy persons. Failure to respond is an indication of adrenal insufficiency. See foregoing cortisol tests for values. This screening test is less time-consuming and can be done on an outpatient basis.

Normal Findings

Cortisol: 20 μg/dL (>552 nmol/L) rise after Cortrosyn administration

Procedure

1. Obtain a 4-mL fasting venous blood sample (red-topped tube) at 8:00 a.m. (0800 hours) Observe standard precautions.
2. Administer Cortrosyn (250-μg dose) intramuscularly or intravenously as prescribed.
3. Obtain additional 4-mL blood specimens 30 and 60 minutes after administration of Cortrosyn. Serum or heparinized blood is acceptable.

Clinical Implications

1. Absent or blunted response to cortisol stimulation occurs in the following conditions:
   a. Addison's disease (adrenal insufficiency)
   b. Hypopituitarism (secondary adrenal insufficiency)
   c. Adrenal carcinoma, adenoma
2. Response to cortisol stimulation: adrenal hyperplasia

Interfering Factors

1. Prolonged steroid administration
2. Estrogens (see Appendix E)

Interventions

Pretest Patient Care

1. Explain test purpose and procedure. Fasting during test is required. Blood specimens are obtained before and after intramuscular (IM) injection of Cortrosyn.
2. Follow guidelines in Chapter 1 for safe, effective, informed *posttest* care.

Posttest Patient Care

1. Have patient resume normal activities.
2. Review test results and monitor appropriately for adrenal insufficiency. Report and record findings. Modify the nursing care plan as needed.
3. Follow guidelines in Chapter 1 for safe, effective, informed *posttest* care.

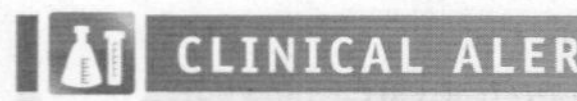

In adrenal hyperplasia, there is an increase of cortisol levels of 3–5 times normal; in adrenal carcinoma, there is no increase.

● Gastrin

Gastrin, a hormone secreted by the antral G cells in stomach mucosa, stimulates gastric acid production and affects antral motility and secretion of pepsin and intrinsic factor. Gastrin values follow a circadian rhythm and fluctuate physiologically in relation to meals. The lowest values are between 3:00 a.m. (0300 hours) and 7:00 a.m. (0700 hours).

Measurement of serum gastrin is generally used to diagnose stomach disorders such as gastrinoma and Zollinger-Ellison syndrome (increased production of gastrin as a result of a tumor in the pancreas) in the presence of hyperacidity. (Gastric hyperacidity must be documented.)

Normal Findings

Adults: <25 to 100 pg/mL or <12 to 48 pmol/L
Children: 10 to 125 pg/mL or 5 to 60 pmol/L
Postprandial: 95 to 140 pg/mL or 46 to 67 pmol/L

Procedure

1. Obtain a 5-mL venous blood sample (red-topped tube) from a fasting patient. Serum is required.
2. Freeze if not tested immediately. If the patient has not been fasting, this must be noted because values are different. Label the specimen with the patient's name, date and time of collection, and test(s) ordered. Place the specimen in a biohazard bag.
3. Observe standard precautions.

Clinical Implications

1. *Increased gastrin levels* are found in the following conditions:
   a. Stomach carcinoma (reduction of gastric acid secretion)
   b. Gastric and duodenal ulcers
   c. Zollinger-Ellison syndrome (>500 pg/mL or >240 pmol/L)
   d. Pernicious anemia
   e. Gastric carcinoma
   f. End-stage renal disease (gastrin metabolized by the kidneys)
   g. Antral G-cell hyperplasia
   h. Vagotomy without gastric resection
   i. Hyperparathyroidism
   j. Pyloric obstruction
2. *Decreased gastrin levels* occur in the following conditions:
   a. Antrectomy with vagotomy
   b. Hypothyroidism

Interfering Factors

Values will be falsely increased in nonfasting patients, older adults, and diabetic patients taking insulin as well as in postgastroscopy patients and those taking H_2 secretion blockers (cimetidine), steroids, and calcium. A protein meal can elevate gastrin markedly.

Interventions

Pretest Patient Care

1. Explain test purpose and procedure.
2. Remind the patient that fasting from food and all beverages except water is required for 12 hours preceding the test. No radioisotopes for 1 week prior to testing.
3. Note if specimen is postprandial. (If after eating, note what was eaten.)
4. Follow guidelines in Chapter 1 for safe, effective, informed *pretest* care.

Posttest Patient Care

1. Have patient resume normal activities.
2. Review test results; report and record findings. Modify the nursing care plan as needed. Follow-up testing using gastric stimulation or gastrin suppression may be indicated.
3. Follow guidelines in Chapter 1 for safe, effective, informed *posttest* care.

● Human Growth Hormone (hGH); Somatotropin

Human growth hormone (somatotropin, hGH) is essential to the growth process and has an important role in the metabolism of adults. It is secreted by the pituitary gland in response to exercise, deep sleep, hypoglycemia, glucagon, insulin, and vasopressin. It also stimulates the production of RNA, mobilizes fatty acids from fat deposits, and is intimately connected with insulinism. If the pituitary gland secretes too little or too much hGH in the growth phase of life, dwarfism or gigantism will result, respectively. An excess of hGH during adulthood leads to acromegaly.

This test confirms hypopituitarism or hyperpituitarism so that therapy can be initiated as soon as possible. Challenge or stimulation tests are generally used to detect hGH deficiency and are more informative. Much controversy surrounds the use of growth hormone stimulation tests, and the diagnosis should be considered in the context of the clinical picture.

Normal Findings

Men: <5 ng/mL or <226 pmol/L
Women: <10 ng/mL or <452 pmol/L
Children: 0 to 20 ng/mL or 0 to 904 pmol/L
Newborns: 5 to 40 ng/mL or 226 to 1808 pmol/L
Stimulation test (using arginine, glucagon, or insulin):
>5 ng/mL or >226 pmol/L (rise from baseline)
>10 ng/mL or >452 pmol/L peak response from baseline
Suppression test (using 100 g of glucose): 0 to 2 ng/mL or 0 to 90 pmol/L or undetectable

NOTE *Because of marked fluctuations in hGH, a random specimen has limited value. Stimulation or inhibitor tests provide more information.*

Procedure

1. Obtain a 5-mL venous blood sample (red-topped tube) from a fasting patient. Serum is best to use. Observe standard precautions. Label the specimen with the patient's name, date and time of collection, and test(s) ordered. Place the specimen in a biohazard bag.
2. Check with your laboratory for specific challenge protocols for stimulation tests such as insulin-induced hypoglycemia, arginine transfusion, glucagon infusion, L-dopa, and propranolol with exercise.

Clinical Implications

1. *Increased hGH levels* are associated with the following conditions:
   a. Pituitary gigantism
   b. Acromegaly
   c. Laron's dwarfism (hGH resistant)
   d. Ectopic GH secretion
   e. Uncontrolled diabetes mellitus
2. *Decreased hGH levels* are associated with the following conditions:
   a. Pituitary dwarfism
   b. Hypopituitarism
   c. Adrenocortical hyperfunction
3. Following stimulation testing, no response (or an inadequate response) is seen in hGH and ACTH deficiencies (hypopituitarism).
   a. Blood glucose must fall to <40 mg/dL (<2.2 mmol/L).
   b. Adrenergic signs must be observed.
4. Following suppression tests, there is no or incomplete suppression in persons with gigantism or acromegaly.
   a. Paradoxical rises in hGH may occur in patients with acromegaly.
   b. Partial suppression is sometimes seen in anorexia nervosa.
   c. In children, rebound-stimulation effect may be seen 2 to 5 hours following administration of glucose (suppression test).

Interfering Factors

1. *Increased levels* are associated with the use of oral contraceptives, estrogens, arginine, glucagon, L-dopa, low glucose, and insulin.
2. Levels will rise to 15 times normal by the second day of starvation; levels also rise after deep sleep, stress, exercise, and anorexia.
3. *Decreased levels* are associated with obesity and the use of corticosteroids.
4. Many drugs interfere with test results (see Appendix E).
5. Recently administered radioisotopes interfere with test results.

Interventions

Pretest Patient Care

1. Explain test purpose and blood-drawing procedure.
2. Remind patient that fasting from food for 8 to 10 hours is required; water is permitted. For accurate levels, the patient should be free of stress and at complete rest in a quiet environment for at least 30 minutes before specimen collection.
3. Note the patient's physiologic state (e.g., feeding, fasting, sleep, activity) at testing in the health care record.
4. For stimulation tests, collect one tube before stimulation and at timed intervals (e.g., 10, 20, 30, 45, and 60 minutes) after stimulation. For suppression tests, collect one tube before suppression and 30, 60, 90, and 120 minutes after suppression.
5. For initial testing of hGH deficiency, a vigorous exercise test is considered to be a simple, risk-free screening test, especially for children.
6. Follow guidelines in Chapter 1 for safe, effective, informed *pretest* care.

Posttest Patient Care

1. Have patient resume normal activities.
2. Review test results; report and record findings. Modify the nursing care plan as needed. A glucose challenge test may be indicated for follow-up.
3. Follow guidelines in Chapter 1 for safe, effective, informed *posttest* care.

● Parathyroid Hormone Assay; Parathyrin; Parathormone (PTH–C-Terminal); Intact PTH

Parathormone (PTH), a polypeptide hormone produced in the parathyroid gland, is one of the major factors in the regulation of calcium concentration in extracellular fluid. Three molecular forms of PTH exist: intact (also called *native* or *glandular hormone*), multiple N-terminal fragments, and C-terminal fragments. PTH follows a circadian rhythm pattern; highest values are between 2:00 and 4:00 p.m. (1400 and 1600 hours), and lowest values are at about 8:00 a.m. (0800 hours).

This test studies altered calcium metabolism, establishes a diagnosis of hyperparathyroidism, and distinguishes nonparathyroid from parathyroid causes of hypercalcemia. A decrease in the level of ionized calcium is the primary stimulus for PTH secretions, whereas a rise in calcium inhibits secretions. This normal relation is lost in hyperthyroidism, and PTH will be inappropriately high in relation to calcium. Acute changes in secretory activity are better reflected by the PTH and N-terminal assay. PTH and N-terminal levels are usually decreased when hypercalcemia is due to neoplastic secretions (prostaglandins). PTH and N-terminal levels may be a more reliable indication of secondary hyperparathyroidism in patients with renal failure. Creatinine level is determined concurrently with all PTH assays to determine kidney function and for meaningful interpretation of results.

Normal Findings

N-terminal: 8 to 24 pg/mL or 8 to 24 ng/L
Intact molecule: 10 to 65 pg/mL or 10 to 65 ng/L
Calcium: 8.5 to 10.9 mg/dL (calcium must be tested to properly interpret results)
C-terminal (biomolecule): 50 to 330 pg/mL or 50 to 330 ng/L

Procedure

1. Obtain a 10-mL venous blood sample (lavender-topped [EDTA] tube) from a patient who has fasted for 10 hours. Collect the sample in chilled vials and keep on ice. Observe standard precautions. Serum or EDTA is used.
2. Immediately take the specimen to the laboratory and centrifuge at 4°C after blood has clotted.

Clinical Implications

1. *Increased PTH values* occur with:
   a. Primary hyperparathyroidism
   b. Pseudohyperparathyroidism when there is a primary defect in renal tubular responsiveness to PTH (secondary hyperparathyroidism)
   c. Hereditary vitamin D dependency
   d. Zollinger-Ellison syndrome (increased production of gastrin as a result of a tumor in the pancreas)
   e. Spinal cord injury
2. *Decreased PTH values* occur in the following conditions:
   a. Hypoparathyroidism (Graves' disease)
   b. Nonparathyroid hypercalcemia
   c. Secondary hypoparathyroidism (surgical)
   d. Magnesium deficiency
   e. Sarcoidosis
   f. Hyperthyroidism
   g. DiGeorge's syndrome (a disorder caused by a defect in chromosome 22 resulting in heart and immune system problems)
3. *Increased PTH–N-terminal values* occur in the following conditions:
   a. Primary hyperparathyroidism
   b. Secondary hyperparathyroidism (more reliable than PTH and C-terminal)

4. *Decreased PTH–N-terminal values* occur in the following conditions:
   a. Hypoparathyroidism
   b. Nonparathyroid hypercalcemia
   c. Aluminum-associated osteomalacia
   d. Severely impaired bone mineralization
5. *Increased PTH–C-terminal values* occur in the following conditions:
   a. Primary hyperparathyroidism (very specific for)
   b. Some neoplasms with elevated calcium
   c. Renal failure (even if parathyroid disease is absent)
6. *Decreased PTH–C-terminal values* occur in the following conditions:
   a. Hypoparathyroidism
   b. Nonparathyroid hypercalcemia

Interfering Factors

1. Elevated blood lipids and hemolysis interfere with test methods.
2. Milk-alkali syndrome (Burnett's syndrome, hypercalcemia) may falsely lower PTH levels.
3. Recently administered radioisotopes (see Appendix E) will alter results.
4. Vitamin D deficiency will increase PTH levels.
5. Many drugs alter results; phosphates raise PTH levels up to 125%, and vitamin A and D overdoses decrease PTH levels (see Appendix E).
6. Lowering plasma calcium by 1.5 mg/dL or 0.38 nmol/L will result in a fourfold increase in PTH levels.

Interventions

Pretest Patient Care

1. Explain test purpose and procedure.
2. Remind the patient that fasting for at least 10 hours is required. Draw blood by 8:00 a.m. (0800 hours) because of circadian rhythm changes. Concurrently, also draw blood for testing of calcium level.
3. Follow guidelines in Chapter 1 for safe, effective, informed *pretest* care.

Posttest Patient Care

1. Have the patient resume normal activities.
2. Review test results; report and record findings. Modify the nursing care plan as needed. Monitor appropriately for calcium imbalance and hypoparathyroidism or hyperparathyroidism.
3. Follow guidelines in Chapter 1 for safe, effective, informed *posttest* care.

● Somatomedin C (SM-C); Insulin-Like Growth Hormone

Somatomedin C (SM-C), a polypeptide hormone produced by the liver and other tissues, mediates growth hormone activity and glucose metabolism. It is carried in the blood and is bound to a protein carrier that prolongs its half-life.

This test is used to monitor the growth of children as well as to diagnose acromegaly and hypopituitarism. Normal SM-C results rule out a deficiency of growth hormone. Testing of SM-C is preferable to growth hormone tests because its levels are more constant. SM-C is also a reliable nutrition index, having a low value for anorexia or malnutrition.

Normal Findings

See Table 6.8.

TABLE 6.8 Values for Somatomedin C

	Male		Female	
Age (yr)	(ng/mL)	(nmol/L)	(ng/mL)	(nmol/L)
0–5	0–103	0–13.5	0–112	0–14.7
6–8	2–118	0.2–15.4	5–128	0.6–16.8
9–10	15–148	2.0–19.4	24–158	3.1–20.7
11–13	55–216	7.2–28.3	65–226	8.5–29.6
14–15	114–232	14.9–30.4	124–242	16.2–31.7
16–17	84–221	11.0–28.9	94–231	12.3–30.3
18–19	56–177	7.3–23.2	66–186	8.6–24.4
20–24	75–142	9.8–18.6	64–131	8.4–17.2
25–50	60–122	7.9–16.0	50–112	6.6–14.7

Levels slowly decrease as person ages.

Procedure

1. Preferably, the patient should be fasting. Obtain a 5-mL plasma venous blood sample using EDTA anticoagulant. Serum may also be used. Observe standard precautions. Label the specimen with the patient's name, date and time of collection, and test(s) ordered. Place the specimen in a biohazard bag.
2. Chill blood-drawing tubes before and place on ice immediately after obtaining the specimen. Spin the sample in a refrigerated centrifuge. Freeze if not analyzing immediately.

Clinical Implications

1. *Increased SM-C levels* are associated with the following conditions:
   a. Acromegaly (some cases), gigantism
   b. Hypoglycemia associated with non–islet cell tumors
   c. Hepatoma
   d. Wilms' tumor (a rare kidney cancer that most commonly occurs in children)
   e. Precocious puberty
2. *Decreased SM-C levels* are associated with the following conditions:
   a. Dwarfism (short stature)
   b. Hypopituitarism
   c. Hypothyroidism
   d. Puberty delay
   e. Laron's dwarfism (autosomal recessive disorder, not responsive to growth hormone)
   f. Cirrhosis of liver and other hepatocellular diseases
   g. Malnutrition and anorexia
   h. Diabetes mellitus (diabetic retinopathy)
   i. Emotional deprivation syndrome (maternal deprivation)

Interfering Factors

1. SM-C levels are *increased* 2 to 3 times in pregnancy.
2. SM-C levels are *decreased* in the following conditions:
   a. Acute illness
   b. Normal aging

Interventions

Pretest Patient Care

1. Explain test purpose and procedure. Fasting is not required.
2. Do not administer radioisotopes within 1 week of testing.
3. Follow guidelines in Chapter 1 for safe, effective, informed *pretest* care.

Posttest Patient Care

1. Have patient resume normal activities.
2. Review test results; report and record findings. Modify the nursing care plan as needed. Monitor appropriately for abnormal growth and development.
3. Follow guidelines in Chapter 1 for safe, effective, informed *posttest* care.

NOTE *Because SM-C is decreased with malnutrition, it can be used to monitor therapy for food deprivation.*

FERTILITY TESTS

Fertility denotes the ability of a man and woman to reproduce; conversely, infertility denotes the lack of fertility—an involuntary reduction in the ability to produce children. When a couple has been engaging in regular, unprotected sexual intercourse for at least 1 year without conceiving, the couple is considered infertile. In about one third of cases, a male factor is the predominant cause; in another one third, the female factor predominates; and in another one third, no cause is found in either partner.

The workup for infertility starts with a complete history and physical exam for both the woman and the man, including their sexual history. A rational approach is to put each partner through a series of tests that generally uncover a vast majority of the contributing factors of infertility. These tests usually take 2 to 3 months to complete.

Standard pretest and posttest care for couples undergoing fertility testing includes the following: Provide information and support. Be sensitive to the couple's need for privacy and confidentiality. Maintain a communication network about new procedures, tests, and treatments. Help couples deal with feelings of sadness and loss. Assist couples to deal with the effects of stress and the financial burden during the diagnostic process. Assist couples in arranging work and testing schedules with the least amount of disruption for the couple. Arrange for counseling with experts who understand the different ways infertility affects someone's life.

Tests include evaluation of amenorrhea, anovulation, sperm count (angiosperm, oligospermia), hormone testing, hysterosalpingogram, laparoscopy, hysteroscopy, fertiloscopy, semen analysis, postcoital test, endometrial biopsy, and chromosome karyotype to exclude Kallmann's syndrome. Hormone testing rules pregnancy in or out (e.g., chorionic gonadotropin, prolactin, luteinizing hormone [LH], follicle-stimulating hormone [FSH], thyroid-stimulating hormone [TSH], postcoital test, and antisperm antibodies). Also, see estrogen testing in Chapter 3.

NOTE *A postcoital examination is done to assess cervical mucus and competent sperm motility. A specimen is obtained from the endocervical canal within 2 to 12 hours of coitus and is examined for viscosity (stretching to 6 cm is normal) and for ferning effect of estrogen. The presence of >50% sperm confirms male competence.*

● Chorionic Gonadotropin; Human Chorionic Gonadotropin (hCG) β Subunit; Pregnancy Test

The glycoprotein hormones human chorionic gonadotropin (hCG), LH, FSH, and TSH are composed of two different subunits. The α subunit is similar in all of the glycoprotein hormones, and the β subunit is unique to each hormone. Highly specific assays allow hCG to be measured in the presence of other glycoprotein hormones. The increased sensitivity of the β-hCG test detects pregnancy as early as 6 to 10 days after implantation of the oocyte. A variety of poorly differentiated or undifferentiated neoplasms may produce ectopic chorionic gonadotropin. Assay for total hCG, both α and β subunits, or β-hCG may detect ectopic tumors (e.g., choriocarcinoma, hydatidiform mole, germinal testicular tumors). In these neoplasms, hCG is usually the product of syncytiotrophoblastic cells.

This qualitative test detects normal pregnancy. It is quicker but less sensitive (sensitivity, 20 to 50 mIU/mL) than the quantitative test. This test can be expected to become positive within 3 days of implantation (i.e., just after the first missed menstrual period). Cross-reactivity with LH is low, and false-positive results are rare. Occasionally, a patient with very high LH levels will give a borderline reaction. The qualitative test is usually done using urine.

The quantitative β-hCG test is used for nonroutine detection of hCG. It is sensitive to 1 to 3 mIU/mL. This test provides the most sensitive and specific test for the detection of early pregnancy, estimation of gestational age, and diagnosis of ectopic pregnancy or threatened spontaneous abortion. This test is also useful in the workup and management of testicular tumors. High levels may be found in choriocarcinoma, embryonal cell carcinoma, and ectopic pregnancy. hCG levels are extremely useful in following germ cell neoplasms that produce hCG, especially trophoblastic neoplasms. There is little cross-reactivity with LH.

Normal Findings

Qualitative (for routine pregnancy tests): urine or serum negative (not pregnant)

Quantitative (for nonroutine detection of hCG)

- Men: <5.0 IU/L or mIU/mL
- Nonpregnant women: <5.0 IU/L or mIU/mL
- Pregnant women:
  - 1 week of gestation: 5 to 50 mIU/mL or IU/L
  - 2 weeks of gestation: 50 to 500 mIU/mL or IU/L
  - 3 weeks of gestation: 100 to 10,000 mIU/mL or IU/L
  - 4 weeks of gestation: 1080 to 30,000 mIU/mL or IU/L
  - 6 to 8 weeks of gestation: 3500 to 115,000 mIU/mL or IU/L
  - 12 weeks of gestation: 12,000 to 270,000 mIU/mL or IU/L
  - 13 to 16 weeks of gestation: up to 200,000 mIU/mL or IU/L
  - 17 to 40 weeks of gestation: gradual fall to 4000 mIU/mL or IU/L

Procedure

1. Obtain a 5-mL venous blood sample. Serum is used for the test.
2. Observe standard precautions. Label the specimen with the patient's name, date and time of collection, and test(s) ordered. Place the specimen in a biohazard bag.
3. Urine may be used for the qualitative test. First morning specimen is recommended.

Clinical Implications

1. *Increased hCG values* occur in the following conditions:
   a. Pregnancy
   b. Successful therapeutic insemination and in vitro fertilization
   c. Hydatidiform mole
   d. Choriocarcinoma
   e. Seminoma
   f. Ovarian and testicular teratomas
   g. Ectopic pregnancy
   h. Certain neoplasms of the lung, stomach, and pancreas
   i. Down syndrome (trisomy 21), midtrimester elevation

2. *Decreased hCG values* occur in:
   a. Threatened spontaneous abortion
   b. Ectopic pregnancy
   c. Trisomy 18, decrease at midtrimester

Interfering Factors

1. Lipemia, hemolysis, and radioisotopes administered within 1 week of testing may affect results.
2. Test results can be positive up to 1 week after complete abortion.
3. False-negative and false-positive results can be caused by many drugs (see Appendix E).
4. Heterophilic antibodies may falsely increase or decrease results.

CLINICAL ALERT

Because there is great variability in hCG concentration among pregnant women, a single test determination cannot be used to accurately date the gestational age. Serial determinations may be helpful when abnormal pregnancy is suspected. Serial values do not double every 48 hr. In normal pregnancy, the hCG level doubles every 48 hr during the first 6 wk of gestation.

Interventions

Pretest Patient Care

1. Explain test purpose and procedure.
2. Determine and record date of last menstrual period in women.
3. Follow guidelines in Chapter 1 for safe, effective, informed *pretest* care.

Posttest Patient Care

1. Have patient resume normal activities.
2. Review test results; report and record findings. Modify the nursing care plan as needed. Counsel appropriately for pregnancy or gestational problems.
3. Follow guidelines in Chapter 1 for safe, effective, informed *posttest* care.

• Follicle-Stimulating Hormone (FSH); Luteinizing Hormone (LH)

FSH and LH are glycoprotein hormones produced and stored in the anterior pituitary. They are under complex regulation by hypothalamic gonadotropin-releasing hormone and by gonadal sex hormones (estrogen and progesterone in females and testosterone in males). FSH acts on granulosa cells of the ovary and Sertoli's cells of the testis, and LH acts on Leydig's (interstitial) cells of the gonads. Normally, FSH increases occur at earlier stages of puberty, 2 to 4 years before LH reaches comparable levels. In males, FSH and LH are necessary for spermatozoa development and maturation. In females, follicular formation in the early stages of the menstrual cycle is stimulated by FSH; then, the midcycle surge of LH causes ovulation of the FSH-ripened ovarian follicles to occur.

This test measures the gonadotropic hormones FSH and LH and may help determine whether a gonadal deficiency is of primary origin or is due to insufficient stimulation by the pituitary hormones.

Evaluation of FSH supports other studies related to determining causes of hypothyroidism in women and endocrine dysfunction in men. In primary ovarian failure or testicular failure, FSH levels are increased. Measuring the levels of FSH and LH is of value in studying children with endocrine problems related to precocious puberty.

In the case of anovulatory fertility problems, the presence or absence of the midcycle peak can be established through a series of daily blood specimens.

Normal Findings

See Table 6.9.

TABLE 6.9 Values for Luteinizing and Follicle-Stimulating Hormones

	Luteinizing Hormone (LH)		Follicle-Stimulating Hormone (FSH)	
	(mIU/mL) or	(IU/L)	(mIU/L) or	(IU/mL)
Female				
Follicular	1.37–9.9	1.37–9.9	1.68–15	1.68–15
Ovulatory peak	6.17–17.2	6.17–17.2	21.9–56.6	21.9–56.6
Luteal	1.09–9.2	1.09–9.2	0.61–16.3	0.61–16.3
Postmenopausal	19.3–100.6	19.3–100.6	14.2–52.3	14.2–52.3
Male	1.42–15.4	1.42–15.4	1.24–7.8	1.24–7.8

Contact your laboratory for reference values in infants and children. Normal values may vary with method of testing and units used.

Procedure

1. Obtain a 5-mL venous blood sample (red-topped tube). Serum is needed for the test. Label the specimen with the patient's name, date and time of collection, and test(s) ordered. Place the specimen in a biohazard bag.
2. In women, record the date of last menstrual period.
3. It is important to measure both FSH and LH.

CLINICAL ALERT

Sometimes, multiple blood specimens are necessary because of episodic releases of FSH from the pituitary gland. An isolated sample may not indicate the actual activity; therefore, pooled blood specimens or multiple single blood specimens may be required.

Clinical Implications

1. *Decreased FSH levels* occur in the following conditions:
   a. Feminizing and masculinizing ovarian tumors when FSH production is inhibited because of increased estrogen secretion.
   b. Failure of hypothalamus to function properly (Kallmann's syndrome)
   c. Pituitary LH or FSH deficiency
   d. Neoplasm of testes or adrenal glands that influences secretion of estrogens or androgens
   e. Polycystic ovary syndrome
   f. Hemochromatosis (increased iron in the body)
   g. Anorexia
2. *Decreased FSH and LH* occur in pituitary or hypothalamic failure.
3. *Increased FSH levels* occur in the following conditions:
   a. Turner's syndrome (ovarian dysgenesis); about 50% of patients with primary amenorrhea have Turner's syndrome.
   b. Hypopituitarism
   c. Sheehan's syndrome (postpartum hypopituitarism)
   d. Precocious puberty, either idiopathic or secondary to a CNS lesion
   e. Klinefelter's syndrome
   f. Castration
   g. Alcoholism
   h. Menopause and menstrual disorders

4. *Both FSH and LH are increased* in the following conditions:
    a. Hypogonadism
    b. Complete testicular feminization syndrome
    c. Gonadal failure
    d. Congenital absence of testicle or testicles (anorchia)
    e. Menopause
5. Elevated basal LH with an LH/FSH ratio >2 and some increase of ovarian androgen in an essentially nonovulatory adult woman is presumptive evidence of Stein-Leventhal syndrome (polycystic ovary syndrome).

Interfering Factors

1. Recently administered radioisotopes
2. Hemolysis of blood sample
3. Estrogens or oral contraceptives, testosterone
4. Several drugs affect test outcomes; see Appendix E.
5. Pregnancy
6. Heterophilic antibodies may falsely increase or decrease results

Interventions

Pretest Patient Care

1. Instruct the patient regarding test purpose and procedure.
2. For women, record date of last menstrual period.
3. Follow guidelines in Chapter 1 for safe, effective, informed *pretest* care.

Posttest Patient Care

1. Review test results; report and record findings. Modify the nursing care plan as needed. Counsel appropriately.
2. Follow guidelines in Chapter 1 for safe, effective, informed *posttest* care.

● Prolactin (hPRL)

Prolactin (hPRL) is a pituitary hormone essential for initiating and maintaining lactation. The gender difference in hPRL does not occur until puberty, when increased estrogen production results in higher hPRL levels in females. Circadian changes in hPRL concentration in adults are marked by episodic fluctuation and a sleep-induced peak in the early morning hours.

This test may be helpful in the diagnosis, management, and follow-up of a hPRL-secreting tumor accompanied by secondary amenorrhea or galactorrhea, hyperprolactinemia, and infertility. It is also useful in the management of hypothalamic disease and in monitoring the effectiveness of surgery, chemotherapy, and radiation treatment of hPRL-secreting tumors.

Normal Findings

Nonpregnant women: 4 to 23 ng/mL or 4 to 23 μg/L
Pregnant women: 34 to 386 ng/mL or 34 to 386 μg/L by third trimester
Men: 3 to 15 ng/mL or 3 to 15 μg/L
Children: 3.2 to 20 ng/mL or 3.2 to 20 μg/L

Procedure

1. Ensure that the patient fasts for 12 hours before testing. Obtain a 5-mL venous blood sample (red-topped tube). Serum is used.

2. Procure specimens in the morning, between 8:00 (0800 hours) and 10:00 a.m. (1000 hours). Draw in chilled tubes and keep specimens on ice.
3. Observe standard precautions. Label the specimen with the patient's name, date and time of collection, and test(s) ordered. Place the specimen in a biohazard bag.

Clinical Implications

1. *Increased hPRL values* are associated with the following conditions:
   a. Galactorrhea or amenorrhea
   b. Diseases of the hypothalamus and pituitary (acromegaly)
   c. hPRL-secreting pituitary tumors
   d. Chiari-Frommel syndrome (abnormal lactation and amenorrhea following pregnancy)
   e. Ectopic production of hPRL from tumors, carcinoma, and leukemia
   f. Hypothyroidism (primary)
   g. Polycystic ovary syndrome
   h. Anorexia nervosa
   i. Insulin-induced hypoglycemia
   j. Adrenal insufficiency
2. *Decreased hPRL values* are found in the following conditions:
   a. Sheehan's syndrome (pituitary apoplexy)
   b. Idiopathic hypogonadotropic hypogonadism

NOTE *The only result of hPRL deficiency in pregnancy is the absence of postpartum lactation.*

Interfering Factors

1. Increased values are associated with newborns, pregnancy, postpartum period, stress, exercise, sleep, nipple stimulation, and lactation (breast-feeding).
2. Drugs (e.g., estrogens, methyldopa, phenothiazines, opiates) may increase values. See Appendix E for other drugs.
3. Dopaminergic drugs inhibit hPRL secretion. Administration of L-dopa can normalize hPRL levels in galactorrhea, hyperprolactinemia, and pituitary tumor. See Appendix E for other drugs.
4. Increased levels are found in cocaine abuse, even after withdrawal from cocaine.
5. Macroprolactin can falsely increase test results.

CLINICAL ALERT

Levels >200 ng/mL or >200 μg/L in a nonlactating female indicate an hPRL-secreting tumor; however, a normal hPRL level does not rule out pituitary tumor.

Interventions

Pretest Patient Care

1. Explain test purpose. Fasting is required. Obtain the blood specimen between 8:00 (0800 hours) and 10:00 a.m. (1000 hours) (3 to 4 hours after patient has awakened). Obtain history of leakage from the breast in nonpregnant females.
2. Have patient avoid stress, excitement, or stimulation; venipuncture itself can sometimes elevate hPRL levels.
3. If possible, discontinue all prescribed medications for 2 weeks before test.
4. Follow guidelines in Chapter 1 for safe, effective, informed *pretest* care.

Posttest Patient Care

1. Have patient resume normal activities.
2. Review test results; report and record findings. Modify the nursing care plan as needed. Counsel regarding repeat testing to monitor treatment. Magnetic resonance imaging may be indicated.
3. Follow guidelines in Chapter 1 for safe, effective, informed *posttest* care.

Progesterone

Progesterone, a female sex hormone, is primarily involved in the preparation of the uterus for pregnancy and its maintenance during pregnancy. The placenta begins producing progesterone at 12 weeks of gestation. Progesterone level peaks in the midluteal phase of the menstrual cycle. In nonpregnant women, progesterone is produced by the corpus luteum. Progesterone is the single best test to determine whether ovulation has occurred.

This test is part of a fertility study to confirm ovulation, evaluate corpus luteum function, and assess risk for early spontaneous abortion. Testing of several samples during the cycle is necessary. Ovarian production of progesterone is low during the follicular (first) phase of the menstrual cycle. After ovulation, progesterone levels rise for 4 to 5 days and then fall. During pregnancy, there is a gradual increase from week 9 to week 32 of gestation, often to 100 times the level in the nonpregnant woman. Levels of progesterone in twin pregnancy are higher than in a single pregnancy. Serum progesterone levels used with β-hCG assist in differentiating normal uterine pregnancy from abnormal uterine or ectopic pregnancy.

Normal Findings

Men: <1.0 ng/mL or <3.2 nmol/L
Women:
Prepubertal: 0.1 to 0.3 ng/mL or 0.3 to 1.0 nmol/L
Follicular: 0.1 to 0.7 ng/mL or 0.5 to 2.3 nmol/L
Luteal: 2 to 25 ng/mL or 6.4 to 79.5 nmol/L
First trimester: 10 to 44 ng/mL or 32.6 to 140 nmol/L
Second trimester: 19.5 to 82.5 ng/mL or 62.0 to 262 nmol/L
Third trimester: 65 to 290 ng/mL or 206.7 to 728 nmol/L

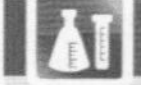

CLINICAL ALERT

Critical Value
Levels <10 ng/mL or <32 nmol/L are associated with abnormal pregnancy outcome.

Procedure

1. Obtain a 5-mL venous blood sample (red-topped tube). Serum is needed for test. Observe standard precautions. Label the specimen with the patient's name, date and time of collection, and test(s) ordered. Place the specimen in a biohazard bag.
2. The test request should include gender, day of last menstrual period, and length of gestation in women.
3. If indicated, a β-hCG may be ordered at the same time.
4. Although urine levels may be tested, serum is preferred.

Clinical Implications

1. *Increased progesterone levels* are associated with the following conditions:
   a. Congenital adrenal hyperplasia
   b. Lipoid ovarian tumor
   c. Molar pregnancy
   d. Chorionepithelioma of ovary
2. *Decreased progesterone levels* are associated with the following conditions:
   a. Threatened spontaneous abortion
   b. Galactorrhea-amenorrhea syndrome (primary or secondary hypogonadism)
   c. Short luteal phase syndrome

Interfering Factors

1. See Appendix E for drugs that affect test outcomes.
2. Progesterone 5 to 10 ng/mL or 16 to 32 nmol/L: pathologic pregnancy
3. Progesterone <5 ng/mL or <16 nmol/L: nonviable pregnancy

Interventions

Pretest Patient Care

1. Explain test purpose and procedure. Note date of last menstrual period and length of gestation.
2. Do not administer radioisotopes within 1 week before the test.
3. Follow guidelines in Chapter 1 for safe, effective, informed *pretest* care.

Posttest Patient Care

1. Have patient resume normal activities.
2. Review test results; report and record findings. Modify the nursing care plan as needed. Counsel and monitor appropriately regarding fertility and pregnancy outcome.
3. Follow guidelines in Chapter 1 for safe, effective, informed *posttest* care.

● Testosterone, Total and Free

Testosterone is responsible for the development of male secondary sexual characteristics. It is secreted by the adrenal glands and testes in men and by the adrenal glands and ovaries in women. Excessive production induces premature puberty in men and masculinity in women. Testosterone exists in serum as both unbound (free) fractions and bound fractions to albumin: sex hormone–binding globulin (SHBG) and testosterone-binding globulin. Unbound (free) testosterone is the active portion. Testosterone levels undergo large and rapid fluctuations; levels peak in early morning in males. Females show a cyclic elevation 1 to 2 days midcycle.

Testosterone measurements in men assess hypogonadism, pituitary gonadotropin function, impotency, and cryptorchidism; these measurements are also useful in the detection of ovarian tumors and hirsutism in women. In prepubertal boys, they can assess sexual precocity. This test may be part of a fertility workup in association with chronic anovulation caused by polycystic ovary syndrome. It can also detect ovarian and adrenal tumors in women with symptoms of hirsutism and amenorrhea.

Normal Findings

Reference values are method dependent.

Total Testosterone

Men: 270 to 1070 ng/dL or 9 to 38 nmol/L (values in older men diminish moderately)

Women: 15 to 70 ng/dL or 0.52 to 2.4 nmol/L

Pregnant women: 3 to 4 times normal
Postmenopausal women: 8 to 35 ng/dL or 0.3 to 1.2 nmol/L (half of normal)
Children:

Age	Female	Male
Premature (26–28 wk)	5–16 ng/dL	59–125 ng/dL
Premature (31–35 wk)	5–22 ng/dL	37–198 ng/dL
Newborn	20–64 ng/dL	75–400 ng/dL
1–5 mo	<20 ng/dL	14–363 ng/dL
6–24 mo	<9 ng/dL	<37 ng/dL
2–3 yr	<20 ng/dL	<15 ng/dL
4–5 yr	<30 ng/dL	<19 ng/dL
6–7 yr	<7 ng/dL	<13 ng/dL
8–9 yr	1–11 ng/dL	2–8 ng/dL
10–11 yr	3–32 ng/dL	2–165 ng/dL
12–13 yr	6–50 ng/dL	3–619 ng/dL
14–15 yr	6–52 ng/dL	31–733 ng/dL
16–17 yr	2–17 ng/dL	158–826 ng/dL
Tanner stage I	2–17 ng/dL	2–15 ng/dL
Tanner stage II	5–40 ng/dL	3–303 ng/dL
Tanner stage III	10–63 ng/dL	10–851 ng/dL
Tanner stage IV–V	11–62 ng/dL	162–847 ng/dL

Free Testosterone
Men: 50 to 210 pg/mL or 174 to 729 pmol/L
Women: 1.0 to 8.5 pg/mL or 3.5 to 29.5 pmol/L
Children:
Boys: 0.1 to 3.2 pg/mL or 0.3 to 11.1 pmol/L
Girls: 0.1 to 0.9 pg/mL or 0.3 to 3.1 pmol/L
Puberty:
Boys: 1.4 to 156 pg/mL or 4.9 to 541 pmol/L
Girls: 1.0 to 5.2 pg/mL or 3.5 to 18.0 pmol/L

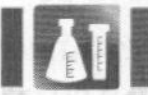

CLINICAL ALERT

Critical Value
Total testosterone >200 ng/dL or >694 pmol/L in females indicates androgenic tumors of the – adrenal or ovaries, especially with severe hirsutism.

Procedure

1. Obtain a 5-mL venous blood sample (red-topped tube); serum is preferred. Observe standard precautions. Label the specimen with the patient's name, date and time of collection, and test(s) ordered. Place the specimen in a biohazard bag.
2. Indicate age and gender on laboratory requisition.

Clinical Implications

1. Males: *decreased total testosterone levels* occur in the following conditions:
   a. Hypogonadism (pituitary failure)
   b. Klinefelter's syndrome

   c. Hypopituitarism (primary and secondary)
   d. Orchidectomy
   e. Hepatic cirrhosis
   f. Down syndrome
   g. Delayed puberty
2. Males: *Decreased free testosterone levels* occur in hypogonadism and older men.
3. Males: *Increased total testosterone levels* occur in the following conditions:
   a. Hyperthyroidism
   b. Syndromes of androgen resistance
   c. Adrenal tumors
   d. Precocious puberty and adrenal hyperplasia in boys
4. Females: *increased total testosterone levels* are associated with the following conditions:
   a. Adrenal neoplasms
   b. Ovarian tumors, benign or malignant (virilizing)
   c. Trophoblastic disease during pregnancy
   d. Idiopathic hirsutism
   e. Hilar cell tumor
5. Females: *increased free testosterone levels* are associated with the following conditions:
   a. Female hirsutism
   b. Polycystic ovary syndrome
   c. Virilization

CLINICAL ALERT

1. Testosterone levels are normal in cryptorchidism, azoospermia, and oligospermia.
2. In general, there appears to be little advantage to doing urine testosterone measurements compared with (or in addition to) serum measurements; the serum test is recommended.

Interfering Factors

1. Alcoholism in males decreases testosterone levels.
2. Estrogen therapy increases testosterone levels (see Appendix E).
3. Many drugs, including androgens and steroids, decrease testosterone levels (see Appendix E).

Interventions

Pretest Patient Care

1. Explain test purpose and procedure. Draw blood at 7:00 a.m. (0700 hours) for highest levels.
2. Draw multiple pooled samples at different times throughout the day if necessary for more reliable results.
3. Do not administer radioisotopes within 1 week before test.
4. Follow guidelines in Chapter 1 regarding safe, effective, informed *pretest* care.

Posttest Patient Care

1. Have patient resume normal activities.
2. Review test results; report and record findings. Modify the nursing care plan as needed. Counsel appropriately regarding hormone dysfunction.
3. Follow guidelines in Chapter 1 for safe, effective, informed *posttest* care.

ENZYME TESTS

Acid Phosphatase; Prostatic Acid Phosphatase (PAP)

Acid phosphatases are enzymes that are widely distributed in tissues, including the bone, liver, spleen, kidney, RBCs, and platelets. However, their greatest diagnostic importance involves the prostate gland, where acid phosphatase activity is 100 times higher than in other tissues. Immunochemical methods are highly specific for determining the prostatic fraction; however, because prostatic acid phosphatase (PAP) is not elevated in early prostatic disease, this test is not recommended for screening.

This test monitors the effectiveness of treatment of cancer of the prostate. Elevated levels of acid phosphatase are seen when prostate cancer has metastasized beyond the capsule to the other parts of the body, especially the bone. Once the carcinoma has spread, the prostate starts to release acid phosphatase, resulting in an increased blood level. The prostatic fraction procedure specifically measures the concentration of prostatic acid phosphatase secreted by cells of the prostate gland. Acid phosphatase is also present in high concentration in seminal fluid. Tests for presence of this enzyme on vaginal swabs may be used to investigate rape.

Normal Findings

Men: <2.5 ng/mL or <2.5 μg/L

Procedure

1. Obtain a 5-mL venous blood sample. Serum may be used, if test is done within 1 hour. EDTA plasma is preferred to stabilize acid phosphatase.
2. Obtaining a specimen in the morning is recommended because diurnal variation exists.
3. Label the specimen with the patient's name, date and time of collection, and test(s) ordered. Place the specimen in a biohazard bag, transport to lab immediately, and place on ice.

Clinical Implications

1. A significantly elevated acid phosphatase value is almost always indicative of metastatic cancer of the prostate. If the tumor is successfully treated, this enzyme level will drop within 3 to 4 days after surgery or 3 to 4 weeks after estrogen administration.
2. Moderately elevated values also occur in the absence of prostate carcinoma in the following conditions:
   a. Niemann-Pick disease (inherited metabolic disorder, a form of sphingolipidosis)
   b. Gaucher's disease (a form of lysosomal storage disease)
   c. Prostatitis (benign prostatic hypertrophy)
   d. Urinary retention
   e. Any cancer that has metastasized to the bone
   f. Myelocytic leukemia

Interfering Factors

1. Various drugs may cause increased or decreased PAP levels.
2. Palpation of the prostate gland and prostate biopsy before testing cause increases in PAP levels.
3. Transurethral resection of the prostate (TURP) and bladder catheterization cause increased levels.

Interventions

Pretest Patient Care

1. Explain test purpose and procedure.
2. No palpation of or procedures on the prostate gland and no rectal examinations should be performed 2 to 3 days before test.
3. Follow guidelines in Chapter 1 for safe, effective, informed *pretest* care.

Posttest Patient Care

1. Have patient resume normal activities.
2. Review test results; report and record findings. Modify the nursing care plan as needed. Counsel appropriately regarding repeat testing. When elevated values are present, retesting and biopsy are considered.
3. Follow guidelines in Chapter 1 for safe, effective, informed *posttest* care.

● Prostate-Specific Antigen (PSA)

Prostate-specific antigen (PSA) is functionally and immunologically distinct from PAP. PSA is localized in both normal prostatic epithelial cells and prostatic carcinoma cells. PSA has proved to be the most prognostically reliable marker for monitoring recurrence of prostatic carcinoma; however, this test does not have the sensitivity or specificity (20% to 40%) to be considered an ideal tumor marker. PSA velocity, the rate of change over time, PSA density, PSA value divided by prostate size, and various PSA isoforms (e.g., bound to protein) are used in an effort to provide better sensitivity and specificity. The gold standard for prostate cancer diagnosis, however, is the prostate tissue biopsy, although it is not 100% correct. PSA detects incidental as well as aggressive carcinomas.

The most useful approach to date may be age-specific PSA reference ranges, which are based on the concept that blood PSA concentration is dependent on patient age. The increase in PSA with advancing age is attributed to four major factors: prostate enlargement, increasing inflammation, presence of microscopic but clinically insignificant cancer, and leakage of PSA into the serum (Table 6.10).

Testing for both PSA and PAP increases detection of early prostate cancer. The American Cancer Society recommends an annual digital rectal examination (DRE) and PSA test starting at age 40 years. PSA testing determines the effectiveness of therapy for prostate cancer and is used as an early indicator of prostate cancer recurrence. The greatest value of PSA is as a marker in the follow-up of patients at high risk for disease progression.

PSA lacks sufficient sensitivity and specificity to be used alone as a screening test for prostatic carcinoma, but in conjunction with a DRE, the detection rate of prostatic carcinoma is greatly increased, although still controversial.

Normal Findings

Serum
PSA <2.5 ng/mL or <2.5 μg/L
cPSA (complexed) <2.2 ng/mL or <2.2 μg/L
Free PSA >25%

TABLE 6.10 Suggested Age-Specific Prostate-Specific Antigen (PSA) Reference Ranges

	PSA Range	
Age (yr)	(ng/mL)	(μg/L)
40–49	0.0–2.5	0.0–2.5
50–59	0.0–3.5	0.0–3.5
60–69	0.0–4.5	0.0–4.5
70–79	0.0–6.5	0.0–6.5

Source: Oesterling JE, Jacobson SJ, Chute CG, et al: Serum prostate-specific antigen in a community-based population of healthy men: Establishment of age-specific reference ranges. JAMA 270(7):860–864, 1993.

Urine

PCA3 score

PCA3 mRNA/PSA mRNA 35 copies/copy of PSA mRNA

(PCA3 is a genetic marker)

Percentage of free PSA = free PSA/total PSA × 100

(Patients with prostate cancer have a lower proportion of free PSA compared with those who have benign conditions.)

Procedure

1. Obtain a 5-mL venous blood serum sample (red-topped tube) or a urine specimen.
2. Observe standard precautions. Place the specimen in a biohazard bag.
3. Record patient's age.

Clinical Implications

1. *PSA increases* occur in prostate cancer (80% of patients).
2. Patients with benign prostatic hypertrophy often demonstrate values between 4.0 and 8.0 ng/mL (4.0 and 8.0 μg/L). Results between 4.0 and 8.0 ng/mL (4.0 and 8.0 μg/L) may represent benign prostatic hypertrophy or possible cancer of the prostate. Results >8.0 ng/mL or >8.0 μg/L are highly suggestive of prostatic cancer.
3. Increases to >4.0 ng/mL or >4.0 μg/L have been reported in about 8% of patients with no prostatic malignancies and no benign diseases.
4. If a prostate tumor is completely and successfully removed, *no* antigen will be detected.
5. If the percentage of free PSA is <25%, there is a high likelihood of prostatic cancer.

Interfering Factors

1. Transient increases in PSA occur following prostate palpation or rectal examination.
2. Increased PSA occurs with urinary retention.
3. Recent exposure to radioisotopes causes test interference.

Interventions

Pretest Patient Care

1. Explain test purpose and procedure.
2. Do not schedule any prostatic examinations, including rectal examination, prostate biopsy, or TURP, for 1 week before the blood test is performed.
3. Follow guidelines in Chapter 1 for safe, effective, informed *pretest* care.

Posttest Patient Care

1. Have patient resume normal activities.
2. Review test results; report and record findings. Modify the nursing care plan as needed. Monitor and counsel as appropriate for response to treatment and progression or remission of prostate cancer.
3. Follow guidelines in Chapter 1 for safe, effective, informed *posttest* care.

CLINICAL ALERT

1. PSA is not a definitive diagnostic marker to screen for carcinoma of the prostate because it is also found in men with benign prostatic hypertrophy.
2. DRE is recommended by the American Cancer Society as the primary test for detection of prostatic tumor. Recent studies indicate that serum PSA may offer additional information. PSA should be used in conjunction with DRE.
3. The value of prostatic cancer screening remains controversial in terms of patient morbidity and longevity outcomes.

● Alanine Aminotransferase (Aminotransferase, ALT); Serum Glutamic-Pyruvic Transaminase (SGPT)

Alanine aminotransferase or ALT is an enzyme with high concentrations found in the liver and relatively low concentrations found in the heart, muscle, and kidney.

This test is primarily used to diagnose liver disease and to monitor the course of treatment for hepatitis, active postnecrotic cirrhosis, and the effects of later drug therapy. ALT is more sensitive in the detection of liver disease than in biliary obstruction. ALT also differentiates between hemolytic jaundice and jaundice due to liver disease.

Normal Findings

Adults:
Males: 10 to 40 U/L or 0.17 to 0.68 μkat/L
Females: 7 to 35 U/L or 0.12 to 0.60 μkat/L
Newborns: 13 to 45 U/L or 0.22 to 0.77 μkat/L

ALT values are slightly higher in males and African Americans. Normal values vary with testing method. Check with your laboratory for reference values.

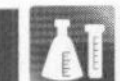

CLINICAL ALERT

Critical Value

Alcohol–acetaminophen syndrome: extremely abnormal ALT/aspartate transaminase (AST) values are found (>9000 U/L [>153 μkat/L]); this extreme level can distinguish this syndrome from alcoholic or viral hepatitis.

Procedure

1. Obtain a 5-mL venous blood sample (red-topped tube). Serum is needed for the test. Observe standard precautions. Label the specimen with the patient's name, date and time of collection, and test(s) ordered. Place the specimen in a biohazard bag.
2. Avoid hemolysis during collection of the specimen. (ALT activity is 6 times higher in RBCs.)

Clinical Implications

1. *Increased ALT levels* are found in the following conditions:
   a. Hepatocellular disease (moderate to high increase)
   b. Alcoholic cirrhosis (mild increase)
   c. Metastatic liver tumor (mild increase)
   d. Obstructive jaundice or biliary obstruction (mild increase)
   e. Viral, infectious, or toxic hepatitis (30 to 50 times normal)
   f. Infectious mononucleosis
   g. Pancreatitis (mild increase)
   h. MI, heart failure
   i. Polymyositis
   j. Severe burns
   k. Trauma to striated muscle
   l. Severe shock
2. AST/ALT comparison
   a. Although the AST level is always increased in acute MI, the ALT level does not always increase unless there is also liver damage.

b. The ALT is usually increased more than the AST in acute extrahepatic biliary obstruction.
c. The AST/ALT ratio is high in alcoholic liver disease; the ALT is more specific than AST for liver disease, but the AST is more sensitive to alcoholic liver disease.

Interfering Factors

1. Many drugs may cause falsely increased or decreased ALT levels (see Appendix E).
2. Salicylates may cause decreased or increased ALT levels.
3. Therapeutic heparin causes increased ALT.
4. Hemolyzed blood causes increases in ALT.
5. Obesity causes increases in ALT.

CLINICAL ALERT

There is a correlation between the presence of elevated serum ALT and abnormal antibodies to the hepatitis B virus core antigen and hepatitis C antigen. Persons with elevated ALT levels should not donate blood.

Interventions

Pretest Patient Care

1. Explain test purpose and blood-drawing procedure.
2. Follow guidelines in Chapter 1 for safe, effective, informed *pretest* care.

Posttest Patient Care

1. Have patient resume normal activities.
2. Review test results; report and record findings. Modify the nursing care plan as needed. Monitor as appropriate for liver disease.
3. Follow guidelines in Chapter 1 for safe, effective, informed *posttest* care.

● Alkaline Phosphatase (ALP), Total; 5′-Nucleotidase

Alkaline phosphatase (ALP) is an enzyme originating mainly in the bone, liver, and placenta, with some activity in the kidney and intestines. It is called *alkaline* because it functions best at a pH of 9. ALP levels are age and gender dependent. Postpuberty ALP is mainly of liver origin.

ALP is used as an index of liver and bone disease when correlated with other clinical findings. In bone disease, the enzyme level rises in proportion to new bone cell production resulting from osteoblastic activity and the deposit of calcium in the bones. In liver disease, the blood level rises when excretion of this enzyme is impaired as a result of obstruction in the biliary tract. Used alone, ALP may be misleading.

Normal Findings

Adults: 52 to 142 U/L

Normal values are higher in pediatric patients and in pregnant women. Values increase up to 3 times in puberty. Check with your laboratory for reference values. Values may vary with method of testing.

Procedure

1. Obtain a 5-mL fasting venous blood sample (red-topped tube). Serum is used for this test. Anticoagulants may not be used. Observe standard precautions. Label the specimen with the patient's name, date and time of collection, and test(s) ordered. Place the specimen in a biohazard bag.
2. Refrigerate sample as soon as possible.
3. Note age and gender on test requisition.

Clinical Implications

1. *Elevated levels of ALP in liver disease* (correlated with abnormal liver function tests) occur in the following conditions:
   a. Obstructive jaundice (gallstones obstructing major biliary ducts; accompanying elevated bilirubin)
   b. Space-occupying lesions of the liver such as cancer (hepatic carcinoma) and malignancy with liver metastasis
   c. Hepatocellular cirrhosis
   d. Biliary cirrhosis
   e. Intrahepatic and extrahepatic cholestasis
   f. Hepatitis, infectious mononucleosis, cytomegalovirus
   g. Diabetes mellitus (causes increased synthesis), diabetic hepatic lipidosis
   h. Chronic alcohol ingestion
   i. Gilbert's syndrome (hyperbilirubinemia)
2. *Bone disease and elevated ALP levels* occur in the following conditions:
   a. Paget's disease (osteitis deformans; levels 10 to 25 times normal)
   b. Metastatic bone tumor
   c. Osteogenic sarcoma
   d. Osteomalacia (elevated levels help differentiate between osteomalacia and osteoporosis, in which there is no elevation), rickets
   e. Healing factors (osteogenesis imperfecta)
3. Other diseases involving *elevated ALP levels* include the following:
   a. Hyperparathyroidism (accompanied by hypercalcemia), hyperthyroidism
   b. Pulmonary and MIs
   c. Hodgkin's disease
   d. Cancer of lung or pancreas
   e. Ulcerative colitis, peptic ulcer
   f. Sarcoidosis
   g. Perforation of bowel (acute infarction)
   h. Amyloidosis
   i. Chronic renal failure
   j. Congestive heart failure
   k. Hyperphosphatasia (primary and secondary)
4. *Decreased levels of ALP* occur in the following conditions:
   a. Hypophosphatasia (congenital)
   b. Malnutrition, scurvy
   c. Hypothyroidism, cretinism
   d. Pernicious anemia and severe anemias
   e. Magnesium and zinc deficiency (nutritional)
   f. Milk-alkali syndrome (Burnett's syndrome)
   g. Celiac sprue

Interfering Factors

1. A variety of drugs produce mild to moderate increases or decreases in ALP levels. See Appendix E for drugs that affect outcomes.
2. Young children, those experiencing rapid growth, pregnant women, and postmenopausal women have physiologically high levels of ALP; this level is slightly increased in older persons.
3. After IV administration of albumin, there is sometimes a marked increase in ALP for several days.
4. ALP levels increase at room temperature and in refrigerated storage. Testing should be done the same day.

5. ALP levels decrease if blood is anticoagulated.
6. ALP levels increase after fatty meals.

Interventions

Pretest Patient Care

1. Explain test purpose and blood-drawing procedure. Fasting is required.
2. Follow guidelines in Chapter 1 for safe, effective, informed *pretest* care.

Posttest Patient Care

1. Have patient resume normal activities.
2. Review test results; report and record findings. Modify the nursing care plan as needed. Monitor appropriately for liver or bone disease and evidence of tumor. Testing for 5′-nucleotidase provides supportive evidence in the diagnosis of liver disease. When ALP and 5′-nucleotidase test results are evaluated, they provide definitive diagnosis of Paget's disease and rickets, in which high levels of ALP accompany normal (0 to 5 U/L or 0 to 0.08 μkat/L) or marginally increased 5′-nucleotidase activity. 5′-Nucleotidase is increased in liver disease (e.g., hepatic carcinoma, biliary cirrhosis, extrahepatic obstruction, metastatic neoplasia of liver). 5′-Nucleotidase level usually does not increase in skeletal disease.
3. A useful test to confirm biliary abnormality is GGT. The GGT test is elevated in hepatobiliary disease, but not in uncomplicated bone disease.
4. Follow guidelines in Chapter 1 for safe, effective, informed *posttest* care.

● Alkaline Phosphatase Isoenzymes (ISO)

The isoenzymes of ALP are produced in various tissues. AP-1, α_2 is produced in the liver and by proliferating blood vessels. AP-2, β_1 is produced by bone and placental tissue. The intestinal isoenzyme AP-3, β_2 is present in small quantities in group O and B individuals who are Lewis-positive secretors. Placental ALP is present in the last trimester of pregnancy.

Any patient with an elevation of serum total ALP is a candidate for ALP isoenzyme (ISO) study. The ALP ISO is mainly used to distinguish between bone and liver elevations of ALP.

Normal Findings

AP-1, α_2: values (liver) reported as weak, moderate, or strong or 24 to 158 U/L (0.40 to 2.64 μkat/L)
AP-2, β_1: values (bone) reported as weak, moderate, or strong or 24 to 146 U/L (0.40 to 2.44 μkat/L)
AP-3, β_2: values (intestines) reported as weak, moderate, or strong or 0 to 22 U/L (0 to 0.36 μkat/L)
AP-4: values (placental) reported as weak, moderate, or strong. Placental AP-4 is found only in pregnant women.

Procedure

1. Obtain a 5-mL fasting venous blood sample in a plain red-topped tube or SST tube. Serum is needed. Centrifuge blood promptly, within 30 minutes after draw.
2. Observe standard precautions. Label the specimen with the patient's name, date and time of collection, and test(s) ordered. Place the specimen in a biohazard bag.
3. Refrigerate if not tested immediately.

Clinical Implications

1. Liver (AP-1, α_2) isoenzymes are elevated in hepatic and biliary diseases such as the following conditions:
   a. Cirrhosis (hepatic)
   b. Hepatic carcinoma
   c. Biliary obstruction, primary biliary cirrhosis

2. Bone (AP-2, β_1) isoenzymes are elevated in the following conditions:
   a. Paget's disease (excessive breakdown and formation of bone tissue)
   b. Hyperparathyroidism
   c. Bone cancer, rickets (all types)
   d. Osteomalacia, osteoporosis
   e. Malabsorption syndrome
   f. Certain renal disorders (uremic bone disease or renal rickets)
3. Intestinal (AP-3, β_2) isoenzymes are elevated in the following conditions:
   a. Intestinal infarction
   b. Ulcerative lesions of stomach, small intestine, and colon
   c. Individuals with blood type O or B secrete intestinal isoenzymes 2 hours after a meal.
4. Placental (AP-4) isoenzymes are increased in the following conditions:
   a. Pregnancy (late in third trimester to onset of labor)
   b. Complications of pregnancy such as hypertension and preeclampsia
5. Placental-like isoenzymes occur in some cancers (unidentified isoenzymes):
   a. Regan's isoenzyme
   b. Nagao's isoenzyme

CLINICAL ALERT

1. This test should not be done if the total ALP level is normal.
2. For evaluation of the biliary tract, alternative tests such as GGT, leucine aminopeptidase (LAP), and 5′-nucleotidase studies are recommended over the ALP ISO test.
3. ALP isoenzymes have little value in children and adolescents because bone and liver fractions are normally elevated.
4. In pregnancy, marked decline of the placental isoenzyme is seen with placental insufficiency and imminent fetal demise.

Interfering Factors

Same as for ALP

Interventions

Pretest Patient Care

1. See total ALP patient pretest care.
2. The same guidelines apply to ALP ISO testing.

Posttest Patient Care

1. See total ALP patient posttest care.
2. The same guidelines apply to ALP ISO testing.

● Angiotensin-Converting Enzyme (ACE)

Angiotensin I is produced by the action of renin on angiotensinogen. Angiotensin I–converting enzyme (ACE) catalyzes the conversion of angiotensin I to the vasoactive peptide angiotensin II. Angiotensin I is concentrated in the proximal tubules.

This test is used primarily to evaluate the severity and activity of sarcoidosis. Serial determinations may be helpful in following the clinical course of the disease with steroid treatment. It is also used in the investigation of Gaucher's disease.

Normal Findings

Angiotensin I: <25 pg/mL or <25 ng/L
Angiotensin II: 10 to 60 pg/mL
ACE: 8 to 53 U/L or 0.14 to 0.88 μkat/L

Check with your laboratory for reference values for infants and children because they are generally higher. Also, check with your laboratory for test method because reference values are based on method used for assay.

Procedure

1. Obtain a 5-mL venous blood sample (red-topped tube). Serum or heparinized plasma is used.
2. Observe standard precautions. Label the specimen with the patient's name, date and time of collection, and test(s) ordered. Place the specimen in a biohazard bag.
3. Freeze the specimen if the test is not performed immediately.

Clinical Implications

1. *Increased ACE levels* are associated with the following conditions:
   a. Sarcoidosis (ACE levels reflect the severity of the disease, with 68% positivity in stage 1 disease, 86% in stage 2, and 92% in stage 3)
   b. Gaucher's disease (lysosomal storage disease)
   c. Leprosy
   d. Acute and chronic bronchitis
   e. Connective tissue diseases
   f. Amyloidosis
   g. Pulmonary fibrosis
   h. Fungal diseases and histoplasmosis
   i. Untreated hyperthyroidism
   j. Diabetes mellitus
   k. Psoriasis
2. *Decreased ACE levels* occur in the following conditions:
   a. Following prednisone treatment for sarcoidosis (steroid therapy)
   b. Advanced lung neoplasms
   c. Starvation

Interfering Factors

1. This test should not be done in persons <20 years of age because they normally have a very high level of ACE.
2. About 5% of the normal adult population has elevated ACE levels.
3. ACE is inhibited by EDTA anticoagulant.
4. Some antihypertensives may cause low ACE values.

Interventions

Pretest Patient Care

1. Explain test purpose and blood-drawing procedure.
2. Follow guidelines in Chapter 1 for safe, effective, informed *pretest* care.

Posttest Patient Care

1. Review test results; report and record findings. Modify the nursing care plan as needed. Monitor as appropriate for sarcoidosis and amyloid disease.
2. Follow guidelines in Chapter 1 for safe, effective, informed *posttest* care.

Amylase and Lipase

Amylase, an enzyme that changes starch to sugar, is produced in the salivary (parotid) glands and pancreas; much lower activities are present in the ovaries, intestines, and skeletal muscle. If there is an inflammation of the pancreas or salivary glands, much amylase enters the blood. Amylase levels in the urine reflect blood changes by a time lag of 6 to 10 hours. (See Urine Amylase Excretion and Clearance [Random, Timed Urine, and Blood] in Chapter 3.) Lipase is a glycoprotein that, in the presence of bile salts and colipase, changes fats to fatty acids and glycerol. The pancreas is the major source of this enzyme. Lipase appears in the blood following pancreatic damage at the same time amylase appears (or slightly later) but remains elevated much longer than amylase (7 to 10 days).

Amylase and lipase tests are used to diagnose and monitor treatment of acute pancreatitis and to differentiate pancreatitis from other acute abdominal disorders (80% of patients with acute pancreatitis will have elevated amylase and lipase levels; lipase stays elevated longer). Lipase assay provides better sensitivity and specificity and is best used with amylase determination.

Normal Findings

Amylase
Newborns: 6 to 65 U/L or 0.1 to 1.1 μkat/L
Adults: 25 to 125 U/L or 0.4 to 2.1 μkat/L
Older adults (>60 years): 24 to 151 U/L or 0.4 to 2.5 μkat/L
Lipase
Adults: 10 to 140 U/L or 0.17 to 2.3 μkat/L
Older adults (>60 years): 18 to 180 U/L or 0.30 to 3.0 μkat/L

Normal values vary widely according to method of testing; check with your laboratory for reference ranges. Amylase levels are low for the first 2 months of life. Most of the activity is of salivary origin. Children up to 2 years of age have virtually no pancreatic amylase.

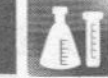
CLINICAL ALERT

Critical Value for Lipase
>600 IU/L or >10 μkat/L

Procedure

1. Obtain a 5-mL venous blood sample (red-topped tube). Serum is used. (EDTA, citrate, and oxalate anticoagulant interfere with lipase testing.)
2. Observe standard precautions. Label the specimen with the patient's name, date and time of collection, and test(s) ordered. Place the specimen in a biohazard bag.

Clinical Implications

1. *Greatly increased amylase levels* occur in acute pancreatitis early in the course of the disease. The increase begins 3 to 6 hours after the onset of pain.
2. *Increased amylase levels* also occur in the following conditions:
   a. Chronic pancreatitis, pancreatic trauma, pancreatic carcinoma, obstruction of pancreatic duct
   b. Partial gastrectomy
   c. Acute appendicitis, peritonitis
   d. Perforated peptic ulcer
   e. Cerebral trauma, shock
   f. Obstruction or inflammation of salivary duct or gland and mumps

g. Acute cholecystitis (common duct stone)
h. Intestinal obstruction with strangulation
i. Ruptured tubal pregnancy and ectopic pregnancy
j. Ruptured aortic aneurysm
k. Macroamylasemia

3. *Decreased amylase levels* occur in the following conditions:
   a. Pancreatic insufficiency
   b. Hepatitis, severe liver disease
   c. Advanced cystic fibrosis
   d. Pancreatectomy
4. *Elevated lipase levels* occur in pancreatic disorders (e.g., pancreatitis, alcoholic and nonalcoholic; pancreatic carcinoma).
5. *Increased lipase values* also are associated with the following conditions:
   a. Cholecystitis
   b. Hemodialysis
   c. Strangulated or infarcted bowel
   d. Peritonitis
   e. Primary biliary cirrhosis
   f. Chronic renal failure
6. Serum lipase levels are normal in patients with elevated amylase who have peptic ulcer, salivary adenitis, inflammatory bowel disease, intestinal obstruction, and macroamylasemia. Coexistence of increased serum amylase and normal lipase levels may be a helpful clue to the presence of macroamylasemia.

Interfering Factors

1. Amylase
   a. Anticoagulated blood gives lower results. Do not use EDTA, citrate, or oxalate.
   b. Lipemic serum interferes with test.
   c. Increased levels are found in alcoholic patients and pregnant women and in diabetic ketoacidosis.
   d. Many drugs can interfere with this test (see Appendix E).
2. Lipase
   a. EDTA anticoagulant interferes with test.
   b. Lipase is increased in about 50% of patients with chronic renal failure.
   c. Lipase increases in patients undergoing hemodialysis.
   d. Many drugs can affect outcomes. See Appendix E.

Interventions

Pretest Patient Care

1. Explain test purpose and procedure. Amylase and lipase testing are done together in the presence of abdominal pain, epigastric tenderness, nausea, and vomiting. These findings characterize acute pancreatitis as well as other acute surgical emergencies.
2. If amylase/creatinine clearance testing is also being done, collect a single, random urine sample at the same time blood is drawn.
3. Follow guidelines in Chapter 1 regarding safe, effective, informed *pretest* care.

Posttest Patient Care

1. Have patient resume normal activities.
2. Review test results; report and record findings. Modify the nursing care plan as needed. Monitor as appropriate for pancreatitis or other acute abdominal conditions.
3. Follow guidelines in Chapter 1 for safe, effective, informed *posttest* care.

● Aspartate Transaminase (Aminotransferase, AST); Serum Glutamic–Oxaloacetic Transaminase (SGOT)

AST is an enzyme present in tissues of high metabolic activity; decreasing concentrations of AST are found in the heart, liver, skeletal muscle, kidney, brain, pancreas, spleen, and lungs. The enzyme is released into the circulation following the injury or death of cells. Any disease that causes change in these highly metabolic tissues will result in a rise in AST levels. The amount of AST in the blood is directly related to the number of damaged cells and the amount of time that passes between injury to the tissue and the test. Following severe cell damage, the blood AST level will rise in 12 hours and remain elevated for about 5 days.

This test is used to evaluate liver and heart disease. The ALT is usually ordered along with the AST.

Normal Findings

Men: 14 to 20 U/L or 0.23 to 0.33 μkat/L
Women: 10 to 36 U/L or 0.17 to 0.60 μkat/L
Newborns: 47 to 150 U/L or 0.78 to 2.5 μkat/L
Children: 9 to 80 U/L or 0.15 to 1.3 μkat/L

Normal values vary widely according to method of testing; check with your laboratory for reference values.

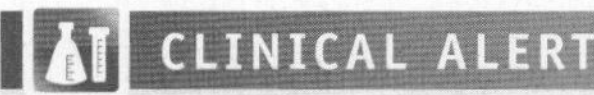

Critical Value
AST is extremely high (>20,000 U/L; >333 μkat/L) in alcohol–acetaminophen syndrome.
AST > ALT, prothrombin time: 100 s
Creatinine: >34 mg/L or >0.30 mmol/L

Procedure

1. Obtain a 5-mL venous sample (red-topped tube). Serum is used. Observe standard precautions. Label the specimen with the patient's name, date and time of collection, and test(s) ordered. Place the specimen in a biohazard bag.
2. Avoid hemolysis.

Clinical Implications

1. *Increased AST levels* occur in MI.
   a. In MI, the AST level may be increased to 4 to 10 times the normal values.
   b. The AST level reaches a peak in 24 hours and returns to normal by post-MI days 3 to 7. Secondary rises in AST levels suggest extension or recurrence of MI.
   c. The AST curve in MI parallels that of creatinine phosphokinase (CPK).
2. *Increased AST levels* occur in liver diseases (10 to 100 times normal).
   a. Acute hepatitis and chronic hepatitis (ALT > AST)
   b. Active cirrhosis (drug induced; alcohol induced: AST > ALT)
   c. Infectious mononucleosis
   d. Hepatic necrosis and metastasis
   e. Primary or metastatic carcinoma
   f. Alcoholic hepatitis
   g. Reye's syndrome

3. Other diseases associate with *elevated AST levels* include the following:
   a. Hypothyroidism
   b. Trauma and irradiation of skeletal muscle
   c. Dermatomyositis
   d. Polymyositis
   e. Toxic shock syndrome
   f. Cardiac catheterization
   g. Recent brain trauma with brain necrosis, cerebral infarction
   h. Crushing and traumatic injuries, head trauma, surgery
   i. Progressive muscular dystrophy (Duchenne's)
   j. Pulmonary emboli, lung infarction
   k. Gangrene
   l. Malignant hyperthermia, heat angiography
   m. Mushroom poisoning
   n. Shock
   o. Hemolytic anemia, exhaustion, heat stroke
4. *Decreased AST levels* occur in the following conditions:
   a. Azotemia
   b. Chronic renal dialysis
   c. Vitamin B_6 deficiency

Interfering Factors

1. Slight decreases occur during pregnancy, when there is abnormal metabolism of pyridoxine.
2. Many drugs can cause elevated or decreased levels (see Appendix E). Alcohol ingestion affects results.
3. Exercise and IM injections do not affect results.
4. False decreases occur in diabetic ketoacidosis, severe liver disease, and uremia.
5. Gross hemolysis causes falsely high levels.

Interventions

Pretest Patient Care

1. Explain test purpose and blood-drawing procedure.
2. Follow guidelines in Chapter 1 for safe, effective, informed *pretest* care.

Posttest Patient Care

1. Review test results; report and record findings. Modify the nursing care plan as needed. Monitor appropriately for heart and liver diseases.
2. Ensure that unexplained AST elevations are further investigated with ALT and GGT tests.
3. Follow guidelines in Chapter 1 for safe, effective, informed *posttest* care.

● Cardiac Troponin T (cTnT); Troponin I (cTnI)

Cardiac troponin is unique to the heart muscle and is highly concentrated in cardiomyocytes. These isoforms show a high degree of cardiac specificity. This protein is released with very small areas of myocardial damage as early as 1 to 3 hours after injury, and levels return to normal within 5 to 7 days. Troponin I (binds to myofilaments of the troponin complex and has an *inhibitory* character) remains increased longer than creatinine kinase-MB (CK-MB) and is more cardiac specific. Troponin T (binds to tropomyosin of the troponin complex) is more sensitive but less specific, being positive with angina at rest. These tests are becoming the most important addition to the clinical assessment of cardiac injury. Cardiac troponin is the preferred test to diagnose MI.

TABLE 6.11 Cardiac Markers

Markers	Time of Initial Elevation	Time of Peak Elevation	Time to Return to Normal
CK-MB	4–8 hr	12–24 hr	72–96 hr
Myoglobin	2–4 hr	8–10 hr	24 hr
Troponin I (cTnI)	4–6 hr	12 hr	3–10 d
Troponin T (cTnT)	4–8 hr	12–48 hr	7–10 d

This test is used in the early diagnosis of small myocardial infarcts that are undetectable by conventional diagnostic methods. Cardiac troponin levels are also used later in the course of MI because they remain elevated for 5 to 7 days after injury. A single sample may be misleading; therefore, serial sampling 0, 4, 8, and 12 hours after chest pains may be ordered to rule out acute MI. See Table 6.11 for a list of cardiac markers.

Normal Findings

Negative (Qualitative)
Reference decision limit is typically >99th percentile cutoff of assay.
Troponin I: <0.12 ng/mL or <0.12 μg/L
Troponin T: <0.01 ng/mL or <0.01 μg/L
Total CK: 0 to 120 ng/mL or 0 to 120 μg/L
CK-MB: 0 to 3 ng/mL or 0 to 3 μg/L
CK index: 0 to 3
Myoglobin: <55 ng/mL or <55 μg/L

Values will vary depending on the testing method used. Check with your laboratory for reference values.

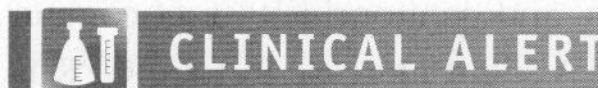

Critical Value

Troponin I: >1.5 ng/mL or >1.5 μg/L

Procedure

1. Obtain a 5-mL venous blood sample in a red-topped tube within hours after onset of chest pain. Observe standard precautions. Label the specimen with the patient's name, date and time of collection, and test(s) ordered. Place the specimen in a biohazard bag.
2. If serial samples are ordered, record date and time of sampling.

Clinical Implications

1. Positive or elevated cTnI levels indicate:
   a. Small infarcts; increases remain for 5 to 7 days.
   b. Myocardial injury during surgery
2. Positive or elevated cardiac troponin T (cTnT) indicates:
   a. Acute MI
   b. Perisurgical MI
   c. Unstable angina

d. Myocarditis
e. Some noncardiac events
   (1) Chronic renal failure
   (2) Acute trauma involving muscle
   (3) Rhabdomyolysis, polymyositis, dermatomyositis

Interfering Factors

1. cTnI levels may be increased in chronic muscle or renal disease and trauma.
2. Levels are not affected by orthopedic or lung surgery.

Interventions

Pretest Patient Care

1. Explain that the test is a sensitive marker for minor myocardial injury in unstable angina.
2. Follow guidelines in Chapter 1 for safe, effective, informed *pretest* care.

Posttest Patient Care

1. Review test results; report and record findings. Modify the nursing care plan as needed. Additional testing may be necessary (e.g., cardiac myosin light classes, glycogen phosphorylcholine BB [GPBB]).
2. Follow guidelines in Chapter 1 for safe, effective, informed *posttest* care.

● Creatine Phosphokinase (CPK); Creatine Kinase (CK); CPK and CK Isoenzymes

Creatine kinase (CPK/CK) is an enzyme found in higher concentrations in the heart and skeletal muscles and in much smaller concentrations in brain tissue. Because CK exists in relatively few organs, this test is used as a specific index of injury to myocardium and muscle. CPK can be divided into three isoenzymes: MM or CK_3, BB or CK_1, and MB or CK_2. CK-MM is the isoenzyme that constitutes almost all the circulatory enzymes in healthy persons. Skeletal muscle contains primarily MM; cardiac muscle contains primarily MM and MB; and brain tissue, GI system, and genitourinary tract contain primarily BB. Normal CK levels are virtually 100% MM isoenzyme. A slight increase in total CPK is reflected from elevated BB from CNS injury. CPK isoenzyme studies help distinguish whether the CPK originated from the heart (MB) or the skeletal muscle (MM).

The CK (CPK) test is used in the diagnosis of MI and as a reliable measure of skeletal and inflammatory muscle diseases. CK levels can prove helpful in recognizing muscular dystrophy before clinical signs appear. CK levels may rise significantly with CNS disorders such as Reye's syndrome. The determination of CK isoenzymes may be helpful in making a differential diagnosis. Elevation of MB, the cardiac isoenzyme, provides a more definitive indication of myocardial cell damage than total CK alone. MM isoenzyme is an indicator of skeletal muscle damage. Newer tests, such as CK isoforms, allow for earlier detection of MI than is possible with CK-MB.

Normal Findings

Men: 38 to 174 U/L (0.63 to 2.90 μkat/L)
Women: 26 to 140 U/L (0.46 to 2.38 μkat/L)
Infants: 2 to 3 times adult values
Isoenzymes
MM (CK_3): 96% to 100% or 0.96 to 1.00
MB (CK_2): 0% to 6% or 0.00 to 0.06
BB (CK_1): 0% or 0.00

NOTE *Normal values may vary with method of testing and reaction temperature. Check with your laboratory.*

NOTE *Healthy African Americans have higher CK levels than do Caucasian and Hispanic persons.*

Procedure

1. Obtain a 5-mL venous blood sample (red-topped tube). Serum must be used.
2. Observe standard precautions. Label the specimen with the patient's name, date and time of collection, and test(s) ordered. Place the specimen in a biohazard bag.
3. If a patient has been receiving multiple IM injections, note this fact on the laboratory requisition.
4. Avoid hemolysis.

Clinical Implications

1. Total CK Levels
   a. *Increased CK/CPK levels* occur in the following conditions:
      (1) Acute MI
         (a) With MI, the rise starts soon after an attack (about 4 to 6 hours) and reaches a peak of at least several times normal within 24 hours. CK returns to normal in 48 to 72 hours.
         (b) CK and CK-MB (CK_2) peak about 1 day after onset, as does AST.
         (c) CK-MB and total CK classically increase with acute MI. CK-MB increase, both in percentage and in absolutely (each isoenzyme percentage times the respective total enzyme), peak, and then decrease.
      (2) Severe myocarditis
      (3) After open heart surgery
      (4) Cardioversion (cardiac defibrillation)
      (5) Myocarditis
   b. Other diseases and procedures that cause increased CK/CPK levels include the following:
      (1) Acute cerebrovascular disease
      (2) Progressive muscular dystrophy (levels may reach 20 to 200 times normal), Duchenne's muscular dystrophy, female carriers of muscular dystrophy
      (3) Dermatomyositis and polymyositis
      (4) Delirium tremens and chronic alcoholism
      (5) Electric shock, electromyography
      (6) Malignant hyperthermia
      (7) Reye's syndrome
      (8) Convulsions, ischemia, or subarachnoid hemorrhage
      (9) Last weeks of pregnancy and during childbirth
      (10) Hypothyroidism
      (11) Acute psychosis
      (12) CNS trauma, extensive brain infarction
      (13) Neoplasms of prostate, bladder, or GI tract
      (14) Rhabdomyolysis with cocaine intoxication
      (15) Eosinophilia–myalgia syndrome
   c. Normal values are found in myasthenia gravis and multiple sclerosis.
   d. Decreased values have no diagnostic meaning and may be caused by low muscle mass and bed rest (overnight values can drop 20%).

2. CK isoenzymes
    a. *Elevated MB (CK_2) isoenzyme levels* occur in the following conditions:
        (1) Myocardial infarct (rises 4 to 6 hours after MI; not demonstrable after 24 to 36 hours; i.e., peak with rapid fall)
        (2) Myocardial ischemia, angina pectoris
        (3) Duchenne's muscular dystrophy
        (4) Subarachnoid hemorrhage
        (5) Reye's syndrome
        (6) Muscle trauma, surgery (postoperative)
        (7) Circulatory failure and shock
        (8) Infections of heart—myocarditis
        (9) Chronic renal failure
        (10) Malignant hyperthermia, hypothermia
        (11) CO poisoning
        (12) Polymyositis
        (13) Myoglobulinemia
        (14) Rocky Mountain spotted fever
    b. BB (CK_1) elevations occur in the following conditions:
        (1) Reye's syndrome
        (2) Some breast, bladder, lung, uterus, testis, and prostate cancers
        (3) Severe shock syndrome
        (4) Brain injury, neurosurgery
        (5) Hypothermia
        (6) Following coronary bypass surgery
        (7) Newborns
    c. MM (CK_3) is elevated in most conditions in which total CK is elevated.
    d. MB (CK_2) is not elevated:
        (1) Exercise (total elevated)
        (2) IM injections (total elevated)
        (3) Strokes, cerebrovascular accident, and other brain disorders in which total CK is elevated
        (4) Pericarditis
        (5) Pneumonia, other lung diseases; pulmonary embolism
        (6) Seizures (CK total may be very high)

CLINICAL ALERT

1. After an MI, MB appears in the serum in 6–12 hr and remains for about 18–32 hr. The finding of MB in a patient with chest pain is diagnostic of MI. In addition, if there is a negative CK-MB for ≥48 hr following a clearly defined episode, it is clear that the patient has not had an MI.
2. CK-MB and total CK classically increase with acute MI. CK-MB and the lactate dehydrogenase isoenzyme LD_1 increase both in percentage and absolutely (each isoenzyme percentage times the respective total enzyme), peak, and then decrease.

Interfering Factors

1. Strenuous exercise, weight lifting, and surgical procedures that damage skeletal muscle may cause increased levels of CK.
2. Alcohol and other drugs of abuse increase CK levels.

3. Athletes have a higher CK value because of greater muscle mass.
4. Multiple IM injections may cause increased or decreased CK levels (see Appendix E).
5. Many drugs may cause increased CK levels.
6. Childbirth may cause increased CK levels.
7. Hemolysis of blood sample causes increased CK levels.

Interventions

Pretest Patient Care

1. Explain test purpose and need for at least three consecutive blood draws following episode.
2. Note on requisition when suspected cardiac episode occurred and dates and times of blood draws.
3. Do not allow exercise before test.
4. Follow guidelines in Chapter 1 for safe, effective, informed *pretest* care.

Posttest Patient Care

1. Have patient resume normal activities.
2. Review test results; report and record findings. Modify the nursing care plan as needed. Monitor as appropriate for MI, muscular dystrophy, and other causes of abnormal test outcomes.
3. High levels of CK/CK-MB may suggest other tests should be done to support diagnosis of acute MI:
   a. Total leukocyte count and differential
   b. Cardiac troponin
   c. Myoglobin
4. Follow guidelines in Chapter 1 for safe, effective, informed *posttest* care.

● Galactose-1-Phosphate Uridyltransferase (GPT); Galactokinase; Galactose-1-Phosphate

The enzyme galactose-1-phosphate uridyltransferase (GPT) is needed in the use of galactose-1-phosphate so that it does not accumulate in the body. A very rare genetic disorder resulting from an inborn (inherited or acquired during intrauterine development) error of galactose metabolism may occur.

This measurement is used to identify galactose defects, which can result in widespread tissue damage and abnormalities such as cataracts, liver disease, and renal disease. It also causes failure to thrive and mental retardation. The screening test should be done immediately to enable diet treatment if testing is positive.

Normal Findings

GPT: 18.5 to 28.5 U/g of hemoglobin (Hb) or 1.19 to 1.84 mU/mol Hb
Galactose-1-phosphate (dried blood spot-screening): <0.74 mmol/L
Galactokinase
Children 0 to 2 years: 11 to 150 mU/g Hb or 183 to 2500 pkat/g Hb
Children 2 to 18 years: 11 to 54 mU/g Hb or 183 to 900 pkat/g Hb
Adults: 12 to 40 mU/g Hb or 200 to 667 pkat/g Hb

Procedure

1. Obtain a 5-mL venous blood sample.
2. Anticoagulate with heparin.
3. Observe standard precautions. Label the specimen with the patient's name, date and time of collection, and test(s) ordered. Place the specimen in a biohazard bag.

Clinical Implications

Decreased values are associated with galactosemia, a rare genetic disorder transmitted in an autosomal recessive fashion. The resulting accumulation of galactitol or galactose-1-phosphate can result in juvenile cataracts, liver failure, failure to thrive, and mental retardation in persons with GTP deficiency.

Interventions

Pretest Patient Care

1. Explain test purpose and procedure. Genetic counseling may be necessary.
2. Follow guidelines in Chapter 1 for safe, effective, informed *pretest* care.

Posttest Patient Care

1. Review test results; report and record findings. Modify the nursing care plan as needed. See newborn screening in Chapter 11.
2. Instruct parents of infants and children with positive test results that the disease can be effectively treated by removing galactose-containing foods, especially milk, from the diet. With dietary galactose restriction, liver and lens changes are reversible.
3. Follow guidelines in Chapter 1 for safe, effective, informed *posttest* care.

● Lactate Dehydrogenase (LD, LDH)

Lactate dehydrogenase (LDH) is an intracellular enzyme that is widely distributed in the tissues of the body, particularly in the kidney, heart, skeletal muscle, brain, liver, and lungs. Increases in the reported value usually indicate cellular death and leakage of the enzyme from the cell.

Although elevated levels of LDH are nonspecific, this test is useful in confirming pulmonary infarction when viewed in relation to other test findings. LDH level is also helpful in the differential diagnosis of muscular dystrophy and pernicious anemia. More specific findings may be found by breaking down the LDH into its five isoenzymes. (When LD values are reported or quoted, *total* LDH is meant.)

Normal Findings

Newborn: 160 to 450 U/L or 2.67 to 7.52 μkat/L
Children: 60 to 170 U/L or 1.00 to 2.84 μkat/L
Adults: 140 to 280 U/L or 2.34 to 4.68 μkat/L

Normal values vary with method of testing. Check with your laboratory for reference values.

Procedure

1. Obtain a 5-mL venous blood sample (red-topped tube). Serum is used. Observe standard precautions.
2. Avoid hemolysis in obtaining blood sample. Label the specimen with the patient's name, date and time of collection, and test(s) ordered. Place the specimen in a biohazard bag.

Clinical Implications

1. *Increased LDH (LD)* occurs in the following conditions:
   a. High levels occur within 36 to 55 hours after MI and continue longer than elevations of serum glutamic–oxaloacetic transaminase (SGOT) or CPK (3 to 10 days). Differential diagnosis of acute MI may be accomplished without LDH isoenzymes.
   b. In pulmonary infarction, increased LDH occurs within 24 hours of pain onset. The pattern of normal SGOT and elevated LDH that levels off 1 to 2 days after an episode of chest pain is indicative of pulmonary infarction.

c. *Elevated levels of LDH* are also observed in various other conditions:
    (1) Congestive heart failure
    (2) Liver diseases (e.g., cirrhosis, alcoholism, acute viral hepatitis)
    (3) Malignant neoplasms, cancer, leukemias, lymphoma
    (4) Hypothyroidism
    (5) Lung diseases
    (6) Skeletal muscle diseases (muscular dystrophy), muscular damage
    (7) Megaloblastic and pernicious anemias, hemolytic anemia, sickle cell disease
    (8) Delirium tremens, seizures
    (9) Shock, hypoxia, hypotension
    (10) Hyperthermia
    (11) Renal infarct
    (12) CNS diseases
    (13) Acute pancreatitis
    (14) Fractures, other trauma including head injury
    (15) Intestinal obstruction
d. Angina and pericarditis do *not* produce LDH elevations.

2. *Decreased LDH levels* are associated with a good response to cancer therapy.

Interfering Factors

1. Strenuous exercise and the muscular exertion involved in childbirth cause increased LDH levels.
2. Skin diseases can cause falsely increased LDH levels.
3. Hemolysis of RBCs due to freezing, heating, or shaking the blood sample will cause falsely increased LDH levels.
4. Various drugs may cause increased or decreased LDH levels (see Appendix E).

CLINICAL ALERT

LDH is found in nearly every tissue of the body; therefore, elevated levels are of limited diagnostic value by themselves. Differential diagnoses may be accomplished with LD isoenzyme determination.

Interventions

Pretest Patient Care

1. Explain test purpose and blood-drawing procedure. Obtain recent history of MI or pulmonary infarction.
2. Follow guidelines in Chapter 1 for safe, effective, informed *pretest* care.

Posttest Patient Care

1. Resume normal activities.
2. Review test results; report and record findings. Modify the nursing care plan as needed. Monitor for myocardial and pulmonary infarction and other diseases related to abnormal results. LD isoenzymes may be ordered.
3. Follow guidelines in Chapter 1 for safe, effective, informed *posttest* care.

● Lactate Dehydrogenase (LDH, LD) Isoenzymes (Electrophoresis)

Electrophoresis, or separation, of LDH identifies the five isoenzymes of fractions of LDH—each with its own physical characteristics and electrophoretic properties. Fractioning the LDH activity sharpens its diagnostic value because LDH is found in many organs. LD isoenzymes are released into the bloodstream when tissue necrosis occurs. The isoenzymes are elevated in terms of the patterns established, not on the basis of the value of a single isoenzyme. The origins of the LDH isoenzymes are as follow: LD_1 and LD_2 are present in cardiac tissue and erythrocytes; LD_3 originates mainly from lung, spleen, pancreas, and placenta; and LD_4 and LD_5 originate from skeletal muscle and liver.

The five isoenzyme fractions of LDH show different patterns in various disorders. Abnormalities in the pattern suggest which tissues have been damaged. This test is useful in the differential diagnosis of megaloblastic anemia (e.g., folate deficiency, pernicious anemia), hemolytic anemia, and, very occasionally, renal infarct. These entities are characterized by LD_1 increases, often with LD_1:LD_2 inversion (flip).

Normal Findings

LD_1: 17% to 27% of total or 0.17 to 0.27
LD_2: 29% to 39% of total or 0.29 to 0.39
LD_3: 19% to 27% of total or 0.19 to 0.27
LD_4: 8% to 16% of total or 0.08 to 0.16
LD_5: 6% to 16% of total or 0.06 to 0.16

Procedure

1. Obtain a 5-mL venous blood sample (red-topped tube). Serum is needed.
2. Avoid hemolysis.
3. Observe standard precautions. Label the specimen with the patient's name, date and time of collection, and test(s) ordered. Place the specimen in a biohazard bag.

NOTE *Serial determinations may be ordered (3 consecutive days).*

Clinical Implications

1. Abnormal LD_1 and LD_2 patterns reflect damaged tissues (Table 6.12).
   a. The appearance of an LD flip (i.e., when LD_1 level is higher than LD_2 level) is helpful in the diagnosis of hemolytic, megaloblastic, and sickle cell anemia. This is because RBCs have an isoenzyme pattern similar to that of heart muscle. The time elapsed to peak values may help to differentiate these conditions.
2. LD_3 increases occur in advanced cancer and malignant lymphoma; this level should decrease following effective therapy. LD_3 is occasionally elevated in pulmonary infarction or pneumonia.

TABLE 6.12 Abnormal Lactate Dehydrogenase Isoenzyme Patterns

Disease	LD_1	LD_2	LD_3	LD_4	LD_5
Myocardial infarction	X	X			
Pulmonary infarction				X	X
Congestive heart failure				X	X
Viral hepatitis				X	X
Toxic hepatitis				X	X
Leukemia, granulocytic		X	X		
Pancreatitis		X	X		
Carcinomatosis (extensive)		X	X		
Megaloblastic anemia	X	X			
Hemolytic anemia	X	X			
Muscular dystrophy	X	X			

3. LD_5 is *increased* in the following conditions:
   a. Liver disease, hepatitis
   b. Congestive heart failure, pulmonary edema
   c. Striated muscle trauma, burns
4. LD_5 increase is more significant when LD_5/LD_4 ratio is increased.
5. In most cancers, one to three of the bands (LD_2, LD_3, and LD_4) are frequently increased. A notable exception is in seminomas and dysgerminomas, in which LD_1 is increased. Frequently, an increase in LD_3 may be the first indication of the presence of cancer.
6. All LD isoenzymes are increased in systemic diseases (e.g., carcinomatosis, collagen vascular disease, disseminated intravascular coagulation, sepsis) (see Table 6.12).
7. Increased total LD with normal distribution of isoenzymes may be seen in coronary artery disease (CAD) with chronic heart failure, hypothyroidism, infectious mononucleosis and other inflammatory states, uremia, and necrosis.

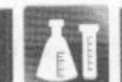

CLINICAL ALERT

LDH isoenzymes should be interpreted in light of clinical findings.

Interventions

Pretest Patient Care

1. Explain test purpose and procedure. Repeat testing on 3 consecutive days is likely. Obtain pertinent clinical signs and symptoms.
2. Follow guidelines in Chapter 1 for safe, effective, informed *pretest* care.

Posttest Patient Care

1. Have patient resume normal activities.
2. Review test results; report and record findings. Modify the nursing care plan as needed. Monitor appropriately for abnormal LD patterns and pulmonary infarction.
3. Follow guidelines in Chapter 1 for safe, effective, informed *posttest* care.

● Renin (Angiotensin); Plasma Renin Angiotensin (PRA)

Renin is an enzyme produced in the kidney that converts angiotensinogen (produced in the liver) to angiotensin I, which is subsequently converted to angiotensin II (in endothelia throughout the body). Angiotensin II is a potent vasopressor agent responsible for hypertension of renal origin and is a powerful releaser of aldosterone from the adrenal cortex. Both angiotensin II and aldosterone increase blood pressure. Renin levels increase when there is decreased renal perfusion pressure. The renin-angiotensin–aldosterone system helps maintain a balance of potassium and sodium blood levels. The renin–aldosterone axis regulates sodium and potassium balance and blood volume and pressure. Renal reabsorption of sodium affects plasma volume. Low plasma volume, low blood pressure, low sodium, and increased potassium induce renin release, causing increased aldosterone through stimulation of angiotensin. Potassium loss, acute blood pressure increases, and increased blood volumes suppress renin release.

This test is most useful in the differential diagnosis of hypertension, whether essential, renal, or renovascular. In primary hyperaldosteronism, the findings will demonstrate that aldosterone secretion is exaggerated and secretion of renin is suppressed. In renal vascular disease, renin is elevated. This test is helpful in identifying renin-producing tumors of the kidney.

Normal Findings

Renin Activity–Plasma Renin Angiotensin (PRA)
Adult (normal-sodium diet):
Supine: 0.2 to 1.6 ng angiotensin I (AI)/mL/h or 0.2 to 1.6 μg AI/h/L
Standing: 0.7 to 3.3 ng AI/mL/h or 0.7 to 3.3 μg AI/h/L
Adult (low-sodium diet):
Supine: renin levels increase 2 times normal
Standing: renin levels increase 6 times normal
Renin Direct
Adult supine: 12 to 79 mU/L or 12 to 79 mU/L
Adult standing: 13 to 114 mU/L or 13 to 114 mU/L

Procedure

1. Obtain a 5-mL venous blood sample (lavender-topped tube). Fasting is required. Collect specimen with scrupulous attention to detail. Use EDTA as the anticoagulant to aid in preservation of any angiotensin formed before examination. Observe standard precautions. Label the specimen with the patient's name, date and time of collection, and test(s) ordered.
2. Draw blood in chilled tubes and place samples on ice. Transport samples to laboratory immediately in a biohazard bag. The sample must be centrifuged in a refrigerated centrifuge.
3. Record posture and dietary status of patient at time of blood drawing.
4. A 24-hour urine sodium should be done concurrently to aid in diagnosis.

Clinical Implications

1. *Increased renin levels* occur in the following conditions:
   a. Secondary aldosteronism with malignant hypertension
   b. Renovascular hypertension
   c. Reduced plasma volume due to low-sodium diet, diuretics, Addison's disease, or hemorrhage
   d. Chronic renal failure
   e. Salt-losing status owing to GI disease (sodium [Na] and potassium [K] wastage)
   f. Renin-producing tumors of kidney
   g. Few patients (15%) with essential hypertension
   h. Bartter's syndrome (high in renin hypertension)
   i. Pheochromocytoma
2. *Decreased renin levels* are found in the following conditions:
   a. Primary aldosteronism
   b. Unilateral renal artery stenosis
   c. Administration of salt-retaining steroids
   d. Congenital adrenal hyperplasia with 17-hydroxylase deficiency
   e. Liddle's syndrome (autosomal dominant disorder resulting in abnormal kidney function and hypertension)

Interfering Factors

1. Levels vary in healthy persons and increase under influences that tend to shrink the intravascular fluid volume.
2. Random specimens may be difficult to interpret unless diet and salt intake of patient are regulated.
3. Values are higher when the patient is in an upright position, when the test is performed early in the day, when the patient is on a low-sodium diet, during pregnancy, and with drugs such as diuretics and antihypertensives and foods such as licorice. See Appendix E for other drugs that affect outcomes.

4. Recently administered radioisotopes interfere with test results.
5. Indomethacin and salicylates decrease renin levels.

Interventions

Pretest Patient Care

1. Explain test purpose and procedure.
2. A regular diet that contains 180 mEq/L (180 mmol/L) of sodium and 100 mEq/L (100 mmol/L) of potassium must be maintained for 3 days before the specimen is obtained. A 24-hour urine sodium and potassium should also be done to evaluate salt balance. The blood test should be drawn at the end of the 24-hour urine test.
3. Instruct the patient that it is necessary to be in a supine position for at least 2 hours before obtaining the specimen. The specimen is drawn with patient in the supine position.
4. Ensure that antihypertensive drugs, cyclic progestogens, estrogens, diuretics, and licorice are terminated at least 2 weeks and preferably 4 weeks before a renin–aldosterone workup.
5. If a standing specimen is ordered, the patient must be standing for 2 hours before testing, and blood should be drawn with the patient in the sitting position.
6. Do not allow caffeine ingestion the morning before or during the test.
7. Follow guidelines in Chapter 1 for safe, effective, informed *pretest* care.

Posttest Patient Care

1. Review test results; report and record findings. Modify the nursing care plan as needed. Counsel appropriately regarding hypertension, further testing, and possible treatment.
2. Have patient resume normal activities.
3. Follow guidelines in Chapter 1 for safe, effective, informed *posttest* care.

● Renin Stimulation/Challenge Test

A challenge test distinguishes primary from secondary hyperaldosteronism on the basis of renin levels. The test is performed with the patient in both the recumbent and upright positions and after the patient has been maintained on a low-salt diet. In normal persons and in those with essential hypertension, renin concentration is increased by the reduction in volume due to sodium restriction and the upright position. In primary aldosteronism, volume depletion does not occur, and renin concentration remains low.

Normal Findings

See challenge test above.

Procedure

1. Admit the patient to the hospital for this test. On admission, obtain and record the patient's weight.
2. Ensure the patient follows a reduced-sodium diet supplemented with potassium for 3 days, along with diuretics (e.g., furosemide, chlorothiazide), as ordered.
3. Weigh patient again on the third day, record data, and ensure that the patient remains upright for 4 hours and participates in normal activities.
4. Obtain a venous heparinized blood sample for renin at 11:00 a.m., when renin is usually at its maximum level. Label the specimen with the patient's name, date and time of collection, and test(s) ordered. Place the specimen on ice and send it immediately to the laboratory in a biohazard bag.

Interpretation of Renin Stimulation Test

In healthy persons and most hypertensive patients, the stimulation of a low-salt diet, a diuretic, and upright posture will raise renin activity to very high levels and result in weight loss. However, in primary aldosteronism, the plasma level is expanded and remains so. In these patients, there is little if any weight loss, and the renin level is very low or undetectable. A response within the normal range can occur in the presence of aldosterone.

Interventions

Pretest Patient Care

1. Explain test purpose and procedure. The purpose of the preparation is to deplete the patient of sodium.
2. Check with individual laboratory for specific practices.
3. Follow guidelines in Chapter 1 for safe, effective, informed *pretest* care.

Posttest Patient Care

1. Resume normal activities.
2. Review test results; report and record findings. Modify the nursing care plan as needed. Counsel appropriately regarding hypertension.
3. Follow guidelines in Chapter 1 for safe, effective, informed *posttest* care.

● Tryptase

Tryptase, an enzyme released from mast cells, is used to help distinguish causes of anaphylaxis or mastocytosis (overproduction of mast cells). This test measures the amount of total tryptase (both the alpha [α] and beta [β] forms) in the blood when mast cells are activated.

Normal Findings

0.4 to 10.9 μg/L (total tryptase)

NOTE *The blood sample should be obtained within 2 hours of suspected event that triggers mast cell activation—for example, allergic immune response.*

Procedure

1. Obtain a 5-mL venous blood sample (serum separator tube).
2. Observe standard precautions. Label the specimen with the patient's name, date and time of collection, and test(s) ordered. Place the specimen in a biohazard bag.

Clinical Implications

Tryptase is increased in:

1. Anaphylaxis and mastocytosis
2. Asthma
3. Myelodysplastic syndrome (bone marrow disorder)
4. Acute myelocytic leukemia
5. End-stage renal failure

Interventions

Pretest Patient Care

1. Explain test purpose and blood-drawing procedure.
2. Follow guidelines in Chapter 1 for safe, effective, informed *pretest* care.

Posttest Patient Care

1. Resume normal activities.
2. Review test results; report and record findings. Modify the nursing care plan as needed.
3. Follow guidelines in Chapter 1 for safe, effective, informed *posttest* care.

● γ-Glutamyltransferase (γ-Glutamyl Transpeptidase, GGT, γGT)

The enzyme γ-glutamyl transpeptidase (γGT) is present mainly in the liver, kidney, and pancreas. Despite the fact that the kidney has the highest level of this enzyme, the liver is considered the source of normal serum activity. γGT has no origin in bone or placenta.

This test is used to determine liver cell dysfunction and to detect alcohol-induced liver disease. Because the GGT is very sensitive to the amount of alcohol consumed by chronic drinkers, it can be used to monitor the cessation or reduction of alcohol consumption in chronic alcoholic patients and early-risk drinkers. GT activity is elevated in all forms of liver disease. This test is much more sensitive than either the ALP test or the transaminase test (i.e., SGOT, serum glutamic-pyruvic transaminase [SGPT]) in detecting obstructive jaundice, cholangitis, and cholecystitis. It is also indicated in the differential diagnosis of liver disease in children and pregnant women who have elevated levels of LDH and ALP. γGT is also useful as a marker for prostatic cancer and hepatic metastasis from breast and colon cancer.

Normal Findings

Men: 7 to 47 U/L (0.12 to 1.80 μkat/L)
Women: 5 to 25 U/L (0.08 to 0.42 μkat/L)

Values are higher in newborns and in the first 3 to 6 months. Values in adult males are 25% higher than in females. Values vary with method (check with your laboratory).

Procedure

1. Obtain a 5-mL venous blood sample. Serum is used.
2. Observe standard precautions. Label the specimen with the patient's name, date and time of collection, and test(s) ordered. Place the specimen in a biohazard bag.

Clinical Implications

1. *Increased γGT levels* are associated with the following conditions:
   a. Liver diseases
      (1) Hepatitis (acute and chronic)
      (2) Cirrhosis (obstructive and familial)
      (3) Liver metastasis and carcinoma
      (4) Cholestasis (especially during or following pregnancy)
      (5) Chronic alcoholic liver disease, alcoholism
      (6) Infectious mononucleosis
   b. γGT levels are also increased in the following conditions:
      (1) Pancreatitis
      (2) Carcinoma of prostate
      (3) Carcinoma of breast and lung
      (4) Systemic lupus erythematosus
      (5) Glycogen storage disease
   c. In MI, γGT is usually normal. However, if there is an increase, it occurs about 4 days after MI and probably implies liver damage secondary to cardiac insufficiency.
   d. Hyperthyroidism
2. *Decreased γGT levels* are found in hypothyroidism.
3. γGT values are normal in bone disorders, bone growth, pregnancy, skeletal muscle disease, strenuous exercise, and renal failure. Children and adolescents are normal.

Interfering Factors

1. Various drugs (e.g., phenothiazines, barbiturates) affect test outcomes (see Appendix E).
2. Alcohol (ethanol)

Interventions

Pretest Patient Care

1. Explain test purpose and blood-drawing procedure. No alcohol is allowed before the test.
2. Follow guidelines in Chapter 1 for safe, effective, informed *pretest* care.

Posttest Patient Care

1. Resume normal activities.
2. Review test results; report and record findings. Modify the nursing care plan as needed. Monitor as appropriate for liver, pancreatic, or thyroid disease and cancer recurrence.
3. Follow guidelines in Chapter 1 for safe, effective, informed *posttest* care.

● Homocysteine (tHcy)

Homocysteine (tHcy) is an amino acid resulting from the synthesis of cysteine from methionine and enzyme reaction of cobalamin and folate. Large quantities of homocysteine are excreted and assimilated in the blood plasma of patients with homocystinemia associated with:

1. Increased risk for vascular disease
2. Increased risk for venous thrombosis
3. Elevated homocysteine with a direct toxic effect on endothelium
4. Elevated in folic acid deficiency and vitamin B_{12} deficiency. Folic acid deficiency is characterized by elevated plasma homocysteine; folic acid supplementation reduces plasma homocysteine. Elevated plasma homocysteine levels due to aberrant vitamin B_{12} respond favorably to vitamin B_{12} supplementation.
5. Increased risk for pregnancy complications and neural tube defects

This test measures the blood plasma level of homocysteine. It is useful for diagnosing individuals with potential increased risk factors for CAD and thromboses, for providing a functional assay for folic acid deficiency, and for diagnosing homocystinemia. Homocysteine is retained by persons with reduced renal function. See Chart 6.3 for testing guidelines.

CHART 6.3 Homocysteine Testing

Reasons to Test for Homocysteine

Unexplained anemia
Peripheral neuropathy or myelopathy
Recurrent spontaneous abortions or infertility
Delayed development or failure to thrive in infants

Whom to Test

Older adults (>75 yr of age)
Vegetarians who are not taking vitamin B_{12} supplement
Patients using drugs that interfere with folate status (e.g., antiepileptics, methotrexate)

How Often to Test

Measured every 3–5 yr
In newborns at 3–5 d

tHcy in Coronary Vascular Disease

In patients <40 yr of age who have coronary vascular disease to exclude homocystinuria
In patients who are at high risk for coronary vascular disease (every 3–5 yr)

Source: Clinical Laboratory News, 2002.

Normal Findings

4 to 17 μmol/L or 0.54 to 2.30 mg/L for fasting specimens

Procedure

1. Obtain a venous blood sample (red-topped tube). Serum or heparinized plasma is needed. Fasting is necessary.
2. Observe standard precautions. Label the specimen with the patient's name, date and time of collection, and test(s) ordered. Place the specimen in a biohazard bag.
3. Place on ice immediately after drawing. Centrifuge immediately and freeze within 1 hour of collection.

Clinical Implications

Increased or elevated homocysteine levels occur in the following conditions:

1. Folic acid deficiency
2. Abnormal vitamin B_{12} metabolism and deficiency
3. Homocystinuria

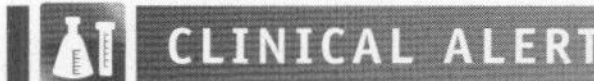

Homocysteine values and their relation to CAD are still being investigated. The methionine load test is also currently investigative and has not yet been approved as a routine test.

Interfering Factors

1. Penicillamine reduces plasma levels of homocysteine.
2. Nitrous oxide, methotrexate deficiency, and azauridine increase plasma levels of homocysteine.

Interventions

Pretest Patient Care

1. Explain test purpose and blood-drawing procedure.
2. The test requires fasting.
3. Evaluate renal function in patients with homocystinuria.
4. Follow guidelines in Chapter 1 for safe, effective, informed *pretest* care.

Posttest Patient Care

1. Allow the patient to eat and drink after blood is drawn.
2. Review test results; report and record findings. Modify the nursing care plan as needed.
3. Evaluate for other cardiovascular risk factors, compare test results, and monitor appropriately. Promote lifestyle changes accordingly.
4. Monitor for folic acid or vitamin B_{12} deficiency and provide supplements as needed.
5. Follow guidelines in Chapter 1 for safe, effective, informed *posttest* care.

● α_1-Antitrypsin (AAT)

α_1-Antitrypsin (AAT) is a protein produced by the liver that inhibits the protease released into body fluids by dying cells. This protein deficiency is associated with pulmonary emphysema and liver disease, both at an early age. Human serum contains at least three inhibitors of protease. Two of the best known are AAT and α_2-macroglobulin. Total antitrypsin levels in blood are composed of about 90% AAT and 10% α_2-macroglobulins.

This is a nonspecific method to diagnose inflammation, severe infection, and necrosis. AAT measurement is important for diagnosing respiratory disease and cirrhosis of the liver because of its direct relation to pulmonary and other metabolic disorders. Pulmonary problems such as emphysema occur when antitrypsin-deficient persons are unable to ward off the action of endoproteases. Those who are deficient in AAT develop emphysema at a much earlier age than do other emphysema patients.

Normal Findings (by Rate Nephelometry)

Adults: 110 to 200 mg/dL or 1.1 to 2.0 g/L
If result is <125 mg/dL (<1.25 g/L), phenotype should be determined to confirm homozygous and heterozygous deficiencies.
Newborn: 145 to 270 mg/dL or 1.45 to 2.70 g/L

Procedure

1. Obtain a 7-mL serum sample. Use a red-topped tube.
2. Observe standard precautions. Label the specimen with the patient's name, date and time of collection, and test(s) ordered. Place the specimen in a biohazard bag.

Clinical Implications

1. Interpretation of AAT levels is based on the following:
   a. High levels are generally found in normal persons.
   b. Intermediate levels are found in persons with a predisposition to pulmonary emphysema.
   c. Low levels are found in persons with obstructive pulmonary disease and in children with cirrhosis of the liver.
2. *Increased AAT levels* occur in the following conditions:
   a. Acute and chronic inflammatory disorders
   b. After injections of typhoid vaccine
   c. Cancer
   d. Thyroid infections
   e. Oral contraceptive use
   f. Stress syndrome
   g. Hematologic abnormalities
3. *Decreased AAT levels* are associated with these progressive diseases:
   a. Adult, early-onset, chronic pulmonary emphysema
   b. Liver cirrhosis in infants (neonatal hepatitis)
   c. Pulmonary disease
   d. Severe hepatic damage
   e. Nephrotic syndrome
   f. Malnutrition

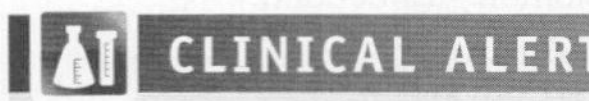

CLINICAL ALERT

Patients with serum levels <70 mg/dL (<0.70 g/L) are likely to have a homozygous deficiency and are at risk for early lung disease.

Interfering Factors

AAT in an acute-phase reactant and any inflammatory process will elevate serum levels.

Interventions

Pretest Patient Care

1. Explain test purpose and procedure. Fasting is required if the patient's history shows elevated cholesterol or triglyceride levels.
2. Follow guidelines in Chapter 1 for safe, effective, informed *pretest* care.

Posttest Patient Care

1. Review test results; report and record findings. Modify the nursing care plan as needed. Advise patients with decreased levels to avoid smoking and, if possible, occupational hazards such as dust, fumes, and other respiratory pollutants.
2. Because AAT deficiencies are inherited, genetic counseling may be indicated. Follow-up AAT phenotype testing can be performed on family members to determine the homozygous or heterozygous nature of the deficiency.
3. Follow guidelines in Chapter 1 for safe, effective, informed *posttest* care.

LIPOPROTEIN TESTS/LIPOPROTEIN PROFILES

Lipoprotein measurements are diagnostic indicators for hyperlipidemia and hypolipidemia. Hyperlipidemia is classified as types I, IIa, IIb, III, IV, and V. Lipids are fatty substances made up of cholesterol, cholesterol esters (liquid compounds), triglycerides, nonesterized fatty acids, and phospholipids. Lipoproteins are unique plasma proteins that transport otherwise insoluble lipids. They are categorized as chylomicrons, β-lipoproteins (low-density lipoproteins [LDLs]), pre-β-lipoproteins (very-low-density lipoproteins [VLDLs]), and α-lipoproteins (high-density lipoproteins [HDLs]). Apolipoprotein A is mainly composed of HDL, chylomicrons, and VLDL. Apolipoprotein B is the main component of LDL. Lipids provide energy for metabolism, serve as precursors of steroid hormones (adrenals, ovaries, testes) and bile acids, and play an important role in cell membrane development. A lipid profile usually includes cholesterol, triglycerides, LDL, and HDL levels.

● Cholesterol (C)

Cholesterol (C) testing evaluates the risk for arthrosclerosis, myocardial occlusion, and coronary arterial occlusion. Cholesterol relates to coronary heart disease (CHD) and is an important screening test for heart disease. It is part of the lipid profile to measure total cholesterol, "bad" cholesterol (LDL-C), good cholesterol (HDL-C), and triglyceride levels. Elevated cholesterol levels are a major component in the hereditary hyperlipoproteinemias. Cholesterol determinations are also frequently a part of thyroid function, liver function, renal function, and diabetes mellitus studies. It is also used to monitor effectiveness of diet, medications, lifestyle changes (e.g., exercise), and stress management.

Normal Findings

Normal values vary with age, diet, gender, and geographic or cultural region.

Adults, fasting:

Desirable level: 140 to 199 mg/dL or 3.63 to 5.15 mmol/L

Borderline high: 200 to 239 mg/dL or 5.18 to 6.19 mmol/L

High: >240 mg/dL or >6.20 mmol/L

Children and adolescents (12 to 18 years):

Desirable level: <170 mg/dL or <4.39 mmol/L

Borderline high: 170 to 199 mg/dL or 4.40 to 5.16 mmol/L

High: >200 mg/dL or >5.18 mmol/L

Procedure

1. Obtain a 5-mL venous blood sample (red-topped tube). Fasting is required. Serum is needed.
2. Observe standard precautions. Label the specimen with the patient's name, date and time of collection, and test(s) ordered. Place the specimen in a biohazard bag.

Clinical Implications

1. Total blood cholesterol levels are the basis for classifying CHD risk.
   a. Levels >240 mg/dL or >6.20 mmol/L are considered high and should include follow-up lipoprotein analysis. Borderline high levels (200 to 239 mg/dL or 5.18 to 6.19 mmol/L) in the presence of CHD or two other CHD risk factors should also include lipoprotein analysis/profiles.
   b. CHD risk factors include male gender, family history, premature CHD (MI or sudden death before age 55 years in a parent or sibling), smoking (>10 cigarettes per day), hypertension, low HDL-C levels (<35 mg/dL or <0.91 mmol/L confirmed by repeat measurement), diabetes mellitus, history of definite cerebrovascular or occlusive peripheral vascular disease, and severe obesity (>30% overweight).
   c. In public screening programs, all patients with cholesterol levels >200 mg/dL or >5.18 mmol/L should be referred to their healthcare providers for further evaluation. Before initiating any therapy, the level should be retested.
2. *Elevated cholesterol levels (hypercholesterolemia)* occur in the following conditions:
   a. Type II familial hypercholesterolemia
   b. Hyperlipoproteinemia types I, IV, and V
   c. Cholestasis
   d. Hepatocellular disease, biliary cirrhosis
   e. Nephrotic syndrome, glomerulonephritis
   f. Chronic renal failure
   g. Pancreatic and prostatic malignant neoplasms
   h. Hypothyroidism
   i. Poorly controlled diabetes mellitus
   j. Alcoholism
   k. Glycogen storage disease (von Gierke's disease)
   l. Werner's syndrome (premature aging; affects 1 in 200,000 in the United States)
   m. Diet high in cholesterol and fats ("dietary affluence")
   n. Obesity
3. *Decreased cholesterol levels (hypocholesterolemia)* occur in the following conditions:
   a. Hypo-α-lipoproteinemia
   b. Severe hepatocellular disease
   c. Myeloproliferative diseases
   d. Hyperthyroidism
   e. Malabsorption syndrome, malnutrition
   f. Megaloblastic or sideroblastic anemia (chronic anemias)
   g. Severe burns, inflammation
   h. Conditions of acute illness, infection
   i. Chronic obstructive lung disease
   j. Mental retardation

Interfering Factors

1. Pregnancy increases cholesterol levels.
2. Certain drugs increase cholesterol levels (oral contraceptives, epinephrine, phenothiazines, vitamins A and D, phenytoin, ACTH, anabolic steroids, β-adrenergic blocking agents, sulfonamides, and thiazide diuretics.

3. Certain drugs decrease cholesterol levels (thyroxine, estrogens, androgens, aspirin, antibiotics (tetracycline and neomycin), nicotinic acid, heparin, colchicine, monoamine oxidase inhibitors, allopurinol, and bile salts.
4. Seasonal variations in cholesterol levels have been observed; levels are higher in fall and winter and lower in spring and summer.
5. Positional variations occur; levels are lower when sitting versus standing and lower when recumbent versus sitting.
6. Plasma (EDTA) values are 10% lower than serum.

Interventions

Pretest Patient Care

1. Explain test purpose and procedure. An overnight fast before testing is recommended, although nonfasting specimens may be taken. Pretest, a normal diet should be consumed for 7 days. The patient should abstain from alcohol for 48 hours before testing. Prolonged fasting with ketosis increases values.
2. Document drugs the patient is taking.
3. Encourage the patient to relax.
4. Follow guidelines in Chapter 1 for safe, effective, informed *pretest* care.

Posttest Patient Care

1. Review test results; report and record findings. Modify the nursing care plan as needed. Cholesterol levels are influenced by heredity, diet, body weight, and physical activity. Some lifestyle changes may be necessary to reduce elevated levels (Chart 6.4).
2. Cholesterol levels >200 mg/dL (or >5.18 mmol/L) should be retested and the results averaged. If the two results differ by >10%, a third test should be done.
3. Once hyperlipidemia has been established, the diet should be lower in animal fats and should replace saturated fats with polyunsaturated fats. Fruits, vegetables (especially greens), and whole-grain products should be increased. Patients with diabetes, as well as others, should seek counsel from a dietitian regarding diet management if necessary. Therapy for hyperlipidemia should always begin with diet modification.
4. The American Heart Association and National Cholesterol Education Program have excellent resources for providing diet and lifestyle management information.
5. At least 6 months of dietary therapy should be tried before initiating cholesterol-reducing drug therapy.
6. Perform a comprehensive lipoprotein analysis if cholesterol levels are not lowered within 6 months after start of therapy.

CLINICAL ALERT

1. Cholesterol measurement should not be done immediately after MI. A 3-mo wait is suggested.
2. Cholesterol >300 mg/dL or >7.8 mmol/L: There is a strong relationship to CHD, but only a fraction of those with CAD have increased cholesterol.

CHART 6.4 Recommendations by the American Heart Association to Lower the Risk for Cardiovascular Disease in Women

- 60–90 min of moderate intensity physical activity most, if not all, days of the week
- Nicotine replacement and other therapy to quit smoking
- Less than 7% daily saturated fat intake of all calories
- Consume oily fish at least twice per week
- Low-dose aspirin therapy should be considered at age 65 or older
- Reduce LDL-C <70 mg/dL or <1.8 mmol/L in very high-risk women

High-Density Lipoprotein Cholesterol (HDL-C)

HDL-C is a class of lipoproteins produced by the liver and intestines. HDL is composed of phospholipids and one or two apolipoproteins. It plays a role in the metabolism of the other lipoproteins and in cholesterol transport from peripheral tissues to the liver. LDL and HDL may combine to maintain cellular cholesterol balance through the mechanism of LDL moving cholesterol into the arteries and HDL removing it from the arteries. Decreased HDL levels are atherogenic, whereas elevated HDL levels protect against arthrosclerosis by removing cholesterol from vessel walls and transporting it to the liver where it is removed from the body. This is known as the "reverse cholesterol transport pathway." There is a strong relationship between HDL-C and CAD.

HDL-C, the good cholesterol, is used to assess CAD risk and monitor persons with known low HDL levels. HDL-C levels are inversely proportional to CHD risk and are a primary independent risk factor. When a slightly increased cholesterol is due to high HDL, therapy is not indicated.

Normal Findings

Men: 35 to 65 mg/dL or 0.91 to 1.68 mmol/L
Women: 35 to 80 mg/dL or 0.91 to 2.07 mmol/L
<25 mg/dL or <0.65 mmol/L of HDL: CHD risk at dangerous level: 2 times the risk
26 to 35 mg/dL or 0.67 to 0.91 mmol/L of HDL: high CHD risk: 1.5 times the risk
36 to 44 mg/dL or 0.93 to 1.14 mmol/L of HDL: moderate CHD risk: 1.2 times the risk
45 to 59 mg/dL or 1.16 to 1.53 mmol/L of HDL: average CHD risk
60 to 74 mg/dL or 1.55 to 1.92 mmol/L of HDL: below-average CHD risk
>75 mg/dL or >1.94 mmol/L of HDL: no risk (associated with longevity)

NOTE *The cholesterol-to-HDL ratio provides more information than does either value alone. The higher the cholesterol-to-HDL ratio, the greater the risk for developing atherosclerosis. This ratio may be reported with total cholesterol values, along with the percentage of HDL-C.*

Procedure

1. Obtain a 5-mL venous blood sample (red-topped tube). Fasting is necessary. The HDL is precipitated out from the total cholesterol for analysis.
2. Calculate a cholesterol-to-HDL-C ratio from these values.

PROCEDURAL ALERT

Cholesterol and HDL-C levels should not be measured immediately after MI. A 3-mo wait is suggested.

Clinical Implications

1. *Increased HDL-C values* occur in the following conditions:
   a. Familial hyper-α-lipoproteinemia (HDL excess)
   b. Chronic liver disease (cirrhosis, alcoholism, hepatitis)
   c. Long-term aerobic or vigorous exercise
2. *Decreased HDL-C values* are associated with increased risk for CHD and premature CHD and occur in the following conditions:
   a. Familial hypo-α-lipoproteinemia (Tangier's disease), apolipoprotein C-III deficiency
   b. α-β-Lipoproteinemia
   c. Hypertriglyceridemia (familial)

   d. Poorly controlled diabetes mellitus
   e. Hepatocellular diseases
   f. Cholestasis
   g. Chronic renal failure, uremia, nephrotic syndrome
   h. In the United States, 3% of men have low HDL levels for unknown reasons, even though cholesterol and triglyceride values are normal, and they are at risk for premature CAD.

Interfering Factors

1. Increased HDL level is associated with estrogen therapy, moderate intake of alcohol and other drugs (especially androgenic and related steroids), and insulin therapy.
2. Decreased HDL levels are associated with the following:
   a. Certain drugs such as steroids, antihypertensive agents, diuretics, β-blockers, triglycerides, and thiazides
   b. Stress and recent illness
   c. Starvation and anorexia
   d. Obesity, lack of exercise
   e. Smoking
   f. Hypertriglyceridemia (>400 mg/dL or >10.36 mmol/L) (retest making sure the patient is properly fasting)

Interventions

Pretest Patient Care

1. Explain test purpose. An 8- to 12-hour fast is recommended. Alcohol should not be consumed for at least 24 hours before test.
2. Ensure that patient is on a stable diet for 3 weeks.
3. If possible, withhold all medication for at least 24 hours before testing. Check with the healthcare provider.
4. Encourage relaxation.
5. Follow guidelines in Chapter 1 for safe, effective, informed *pretest* care.

Posttest Patient Care

1. Review test results; report and record findings. Modify the nursing care plan as needed.
2. Low HDL levels can be raised by diet management, exercise, weight loss, and smoking cessation. Many resources are available through the American Heart Association and other organizations.
3. Drug therapy may be necessary if other methods fail to raise HDL levels.
4. Follow guidelines in Chapter 1 for safe, effective, informed *posttest* care.

● Very-Low-Density Lipoprotein (VLDL); Low-Density Lipoprotein (LDL)

Sixty percent to 70% of the total serum cholesterol is present as LDL. LDLs are the cholesterol-rich remnants of the VLDL lipid transport vehicle. Because LDL has a longer half-life (3 to 4 days) than its precursor VLDL, LDL is more prevalent in the blood. It is mainly catabolized in the liver and possibly in nonhepatic cells as well. The VLDLs are major carriers of triglycerides. Degradation of VLDL is a major source of LDL. Circulating fatty acids form triglycerides in the liver, and these are packaged with apoprotein and cholesterol to be exported into the blood as VLDLs. Recently, studies have shown that not only is the amount of cholesterol present in LDL of importance but also of importance are the number of LDL particles (LDL-P). It has been shown that the higher the number of LDL particles, the higher is the risk for heart disease.

This test is specifically done to determine CHD risk. LDL, "the bad cholesterol," is closely associated with increased incidence of atherosclerosis and CHD. The test of choice is LDL because it has a longer half-life and it is easier to measure.

Normal Findings

Adults:

Optimal: <100 mg/dL or <2.6 mmol/L
Near optimal: 100 to 129 mg/dL or 2.6 to 3.3 mmol/L
Borderline high: 130 to 159 mg/dL or 3.4 to 4.1 mmol/L
High: 160 to 189 mg/dL or 4.2 to 4.9 mmol/L
Very high: ≥190 mg/dL or ≥5.0 mmol/L

Children and adolescents:

Desirable: <110 mg/dL or <2.8 mmol/L
Borderline high risk: 110 to 129 mg/dL or 2.8 to 3.4 mmol/L
High risk: >130 mg/dL or >3.4 mmol/L

LDL-P

Optimal: <1000 nmol/L
Borderline: 1300 to 1600 nmol/L
High risk: >1600 nmol/L

Procedure

1. Use the following equation for VLDL calculation (estimation): triglycerides ÷ 5.
2. Calculate LDL-C levels by using Friedwald's formula:

$$\text{LDL-C} = \text{total cholesterol} - \text{HDL-C} - \frac{(\text{triglycerides})}{5}$$

3. The formula is valid only if the cholesterol and triglyceride values are from a fasting specimen and the triglyceride value is >400 mg/dL or >10.4 mmol/L.
4. Lipoprotein analysis measures fasting levels of total cholesterol, total triglycerides, and HDL-C. Calculate LDL-C from these values.
5. There is a direct test for LDL that may be ordered if triglycerides are >400 mg/dL or >10.4 mmol/L.

Clinical Implications

1. *Increased LDL levels* are caused by the following conditions:
   a. Familial type II hyperlipidemia, familial hypercholesterolemia
   b. Secondary causes include the following:
      (1) Diet high in cholesterol and saturated fat
      (2) Hyperlipidemia secondary to hypothyroidism
      (3) Nephrotic syndrome
      (4) Multiple myeloma and other dysglobulinemias
      (5) Hepatic obstruction or disease
      (6) Anorexia nervosa
      (7) Diabetes mellitus
      (8) Chronic renal failure
      (9) Porphyria (inherited or acquired disorders of certain enzymes that affect the nervous system)
      (10) Premature CHD
2. *Decreased LDL levels* occur in the following conditions:
   a. Hypolipoproteinemia
   b. Tangier's disease (autosomal recessive disease resulting in low levels of HDL-C and accumulation of cholesterol)

c. Type I hyperlipidemia
d. Apolipoprotein C-II deficiency
e. Hyperthyroidism
f. Chronic anemias
g. Severe hepatocellular disease
h. Reye's syndrome
i. Acute stress (burns, illness)
j. Inflammatory joint disease
k. Chronic pulmonary disease

Interfering Factors

1. Increased LDLs are associated with pregnancy and certain drugs such as steroids, progestins, and androgens (see Appendix E).
2. Not fasting may cause false elevation.
3. Decreased LDLs are found in women taking oral estrogen therapy.

Interventions

Pretest Patient Care

1. Explain test purpose. A 9- to 12-hour fast is recommended. Alcohol should not be consumed for at least 24 hours before test.
2. The patient should ideally be on a stable diet for 3 weeks.
3. If possible, withhold all medication for at least 24 hours before testing. Check with the healthcare provider.
4. Encourage relaxation.
5. Follow guidelines in Chapter 1 for safe, effective, informed *pretest* care.

Posttest Patient Care

1. Review test results; report and record findings. Modify the nursing care plan as needed. Counsel appropriately about results and need for further testing.
2. If patient has high LDH levels, repeat the test in 2 to 8 weeks and average the values to establish an accurate baseline from which to devise a treatment plan (Table 6.13).
3. A comprehensive history and physical exam, together with analysis of test results, determine whether high LDL-C is secondary to another disease or drug or is the result of a familial lipid disorder. The patient's total coronary risk profile, clinical status, age, and gender are considered when prescribing a cholesterol-lowering treatment program (Table 6.14 shows LDL-C/HDL-C ratios).
4. Treatment may include one of the statins (e.g., Lipitor [atorvastatin]), niacin (e.g., Niaspan), fibrates (e.g., Lopid [gemfibrozil]), or a cholesterol absorption inhibitor (e.g., Zetia [ezetimibe]).

TABLE 6.13 Stages of Treatment for High Lactate Dehydrogenase Levels

	Initiation Level	Minimal Goal
Dietary Treatment		
Without CHD or two other risk factors	>160 mg/dL (>4.1 mmol/L)	<160 mg/dL (<4.1 mmol/L)
With CHD or two other risk factors	>130 mg/dL (>3.4 mmol/L)	<130 mg/dL (<3.4 mmol/L)
Drug Treatment		
Without CHD or two other risk factors	>190 mg/dL (>4.9 mmol/L)	<160 mg/dL (<4.1 mmol/L)
With CHD or two other risk factors	>160 mg/dL (>4.1 mmol/L)	<130 mg/dL (<3.4 mmol/L)

CHD, coronary heart disease.

TABLE 6.14 LDL-C/HDL-C Ratio

Risk Level	Men	Women
Low	1.00	1.47
Average	3.55	3.22
Moderate	6.25	5.03
High	7.99	6.14

C, cholesterol; HDL, high-density lipoprotein; LDL, low-density lipoprotein.

NOTE *Patients need a lower initiation level and goal if they are at high risk because of existing CHD or any two of the following risk factors: male gender, family history of premature CHD, smoking, hypertension, low HDL-C, diabetes mellitus, cerebrovascular or peripheral vascular disease, or severe obesity.*

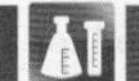

CLINICAL ALERT

Another method for assessing CAD/CHD risk is by calculating the LDH/HDL ratio (LDL-C ÷ HDL-C).

Apolipoprotein A and B (Apo A-I, Apo B)

Hypolipoproteins and apolipoproteins are surface proteins of lipoprotein particles and are important in the study of atherosclerosis. Apolipoprotein A (Apo A) is the main (90%) component of HDL. Apolipoprotein B (Apo B) is the main component of LDL and VLDL and is important in regulating cholesterol synthesis and metabolism.

This test is used to evaluate the risk for CAD. Apo A-I deficiencies are often associated with premature cardiovascular disease. Apo B plays an important role in LDL catabolism. The ratio of Apo A to Apo B correlates more closely with increased risk for CAD than do cholesterol levels or the LDL/HDL ratio. The lower the ratio, the higher the risk.

Normal Findings

Apo A-I
Men: 110 to 180 mg/dL or 1.1 to 1.8 g/L
Women: 110 to 205 mg/dL or 1.1 to 2.0 g/L

Apo B
Men: 55 to 100 mg/dL or 0.55 to 1.00 g/L
Women: 45 to 110 mg/dL or 0.45 to 1.10 g/L

Apo A-I/Apo B Ratio
Men: 0.80 to 1.33
Women: 0.94 to 2.63

Procedure

1. Obtain a 5-mL venous blood sample (red-topped tube). Serum is needed.
2. Do not freeze the specimen. Label the specimen with the patient's name, date and time of collection, and test(s) ordered. Place the specimen in a biohazard bag.
3. Fasting for 12 hours is needed.

Clinical Implications

1. *Increased Apo A-I* is associated with familial (inherited) hyper-α-lipoproteinemia.
2. *Decreased Apo A-I* is associated with the following conditions:
   a. Tangier's disease (extremely low), hypo-α-lipoproteinemia
   b. β-Lipoproteinemia
   c. Apo C-II deficiency
   d. Apo A-I Milano disease
   e. Apo A-I–C-III deficiency
   f. Hypertriglyceridemia (familial)
   g. Poorly controlled diabetes
   h. Premature CHD
   i. Hepatocellular disease
   j. Nephrotic syndrome and renal failure
3. *Increased Apo B* is associated with the following conditions:
   a. Hyperlipoproteinemia types IIa, IIb, and V
   b. Premature CHD Fredrickson type IIa
   c. Diabetes mellitus
   d. Hypothyroidism
   e. Nephrotic syndrome, renal failure
   f. Hepatic disease and obstruction
   g. Dysglobulinemia
   h. Porphyria
   i. Cushing's syndrome
   j. Werner's syndrome (rare autosomal recessive progeroid syndrome, premature aging)
4. *Decreased Apo B* occurs with the following conditions:
   a. α-β-Lipoproteinemia
   b. Hypo-α-lipoproteinuria (Tangier's disease)
   c. Hypo-β-lipoproteinemia
   d. Type I hyperlipidemia
   e. Apo C-II deficiency
   f. Hypothyroidism
   g. Malnutrition/malabsorption
   h. Reye's syndrome

Interfering Factors

1. *Decreased Apo A-I* is associated with a diet high in polyunsaturated fats, smoking, and some drugs (see Appendix E).
2. *Decreased Apo B* is associated with a diet high in polyunsaturated fats and low-cholesterol diets and many drugs.
3. *Increased apolipoprotein levels* can be caused by various drugs.
4. Apolipoproteins are acute-phase reactants and should not be measured in ill patients (e.g., acute stress, burns, major illness, inflammatory diseases).

CLINICAL ALERT

An adverse Apo A-I/Apo B ratio in early life is a potential marker for CHD risk. Apo A-I values <90 mg/dL or <0.90 g/L indicate increased CAD risk. Apo B values >110 mg/dL or >1.10 g/L indicate increased CAD risk.

Interventions

Pretest Patient Care

1. Explain test purpose and procedure. A 12-hour fast is required, but water may be taken. Smoking is prohibited. Alcohol is prohibited.
2. Encourage relaxation.
3. Follow guidelines in Chapter 1 for safe, effective, informed *pretest* care.

Posttest Patient Care

1. Resume normal activities.
2. Review test results; report and record findings. Modify the nursing care plan as needed. Counsel appropriately regarding CAD risk and potential lifestyle changes.
3. Follow guidelines in Chapter 1 for safe, effective, informed *posttest* care.

● Triglycerides

Triglycerides account for >90% of dietary fat intake and comprise 95% of fat stored in tissues. Because they are insoluble in water, they are the main plasma glycerol ester. Normally stored in adipose tissue as glycerol, fatty acids, and monoglycerides, the liver reconverts these to triglycerides. Of the total, 80% of triglycerides are in VLDL, and 15% are in LDL.

This test evaluates suspected atherosclerosis and measures the body's ability to metabolize fat. Elevated triglycerides, together with elevated cholesterol, are atherosclerotic disease risk factors. Because cholesterol and triglycerides can vary independent of each other, measurement of both values is more meaningful. Triglyceride level is needed to calculate the LDL-C and is also used to evaluate turbid samples of blood and plasma.

Normal Findings

Desirable: <150 mg/dL or <1.70 mmol/L
Borderline high: 150 to 199 mg/dL or 1.70 to 2.25 mmol/L
High: 200 to 499 mg/dL or 2.26 to 5.64 mmol/L
Very high: ≥500 mg/dL or ≥5.65 mmol/L
Table 6.15 lists specific values.

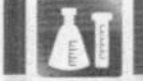

CLINICAL ALERT

Critical Value

Values >500 mg/dL (>5.6 mmol/L) indicate hypertriglyceridemia in the presence of diagnosed pancreatitis.

TABLE 6.15 Values for Triglycerides

Age (yr)	Males	Females
0–9	30–100 mg/dL (0.34–1.13 mmol/L)	35–110 mg/dL (0.40–1.24 mmol/L)
10–14	32–125 mg/dL (0.36–1.41 mmol/L)	37–131 mg/dL (0.42–1.48 mmol/L)
15–20	37–148 mg/dL (0.42–1.67 mmol/L)	39–124 mg/dL (0.44–1.40 mmol/L)
20–24	34–137 mg/dL (0.38–1.55 mmol/L)	32–100 mg/dL (0.36–1.13 mmol/L)

Adults: <250 mg/dL or <2.82 mmol/L.

Values are related to age, diet, gender, and race.

Procedure

1. Obtain a 5-mL venous blood sample. Serum is used, but many labs use EDTA anticoagulant plasma levels, which are slightly lower. Fasting for 12 to 14 hours is required.
2. Observe standard precautions. Do not use glycerinated tubes. Label the specimen with the patient's name, date and time of collection, and test(s) ordered. Place the specimen in a biohazard bag.

Clinical Implications

1. *Increased triglycerides* occur with the following conditions:
   a. Hyperlipoproteinemia types I, IIb, III, IV, and V
   b. Liver disease, alcoholism (can be extremely high with alcoholism)
   c. Nephrotic syndrome, renal disease
   d. Hypothyroidism
   e. Poorly controlled diabetes mellitus
   f. Pancreatitis
   g. Glycogen storage disease (von Gierke's disease)
   h. MI (elevated levels may persist for several months)
   i. Gout
   j. Werner's syndrome (rare autosomal recessive progeroid syndrome, premature aging)
   k. Down syndrome
   l. Anorexia nervosa
2. *Decreased triglyceride* levels occur with the following conditions:
   a. Congenital α-β-lipoproteinemia
   b. Malnutrition, malabsorption syndromes
   c. Hyperthyroidism, hyperparathyroidism
   d. Brain infarction
   e. Chronic obstructive lung disease

NOTE *Certain levels of triglycerides are associated with certain disorders:*

1. *Desirable: 150 mg/dL (<1.70 mmol/L)—not associated with a disease state*
2. *Borderline: 150 to 500 mg/dL (1.70 to 5.65 mmol/L)—associated with peripheral vascular disease and may be a marker for genetic forms of hyperlipoproteinemias that need specific therapy*
3. *Hypertriglyceridemia*
   a. *>500 mg/dL (>5.6 mmol/L)—associated with risk for pancreatitis*
   b. *>1000 mg/dL (>11.3 mmol/L)—associated with type I or V hyperlipidemia and substantial risk for pancreatitis*
   c. *>5000 mg/dL (>56.5 mmol/L)—associated with eruptive xanthoma, corneal arcus, lipemia retinalis, and enlarged liver and spleen*

CLINICAL ALERT

Chylomicronemia, although associated with pancreatitis, is not accompanied by increased atherogenesis. Chylomicrons are not seen in normal fasting serum but instead are found as exogenous triglycerides in healthy persons after a fatty meal has been eaten. After refrigeration, chylomicrons float to the surface of a blood sample.

Interfering Factors

1. A transient increase occurs following a heavy meal or alcohol ingestion.
2. Transient decrease occurs after strenuous exercise, permanent decrease with weight loss.

3. Increased values are associated with pregnancy and oral contraceptive use.
4. Values may be increased in acute illness, colds, or flu.
5. Many drugs cause increases or decreases (see Appendix E).
6. Values are increased with obesity, physical inactivity, and smoking.

Interventions

Pretest Patient Care

1. Explain test purpose and procedure. Fasting for at least 12 hours overnight is required, but water may be ingested.
2. Ask the patient to follow a normal diet for 1 week before the test. No alcohol is permitted for at least 24 to 48 hours before testing.
3. Follow guidelines in Chapter 1 for safe, effective, informed *pretest* care.

Posttest Patient Care

1. Review test results (Chart 6.5); report and record findings. Modify the nursing care plan as needed. Weight reduction, a low-fat diet, and an exercise program can reduce high triglyceride levels.
2. Advise that triglycerides are not a strong predictor of CHD and, as such, are not an independent risk factor if <250 mg/dL (<2.8 mmol/L). However, increased levels may increase cardiovascular disease risk.
3. Follow guidelines in Chapter 1 for safe, effective, informed *posttest* care.

● Lipoprotein Electrophoresis

Lipoproteins are composed of hydrophobic lipids bound to protein, which produces a liquid-soluble complex. Chylomicrons primarily transport dietary triglycerides from the intestines. They are proteins derived from dietary sources and, if significantly increased, they can extend into the pre-β area. In hyperchylomicronemia, chylomicrons represent dietary fat in transport. The standing plasma contains a cream layer over a clear layer in type I hyperlipidemia (where chylomicrons are elevated) but not in type IV (where both chylomicrons and triglycerides are elevated). VLDLs transport cholesterol and triglycerides that have been synthesized in the liver. LDLs are the major cholesterol-transporting lipoproteins. Atherosclerotic plaque cholesterol is derived from LDLs, and LDL elevations are associated with an increased CAD risk. Conversely, HDLs provide protection against atherosclerosis by reversing cholesterol transport mechanisms. Levels of plasma HDL-C are inversely proportional to the risk for heart disease.

Lipoprotein electrophoresis evaluates hyperlipidemia and determines abnormal serum lipoprotein distribution and concentration. Quantitation is not available with this procedure. Visual estimates of stain density in comparison to normal patterns are usually done. Serum cholesterol and triglyceride levels should also be done at the same time.

Normal Findings

For 12- to 14-hour fasting specimen:
Chylomicrons: 0% to 2% or 0.00 to 0.02 (about 90% triglycerides)
β or LDL: 33% to 52% or 0.33 to 0.52 (mass fraction of total lipoprotein)—cholesterol, triglyceride, phospholipid
Pre-β or VLDL: 7% to 28% or 0.07 to 0.28 (mass fraction of total lipoprotein)—triglyceride, phospholipid, cholesterol
α or HDL: 10% to 30% or 0.10 to 0.30 (mass fraction of total lipoprotein)—protein, phospholipid, cholesterol
Plasma appearance: clear

CHART 6.5 Example of Lipid Test Outcomes, Interpretation, and Intervention

A 63-yr-old woman, on annual exam, had the following findings: moderately overweight, height 5′6″ (167 cm), weight 170 pounds (77 kg), blood pressure 126/72 mm Hg, pulse 72 regular, moderately active lifestyle, and family (father and mother) history of coronary artery and vascular diseases. Fasting lipid panel was ordered and done in the clinic July 10, 2012. Results were:

Results of First Testing[a]

Cholesterol (C)	320 mg/dL (8.3 mmol/L)
Triglycerides	414 mg/dL (4.68 mmol/L)
HDL-C (good) cholesterol	38 mg/dL (0.99 mmol/L)
LDL-C (bad) cholesterol	Unable to calculate
Cholesterol/HDL ratio	8.4

[a]For reference ranges, see table below.

Because the triglycerides were high, glucose and HbA_{1C} was ordered, and the results were within normal limits. A screening TSH was then done, with results of 6.4 mIU/L (normal, 0.40–5.50), and treatment with oral levothyroxine (Levoxyl) 50 mg (synthetic thyroid) every day for 2 mo.

On September 10, 2012, a fasting lipid panel and TSH tests were repeated. Results are reported in the following table:

Chemistry	Result	Units	Ref. Range
Cholesterol	333 H	mg/dL	<200
Triglycerides	496 H	mg/dL	35–160
HDL-C (good)	44	mg/dL	>40
LDL-C (bad)[a]	—	mg/dL	70–130
Chol/HDL ratio	7.6 H	—	3.0–6.0

H, high.

[a]Unable to calculate owing to triglycerides greater than 400 mg/dL.

Elevated triglycerides were treated by administering gemfibrozil 600 mg twice a day for 3 mo and a low-cholesterol diet. Levothyroxine was continued to maintain TSH levels within normal limits.

Repeat lipid panels were done at a community testing at a local drugstore on December 15, 2013, with the following results given to the healthcare provider at the next follow-up office visit. Gemfibrozil was discontinued and atorvastatin (Lipitor) 200 mg (1 tablet daily)s at 8 p.m., was begun for 2 mo, and then follow-up lipid panel was ordered.

Results of Second Testing

Total blood cholesterol	289 mg/dL (7.5 mmol/L)
HDL-C (good)	30 mg/dL (0.78 mmol/L)
Total C/HDL ratio	9.6
LDL-C (bad)	92 mg/dL (2.4 mmol/L)
Triglycerides	100 mg/dL (1.13 mmol/L)

continues on pg. 436 >

CHART 6.5, continued

Lipids	Age (yr)	Excellent Protection M	Excellent Protection F	Moderate Risk M	Moderate Risk F	High Risk M	High Risk F	Very High Risk M	Very High Risk F
Total	20–39	≤179	≤176	180–202	177–197	203–225	198–220	>223	>220
Cholest.	40–59	≤209	≤209	210–233	210–236	234–257	236–259	>257	>259
(mg/dL)	60+	≤213	≤227	214–240	228–252	241–262	253–278	>262	>275
LDL-C (bad)	20–39	≤117	≤108	118–137	109–127	138–159	128–149	>169	>149
(mg/dL)	40–59	≤140	≤128	141–162	129–155	163–183	156–181	>183	>181
	60+	≤143	≤149	144–165	150–175	166–190	176–198	>190	>198
HDL-C	20–39	>51	>63	51–37	63–45	<37	<45	—	—
(good)	40–59	>52	>69	52–37	69–49	<37	<49	—	—
(mg/dL)	<60+	>60	>74	60–40	74–50	<40	<50	—	—
Triglyc.	20–39	≤93	≤77	94–133	78–106	134–195	107–146	>195	>146
(mg/dL)	40–59	≤121	≤98	122–170	99–140	171–231	144–190	>231	>190
	60+	≤110	≤110	111–154	111–146	155–206	147–206	>206	>206
Total	20–39	≤3.6	≤2.8	3.7–5.1	2.9–3.8	5.2–6.1	3.7–4.2	>6.1	>4.2
Cholest./	40–59	≤4.2	≤3.0	4.3–6.0	3.1–4.0	6.1–7.4	4.1–4.9	>7.4	>4.9
HDL ratio	60+	≤4.0	≤3.2	4.1–6.0	3.3–4.6	6.1–6.9	4.9–5.5	>6.9	>5.5

These test results were given to the healthcare provider at the next follow-up office visit. On February 20, 2013, the lipid panel results were:

Total cholesterol	190 mg/dL (4.9 mmol/L)
Triglycerides	207 mg/dL (2.34 mmol/L)
HDL	45 mg/dL (1.17 mmol/L)
LDL	104 mg/dL (2.7 mmol/L)

Because the patient had arthritis, she was treated with rofecoxib (Vioxx) 25 mg every day and ranitidine 150 mg twice daily. Liver studies were indicated. Results of the ALT were 28 (normal, 10–60 U/L or 0.17–1.02 mkat/L). As a result of these testings, Lipitor and arthritis medications were continued until the next healthcare provider visit in 6 months.

Procedure

1. Obtain a 5-mL sample of serum or plasma. Fasting 12 to 14 hours is required. Do not freeze.
2. Observe standard precautions. Label the specimen with the patient's name, date and time of collection, and test(s) ordered. Place the specimen in a biohazard bag. To aid in the classification, the blood sample is refrigerated overnight, and the serum or plasma is observed for any creamy layers, turbidity, or color change.

Clinical Implications

1. Patients may be phenotyped (i.e., physical appearance or classification makeup) using Frederickson's classification system. Triglyceride, cholesterol, and lipoprotein levels are considered in this system.
2. Lipoproteins are decreased in the following conditions:
   a. β-Lipoproteinemia
   b. Tangier's disease
   c. Hypo-β-lipoproteinemia

3. Lipoproteins are increased in the following conditions:
    a. Hyper-β-lipoproteinemia
    b. Hypercholesterolemia
    c. Hyper-α-lipoproteinemia
    d. Hyper pre-β-lipoproteinemia

Interfering Factors

1. Lipid phenotypes are affected by stress or dietary changes.
2. Phenotyping is invalid in the presence of secondary disorders, such as diabetes mellitus, renal failure, or nephritis.
3. Certain drugs may alter electrophoretic mobilizing of lipoproteins.
4. Heparinized blood is not acceptable; test results are not reliable during heparin therapy.

NOTE *A clear distinction must be made between primary (inherited) and secondary (liver disease, alcoholism, metabolic diseases) causes.*

Interventions

Pretest Patient Care

1. Explain test purpose and blood-drawing procedure. A 12-hour fast is required before blood is drawn.
2. Ask the patient to follow a normal diet for 2 weeks before test.
3. Follow guidelines in Chapter 1 for safe, effective, informed *pretest* care.

Posttest Patient Care

1. Review test results; report and record findings. Modify the nursing care plan as needed. Counsel appropriately regarding dietary and drug therapy. The National Cholesterol Education Program and other organizations have many resources available (National Cholesterol Education Program, National Institutes of Health, 9000 Rockville Pike, Bethesda, MD 20184).
2. Follow guidelines in Chapter 1 for safe, effective, informed *posttest* care.

NOTE *This test has been largely replaced with the lipid profile panel.*

● Free Fatty Acids; Fatty Acid Profile

Free fatty acids are formed by lipoprotein and triglyceride breakdown. The amount of free fatty acids and triglycerides present in blood comes from dietary sources or fat deposits or is synthesized by the body. Carbohydrates can be converted to fatty acids and then stored in fat cells as triglycerides. Fatty acid and carbohydrate metabolism is altered in the fat breakdown process (e.g., when fasting). Unusually high levels are associated with untreated diabetes.

Specific fatty acid measurement can be useful for monitoring nutritional status in the presence of malabsorption, starvation, and long-term parenteral nutrition. It is also valuable for the differential diagnosis of polyneuropathy when Refsum's disease is suspected. In this disease, the enzyme that degrades phytanic acid is lacking. Free fatty acids are also useful in detecting pheochromocytoma and glucagon thyrotropin and adrenocorticotropin-secreting tumors.

Normal Findings

Adults: 8 to 25 mg/dL or 0.28 to 0.89 mmol/L
Children (or obese adults): <31 mg/dL or <1.0 mmol/L

Fatty Acid Profile
Linoleate: >25% or >0.25 of total fatty acids
Arachidate: 0% to 6% or 0.00 to 0.06
Oleic: 26% to 35% or 0.26 to 0.35
Linoleic: 8% to 16% or 0.08 to 0.16
Steric: 10% to 14% or 0.10 to 0.14
Phytanic Acid
Normal: 0.3% or 0.003
Borderline: 0.3% to 0.5% or 0.003 to 0.005

Procedure

1. Obtain a 5-mL blood sample and place on ice. Serum or EDTA plasma may be used.
2. Fasting is required.
3. The blood serum should be separated from blood cells within 45 minutes of collection and should be placed on ice. Observe standard precautions. Label the specimen with the patient's name, date and time of collection, and test(s) ordered. Place the specimen in a biohazard bag.

Clinical Implications

1. *Increased free fatty acid values* are associated with the following conditions:
   a. Poorly controlled diabetes mellitus
   b. Pheochromocytoma
   c. Hyperthyroidism
   d. Huntington's disease (neurodegenerative genetic disorder)
   e. von Gierke's disease (glycogen storage disease due to deficiency of glucose-6-phosphatase)
   f. Alcoholism
   g. Acute MI
   h. Reye's syndrome
2. *Increased phytanic acid* occurs in the following conditions:
   a. Refsum's disease (autosomal recessive neurologic disease); if >50%, repeat the test to confirm
   b. β-Lipoproteinemia
3. *Decreased fatty acids* are found in:
   a. Cystic fibrosis
   b. Malabsorption (acrodermatitis enteropathica)
   c. Zinc deficiency (linoleate and arachidate low)

Interfering Factors

1. Values are elevated by strenuous exercise, anxiety, hypothermia, certain drugs (see Appendix E), and long-term fasting.
2. Values are decreased by long-term IV or parenteral nutrition therapy and certain drugs (see Appendix E).
3. Prolonged fasting or starvation affects levels (rise as much as 3 times normal).

Interventions

Pretest Patient Care

1. Explain test purpose and blood-drawing procedure. Fasting is required, but water may be taken.
2. Do not test patients receiving heparin therapy. For free fatty acids, no alcohol may be taken within 24 hours.
3. Discontinue strenuous exercise before the test. Encourage relaxation.
4. Follow guidelines in Chapter 1 for safe, effective, informed *pretest* care.

Posttest Patient Care

1. Have patient resume normal activities.
2. Review test results; report and record findings. Modify the nursing care plan as needed.
3. Follow guidelines in Chapter 1 for safe, effective, informed *posttest* care.

See Figure 6.4 for a complete laboratory test.

```
   Home:                          Work:
LIVER PANEL [80076]  Order #: 5830357  Spec. #: M4742          Details:5830357
    Final result: 8/5/2002, Ordered                            Routing:5830357

Order/Component             Result   Flag   Ref. Range   Units    Status
ALBUMIN                     3.5             3.5 - 5.0    g/dL     Final
TOTAL BILIRUBIN             0.5             0.2 - 1.3    mg/dL    Final
DIRECT BILIRUBIN            0.1             0.0 - 0.4    mg/dL    Final
AST/SGOT                    27              14 - 36      U/L      Final
ALT/SGPT                    38              9 - 52       U/L      Final
ALK PHOSPHATASE             80              38 - 126     U/L      Final
TOTAL PROTEIN               6.7             6.3 - 8.2    g/dL     Final

  Flag Codes:
  L - Below low reference range  H - Above high reference range

Resulting Tech: 135

Provider Status: Ordered
BASIC METABOLIC PANEL [80048]  Order #: 5830359  Spec. #: M4742 Details:5830359
    Final result: 8/5/2002-Abnormal, Ordered                    Routing:5830359

Order/Component             Result   Flag   Ref. Range   Units    Status
FASTING STATUS              FASTING                               Final
GLUCOSE                     85              65 - 110     mg/dL    Final
SODIUM                      140             137 - 145    mmol/L   Final
POTASSIUM                   4.6             3.6 - 5.0    mmol/L   Final
CHLORIDE                    109      H      98 - 107     mmol/L   Final
ECO2                        22              22 - 30      mmol/L   Final
BUN                         15              7 - 17       mg/dL    Final
CREATININE                  0.7             0.7 - 1.2    mg/dL    Final
CALCIUM                     8.9             8.3 - 10.7   mg/dL    Final

  Flag Codes:
  L - Below low reference range  H - Above high reference range

Resulting Tech: 135

Provider Status: Ordered
LIPID PANEL [80061]  Order #: 5830356  Spec. #: M4742          Details:5830356
    Final result: 8/5/2002-Abnormal, Ordered                   Routing:5830356

Order/Component             Result   Flag   Ref. Range   Units    Status
FASTING STATUS              FASTING                               Final
CHOLESTEROL                 172             100 - 199    mg/dL    Final
              Comment: Desirable ............. <200 mg/dL
                         Borderline-High ..... 200-239 mg/dL
                         High ................. >=240 mg/dL
TRIGLYCERIDE                193      H      35 - 149     mg/dL    Final
              Comment:
                         Desirable ............. <150 mg/dL
                         Borderline-High ..... 150-199 mg/dL
                         High ............... 200-499 mg/dL
                         Very High ............ >=500 mg/dL
                         **9/1/01 New NCEP Lipid Guidelines**
HDL                         63              40 - 200     mg/dL    Final
              Comment:
                         Desirable .............. >40 mg/dL
                         **9/1/01 New NCEP Lipid Guidelines**
CHOL/HDL                    2.74                                  Final
CALCULATED LDL              71              0 - 99       mg/dL    Final
```

FIGURE 6.4. Example of laboratory test results (54-year-old female, annual physical examination). Includes lipid panel, liver panel, and basic metabolic panel.

```
                Comment:
                          Optimal ................ <100 mg/dL
                          Above Optimal ....... 100-129 mg/dL
                          Borderline-High ..... 130-159 mg/dL
                          High ................ 160-189 mg/dL
                          Very High ............. >=190 mg/dL
                          **9/1/01 New NCEP Lipid Guidelines**
   LDL/HDL                    1.13                                Final
                Comment:                  LDL/HDL    CHOL/HDL
                          1/2 Avg Risk      1.47         3.27
                              Avg Risk      3.22         4.44
                           2x Avg Risk      5.03         7.05
                           3x Avg Risk      6.14        11.04
                          **NOT INCLUDED IN NCEP GUIDELINES**

     Flag Codes:
     L - Below low reference range  H - Above high reference range

   Resulting Tech: 135

   Provider Status: Ordered

   Status of other order(s) for this encounter:
   ECHO HEART, STRESS [93350]  Order #: 5830102
       No Result, Ordered
   X-RAY CHEST 2 VW [71020]  Order #: 5830358
       No Result, Ordered

      From: User Lab
      Sent: Aug 5, 2002   4:00 PM
```

FIGURE 6.4. continued

THYROID FUNCTION TESTS

Laboratory determinations of thyroid function are useful in distinguishing patients with euthyroidism (normal thyroid gland function) from those with hyperthyroidism (increased function) or hypothyroidism (decreased function).

● Patient Care for Thyroid Testing

Pretest Patient Care

1. Explain test purpose and blood specimen collection procedure. To understand the thyroid function tests, it is necessary to understand the following basic concepts. The thyroid gland takes iodine from the circulating blood, combines it with the amino acid tyrosine, and converts it to the thyroid hormones thyroxine (T_4) and triiodothyronine (T_3). Iodine composes about two thirds of the weight of the thyroid hormones. The thyroid gland stores T_3 and T_4 until they are released into the bloodstream under the influence of TSH from the pituitary gland. Only a small amount of the hormone is not bound to protein. However, it is the free portion of the thyroid hormones that is the true determinant of the thyroid status of the patient.
2. Assess for signs and symptoms of thyroid disease and note thyroid and iodine medications. Fasting is required for some tests.
3. A typical thyroid panel may include the following tests:
   a. T_3 uptake (T_3 U)
   b. Free T_4 (FT_4)
   c. Total T_4
   d. T_3 total
   e. Free thyroxine index (FTI, T_7)
   f. TSH

4. The most useful laboratory tests to confirm or exclude hyperthyroidism are total T_4, FTI, total T_3, and TSH. The most useful tests to detect hypothyroidism are total T_4, FTI, and TSH. A thyrotropin-releasing hormone (TRH) stimulation test can be valuable in establishing the thyroid status in some patients with equivocal signs of thyroid dysfunction and borderline laboratory values. It should be kept in mind that values obtained for the assessment of thyroid function can be influenced by factors other than disease, such as age, current illness, binding capacity of serum proteins, and some drugs.
5. In patients with stable thyroid status, TSH is more sensitive than an FT_4 measurement for detecting mild thyroid hormone deficiency or excess. In patients with unstable thyroid status, FT_4 is a better indicator of posttreatment status than TSH.
6. Follow guidelines in Chapter 1 for safe, effective, informed *pretest* care.

Posttest Patient Care

1. Review test results; report and record findings. Modify the nursing care plan as needed. Counsel and monitor appropriately for abnormal thyroid function and disease. Follow-up testing may be required.
2. Thyroid antibody testing can also be done for diagnosis of autoimmune thyroid disease.
3. Follow guidelines in Chapter 1 for safe, effective, informed *posttest* care.

● Calcitonin

Calcitonin, a hormone secreted by the C cells (parafollicular) of the thyroid gland, inhibits bone resorption by regulating the number and activity of osteoblasts. Calcitonin is secreted in direct response to high blood calcium levels and helps to prevent abrupt changes in calcium levels and the excessive loss of calcium.

Measurement of calcitonin is used to diagnose familial medullary thyroid carcinoma (MTC) and postoperatively to detect recurrence or metastasis of thyroid carcinoma. This test is done to measure increases in immunoreactive calcitonin after stimulation with calcium or pentagastrin. Early detection of elevated calcitonin leads to diagnosis of tumor or abnormally secreting C cells before cancer spreads. (Doubling of serum levels correlates with recurrence.) Calcitonin levels are also used in the investigation of families (of a patient with MTC) to detect early subclinical cases of MTC that may exist as C-cell hyperplasia or microscopic MTC.

Normal Findings

Men: 0.0 to 8.4 pg/mL or 0.0 to 8.4 ng/L
Women: 0.0 to 5.0 pg/mL or 0.0 to 5.0 ng/L
Calcium Infusion (2.4 mg/kg)
Men: ≤190 pg/mL or ≤190 ng/L
Women: ≤130 pg/mL or ≤130 ng/L
Pentagastrin Injection (0.5 μg/kg)
Men: <110 pg/mL or <110 ng/L
Women: <35 pg/mL or <35 ng/L

Reference values may differ depending on whether serum or plasma was used. Check with your laboratory.

Procedure

1. Obtain a 5-mL venous blood specimen in a green-topped tube. Fasting is necessary.
2. Heparinize and chill the blood immediately. If testing is not performed immediately, blood should be frozen. Label the specimen with the patient's name, date and time of collection, and test(s) ordered. Place the specimen in a biohazard bag.

Clinical Implications

1. *Increased levels of calcitonin* are associated with the following conditions:
   a. MTC
   b. C-cell hyperplasia
   c. Chronic renal failure
   d. Pernicious anemia
   e. Zollinger-Ellison syndrome (increased production of gastrin as a result of a tumor in the pancreas)
   f. Cancer of lung (oat cell lung cancer marker), breast, or pancreas (ectopic calcitonin)
   g. Carcinoid syndrome
   h. Alcoholic cirrhosis
   i. Patients with pancreatitis and thyroiditis
   j. Hypercalcemia of any etiology
2. In a small proportion of patients who do have medullary cancer, the fasting level of calcitonin is normal. In these instances, a provocative test using calcium or pentagastrin should be done.
   a. Very high levels (i.e., 5- to 30-fold increase over basal levels) are evidence of MTC but are not diagnostic.
   b. These stimulation tests are not needed if the basal calcitonin test is diagnostically high.
   c. In patients with elevated calcitonin levels who do not have MTC, the response is not as vigorous.

Interfering Factors

1. Levels are normally increased in pregnancy at term and in newborns.
2. Gross lipemia and hemolysis interfere with test.

CLINICAL ALERT

1. Screening families of patients with proven medullary cancer of the thyroid with the calcitonin test is recommended because the tumor has both sporadic and familial incidence.
2. If the calcitonin test is normal in family members, it is advisable to repeat the calcium provocative test periodically (over a period of months or years).
3. Some patients who have MTC do not respond to the stimulation test.

Interventions

Pretest Patient Care

1. Explain test purpose and procedure.
2. Remind patient that fasting from food overnight is required. Water is permitted.
3. Be aware that if the provocative tests using calcium and pentagastrin are to be done, the patient is to be fasting also.
   a. Inject *pentagastrin* 0.5 μg/kg IV push. Draw blood samples before the injection to determine baseline value of calcitonin. Draw a blood sample 1.5, 2, and 5 minutes after the injection.
   b. Inject *calcium*, 2.0 mg/kg, after baseline sample is drawn. Draw a blood sample 5 and 10 minutes after injection.
4. Follow guidelines in Chapter 1 for safe, effective, informed *pretest* care.

NOTE *A combined calcium and pentagastrin test may be more effective and reliable than either test by itself.*

Posttest Patient Care

1. Review test outcome; report and record findings. Modify the nursing care plan as needed. Monitor side effects of injection.
2. The patient may experience transient nausea or fatigue after injection and may experience chest pain for a short time.
3. Resume normal activities when symptoms abate.
4. Follow guidelines in Chapter 1 for safe, effective, informed *posttest* care.

● Free Thyroxine (FT_4)

FT_4 comprises a small fraction of total T_4. The FT_4 is unbound to protein and available to the tissues, and it is the metabolically active form of this hormone. This fraction constitutes about 5% of the circulatory T_4.

FT_4 has diagnostic value in situations in which total hormone levels do not correlate with the thyrometabolic state and there is suspected abnormality in thyroxine-binding globulin (TBG) levels. It provides a more accurate picture of the thyroid status in persons with abnormal TBG levels in pregnancy and in those who are receiving estrogens, androgens, phenytoin, or salicylates.

Normal Findings

0.7 to 2.0 ng/dL or 10 to 26 pmol/L
For patients taking levothyroxine (Synthroid), up to 5.0 ng/dL or 64 pmol/L

Procedures

1. Obtain a 5-mL venous blood sample. Accurate results can be obtained with as little as 0.5 mL of blood in pediatric cases. Serum is needed for this test.
2. Observe standard precautions. Label the specimen with the patient's name, date and time of collection, and test(s) ordered. Place the specimen in a biohazard bag.

Clinical Implications

1. *Increased FT_4 levels* are associated with the following conditions:
   a. Graves' disease (hyperthyroidism)
   b. Hypothyroidism treated with T_4
   c. Euthyroid sick syndrome
2. *Decreased FT_4 levels* are associated with the following conditions:
   a. Primary hypothyroidism
   b. Secondary hypothyroidism (pituitary)
   c. Tertiary hypothyroidism (hypothalamic)
   d. Hypothyroidism treated with T_3

Interfering Factors

1. Values are increased in infants at birth and rise even higher after 2 to 3 days of life.
2. Many drugs affect test outcomes (see Appendix E).
3. Heparin causes falsely elevated FT_4 values.
4. Levels can fluctuate in patients with severe or chronic illness.
5. Levels fluctuate in pregnancy (low in late pregnancy).

Interventions

Refer to Patient Care for Thyroid Testing on pages 440–441.

Free Triiodothyronine (FT_3)

This is one of the determinations used to evaluate thyroid function and measure that fraction of the circulatory T_3 that exists in the free form in the blood unbound to protein. Free T_3 (FT_3)is done to rule out T_3 toxicosis, to evaluate thyroid replacement therapy, and to clarify protein-binding abnormalities.

Normal Findings

Adults: 260 to 480 pg/dL or 4.0 to 7.4 pmol/L

Procedure

1. Obtain a 5-mL venous blood sample.
2. Observe standard precautions. Label the specimen with the patient's name, date and time of collection, and test(s) ordered. Place the specimen in a biohazard bag.

Clinical Implications

1. *Increased FT_3 values* are associated with the following conditions:
   a. Hyperthyroidism
   b. T_3 toxicosis
   c. Peripheral resistance syndrome
2. *Decreased FT_3 values* are associated with the following conditions:
   a. Hypothyroidism (primary and secondary)
   b. Third trimester of pregnancy

NOTE *In nonthyroidal illness, a low FT_3 level is a nonspecific finding.*

Interfering Factors

1. Recently administered radioisotopes and some drugs (see Appendix E)
2. High altitude: FT_3 levels are higher.

Interventions

Pretest Patient Care

1. See Patient Care for Thyroid Testing on pages 440–441. The same protocols prevail for FT_3.
2. Follow Chapter 1 guidelines for safe, effective, informed *pretest* care.

Posttest Patient Care

1. See Patient Care for Thyroid Testing on page 441. The same protocols prevail in FT_3 testing.
2. Follow Chapter 1 guidelines for safe, effective, informed *posttest* care.

Free Thyroxine Index (FTI, T_7)

The FTI is a mathematical calculation used to correct the estimated total T_4 for the amount of TBG present. To perform this calculation, two results are needed: the T_4 value and the T_3 uptake ratio. The product of these two values is the FTI. The FTI is useful in the diagnosis of hyperthyroidism and hypothyroidism, especially in patients with known or suspected abnormalities in T_4-binding protein levels. In such cases, blood levels and clinical signs may seem contradictory unless both T_4 and TBG are considered as interrelated parameters of thyroid status. Measurement of FT_4 also gives a more accurate picture of the thyroid status when the TBG is abnormal in pregnant women or persons being treated with estrogen, androgens, phenytoin, or salicylates.

Normal Findings

Adults: 1.5 to 3.8 index (these are arbitrary units)
Check with your laboratory for their normal values.

Procedure

1. Make a calculation based on results of T_3 uptake and T_4 total, as follows:

$$\text{FTI} = T_4 \text{ total} \times T_3 \text{ U}(\%)100$$

2. The FTI permits meaningful interpretation by balancing out most nonthyroidal factors. In recent years, this parameter has lost popularity and is of dubious value.

Clinical Implications

Application of the equation for the FTI includes the information presented in Table 6.16. This is a mathematical calculation that does not involve the patient.

Interfering Factors

1. Levels fluctuate in pregnancy.
2. See Appendix E for drugs that affect test outcomes.

Interventions

Pretest Patient Care

1. Inform the patient about the test purpose and method of calculation.
2. Follow Chapter 1 guidelines for safe, effective, informed *pretest* care.

Posttest Patient Care

1. Be prepared to counsel patient if treatment is required. Review test results; report and record findings. Modify the nursing care plan as needed.
2. Follow Chapter 1 guidelines for safe, effective, informed *posttest* care.

● Neonatal Thyroid-Stimulating Hormone (TSH)

Signs of congenital hypothyroidism are minimal at birth. Congenital hypothyroidism has an incidence of 1:3600 to 1:5000 in the United States.

This measurement is used as a confirmatory test or in conjunction with neonatal T_4, for infants with positive T_4 screens or low blood serum T_4 levels, and for screening in all U.S. states. See newborn screening in Chapter 11 for more information.

TABLE 6.16 Application of Equation to Determine Thyroxine Uptake

Status	TBG	T_3 Uptake	×	T_4	=	FTI
Euthyroid	Normal	35%		9.0		3.1
Euthyroid	Low	52%		4.0		2.1
Euthyroid	High	13%		16.0		2.1
Hypothyroid	High	24%		4.0		0.9
Hypothyroid	Low	46%		13.0		6.0

T_3, triiodothyronine; T_4, thyroxine; FTI, free thyroxine index; TBG, thyroxine-binding globulin.

Normal Findings

Newborn screen: <20 μU/mL or <20 mU/L by third day of life

TSH surges at birth, peaking at 30 minutes of life at a level of 25 to 160 μU/mL or 25 to 160 mU/L. It declines and reaches adult levels by the first week to 10 days of life.

Procedure

1. Cleanse the infant's heel with an antiseptic and puncture with a sterile disposable lancet. Collect this whole blood specimen 3 to 7 days after birth.
2. If bleeding is slow, it helps to hold the leg dependent for a short time before blotting the blood on the filter paper. Do not use pipettes or capillary tubes to collect blood.
3. Completely fill in the circles on the filter paper. This can best be done by placing one side of the filter paper against the infant's heel and watching for the blood to appear on the front side of the paper and to fill the circle completely. The filter paper is a special filter paper card obtained from the laboratory.
4. Air-dry the filter paper for 1 hour, fill in all information, and send to the laboratory immediately. Do not expose samples to extreme heat or light.

Clinical Implications

An elevated neonatal TSH test is associated with neonatal hypothyroidism, a confirmatory test.

Interventions

Pretest Patient Care

1. Inform the parents about the test purpose and method of specimen collection.
2. See Patient Care for Thyroid Testing on pages 440–441.
3. See Chapter 1 guidelines for safe, effective, informed *pretest* care.

Posttest Patient Care

1. Be prepared to counsel parents regarding steps to take if the TSH test is abnormal and type of treatment required. See newborn screening in Chapter 11. Review test results; report and record findings. Modify the nursing care plan as needed.
2. See Chapter 1 guidelines for safe, effective, informed *posttest* care.

• Neonatal Thyroxine (T_4); Neonatal Screen for Hypothyroidism

Normal brain growth and development cannot take place without adequate thyroid hormone. Congenital hypothyroidism (cretinism) is characterized by low levels of T_4 and elevated levels of TSH. Screening for congenital hypothyroidism is done in all 50 states. If hypothyroidism is undetected, growth and mental retardation occur and, in some cases, death occurs.

This is a screening test of T_4 activity to detect neonatal hypothyroidism. Specimens should be obtained after the first 24 hours of protein feeding or within the first week of life. T_4 is obtained from whole blood blotted on filter paper using a radioimmunoassay technique.

Normal Findings

Peaks in 24 hours then decreases
Neonates (1 to 3 days): 12 to 22 μg/dL or 152 to 292 nmol/L
Neonates (1 to 2 weeks): 10 to 17 μg/dL or 126 to 214 nmol/L

CLINICAL ALERT

Critical Value

7 d or younger: T_4 <6.5 μg/dL or <84 nmol/L
8 d and older: T_4 <5.0 μg/dL or <64 nmol/L

Procedure

1. Cleanse the infant's heel with an antiseptic and puncture the skin with a sterile disposable lancet. To help blood flow, warm the foot or massage the leg.
2. If bleeding is slow, it helps to hold the leg dependent for a short time before blotting the blood on the filter paper. Wipe away the first drop of blood.
3. Completely fill in the circles on the filter paper. This can best be done by placing one side of the filter paper against the infant's heel and watching for the blood to appear on the front side of the paper and to fill the circle completely. Do not damage filter paper. Apply a sterile dressing to the wound.
4. Air-dry for 1 hour, fill in all requested information, and send to the laboratory immediately. Protect specimen from extreme heat and light.

Clinical Implications

1. Low values are associated with hypothyroidism.
2. A number of nonthyroid conditions can result in depressed T_4 levels (e.g., low birth weight, prematurity, twinning, fetal distress, deficient TBG levels).

Interventions

Pretest Patient Care

1. Refer to neonatal TSH testing for care. The same protocols prevail for neonatal T_4.
2. Be aware that T_4 is usually collected at the same time as the phenylketonuria (PKU) specimen.
3. The optimal collection time is 3 to 7 days after birth; the baby must be on protein feeding for at least 24 hours. For low-birth-weight or premature babies, the recommended time is 4 to 10 days old.

Posttest Patient Care

1. Refer to neonatal TSH testing for care. The same protocols prevail for neonatal T_4. Also, see newborn screening in Chapter 11. Review test results; report and record findings. Modify the nursing care plan as needed.
2. If the baby is released early, the baby must be brought back for testing.

CLINICAL ALERT

1. Do not interpret this test in terms of the adult serum T_4 values. This is an entirely different procedure using a different type of specimen.
2. Notify the attending healthcare provider and the infant's parent or parents of positive results within 24 hr.
3. If T_4 results are abnormal, a TSH test should be done.
4. Normal T_4 and, in some cases, normal TSH screening results do not ensure against failure of normal development because of the presence of hypothyroidism. Of all cases of infantile hypothyroidism, 6%–12% have normal screening hormone levels.

● Thyroglobulin (Tg)

Thyroglobulin (Tg) is composed of glycoprotein and the iodinated secretions of epithelial cells of the thyroid. These iodinated secretions contain both the precursors of T_3 and T_4 and the hormones themselves.

This test is helpful in the differential diagnosis of hyperthyroidism and in monitoring the course of differentiated or metastatic thyroid cancer. It is not useful in the diagnosis of thyroid cancer. Levels decrease following successful initial treatment, and in recurrence of metastases, the level will again rise. Lack of sensitivity and specificity limits the value of this test.

Normal Findings

Adults: 2 to 55 ng/mL or 2 to 55 μg/L
Newborns (48 hours): 36 to 48 ng/mL or 36 to 48 μg/L

NOTE *Eighty-seven percent of normal adults have serum values of Tg <10 ng/mL or <10 mg/L. Athyrotic patients have values <5 ng/mL or <5 mg/L.*

Procedure

1. Obtain a 5-mL venous blood sample. Serum is needed.
2. Observe standard precautions. Label the specimen with the patient's name, date and time of collection, and test(s) ordered. Place the specimen in a biohazard bag.

Clinical Implications

1. *Increased Tg levels* are associated with the following conditions:
   a. Untreated and metastatic differentiated thyroid cancers (not MTC)
   b. Hyperthyroidism (not good correlation with elevated T_4)
   c. Subacute thyroiditis, thyrotoxicosis
   d. Benign adenoma (some cases)
   e. Occurrence of metastases after initial treatment (thyroid carcinoma)
2. *Decreased Tg levels* are associated with the following conditions:
   a. Thyrotoxicosis factitia
   b. Infants with goitrous hypothyroidism

Interfering Factors

1. Newborns have high Tg levels that drop to adult levels by 2 years of age.
2. Autoantibodies to Tg cause decreased values. Tg antibody test may have to be done to confirm decreased levels.

NOTE *Normal reference value for Tg antibody is <40 IU/mL.*

Interventions

Pretest Patient Care

1. See Patient Care for Thyroid Testing on pages 440–441.
2. Ensure that patient is off thyroid medication for 6 weeks before specimen collection. The TSH should be elevated before testing for Tg.
3. Determination of Tg levels may be substituted for ^{131}I scans in patients at low risk for thyroid cancer.
4. Follow guidelines in Chapter 1 for safe, effective, informed *pretest* care.

Posttest Patient Care

1. Resume thyroid medication and have patient resume normal activities. Review test results; report and record findings. Modify the nursing care plan as needed.
2. Monitor as appropriate for metastatic thyroid cancer.
3. Refer to patient aftercare instructions for thyroid testing on page 441. The same protocols prevail for Tg testing. Follow guidelines in Chapter 1 for safe, effective, informed *posttest* care.

● Thyroid-Stimulating Hormone (TSH; Thyrotropin)

The thyroid is unique among the endocrine glands because it has a large store of hormone and a slow rate of normal turnover. Stimulation of the thyroid gland by TSH, which is produced by the anterior pituitary gland, causes the release and distribution of stored thyroid hormones. TSH stimulates secretion of T_4 and T_3. TSH secretion is physiologically regulated by T_3 and T_4 (feedback inhibition) and is stimulated by TRH from the hypothalamus. TSH is the single most sensitive test for primary hypothyroidism. If there is clear evidence of hypothyroidism and the TSH is not elevated, then an implication of possible hypopituitarism exists.

This measurement is used in the diagnosis of primary hypothyroidism when there is thyroid gland failure owing to intrinsic disease, and it is used to differentiate primary from secondary hypothyroidism by determining the actual circulatory level of TSH. TSH levels are high in primary hypothyroidism. Low TSH levels occur in hyperthyroidism.

TSH measurements with sufficient sensitivity to distinguish low levels from normal levels have become the preferred test for hyperthyroidism. The third-generation TSH test is useful for diagnosing sick euthyroid patients and in differentiating mild hyperthyroidism from Graves' disease. With the new, sensitive assays, a TRH stimulation test is no longer necessary.

Normal Findings

Adults: 0.45 to 4.5 μU/mL or 0.45 to 4.5 mU/L
Children (6 to 10 years): 0.66 to 4.14 μU/mL or 0.66 to 4.14 mU/L
Adolescents (11 to 19 years): 0.53 to 3.59 μU/mL or 0.53 to 3.59 mU/L
Neonates (1 to 3 days): 5.17 to 14.6 μU/mL or 5.17 to 14.6 mU/L

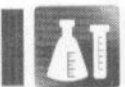

CLINICAL ALERT

Critical Values

Values <0.1 mU/L are an indication of primary hyperthyroidism or exogenous thyrotoxicosis. Risk exists for atrial fibrillation at TSH levels <0.1 mU/L (major risk factor for stroke).

Procedure

1. Obtain a 5-mL venous blood sample (red-topped tube). Serum is needed.
2. Observe standard precautions. Label the specimen with the patient's name, date and time of collection, and test(s) ordered. Place the specimen in a biohazard bag.

Clinical Implications

1. *Increased TSH levels* are seen in the following conditions:
   a. Adults and neonates with primary hypothyroidism
   b. Thyrotropin-producing tumor (e.g., ectopic TSH secretion from lung, breast tumors)
   c. Hashimoto's thyroiditis
   d. Thyrotoxicosis due to pituitary tumor
   e. TSH antibodies (rare)
   f. Hypothyroid patients receiving insufficient thyroid replacement hormone or with thyroid hormone resistance
2. *Decreased TSH levels* are associated with the following conditions:
   a. Primary hyperthyroidism
   b. Secondary and tertiary hypothyroidism
   c. Treated Graves' disease
   d. Euthyroid sick syndrome
   e. Over-replacement of thyroid hormone in treatment of hypothyroidism

Interfering Factors

1. Values are normally high in neonatal cord blood. There is hypersecretion of TSH in newborns up to 2 to 3 times normal. The TSH level approaches normal by the first week of life.

2. Values are suppressed during treatment with T_4 and corticosteroids. See Appendix E for other drugs.
3. Values are abnormally increased with lithium, potassium iodide, amphetamine abuse, and iodine-containing drugs.
4. Radioisotopes administered within 1 week before test invalidate the result.
5. Values may be decreased in the first trimester of pregnancy.
6. Values are increased in older adult patients (>80 years old); upper limit for these patients is 10 μU/mL or 10 mU/L.
7. Heterophilic antibodies may falsely increase or decrease test results.

Interventions

Pretest Patient Care

1. Explain test purpose and procedure.
2. Follow guidelines in Chapter 1 for safe, effective, informed *pretest* care.

Posttest Patient Care

1. Have patient resume normal activities.
2. Review test results; report and record findings. Modify the nursing care plan as needed. Counsel as appropriate for hypothyroidism or hyperthyroidism.
3. Follow guidelines in Chapter 1 for safe, effective, informed *posttest* care.

● Thyroxine-Binding Globulin (TBG)

Almost all of the thyroid hormones in the blood are protein bound: albumin, thyroid-binding PAB, and, most important, TBG. Variations in TBG levels have a major effect on bound and free (metabolically active) forms of T_4 and T_3. Before considering this test, TSH, FTI, and total T_4 should be measured.

The TBG measurement is useful to distinguish between hyperthyroidism causing high T_4 levels and euthyroidism with increased binding by TBG, increased T_4, and normal levels of free hormones; to identify hereditary deficiency or increase of TBG; and to work up thyroid disease in hypothyroid populations, when the mean TBG concentration is significantly higher than the mean level in normal thyroid populations. In hyperthyroid populations, the mean TBG level concentration is lower than the mean level in normal thyroid populations.

Normal Findings

Infants: 3 to 6 mg/dL or 30 to 60 mg/L
Men: 1.2 to 2.5 mg/dL or 12 to 25 mg/L
Women: 1.4 to 3.0 mg/dL or 14 to 30 mg/L
On oral contraceptives: 1.5 to 5.5 mg/dL or 15 to 55 mg/L
Third trimester of pregnancy: 4.7 to 5.9 mg/dL or 47 to 59 mg/L

Procedure

1. Obtain a 5-mL venous blood specimen (red-topped tube). Serum is needed.
2. Observe standard precautions. Label the specimen with the patient's name, date and time of collection, and test(s) ordered. Place the specimen in a biohazard bag.

Clinical Implications

1. *TBG is increased* in the following conditions:
   a. Genetically determined high TBG
   b. Hypothyroidism (some cases)
   c. Infectious hepatitis

d. Acute intermittent porphyria
e. Estrogen-producing tumors (endogenous or exogenous)
f. Late-stage HIV infections

2. *TBG is decreased* in the following conditions:
a. Genetic deficiency of TBG
b. Nephrotic syndrome
c. Major illness, surgical stress
d. Ovarian hypofunction
e. Acromegaly
f. Chronic liver disease
g. Marked hypoproteinemia, malnutrition

Interfering Factors

1. Many drugs increase (e.g., estrogens, oral contraceptives) or decrease (e.g., nicotinic acid, phenytoin, steroids) values (see Appendix E).
2. Neonates have higher values.
3. Recently administered radioisotopes affect results.
4. Pregnancy increases levels.
5. Prolonged heroin use or methadone increases levels.

Interventions

Pretest Patient Care

1. See Patient Care for Thyroid Testing on pages 440–441.
2. Follow Chapter 1 guidelines for safe, effective, informed *pretest* care.

Posttest Patient Care

1. See Patient Care for Thyroid Testing on page 441.
2. Follow Chapter 1 guidelines for safe, effective, informed *posttest* care.

● Thyroxine (T_4), Total

Thyroxine is the thyroid hormone with four atoms of iodine; hence, it is called T_4. The combination of the serum T_4 and T_3 uptake as an assessment of TBG helps to determine whether an abnormal T_4 value is due to alterations in serum TBG or to changes in thyroid hormone levels. Deviations of both tests in the same direction usually indicate that an abnormal T_4 level is due to abnormalities in thyroid hormone. Deviations of the two tests in opposite directions provide evidence that an abnormal T_4 may relate to alterations in TBG.

T_4, one of the thyroid function panel tests, is a direct measurement of the concentration of T_4 in the blood serum. Total T_4 level is a good index of thyroid function when the TBG is normal. The increase in TBG levels normally seen in pregnancy and with estrogen therapy increases total T_4 levels. The decrease of TBG levels in persons receiving anabolic steroids, in chronic liver disease, and in nephroses decreases the total T_4 value. This test is commonly done to rule out hyperthyroidism and hypothyroidism. The T_4 test also can be used as a guide in establishing maintenance doses of thyroid hormone in the treatment of hypothyroidism. In addition, it can be used in hyperthyroidism to follow the results achieved with antithyroid drug administration.

Normal Findings

Adults: 5.4 to 11.5 μg/dL or 57 to 148 nmol/L
Children: 6.4 to 13.3 μg/dL or 83 to 172 nmol/L
Neonates: 11.8 to 22.6 μg/dL or 152 to 292 nmol/L

If testing is done by radioimmunoassay, it is reported as T_4 RIA.

CLINICAL ALERT

Critical Values

>20 μg/dL or >258 nmol/L: Thyroid storm is possible.

<2.0 μg/dL or <26 nmol/L: Myxedema coma is possible.

Procedure

1. Obtain a 5-mL venous blood sample. Serum is used. If the patient is already receiving thyroid treatment, it must be discontinued 1 month before the test.
2. Observe standard precautions. Label the specimen with the patient's name, date and time of collection, and test(s) ordered. Place the specimen in a biohazard bag.

Clinical Implications

1. *Increased T_4 values* are found in the following conditions:
   a. Hyperthyroidism (Graves' disease, goiter)
   b. Clinical status that increases TBG
   c. Thyrotoxicosis factitia
   d. Acute thyroiditis
   e. Hepatitis, liver disease
   f. Lymphoma
2. *Decreased T_4 values* are found in the following conditions:
   a. Hypothyroidism
   b. Disorders of decreased TBG
   c. Hypoproteinemia
   d. Treatment with T_3
   e. Nephrotic syndrome

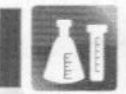

CLINICAL ALERT

T_4 values are higher in neonates due to elevated TBG. Values rise abruptly in the first few hours after birth and decline gradually until the age of 5 yr.

Interfering Factors

1. Total T_4 levels increase during the second or third month of pregnancy as a result of increased estrogen production. Normal range: 5.5 to 16.0 μg/dL or 71 to 206 nmol/L.
2. Total T_4 levels increase with the use of drugs such as estrogens, heroin, and methadone and excess iodine (see Appendix E).
3. Contrast agents used for x-rays and other diagnostic procedures affect results.
4. Values are decreased with salicylates, anticonvulsants, and steroids.

Interventions

Pretest Patient Care

1. Explain test purpose and procedure. T_4 is usually the first test used in the diagnosis of hypothyroidism or hyperthyroidism, along with the TSH.
2. Have patient avoid strenuous exercise.
3. Do not administer radiopaque contrast for 1 week before testing.

4. If patient is on thyroid therapy, discontinue treatment for 1 month before testing to determine baseline values.
5. Follow guidelines in Chapter 1 for safe, effective, informed *pretest* care.

Posttest Patient Care

1. Have patient resume normal activities.
2. See Patient Care for Thyroid Testing on page 441.
3. Follow guidelines in Chapter 1 for safe, effective, informed *posttest* care.

● Triiodothyronine (T_3), Total

T_3 has three atoms of iodine, compared with four atoms in T_4. T_3 is more active metabolically than T_4, but its effect is shorter. There is much less T_3 than T_4 in the serum, and it is bound less firmly to TBG.

This measurement is a quantitative determination of the total T_3 concentration in the blood and is the test of choice in the diagnosis of T_3 thyrotoxicosis. *It is not the same as the T_3 uptake test that measures the unsaturated TBG in serum.* It can also be very useful in the diagnosis of hyperthyroidism. T_3 thyrotoxicosis refers to a variant of hyperthyroidism in which a thyrotoxic patient has elevated T_3 values and normal T_4 values. This test is not reliable in diagnosing hypothyroidism.

Normal Findings

Adults: 80 to 200 ng/dL or 1.2 to 3.1 nmol/L
Adolescents (12 to 23 years): 82 to 213 ng/dL or 1.3 to 3.28 nmol/L
Children (1 to 14 years): 105 to 245 ng/dL or 1.6 to 3.8 nmol/L
Neonates (1 to 3 days): 96 to 292 ng/dL or 1.4 to 4.4 nmol/L
Pregnancy: 116 to 247 ng/dL or 1.8 to 3.8 nmol/L

If radioimmunoassay is used, the result is reported as T_3 RIA.

CLINICAL ALERT

Critical Values
<50 ng/dL (<0.77 nmol/L) or >300 ng/dL (>4.62 nmol/L)

Procedure

1. Obtain a 5-mL venous blood sample. Serum is needed.
2. Observe standard precautions. Label the specimen with the patient's name, date and time of collection, and test(s) ordered. Place the specimen in a biohazard bag.

Clinical Implications

1. *Increased T_3 values* are associated with the following conditions:
   a. Hyperthyroidism
   b. T_3 thyrotoxicosis (Graves' disease)
   c. Daily dosage >25 μg of T_3 (Cytomel [lyothyronine])
   d. Acute thyroiditis
   e. TBG elevation from any cause
   f. Daily dosage >300 μg of T_4
   g. Early thyroid failure
   h. Thyrotoxicosis factitia
   i. Iodine deficiency goiter

2. *Decreased T_3 values* are associated with the following conditions:
   a. Hypothyroidism; however, some clinically hypothyroid patients will have normal levels.
   b. Starvation and state of nutrition subacute nonthyroid illness
   c. TBG decrease from any cause

Interfering Factors

1. Values are increased in pregnancy and with the use of drugs such as estrogens, methadone, and heroin (see Appendix E).
2. Values are decreased with the use of drugs such as anabolic steroids, androgens, large doses of salicylates, phenytoin, and nicotinic acid (see Appendix E).
3. Fasting causes T_3 level to decrease.

Interventions

Pretest Patient Care

1. Care is the same as for T_4 testing.
2. Follow Chapter 1 guidelines for safe, effective, informed *pretest* care.

Posttest Patient Care

1. Care is the same as for T_4 testing.
2. Follow Chapter 1 guidelines for safe, effective, informed *posttest* care.

● Triiodothyronine Uptake (T_3 U)

This test is an indirect measurement of unsaturated TBG in blood. This determination, expressed in arbitrary terms, is inversely proportional to the TBG. For this reason, low T_3 U levels are indicative of situations that result in elevated levels of TBG uptake. For example, in hypothyroidism, when insufficient T_4 is available to produce saturation of TBG, unbound TBG (UTBG) is elevated, and T_3 U values are low. Similarly, in pregnant patients or those receiving estrogen, TBG levels are increased proportionately more than are T_4 levels, resulting in high levels of UTBG, which are reflected in low T_3 U results. This test should not be ordered alone—it is useful only when T_4 is done. It is also used to calculate the T_7 or FTI. With the improvements in other thyroid function assays, this test does not provide much utility.

Normal Findings

0.9 to 1.10 (ratio between patient specimen and the standard control)
25% to 35% or 25 to 37 AU (arbitrary units)

Procedure

1. Obtain a 5-mL venous blood sample. Serum is needed.
2. Observe standard precautions. Label the specimen with the patient's name, date and time of collection, and test(s) ordered. Place the specimen in a biohazard bag.

Clinical Implications

See Table 6.17 for implications of clinical conditions for test results.

Interfering Factors

1. *Decreased T_3 U levels* occur in normal pregnancy and with drugs such as estrogens, antiovulatory drugs, methadone, and heparin.
2. *Increased T_3 U levels* occur with drugs such as dicumarol, heparin, androgens, anabolic steroids, phenytoin, and large doses of salicylates.

TABLE 6.17 Implications of Conditions for T_3 (T_3 U) Testing

Clinical Condition	T_4	T_3 U	FTI
Normal	Normal	Normal	Normal
Hyperthyroid	Increased	Increased	Increased
Hypothyroid	Decreased	Decreased	Decreased
Increased TBG, as in pregnancy	Increased	Decreased	Normal
Decreased TBG, as in nephrotic syndrome	Decreased	Increased	Normal

T_3 U, triiodothyronine uptake; T_4, thyroxine; FTI, free thyroxine index.

Interventions

Pretest Patient Care

1. See Patient Care for Thyroid Testing on pages 444–441.
2. *Pretest* care is the same as for T_4 testing.

Posttest Patient Care

1. See Patient Care for Thyroid Testing on page 445.
2. *Posttest* care is the same as for T_4 testing.

CLINICAL ALERT

1. This test has nothing to do with the actual T_3 blood level despite its name, which is sometimes confusingly abbreviated to the T_3 test. It is emphasized that the T_3 U and the true T_3 are entirely different tests. The T_3 U gives only an indirect measurement of overall binding.
2. This test should be used only in conjunction with the T_4 test to calculate the FTI.
3. Some methods of determining T_3 U have a direct relation with T_4. Check the reference values of your laboratory.

BIBLIOGRAPHY

American Academy of Pediatrics: Clinical Practice Guidelines: Phototherapy to prevent severe neonatal hyperbilirubinemia in the newborn infant 35 or more weeks of gestation. Pediatrics 128(4):e1406, 2011

American Association of Clinical Endocrinologists: Medical guidelines for clinical practice for the evaluation and treatment of hyperthyroidism and hypothyroidism. Endocrine Practice 8:458–469, 2002. 2006 amended version, erratum in Endocrine Practice 14(6):802–803, 2008

American College of Cardiology: ACCF 2012 expert consensus document on practical clinical considerations in the interpretation of troponin elevations. J Am Coll Cardiol 60(23):2427–2463, 2012

American College of Endocrinology and American Diabetes Association: Consensus statement on inpatient diabetes and glycemic control. Diabetes Care 29:1955–1962, 2006

American Diabetes Association: Diagnosis and classification of diabetes mellitus. Diabetes Care 33:S62–S69, 2010

American Diabetes Association: Standards of medical care in diabetes—2010. Diabetes Care 33:S11–S61, 2010.

American Diabetes Association: Standards of medical care in diabetes—2017: Summary of revisions. Diabetes Care 40(Suppl 1): S4–S5, 2017. doi: 10.2337/dc17-S003

Burtis C, Ashwood E, Bruns D: Tietz Textbook of Clinical Chemistry and Molecular Diagnostics, 5th ed. St. Louis, MO, Elsevier Saunders, 2012

Crawford ED, Higano CS, Roach M: Complete Guide to Prostate Cancer. Atlanta, GA, American Cancer Society, 2005

Durkin S: C-reactive protein: Inflammatory marker or predictor of outcomes? Advance for Nurses 23–24, May 16, 2005

Hanas R, John G: 2010 Consensus statement on the worldwide standardization of the hemoglobin A1C measurement. Diabetes Care 33(8):1903–1904, 2010

Hortin GL: Estimated glomerular filtration rates: A key role in addressing the epidemic of chronic kidney disease. Clin Lab News 32(11), 2006

Kiechle FL, Leon S, Severyn W: Tight glycemic control: Overcoming barriers to implementation in the intensive care unit. Clin Lab News 33(2), 2007

Leavelle D (ed): Mayo Clinic Interpretive Handbook. Rochester, MN, Mayo Medical Laboratories, 2017

Lingvay IL, Kaloyanova PF, Adams-Huet B, et al: Insulin as initial therapy in type 2 diabetes: Effective, safe, and well accepted. J Invest Med 55(2):62–68, 2007

MacKenzie HA: Recent advances in photoacoustic, non-invasive disease testing: Oak Ridge Conferences, April 23 and 24, 1999. Sponsor: American Association for Clinical Chemistry.

McPherson RA, Pincus MR: Henry's Clinical Diagnosis and Management by Laboratory Methods, 22nd ed. Philadelphia, Saunders Elsevier, 2011

Morrison F, Shubina M, Turchin A: Lifestyle counseling in routine care and long-term glucose, blood pressure, and cholesterol control in patients with diabetes. Diabetes Care 35:334–341, 2012

Nathan DM, Buse JB, Davidson MB, et al: Management of hyperglycemia in type 2 diabetes: A consensus algorithm for the initiation and adjustment of therapy. Diabetes Care 32(1):193–203, 2009

National Academy of Clinical Biochemistry: Laboratory medicine practice guidelines: Clinical characteristics and utilization of biochemical markers in acute coronary syndromes. Clin Chem 53(4):552–574, 2007

National Institutes of Health: National Cholesterol Education Program: Detection, evaluation, and treatment of high blood cholesterol in adults. NIH Publication no. 01-3670, 2001

Rohling CL, Wiedmeyer HM, Little RR, et al: Defining the relationship between plasma glucose and Hb A_{1c}. Diabetes Care 25:275–278, 2002

Sacks DB, Arnold M, Bakris GL, et al: Guidelines and recommendations for laboratory analysis in the diagnosis and management of diabetes mellitus. Clin Chem 57(6):e1–e47, 2011

Scirica BM, Morrow DA, Cannon CP, et al: Clinical application of c-reactive protein across the spectrum of acute coronary syndromes. Clin Chem 53(10):1800–1807, 2007

Smith RA, Brooks D, Cokkinides V, et al: Cancer screening in the United States, 2013: A review of current American Cancer Society guidelines, current issues in cancer screening, and new guidance on cervical cancer screening and lung cancer screening. CA Cancer J Clin 63:87–105, 2013. Available at: http://onlinelibrary.wiley.com/doi/10.3322/caac.21174/full

Soldin SJ, Wong EC, Brugnara C, et al: Pediatric Reference Intervals, 7th ed. Washington, DC, AACC Press, 2011

U.S. Department of Health and Human Services: Substance Abuse and Mental Health Administration. Drug Abuse Warning Network. Available at: http://www.samhsa.gov/data/2k13/DAWN2k11ED/rpts/DAWN2K11-Trend-Tables.htm

U.S. Preventive Services Task Force: Clinical summary screening for osteoporosis. Ann Intern Med, Jan 18, 2011

U.S. Preventive Services Task Force: Screening for thyroid disease. Ann Intern Med 140:125–127, 2004

U.S. Preventive Services Task Force: Screening for thyroid dysfunction in nonpregnant, asymptomatic adults. Available at: https://www.uspreventiveservicestaskforce.org/Page/Document/UpdateSummaryFinal/thyroid-dysfunction-screening?ds=1&s=thyroid%20screening

Williamson MA, Snyder LM (eds): Wallach's Interpretation of Diagnostic Tests, 10th ed. Philadelphia, Lippincott Williams & Wilkins, 2014

Worsley GJ, Tourniaire GA, Medlock KES, et al: Continuous blood glucose monitoring with a thin-film optical sensor. Clin Chem 53(10):1820–1826, 2007

Wu AHB: Tietz Clinical Guide to Laboratory Tests, 4th ed. Philadelphia, Saunders Elsevier, 2006

Young DS: Effects of Drugs on Clinical Laboratory Tests, 5th ed. Washington, DC, AACC Press, 2000

Young DS: Effects of Preanalytical Variables on Clinical Laboratory Tests, 3rd ed. Washington, DC, AACC Press, 2007

7 Microbiologic Studies

OVERVIEW OF MICROBIOLOGIC STUDIES

Diagnostic Testing and Microbes

Microorganisms that cause infectious disease are defined as *pathogens*. Organisms that are pathogenic under one set of conditions may, under other conditions, reside within or on the surface of the body without causing disease. When organisms are present but do not cause harm to the host, they are considered commensals. When organisms multiply and cause tissue damage, they are considered pathogens, with the potential for causing or increasing a pathogenic process (Chart 7.1). Some organisms that were formerly considered insignificant contaminants or commensals have taken on roles as causative agents for opportunistic diseases in patients with HIV infection or other immunodeficiency syndromes or diseases associated with a compromised health status. Consequently, virtually any organism recovered in pure culture from a body site must be considered a *potential pathogen*.

Basic Concepts of Infectious Disease

Infectious processes demonstrate observable physiologic responses to the invasion and multiplication of the offending microorganisms. Once an infectious disease is suspected, appropriate cultures should be done or nonculture techniques should be used, such as serologic testing for antigens and antibodies, monoclonal antibodies, and DNA probes. Proper specimen collection and appropriate blood and skin tests are necessary to detect and diagnose the presence of the microorganism.

Opportunity for infection depends on host resistance, organism volumes, and the ability of the organism to find a portal of entry and to overcome host defenses, invade tissues, and produce toxins. Organisms may become seated in susceptible persons through inhalation, ingestion, direct contact, inoculation, breaks in natural skin or mucous membrane barriers, changes in organism volumes, alterations in normal flora balances, or changes in other host defense mechanisms.

Host Factors

The development of an infectious disease is influenced by the patient's general health, normal defense mechanisms, previous contact with the offending organism, past clinical history, and type and location of infected tissue. Mechanisms of host resistance are detailed in the following lists:

1. Primary host defenses
   a. Anatomic barriers
      (1) Intact skin surfaces
      (2) Nose hairs
      (3) Respiratory tract cilia
      (4) Coughing and flow of respiratory tract fluids and mucus
      (5) Swallowing and gastrointestinal (GI) tract peristalsis
   b. Physiologic barriers
      (1) High or low pH and oxygen tension (prevents proliferation of organisms)
      (2) Chemical inhibitors to bacterial growth (e.g., proteases)
      (3) Bile acids
      (4) Active lysozymes in saliva and tears
      (5) Fatty acids on skin surfaces
2. Secondary host defenses (physiologic barriers)
   a. Responses of complement, lysozymes, opsonins, and secretions
   b. Phagocytosis

CHART 7.1 Some Common Pathogens Detectable in Body Tissues and Fluids by Diagnostic Methods

Nasopharyngeal and Oropharyngeal Specimens	Sputum	Feces
β-Hemolytic streptococci	*Blastomyces dermatitidis*	*Campylobacter jejuni*
Bordetella pertussis	*Bordetella pertussis*	*Clostridium botulinum*
Mycoplasma spp.	*Candida albicans*	*Entamoeba histolytica*
Moraxella catarrhalis	*Coccidioides immitis*	*Escherichia coli*
Herpes simplex virus	Influenza viruses	*Salmonella* spp.
Pseudomonas spp.	*Streptococcus pneumoniae*	*Shigella* spp.
Candida albicans	*Pseudomonas* spp.	*Staphylococcus aureus*
Corynebacterium diphtheriae	*Haemophilus influenzae*	*Vibrio cholerae*
Haemophilus influenzae	β-Hemolytic streptococci	*Vibrio vulnificus*
Neisseria meningitidis	*Histoplasma capsulatum*	*Vibrio parahaemolyticus*
Streptococcus pneumoniae	*Klebsiella* spp.	*Yersinia enterocolitica*
Staphylococcus aureus	*Mycobacterium* spp.	*Clostridium difficile*
Enterobacteriaceae	*Yersinia pestis*	Rotavirus
Cryptococcus neoformans	*Francisella tularensis*	Hepatitis A, B, and C
Respiratory syncytial virus	*Staphylococcus aureus*	*Giardia lamblia*
Influenza viruses	*Mycoplasma* spp.	*Cryptosporidium* spp.
Parainfluenza viruses	*Legionella* spp.	Norovirus
Adenovirus	*Chlamydophila pneumoniae*	*Aeromonas* sp.
Rhinovirus	*Pneumocystis* spp.	*Plesiomonas* sp.
Coronavirus		*Leptospira* spp.

Urine	
Streptococcus agalactiae	*Pseudomonas aeruginosa*
Escherichia coli, other	*Staphylococcus aureus*
Enterobacteriaceae	*Staphylococcus saprophyticus*
Enterococcus spp.	*Salmonella* and *Shigella* spp.
Neisseria gonorrhoeae	*Trichomonas vaginalis*
Mycobacterium tuberculosis	*Candida albicans* and other yeasts
	Staphylococcus epidermidis

Skin	Ear
Bacteroides spp.	*Aspergillus fumigatus*
Clostridium spp.	*Candida albicans* and other yeast
Fungi	Enterobacteriaceae
Pseudomonas spp.	β-Hemolytic streptococci
Staphylococcus aureus	*Streptococcus pneumoniae*
Streptococcus pyogenes	*Pseudomonas aeruginosa*
Varicella zoster virus	*Staphylococcus aureus*
Sarcoptes scabiei	*Moraxella catarrhalis*
Herpes simplex virus	*Mycoplasma pneumoniae*
Bacillus anthracis	*Peptostreptococcus* spp.
Treponema pallidum	*Bacteroides fragilis*
	Fusobacterium nucleatum
	Influenza virus
	Respiratory syncytial virus (RSV)

continues on pg. 460 >

CHART 7.1, continued

Cerebrospinal Fluid	Vaginal Discharge	Urethral Discharge
Bacteroides spp.	β-Hemolytic streptococci	*Chlamydia trachomatis*
Cryptococcus neoformans	*Candida albicans*	Coliform bacilli
Haemophilus influenzae	*Gardnerella vaginalis*	Herpes simplex virus
Mycobacterium tuberculosis	*Listeria monocytogenes*	*Neisseria gonorrhoeae*
Neisseria meningitidis	*Mycoplasma* spp.	*Treponema pallidum*
Streptococcus pneumoniae	Human papilloma virus	*Trichomonas vaginalis*
Enteroviruses	*Neisseria gonorrhoeae*	*Mycoplasma* spp.
Listeria monocytogenes	*Treponema pallidum*	*Ureaplasma urealyticum*
Streptococcus agalactiae (Group B)	Herpes simplex virus	Human papillomavirus
Staphylococcus spp.	*Trichomonas vaginalis*	*Mobiluncus* spp. and other anaerobes
Escherichia coli	*Chlamydia trachomatis*	
Herpes simplex virus		
Mycoplasma spp.		

   c. Immunoglobulin A (IgA), immunoglobulin G (IgG), and immunoglobulin M (IgM) antibody formation
   d. Cell-mediated immune responses
3. Factors decreasing host resistance
   a. Age (very young or very old)
   b. Presence of chronic disease (e.g., cancer, cardiovascular disease, diabetes)
   c. Use or history of certain therapeutic modalities, such as radiation, chemotherapy, corticosteroids, antibiotics, or immunosuppressants
   d. Toxins, including alcohol; drugs (including legal, illegal, prescription, and nonprescription); venom or toxic secretions from a reptile or insect; or other nonhuman bites or punctures
   e. Others, including excessive physical or emotional stress states, nutritional state, and presence of foreign material at the site

COLLECTION AND TRANSPORT OF SPECIMENS

General Principles

The healthcare provider is responsible for collecting specimens for diagnostic examinations. Because procedures vary, check institutional protocols for specimen retrieval, transport, and preservation, and reporting of test results.

Specimens for bacterial culture should be representative of the disease process. Also, sufficient material must be collected to ensure an accurate examination. As an example, serous drainage from a diabetic foot ulcer with possible osteomyelitis may yield inaccurate results. In this case, a bone biopsy or purulent drainage of infected tissue would be a better specimen. Likewise, if there is a lesion of the skin and subcutaneous tissue, material from the margin of the lesion rather than the central part of the lesion would be more desirable. If a purulent sputum sample cannot be obtained to aid in the diagnosis of pneumonia, blood cultures, pleural fluid examination, and bronchoalveolar lavage (BAL) specimens are also acceptable.

It is imperative that material be collected where the suspected organism is most likely to be found, with as little contamination from normal flora as possible. For this reason, certain precautions must be followed routinely:

1. Observe standard precautions. Clean the skin starting centrally and going out in larger circles. Repeat several times, using a clean swab or wipe each time. If 70% alcohol is used, it should be applied for 2 minutes. Tincture of iodine requires only 1 minute of cleansing.
2. Bypass areas of normal flora; culture only for a specific pathogen.
3. Collect fluids, tissues, skin scrapings, and urine in sterile containers with tight-fitting lids. Polyester-tipped swabs in a collection system containing an ampule of Stuart's transport medium ensure adequacy of the specimen for 72 hours at room temperature.
4. Label specimen with the patient's name, date, and test(s) ordered and place the specimen in a biohazard bag.

PROCEDURAL ALERT

1. Without routine precautions for collecting and handling specimens, the patient's condition may be incorrectly diagnosed, laboratory time may be wasted, effective treatment may be delayed, or pathogenic organisms may be transmitted to healthcare workers and other patients.
2. It is important to report all identified diseases, conditions, and outbreaks according to state and federal guidelines.

Collection Procedures

Microbiologic specimens may be collected from many sources, such as blood, tissue, pus or wound exudates or drainage, urine, sputum, feces, genital discharges or secretions, cerebrospinal fluid (CSF), and eye or ear drainage. During specimen collection, these general procedures should be followed:

1. Label specimens properly with the following information (institutional requirements may vary):
   a. Patient's name, age, gender, address, hospital identification number, and healthcare provider's full name
   b. Specimen source (e.g., throat, conjunctiva)
   c. Date and time of collection
   d. Specific studies ordered
   e. Clinical diagnosis; suspected microorganisms
   f. Patient's history
   g. Patient's immune status
   h. Previous and current infections
   i. Previous or current antibiotic therapy
   j. Isolation status (e.g., contact, respiratory, wound)
   k. Other requested information pertinent to testing
2. Avoid contaminating the specimen; maintain aseptic or sterile technique as required:
   a. Special supplies may be required:
      (1) For anaerobes, sterile syringe aspiration of pus or other body fluid
      (2) Anaerobic transport containers for tissue specimens
   b. Sterile specimen containers
   c. Precautions to take during specimen collection include:
      (1) Observe standard precautions.
      (2) Take care to maintain cleanliness outside container surfaces.
      (3) Use appropriately fitting covers or plugs for specimen tubes and bottles.
      (4) Replace sterile plugs and caps that have become contaminated.

3. Ensure the preservation of specimens by delivering them promptly to the laboratory. Many specimens may be refrigerated (not frozen) for a few hours without any adverse effects. Note the following exceptions:
   a. Urine culture samples must be refrigerated unless a preservative that allows for short-term storage at room temperature is used.
   b. CSF specimens should be transported to the laboratory as soon as possible. If this is problematic, the culture should be incubated (meningococci do not withstand refrigeration). Both culture bottles must be maintained at room temperature prior to being placed in the analyzer.
   c. Blood culture bottles must be maintained at room temperature.
4. Transport specimens quickly to the laboratory to prevent desiccation of the specimen and death of the microorganisms.
   a. For anaerobic cultures, no more than 10 minutes should elapse between time of collection and culture. Anaerobic specimens should always be placed into an anaerobic transport container.
   b. Feces suspected of harboring *Salmonella* or *Shigella* organisms should be placed in a special transport medium, such as Cary-Blair, if culturing of the specimen will be delayed longer than 30 minutes.
5. Ensure that specimen quantity is adequate. With few exceptions, the quantity of the specimen should be as large as possible. When only a small quantity is available, swabs should be moistened with sterile saline just before collection, especially for nasopharyngeal cultures.
6. Handle specimen collection in the following way:
   a. Submit entire fluid specimen collected. Do not submit fluids on swabs.
   b. Whenever possible, specimens should be collected before antibiotic regimens are instituted; for example, complete all blood culture sampling before starting antibiotic therapy.

Transport of Specimens by Mail

Several kits containing transport media are available for use when there is a significant delay between collection and culturing. Culture swabs (containing transport medium) are available for bacterial, viral, and anaerobic collection of specimens. Some laboratories provide Cary-Blair and polyvinyl alcohol (PVA) or non–mercury-based fixative transport vials for stool collection for culture and ova and parasite examination, respectively. Depending on the request, some specimens may have to be shipped in a Styrofoam box with refrigerant packs. This is especially true for specimens to be tested for viral examination. It is prudent to consult the reference laboratory to which specimens will be sent for information on proper collection and shipment.

According to the Code of Federal Regulations (49 CFR Part 173), a viable organism or its toxin or a diagnostic specimen (volume <50 mL) must be placed in a secure, closed, watertight container that is then enclosed in a second secure, watertight container. Biohazard labels should be placed on the outside of the container.

Specimens that are to be transported within an institution should be placed in a sealed biohazard bag. Ideally, the requisition should accompany the specimen but not be sealed inside the bag.

DIAGNOSTIC TESTING PROCEDURES

Five different categories of laboratory tests are used for the diagnosis of infections: smears and stains, cultures, tissue biopsy, serologic testing, and skin testing. Cultures and skin testing are described in detail in this chapter; serologic testing is described in Chapter 8. A brief description of each of these procedures follows.

The Smear and Stain

A smear specimen for microscopic study is usually prepared by rolling a small quantity of the specimen material across a glass slide. A drop of saline in which the specimen has been emulsified can also be used. If the slide is also to be stained, it is generally fixed by rinsing in methanol. For direct examination of unstained material, phase-contrast microscopy can be used.

Smears are most often observed after they have been stained. Stains are salts composed of a positive and a negative ion, one of which is colored. Structures present in the specimen pick up the stain and make the organism visible under the light microscope. One staining procedure, called the *negative stain*, colors the background but leaves the organisms themselves uncolored. The gross structure of the organisms can then be studied.

Bacterial stains are of two major types: simple and differential. A *simple stain* consists of a coloring agent such as gentian violet, crystal violet, carbol-fuchsin, methylene blue, or safranine O. A thin smear of sampled organisms is stained and then observed under an oil-immersion lens. A *differential stain* is one in which two chemically different stains are applied to the same smear. Organisms that are physiologically different pick up different stains.

The *Gram stain* is the most important of all bacteriologic differential stains. It divides bacteria into two physiologic groups: gram-positive and gram-negative organisms. The staining procedure consists of four major steps: (1) staining the smear with gentian or crystal violet; (2) washing off the violet stain and flooding the smear with an iodine solution; (3) washing off the iodine solution and flooding the smear with 95% alcohol or an acetone-alcohol mixture; and (4) counterstaining the smear with safranine O, a red dye. The Gram stain permits morphologic study of the sampled bacteria and divides all bacteria according to their ability or inability to pick up one or both of the stains. Gram-positive and gram-negative bacteria exhibit different properties, which helps to identify and differentiate them.

Stains other than the Gram stain are used for examining bacteriologic smears. Some, such as the *acid-fast stain*, can identify organisms of the genus *Mycobacterium*. Other stains differentiate certain structures, such as capsules, endospores, or flagella.

Cultures

Preparation of a culture involves growing microorganisms or living tissue cells on a special medium that supports the growth of a given material. Cultures may be maintained in test tubes or Petri dishes. The container holds the *culture medium*, which is either solid, semisolid, or liquid. Each organism has its own special requirements for growth (proper combination of nutritive ingredients, temperature, and presence or absence of oxygen). The culture is prepared in accordance with the needs of the organism. Later, it is usually incubated to enhance growth. Acid-fast bacilli (AFB) cultures, to determine whether an individual has an active *Mycobacterium tuberculosis* infection, can take up to 6 weeks.

Tissue Biopsy

At times, microorganisms are isolated from small quantities of body tissue that have been surgically removed. Such tissue is removed aseptically and transferred to a sterile container to be rapidly transported to the laboratory for analysis. Generally, the specimens are finely ground in a sterile homogenizer and then stained and cultured.

Serologic Testing

Infections can be diagnosed by detection of an immunologic response specific to an infecting agent in a patient's serum. Normal humans produce both IgM (first-response antibodies) and IgG (antibodies that may persist long after an infection) to most pathogens. For most pathogens, detection of IgM antibodies or a fourfold increase in the patient's antibody titer is considered to be diagnostic of current infection. If the infecting agent is rare or previous exposure is unlikely (e.g., rabies virus, botulin), the presence of specific IgG antibody in a single serum specimen can be diagnostic. Methods for detecting the presence of antibodies include immunodiffusion assay, complement fixation, enzyme-linked immunosorbent assay (ELISA), indirect or direct fluorescent antibody, radioimmunoassay, and Western blot immunoassay (see Chapter 8).

Skin Testing

Skin testing determines hypersensitivity to the toxic products formed in the body by pathogens. In general, three types of skin tests are performed: scratch tests, patch tests, and intradermal tests.

BLOOD, URINE, EYE, AND EAR CULTURES

● Blood Cultures

Blood cultures are collected whenever there is reason to suspect bacteremia or septicemia. Although mild transitory bacteremia is a frequent finding in many infections, a persistent, continuous, or recurrent bacteremia indicates a more serious condition that may require immediate treatment. The expeditious detection and identification of pathogens (bacteria, fungi, viruses, and parasites) in the blood may aid in making a clinical and etiologic diagnosis.

Indications for Blood Culture

1. Bacteremia
2. Septicemia
3. Shock
4. Unexplained postoperative shock
5. Postoperative shock after genitourinary tract manipulation or surgery
6. Unexplained fever of several days' duration
7. Chills and fever in patients with:
    a. Infected burns
    b. Urinary tract infection
    c. Rapidly progressing tissue infection
    d. Postoperative wound sepsis
    e. Indwelling venous or arterial catheter
8. Debilitated patients receiving:
    a. Antibiotics
    b. Corticosteroids
    c. Immunosuppressives
    d. Antimetabolites
    e. Parenteral hyperalimentation
9. Following body piercing (nose, tongue, nipples, umbilicus) with signs of infection and bacteremia

NOTE

1. *During an acute febrile illness, immediately draw two separate blood samples from separate sites. Obtain cultures prior to starting antimicrobial therapy because antimicrobial therapy may interfere with bacterial growth.*
2. *For fever of unknown origin, two blood cultures can be initially drawn 45 to 60 minutes apart. If necessary, two more sets of samples can be drawn 24 to 48 hours later.*
3. *In cases of acute endocarditis, draw blood cultures as stated earlier. If results are negative, two more sets of samples may be obtained on subsequent days.*
4. *Parasites in the blood* (Plasmodium, Trypanosoma, *and* Babesia) *are usually detected by direct microscopic observation.*
5. *For infants and small children, only 1 to 5 mL of blood can safely be drawn for culture. Quantities <1 mL may be insufficient to detect bacterial organisms. In adults, cultures should optimally be 20 to 30 mL of blood.*

Reference Values

Normal

Negative for pathogens

Procedure for Blood Culture

During venipuncture, because of the high potential for infecting the patient, aseptic technique must be used. Key points are listed as follows:

1. Observe standard precautions. The proposed puncture site should be scrubbed with an antiseptic agent such as chlorhexidine. Allow to dry for 1 to 2 minutes.
2. Cleanse the rubber stoppers of culture bottles with chlorhexidine and allow to air-dry.
3. Perform venipuncture with a sterile syringe and needle; avoid contamination of the cleansed puncture site.
4. Withdraw about 10 to 30 mL of blood into a 20-mL syringe or directly into the culture tubes. Because of the danger of accidental needle sticks, the practice of changing needles to transfer the specimen into blood culture bottles has been replaced by direct injection with the original phlebotomy needle.
5. If two culture bottles are to be inoculated (one anaerobic and one aerobic), first inoculate the aerobic bottle with the optimal, manufacturer-recommended volume and then inoculate the anaerobic bottle with the remaining, being careful not to over-inoculate. Be certain to inoculate each bottle with the optimum blood volume.
6. Mix both bottles gently.
7. Label specimens with the patient's name, date, and tests ordered and immediately transfer them to the laboratory.
8. Cleanse the site with alcohol after the venipuncture because some patients are sensitive to iodine.

PROCEDURAL ALERT

1. Handle all blood specimens according to standard precautions.
2. After disinfection, *do not* palpate the venipuncture site unless sterile gloves are worn. Palpation is the greatest potential cause of blood culture contamination.
3. Specimens can be drawn from two or three different sites to exclude a skin-contaminating organism.
4. Collection of more than three blood cultures in a 24-hr period does not improve the detection of bacteria.
5. It is recommended to draw blood below an intravenous line (if possible) to prevent dilution of the sample.

Clinical Implications

1. *Negative* cultures: If all cultures, subcultures (if performed), and Gram-stained smears are negative, the blood culture may be reported as no growth after 5 to 7 days of incubation.
2. *Positive* cultures: Pathogens most commonly found in blood cultures include:
   a. *Bacteroides* spp.
   b. *Brucella* spp.
   c. Enterobacteriaceae
   d. *Pseudomonas aeruginosa*
   e. *Haemophilus influenzae*
   f. *Listeria monocytogenes*
   g. *Streptococcus pneumoniae*

h. *Enterococcus* spp.
i. *Staphylococcus aureus*, *Staphylococcus epidermidis*
j. *Streptococcus* spp. including β-hemolytic streptococci
k. *Candida albicans*
l. *Clostridium perfringens*

Interfering Factors

Blood cultures are subject to contamination, especially by skin bacteria. These skin organisms should be identified if possible.

Interventions

Pretest Patient Care

1. Explain purpose of and procedure for culture. Obtain and document pertinent history of signs and symptoms of infection.
2. Follow guidelines in Chapter 1 for safe, effective, informed *pretest* care.

Posttest Patient Care

1. Review test results; report and record findings. Modify the nursing care plan as needed. Monitor for bacteremia, septicemia, and other febrile illness. Counsel the patient appropriately about treatment (triple antibiotic therapy).
2. Follow guidelines in Chapter 1 for safe, effective, informed *posttest* care.

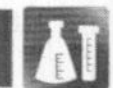

CLINICAL ALERT

The healthcare provider should be notified immediately about positive culture results so that appropriate treatment may be started.

• Urine Cultures

Urine cultures are most commonly used to diagnose bacterial urinary tract infection (kidneys, ureter, bladder, and urethra). Urine is an excellent culture and growth medium for most organisms that infect the urinary tract. The combination of pyuria (pus in the urine) and significant bacteriuria strongly suggests the presence of a urinary tract infection.

General Collection Procedures for Urine Culture

1. Early-morning specimens should be obtained whenever possible because bacterial counts are highest at that time.
2. A clean-voided urine specimen of at least 3 to 5 mL should be collected into a sterile container. Catheterization and aspiration of a suprapubic or indwelling catheter are alternative methods for procuring urine specimens.
3. Urine specimens for culture must never be retrieved from a urine collection bag that is part of an indwelling catheter drainage system.
4. Ideally, urine should be transported to the laboratory and examined as soon as possible. When this is not possible, the urine can be refrigerated for up to 24 hours before being cultured.
5. Whenever possible, specimens should be obtained before antibiotic or antimicrobial therapy begins.
6. Professional health personnel should instruct the patient concerning proper specimen collection technique. Failure to isolate a causative organism is frequently the result of faulty cleansing or collection techniques that can come from lack of information about the proper collection procedure.

7. Provide proper supplies and privacy for cleansing and urine collection. Instruct patients in proper cleansing techniques. The patient who is unable to comply with instructions should be assisted by healthcare personnel.
8. The urine specimen should be properly labeled. Pertinent information includes:
   a. Patient's identification information
   b. Healthcare provider's name
   c. Suspected clinical diagnosis
   d. Method of collection
   e. Date and time obtained
   f. Specific chemotherapeutic agents being administered

CLINICAL ALERT

Catheterization heightens the risk for introducing bacteria.

CLINICAL ALERT

1. Urine is an excellent culture medium. At room temperature, it promotes the growth of many organisms. Specimen collection should be as aseptic as possible. Samples should be transported to the laboratory and examined as soon as possible. The specimen must be refrigerated or placed in a preservative if there is a delay in examination.
2. In the case of suspected urinary tract tuberculosis (TB), three consecutive early-morning specimens should be collected. Special care should be taken when cleaning the external genitalia to reduce the risk for contamination with commensal acid-fast *Mycoplasma* or *Mycobacterium smegmatis.*

Reference Values

Normal

Negative

Procedure for Clean-Catch (Midstream) Urine Specimen

1. For women
   a. Wash and dry hands thoroughly.
   b. Remove the cap from the sterile container and place it so that only the outer surface touches whatever it is placed on.
   c. Cleanse the area around the urinary meatus from front to back with an antiseptic wipe or sponge.
   d. Spread the labia apart with one hand. Hold the sterile container in the other hand, using care not to contaminate the inside surface.
   e. Void the first 25 mL into the toilet and then catch the rest of the urine directly into the sterile container without stopping the urine stream until sufficient quantity is collected. Hold the collection cup in such a way that it avoids contact with the legs, vulva, or clothing. Keep fingers away from the rim and inner surface of the container.
   f. Recap the specimen container, taking care not to contaminate the inside surface of the cap.
   g. Wash and dry hands thoroughly.
   h. Observe standard precautions when handling specimens.
2. For men
   a. Wash and dry hands thoroughly.
   b. Remove the cap from the sterile container and place it so that only the outer surface touches whatever it is placed on.

c. Retract the foreskin completely to expose the glans.
d. Cleanse the area around the meatus with antiseptic wipe or sponge.
e. Void the first 25 mL of urine directly into the toilet and then void a sufficient amount of urine into the sterile specimen container. Do not collect the last few drops of urine.
f. Recap the specimen container, taking care not to contaminate the inside surface of the cap.
g. Wash and dry hands thoroughly.
h. Observe standard precautions when handling specimens.

3. For infants and young children
   a. Use a suitable plastic collection apparatus to collect urine. Because the collection bag touches skin surfaces and picks up commensal organisms, the specimen must be analyzed as soon as possible.
   b. Cleanse and dry the urethral area thoroughly before applying the collection bag.
   c. Cover collection bag with a diaper or undergarment to prevent dislodging.
   d. Be aware that specimens collected by catheterization may be necessary to detect a urinary tract infection because of the contamination associated with collection bags.

Clinical Implications

1. A bacterial count of >100,000 colony forming units (CFU)/mL indicates infection. A mixed bacterial count of <10,000 CFU/mL does not necessarily indicate infection but rather indicates possible contamination. However, growth of a single potential pathogen to >10,000 CFU/mL may be clinically significant in a symptomatic patient.
2. The following organisms, when present in the urine in sufficient quantity, may be considered pathogenic:
   a. *Escherichia coli* and other Enterobacteriaceae
   b. *Enterococcus* spp.
   c. *Neisseria gonorrhoeae*
   d. *M. tuberculosis* (requires special culture media)
   e. *P. aeruginosa*
   f. *S. aureus*
   g. *Staphylococcus saprophyticus*
   h. Streptococci (β-hemolytic, usually group B)
   i. *C. albicans* and other yeasts
3. Urine samples obtained by straight catheterization, suprapubic aspiration, or cystoscopy or during surgery represent bladder urine. Growth of *any* isolate is considered clinically significant.

Interfering Factors

1. Patients who are receiving forced fluids may have urine that is sufficiently dilute to reduce the bacterial count to <100,000 CFU/mL.
2. Bacterial contamination comes from sources such as:
   a. Perineal hair
   b. Bacteria beneath the prepuce in male patients
   c. Bacteria from vaginal secretions, from the vulva, or from the distal urethra in female patients
   d. Bacteria from the hands, skin, or clothing

Interventions

Pretest Patient Care

1. Explain purpose of test, procedure for urine collection, and interfering factors.
2. Ensure that the cleansing procedure is done correctly to remove contaminating organisms from the vulva, urethral meatus, and perineal area so that any bacteria found in the urine can be assumed to have come only from the bladder and urethra.
3. Follow guidelines in Chapter 1 for safe, effective, informed *pretest* care.

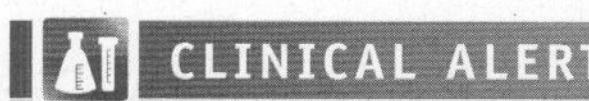

The urine culture sample should *not* be taken from a urinal or bedpan and should *not* be brought from home. The urine should be collected directly into the sterile container that will be used for culture.

Posttest Patient Care

1. Review test results; report and record findings. Modify the nursing care plan as needed. Monitor for urinary tract infection. Counsel the patient appropriately about treatment and possible further testing.
2. Follow guidelines in Chapter 1 for safe, effective, informed *posttest* care.

● Eye and Ear Cultures

Bacterial conjunctivitis, caused by *S. pneumoniae, S. aureus,* and *H. influenzae*, is the most common type of infectious conjunctivitis. Inflammation of the cornea usually follows some type of trauma to the ocular surface. Postsurgical and posttraumatic endophthalmitis is often associated with *Bacillus* spp. and Enterobacteriaceae in addition to the aforementioned organisms.

Acute otitis media occurs in the form of a pustule and is often caused by *S. aureus.* Swimmer's ear is related to maceration of the ear from swimming or hot, humid weather; it often is caused by *P. aeruginosa*. Otitis media often begins as a viral infection, with a bacterial infection occurring soon afterward. In children, the most common pathogens are *S. pneumoniae, H. influenzae*, and *Moraxella catarrhalis*.

Reference Values

Normal

Low counts of *S. epidermidis*, *Lactobacillus* spp., and *Propionibacterium acnes* may be found in eye cultures and in the flora of the external ear.

Procedure for Eye Cultures

1. Observe standard precautions. Purulent material from the lower conjunctival sac or inner canthus of the eye is collected on a sterile swab and placed in transport medium. Each eye should be cultured separately.
2. Scrapings of the cornea with a heat-sterilized platinum spatula directly onto the medium (blood or chocolate agar, brain-heart infusion medium for fungi, or thioglycolate broth) in cases of keratitis should be obtained by an ophthalmologist. For viral culture, the material is placed into viral transport broth.
3. Do not refrigerate specimens or transport on ice. Deliver to the laboratory as soon as possible.

Procedure for Ear Cultures

1. Cleanse the ear with a mild germicide to exclude contaminating skin flora in cases of external otitis.
2. Use a sterile swab or syringe and needle to collect middle ear fluid. Cultures from the mastoid usually are taken during surgery.
3. Do not refrigerate specimens. Label specimens with the patient's name, date, and test(s) ordered and deliver to the laboratory as soon as possible.

Interventions

Pretest Patient Care

1. Explain purpose of and procedure for the culture. Record signs and symptoms of ear infection, pain, redness, and drainage.
2. Follow guidelines in Chapter 1 for safe, effective, informed *pretest* care.

Posttest Patient Care

1. Review test results; report and record findings. Modify the nursing care plan as needed. Monitor the site of infection. Counsel the patient appropriately.
2. Follow guidelines in Chapter 1 for safe, effective, informed *posttest* care.

RESPIRATORY TRACT CULTURES

Three types of culture may be used to diagnose respiratory tract infections: sputum, throat swabs, and nasopharyngeal swabs. At times, the purposes for which certain tests are ordered overlap.

Reference Values

The following organisms may be present in the nasopharynx of apparently healthy persons:

1. *C. albicans*
2. *Corynebacterium* spp.
3. *Haemophilus hemolyticus, Haemophilus parainfluenzae*
4. Staphylococci (coagulase negative)
5. Streptococci (α-hemolytic)
6. Streptococci (nonhemolytic)
7. Micrococci
8. *Lactobacillus* spp.
9. *Veillonella* spp.

CLINICAL ALERT

1. Twenty percent of normal adults carry *S. aureus*; 10% are carriers of group A hemolytic streptococci.
2. A rapid strep test gives results after 10 min instead of 24–48 hr. It has a false-negative rate of 5%–10%, about the same as traditional methods. It permits rapid diagnosis and treatment.
3. Both throat and urine cultures are done to detect cytomegalovirus (CMV).

● Sputum Cultures

Sputum is *not* material from the postnasal region and is *not* spittle or saliva. A sputum specimen comes from deep within the bronchi. Effective coughing usually enables the patient to produce a satisfactory sputum specimen.

Indications for Collection

Sputum cultures are important for diagnosis of the following conditions:

1. Bacterial pneumonia
2. Pulmonary tuberculosis (TB)
3. Chronic bronchitis
4. Bronchiectasis
5. Suspected pulmonary mycotic infections
6. Mycoplasmal pneumonia
7. Suspected viral pneumonia

Reference Values

Normal

Negative: normal oral flora

Procedure

1. Instruct patients to provide a deep-cough specimen into a sterile container. Often, an early-morning specimen is best. Expectorated material of 1 to 3 mL is sufficient for most examinations. Remember that good sputum samples depend on thorough healthcare worker education and patient understanding during the collection process.
2. Label specimens with the patient's name, date, and test(s) ordered and note the suspected infection on the accompanying requisition.
3. Do not refrigerate specimens; deliver to the laboratory as soon as possible.

Interventions

Pretest Patient Care

1. Assess for and document signs and symptoms of infection (coughing, productive sputum, blood in sputum).
2. Instruct the patient that this test requires tracheobronchial sputum from deep in the lungs. Instruct the patient to take two or three deep breaths and then to take another deep breath and forcefully cough with exhalation.
3. Ask respiratory therapy personnel to assist the patient in obtaining an "aerosol-induced" specimen if the cough is not productive. Patients breathe aerosolized droplets of a sodium chloride–glycerin solution until a strong cough reflex is initiated. The specimen often appears watery but is in fact material directly from alveolar spaces. It should be noted on the requisition as being aerosol induced.
4. Remember that when pleural empyema is present, thoracentesis fluid and blood culture are excellent diagnostic specimens. Bronchial washings, BAL, and bronchial brush cultures are excellent for detecting most major pathogens of the respiratory tract.
5. Follow guidelines in Chapter 1 for safe, effective, informed *pretest* care.

Posttest Patient Care

1. Review test results; report and record findings. Modify the nursing care plan as needed. Monitor for respiratory tract infections. Counsel the patient about treatment.
2. Follow guidelines in Chapter 1 for safe, effective, informed *posttest* care.

● Throat Cultures (Swab or Washings)

1. Throat cultures are important for diagnosis of the following conditions:
   a. Streptococcal sore throat
   b. Diphtheria (obtain both throat and nasopharyngeal cultures)
   c. Thrush (candidal infection)
   d. Viral infection
   e. Tonsillar infection
   f. Gonococcal pharyngitis
   g. *Bordetella pertussis*
2. Throat cultures can establish the focus of infection in:
   a. Scarlet fever
   b. Rheumatic fever
   c. Acute hemorrhagic glomerulonephritis
3. Throat cultures can be used to detect the carrier state of persons harboring such organisms as:
   a. β-Hemolytic streptococcus
   b. *Neisseria meningitidis*
   c. *Corynebacterium diphtheriae*
   d. *S. aureus*

Reference Values

Normal

Negative: normal oral flora

Procedure

1. For adult patients
   a. Place the patient's mouth in good visual light.
   b. Use a sterile throat culture kit with a polyester-tipped applicator or swab and a sterile container or tube of culture medium.
   c. Tilt head back. Depress the patient's tongue with a tongue blade and visualize the throat as well as possible. Rotate the swab firmly and gently over the back of the throat, around both tonsils or fossae, and on areas of inflammation, exudation, or ulceration.
      (1) Avoid touching the tongue or lips with the swab.
      (2) Because most patients gag or cough, the collector should wear a facemask for protection.
   d. Place the swab into the designated receptacle so that it comes in contact with the culture medium. Label specimen with the patient's name, date, and test(s) ordered and immediately send the specimen to the laboratory.
   e. Refrigerate the throat culture if examination is delayed.
2. For pediatric patients
   a. Seat the patient in the adult's lap.
   b. Have the adult encircle the child's arms and chest to prevent the child from moving.
   c. Place one hand on the child's forehead to stabilize the head and to prevent movement.
   d. Proceed with the technique used for collection of the throat and nose culture as described for adults.
3. For throat washings
   a. Have the patient gargle with 5 to 10 mL of sterile saline solution and then expectorate it into a sterile cup.
   b. Remember that this method provides more specimen than a throat swab and is more definitive for viral isolation.

Clinical Implications

Positive findings are associated with infection in the presence of:

1. Group A hemolytic streptococci
2. *N. gonorrhoeae*
3. *C. diphtheriae*
4. *B. pertussis*
5. Adenovirus and herpesvirus
6. *Mycoplasma* and *Chlamydia*

Interventions

Pretest Patient Care

1. Explain purpose of and procedure for the text to patient or parents. Assess for and document signs and symptoms of infection (pain, redness, inflammation, and/or presence of exudates).
2. Follow guidelines in Chapter 1 for safe, effective, informed *pretest* care.

Posttest Patient Care

1. Review test results; report and record findings. Modify the nursing care plan as needed. Monitor for throat infection. Counsel the patient appropriately. Assess for and document any change in signs and symptoms.

2. For treatment of *B. pertussis* (whooping cough), macrolide antibiotics (e.g., erythromycin, clarithromycin, and azithromycin) are preferred in individuals older than 1 month. An alternative is trimethoprim-sulfamethoxazole (TMP-SMX) in patients older than 2 months who cannot tolerate macrolides or are infected with a macrolide-resistant strain of *B. pertussis*. The Tdap vaccine protects against tetanus, diphtheria, and pertussis; the vaccine is usually given in a scheduled series of doses from birth to 6 years of age and one booster dose at age 11 years.
3. Follow guidelines in Chapter 1 for safe, effective, informed *posttest* care.

● Nasopharyngeal Cultures (Swab)

Nasopharyngeal swabs are the optimal specimen for detection of *B. pertussis*. Nasopharyngeal swabs, aspirates, and washes are better suited for recovery of respiratory syncytial virus, parainfluenza virus, and viruses causing rhinitis.

Indications for Collection

1. Submitted primarily for viral cultures
2. *B. pertussis*
3. *C. diphtheriae*

Reference Values

Normal

Negative: normal oral flora

Procedure

1. Tip the patient's head back to collect a nasopharyngeal specimen.
2. Insert a flexible, calcium alginate–tipped swab carefully through the nose into the posterior nasopharynx and rotate the swab.
3. Pass two swabs simultaneously through one nostril and leave in nasopharynx for 15 to 30 seconds. Repeat procedure on other nostril with same two swabs. Although the calcium alginate–tipped swabs are most commonly used, aspirated nasopharyngeal specimens, obtained through a soft rubber bulb or plastic-tipped catheter, can be used.
4. Take specimens from both the nasopharyngeal area and the throat for *C. diphtheriae* confirmation.
5. In some cases, vacuum-assisted or bulb-collected nasopharyngeal specimens may be necessary.
6. Handle specimens as follows:
   a. Transport specimens for viral infection in appropriate transport media and refrigerate if not cultured within a few hours.
   b. Do not refrigerate samples unless for diphtheria or pertussis (whooping cough).

OTHER CULTURES AND SMEARS

● Wound and Abscess Cultures

Wound infections and abscesses occur as complications of surgery, trauma, or infection that interrupts a skin surface. Material from infected wounds reveals a variety of aerobic and anaerobic microorganisms. Because anaerobic microorganisms are the preponderant microflora in humans and are consistently present in the upper respiratory, GI, and genitourinary tracts, they are also likely to invade other parts of the body to cause severe, and sometimes fatal, infections. Blood cultures should always be drawn from patients with bullous lesions, burn infections, or significant myonecrosis. Infections can also occur when individuals with open wounds are exposed to *Vibrio vulnificus*, a bacterium present in warm coastal waters. *V. vulnificus* wound infections are of serious concern in hurricane-affected areas that experience coastal flooding.

Reference Values

Normal

Clinical specimens taken from wounds can harbor any of the following microorganisms. Pathogenicity depends on the quantity of organisms present. Quantitative or semiquantitative reporting of culture results may provide information on the relative importance of the various organisms present in the lesion and also the response of the infection to antibiotic therapy.

Potential pathogens:

1. *Actinomyces* spp.
2. *Bacteroides* and *Fusobacterium* spp.
3. *C. perfringens* and other species
4. *E. coli*
5. Other gram-negative enteric bacilli
6. *Mycobacterium marinum*
7. *Nocardia* spp.
8. *Pseudomonas* spp.
9. *S. aureus*
10. *Corynebacterium jeikeium*
11. *Enterococcus* spp.
12. Streptococci (β-hemolytic)
13. *Candida* spp.
14. *V. vulnificus*

Procedure

1. Procedure for wound culture
   a. Observe standard precautions.
   b. Most wounds need some form of preparation to reduce the risk for introducing extraneous organisms into the collected specimen. In the presence of moderate to heavy pus or drainage, irrigate the wound with sterile saline until all visible debris has been washed away. When culturing chronically present wounds (pressure sores), débride the wound surface of any loose necrotic, sloughed material before culturing. Cultures of the surface alone may be misleading; biopsies of deeper tissue are recommended.
   c. Disinfect the surface of the wound with 70% alcohol or an iodine solution.
   d. Apply sterile gauze pads to absorb excess saline and to expose the culture site. Always culture highly vascular areas of granulation tissue. Wearing sterile gloves, separate margins of deep wounds with thumb and forefinger to permit insertion of the swab deep into the wound cavity. Press and rotate the swab several times over the clean wound surfaces to extract tissue fluid containing the potential pathogen. Avoid touching the swab to intact skin at the wound edges. Whenever possible, submit tissue or an aspirate of the pus.
   e. Immediately place the swab into the appropriate transport container.
2. Procedure for anaerobic collection of aspirated material
   a. Decontaminate the culture site with surgical soap and 70% ethyl or isopropyl alcohol.
   b. Aspirate at least 1 mL of fluid using a sterile 3-mL syringe and a needle of appropriate gauge. Immediately transfer the aspirate to an anaerobic transport medium.
   c. Aspiration cultures are commonly done for closed wounds, such as soft tissue abscesses, cellulitis, or infected skin flaps. Tissue biopsies are more often performed during surgery, when infected tissue is more easily accessible.
   d. Never submit a swab when a tissue sample can be obtained.

Properly label the specimen for the microbiology laboratory with the following information:

1. Patient identification information
2. Healthcare provider's name

3. Date and time the specimen was collected
4. Anatomic site or specific source of the specimen
5. Type of specimen (e.g., granulation tissue, abscess fluid, postsurgical wound)
6. Examination requested
7. Patient's diagnosis
8. Current antibiotic therapy, if any

Clinical Implications

Clinically significant pathogens are likely to be present in the following specimens:

1. Pus from deep wounds or abscesses, especially if associated with a foul odor
2. Necrotic tissue or débrided material from suspected gas gangrene (also known as *clostridial myonecrosis* and *myonecrosis*) infection
3. Samples from infections bordering mucous membranes
4. Postoperative wound drainage
5. Lower extremity ulcers from diabetic patients
6. Decubitus ulcers from elderly or bedridden patients

CLINICAL ALERT

A microscopic examination of pus and wound exudates can be very helpful in diagnosing a pathogenic organism. Consider the following:

1. Pus from streptococcal infections is thin and serous.
2. Pus from staphylococcal infections is gelatinous.
3. Pus from *P. aeruginosa* infections is blue-green.
4. Actinomycosis infections show "sulfur" granules.
5. Bronze discoloration of the skin and fluid-filled blisters are present in gas gangrene.

Interventions

Pretest Patient Care

1. Explain purpose of and procedure for wound culture. Assess for and document signs and symptoms of wound infection (redness, inflammation, presence and type of drainage, and/or fever).
2. Follow guidelines in Chapter 1 for safe, effective, informed *pretest* care.

Posttest Patient Care

1. Review test results; report and record findings. Modify the nursing care plan as needed. Monitor the site of infection. Counsel the patient appropriately about treatment.
2. Follow guidelines in Chapter 1 for safe, effective, informed *posttest* care.

● Skin Cultures

The most common bacteria implicated in skin infections are *Staphylococcus aureus* and *Streptococcus pyogenes* (group A). The common abnormal skin conditions include:

1. Pyoderma
   a. Staphylococcal impetigo, characterized by bullous lesions with thin, amber, varnish-like crusts
   b. Streptococcal impetigo, characterized by thick crusts
2. Erysipelas
3. Folliculitis
4. Furuncles
5. Carbuncles

6. Secondary invasion of burns, scabies, and other skin lesions
7. Dermatophytoses, especially athlete's foot, scalp and body ringworm, and jock itch

Reference Values

Normal

The following organisms may be present on the skin of a healthy person. When present in low numbers, some of these organisms may be considered normal commensals; at other times, when they multiply to excess, these same organisms may become pathogens.

1. *Clostridium* spp.
2. *Enterobacteriaceae*
3. *Corynebacterium* spp.
4. Enterococci
5. Mycobacteria
6. Staphylococci
7. Streptococci
8. Yeasts and fungi

Procedure

To obtain scrapings from vesicular lesions or skin:

1. Observe standard precautions.
2. Clean the affected site with sterile saline, wipe gently with alcohol, and allow it to air-dry.
3. Aspirate a fluid sample from fresh, intact vesicles with a 25-gauge needle attached to a tuberculin syringe, and transfer the specimen to the transport medium by ejecting it from the syringe.
4. If fluid cannot be aspirated, open the vesicles and use a cotton-, rayon-, or Dacron-tipped applicator to swab the base of the lesion to collect infected cells. Place the swab directly into transport medium (e.g., self-contained foam pad with Stuart's media).
5. To make smears for stains, use a scalpel blade to scrape the base of the lesion, taking care not to macerate the cells. Spread scraped material in a thin layer on a slide.
6. Label specimen with the patient's name, date, and tests ordered and place the specimen in biohazard bag; do not refrigerate. Immediately transport the specimen to the laboratory for bacterial, fungal, or viral cultures.

CLINICAL ALERT

The most useful and common specimens for detection of fungal infection are skin scrapings, nail scrapings, and hair.

Clinical Implications

When present on the skin in significant quantities, the following organisms may be considered pathogenic and indicative of an abnormal condition:

1. Enterobacteriaceae
2. Fungi (*Sporotrichum*, *Actinomyces*, *Nocardia*, *C. albicans*, *Trichophyton*, *Microsporum*, *Epidermophyton*)
3. *Staphylococcus aureus*
4. *Streptococcus pyogenes*
5. *P. aeruginosa*
6. Varicella-zoster virus
7. Herpes simplex virus

Interventions

Pretest Patient Care

1. Explain purpose of and procedure for skin culture.
2. Follow guidelines in Chapter 1 for safe, effective, informed *pretest* care.

Posttest Patient Care

1. Review test results; report and record findings. Modify the nursing care plan as needed. Monitor site of infection. Counsel the patient appropriately about treatment. Report rashes and/or fever.
2. Follow guidelines in Chapter 1 for safe, effective, informed *posttest* care.

● Stool and Anal Cultures and Smears

Stool cultures are commonly done to identify bacteria associated with enteric infection. Of all specimens collected, feces are likely to contain the greatest number and greatest variety of organisms. For a routine stool culture, the stool is examined to detect and to rule out *Salmonella*, *Shigella*, *Campylobacter*, *Aeromonas*, *Plesiomonas*, and predominating numbers of *Staphylococcus* organisms; cultures for yeast, *Pseudomonas*, *Yersinia*, *Vibrio*, and Shiga toxin–producing *E. coli* have to be specifically requested, depending on laboratory practice. *Clostridium difficile* causes antibiotic-associated colitis. It is diagnosed by detection of the toxins.

A single negative stool culture should not be considered the end point in testing. At least three stool cultures collected on separate days are recommended if the patient's clinical picture suggests bacterial involvement despite previous negative cultures. Moreover, once a positive diagnosis has been made, the patient's personal contacts should also be tested to prevent a potential spread of infection.

Reference Values

Normal

The following organisms may be present in the stool of apparently healthy people:

1. *C. albicans*
2. *Enterococcus* spp.
3. *E. coli*
4. *Proteus* spp.
5. *P. aeruginosa*
6. *Streptococcus* spp.
7. *Staphylococcus* spp.

Procedure

1. Procedure for stool specimen collection
   a. Observe standard precautions.
   b. Use a dry container or a clean, dry bedpan to collect feces. Do not contaminate stool specimen with urine, water, soap, or disinfectants.
   c. Remember that a freshly passed stool is best. Diarrheal stool usually gives acceptable results.
   d. Select portions containing pus, blood, or mucus; 1 to 2 grams is sufficient.
   e. Do not retrieve stool from the toilet for specimen use.
   f. Do not place toilet tissue or diapers with the specimen. Either may contain bismuth, which interferes with laboratory tests.
   g. Transfer stool specimens from the bedpan to the container with tongue blades.
   h. Label the sealed specimen container with the patient's name, date, and tests ordered and immediately send it to the laboratory.
   i. Place the specimen in a transport medium, such as Cary-Blair medium, if a delay of longer than 2 hours for stool culture is anticipated (from time of collection until receipt in the laboratory). Specimens processed within 2 hours of collection do not require added preservatives.

2. Procedure for obtaining a rectal swab
   a. Observe standard precautions.
   b. Insert the swab gently into the rectum (to a depth of at least 3 cm) and rotate it to retrieve a visible amount of fecal material (Fig. 7.1).
   c. Place the swab into the receptacle containing transport medium, such as Cary-Blair medium.
   d. Label specimen with the patient's name, date, and test(s) ordered. Send it in a biohazard bag to the laboratory as soon as possible.
   e. Rectal swab may not contain sufficient sample to detect enteric pathogens. Whenever possible, stool should be submitted.
3. Procedure for performing cellophane tape test for pinworm (*Enterobius vermicularis*)
   a. Observe standard precautions. The tape test is indicated in cases of suspected enterobiasis (pinworms).
   b. Apply a strip of clear cellophane tape (not micropore or adhesive-type tape) to the perineal region. Remove and spread the tape on a slide for microscopic examination.
   c. Remember that a paraffin-coated swab can be used in place of the cellophane tape test. If used, place the swab within a stoppered test tube.
   d. Be aware that it may be necessary to make four to six examinations on consecutive days before ruling out the presence of pinworms.
   e. Test for pinworm eggs in the morning, before the patient has defecated or bathed.

CLINICAL ALERT

Stool specimens are far superior to rectal swab specimens. Often, rectal swabs reach only the anal canal and provide material of limited diagnostic significance.

Clinical Implications

1. *C. albicans*, *S. aureus*, and *P. aeruginosa*, found in large numbers in the stool, are considered pathogenic in the setting of previous antibiotic therapy. Alterations of normal flora by antibiotics often change the environment so that normally harmless organisms become pathogens.
2. *Cryptosporidiosis* is a cause of severe, protracted diarrhea in immunosuppressed patients. *Cryptosporidium* organisms can be detected by ova and parasite examination.

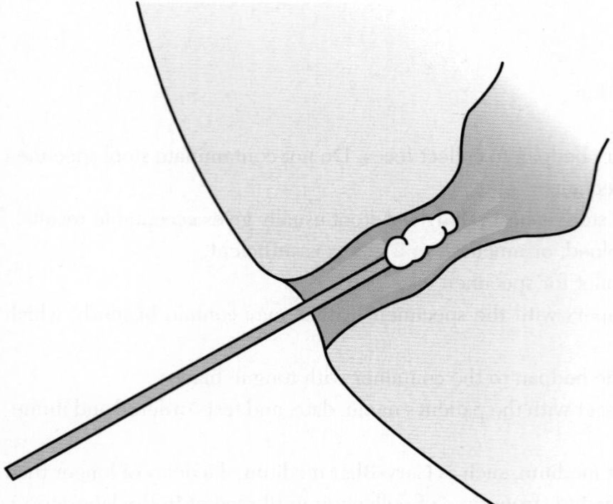

FIGURE 7.1. Method for obtaining the rectal culture.

3. *Helicobacter pylori* has been associated with gastritis and peptic ulcer disease. *H. pylori* is found only on the mucus-secreting epithelial cells of the stomach. Detection of *H. pylori* in gastric biopsy specimens necessitates collection of the specimens in sterile containers. Smears and cultures should be examined for the presence of this organism. Initial culture incubation requires 7 days. Therefore, results of gastric biopsy specimen cultures may take 8 to 10 days to obtain. A test for *H. pylori* antigen in the stool provides rapid detection of *H. pylori*.
4. *C. difficile*: Whenever normal flora are reduced by antibiotic therapy or other host factors, the syndrome known as *pseudomembranous colitis* can occur. This condition is caused by *C. difficile*. It may be present in small numbers in the normal person, or it may occur in the hospital environment. When normal flora are reduced, *C. difficile* can multiply and produce its toxins.

The definitive diagnosis of *C. difficile*–associated diarrhea is based on clinical criteria. Endoscopic visualization of a characteristic pseudomembrane or plaque, together with a history of antibiotic therapy, is diagnostic of *C. difficile*. Three laboratory tests are also available. These include stool culture for *C. difficile* (nonspecific; requires at least 48 hours); tissue culture for detection of cytotoxin (requires 48 hours); and rapid tests that are sensitive and specific for *C. difficile* antigens and toxins.

Interfering Factors

Stool from patients receiving barium, bismuth, mineral oil, or antibiotics is not satisfactory a specimen for identifying protozoa.

Interventions

Pretest Patient Care

1. Explain purpose of test, procedure for stool collection, and interfering factors. Assess for and document history of diarrhea, including type and length of time. Instruct the patient to defecate into a clean, dry bedpan or large-mouthed container.
2. Do not allow patient to defecate into the toilet bowl or urinate into the bedpan or collecting container because urine has an adverse effect on protozoa.
3. Do not place toilet paper into the bedpan or collection container; it may contain bismuth, which can interfere with testing.
4. Follow guidelines in Chapter 1 for safe, effective, informed *pretest* care.

Posttest Patient Care

1. Review test results; report and record findings. Modify the nursing care plan as needed. Monitor for intestinal infection. Counsel the patient appropriately about treatment and possible further testing. Assess for and report any change in signs and symptoms.
2. Follow guidelines in Chapter 1 for safe, effective, informed *posttest* care.

CLINICAL ALERT

1. In the institutional setting, patients with diarrhea should remain in isolation until the cause for the diarrhea is determined.
2. When pathogens are found in the diarrheic stool, the patient usually remains isolated until the stool becomes formed and antibiotic therapy is completed.

● Cerebrospinal Fluid (CSF) Cultures and Smears

Bacteriologic examination of CSF is an essential step in the diagnosis of any case of suspected meningitis. Acute bacterial meningitis is an infection of the meninges. It is a rapidly progressive, fatal infection if left untreated or if treated inadequately. Death can occur within hours of symptom onset. Prompt identification of the causative agent is necessary for appropriate antibiotic therapy and aggressive treatment. Meningitis is caused by a variety of gram-positive and gram-negative microorganisms. Bacterial meningitis also can be secondary to infections in other areas of the body.

A smear and culture should be performed on all CSF specimens obtained from persons with suspected meningitis, whether the CSF appears clear (normal) or cloudy.

In bacterial meningitis (except TB meningitis), the CSF shows the following characteristics:

1. Purulence (usually)
2. Increased numbers of leukocytes
3. Preponderance of polymorphonuclear cells
4. Decreased CSF glucose concentration in relation to serum glucose
5. Elevated CSF protein concentration

In meningitis caused by the tubercle bacillus, viruses, fungi, or protozoa, the CSF shows the following characteristics:

1. Nonpurulent (usually)
2. Decreased mononuclear white cell count; increased lymphocytes
3. Normal or decreased CSF glucose concentration
4. Elevated CSF protein concentration

In those persons with suspected meningitis, the CSF is generally submitted for chemical and cytologic examinations as well as culture.

Indications for Collection

1. Viral meningitis
2. Pyogenic meningitis
3. TB meningitis
4. Chronic meningitis

Reference Values

Normal

1. Negative: no growth
2. Bacteria are not normally present in CSF. However, the specimen may be contaminated by normal skin flora during the process of CSF collection.

Procedure

1. Collect the specimen under sterile conditions. Three or four tubes (1 mL per tube) of CSF should be collected. The third tube is used for cell count and differential; the others can be used for microbiologic and chemical studies.
2. Seal immediately to prevent leakage or contamination. Label the specimen with the patient's name, date, and tests ordered and send the specimen to the laboratory without delay.
3. Properly label the specimen. Alert laboratory staff so that the specimen can be examined immediately.
4. Notify the healthcare provider as soon as results are obtained so that appropriate treatment can be started in a timely fashion.
5. If the CSF specimen cannot be delivered to the laboratory immediately, the container should be stored at room temperature.
6. No more than 4 hours should elapse before laboratory analysis takes place because of the low survival rates of the organisms causing meningitis (especially *H. influenzae* and *N. meningitidis*).

CLINICAL ALERT

In cases of suspected meningitis, a culture should be done and a diagnosis made as quickly as possible. This is important because some causative organisms cannot tolerate temperature changes. If a viral cause is suspected, a portion of the CSF should be refrigerated (0°C–4°C). Freezing is not recommended unless inoculation into tissue culture will take longer than 5 d. If polymerase chain reaction (PCR) testing is to be performed, specimens may need to be frozen immediately.

CLINICAL ALERT

Newborns have the highest prevalence of meningitis of any age group. Organisms causing infection in the newborn (usually acquired during the birth process) include group B streptococcus, *E. coli*, and *L. monocytogenes*.

CLINICAL ALERT

CSF findings may not differentiate between bacterial and viral meningitis. Generally, however, white blood cell counts of 1000–10,000 cells/μL are associated with a bacterial cause, whereas counts from <100–1000 cells/μL are associated with an underlying viral origin.

Clinical Implications

1. Pathogens found in CSF include:
   a. *Cryptococcus* and other fungi
   b. *H. influenzae*
   c. *Naegleria* or *Acanthamoeba* spp.
   d. Viruses (usually enteroviruses) or herpes simplex virus
   e. *L. monocytogenes*
   f. *M. tuberculosis*
   g. *N. meningitidis*
   h. *Streptococcus pneumoniae*
   i. *Staphylococcus aureus*
   j. *Staphylococcus epidermidis*
   k. *Streptococcus* (group B)
   l. *Treponema pallidum*
   m. *Toxoplasma gondii*
2. Positive CSF cultures occur in:
   a. Meningitis
   b. Trauma
   c. Abscess of brain or ependyma of spine
   d. Septic thrombophlebitis of venous sinuses

Interventions

Pretest Patient Care

1. Explain purpose of and procedure for lumbar puncture (see Chapter 5).
2. Follow guidelines in Chapter 1 for safe, effective, informed *pretest* care.

Posttest Patient Care

1. Review test results; report and record findings. Modify the nursing care plan as needed. Monitor for meningitis. Counsel the patient appropriately (see Chapter 5).
2. Follow guidelines in Chapter 1 for safe, effective, informed *posttest* care.

Cervical, Urethral, Anal, and Oropharyngeal Cultures and Smears for Gonorrhea and Other Sexually Transmitted Infections (STIs)

These tests are done for patients with genital ulcers, vaginal lymphadenopathy, bacterial vaginosis (pathogens such as *Gardnerella*, *Bacteroides*, *Prevotella*, and *Mobiluncus*), lesions affecting epithelial surfaces, signs and symptoms of bacterial sexually transmitted infections (STIs), pelvic inflammatory disease, urethritis, or abnormal discharge and itching.

Reference Values

Normal

Negative: normal flora; negative for pathogenic antigens

Procedure

1. For cervical specimens
   a. Be aware that the cervix is the best site from which to obtain a culture specimen.
   b. Observe standard precautions.
   c. Moisten the vaginal speculum with warm water; *do not* use a lubricant. Remove cervical mucus, preferably with a cotton ball held in a ring forceps.
   d. Insert a sterile, cotton-tipped swab into the endocervical canal; move the swab from side to side; allow 30 seconds for absorption of organisms by the swab (Fig. 7.2).

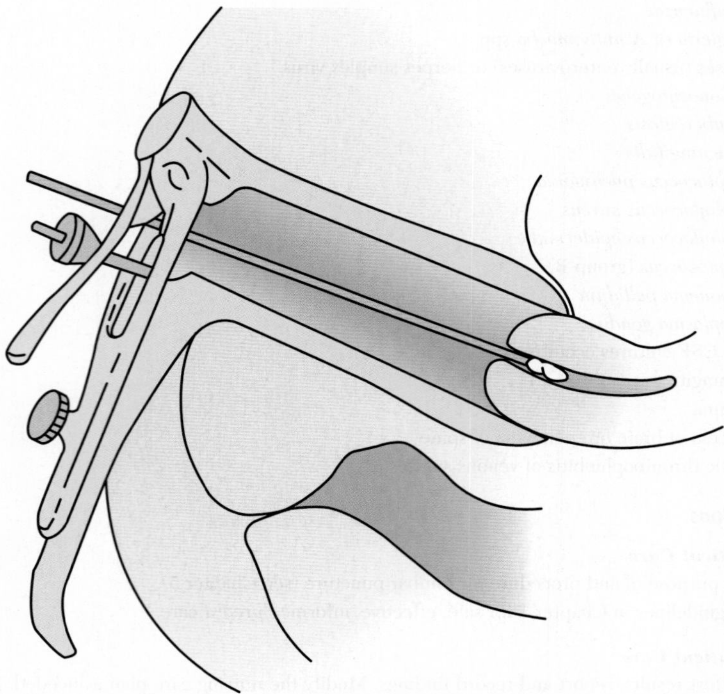

FIGURE 7.2. Method for obtaining the endocervical specimen.

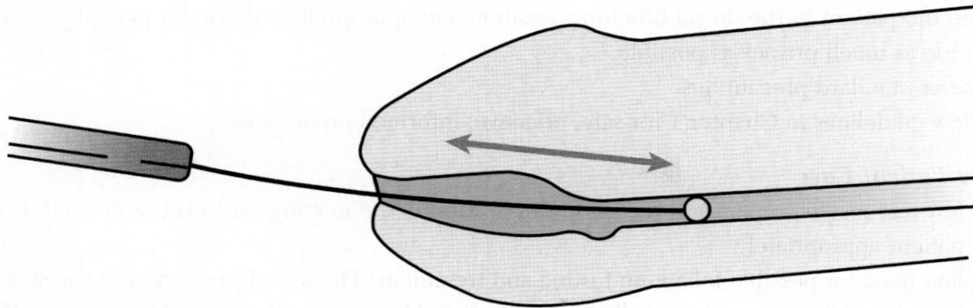

FIGURE 7.3. Method for obtaining the urethral specimen.

2. For vaginal specimens
   a. A vaginal fluid sample is collected on a swab by contacting the lower one third of the vaginal wall. The swab is placed for 10 minutes in a test vessel to which a developer solution has been added. The solution will turn blue or green if positive (OSOM BVBLUE Test, Sekisui Diagnostics, Lexington, MA).
   b. Using an immunographic assay, a vaginal fluid sample is obtained by a swab that is subsequently placed in a test tube to which a sample buffer has been added. The results are read after 10 minutes (OSOM Trichomonas Rapid Test, Sekisui Diagnostics, Lexington, MA).
3. For urethral specimens (male patients)
   a. Use a sterile swab to obtain the specimen from the anterior urethra by gently scraping the urethral mucosa (Fig. 7.3).
   b. Rotate the swab 360° to dislodge some of the epithelial cells for *Chlamydia trachomatis*. *N. gonorrhoeae* organisms inhabit the exudate, whereas *C. trachomatis* organisms are intracellular (within the epithelial cells).
4. For anal canal specimens
   a. Insert a sterile, cotton-tipped swab approximately 2.5 cm into the anal canal. (If the swab is inadvertently pushed into feces, use another swab to obtain the specimen.)
   b. Move the swab from side to side in the anal canal to sample the crypts; allow several seconds for absorption of organisms by the swab.
   c. Remember that this site is likely to be positive in a patient with STI, when a cervical specimen is negative.
5. Swabs for culture should be transported to the laboratory in Stuart's transport medium and should be held at room temperature until processed.
6. If specimens are not processed within 12 hours, they should be refrigerated. Recovery of a pathologic organism may be more difficult because of delay in processing.

PROCEDURAL ALERT

1. If the male urethral culture is negative but gonorrhea is still suspected, prostatic massage may produce an increased number of organisms in the urethral discharge. The first morning specimen before urination may be the best.
2. In a female patient, the anal canal specimen can be obtained after the cervical specimen without changing the patient's position and without using the anoscope. Observe standard precautions.

Interventions

Pretest Patient Care

1. Explain purpose of and procedure for specimen collection. Assess for and document signs and symptoms of infection (drainage, pain, itching).

2. Place the patient in the dorsal lithotomy position and appropriately drape for genital procedures. Provide as much privacy as possible.
3. Observe standard precautions.
4. Follow guidelines in Chapter 1 for safe, effective, informed *pretest* care.

Posttest Patient Care

1. Review test results; report and record findings. Modify the nursing care plan as needed. Counsel the patient appropriately.
2. Explain need for possible follow-up testing and treatment. The use of pre-exposure vaccines (e.g., hepatitis A and B [frequently sexually transmitted] and human papillomavirus) is the most effective means of preventing STIs.
3. Follow guidelines in Chapter 1 for safe, effective, informed *posttest* care.

CLINICAL ALERT

The finding of repeated negative cultures for gonococci does not always exclude a diagnosis of gonorrhea.

● Tissue, Bone, and Body Fluid Cultures

Types of fluid collected for bacterial, viral, or fungal culture include pleural, ascitic, synovial, and pericardial fluid. Tissues may have to be minced or ground to release trapped bacteria before culturing.

Reference Values

Normal

Negative for pathogens

Procedure

1. Transport body fluids to the laboratory in a sterile tube or sterile-capped syringe. Ten to 20 mL of fluid is adequate for culture examination.
2. Collect bone during surgery and send to the laboratory in a sterile container. Place fragments directly onto the agar surface or into enrichment broth.
3. Collect pieces of tissue during surgery or during needle biopsy procedures. They should be collected in a sterile specimen cup. Add a small amount of sterile, nonbacteriostatic saline to keep specimen moist.

Interventions

Pretest Patient Care

1. Explain purpose of and procedure for the culture.
2. Follow guidelines in Chapter 1 for safe, effective, informed *pretest* care.

Posttest Patient Care

1. Review test results; report and record findings. Modify the nursing care plan as needed. Monitor the site of collection, and counsel the patient appropriately.
2. Follow guidelines in Chapter 1 for safe, effective, informed *posttest* care.

SKIN TESTS

Skin testing is done for three major reasons: (1) to detect sensitivity to allergens such as dust and pollen, (2) to determine sensitivity to microorganisms believed to cause infection, and (3) to determine whether cell-mediated immune functions are normal. This chapter only briefly discusses the test that detects sensitivity to allergens; most of the discussion in this chapter focuses on skin tests used to determine sensitivity to pathogens.

Reference Values

Normal

Negative reactions indicate lack of exposure to a specific infection (e.g., TB-producing agent) or sensitivity to a specific allergen (e.g., mold).

Intradermal Tests

The substance being tested is injected into the layers of skin with a tuberculin syringe fitted with a short-bevel, 26- or 27-gauge needle. A positive reaction produces a red, inflamed area at the site of the injection within a given time period (e.g., 48 to 72 hours for the Mantoux test for TB).

Skin tests that indicate hypersensitivity to a toxin from an infection-producing agent may also signal immunity to the infectious agent. Positive reactions may also indicate an active or inactive phase of the infection under study. Skin tests can be categorized according to their nature and purpose as follows:

1. Tests to reveal a present or past exposure to the infectious agent, for example, tuberculin test (positive reaction indicates presence of active or inactive TB)
2. Tests to show sensitivity to materials toward which a person may react in an exaggerated manner; for example, allergenic extracts such as house dust and pollen (positive reaction indicates sensitivity to allergen extracts)
3. Tests to detect impaired cellular immunity. Intradermal skin testing with several common antigenic microbial substances (e.g., purified protein derivative [PPD] tuberculin, mumps virus, *C. albicans*, streptokinase-streptodornase) can determine whether immune function is normal. This would be important in treating leukemia and cancer with chemotherapy. (Negative reaction to any intradermal antigen indicates impaired immunity.)

Procedure

1. Follow the manufacturer's instructions for the diagnostic skin tests. Most are prepackaged as sterile kits.
2. Inject the ordered amount of the test material intradermally on the volar aspect of the forearm.
3. A positive reaction is generally manifested by redness or swelling >1 cm in diameter at the injection site. A central area of necrosis is a highly significant finding.

CLINICAL ALERT

Material for diagnostic skin tests may be inadvertently injected into subcutaneous tissue rather than intradermal tissue. A subcutaneous injection yields a false-negative result. See individual skin tests for pretest and posttest interventions.

● Tuberculin Skin Test (TB Test); Two-Step TB Test

The intradermal tuberculin skin test detects TB infection; it does not distinguish active TB from dormant TB. PPD tuberculin is a protein fraction of the tubercle bacilli; when it is introduced into the skin of a person with active or dormant TB infection, it causes a localized skin erythema and induration at the injection site because of accumulated small, sensitized lymphocytes.

The Mantoux test is the TB skin test of choice. The tuberculin is injected into the intradermal skin layer with a syringe and fine-gauge needle. The multiple puncture test (tine test) is used for screening purposes for asymptomatic persons, but the Mantoux test is far more accurate.

The two-step TB skin test is done to reduce the likelihood that a “boosted” reaction will be interpreted as a recent infection. The two-step skin test is not routine for contact case investigation.

Indications for Testing

1. Persons who exhibit signs (x-ray film abnormality) or symptoms (e.g., cough, hemoptysis, weight loss) suggestive of TB
2. Recent close contacts with persons known to have or suspected of having TB
3. Persons who show abnormal chest radiographs compatible with past TB exposure
4. Members of groups at high risk for *M. tuberculosis* infection, such as immigrants from countries where TB is common (Africa, Asia, the Caribbean, Eastern Europe, Latin America, and Russia) or those who live or work in long-term care settings, correctional institutions, or homeless shelters.
5. The two-step test is indicated for individuals who will be subject to periodic retesting (such as employees or residents of long-term care facilities). Using the two-step test reduces the change that a subsequent skin test will result in a boosted reaction that could be misinterpreted as a recent TB infection.

Reference Values

Normal

Reaction negative or not significant

Procedure for Intradermal Skin Test (Mantoux)

1. Observe standard precautions. Draw up PPD tuberculin into a tuberculin syringe (follow manufacturer's directions carefully). Use 0.1 mL for each test.
2. Cleanse the skin on the volar or dorsal aspect of the forearm with alcohol and allow it to dry.
3. Stretch the skin taut.
4. Hold the tuberculin syringe close to the skin so that the hub of the needle touches the skin as the needle is introduced, bevel side facing up, under the skin. A discrete, pale elevation of the skin (wheal) 6 to 10 mm in diameter should be produced when the prescribed amount of PPD tuberculin is injected into the intradermal skin layer.
5. For the *two-step test*, administer the Mantoux intradermal skin test, as described, for all persons for whom testing is indicated. Strictly enforce reading of results in 48 to 72 hours. If the result is positive, do not administer a second PPD dose but refer the patient for follow-up. If induration is present but does not classify as positive, retest immediately on the patient's other arm and read the results in 48 to 72 hours. If the result of the first Mantoux test is negative, retest in 1 to 2 weeks, using the same PPD dose and the same arm as for the first test. Read the results in 48 to 72 hours. If the reaction at second test is negative (no induration), perform no further testing. Make plans to administer the one-step Mantoux test annually.
6. Document site of test for follow-up reading of results.

Clinical Implications

1. The test should be read 48 to 72 hours after injection. The larger the area of the skin reaction, the more likely it is to represent TB infection. An indurated area of 5 mm or more is positive in people with HIV, with organ transplants, or with recent close contact with a person who has TB. An indurated area of 10 mm or more is positive in recent immigrants, intravenous drug users, employees and residents of high-risk settings, children younger than 4 years of age, and others in high-risk categories. An induration of 15 mm or more is positive in any other person. False-positive reactions can occur from previous bacillus Calmette-Guérin (BCG) vaccination, or problems with administration of or reading the skin test.
2. A significant reaction does not distinguish between active and dormant TB infection; the stage of infection can be determined from the results of clinical bacteriologic sputum tests and chest roentgenograms.

3. A significant reaction in a clinically ill patient means that active TB should be considered as a cause for illness. With HIV infection, a reaction of 5 mm or more is considered positive.
4. A significant reaction in a healthy person usually signifies either healed TB or an infection caused by a different mycobacterium. Chest x-rays can confirm the absence of an active infectious process.

Interfering Factors

False-negative results may occur even in the presence of active TB or whenever sensitized T lymphocytes are temporarily depleted in the body.

Reading the Test Results

1. The test should be read 48 to 72 hours after injection.
2. Examine the injection site in good light.
3. The patient should flex the forearm at the elbow.
4. Inspect the skin for induration (hardening or thickening).
5. Rub finger lightly from the normal skin area to the indurated zone (if present).
6. Circle the zone of induration with a pencil and measure the diameter in millimeters perpendicularly to the long axis of the forearm. Disregard erythema if it occurs without induration; it is clinically insignificant.
7. Large reactions may still be evident 7 days after the test.

CLINICAL ALERT

1. Tuberculin test material should never be transferred from one container to another.
2. Intradermal skin tests should be given immediately after the tuberculin is drawn up.
3. The greatest value of tuberculin skin testing is in the negative results; a negative test result in the presence of signs and symptoms of lung infection is strong evidence against active TB in most cases.
4. A presumptive diagnosis of TB must be bacteriologically confirmed.
5. In the United States, the incidence of TB is highest among foreign-born persons. The rate of TB has steadily declined in the United States since a peak in 1992.
6. TB is acquired through close, frequent, and prolonged exposure to infected persons.
7. Persons who have received BCG vaccine prophylactically or for bladder cancer treatment have a false-positive result on a TB skin test. Reactions of 5–10 mm may be caused by BCG vaccination. However, unless the vaccination was very recent, tuberculin reactions >10 mm should not be attributed to BCG.
8. Periodic chest x-ray films are valuable adjuncts for monitoring patients who test positive because there is no sure way of predicting who will develop active TB.
9. BCG is a freeze-dried preparation of a live, attenuated bovine strain of mycobacteria. It is used for TB immunization in children (e.g., infant with a negative TB test who lives in a household with untreated or ineffectively treated cases of TB) in countries with a high incidence of TB.
10. Healthcare providers in contact with suspected or confirmed TB must wear a properly fitted, high-efficiency, dust- and mist-proof mask.

Interpreting the Test Results

1. The test interpretation is based on the presence or absence of induration.
2. Negative or insignificant reaction: zone of induration <5 mm in diameter, unless the patient has HIV, organ transplant, or recent close contact with a person who has TB; positive or significant reaction: zone of induration >10 mm in diameter in persons at high risk.

3. For persons in good health with no risk factors, an induration of 15 to 20 mm usually is considered positive. However, because those who are at increased risk for TB (in poor health) have decreased hypersensitivity, a 5-mm induration may be considered positive. Retest within 3 weeks. See Chart 7.2 for classification of test results.

Potential Causes of False-Negative Results

Reactions can be categorized according to the following factors:

1. Factors related to person being tested
   a. Viral infections (measles, mumps, chickenpox)
   b. Live virus vaccinations (measles, mumps, polio)
   c. Nutritional factors (severe protein depletion)
   d. Diseases affecting lymphoid organs (Hodgkin's disease, lymphoma, chronic lymphocytic leukemia, sarcoidosis)
   e. Drugs (corticosteroids, other immunosuppressive agents)
   f. Age (newborns, elderly patients with waned sensitivity)
   g. Recent or overwhelming *M. tuberculosis* infection
2. Factors related to tuberculin injected
   a. Improper storage (exposure to light, heat)
   b. Improper dilution
   c. Chemical denaturation
   d. Contamination
   e. Absorption (partially controlled by adding Tween-80)
   f. Outdated material

CHART 7.2 Classification of the Tuberculin Skin Test Reaction

An induration of **5 or more millimeters** is considered positive for:

- HIV-infected persons
- Close contacts of a person with infectious TB
- Persons who have abnormal chest radiographs
- Persons who inject drugs and whose HIV status is unknown

An induration of **10 or more millimeters** is considered positive for:

- Foreign-born persons
- HIV-negative persons who inject drugs
- Medically underserved, low-income populations
- Residents of long-term care facilities
- Persons with certain medical conditions[a]
- Children <4 yr old without any other risk factors
- Staff of long-term care facilities and healthcare facilities

An induration of **15 or more millimeters** is considered positive for:

- Persons who do not have any risk factors for TB

[a]For example, diabetes mellitus, prolonged corticosteroid therapy, immunosuppressive therapy, gastrectomy, some hematologic and reticuloendothelial diseases, end-stage renal disease, silicosis, and body weight that is 10% or more below ideal.
From Centers of Disease Control and Prevention (CDC), Tuberculosis Training and Education Resource Guide, 2003

3. Factors related to method of administration
   a. Injection of too little or too much antigen
   b. Delayed administration after drawing up dose
   c. Injection too deep or too shallow
4. Factors related to test interpretation and recording of results
   a. Test not read within prescribed time frame
   b. Inexperienced or improperly trained reader
   c. Conscious or unconscious bias
   d. Recording error
   e. Measurement error

Interventions

Pretest Patient Care

1. Explain purpose of and procedure for TB skin test; convey the importance and necessity of returning for reading of the skin reaction. Obtain history of occupation, living conditions, and reason for testing.
2. Follow guidelines in Chapter 1 for safe, effective, informed *pretest* care.

Posttest Patient Care

1. Review test results within the prescribed time; report and record findings. Modify the nursing care plan as needed. Monitor and counsel the patient appropriately about the need for chest radiograph and sputum cultures for those with positive TB skin tests. Discuss initial and continued therapy and institute infection and case control as required. The possibility of TB infection must be ruled out before preventive therapy can start. TB is a reportable infection to local, state, and federal authorities.
2. Follow guidelines in Chapter 1 for safe, effective, informed *posttest* care.

● Mumps Test

Mumps, the common disease that produces swelling and tenderness of the parotid glands, is caused by a myxovirus.

An antigen made from infected monkeys or chickens is injected intradermally. A positive mumps skin test may indicate either a previous infection or an existing infection; therefore, it is not very effective as a diagnostic tool. The test is used primarily as part of a battery of skin tests to determine immunocompetence.

Reference Values

Normal

Reaction negative or not significant

Procedure

1. Observe standard precautions. Before injecting antigen, assess for allergy to eggs. Persons who are allergic to eggs are at risk for an anaphylactic reaction to mumps antigen.
2. Inject mumps antigen intradermally.

Clinical Implications

1. A positive reaction indicates resistance to the mumps virus.
2. A negative reaction indicates susceptibility to mumps virus.

Interpreting the Test Results

1. Read the test 48 hours after the time of injection.
2. Positive reaction: erythema and a lesion >10 mm in diameter.
3. Negative reaction: no erythema and a lesion <10 mm in diameter.

Interventions

Pretest Patient Care

1. Explain purpose of and procedure for skin test.
2. Follow guidelines in Chapter 1 for safe, effective, informed *pretest* care.

> **CLINICAL ALERT**
>
> The Advisory Committee on Immunization Practices (ACIP) recommends mumps vaccination as follows: the first dose of the measles, mumps, rubella (MMR) vaccine should be given at ages 12–15 mo, followed by a second dose at ages 4–6 yr. The ACIP also recommends two doses of MMR for students attending college and other post–high school institutions. Unvaccinated healthcare workers born before 1957 should have one dose of a live mumps virus vaccine, whereas healthcare workers born after 1957 should have two doses (minimum interval of 28 d between doses).

Posttest Patient Care

1. Review test results regarding immunocompetence; report and record findings. Modify the nursing care plan as needed.
2. Follow guidelines in Chapter 1 for safe, effective, informed *posttest* care.

● *Candida* and Tetanus Toxoid Tests

Candida and tetanus toxoid are additional skin tests that can be done to detect delayed-type hypersensitivity. The *Candida* antigen is a mixture of trichophytin and *Oidium*. Both antigens are administered in a manner similar to the tuberculin skin test.

Interpretation of absence of normal immune response:

1. For high-risk patients (HIV infection, intravenous drug abuse, immunocompromise), an induration area >5 mm is considered positive.
2. For patients at moderate risk (institutionalized patients, healthcare workers), an indurated area >10 mm is significant.
3. In patients with no significant risk factors, an indurated area of 15 mm or larger is considered positive.

These additional skin tests are helpful in evaluating a negative PPD test in an immunosuppressed person. No reaction to mumps, tetanus, or *Candida* testing may indicate a false-negative PPD test. However, an induration >2 mm with the mumps, *Candida*, or tetanus antigen confirms the negative PPD result.

DIAGNOSIS OF MICROBIAL DISEASE

● Diagnosis of Bacterial Disease

Bacteriologic studies attempt to identify the specific organism causing an infection (Table 7.1). This organism may be specific to one disease, such as *M. tuberculosis* for TB, or it may cause a variety of infections, such as those associated with *S. aureus*. Antibiotic susceptibility studies then determine the

TABLE 7.1 Bacterial Infections and Their Laboratory Diagnosis

Infection	Causative Organism	Source(s) of Specimen	Diagnostic Test(s)
Anthrax	*Bacillus anthracis*	Blood, sputum, skin	Gram stain, smear and culture
Brucellosis (undulant fever)	*Brucella melitensis, Brucella abortus, Brucella suis*	Blood, bone marrow, CSF, tissue, lymph node, urine	Culture, serology
Bubonic plague	*Yersinia pestis*	Buboes (enlarged and inflamed lymph nodes), blood, sputum	Skin, blood, and sputum smear; culture
Chancre	*Haemophilus ducreyi*	Genital lesion biopsy	Lesion smear and culture; biopsy
Cholera	*Vibrio cholerae*	Feces	Stool smear and culture
Diphtheria	*Corynebacterium diphtheriae*	Nasopharynx	Nasopharyngeal smear and culture
Erysipeloid	*Erysipelothrix rhusiopathiae*	Lesion, blood	Smear and culture
Gastritis, gastric ulcer	*Helicobacter pylori*	Gastric tissue biopsy	Culture, biopsy, with histopathologic exam
Gonorrhea	*Neisseria gonorrhoeae*	Cervix, urethra, CSF, blood, joint fluid, throat	Smear and culture, nucleic acid amplification assay
Granuloma inguinale (donovanosis)	*Calymmatobacterium granulomatis*	Groin lesion	Smear
Legionnaires' disease	*Legionella pneumophila*	Sputum	Culture, direct fluorescent antibody; serologic test, urine antigen test, nucleic acid amplification assay
Leprosy (Hansen's disease)	*Mycobacterium leprae*	Skin scrapings	Acid fast smear, biopsy with histopathologic exam
Listeriosis	*Listeria monocytogenes*	Blood, CSF, amniotic fluid, placenta, vagina	Smears and culture, serologic test
Lyme disease	*Borrelia burgdorferi*	Blood	Serologic test
Lymphogranuloma venereum	*Chlamydia trachomatis*	Genitalia, conjunctiva, urethra, urine	Culture, DNA probe, amplified test
Mycoplasma	*Mycoplasma pneumoniae*	Sputum, nasopharyngeal and throat swabs	Serology, culture, PCR
Nocardiosis	*Nocardia asteroides*	Sputum, lesion	Smear and culture
Pneumonia	*Haemophilus influenzae, Klebsiella pneumoniae, Staphylococcus aureus, Streptococcus pneumoniae*	Bronchoscopy, secretions, sputum, blood, lung aspirate or biopsy, pleural fluid	Smear and culture

table continues on pg. 492 >

TABLE 7.1, continued

Infection	Causative Organism	Source(s) of Specimen	Diagnostic Test(s)
Psittacosis	*Chlamydia psittaci*	Blood, sputum, lung tissue	Culture, smear, serologic tests
Relapsing fever	*Borrelia recurrentis*	Peripheral blood	Direct examination, serology
Strep throat, scarlet fever, impetigo	*Streptococcus pyogenes*	Throat, lesion	Culture, serologic test
Tetanus	*Clostridium tetani*	Wound	Smear and culture
Toxic shock syndrome	*Staphylococcus aureus*	Tissue	Culture
Tuberculosis	*Mycobacterium tuberculosis*	Sputum, gastric washings, urine, CSF	Smear and culture of sputum, gastric washings, urine, and CSF; skin test, QuantiFERON-TB assay
Tularemia	*Francisella tularensis*	Skin, lymph node, ulcer tissue biopsy, sputum, bone marrow	Serologic test, smear and culture
Typhoid	*Salmonella typhi*	Blood (after first week of infection); feces (after second week of infection)	Culture and serologic test
Whooping cough	*Bordetella pertussis*	Nasopharyngeal swab	Culture, fluorescent antibody test, nucleic acid amplification assay, serologic test

CSF, cerebrospinal fluid; PCR, polymerase chain reaction.

responses of the specific organism to various classes and types of antibiotics. An antibiotic that inhibits bacterial growth is the logical choice for treating the infection.

Some questions that need to be asked when searching for bacteria as the cause of a disease process include the following: (1) Are bacteria responsible for this disease? (2) Is antimicrobial therapy indicated? Most bacteria-related diseases have a febrile course. From a practical standpoint during evaluation of the febrile patient, the sooner a diagnosis can be reached and the sooner a decision can be made concerning antimicrobial therapy, the less protracted the period of recovery.

Anaerobic bacterial infections are commonly associated with localized necrotic abscesses: They may yield several different strains of bacteria. Because of this, the term *polymicrobic disease* is sometimes used to refer to anaerobic bacterial diseases. This view is in sharp contrast to the "one organism, one disease" concept that characterizes other infections, such as typhoid fever, cholera, or diphtheria. Isolation and identification of the different strains of anaerobic bacteria and susceptibility studies may be desirable so that appropriate therapy may be given.

● Studies of the Susceptibility of Bacteria to Antimicrobial Agents

The susceptibility test detects the type and amount of antibiotic or chemotherapeutic agent required to inhibit bacterial growth. Often, culture and susceptibility tests are ordered together. Susceptibility studies also may be indicated when an established regimen or treatment is to be altered.

A common and useful test for evaluating antibiotic susceptibility is the disk diffusion method (Fig. 7.4). A set of antibiotic-impregnated disks on agar is inoculated with a culture derived from the specific bacteria being tested. After a suitable period of incubation, the degree of bacterial growth within the different antibiotic zones on the disks is determined and measured. Growth zone diameters, measured in millimeters, are correlated to the minimum inhibitory concentration (MIC) to determine whether the organism is truly susceptible to the antibiotic. Another method is a broth dilution test (Fig. 7.5). The organism is grown in the presence of doubling dilutions of the antibiotic. The lowest concentration of the antibiotic that inhibits the organism's growth is the MIC. Many commercial systems are based on this method.

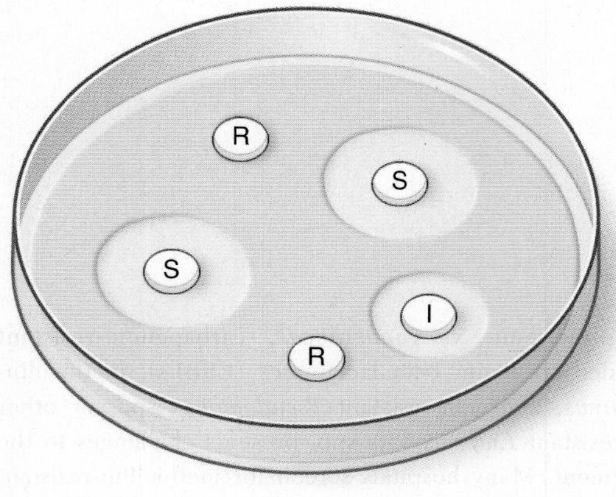

FIGURE 7.4. Disk diffusion method for evaluation of antibiotic susceptibility. (From Aschenbenner D, Venable S: Drug Therapy in Nursing, 4th ed. Philadelphia, Wolters Kluwer, 2013)

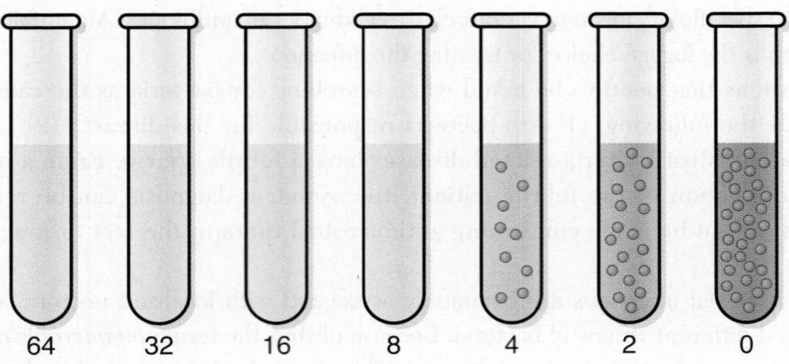

FIGURE 7.5. Broth dilution method for determining the minimal inhibitory concentration necessary to fight infection. (From Aschenbenner D, Venable S: Drug Therapy in Nursing, 4th ed. Philadelphia, Wolters Kluwer, 2013)

Clinical Implications

1. The terms *sensitive* and *susceptible* imply that an infection caused by the bacterial strain tested is likely to respond favorably in the presence of the indicated antimicrobial agent.
2. The terms *intermediate*, *partially resistant*, and *moderately susceptible* mean that the bacterial strain tested is not completely inhibited by therapeutic concentrations of a test drug.
3. *Indeterminate* means that the bacterium has an MIC that approaches achievable blood and tissue concentrations. It implies clinical efficacy in body sites where the antibiotic is physiologically concentrated. The intermediate category also includes a buffer zone, which should prevent major errors due to technical factors.
4. The term *resistant* implies that the organism is not inhibited by the antibiotic. This infection is not likely to respond to treatment.
5. Some antimicrobial agents act in a *bactericidal* manner, meaning that they kill the organism. Others act in a *bacteriostatic* manner, meaning that they inhibit growth of the organism but do not necessarily kill it.
   a. Bactericidal agents
      (1) Aminoglycosides
      (2) Cephalosporins
      (3) Metronidazole
      (4) Penicillins
      (5) Quinolones
      (6) Rifampin
      (7) Vancomycin
   b. Bacteriostatic agents
      (1) Chloramphenicol
      (2) Erythromycin
      (3) Sulfonamides
      (4) Tetracycline
6. Emergence of strains of penicillin-resistant *N. gonorrhoeae*, carbapenem-resistant Enterobacteriaceae (CRE) and extended spectrum beta lactamases (ESBLs), methicillin-resistant (or oxacillin-resistant) *S. aureus*, amikacin-resistant *Pseudomonas* spp. or other gram-negative rods, and vancomycin-resistant *Enterococcus* spp. presents challenges to the healthcare provider in regard to treatment. Many hospitals screen for methicillin-resistant *S. aureus* (MRSA) and vancomycin-resistant *Enterococcus* spp. (VRE) so as to isolate patients infected with these organisms.

Diagnosis of Mycobacterial Infections

The genus *Mycobacterium* contains several species of bacteria that are pathogenic to humans (Table 7.2). For example, *M. tuberculosis* is spread from person to person through inhalation of airborne respiratory secretions containing mycobacteria expelled during coughing, sneezing, or talking. In patients with AIDS, *Mycobacterium avium–intracellulare* (MAI) complex is acquired through the GI tract, often through ingestion of contaminated water or food.

The disease progression of mycobacteriosis, particularly in patients with AIDS, is rapid (a few weeks). This short time span has required new methods for rapid recovery and identification of mycobacteria so that antibiotic therapy can be instituted promptly. These techniques involve the use of instruments that shorten the growth period for mycobacteria to 1 to 2 weeks. Isotopic nucleic acid probes are available for culture identification of *M. tuberculosis*, MAI complex, *Mycobacterium kansasii*, and *Mycobacterium gordonae*. Nucleic acid amplification assays, which use DNA technology to detect mycobacteria directly in clinical specimens, are also available to clinical laboratories.

Multidrug-resistant TB (MDR TB) describes TB that is resistant to the two most powerful anti-TB drugs: isoniazid and rifampin. Extensively drug resistant TB (XDR TB) is a rare subset of MDR TB, which is especially concerning to persons with HIV or severely depressed immune systems. Since 2012, MDR TB detection and diagnosis is increasing with the use of Xpert MTB/RIF assay (Cepheid, Sunnyvale, CA) in 77 countries.

Reference Values

Normal

Negative results on AFB smear or culture

Collection of Specimens

1. Sputum and bronchial aspirates and lavages are the best samples for diagnosis of pulmonary infection. Purulent sputum (5 to 10 mL) from the first productive cough of the morning should be expectorated into a sterile container. If the specimen is not processed immediately, it should be refrigerated. Pooled specimens collected over several hours are not acceptable. For best results,

TABLE 7.2 Mycobacterial Infections and Their Laboratory Diagnosis

Causative Organism	Source(s) of Specimen	Diagnostic Test(s)
Mycobacterium avium–intracellulare	Sputum, stool, CSF, tissue, blood, semen, lymph nodes	Culture and smear; DNA probe
Mycobacterium chelonae	Surgical wound, sputum, tissue	Culture and smear
Mycobacterium fortuitum	Surgical wound, bone, joint, tissue, sputum	Culture and smear
Mycobacterium kansasii	Skin, joint, lymph nodes, sputum, tissue	Culture and smear
Mycobacterium leprae	CSF, skin, bone marrow, lymph nodes	Histopathologic examination of lesion
Mycobacterium marinum	Joint lesion, skin	Culture and smear
Mycobacterium tuberculosis	Sputum, urine, CSF, tissue, bone marrow	Culture and smear; skin test; DNA probe; nucleic acid amplification assay
Mycobacterium xenopi	Sputum	Culture and smear

CSF, cerebrospinal fluid.

three specimens should be collected over several days. A prerequisite of good specimen collection is the use of sterile, sturdy, leak-proof containers placed into biohazard bags.

2. AFB smears and cultures are done to determine whether TB-like symptoms are due to *M. tuberculosis* infection or infection from another mycobacterium and to aid in determining whether TB is intrapulmonary or extrapulmonary.
3. If the patient is unable to produce sputum, an early-morning gastric sample may be aspirated and cultured. This specimen must be hand-delivered to the laboratory to be processed or neutralized immediately.
4. Patients with suspected renal disease should provide early-morning urine specimens collected for 3 days in a row. Pooled 24-hour urine collections are not recommended. Unless processed immediately, the specimen should be refrigerated.
5. If TB meningitis is suspected, at least 10 mL (2 mL in children) of CSF should be obtained.
6. Sterile body fluids, tissue biopsy samples, and material aspirated from skin lesions are acceptable specimens for mycobacterial cultures. Tissue should be placed in a neutral transport medium to avoid desiccation. Swab specimens are not suitable for mycobacterial culture.
7. Feces are commonly the first specimens from which MAI complex can be isolated in a patient with disseminated disease. An acid-fast stain can be performed directly.
8. MAI complex organisms can also be isolated from the blood of immunosuppressed patients.

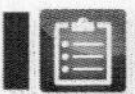

PROCEDURAL ALERT

Acid-fast organisms stain red; however, not all mycobacteria take up the stain, and cultures may need to be done.

Diagnosis of *Mycobacterium tuberculosis*

These tests diagnose TB-infected persons who are at increased risk for TB development and who will benefit from treatment. The QuantiFERON-TB Gold test (QFT-G; Qiagen, Germantown, MD) is a test used to detect latent TB. The QFT-G measures interferon-gamma (IFN-γ), a component of cell-mediated immune activity to TB response. Tuberculin skin testing (TST) screens for new or latent TB infection in high-risk groups. The TST measures lymphocyte response to TB in persons sensitized to the TB antigen. This test has been used for years and measures a delayed hypersensitivity response (48 to 72 hours).

Reference Values

Normal

QFT-G:

Negative: <0.35 IU/mL IFN-γ

Positive: ≥0.35 IU/mL IFN-γ

TST: negative for cutaneous hypersensitivity—area of induration, <10 mm (unless person is HIV positive, had recent contact with person with TB, had an organ transplant, or is immunosuppressed, in which case <5 mm)

Procedure

1. Obtain a 5-mL venous blood sample (dark-green topped [sodium heparin] tube) for the QFT-G.
2. See description in Tuberculin Skin Test (TB Test); Two-Step TB Test section.

Clinical Implication

1. A positive QFT-G result indicates that TB infection is likely.
2. A negative QFT-G result indicates that TB infection is unlikely but cannot be excluded.

Interfering Factors

1. Diabetes, silicosis, and chronic renal failure may decrease responsiveness to both the TST and QFT-G tests.
2. Treatment with immunosuppressive drugs has been shown to decrease the response to the TST.
3. Some of the hematologic disorders, such as leukemia and lymphoma, may decrease response to the TST and QFT-G test.

Interventions

Pretest Patient Care

1. Explain purpose of test, procedure for specimen collection, and interfering factors.
2. Follow guidelines in Chapter 1 for safe, effective, informed *pretest* care.

Posttest Patient Care

1. Review test results; report and record findings. Modify the nursing care plan as needed. Counsel the patient appropriately.
2. Follow guidelines in Chapter 1 for safe, effective, informed *posttest* care.

● Diagnosis of Rickettsial Disease

Rickettsiae are small, gram-negative coccobacilli that structurally resemble bacteria but are one tenth to one half as large. Polychromatic stains (Giemsa stain) are better than simple stains or the Gram stain for demonstrating rickettsiae in cells.

Rickettsiosis is the general name given to any disease caused by rickettsiae (Table 7.3). These organisms are considered to be *obligate intracellular parasites*; that is, they cannot exist anywhere except inside the bodies of living organisms. Diseases caused by rickettsiae are transmitted by *arthropod vectors*, such as lice, fleas, ticks, or mites. Rickettsial diseases are divided into the following general groups:

1. Typhus-like fevers
2. Rocky Mountain spotted fever (caused by *Rickettsia rickettsia*; transmitted by ixodid [hard] ticks)
3. Scrub typhus (caused by *Orientia tsutsugamushi*; transmitted by mites)
4. Q fever (caused by rickettsial-like bacillus *Coxiella burnetii*; chronic or acute)
5. Other rickettsial diseases

Q fever, caused by *C. burnetii*, is characterized by an acute febrile illness, severe headache, rigors, and possibly pneumonia or hepatitis. It can cause encephalitis in children and has been isolated in breast milk and in the placenta of infected mothers, making it possible for a fetus to be infected in utero. Both complement fixation and fluorescent antibody tests can detect antibodies to the organism. *C. burnetii* displays an antigenic variation during an infection. Phase I antibodies are preponderant during the chronic phase, whereas phase II antibodies predominate during the acute phase. A diagnosis is made when the phase I titer in a convalescent serum specimen is four times greater than that in an acute serum specimen.

Early diagnosis of rickettsial infection is usually based on observation of clinical symptoms such as fever, rash, and exposure to ticks. Biopsy specimens of skin tissue from a patient with suspected Rocky Mountain spotted fever can be tested with an immunofluorescent stain and diagnosed 3 to 4 days after symptoms appear. Signs and symptoms include the following:

1. Fever
2. Skin rashes
3. Parasitism of blood vessels
4. Extreme exhaustion

TABLE 7.3 Rickettsial Diseases and Their Laboratory Diagnosis

Disease		Geographic	Natural Cycle			
Group/Type	**Agent**	**Distribution**	**Arthropod**	**Mammal**	**Transmission to Humans**	**Serologic Diagnosis**
Boutonneuse fever	*Rickettsia conorii*	Africa, Europe, Mideast, India	Ticks	Wild rodents	Tick bite	Positive group- and type-specific serologic test
Ehrlichiosis	*Ehrlichia canis, Ehrlichia sennetsu*	Southeast Asia	Ticks	Human	Tick bite	PCR amplification, peripheral blood smears
Endemic (murine) typhus	*Rickettsia typhi*	Worldwide	Flea	Rodents	As above	Positive group- and type-specific serologic test
Epidemic typhus[a]	*Rickettsia prowazekii*	Worldwide	Body louse	Human	Infected louse feces into broken skin	Positive group- and type-specific serologic test
North Asian tick-borne rickettsiosis	*Rickettsia sibirica*	Siberia, Mongolia	Ticks	Wild rodents	Tick bite	Complement fixation
Oroya fever	*Bartonella bacilliformis*	Peru, Ecuador, Columbia, Brazil	Sand fly	Human	Bite of sand fly	PCR, culture, serologic tests
Q fever	*Coxiella burnetii*	Worldwide	Ticks	Small mammals, cattle, sheep, and goats	Inhalation of dried, infected material, milk, products of conception	Positive for complement fixation phases I and II
Queensland tick typhus	*Rickettsia australis*	Australia	Ticks	Marsupials, wild rodents	Tick bite	Complement fixation
Rickettsial pox	*Rickettsia akari*	North America, Europe	Blood-sucking	Mouse, other rodents	Mite bite	Microimmunofluorescence
Spotted fever, Rocky Mountain spotted fever	*Rickettsia rickettsii*	Western hemisphere	Ticks	Wild rodents, dogs	Tick bite	Serologic tests—IFA or latex agglutination
Scrub typhus	*Rickettsia tsutsugamushi*	Asia, Australia, Pacific Islands	Trombiculid	Wild rodents	Mite bite	Specific complement fixation positive in about 50% of patients, and indirect immunofluorescence
Trench fever	*Rochalimaea quintana*	Europe, Africa, North America	Body louse	Human	Infected louse feces into broken skin	PCR, culture and serologic tests

IFA, immunofluorescence assay; PCR, polymerase chain reaction.

[a]Recurrence years after original attack of epidemic typhus.

5. Stupor and coma
6. Headache
7. Ringing in the ears
8. Dizziness

NOTE *Rickettsial diseases are often characterized by an incubation period of 10 to 14 days, followed by an abrupt onset of the signs and symptoms listed, in a patient with a history of arthropod bites. Cultures of rickettsia are performed only in reference laboratories. Rickettsial infections usually are diagnosed by serologic methods, using acute and convalescent serum specimens. A fourfold rise in serum antibody titer is preferable, but a single titer greater than 1:64 is highly suggestive of infection (see Chapter 8).*

• Diagnosis of Parasitic Disease

About 70 species of animal parasites commonly infect the human body (Table 7.4). More than half of these can be detected by examination of stool specimens because the parasites inhabit the GI tract and its environs. Of the parasites that can be diagnosed by stool examinations, about one third are single-celled protozoa, and two thirds are multicellular worms. Only six or seven types of intestinal protozoa are clinically important, but almost all of the worm classes are potentially pathogenic.

Diagnosis of parasites begins with ova and parasite examination. Other diagnostic options include sigmoidoscopy smears, biopsies, barium radiologic studies, and serologic tests. Collection of fecal specimens for parasites should be done before administration of barium sulfate, mineral oil, bismuth, antimalarial drugs, and some antibiotics (e.g., tetracycline). For ova and parasite examination, ideally, one specimen should be collected every other day for a total of three specimens. At the most, these specimens should be gathered within 10 days.

For detection of *Giardia*, other diagnostic tests such as the Entero-Test (string test) and duodenal aspiration or biopsy may be necessary. The Entero-Test consists of a gelatin capsule containing a coiled length of nylon yarn. The capsule is swallowed, the gelatin dissolves, and the weighted string is carried into the duodenum. After about 4 hours, the string is withdrawn, and the accompanying mucus is examined microscopically for *Giardia*. Duodenal fluid also can be submitted to be examined for *Giardia* and *Strongyloides stercoralis*. The specimen should contain no preservatives and should be examined for organisms within 1 hour after collection.

Cryptosporidium parvum has long been recognized as an animal parasite but is also capable of infecting humans, especially physiologically compromised patients. Organisms have been recovered from the gallbladder, lungs, and stool.

CLINICAL ALERT

In the diagnosis of parasitic worms, the most important factor is the number of worms harbored.

Collection of Specimens

1. Multiple specimens may be necessary to detect a parasitic infection.
2. Most parasites found in humans are identified in blood or feces but may also be evident in urine, sputum, tissue fluids, or biopsy tissues.
3. Fecal specimens should not be contaminated with water or urine. All specimens should be labeled with the patient's name, healthcare provider's name, identification number (if applicable), and date and time collected. Various commercial collection systems are available to allow collection of specimens at home, in a nursing institution, or in a hospital setting. Clear instructions should be

TABLE 7.4 Parasitic Diseases and Their Laboratory Diagnosis

Disease	Causative Organism(s)	Source(s) of Specimen	Diagnostic Test(s)
Acanthamoebiasis	*Acanthamoeba culbertsoni*	CSF, corneal biopsy or scraping	Smear and tissue culture
Amebiasis	*Entamoeba histolytica*	Stool, liver	Stool smear, rectal biopsy, serologic test, antigen test
Ascariasis	*Ascaris lumbricoides*	Stool, sputum	Ova and parasite examination, antigen test, rectal biopsy, serologic test
Blastocystis	*Blastocystis hominis*	Stool	Ova and parasite examination
Cestodiasis of intestine (tapeworm disease)	*Taenia saginatus, Taenia solium, Diphyllobothrium, Hymenolepis nana, Hymenolepis diminuta*	Stool	Ova and parasite examination, Scotch tape test for *Enterobius vermicularis*
Chagas' disease	*Trypanosoma cruzi*	Blood, spinal fluid	Giemsa- or Wright-Giemsa–stained smear
Cryptosporidiosis	*Cryptosporidium parvum*	Stool, lung, gallbladder	Ova and parasite examination, antigen test, direct fluorescent antibody test
Cysticercosis	*Taenia solium* larvae	Muscle and brain	Muscle and brain cyst biopsy, serology
Echinococcosis	*Echinococcus granulosus*	Sputum and urine, liver, spleen	Ova and parasite examination, direct microscopic examination, serologic test, Casoni's skin test; liver and bone biopsy
Enterobiasis (pinworm disease)	*Enterobius vermicularis*	Stool	Scotch tape test
Filariasis	*Wuchereria bancrofti, Brugia malayi, Loa loa*	Blood	Blood smear, lymph node biopsy, serologic test
Giardiasis	*Giardia lamblia*	Stool, duodenal aspirate or biopsy	Ova and parasite examination, antigen test, direct fluorescent antibody test, microscopic examination of Entero test
Hookworm	*Ancylostoma duodenale, Necator americanus*	Stool	Ova and parasite examination
Isosporiasis	*Isospora belli*	Stool	Ova and parasite examination
Kala-azar	*Leishmania donovani*	Liver, bone marrow, blood	Giemsa- or Wright-Giemsa–stained smear and culture, lymph node and spleen biopsy

Malaria	*Plasmodium falciparum, Plasmodium malariae, Plasmodium vivax, Plasmodium ovale*	Blood, bone marrow	Giemsa- or Wright-Giemsa–stained smear
Naegleriasis	*Naegleria fowleri*	CSF	Smear
Onchocerciasis	*Onchocerca volvulus*	Skin	Skin biopsy with histopathologic exam
Paragonimiasis	*Paragonimus westermani*	Sputum, stool	Ova and parasite examination, serologic test, skin test
Sarcocystis	*Sarcocystis hominis* or *Sarcocystis suihominis*	Stool	Ova and parasite examination
Scabies	*Sarcoptes scabiei*	Skin	Skin smear, direct examination
Schistosomiasis of intestine and bladder	*Schistosoma mansoni, Schistosoma japonicum, Schistosoma haematobium*	Stool, urine	Ova and parasite examination, serologic test, skin test, rectal, bladder, and liver biopsy
Strongyloidiasis	*Strongyloides stercoralis*	Stool, duodenal aspirate	Ova and parasite examination, serologic test
Toxoplasmosis	*Toxoplasma gondii*	Blood, tissue, CSF	Serologic test, tissue smear, biopsy
Trematodes	*Fasciola hepatica, Clonorchis sinensis, Fasciolopsis buski*	Stool	Ova and parasite examination
Trichinosis	*Trichinella spiralis*	Muscle	Serologic test, skin test, muscle biopsy
Trichomoniasis	*Trichomonas vaginalis*	Vagina, bladder, urethra	Vaginal and urethral smear and culture, DNA probe
Trichuriasis	*Trichuris trichiura*	Stool	Ova and parasite examination
Trypanosomiasis	*Trypanosoma rhodesiense, Trypanosoma gambiense*	Blood, spinal fluid, lymph node	Blood, spinal fluid and lymph node smear, serologic test
Visceral larva migrans	*Toxocara canis, Toxocara cati*	Liver	Serologic test, skin test, liver biopsy

CSF, cerebrospinal fluid.

communicated and given in writing to the patient to ensure proper collection. See Chapter 4, Stool Studies, for more information.

4. When sputum is collected for ova and parasites, it should be "deep sputum" from the lower respiratory tract. It should be collected early in the morning, before the patient eats or brushes the teeth, and it should be immediately delivered to the laboratory. See Appendix B, Guidelines for Specimen Transport and Storage, for more information.

Clinical Implications

1. General considerations
   a. *Eosinophilia* may be an indicator of parasitic infection.
   b. Protozoa and helminths, particularly larvae, may be found in organs, tissues, and blood.
2. Specimen-related considerations
   a. *Hepatic puncture* can reveal visceral leishmaniasis. Liver biopsy may yield toxocaral larvae and schistosomal worms and eggs. Hepatic abscess material from the peripheral area may reveal more organisms than the necrotic center.
   b. *Bone marrow* may be positive for trypanosomiasis and malaria when blood samples produce negative results. Bone marrow specimens are obtained through puncture of the sternum, iliac crest, vertebral processes, trochanter, or tibia.
   c. Puncture or biopsy samples from a *lymph node* may be examined for the presence of trypanosomiasis, leishmaniasis, toxoplasmosis, and filariasis.
   d. *Mucous membrane* lesion or *skin samples* may be obtained through scraping, needle aspiration, or biopsy.
   e. *CSF* may contain trypanosomes and toxoplasma organisms.
   f. *Sputum* may reveal *Paragonimus westermani* (lung fluke) eggs. Occasionally, the larvae and hookworm of *S. stercoralis* or *Ascaris lumbricoides* may be expectorated during pulmonary migration. In pulmonary *echinococcosis* (hydatid disease), hydatid cyst contents may be found in sputum.
   g. Specimens taken from *cutaneous ulcers* should be aspirated below the ulcer bed rather than at the surface. A few drops of saline may be introduced by needle and syringe to aspirate intracellular leishmanial organisms.
   h. *Corneal* scrapings or biopsy specimens can be examined histologically or cultured for the presence of *Acanthamoeba*. This organism is rare but can cause keratitis among contact lens wearers.
   i. Films for *blood parasites* are usually prepared when the patient is admitted. Samples should be taken at 6- to 18-hour intervals for at least 3 successive days.

• Diagnosis of Fungal Disease

Fungal diseases, also known as *mycoses*, are common in healthcare settings. According to the Centers for Disease Control and Prevention (CDC), *Candida* is the most common cause of healthcare-associated bloodstream infections. Like some antibiotics, some antifungal medications are becoming resistant to first- and second-line medications (fluconazole and echinocandins). Some studies indicate that use of antibiotics contributes to antifungal resistance (Table 7.5). Fungi prefer the debilitated host, the person with chronic disease or impaired immunity, or a patient who has been receiving prolonged antibiotic therapy.

Of more than 200,000 species of fungi, approximately 200 species are generally recognized as being pathogenic for humans. Fungi live in soil enriched by decaying nitrogenous matter and are capable of maintaining a separate existence through a parasitic cycle in humans or animals. The systemic mycoses are not communicable in the usual sense of human-to-human or animal-to-animal transfer. Humans become accidental hosts through inhalation of spores or by introduction of spores into tissues through trauma.

TABLE 7.5 Fungal Diseases and Their Laboratory Diagnosis

Disease	Causative Organism(s)	Source(s) of Specimen	Diagnostic Test(s)
Aspergillosis	*Aspergillus fumigatus, Aspergillus flavus, Aspergillus terreus*	Sputum, tissue, ear, corneal scraping	Smear and culture, serologic test, chest x-ray, computed tomography
Blastomycosis	*Blastomyces dermatitidis*	Skin lesion, sputum, bone, joint	Smear and culture, serologic test, skin biopsy, urine antigen test
Candidiasis	*Candida albicans*	Mucous membrane, sputum, blood, tissue, urine, CSF	Smear and culture
Coccidioidomycosis	*Coccidioides immitis*	Sputum, bone, skin, joint, CSF	Smear and culture, serologic skin test, biopsy
Cryptococcosis	*Cryptococcus neoformans*	CSF, sputum, urine	Smear and culture, serologic test, antigen detection
Histoplasmosis	*Histoplasma capsulatum*	Sputum, urine, blood, bone marrow	Smear and culture, serologic test, biopsy, urine antigen test
Mucormycosis	Members of order Mucorales (*Absidia, Rhizopus, Mucor*)	Nose, pharynx, stool, CSF, sputum, ear	Smear and culture, biopsy
Paracoccidioidomycosis	*Paracoccidioides*	Lung tissue, sputum, bone, CSF	Smear and culture, serologic test, biopsy
Pseudallescheriasis	*Allescheria boydii*	Lesions of skin, bone, brain, joint	Smear and culture, biopsy
Sporotrichosis	*Sporothrix schenckii*	Skin lesion, CSF, bone marrow, ear	Smear and culture, biopsy, serologic test
Tinea pedis (athlete's foot)	*Epidermophyton* spp. and *Candida albicans, Trichophyton mentagrophytes, Trichophyton rubrum*	Skin	Skin scrapings for smear and culture
Tinea capitis (ringworm of scalp)	*Microsporum* (any spp.) and *Trichophyton* (all except *T. concentricum*)	Skin, hair	Hair, skin scrapings for smear and culture
Tinea barbae (ringworm of beard, barber's itch)	*Trichophyton* and *Microsporum* spp.	Skin, hair	Hair, skin scrapings for smear and culture
Tinea cruris (jock itch)	*Epidermophyton* spp. and *Candida albicans*	Skin	Skin scrapings for smear and culture
Tinea corporis (ringworm of the body)	*Trichophyton rubrum, Trichophyton tonsurans*	Skin	Skin scrapings for smear and culture
Tinea unguium (nail)	*Trichophyton rubrum, Trichophyton tonsurans, Trichophyton verrucosum, Epidermophyton* spp.	Nail	Nail culture

CSF, cerebrospinal fluid.

Altered susceptibility may result in fungal lesions; this frequently occurs in patients who have a debilitating disease, diabetes, or impaired immunologic responses due to steroid or antimetabolite therapy. Prolonged administration of antibiotics can result in a fungal superinfection.

Fungal diseases may be classified according to the type of tissues involved:

1. Dermatophytoses include superficial and cutaneous mycoses, such as athlete's foot, ringworm, and jock itch. Species of *Microsporum*, *Epidermophyton*, and *Trichophyton* are the causative organisms.
2. Subcutaneous mycoses involve the subcutaneous tissues and muscles.
3. Systemic mycoses involve the deep tissues and organs and are the most serious of the three groups.

Amphotericin B, introduced into practice in 1958, was for many years the only drug available to treat invasive fungal infections. Now ketoconazole, fluconazole, itraconazole, and lipid formulations of amphotericin B provide alternative choices when treatment of fungal disease is warranted.

Collection of Hair and Skin Specimens

1. Clean the suspected area with 70% alcohol to remove bacteria. Use sterile techniques and standard precautions.
2. Scrape the peripheral erythematous margin of putative ringworm lesions with a sterile scalpel or wooden spatula and place the scrapings in a covered sterile container.
3. Clip samples of infected scalp or beard hair and place in a covered sterile container.
4. Pluck hair stubs out with tweezers because the fungus is usually found at the base of the hair shaft. Use of a Wood's light in a darkened room helps identify the infected hairs.
5. Samples from infected nails should be procured from beneath the nail plate to obtain softened material from the nail bed. If this is not possible, collect shavings from the deeper portions of the nail and place them in a covered sterile container.

Common Diagnostic Methods for Fungal Diseases

1. A Wood's light is used to determine presence of a fungus directly on hair. A Wood's light is a lamp that uses ultraviolet rays of 3660 A. In a darkened room, infected hairs fluoresce a bright yellow-green under the Wood's light.
2. Direct microscopic examination of tissue samples placed on a slide is performed to determine whether a fungus is actually present. The potassium hydroxide (KOH) test or Calcofluor white stain test is used to detect the presence of mycelial fragments, arthrospores, spherules, or budding yeast cells and involves mixing the specimen with the reagent on a glass slide. The slide is then microscopically examined for fungal elements.
3. A fluorescent brightener, Calcofluor white, fluoresces when exposed to ultraviolet light. This reagent stains the fungi, causing them to exhibit a fluorescence that can be detected microscopically. It can be used on tissue and has the same sensitivity as KOH. Moreover, it allows for easier and faster detection of fungal elements. Calcofluor white–stained specimens can also be examined under bright-field or phase-contrast microscopy.
4. Cultures are done to identify the specific type of fungus. Fungi are slow growing and are subject to overgrowth by contaminating and more rapidly growing organisms. Fungemia (fungus in the blood) is an opportunistic infection, and often, a blood culture reveals the earliest suggestion of the causative organism.
5. For fungal serology tests, single titers greater than 1:32 usually indicate the presence of disease. A fourfold or greater rise in titer of samples drawn 3 weeks apart is significant. However, serologic diagnosis of *Candida* and *Aspergillus* species can be disappointing. Complement fixation tests for *histoplasmosis* and *coccidioidomycosis* can aid in the diagnosis of these diseases. The immunodiffusion test is helpful for the diagnosis of *blastomycosis*.
6. Antigen tests performed on urine specimens are available for the detection of disseminated *Histoplasma capsulatum* and *Blastomyces dermatitidis*. The urinary antigen test has a 92% sensitivity.

Types of Specimens

1. Skin
2. Nails
3. Hair
4. Ulcer scrapings
5. Pus
6. CSF
7. Urine
8. Blood
9. Bone marrow
10. Stool
11. Bronchial washings
12. Tissue biopsy specimens
13. Prostatic secretions
14. Sputum

● Diagnosis of Spirochetal Disease

Spirochetes appear as spiral and curved bacteria. The four genera of spiral and curved bacteria—*Borrelia*, *Treponema*, *Leptospira*, and *Spirillum* (Table 7.6)—include several human pathogens. Most spirochetes multiply within a living host. Pathogenic *Treponema* organisms are transmitted from person to person through direct contact. *Borrelia* pass through an arthropod vector. *Leptospira* are usually contracted accidentally by humans through water contaminated with animal urine or a bite by an infected animal.

Clinical Implications

1. *Borrelia* appear in the blood at the onset of relapsing fever. Louse-borne relapsing fever is caused by *Borrelia recurrentis*, tick-borne relapsing fever by several other *Borrelia* species, and Lyme disease by *Borrelia burgdorferi*. To date, there is no evidence that Lyme disease is transmitted by person-to-person contact.
2. *Treponema (Borrelia) vincentii* is the species responsible for ulcerative gingivitis (trench mouth).
   a. *T. pallidum* subsp. *pallidum* causes venereal syphilis in humans.
   b. *T. pallidum* subsp. *pertenue* causes yaws (a chronic skin disease affecting children under age 15 years in poverty-stricken areas).
   c. *Treponema carateum* causes pinta (also known as *carate*, a chronic, nonvenereal infection spread through contact with open skin).
   d. *T. pallidum* subsp. *endemicum* causes bejel (nonvenereal syphilis).
3. *Leptospira* is the genus of microorganism responsible for Weil's disease (infectious jaundice), swamp fever, swineherd's disease, and canicola fever.
   a. The organism is widely distributed in the infected person and appears in the blood early in the disease process.
   b. After 10 to 14 days, the organisms appear in considerable numbers in the urine.
   c. Patients with Weil's disease show striking antibody responses; serologic testing is useful for diagnosis of this disease.
4. *Streptobacillus moniliformis* and *Spirillum minor* are the species responsible for rat-bite fever. Although this condition occurs worldwide and is common in Japan and Asia, it is uncommon in North and South America and most European countries. Cases in the United States have been linked to bites or scratches by infected rodents (such as rats, mice, and gerbils). The case fatality rate is 7% to 10% among untreated patients.

TABLE 7.6 Spirochetal Diseases and Their Laboratory Diagnosis

Disease	Causative Organism(s)	Source(s) of Specimen	Diagnostic Test(s)
Lyme disease	*Borrelia burgdorferi*	Skin lesion, blood, CSF	Serologic test
Nonvenereal syphilis	*Treponema endemicum*	Skin, blood	Serologic test
Pinta	*Treponema carateum*	Skin	Skin smear, serologic test
Rat-bite fever	*Spirillum minor, Streptobacillus moniliformis*	Blood, joint fluid, abscess	Culture, serology
Relapsing fever	*Borrelia recurrentis*	Blood	Blood smear
Syphilis	*Treponema pallidum*	Skin lesion	Skin smear, nonspecific treponemal (VDRL, RPR) and specific treponemal (FTA-ABS) serologic tests
Weil's disease (leptospiral jaundice)	*Leptospira interrogans*	Urine, blood, CSF	Culture, serologic test
Yaws	*Treponema pertenue*	Skin	Culture, serologic test

CSF, cerebrospinal fluid; FTA-ABS, fluorescent treponemal antibody absorption test; RPR, rapid plasma reagin; VDRL, Venereal Disease Research Laboratory.

NOTE *The deer tick can carry Lyme disease, whereas the wood tick carries Rocky Mountain spotted fever.*

Reference Values

Normal

Negative ELISA or immunofluorescence assay (IFA) for the antibody to *B. burgdorferi*

Procedure

1. Obtain a 2-mL blood specimen in a red-topped tube.
2. For Lyme disease, a two-step process is used. The first step uses either ELISA or IFA. A second step, using a Western blot test, is performed to confirm a positive ELISA or IFA result. If the Western blot is negative, it suggests that step 1 was a false positive. (Ten proteins are used in the serodiagnosis of Lyme disease.)

Interventions

Pretest Patient Care

1. Explain purpose and procedure. Assess for and document signs and symptoms of Lyme disease (rash [erythema migrans], arthritis, facial paralysis, tingling or burning sensations in the extremities, and meningitis).
2. Follow guidelines in Chapter 1 for safe, effective, informed *pretest* care.

Posttest Patient Care

1. Review test results; report and record findings. Modify the nursing care plan as needed. Monitor and counsel the patient appropriately. Recommended treatment for patients with Lyme disease includes antibiotics (e.g., amoxicillin, doxycycline, and cefuroxime axetil).
2. Follow guidelines in Chapter 1 for safe, effective, informed *posttest* care.

● Diagnosis of Viral and Mycoplasmal Infection

Viral infections are the most common of all human infections. Once thought to be confined to the childhood years, viral infections in adults have increasingly been recognized as the cause of significant morbidity and mortality. They also affect immunosuppressed and elderly patients (Chart 7.3). Viruses are responsible for hepatitis, AIDS, and other STIs.

Viruses are submicroscopic, filterable, infectious organisms that exist as intracellular parasites. They are divided into two groups according to the type of nucleic acid they contain: RNA or DNA.

CHART 7.3 Viral Infections in Infants, Children, and Adults

Infection or Syndrome	Suspected Viral Agents
Infants and Children	
Upper respiratory tract infection	Rhinovirus, coronavirus, parainfluenza, adenovirus, respiratory syncytial virus, influenza, human metapneumovirus
Pharyngitis	Adenovirus, Coxsackie A, herpes simplex, Epstein-Barr, rhinovirus, parainfluenza, influenza
Croup	Parainfluenza, respiratory syncytial, human metapneumovirus
Bronchitis	Parainfluenza, respiratory syncytial, human metapneumovirus
Bronchiolitis	Respiratory syncytial, parainfluenza, human metapneumovirus
Pneumonia	Respiratory syncytial, adenovirus, influenza, parainfluenza
Gastroenteritis	Rotavirus, adenoviruses 40–41, calicivirus, astrovirus, Norovirus
Adults	
Upper respiratory tract infection	Rhinovirus, coronavirus, adenovirus, influenza, parainfluenza
Pneumonia	Coxsackie B
Gastroenteritis	Norovirus
All Persons	
Parotitis	Mumps, parainfluenza
Myocarditis/pericarditis	Coxsackie and echoviruses
Keratitis/conjunctivitis	Herpes simplex, varicella-zoster, adenovirus
Pleurodynia	Coxsackie B
Herpangina	Coxsackie A
Febrile illness with rash	Enteroviruses
Infectious mononucleosis	Epstein-Barr, cytomegalovirus
Meningitis	Enteroviruses, lymphocytic choriomeningitis, herpes simplex virus
Encephalitis	Herpes simplex, togaviruses, bunyaviruses, flaviviruses, rabies, enteroviruses, measles, HIV, JC virus
Hepatitis	Hepatitis A, B, C, non-A, non-B; delta agent; E
Hemorrhagic cystitis	Adenovirus, BK virus
Cutaneous infection with rash	Herpes simplex, varicella-zoster, enteroviruses, Epstein-Barr, measles, rubella, parvovirus, human herpesvirus 6
Hemorrhagic fever	Ebola, Marburg, Lassa, hantavirus
Acute respiratory failure	Hantavirus

The *mycoplasmas* are Scotobacteria without cell walls that are surrounded by a single triple-layered membrane; they are also known as pleuropneumonia-like organisms (PPLOs). Physiologically, mycoplasmal infections are considered to be intermediate between those caused by bacteria and those caused by rickettsiae. One species, *Mycoplasma pneumoniae*, is recognized as the causative agent of primary atypical pneumonia and bronchitis. Other species are suspected as possible causal agents for urethritis, infertility, early-term spontaneous abortion, rheumatoid arthritis, myringitis, and erythema multiforme.

Viruses and mycoplasmas are infectious agents small enough to pass through bacteria-retaining filters. Although small size is the only property they have in common, viruses and mycoplasma cause illnesses that are often indistinguishable from each other in terms of clinical signs and symptoms; in addition, both frequently occur together as dual infections. Therefore, the serologic (antigen-antibody) procedures commonly used for diagnosing viral infection are also used for diagnosing mycoplasmal infections (Table 7.7).

Approach to Diagnosis

1. Isolation of the virus in tissue culture remains the gold standard for detection of many common viruses. Diagnostic modalities include the following:
   a. Tissue culture
   b. Direct detection in specimens
   c. Identification through specific cytopathic effect
   d. Use of immunofluorescence and immunoperoxidase, latex agglutination, or ELISA to identify
   e. Visualization through an electron microscope
   f. Direct nucleic acid hybridization probe and nucleic acid amplification assay
2. Serologic studies for antigen-antibody detection are valuable in regard to viral disease. Epstein-Barr virus (EBV) and human hepatitis viruses are routinely serodiagnosed. Classically, a fourfold rise in antibody titer is used to identify a particular infectious agent, provided that the pathogenesis of the agent agrees with the symptoms of the infected patient. An acute-phase serum is collected within the first several days after symptom onset. A convalescent-phase serum is collected 2 to 4 weeks later. A fourfold difference in antibody titer between the two sera is statistically significant. Alternatively, detection of specific IgM suggests acute infection. IgG antibody without IgM suggests infection sometime in the past.
3. Available cell cultures vary greatly in their sensitivity to different viruses. One cell type or species may be more sensitive than another for detecting the virus in low titers. For example, human embryonic kidney (HEK) can be used for adenovirus, enterovirus, herpes simplex, measles, influenza, parainfluenza, and rubella; however, HEK cannot be used for cytomegalovirus (CMV) or influenza.
4. The critical first step in successful viral diagnosis is the timely and proper collection of specimens. The choice of which specimen to collect depends on typical signs and symptoms and the suspected virus. Improper specimen choice and collection is one of the biggest factors in diagnostic delays.

Specimen Collection

1. Collect specimens for viruses as early as possible during the course of the illness, preferably within the first 4 days after symptom onset. If specimen collection is delayed for 7 or more days after symptoms appear, diagnosis will be compromised. Virus titers are highest in the early part of the illness, when the host has not yet mounted a robust immune response. Little neutralizing antibody is present. Detection of a virus by culture, direct detection, or serology is greatly enhanced when the virus titers are high.
2. Sampling procedure
   a. For localized infection
      (1) Direct sampling of affected site (e.g., throat swab, skin scraping)
      (2) Indirect sampling. For example, if CSF is the target sample in a central nervous system infection, the indirect approach would involve obtaining throat or rectal swabs for culture.

TABLE 7.7 Viral Infections and Their Laboratory Diagnosis

Infection Type and Virus Information	Throat	Stool/Rectal Swab	CSF	Urine	Vesicle Fluid/ Swab	Conjunctival Swab/ Scraping	Other	Blood Serology	Additional Information
Respiratory									
Adenovirus	X						Nasopharyngeal swab	Yes	
Enterovirus	X							No[a]	
Herpes simplex virus (HSV)	X						Nasopharyngeal swab	Yes	
Influenza virus	X							Yes	
Mumps virus	X			X				Yes	
Parainfluenza virus	X						Nasopharyngeal swab	Yes	
Respiratory syncytial virus (RSV)	X						Nasopharyngeal aspirate or swab	Yes	
Rhinovirus	X						Nasal		Nasal specimen preferred
Rash									
Maculopapular									
Adenovirus	X	X					Nasopharyngeal swab	Yes	
Enterovirus	X	X						No[a]	
Rubella virus	X			X			Viral culture rarely done	Yes	Special culture required
Measles (rubeola)	X						Viral culture rarely done	Yes	Special culture required

table continues on pg. 510 >

TABLE 7.7, continued

Infection Type and Virus Information	Throat	Stool/Rectal Swab	CSF	Urine	Vesicle Fluid/ Swab	Conjunctival Swab/ Scraping	Other	Blood Serology	Additional Information
Vesicular									
Coxsackievirus A or echovirus	X	X		X				No[a]	Many strains of type A Coxsackievirus do not grow in tissue culture.
HSV				X				Yes	
Varicella-zoster virus (VZV)				X				Yes	
Vaccinia and other poxviruses				X				No	
Central Nervous System (Aseptic Meningitis, Encephalitis)									
Arbovirus	X						Blood CSF-PCR is useful	Yes	
Enterovirus	X	X	X	X				No[a]	
HSV			X		X		Brain biopsy CSF-PCR is test of choice	Yes	Recovery of HSV type 1 from CSF is rare except in neonates.
Mumps virus	X			X	X			Yes	
Rabies virus							Blood	Yes	Skin biopsy of neck for fluorescent assay

Congenital and Perinatal							
Cytomegalovirus (CMV)	X			X	Blood (leukocytes)	Yes	
Enterovirus	X	X	X (PCR)		Blood	No[a]	
HSV	X		X (PCR)		Blood	Yes	
Gastrointestinal							
Adenovirus		X				Yes	
Norovirus						Research laboratories only	Parvoviruses and rotaviruses cannot be cultivated in the usual cell cultures used for diagnostic virology but can be seen with electron microscopy or detected immunologically.
Rotavirus		X (antigen test)				Research laboratories only	
Eye							
Adenovirus	X					Yes	Other viruses that can cause infections: CMV and VZV
Enterovirus	X					No[a]	
HSV	X					Yes	
Heart							
Coxsackievirus B	X	X			Pericardial fluid	No[a]	Mumps, measles (rubeola) are rare causes of heart disease.
CMV	X		X		Pericardial fluid	Yes	

table continues on pg. 512 >

TABLE 7.7, continued

Infection Type and Virus Information	Throat	Stool/ Rectal Swab	CSF	Urine	Vesicle Fluid/ Swab	Conjunctival Swab/ Scraping	Other	Blood Serology	Additional Information
Heart									
Influenza A, V	X							Yes	
Infectious mononucleosis	X			X			Blood (leukocytes)	Yes	
Epstein-Barr virus (EBV)								Yes	
Immunodeficient patient CMV	X			X			Blood (leukocytes)	Yes	Many other viruses, such as adenovirus and enterovirus, can cause severe disease in immunologically compromised patients.
Hepatitis									
CMV	X			X			Liver	Yes	
EBV								Yes	
Hepatitis A, B, and C							Liver biopsy	Yes	See Chapter 8
Genital									
HSV					X		Endocervical swab	Yes	See Chapter 8
Urinary									
Adenovirus				X				Yes	

CSF, cerebrospinal fluid; PCR, polymerase chain reaction.

[a]Enterovirus serology is not routinely available but can be performed with selected antigens under special circumstances.

   b. Sampling from more than one site, for example, in disseminated infection or with nonspecific clinical findings
   c. The type of applicator used to obtain specimens may affect accuracy of results. Do not use wooden applicators or cotton swabs because they are toxic to viruses. A self-contained transport system is recommended to ensure that the specimen remains moist.
3. When transporting specimens:
   a. Viral specimens are unstable and rapidly lose infectivity outside of living cells. Prompt delivery to the laboratory is essential. Samples must be refrigerated or placed on ice or cold packs while in transit.
   b. Freezing and thawing of specimens diminishes the quantity of available viable virus.
4. Accurate patient information must accompany the specimen to the laboratory. In addition to the required patient identification information, the requisition should include:
   a. Pertinent information that would influence processing of the specimen (e.g., patient is immunocompromised owing to renal transplantation)
   b. Exact nature of the specimen
   c. Patient demographics
   d. Contact person or clinic so as to expedite notification of abnormal results
5. Specimens of small volume (e.g., vesicular fluid, fine-needle aspiration, biopsy samples) should be transported in a liquid medium. Suggested viral transport media are Hank's balanced salt solution or 0.2 mol/L sucrose phosphate. Several commercially available viral transport media can be used.

Often, a complete microbiologic workup of a specimen (tissue, bronchoscopy) is requested along with a viral workup. Because viral transport media contain antibiotics, sterile saline is recommended. Personnel in the laboratory can then divide the specimen for workup within the microbiology subsections.

Specimens of a liquid nature (urine, CSF, sputum, body fluids) are collected in a sterile container. For patients with suspected viremia, a viral culture of the buffy coat of peripheral blood is submitted. Blood specimens are collected in evacuated tubes containing heparin or ethylenediaminetetraacetic acid (EDTA).

Clinical Implications

1. Herpes simplex is the virus most frequently isolated and diagnosed virus in the laboratory.
2. Viral culture results are normally available within 3 to 5 days, although rapid test results (24 hours) are accurate and available for certain viruses, such as CMV.
3. Significance of viral cultures
   a. Positive viral culture results from the following sources are *diagnostically accurate*:
      (1) Autopsy specimens
      (2) Blood (buffy coat)
      (3) Biopsy
      (4) CSF
      (5) Other body fluids
      (6) Cervix
      (7) Eye
      (8) Skin lesions
      (9) Fine-needle aspirates
      (10) Bronchial alveolar wash brushing
   b. *Probably diagnostically accurate* are:
      (1) Throat
      (2) Urine
      (3) Sputum
      (4) Genital (cervical, penile)
      (5) Nasal aspirates or washes

(6) Vesicular
(7) Skin (mouth, lip)

c. *Possibly diagnostically accurate* is stool or rectal swab.
d. Viruses do not comprise normal flora in the body. However, bacterial or fungal contamination of specimens can occur.

Diagnosis of West Nile Virus (WNV), West Nile Fever, and West Nile Encephalitis

The West Nile virus (WNV) is a single-stranded RNA flavivirus first isolated in Uganda in 1937. The virus first appeared in the United States in 1999 and, to date, has been documented in almost every state. The routes of transmission include the mosquito, which serves as the vector, and birds (e.g., crows, sparrows, jays), which are the reservoir hosts. The infected mosquito can then carry the virus particles in its salivary glands and infect susceptible bird species as well as humans. Transmission can also occur during blood transfusions, organ transplants, exposure in a laboratory setting, or from mother to baby. There is no evidence that the virus can be spread by human-to-human casual contact or from handling infected birds. Symptoms of WNV include fever, headache, neck stiffness, and skin rash. West Nile fever is the mild form of the infection, characterized by flu-like symptoms lasting only a few days with no long-term effects. West Nile encephalitis is the more severe form of the infection, characterized by encephalitis, meningitis, or both, which can lead to stupor, disorientation, coma, convulsions, and occasionally death.

Enzyme immunoassay is used to measure the antibodies IgM, which are produced early in the course of the infection, and IgG, which may not, however, be detectable for 4 to 5 days into the illness.

Reference Values

Normal

Negative for the WNV IgM antibody by ELISA
Negative for the WNV IgG antibody by ELISA

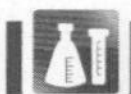

CLINICAL ALERT

The blood test may be negative early in the course of the infection; however, within 8 d of the onset of symptoms, 90% of infected people will become positive.

Procedure

Collect either a blood or CSF sample. Not all laboratories are equipped to measure the antibody, and the sample may have to be forwarded to a commercial or public health laboratory.

PROCEDURAL ALERT

1. The ELISA test can cross-react with other flaviviruses, such as yellow fever; therefore, additional serologic testing may be necessary to confirm a positive sample.
2. The CDC has made recommendations for both the employer and the employee (healthcare worker) when handling potentially infectious materials. The employer should provide training that addresses and reinforces how WNV is transmitted and the potential risks of exposure as well as personal protective equipment (PPE). The healthcare worker should use the PPE provided, minimize aerosol generation when handling specimens, and report any needlestick or sharps-related injury.

Interfering Factors

Exposure to the St. Louis encephalitis virus may result in a false-positive test result for WNV.

CLINICAL ALERT

In 2003, the CDC reported that 1000 blood donors tested positive for WNV, and as a result, about 24 people were infected from transfusions. All donated blood is now tested for WNV to detect and remove infected donations from the blood supply.

Interventions

Pretest Patient Care

1. Explain purpose of and procedure for test.
2. Follow guidelines in Chapter 1 for safe, effective, informed *pretest* care.

Posttest Patient Care

1. Review test results; report and record findings. Modify the nursing care plan as needed. Monitor and counsel the patient appropriately.
2. Follow guidelines in Chapter 1 for safe, effective, informed *posttest* care.

CLINICAL ALERT

Currently, there is no vaccination against WNV. Treatment is aimed at prevention of secondary infections (e.g., pneumonia and urinary tract infection), airway management, and supportive care.

● Diagnosis of Human Monkeypox Virus

In 2003, the monkeypox virus was identified in the United States, the first time the disease was seen outside of Africa. The virus was introduced into the United States through a shipment of animals, including sick prairie dogs eventually sold as pets, and some individuals who had contact with the pets became ill. The primary route of transmission is through close contact with, bite or scratch, from an infected animal. Symptoms include fever (>99.3°F or >37.4°C), headache, backache, muscular pain or tenderness, and a papular rash.

Reference Values

Normal

Negative for the monkeypox virus

Procedure

1. Oropharyngeal, scab lesion, or blood specimen can be used.
2. An oropharyngeal specimen can be obtained by swabbing or brushing the posterior tonsillar tissue. The swab should then be placed into a 2-mL screw-capped tube.
3. For a scab lesion, cleanse site with an alcohol wipe. Using either a scalpel or sterile 26-gauge needle, remove the top of the vesicle or pustule. Place specimen in a 2-mL sterile screw-capped plastic tube. Also, the base of the vesicle or pustule should be scraped with a swab or wooden end of an applicator stick and smeared onto a glass microscope slide.
4. For a serum sample, obtain 7 to 10 mL of venous blood in a marble-topped or yellow-topped serum separator tube, centrifuge, and collect the serum.

5. For a whole blood sample, obtain 3 to 5 mL of venous blood in a purple-topped tube and mix with anticoagulant.
6. Label specimens with the patient's name, date, and test(s) ordered, and place specimens in a biohazard bag.
7. Assays for the monkeypox virus include immunohistochemical testing methods, polymerase chain reaction (PCR) for DNA, or morphologic identification by electron microscopy.

NOTE *The microscope slide can be applied directly to the vesicular fluid for a touch preparation.*

PROCEDURAL ALERT

Use either polyester or Dacron swabs. No transport medium should be added to the tube for either an oropharyngeal or scab lesion specimen.

Clinical Implications

Detection of the virus after onset of symptoms is evidence of the infection.

NOTE *The clinical features of monkeypox virus are similar to smallpox. However, with human monkeypox virus, there is enlargement of lymph nodes.*

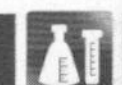

CLINICAL ALERT

Report cases of human monkeypox virus to local, state, and federal health departments.

● Diagnosis of Severe Acute Respiratory Syndrome (SARS)

Severe acute respiratory syndrome (SARS) is linked to a coronavirus (SARS-CoV). It is an atypical pneumonia that was first identified in Guangdong Province, China, in 2002, but since then has been seen in Asia, Europe, and North America. SARS is spread by person-to-person contact or contact with infectious material (e.g., respiratory secretions). Symptoms include fever (>100.4°F or >38°C), headache, cough, shortness of breath, muscular weakness, malaise, confusion, and diarrhea.

Reference Values

Normal

Negative for SARS-CoV antibody in a convalescent-phase serum obtained more than 28 days after onset of symptoms

Procedure

1. Collect a respiratory tract specimen, blood sample, or stool specimen.
2. Respiratory specimens may be collected from nasopharyngeal aspirates or swabs or oropharyngeal swabs.
   a. Nasopharyngeal aspirates are collected by instilling 1 to 1.5 mL of nonbacteriostatic saline into one nostril and then subsequently aspirating, through a plastic catheter, into a sterile vial.
   b. Nasopharyngeal or oropharyngeal specimens can be obtained by inserting a swab into the nostril or posterior pharynx, respectively. The swabs should then be placed into sterile vials containing 2 mL of viral media.

3. Obtain 5 to 10 mL (at least 1 mL in pediatric cases) of whole blood in a serum separator tube, or in an EDTA tube. If collected in a serum separator tube, the blood is allowed to clot and then centrifuged.
4. Collect 10 to 50 mL of stool, place in a leak-proof stool cup, and cap securely.
5. Label specimens with the patient's name, date, and test(s) ordered and place specimens in a biohazard bag.
6. Assays for the SARS-CoV infection include:
   a. ELISA
   b. Reverse transcriptase PCR (RT-PCR)
   c. Indirect fluorescent antibody
7. If the sample is to be shipped, it should be either packed in cold packs (4°C) for domestic travel or in dry ice if being shipped internationally.

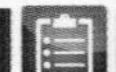

PROCEDURAL ALERT

Do not use swabs with wooden sticks or calcium alginate because they may contain substances that can interfere with the analysis.

Clinical Implications

Detection of the antibody to SARS-CoV in a convalescent-phase serum obtained more than 28 days after onset of symptoms is evidence of the infection.

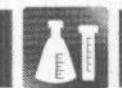

CLINICAL ALERT

Evidence of SARS should be reported to local, state, and federal health departments.

Interventions

Pretest Patient Care

1. Explain necessity, purpose, and procedure of testing. Assess for and document signs and symptoms of infection (fever, cough, shortness of breath, muscular weakness). Ask the patient about travel (especially travel within the last 10 days to a SARS-affected area), living accommodations, and contact with suspected cases. Also, ascertain whether the individual is a healthcare worker who may have been in direct contact with patients.
2. Close contact (e.g., living with or taking care of a person with SARS), sharing eating or drinking utensils, or close conversation (<3 feet) may result in transmission of the infection.
3. Follow guidelines in Chapter 1 for safe, effective, informed *pretest* care.

Posttest Patient Care

1. Review test results; report and record findings. Modify the nursing care plan as needed. Assess for and document any change in signs and symptoms.
2. Follow guidelines in Chapter 1 for safe, effective, informed *posttest* care.

CLINICAL ALERT

1. **If you are caring for someone with SARS, you should protect yourself by wearing disposable gloves; do not use silverware, towels, bedding, or other items that have been used by the person with SARS until thoroughly washed; make sure the individual covers his or her nose and mouth with a tissue before coughing or sneezing.**
2. **Clean all contaminated surfaces with household disinfectant.**

● Diagnosis of Highly Pathogenic Asian Avian Influenza A (H5N1) ("Bird Flu")

Asian highly pathogenic avian influenza (HPAI), commonly called "bird flu," is an infectious disease of birds caused by influenza A viruses. Bird flu viruses typically do not infect humans; however, in 1997, several cases of human infection were reported. Since 2003, the most human Asian HPAI cases have been reported from Indonesia, Vietnam, and Egypt. The first report in North America was in in Canada in 2014 after a person traveled to China. There are 16 different hemagglutinin (H) and 9 different neuraminidase (N) protein subtypes of influenza A virus, with many different combinations possible. These viruses are constantly changing, and over time, it has become apparent that they can infect and spread among humans. Influenza H5N1 virus has now been associated with human infection and death. Person-to-person spread is inefficient and, therefore, rare; however, because viruses have the ability to change, this may be a concern in the future.

Reference Values

Normal

Negative by hemagglutination inhibition (HAI), IFA staining, or RT-PCR

Procedure

1. Blood specimen: Obtain 5 to 10 mL of blood in a serum separator tube.
2. Nasal specimen: Instill 1 to 1.5 mL of nonbacteriostatic saline into one nostril and subsequently aspirate with a plastic catheter or tubing. A nasal swab can also be used to obtain a specimen by swabbing both nostrils and placing into a sterile vial.
3. Sputum specimen: Have patient rinse mouth with water and then expectorate deep-cough sputum into a sterile screw-cap sputum container.
4. Label specimen with the patient's name, date, and test(s) ordered and place specimen in biohazard bag and transport to laboratory.

PROCEDURAL ALERT

Growing the virus in culture is the gold standard for influenza diagnostics. If influenza A H5N1 is suspected, the virus should be cultured under Biosafety Level 3 (BSL-3) conditions with enhancements for positive identification of subtype.

Clinical Implications

A positive test is consistent with infection; however, identification of the viral subtype is necessary to confirm avian influenza.

Interventions

Pretest Patient Care

1. Explain necessity, purpose, and procedure of testing. Assess for and document signs and symptoms of infection (fever, cough, sore throat, and muscular weakness). Note recent travel history to areas known to have avian flu outbreaks or possible exposure to migratory waterfowl, especially wild ducks or domestic poultry, such as chickens or turkeys.
2. Follow guidelines in Chapter 1 for safe, effective, informed *pretest* care.

Posttest Patient Care

1. Review test results; report and record findings. Modify the nursing care plan as needed. Counsel the patient as appropriate.

2. There are no vaccines available to the general public. The antiviral medications oseltamivir and zanamivir may be effective treatments for H5N1 influenza; however, additional studies are necessary to demonstrate current and future efficacy.
3. Follow guidelines in Chapter 1 for safe, effective, informed *posttest* care.

● Diagnosis of Sexually Transmitted Infections (STIs)

STIs present a serious and increasing public health problem. They are caused by a variety of etiologic agents (Table 7.8). Some conditions, such as chlamydial and nongonococcal urethritis, have reached epidemic proportions. Although nongonococcal urethritis is a nonreportable infection in the United States, it is estimated that more than 2 million new cases occur each year. Manifestations of these infections range from the carrier state (asymptomatic) to infections with obvious symptoms such as cervicitis, conjunctivitis, endometritis, epididymitis, infertility, pharyngitis, proctitis, lymphogranuloma venereum, salpingitis, trachoma, urethritis, and, in the neonate, conjunctivitis and pneumonia.

Suggested Specimens

1. Urethral, vaginal, and cervical swabs
2. Semen
3. Urine
4. Prostatic secretion
5. Tissue biopsy
6. Swabs of oral lesions
7. Blood for serologic tests

Common Diagnostic Methods

1. Viral isolation in tissue cell cultures
2. Specific serologic antibody assays and syphilis detection tests
3. Cytologic techniques, such as Papanicolaou (Pap) and Tzanck tests, to demonstrate giant cells associated with herpesvirus infection
4. Gram stain and bacterial culture; saline wet prep
5. ELISA and immunoperoxidase assay to detect etiologic agent
6. Fluorescein or enzyme-tagged monoclonal antibodies to detect and identify etiologic agents
7. DNA probe
8. Nucleic acid amplification test (NAAT)

Clinical Considerations

1. Patients presenting with one STI may also be infected with other types of sexually transmitted pathogens.
2. Asymptomatic carriers are common.
3. Tracing and testing of sexual partners is a very important part of diagnosis and treatment.
4. The infection may recur if the patient is reinfected by the nontreated sexual partner.
5. Genital tract infections caused by sexually transmitted organisms in children are often the result of sexual abuse. Cultures should always be obtained, especially for *Chlamydia*, when required as legal evidence.
6. For suspected herpetic lesions, the virus is best recovered from the base of an active lesion. The older the lesion, the less likely it is to yield viable virus. Open the vesicle with a small-gauge needle or Dacron swab. Rub the base of the lesion vigorously to recover infected cells onto the swab, and place the swab in a viral transport medium. If large vesicles are present, aspirate material directly by needle and syringe. A separate swab can be collected for a Tzanck preparation (histology stain).

TABLE 7.8 Sexually Transmitted Infections and Their Laboratory Diagnosis

Infection	Causative Agent(s)[a]	Diagnosis
Chancroid	*Haemophilus ducreyi*	Culture of lesion or aspirate. Differential diagnosis should include syphilis, herpes, and lymphadenopathy-associated virus (LAV) monoclonal antibody test.
Gonorrhea	*Neisseria gonorrhoeae*	Gram stain of male urethra; culture or PCR of male urethra or female cervix, rectum, or pharynx; DNA probe; PCR of urine
Granuloma inguinale (donovanosis)	*Calymmatobacterium granulomatis* (formerly *Donovania granulomatis*)	Wright-Giemsa stain of lesion, tissue biopsy
Hepatitis B	Hepatitis B virus (HBV)	Serologic testing, hepatitis B antigen and antibody
Genital herpes	Herpes simplex virus (HSV) types 1 and 2	Viral culture from unroofed blister, scrapings examined by fluorescent microscopy or cytologic stains
Lymphogranuloma venereum (LGV)	*Chlamydia trachomatis* serotypes L_1, L_2, and L_3	Culture of aspirate of bubo, serologic test
Molluscum contagiosum	Molluscum contagiosum virus	Clinical appearance of lesions (pearly white, painless, umbilicated papules), microscopic examination of scrapings
Chlamydia	*Chlamydia trachomatis* serotypes D–K	Cell culture, urogenital swabs for direct antigen test, DNA probe technology, nucleic acid amplification test
Candidosis (moniliasis)	*Candida albicans*	Culture, potassium hydroxide (KOH) wet mount, Gram stain, DNA probe
Pelvic inflammatory disease (PID)	*Neisseria gonorrhoeae, Chlamydia trachomatis*	Clinical symptoms, cervical culture, DNA probe, PCR, laparoscopy or culdocentesis
Pediculosis pubis	*Phthirus pubis* (pubic or crab louse)	Adult lice or nits appear on body hairs
Scabies	*Sarcoptes scabiei*	Characteristic lesions, scrapings for microscopy
Syphilis	*Treponema pallidum*	Darkfield microscopy, serologic test
Trichomoniasis	*Trichomonas vaginalis*	Vaginal, urethral, or prostatic secretion examined microscopically, culture; antigen test; DNA probe
Nonspecific urethritis (nongonococcal urethritis—NGU)	*Chlamydia trachomatis* (50% of cases), *Ureaplasma urealyticum*, a human T-strain mycoplasma (*Mycoplasma hominis*), *Trichomonas vaginalis, Candida albicans,* herpes simplex virus	Identification by smear, culture, or molecular tests of specific etiologic agent

table continues on pg. 521 >

TABLE 7.8, continued

Infection	Causative Agent(s)[a]	Diagnosis
Nonspecific vaginitis	*Gardnerella vaginalis, Mobiluncus curtisii, Mobiluncus mulieris*	Wet mount for "clue" cells or Papanicolaou test; fishy smell is released when specimen fluid is mixed with 10% KOH; culture; DNA probe; culture or enzyme immunoassay to rule out gonorrhea
Condylomata acuminata (venereal warts)	Human papilloma DNA virus	Typical clinical lesion: cauliflower-like, soft, pink growth around vulva, anus, labia, vagina, glans penis, urethra, and perineum; rule out syphilis
AIDS	HIV	Serologic tests
Gastrointestinal (giardiasis, amebiasis, shigellosis, campylobacteriosis, and anorectal infections)	Enteric infections: *Giardia lamblia, Entamoeba histolytica,* and *Cryptosporidium* spp.	Ova and parasite examination
	Shigella spp.	Stool culture
	Campylobacter fetus	Stool culture
	Strongyloides spp. (worms)	Ova and parasite examination
	Anorectal:	
	Neisseria gonorrhoeae	Anal swab specimen, culture, DNA probe
	Chlamydia trachomatis	Anal swab culture, DNA probe
	Treponema pallidum	Darkfield microscopy plus serologic test
	Herpes simplex virus	Tissue culture
	Human papillomavirus	Signs and symptoms, DNA probe

PCR, polymerase chain reaction.

[a]The pathogens causing sexually transmitted infections span the full range of medical microbiology; their only common characteristic is that they may cause genital infection or be transmitted by genital contact.

7. For darkfield examination (e.g., syphilis), cleanse the area around the lesion with sterile saline. Abrade the surface with sterile dry gauze until blood is expressed. Continue to blot until blood ceases; squeeze the area until serous fluid is expressed. Touch the material to a clean glass slide, add a cover slip, and examine the specimen immediately for motile spirochetes.
8. Complications of untreated STIs include ectopic (tubal) pregnancy, infertility, chronic pelvic pain, and poor pregnancy outcomes.

● Diagnosis of Foodborne Illness (Food Poisoning)

Most cases of foodborne illness (food poisoning) in the United States are associated with various types of bacteria found in soil, water, airborne dust, vegetation, cereals, pasteurized food, and powdered milk. GI anthrax, due to ingestion of contaminated meat from an infected animal, has been reported in developing nations but rarely in the United States. Spices in meat have been reported to be contaminated with *Bacillus* spores. *Bacillus cereus* produces two toxins: an emetic toxin that causes vomiting and an enterotoxin that causes diarrhea. Unrefrigerated fried rice has been associated with the emetic toxin, whereas poultry, cooked meats, mashed potatoes, soups, and desserts have been associated with the enterotoxin. *Salmonella,* norovirus, *C. perfringens*, and *E. coli* are commonly associated with outbreaks of foodborne illnesses. The CDC estimates that 48 million people in the United States become sick each year due to foodborne illnesses, resulting in 128,000 hospitalizations and 3000 deaths. *E. coli* can be found in ground beef, leafy greens, and dairy. Changes in eating habits (e.g., raw natural diets) may contribute to increases in food-borne illnesses.

This test is used to detect one of the two toxins produced by *B. cereus*.

Reference Values

Normal

Negative for culture of *B. cereus* colonies by DNA probe or other microbiologic tests

Procedure

Collect stool specimens (25 to 50 g) for culture. Call your laboratory or public health department about special stool culture collection.

PROCEDURAL ALERT

- Suspected food specimens may also be tested.
- Refrigerate specimen in clean, sealed, leak-proof containers.
- If a delay of more than 2 hr is anticipated, the specimen should be placed in a Cary-Blair transport medium.

Clinical Implications

Positive abnormal findings of the special characteristics of *B. cereus* are consistent with food poisoning.

Interventions

Pretest Patient Care

1. Explain purpose and procedure for diagnosing food poisoning. Assess for and document signs and symptoms of infection (diarrhea, fever, abdominal cramps). Document history of recently ingested foods.
2. Follow guidelines in Chapter 1 for safe, effective, informed *pretest* care.

Posttest Patient Care

1. Review test results; report and record findings. Modify the nursing care plan as needed. Monitor prescribed drug treatment (vancomycin, erythromycin).
2. Follow guidelines in Chapter 1 for safe, effective, informed *posttest* care.

BIOTERRORISM AND EMERGENCY RESPONSE: INFECTIOUS AGENTS

Bioterrorism is the intentional release of a biologic agent through air, water, or food to cause illness or death to people, animals, and/or vegetation. The CDC has placed bioterrorism agents into three categories. Category A includes anthrax, botulism, plague, smallpox, tularemia, and the viral hemorrhagic fevers. Category B includes, among other things, *C. perfringens* epsilon toxin, Q fever, ricin toxin, *Staphylococcus* enterotoxin B, and food and water safety threats. Category C includes emerging infections such as hantaviruses and Nipah virus.

Diagnosis of Anthrax Infection

Anthrax is a communicable infectious disease transmitted from animals to humans. Humans can contact *Bacillus anthracis* (encapsulated, aerobic, spore-forming, rod-shaped, gram-positive bacillus) from handling or consuming undercooked meat from infected animals. The organism can also be inhaled from animal products (e.g., wool) or during intentional release of spores (i.e., bioterrorism). There are four forms of anthrax: cutaneous, GI, oropharyngeal, and inhalational. The incubation period for cutaneous anthrax is usually immediate or within 24 hours. There is localized skin involvement with papular lesions that turn vesicular and subsequently develop into black eschar within 7 to 10 days. GI anthrax usually requires an incubation period of 1 to 7 days. Two to 4 days after the onset of symptoms, ascites develops, which can soon be followed by shock and death. The incubation period for oropharyngeal anthrax is generally about 1 to 7 days marked by severe sore throat, dysphagia, and fever. Although the incubation period for inhalational anthrax (results from inspiration of 8000 to 50,000 spores) typically ranges from 1 to 7 days, it can be prolonged up to 2 months. Typically, the symptoms are abrupt in onset with a high fever and severe respiratory distress. Shock and death can occur within 24 to 36 hours.

PROCEDURAL ALERT

1. As soon as anthrax is suspected, notify the state public health laboratory and CDC.
2. Take precautions to avoid production of aerosols of infected material.
3. If GI anthrax is suspected, collect samples of gastric aspirate, feces, or food along with three blood cultures.
4. Household bleach solutions (5.25% hypochlorite) diluted 1:10 can be used to decontaminate surfaces. Contaminated instruments should be autoclaved after immersion in decontamination solution.
5. Proper immunization is required for persons who work directly with contaminated animal hides or animal tissues or spores.
6. Skin infections constitute 95% of anthrax infections, with a 20% death rate in untreated skin (cutaneous) anthrax.
7. Abnormal chest x-ray findings show widening of the mediastinum due to hemorrhage.
8. Person-to-person transmission of inhalation anthrax infection has not been observed.

Reference Values

Normal

Negative for the *B. anthracis* organism (appears as two to four encapsulated cells)

Procedure

1. Use sputum, throat cultures, blood, skin, stool, pleural fluid, CSF, or ascitic fluid specimens to isolate *B. anthracis*. Laboratory methods include Gram stain, culture, and PCR. Collect the appropriate blood volume (usually 8 to 10 mL) and number of tubes per laboratory protocol. For PCR, collect 10 mL of blood in a purple-topped tube (anticoagulant, EDTA). For both CSF and pleural fluid, collect >1 mL into a sterile container. For skin lesions, two swabs are taken: one for Gram stain and culture and the other for PCR.
2. Perform procedure in a Biosafety Level 2 (BSL-2) microbiologic laboratory. BSL-2 practices are used in laboratories in which human-derived blood or other body fluids are being tested for infectious agents.
3. Analyze samples in a certified class II biological safety cabinet (BSC) (Fig. 7.6).
4. Subculture a routine sputum, blood, or stool sample to sheep blood agar (SBA), MacConkey agar, or phenylethyl alcohol (PEA) plates.

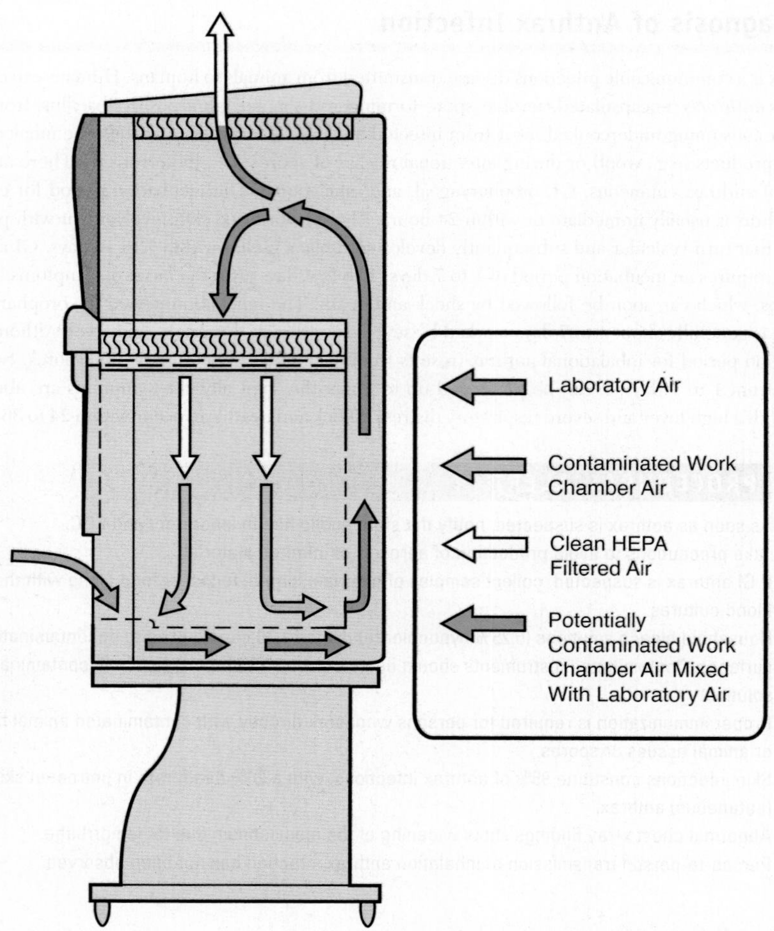

FIGURE 7.6. Class II, type A2 biological safety cabinet. *HEPA*, high-efficiency particulate air. (Reprinted with permission from Microzone Corp., Ottawa, Ontario, Canada.)

5. Incubate cultures at 35° to 37°C and examine within 18 to 24 hours of incubation.
6. Test isolates for motility, morphology, beta hemolysis, and Gram stain to differentiate colonies of *B. anthracis* from other bacilli.
7. Remember that *B. anthracis* is an encapsulated gram-positive rod—with oval-shaped, nonswelling spores, and ground-glass appearance of colonies—and is nonmotile and nonhemolytic.
8. Soak two dry sterile swabs in vesicular fluid (previously unopened vesicle) for cutaneous anthrax.
9. Use a stool specimen for GI anthrax.
10. Use a sputum specimen for inhalation anthrax; in the later stages, collect a blood sample.
11. See Chart 7.4 for the collection of specimens for inhalation and cutaneous anthrax.

PROCEDURAL ALERT

B. anthracis grows well in SBA plates but does not grow on MacConkey agar.

CHART 7.4 Collecting Specimens for Inhalation and Cutaneous Anthrax

Inhalation Anthrax	Cutaneous Anthrax
• Collect blood, pleural fluid (if patient has pleural effusion), or cerebrospinal fluid (if patient has signs or symptoms of meningitis) specimen for Gram stain, culture, and polymerase chain reaction (PCR) • Bronchial or pleural biopsy for immunohistochemistry • Use acute and convalescent (14–35 d after onset of symptoms) sera for serology • The Inova Fairfax protocol and the three-tier screening protocol outline alternative screening algorithms for use in evaluating large numbers of patients in emergency situations.	• Swab the lesion for Gram stain, culture, and PCR, or obtain a blood specimen if patient has signs of systemic infection • Skin biopsy for immunohistochemistry • Use acute and convalescent sera for serology

From Centers for Disease Control and Prevention: Recommended specimens for microbiology and pathology of diagnosis of anthrax. Available at: https://www.cdc.gov/anthrax/specificgroups/lab-professionals/recommended-specimen.html; last reviewed and updated January 30, 2017.

Clinical Implications

The isolation of *B. anthracis* rods confirms the diagnosis of anthrax.

NOTE *If B. anthracis is not identified, perform supportive tests: PCR, immunohistochemistry, and serology (see Chart 7.4). If any two of three are positive, this is confirmation of anthrax. If any one of three is positive, this is considered a suspected case of anthrax; if not linked to a confirmed environmental exposure, then it is not anthrax.*

Interventions

Pretest Patient Care

1. Explain the purpose, procedure, and risks of obtaining a specimen.
2. Obtain and record current occupation and history of occupations. Assess for and document signs and symptoms of anthrax (fever, dyspnea, coughing, chest pain, heavy perspiration, and bluish skin due to lack of oxygen).
3. Avoid direct contact with lesions.
4. Follow guidelines in Chapter 1 for safe, effective, informed *pretest* care.

Posttest Patient Care

1. Contact the Federal Bureau of Investigation (FBI), CDC, and state public health department if *B. anthracis* is identified.
2. Review test results; report and record findings. Modify the nursing care plan as needed. Monitor treatment. Report signs and symptoms.
3. Postexposure prophylaxis for anthrax includes ciprofloxacin (500 mg twice daily) or doxycycline (100 mg twice daily) for 60 days.
4. Follow guidelines in Chapter 1 for safe, effective, informed *posttest* care.

NOTE *Do not use extended-spectrum cephalosporins or TMP-SMX because anthrax has been shown to be resistant to some of these classes of drugs.*

Diagnosis of Botulism Infection

Human botulism is caused by the spore-forming, obligate anaerobe, rod-shaped bacterium *Clostridium botulinum*. *C. botulinum* produces the botulinum toxin, which is the most poisonous biologic substance known. There are seven distinct antigenic types of the botulinum toxin designated types A through G. All forms of botulism are the result of absorption from a mucosal surface (e.g., GI tract or lung) or a wound into the circulatory system. *C. botulinum* can be found in the soil and in undercooked food that is not kept hot. Cases of water-borne botulism have not been documented, although aerosolization of the toxin and subsequent inhalation has been done experimentally. Foil-wrapped potatoes held at room temperature after baking can cause botulism, as can contaminated condiments, such as sautéed onions or cheese sauce. Botulism has been divided into four naturally occurring forms: (1) food-borne, (2) wound, (3) infant (up to 8 months of age), and (4) unclassified (no food or wound source has been identified).

NOTE *Inhalational botulism does not occur naturally.*

This test is used to confirm the presence of *C. botulinum*, which produces the botulinum toxin.

Reference Values

Normal

Absence of botulinum toxin

Absence of incremental response to repetitive nerve stimulation on an electromyogram

Procedure

1. Obtain specimens from blood, stool, gastric aspirates or vomitus, and, if available, suspected food.
2. Obtain at least 30 mL of venous blood in a red-topped Vacutainer.
3. Use an enema (with sterile water) to obtain an adequate fecal sample if the patient is constipated.
4. Refrigerate all samples.
5. Use the mouse lethality bioassay to determine whether there is any botulinum toxin present.

NOTE *Sterile water, not saline, should be used for the enema solution because saline will interfere with the bioassay.*

NOTE *The Laboratory Response Network (LRN), which is overseen by the CDC, is a network of more than 150 laboratories that are capable of responding to bioterrorism and public health emergencies.*

PROCEDURAL ALERT

In some cases, an electromyogram is performed to differentiate cause of acute flaccid paralysis.

Clinical Implications

1. The identification of botulism neurotoxin is evidence of botulism poisoning.
2. Mortality rates vary depending on the type of botulism poisoning (foodborne, 5% to 10% with treatment in developed countries; wound botulism, 1% to 15% depending on amount of wound contamination; infant botulism, 2%). Severe respiratory distress due to paralysis of muscles can lead to death.

Interfering Factors

The use of anticholinesterases (e.g., physostigmine salicylate or pralidoxime chloride) by the patient can interfere with the bioassay.

Interventions

Pretest Patient Care

1. Explain the purpose, procedure, and risks of obtaining a specimen.
2. Follow guidelines in Chapter 1 for safe, effective, informed *pretest* care.

Posttest Patient Care

1. Do not isolate patients diagnosed with botulism because it is not contagious and cannot be transmitted from person to person.
2. Review test results; report and record findings. Modify the nursing care plan as needed. Provide supportive care to patient and monitor appropriately.
3. Administer an antitoxin (i.e., equine antitoxin) in a timely manner to minimize subsequent nerve damage. In the United States, the botulinum antitoxin is stored in the National Strategic Stockpile and is available from the CDC.
4. Antibiotics can be used to treat secondary infections; however, they do not have a direct effect on the botulinum toxin.
5. Monitor the patient for impending respiratory failure.
6. Follow Chapter 1 guidelines for safe, effective, informed *posttest* care.

CLINICAL ALERT

1. Postexposure prophylaxis is limited owing to antitoxin scarcity and reactogenicity.
2. By law, in most areas of the country, suspected botulism must be reported to local public health authorities.

CLINICAL ALERT

1. Laboratory personnel should observe standard precautions.
2. Decontaminate surfaces with 0.1% hypochlorite bleach solution.
3. Contaminated clothing should be washed with soap and water.

● Diagnosis of Hemorrhagic Fever, Hantavirus, Ebola Virus, Marburg Virus, and Yellow Fever Infection

These tests are done to diagnose hemorrhagic fever (HF; with renal symptoms, HFRS), an endemic threat in the United States, and yellow fever associated with hepatitis. Signs and symptoms include fever, thrombocytopenia, renal failure, shock, multiorgan failure, and lung edema. Jaundice occurs in yellow fever. Heavy rains are associated with an increase in number of rodents (which are the vectors in HF) and mosquitoes in yellow fever. The hantavirus Sin Nombre is responsible for hantavirus pulmonary syndrome (HPS). The deer mouse is the major reservoir for the hantavirus Sin Nombre. The mortality rate associated with HPS can be as high as 5% to 15%. Marburg HF is caused by an animal-borne RNA virus and is found in the Filovirus family (also includes the Ebola virus). Individuals handling infected green monkeys are at risk, as are people in close contact with infected individuals such as in a healthcare setting or family members.

Reference Values

Normal

No evidence of hantavirus, Ebola virus, or 17 other viruses that may cause HF
No evidence of yellow fever virus that may cause hepatitis
Negative for presence of antibodies to hantavirus
Negative antigen-detection ELISA for Marburg virus

Procedure

1. Obtain specimen of blood (red-topped tube), sputum, tissue, and possibly urine following standard precautions.
2. Label specimens with the patient's name, date, and test(s) ordered and place specimens in biohazard bags. All specimens are considered infectious.
3. Antigen-capture ELISA, IgM-capture ELISA, PCR, or virus isolation methods are used on specimens collected.

PROCEDURAL ALERT

1. Follow airborne precautions with negative-pressure rooms if available.
2. Use personal protective equipment.

Clinical Implications

Growth of hantavirus (or any of the other 17 causative viruses) in culture or presence of hantavirus antigens is evidence of infection. Thrombocytopenia is present in blood samples.

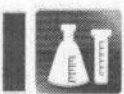

CLINICAL ALERT

Evidence of HF is reported to local, state, and federal authorities.

Interventions

Pretest Patient Care

1. Explain necessity, purpose, and procedure of testing. Assess for and document signs and symptoms of infection (headache, pneumonia, fever, vomiting, cough, muscular pain, jaundice, hemorrhage from nose or GI tract, facial swelling). HPS is characterized by a fever (temperature >101°F) with bilateral diffuse interstitial pulmonary edema. Questions regarding occupation, living accommodations, and circumstances (e.g., recent heavy rains, mosquitoes, tropical climate, port city) are important.
2. In most cases, no person-to-person transmission has been described; however, close contact with infected individuals poses a higher risk.
3. Follow guidelines in Chapter 1 for safe, effective, informed *pretest* care.

Posttest Patient Care

1. Review test results; report and record findings. Modify the nursing care plan as needed. Counsel, monitor, and treat the patient appropriately. Report signs and symptoms. Patients are usually very ill. If the HF viruses are isolated or the hantavirus antigens (or other causative viruses) are identified, supportive therapy (e.g., supplemental oxygen, mechanical ventilation, maintaining blood pressure through volume control) and antibiotics are used to treat secondary bacterial infections. Correct dehydration and electrolyte imbalance and treat acidosis and blood cell abnormalities.
2. Immunity to yellow fever occurs after recovery.

3. Recovery from Marburg virus HF can be prolonged. Some complications include testicular inflammation, recurrent hepatitis, inflammation of the parotid gland, or uveitis (intraocular inflammation).
4. Follow guidelines in Chapter 1 for safe, effective, informed *posttest* care.

CLINICAL ALERT

1. Monitor close and high-risk contact for 21 d.
2. There is no known cure, vaccine, or treatment, other than supportive care, for HPS.

● Diagnosis of Plague, Bubonic Plague, Pneumonic Plague, and Primary Septicemic Plague Infection

This test is done to diagnose plague. Plague (enzootic infection of rats, squirrels, prairie dogs, and other rodents caused by the bacteria *Yersinia pestis*) can be found on every continent except Australia. Plague is transmitted by the bite of an infected flea, or from direct contact from body fluid or tissues or inhaling droplets from an infected person or animal. Signs and symptoms include a sudden onset of fever, chills, generalized weakness, and buboes (swollen tender lymph nodes). Buboes typically develop in the axilla, cervical, or groin regions.

There are three forms of the infection: bubonic (regional lymph node involvement), pneumonic (lung involvement), and septicemic (primarily after skin inoculation). Bubonic plague has an incubation period of 2 to 6 days, with 80% of cases going on to become septicemic plague, which carries a 100% mortality rate if not treated. Septicemic plague occurs after a skin inoculation or progression of bubonic plague and, like pneumonic plague, if left untreated results in 100% mortality.

Reference Values

Normal

Negative for the presence of *Y. pestis*
Titer <1:16 using passive hemagglutination on acute and convalescent serum
Titer >1:256 is presumptive of immunologic response.

Procedure

1. Obtain specimens of blood, sputum, or a lymph node aspirate following standard precautions.
2. Transport specimens per laboratory protocol.

PROCEDURAL ALERT

Specimens should be taken prior to treatment if at all possible, but antibiotic treatment should not be delayed. Specimens should be processed using BSL-2 practices or BSL-3 if there is a high potential for aerosolization (e.g., centrifugation procedures). BSL-2 and -3 practices include controlled access and decontamination of all waste and laboratory clothing before laundering.

Clinical Implications

A positive culture for *Y. pestis* is evidence of the infection, and antibiotic treatment should begin immediately. If test results are negative but clinical manifestations still point to plague, further serologic testing should be done.

CLINICAL ALERT

1. Evidence of plague must be reported to the local, state, and federal authorities.
2. Persons having close contact (<2 m) with an infected individual should receive postexposure antibiotic prophylaxis for 7 d.

Interventions

Pretest Patient Care

1. Explain necessity, purpose, and procedure of testing. Assess for and document signs and symptoms of infection (sudden onset of fever, chills, headache, weakness).
2. There is limited evidence of person-to-person spread. Observe standard precautions in bubonic plague; observe droplet precautions in pneumonic plague.
3. Follow guidelines in Chapter 1 for safe, effective, informed *pretest* care.

Posttest Patient Care

1. Review test results; report and record findings. Modify the nursing care plan as needed. Counsel, monitor, and treat the patient appropriately. Evidence does not support that residual *Y. pestis* poses an environmental threat, and the organism does not survive long outside the host. For prophylaxis of bubonic or pneumonic plague, oral doxycycline, tetracycline, or TMP-SMX should be considered.
2. Notify the CDC if results are positive.
3. Follow guidelines in Chapter 1 for safe, effective, informed *posttest* care.

● Diagnosis of Smallpox Infection

Smallpox, an infectious disease caused by the variola virus, was once worldwide in scope; however, vaccination has all but eliminated the virus, with the exception of existence of the variola virus in laboratory reserves. Since 2001, concerns about its use as a biologic weapon have prompted medical and public healthcare professionals to make recommendations for steps to be taken in case of exposure and outbreak. There are two principal forms of smallpox: variola minor and variola major. Smallpox is spread from person to person by means of coughing; direct contact; or contaminated clothing, bedding, or infected bodily fluids. A person sometimes is infectious to others at the onset of fever but is always infections to others by the time of rash onset until smallpox scabs have completely disappeared. This test is used to determine the presence of the DNA virus responsible for smallpox.

Reference Values

Normal

No Guarnieri's bodies isolated in scrapings of skin lesions
Absence of brick-shaped virions (i.e., variola virus) by electron microscopy
Low levels of neutralizing, hemagglutinin-inhibiting or complement-fixing antibodies

Procedure

1. Open skin lesions with a blunt instrument (e.g., blunt edge of a scalpel) and collect the vesicular or pustular fluid on a cotton swab.
2. Remove scabs with a forceps; they can also be used.
3. Place specimens in a Vacutainer tube; re-stopper and seal it with adhesive tape.
4. Place the Vacutainer tube in a durable, watertight container for transport.
5. Ensure that the laboratory examining the specimens is a Biosafety Level 4 laboratory.
6. Confirm smallpox infection by the appearance of brick-shaped virions under the electron microscope.
7. Definitive laboratory identification requires growth of the virus in cell culture.
8. Use a cotton swab to obtain specimens from the oral cavity or oropharynx if necessary.

PROCEDURAL ALERT

1. Observe standard precautions (i.e., gloves, gowns, and mask should be worn by laboratory personnel). All laundry and waste should be transported in biohazard bags and autoclaved before being laundered or incinerated.
2. Specimen collection and examination should be performed by laboratory personnel who have recently been vaccinated.
3. All surfaces should be cleaned with bleach or quaternary ammonia.

Clinical Implications

1. Evidence of virions or Guarnieri's bodies indicates presence of smallpox infection.
2. High levels of antibodies indicate infection.

Interventions

Pretest Patient Care

1. Explain the purpose, procedure, and risks of obtaining a specimen. Assess for and document signs and symptoms of infection (chills, high fever, backache, pustules that leave a pockmark).
2. Follow guidelines in Chapter 1 for safe, effective, informed *pretest* care.

Posttest Patient Care

1. Review test results; report and record findings. Modify the nursing care plan as needed. Isolate the individual immediately if the smallpox virus is identified.
2. Report signs and symptoms.
3. Smallpox vaccination within 3 days after exposure may prevent or significantly decrease severity of symptoms. After 3 days and up to 7 days after exposure, vaccination offers some protection or may modify infection severity. Adverse effects range from mild and self-limited to severe and life-threatening events.
4. Follow guidelines in Chapter 1 for safe, effective, informed *posttest* care.

CLINICAL ALERT

1. A confirmed case of smallpox should be brought to the attention of local, state, and federal health authorities.
2. Because there are no antiviral drugs for smallpox, supportive therapy and antibiotics for secondary bacterial infections should be offered to the patient.
3. Household members should be vaccinated and monitored closely.

● Diagnosis of Tularemia Infection

Tularemia, also known as "rabbit fever," is primarily found in rural areas, although occasionally it occurs in urban and suburban areas. Tularemia is caused by the bacterium *Francisella tularensis*, an intracellular parasite (aerobic, gram-negative coccobacillus) that is spread to humans by infected animals (e.g., mice, squirrels, rabbits) or contaminated water, soil, and vegetation. Animals become infected through tick, fly, and mosquito bites. Once infected, person-to-person transmission has not been documented. Two major subspecies of *F. tularensis* have been identified: type A (*F. tularensis* biovar. *tularensis*), which is highly virulent in humans, and type B (*F. tularensis* biovar. *palaearctica*), which is relatively avirulent.

Humans can contract *F. tularensis* through the skin, mucous membranes, lungs, and GI tract. Because *F. tularensis* is highly infectious (10 to 50 organisms can cause disease), its use in biologic terrorism cannot be overlooked. The incubation period is usually 3 to 5 days but can be as long as 14 days, followed by an abrupt onset of symptoms, including fever, chills, and headaches. Mortality can be as high as 30% if not treated and 10% if treated.

This test is used to determine the presence of the *F. tularensis* organism.

Reference Values

Normal

Absence of the *F. tularensis* organism
Negative serum antibody titers

Procedure

1. Obtain specimens of respiratory secretions (i.e., sputum), blood, lymph node biopsy samples, or scrapings from infected ulcers.
2. Collect sputum samples after a forced deep cough and place in a sterile, screw-top container.
3. Obtain a 5- to 7-mL Vacutainer from a venipuncture for blood samples.
4. Obtain a skin scraping at the leading edge of a lesion from an infected ulcer and place in a clean, screw-top tube.
5. Perform presumptive identification of *F. tularensis* in a BSL-2 laboratory.
6. Ensure that confirmation of the organism is done in a BSL-3 clinical laboratory. BSL-3 laboratories process indigenous or exotic agents with a potential for respiratory transmission and causation of serious or lethal infection.

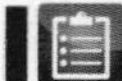

PROCEDURAL ALERT

1. Observe standard precautions.
2. Contaminated clothing or linens should be disinfected per standard precautions protocols.
3. Decontaminate surfaces with a 10% bleach solution.
4. Laboratory personnel who may have had a potential infective exposure should be given prophylactic antibiotics if the risk for infection is high (e.g., needlestick).

Clinical Implications

Identification of *F. tularensis* and/or increased antibody titers indicate the presence of tularemia. Antibodies do not appear until 2 to 3 weeks after exposure and peak at about 5 weeks.

Interventions

Pretest Patient Care

1. Explain the purpose, procedure, and risks of obtaining a specimen. Assess for and document signs and symptoms of infection (ulcer at site of infection, swollen lymph nodes, fever, chills, headache, fatigue), history of urban or rural living, and occupation (e.g., handling infected animal carcasses).
2. Follow guidelines in Chapter 1 for safe, effective, informed *pretest* care.

Posttest Patient Care

1. If the *F. tularensis* organism is cultured from the patient, isolation is not recommended because human-to-human transmission has not been documented.
2. Postexposure treatment includes antibiotics such as streptomycin, gentamicin, or ciprofloxacin.
3. Review test results; report and record findings. Modify the nursing care plan as needed. Counsel the patient and monitor appropriately.
4. Follow guidelines in Chapter 1 for safe, effective, informed *posttest* care.

CLINICAL ALERT

1. Postexposure prophylactic antibiotic treatment of persons in close contact with the infected patient is not recommended because person-to-person transmission has not been documented.
2. Pregnant women should be treated with ciprofloxacin because rare cases of fetal nerve deafness and renal damage have been reported with some of the aminoglycosides.
3. Suspicion of inhalational tularemia (i.e., signs and symptoms) must be reported to local or state public health authorities and the CDC.

BIBLIOGRAPHY

Centers for Disease Control and Prevention: Avian influenza in birds. Available at: https://www.cdc.gov/flu/avianflu/avian-in-birds.htm

Centers for Disease Control and Prevention: Emergency preparedness and response, bioterrorism agents/disease, A–Z, by category. Available at: http://emergency.cdc.gov/agent/agentlist-category.asp

Centers for Disease Control and Prevention: Epidemic/Epizootic West Nile Virus in the United States: Guidelines for Surveillance, Prevention, and Control, 4th ed. Fort Collins, CO, Division of Vector-Borne Infectious Diseases, 2013

Centers for Disease Control and Prevention: Get Smart for Health Care, Clinician Guide, August 9, 2012

Centers for Disease Control and Prevention: Guidelines for using the QuantiFERON-TB gold test for detecting *Mycobacterium tuberculosis* infection, United States. MMWR Recomm Rep 54(RR-15):49–55, 2005

Centers for Disease Control and Prevention: Health care-associated infections (HAIs). Carbapenem-resistant Enterobacteriaceae (CRE). Available at: http://www.cdc.gov/HAI/organisms/cre/index.html

Centers for Disease Control and Prevention: Interim guidelines for investigation of and response to *Bacillus anthracis*. MMWR 50(44):987–990, 2001

Centers for Disease Control and Prevention: Investigation of anthrax associated with intentional exposure and interim public health guidelines. MMWR 50(41):889–893, 2001

Centers for Disease Control and Prevention: Investigation of bioterrorism-related anthrax and interim guidelines for clinical evaluation of persons with possible anthrax. MMWR 50(43):941–948, 2001

Centers for Disease Control and Prevention: Prevention and control of seasonal influenza with vaccines; Recommendations of the Advisory Committee on Vaccination Practices, United States, 2016–17 influenza seasons. MMWR Recomm Rep 65(5):1–54, 2017

Centers for Disease Control and Prevention: Recommended antimicrobial agents for the treatment and postexposure prophylaxis of pertussis, 2005 CDC guidelines. MMWR Recomm Rep 54(RR-14):1–16, 2005

Centers for Disease Control and Prevention: Rodents, diseases directly transmitted by rodents. Available at: http://www.cdc.gov/rodents/diseases/direct.html; last updated January 20, 2017

Centers for Disease Control and Prevention: Sexually transmitted diseases treatment guidelines, 2015. MMWR Recomm Rep 55(RR3):1–137, 2015

Centers for Disease Control and Prevention: Surveillance guidelines for smallpox vaccine (vaccinia) adverse reactions. MMWR Recomm Rep 55(RR-1):1–16, 2006

Centers for Disease Control and Prevention: Updated recommendations of the Advisory Committee on Immunization Practices for the control and elimination of mumps. MMWR Morb Mortal Wkly Rep 55(RR22):629–630, 2006

Code of Federal Regulations, 49 CFR 173.134

Inglesby TV, Dennis DT, Henderson DA, et al: Plague as a biological weapon: Medical and public health management. JAMA 283:2281–2290, 2000

Miller J, Engelberg S, Broad W: Germs: Biological weapons and America's secret war. New York, Touchstone/Simon & Schuster, 2002

Stern EJ, Uhde KB, Shadomy SV, et al: Conference report on public health and clinical guidelines for anthrax. Emerg Infect Dis 14(4), 2008. Available at: http://wwwnc.cdc.gov/eid/article/14/4/07-0969.htm

Tille PM: Bailey and Scott's Diagnostic Microbiology, 13th ed. St. Louis, Mosby, 2013

U.S. Department of Health and Human Services: Primary Containment for Biohazards: Selection, Installation and Use of Biological Safety Cabinets, 3rd ed. Atlanta, GA, Centers for Disease Control and Prevention, 2007

U.S. Preventive Services Task Force: Guide to Clinical Preventive Services, Rockville, MD, Agency for Health Care Research and Quality, 2014

Versalovic J, Carroll KC, Funke G, et al (eds): Manual of Clinical Microbiology, 11th ed. Washington, DC, ASM Press, 2015

Winn W, Allen S, Janda W, et al: Color Atlas and Textbook of Diagnostic Microbiology, 6th ed. Philadelphia, Lippincott Williams & Wilkins, 2005

Wormser GP, Dattwyler RJ, Shapiro ED, et al: The clinical assessment, treatment, and prevention of Lyme disease, human granulocytic anaplasmosis, and babesiosis: Clinical practice guidelines by the Infectious Diseases Society of America. Clin Infect Dis 43(9):1089–1134, 2006. doi:10.1086/508667. Available at: http://www.idsociety.org/uploadedFiles/IDSA/Guidelines-Patient_Care/PDF_Library/Lyme%20Disease.pdf

Wu AHB: Tietz Clinical Guide to Laboratory Tests, 4th ed. Philadelphia, Saunders Elsevier, 2006

Immunodiagnostic Studies

8

OVERVIEW OF IMMUNODIAGNOSTIC STUDIES

Immunodiagnostic or serodiagnostic testing studies antigen–antibody reactions for diagnosis of infectious disease, autoimmune disorders, immune allergies, and neoplastic disease. These modalities also test for blood groups and types, tissue and graft transplant matching, and cellular immunology. Blood serum is tested for antibodies against particular antigens—hence, the term *blood serology testing*.

Antigens are substances that stimulate and subsequently react with the products of an immune response. They may be enzymes, toxins, microorganisms (e.g., bacterial, viral, parasitic, fungal), tumors, or autoimmune factors. *Antibodies* are proteins produced by the body's immune system in response to an antigen or antigens. The antigen–antibody response is the body's natural defense against invading organisms. Red blood cell groups contain almost 400 antigens. Immune reactions to these antigens result in a wide variety of clinical disorders, which can be tested (e.g., Coombs' test).

Pathologically, *autoimmune disorders* are produced by autoantibodies—that is, antibodies against *self*. Examples include systemic rheumatic diseases (SRDs), such as rheumatoid arthritis (RA) and lupus erythematosus.

Immunodeficiency diseases exhibit a lack of one or more basic components of the immune system, which includes B lymphocytes, T lymphocytes, phagocytic cells, and the complement system. These diseases are classified as primary (e.g., congenital, DiGeorge syndrome) and secondary (e.g., AIDS).

Hypersensitivity reactions are documented using immediate hypersensitivity tests and are defined as abnormally increased immune responses to some allergens (e.g., allergic reaction to bee stings or pollens). Delayed hypersensitivity skin tests are commonly used to evaluate cell-mediated immunity. Histocompatibility antigens (transplantation antigens) and tests for human leukocyte antigen (HLA) are important diagnostic tools to detect and prevent immune rejection in transplantation.

Types of Tests

Many methods of varying sophistication are used for immunodiagnostic studies (Table 8.1).

Collection of Serum for Immunologic Tests

Specific antibodies can be detected in serum and other body fluids (e.g., synovial fluid, cerebrospinal fluid [CSF]).

1. *Procure samples.* For diagnosis of infectious disease, a blood sample (serum preferred) using a 7-mL red-topped tube should be obtained at illness onset (acute phase), and the other sample should be drawn 3 to 4 weeks later (convalescent phase). In general, serologic test usefulness depends on a titer increase in the time interval between the acute and the convalescent phase. For some serologic tests, one serum sample may be adequate if the antibody presence indicates an abnormal condition or the antibody titer is unusually high. See Appendix A for standard precautions.
2. *Perform the serologic test before doing skin testing.* Skin testing often induces antibody production and could interfere with serologic test results.
3. *Label the specimen with the patient's name, date, and tests ordered and place in a biohazard bag.* Send samples to the laboratory promptly. Hemolyzed samples cannot yield accurate results. Hemoglobin in the serum sample can interfere with complement-fixing antibody values.

Interpreting Results of Immunologic Tests

The following factors affect test results:

1. History of previous infection by the same organism
2. Previous vaccination (determine time frame)
3. Anamnestic reactions caused by heterologous antigens: An *anamnestic reaction* is the appearance of antibodies in the blood after administration of an antigen to which the patient has previously developed a primary immune response.
4. Cross-reactivity: Antibodies produced by one species of an organism can react with an entirely different species (e.g., *Tularemia* antibodies may agglutinate *Brucella*, and vice versa, rickettsial infections may produce antibodies reactive with *Proteus* OX19).
5. Presence of other serious illness states (e.g., lack of immunologic response in agammaglobulinemia, cancer treatment with immunosuppressant drugs)
6. Seroconversion: the detection of specific antibody in the serum of an individual when this antibody was previously undetectable

TABLE 8.1 Some Tests That Determine Antigen–Antibody Reactions

Name of Test	Observable Reaction	Visible Change	Tests for
Agglutination, hemagglutination (HA), immune hemagglutination assay (IHA)	Particulate antigen reacts with corresponding antibody; antigen may be in form of red blood cells (hemagglutination, latex, or charcoal coated with antigen).	Clumping	Treponemal, heterophile, and cold agglutinin antibodies
Precipitation (e.g., immunodiffusion [ID], counterimmunoelectrophoresis [CIE])	Soluble antigen reacts with corresponding antibody by ID or count.	Precipitates	Fungal antibodies, food poisoning
Complement fixation (CF)	Competition between two antigen–antibody systems (test and indicator systems)	Complement activation, hemolysis	Viral antibodies
Immunofluorescence (e.g., indirect fluorescent antibody [IFA])	Fluorescent-tagged antibody reacts with antigen–antibody complex in the presence of ultraviolet light.	Visible microscopic fluorescence	Antinuclear antibodies (ANAs); antimitochondrial antibodies (AMAs)
Enzyme immunoassay (EIA)	Enzymes are used to label induced antigen–antibody reactions.	Chromogenic fluorescent or luminescent change in substrate	Hepatitis and HIV (screening)
Enzyme-linked immunosorbent assay (ELISA)	Indirect EIA for quantification of an antigen or antibody enzyme and substrate	Color change indicates enzyme substrate reaction.	Lyme disease, Epstein-Barr virus, extractable nuclear antibodies (connective tissue/systemic rheumatic disease)
Immunoblot (e.g., Western blot [WB])	Electrophoresis separation of antigen subspecies	Detection of antibodies of specific mobility	Confirms HIV-1
Polymerase chain reaction (PCR)	Amplifies low levels of specific DNA sequences; each cycle doubles the amount of specific DNA sequence.	Exponential accumulation of DNA fragment being amplified; defects in DNA appear as mutations.	Slightest trace of infection can be detected; more accurate than traditional tests for chlamydia; genetic disorders

table continues on pg. 539 >

TABLE 8.1, continued

Name of Test	Observable Reaction	Visible Change	Tests for
Rate nephelometry	Measures either antigen or antibody in solution through the scattering of a light beam; antibody reagent used to detect antigen IgA, IgG, IgM; concurrent controls are run to establish amount of background scatter in reagents and test samples.	Light scatter proportionately increases as numbered size of immune complexes increases.	Quantitative immunoglobulins IgA, IgM, C-reactive protein, anti-streptolysin O recorded in mg/dL or IU/mL
Flow cytometry	Blood cell types are identified with monoclonal antibodies (mABs) specific for cell markers by means of a flow cytometer with an argon laser beam; as the cells pass the beam, they scatter the light; light energy is converted into electrical energy cells and stained with green (fluorescence) or orange (phycoerythrin).	Light scatter identifies cell size and granularity of lymphocytes, monocytes, and granulocytes; color fluorochromes tagged to monoclonal antibodies bind to specific surface antigens for simultaneous detection of lymphocyte subsets.	Lymphocyte immunophenocytology differentiates B cells from T cells and T-helper cells from T-suppressor cells.
Restriction fragment length polymorphism (RFLP)	DNA-based typing technique	—	Epidemiology of nosocomial and community-acquired infections
Complementary DNA (cDNA) probes	Uses cDNA probes directed against ribosomal RNA	Amplifies nucleic acid to identify presence of bacterial or viral load	Infectious disease such as tuberculosis, hepatitis C virus, and HIV

IgA, immunoglobulin A; IgG, immunoglobulin G; IgM, immunoglobulin M.

Serologic Versus Microbiologic Methods

Serologic testing for microbial immunology evaluates the presence of antibodies produced by antigens of bacteria, viruses, fungi, and parasites. The best means of establishing infectious disease etiology is by isolation and confirmation of the involved pathogen. Serologic methods can assist or confirm microbiologic analysis when the patient is tested late in the disease course, antimicrobial therapy has suppressed organism growth, or culture methods cannot verify a causative agent.

BACTERIAL TESTS

● Syphilis Detection Tests

Syphilis is a venereal disease caused by *Treponema pallidum*, a spirochete with closely wound coils approximately 8 to 15 μm long. Untreated, the disease progresses through three stages that can extend over many years.

Antibodies to syphilis begin to appear in the blood 4 to 6 weeks after infection (Table 8.2). Nontreponemal tests determine the presence of reagin, which is a nontreponemal autoantibody directed against cardiolipin antigens. These tests include the rapid plasma reagin (RPR) and Venereal Disease Research Laboratory (VDRL) tests. The U.S. Centers for Disease Control and Prevention (CDC) recommend these tests for syphilis screening; however, they may show negative results in some cases of late syphilis. Biologic false-positive results can also occur (Table 8.3).

Conversely, treponemal (i.e., specific) tests detect antibodies to *T. pallidum*. These tests include the passive particle agglutination *T. pallidum* test (TP-PA) and the fluorescent treponemal antibody absorption test (FTA-ABS). These tests confirm syphilis when a positive nontreponemal test result is obtained. Because these tests are more complex, they are not used for screening. Certain states require automatic confirmation for all reactive screening tests by using a treponemal test such as the TP-PA or FTA-ABS.

Normal Findings

Nonreactive, negative for syphilis

TABLE 8.2 Sensitivity of Commonly Used Serologic Tests for Syphilis

Test	Stage: Primary (%)	Stage: Secondary (%)	Stage: Late (%)
Nontreponemal (Reagin) Tests			
Venereal Disease Research Laboratory (VDRL) test	70	99	1[a]
Rapid plasma reagin (RPR) card test; automated reagin test (ART)	80	99	0
Specific Treponemal Tests			
Fluorescent treponemal antibody absorption test (FTA-ABS)	85	100	98
Treponema pallidum particle agglutination (TP-PA)	65	100	95
(This new procedure has sensitivity similar to MHA-TP.)			

[a]Treated late syphilis.

Modified from Tramont EC: *Treponema pallidum* (syphilis). In Mandell GL, Douglas RE, Bennett JE (eds): Principles and Practice of Infectious Diseases, 7th ed., Vol. 2, Philadelphia, Elsevier Health Services, 2010. Also product insert Serodia TP-PA, Fujirebio, Inc., Tokyo, Japan, 2000.

TABLE 8.3 Nonsyphilitic Conditions Giving Biologic False-Positive Results Using Venereal Disease Research Laboratory and Rapid Plasma Reagin Tests

Disease	Approximate Percentage BFPs
Malaria	100
Leprosy	60
Relapsing fever	30
Active immunization in children	20
Infectious mononucleosis	20
Lupus erythematosus	20
Lymphogranuloma venereum	20
Pneumonia, atypical	20
Rat-bite fever	20
Typhus fever	20
Vaccinia	20
Infectious hepatitis	10
Leptospirosis (Weil's disease)	10
Periarteritis nodosa	10
Trypanosomiasis	10
Chancroid	5
Chickenpox	5
Measles	5
Rheumatoid arthritis	5–7
Rheumatic fever	5–6
Scarlet fever	5
Subacute bacterial endocarditis	5
Pneumonia, pneumococcal	3–5
Tuberculosis, advanced pulmonary	3–5
Blood loss, repeated	? (low)
Common cold	? (low)
Pregnancy	? (low)

BFPs, biologic false-positive results.

Sensitivity of FTA-ABS

Primary syphilis: 84%
Secondary syphilis: 100%
Latent syphilis: 100%
Late syphilis: 96%

Sensitivity of TP-PA

Primary syphilis: 86%
Secondary syphilis: 100%
Latent syphilis: 100%

NOTE *A reactive RPR or VDRL test should be confirmed with an FTA-ABS or TP-PA.*

Procedure

1. Collect a 7-mL blood serum sample in a red-topped tube. Observe standard precautions. Fasting is usually not required.
2. Label the specimen with the patient's name, date, and tests ordered and place in a biohazard bag for transport to the laboratory.

PROCEDURAL ALERT

If the RPR test is used, the following need to be observed:

1. Excess chyle released into the blood during digestion interferes with test results; therefore, the patient should fast for 8 hr.
2. Alcohol decreases reaction intensity in tests that detect reagin; therefore, alcohol ingestion should be avoided for at least 24 hr before blood is drawn.

Clinical Implications

1. Diagnosis of syphilis requires correlation of patient history, physical findings, and results of syphilis antibody tests. *T. pallidum* is diagnosed when *both* the screening and the confirmatory tests are reactive.
2. Treatment of syphilis may alter both the clinical course and the serologic pattern of the disease. Treatment related to tests that measure *reagin* (RPR and VDRL) includes the following measures:
   a. If the patient is treated at the seronegative primary stage (e.g., after the appearance of the syphilitic chancre but before the appearance of reaction or reagin), the VDRL remains nonreactive.
   b. If the patient is treated in the seropositive primary stage (e.g., after the appearance of a reaction), the VDRL usually becomes nonreactive within 6 months of treatment.
   c. If the patient is treated during the secondary stage, the VDRL usually becomes nonreactive within 12 to 18 months.
   d. If the patient is treated >10 years after the disease onset, the VDRL usually remains unchanged.
3. A negative serologic test may indicate one of the following circumstances:
   a. The patient does not have syphilis.
   b. The infection is too recent for antibodies to be produced. Repeat tests should be performed at 1-week, 1-month, and 3-month intervals to establish the presence or absence of disease.
   c. The syphilis is in a latent or inactive phase.
   d. The patient has a faulty immunodefense mechanism.
   e. Laboratory techniques were faulty.

False-Positive and False-Negative Reactions

A positive reaction is not conclusive for syphilis. Several conditions produce biologic false-positive results for syphilis. Biologic false-positive reactions are by no means "false." They may reveal the presence of other serious diseases. It is theorized that reagin (reaction) is an antibody against tissue lipids. Lipids are presumed to be liberated from body tissue in the normal course of activity. These liberated lipids may then induce antibody formation. Nontreponemal biologic false-positive reactions can occur in the presence of drug abuse, lupus erythematosus, mononucleosis, malaria, leprosy, viral pneumonia, recent immunization, or, on rare occasions, pregnancy. False-negative reactions may occur early in the disease course or during inactive or later stages of disease.

Interfering Factors

1. Hemolysis can cause false-positive results.
2. Hepatitis can result in a false-positive test.
3. Testing too soon after exposure can result in a false-negative test.

Interventions

Pretest Patient Care

1. Explain test purpose and procedure. Assess for interfering factors. Instruct the patient to abstain from alcohol for at least 24 hours before the blood sample is drawn.
2. Follow guidelines in Chapter 1 for safe, effective, informed *pretest* care.

Posttest Patient Care

1. Review test results; report and record findings. Modify the nursing care plan as needed. Counsel the patient regarding abnormal findings. Explain biologic false-positive or false-negative reactions. Explain the need for possible follow-up testing.
2. Follow guidelines in Chapter 1 for safe, effective, informed *posttest* care.

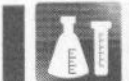

CLINICAL ALERT

1. **Sexual partners of patients with syphilis should be evaluated for the disease.**
2. **After treatment, patients with early-stage syphilis should be tested at 3-mo intervals for 1 yr to monitor for declining reactivity.**

● Lyme Disease Tests

Lyme disease is a multisystem disorder caused by the spirochete *Borrelia burgdorferi*. It is transmitted by the bite of tiny deer ticks, which reside on deer and other wild animals. Lyme disease is present worldwide, but certain geographic areas show higher incidences. Transmission to humans is highest during the spring, summer, and early fall months. The tick bite usually produces a characteristic rash, termed *erythema chronicum migrans*. If untreated, sequelae lead to serious joint, cardiac, and CNS symptoms.

Serologic testing for antibodies to Lyme disease includes enzyme-linked immunosorbent assay (ELISA) and Western blot analysis. Antibody formation takes place in the following manner: Immunoglobulin M (IgM) is detected 3 to 4 weeks after Lyme disease onset, peaks at 6 to 8 weeks after onset, and then gradually disappears. Immunoglobulin G (IgG) is detected 2 to 3 months after infection and may remain elevated for years. Current CDC recommendations for the serologic diagnosis of Lyme disease are to screen with a polyvalent ELISA (IgG and IgM) and to perform supplemental testing (Western blot) on all equivocal and positive ELISA results.

Western blot assays for antibodies to *B. burgdorferi* are supplemental rather than confirmatory because their specificity is less than optimal, particularly for detecting IgM. Two-step positive results provide supportive evidence of exposure to *B. burgdorferi*, which could support a clinical diagnosis of Lyme disease but should not be used as a criterion for diagnosis.

Normal Findings

Negative for both IgG and IgM Lyme antibodies by ELISA and Western blot

Procedure

1. Collect a 7-mL blood serum sample in a red-topped tube. CSF may also be used for the test.
2. Observe standard precautions. Label the specimen with the patient's name, date, and tests ordered and place in a biohazard bag.

Clinical Implications

1. Ten proteins are useful in the serodiagnosis of Lyme disease. Positive blots are:
   a. IgM: two of three of the following bands: 21/25, 39, and 41
   b. IgG: five of the following bands: 18, 21/25, 28, 30, 39, 41, 45, 58, 66, and 93
2. Serologic tests lack the degree of sensitivity, specificity, and standardization necessary for diagnosis in the absence of clinical history. The antigen detection assay for bacterial proteins is of limited value in early stages of disease.
3. In patients presenting with a clinical picture of Lyme disease, negative serologic tests are inconclusive during the first month of infection.

4. Repeat paired testing should be performed if borderline values are reported.
5. The CDC states that the best clinical marker for Lyme disease is the initial skin lesion erythema migrans (EM), which occurs in 60% to 80% of patients.
6. CDC laboratory criteria for the diagnosis of Lyme disease include the following factors:
   a. Isolation of *B. burgdorferi* from a clinical specimen
   b. IgM and IgG antibodies in blood or CSF
   c. Paired acute and convalescent blood samples showing significant antibody response to *B. burgdorferi*

Interfering Factors

1. False-positive results may occur with high levels of rheumatoid factors or in the presence of other spirochete infections, such as syphilis (cross-reactivity).
2. Asymptomatic individuals who spend time in endemic areas may have already produced antibodies to *B. burgdorferi*.

Interventions

Pretest Patient Care

1. Assess patient's clinical history, exposure risk, and knowledge regarding the test. Explain test purpose and procedure as well as possible follow-up testing.
2. Follow guidelines in Chapter 1 for safe, effective, informed *pretest* care.

Posttest Patient Care

1. Review test results; report and record findings. Modify the nursing care plan as needed. Explain the need for possible follow-up treatment and testing to monitor response to antibiotic therapy.
2. Unlike other diseases, people do not develop resistance to Lyme disease after infection and *may continue to be at high risk,* especially if they live, work, or recreate in areas where Lyme disease is present.
3. If Lyme disease has been ruled out, further testing may include *Babesia microti*, a parasite transmitted to humans by a tick bite. Symptoms include loss of appetite, fever, sweats, muscle pain, nausea, vomiting, and headaches.
4. Follow guidelines in Chapter 1 for safe, effective, informed *posttest* care.

● Legionnaires' Disease Antibody Test

Legionnaires' disease is a respiratory condition caused by *Legionella pneumophila*. It is best diagnosed by organism culture; however, the organism is difficult to grow.

Detection of *L. pneumophila* in respiratory specimens by means of direct fluorescent antibody (DFA) technique is useful for rapid diagnosis but lacks sensitivity when only small numbers of organisms are available. Serologic tests should be used only if specimens for culture are not available or if culture and DFA produce negative results.

Normal Findings

Negative for Legionnaires' disease by indirect fluorescent antibody (IFA) test or ELISA

Procedure

1. Collect a 7-mL blood serum sample in a red-topped tube. Observe standard precautions. Label the specimen with the patient's name, date, and tests ordered and place in a biohazard bag for transport to the laboratory.

2. Follow-up testing is usually requested 3 to 6 weeks after initial symptom appearance.
3. Alert the patient that a urine specimen may be required if antigen testing is indicated.

Clinical Implications

1. A dramatic rise of titer levels to more than 1:128 in the interval between acute- and convalescent-phase specimens occurs with recent infections.
2. Serologic tests, to be useful, must be performed on an acute (within 1 week of onset) and convalescent (3 to 6 weeks later) specimen.
3. Serologic testing is valuable because it provides a confirmatory diagnosis of *L. pneumophila* infection when other tests have failed. IFA is the serologic test of choice because it can detect all classes of antibodies.
4. Demonstration of *L. pneumophila* antigen in urine by ELISA is indicative of infection.

Interventions

Pretest Patient Care

1. Assess clinical history and knowledge about the test. Explain purpose and procedure of blood test.
2. Follow guidelines in Chapter 1 for safe, effective, informed *pretest* care.

Posttest Patient Care

1. Review test results; report and record findings. Modify the nursing care plan as needed. Counsel the patient regarding abnormal findings; explain the need for possible follow-up testing, because negative results do not rule out *L. pneumophila*.
2. Follow guidelines in Chapter 1 for safe, effective, informed *posttest* care.

● Chlamydia Nucleic Acid Amplification Test (NAAT)

Chlamydia is caused by a genus of bacteria (*Chlamydia* spp.) that require living cells for growth and are classified as obligate cell parasites. Recognized species include *Chlamydia psittaci*, *Chlamydia pneumoniae*, and *Chlamydia trachomatis*. *C. psittaci* causes psittacosis in birds and humans, and *C. pneumoniae* is responsible for approximately 10% of cases of community-acquired pneumonia. *C. trachomatis* is grouped into three serotypes. One group causes lymphogranuloma venereum (LGV), a venereal disease. Another group causes trachoma, an eye disease. The third group causes genital tract infections different from LGV. Culture of the organism is definitive for chlamydiae. *C. trachomatis* infection is the most common reportable sexually transmitted infection (STI) in the United States, and reporting has been required in all 50 states and the District of Columbia since 2000. The national infection rate for *C. trachomatis* has increased from 2000 to 2015, with the exception of a slight decrease during 2011 to 2013. In 2015, there were 478.8 reported cases per 100,000 people.

Screening for chlamydia is particularly important because it is such a common sexually transmitted disease (STD), which is often asymptomatic, but which can cause serious complications if left untreated. Annual screening for chlamydia is recommended for all sexually active women under the age of 25, for women older than 25 if they have new or multiple sex partners or a sex partner with a diagnosed STD, and for men who have sex with other men. Pregnant women who are at risk should also be screened for chlamydia early in pregnancy.

Although methods such as culture, direct fluorescent antibody stain and DNA probe are available to test for chlamydia, the nucleic acid amplification test (NAAT) (which detects the genetic material of *chlamydia trachomatis*), is recommended because it is more sensitive and specific and can be done without a pelvic exam for women.

Normal Findings

Negative for chlamydia DNA

Procedure

For females:

1. Use a collection swab with a plastic or wire shaft and rayon, dacron or cytobrush tip to swab the vagina.
2. Use a sucrose phosphate glutament buffer or M4 media to store and transport the specimen to the lab at ≤4 °C within 24 hours. If the sample cannot be transported to the lab within 24 hours, store at −70 °C.

For males:

1. Obtain a first morning urine sample.
2. Place specimen in a biohazard bag for transport to the laboratory.

Clinical Implications

1. The NAAT test detects the presence of chlamydia DNA, but does not measure whether antibiotic treatment is effective. In those cases, bacterial culture using antibody testing is needed to determine the correct antibiotic therapy.

Interventions

Pretest Patient Care

1. Assess patient knowledge regarding the test and explain purpose and procedure. Elicit history regarding possible exposure to organism.
2. Follow guidelines in Chapter 1 for safe, effective, informed *pretest* care.

Posttest Patient Care

1. Review test results; report and record findings. Modify the nursing care plan as needed.
2. Follow guidelines in Chapter 1 for safe, effective, informed *posttest* care.

● Streptococcal Antibody Tests: Antistreptolysin O Titer (ASO), Streptozyme, Antideoxyribonuclease-B Titer (Anti-DNase-B, ADNase-B) (ADB, Streptodornase)

Group A β-hemolytic streptococci are associated with streptococcal infections or illness.

These tests detect antibodies to enzymes produced by organisms. Group A β-hemolytic streptococci produce several enzymes, including streptolysin O, hyaluronidase, and DNase B. Serologic tests that detect these enzyme antibodies include antistreptolysin O titer (ASO), which detects streptolysin O; streptozyme, which detects antibodies to multiple enzymes; and anti-DNase B (ADB), which detects DNase B. Serologic detection of streptococcal antibodies helps to establish prior infection but is of no value for diagnosing acute streptococcal infections. Acute infections should be diagnosed by direct streptococcal cultures or the presence of streptococcal antigens.

The ASO test aids in the diagnosis of several conditions associated with streptococcal infections, such as rheumatic fever, glomerulonephritis, endocarditis, and scarlet fever. Serial rising titers over several weeks are more significant than a single result. ADB antibodies may appear earlier than ASO in streptococcal pharyngitis, and this test is more sensitive for streptococcal pyoderma.

Normal Findings

ASO titer:

Adult: <160 Todd units/mL or <200 IU

Child (5 to 12 years of age): 170 to 330 Todd units/mL

ADB: A negative test is normal.

Preschool-age children: <60 Todd units/mL

School-age children: <170 Todd units/mL

Adults: <85 Todd units/mL

Streptozyme: negative for streptococcal antibodies

Procedure

1. Collect a 7-mL blood serum sample in a red-topped tube. Observe standard precautions. Label the specimen with the patient's name, date, and tests ordered and place in a biohazard bag for transport to the laboratory.
2. Repeat testing is recommended 10 days after the first test.

Clinical Implications

1. In general, a titer >160 Todd units/mL is considered a definite elevation for the ASO test.
2. The ASO or the ADB test alone is positive in 80% to 85% of group A streptococcal infections (e.g., streptococcal pharyngitis, rheumatic fever, pyoderma, glomerulonephritis).
3. When ASO and ADB tests are run concurrently, 95% of streptococcal infections can be detected.
4. A repeatedly low titer is good evidence for the absence of active rheumatic fever. Conversely, a high titer does not necessarily mean rheumatic fever of glomerulonephritis is present; however, it does indicate the presence of a streptococcal infection.
5. ASO production is especially high in rheumatic fever and glomerulonephritis. These conditions show marked ASO titer increases during the symptomless period preceding an attack. Also, ADB titers are particularly high in pyoderma.

Interfering Factors

1. An increased titer can occur in healthy carriers.
2. Antibiotic therapy suppresses streptococcal antibody response.
3. Increased B-lipoprotein levels inhibit streptolysin O and produce falsely high ASO titers.

CLINICAL ALERT

The ASO test is impractical in patients who have recently received antibiotics or who are scheduled for antibiotic therapy because the treatment suppresses the antibody response.

Interventions

Pretest Patient Care

1. Assess patient's clinical history and test knowledge. Explain test purpose and procedure.
2. Follow guidelines in Chapter 1 for safe, effective, informed *pretest* care.

Posttest Patient Care

1. Review test results; report and record findings. Modify the nursing care plan as needed. Counsel the patient regarding abnormal findings; explain the need for possible follow-up testing. See Interpreting Results of Immunologic Tests on page 537.
2. Follow guidelines in Chapter 1 for safe, effective, informed *posttest* care.

Helicobacter pylori (HPY) IgG Antibody Serum, Stool, and Breath (PY) Test

Helicobacter pylori (previously known as *Campylobacter pylori*) is a bacterium associated with gastritis, duodenal and gastric ulcers, and possibly gastric carcinoma. The healthcare provider orders this test when screening a patient for possible *H. pylori* infection. The organism is present in 95% to 98% of patients with duodenal ulcers and 60% to 90% of patients with gastric ulcers. A person with gastrointestinal symptoms with evidence of *H. pylori* colonization (e.g., presence of specific antibodies, positive breath test, positive culture, positive biopsy) is considered to be infected with *H. pylori*. A person without gastrointestinal symptoms having evidence of the presence of *H. pylori* is said to be colonized rather than infected.

This test detects *H. pylori* infection of the stomach. Traditionally, the presence of *H. pylori* has been detected through biopsy specimens obtained by endoscopy. As with any invasive procedure, there is risk and discomfort to the patient. Noninvasive methods of detection include the following:

1. Breath: measures isotopically labeled CO_2 in breath specimens
2. Stool: *H. pylori* stool antigen test (HpSa)

The presence of *H. pylori*–specific IgG antibodies has been shown to be an accurate indicator of *H. pylori* colonization. ELISA testing relies on the presence of *H. pylori* IgG-specific antibody to bind to antigen on the solid phase, forming an antigen–antibody complex that undergoes further reactions to produce a color indicative of the presence of antibody and is quantified using a spectrophotometer or ELISA microweld plate reader. The sensitivity is 94% and specificity 78%, compared with an invasive procedure, such as biopsy, for which the sensitivity is 93% and specificity 99%.

Normal Findings

Negative for *H. pylori* by ELISA indicates no detectable IgG antibody in serum or stool.
A positive result indicates the presence of detectable IgG antibody in serum or stool.

Breath

Negative: <50 disintegrations per minute (DPM) for *H. pylori*
50 to 199 DPM indeterminate for *H. pylori*
>200 DPM positive for *H. pylori*

Procedure

1. Collect a 7-mL blood serum sample in a red-topped tube. Observe standard precautions. Label the specimen with the patient's name, date, and test(s) ordered and place in a biohazard bag for transport to the laboratory.
2. Be aware that a random stool specimen may be ordered to test for the presence of *H. pylori* antigen.
3. The breath test is a complex procedure and requires a special kit. Ensure that the collection balloon is fully inflated. Transfer the breath specimen to the laboratory. Keep at room temperature.
4. The ^{13}C-urea breath test (^{13}C-UBT) requires the patient to swallow an isotopically labeled (^{13}C) urea tablet. The urea is subsequently hydrolyzed to ammonia and labeled CO_2 by the presence of *H. pylori* urease activity. After approximately 30 minutes, an exhaled breath sample is collected, and $^{13}CO_2$ levels are assessed using isotope ratio mass spectrometry.

PROCEDURAL ALERT

1. The patient should have no antibiotics and bismuth for 1 mo and no proton pump inhibitors and sucralfate for 2 wk before test.
2. Instruct the patient not to chew the capsule.
3. The patient should be at rest during breath collection.

Clinical Implications

1. This assay is intended for use as an aid in the diagnosis of *H. pylori*, and additionally, false-negative results may occur. The clinical diagnosis should not be based on serology alone but rather on a combination of serology (and breath or stool tests), symptoms, and gastric biopsy–based tests as warranted.
2. The stool antigen test is used to monitor response during therapy and to test for cure after treatment.

Interventions

Pretest Patient Care

1. Explain test purpose, procedure, and knowledge of signs and symptoms and risk factors for transmission: close living quarters, many persons in household, and poor household sanitation and hygiene. The patient swallows a capsule before a breath specimen is obtained. The serum antibody test would be appropriate for a previously untreated patient with a documented history of gastroduodenal ulcer disease and unknown *H. pylori* infection status.
2. Follow guidelines in Chapter 1 for safe, effective, informed *pretest* care.

Posttest Patient Care

1. Review test results; report and record findings. Modify the nursing care plan as needed. Counsel the patient regarding abnormal findings; explain the need for possible follow-up testing and treatment, which may entail 4 to 6 weeks of antibiotics to eradicate *H. pylori* and medication to suppress acid production. Many persons may be infected with *H. pylori* but are asymptomatic.
2. Follow guidelines in Chapter 1 for safe, effective, informed *posttest* care.

VIRAL TESTS

● Epstein-Barr Virus (EBV) Antibody Tests: Infectious Mononucleosis (IM) Slide (Screening) Test, Heterophile Antibody Titer, Epstein-Barr Antibodies to Viral Capsid Antigen and Nuclear Antigen

Epstein-Barr virus (EBV) is a herpesvirus found throughout the world. The most common symptomatic manifestation of EBV infection is a disease known as *infectious mononucleosis* (IM). This disease induces formation of increased numbers of abnormal lymphocytes in the lymph nodes and stimulates increased heterophile antibody formation. IM occurs most often in young adults who have not been previously infected through contact with infectious oropharyngeal secretions. Symptoms include fever, pharyngitis, and lymphadenopathy. EBV is also thought to play a role in the etiology of Burkitt's lymphoma, nasopharyngeal carcinoma, and chronic fatigue syndrome.

The most common test for EBV is the rapid slide test (Monospot) for heterophile antibody agglutination. The heterophile antibody agglutination test is not specific for EBV and therefore is not useful for evaluating chronic disease. If the heterophile test is negative in the presence of acute IM symptoms, specific EBV antibodies should be determined. These include antibodies to viral capsid antigen (anti-VCA) and antibodies to EBV nuclear antigen (EBNA) using IFA and ELISA tests.

Diagnosis of IM is based on the following criteria: clinical features compatible with IM, hematologic picture of relative and absolute lymphocytosis, and presence of heterophile antibodies.

Normal Findings

Negative for IM by latex agglutination (LA)
Negative for EBV antibodies by IFA or ELISA

NOTE *Heterophile antibodies are present within 14 to 21 days in 60% of patients and within 30 days in 85% of patients.*

Procedure

1. Collect a 7-mL blood serum sample in a red-topped tube. Observe standard precautions.
2. Label the specimen with the patient's name, date, and tests ordered and place in a biohazard bag for transport to the laboratory.

Clinical Implications

1. The presence of heterophile antibodies (Monospot), along with clinical signs and other hematologic findings, is diagnostic for IM.
2. Heterophile antibodies remain elevated for 8 to 12 weeks after symptoms appear.
3. Approximately 90% of adults have antibodies to the virus.
4. The Monospot test is negative more frequently in children and almost uniformly in infants with primary EBV infection.

Interventions

Pretest Patient Care

1. Assess patient's clinical history, symptoms, and test knowledge. Explain test purpose and procedure. If preliminary tests are negative, follow-up tests may be necessary.
2. Follow guidelines in Chapter 1 for safe, effective, informed *pretest* care.

Posttest Patient Care

1. Review test results; report and record findings. Modify the nursing care plan as needed.
2. Counsel the patient regarding abnormal findings; explain the need for possible follow-up testing and treatment, such as intravenous fluids. See Interpreting Results of Immunologic Tests on page 537.
3. Tell the patient that, after primary exposure, a person is considered immune. Recurrence of IM is rare.
4. Resolution of IM usually follows a predictable course: Pharyngitis disappears within 14 days after onset; fever subsides within 21 days; and fatigue, lymphadenopathy, and liver and spleen enlargement regress by 21 to 28 days.
5. Follow guidelines in Chapter 1 for safe, effective, informed *posttest* care.

Hepatitis Tests: Hepatitis A (HAV), Hepatitis B (HBV), Hepatitis C (HCV), Hepatitis D (HDV), Hepatitis E (HEV), Hepatitis G (HGV)

Hepatitis can be caused by viruses and several other agents, including drugs and toxins. Approximately 95% of hepatitis cases are due to five major virus types: hepatitis A, B, C, D, and E (Table 8.4). Diagnosing the specific virus is difficult because the symptoms (e.g., chills, weight loss, fever, distaste for cigarettes and food, darker urine and lighter stool) presented by each viral type are similar. Additionally, some individuals may be asymptomatic or have very mild symptoms that are ascribed to the "flu." Serologic tests for hepatitis virus markers have made it easier to define the specific type.

Hepatitis A virus (HAV), which is acquired through enteric transmission, infects the gastrointestinal tract and is eliminated through the feces. Serologically, the presence of the IgM antibody to HAV (IgM anti-HAV) and the total antibody to HAV (total anti-HAV) identifies the disease and determines previous exposure to or recovery from HAV.

Hepatitis B virus (HBV) demonstrates a central core containing the core antigen and a surrounding envelope containing the surface antigen: <0.01 pg/mL for viral load. Detection of hepatitis B core antigen (HBcAg), envelope antigen (HBeAg), and surface antigen (HBsAg) or their corresponding antibodies constitutes hepatitis B serologic or plasma assessment. Viral transmission occurs through exposure to contaminated blood or blood products through an open wound (e.g., needlesticks, lacerations). Hepatitis monitoring panel for serial testing includes four B markers: HBsAg, HBeAg, anti-HBe, and anti-HBs. Interpretation depends on clinical setting. Hepatitis B DNA ultrasensitive quantitative PCR is the most sensitive test available for hepatitis B viral load.

TABLE 8.4 Hepatitis Test Findings in Various Stages

Disease	Viral Specific and Serologic Tests				
Stages	HAV	HBV	HCV	HDV	HEV
Acute	IgM anti-HAV	IgM anti-HBc, HBsAg	Anti-HCV	HDAg	IgM anti-HEV
Chronic	Fecal HAV 1–2 wk before symptoms	2%–10% of all persons >5 yr will progress to chronic infection	85% Anti-HCV	6% total anti-HDV	None
Infectivity	None	HBeAg, HBsAg, HBV-DNA	Anti-HCV	Total anti-HDV	None
Recovery	None	Anti-HBe, anti-HBs	None	None	None
Viral load (viral genome)		HBV DNA	HCV RNA		
Carrier state	None	HBsAg	None	HBAg, anti-HDV	None
Immunity	Total anti-HAV	Anti-HBs, total anti-HBc	None	None	Uncertain
Acute viral panel	IgM anti-HAV	HBsAg	Anti-HCV, HIV test also		

HAV, hepatitis A; anti-HBc, antibody to hepatitis B core antigen; HBeAg, hepatitis B envelope antigen; HBsAg, hepatitis B surface antigen; HBV, hepatitis B; HCV, hepatitis C; HDV, hepatitis D; HEV, hepatitis E; IgM, immunoglobulin M.

Hepatitis C virus (HCV), formerly known as non-A, non-B hepatitis, is also transmitted parenterally. HCV infection is characterized by presence of antibodies to HCV (anti-HCV) and levels of alanine aminotransferase (ALT) that fluctuate between normal and markedly elevated. Levels of anti-HCV remain positive for many years; therefore, a reactive test indicates infection with HCV or a carrier state but not infectivity or immunity. PCR or reverse transcriptase PCR (RT-PCR) (viral load), which detects HCV RNA, should be used to confirm infection when acute hepatitis C is suspected. A negative hepatitis C antibody (recombinant immunoblot assay [RIBA]) does not exclude the possibility of HCV infection because seroconversion may not occur for up to 6 months after exposure.

Hepatitis D virus (HDV) is encapsulated by the HBsAg. Without the HBsAg coating, HDV cannot survive. Because HDV can cause infection only in the presence of active HBV infection, it is usually found where a high incidence of HBV occurs. Transmission is parenteral. Serologic HDV determination is made by detection of the hepatitis D antigen (HDAg) early in the course of the infection and by detection of anti-HDV antibody (anti-HDV) in the later stages of the disease.

Hepatitis E virus (HEV) is transmitted enterically and is associated with poor hygienic practices and unsafe water supplies, especially in developing countries. It is quite rare in the United States. Specific serologic tests include detection of IgM and IgG antibodies to HEV (anti-HEV).

Hepatitis G virus (HGV) is transmitted by contaminated blood supply and is seen when HCV and HBV are detected together. See Table 8.5 for a summary of the features of the different hepatitis agents.

The following terms are used:

ALT (alanine aminotransferase): an enzyme normally produced by the liver; blood levels may increase in cases of liver damage

Anti-HBc: antibody to hepatitis B core antigen

Anti-HBe: antibody to hepatitis B envelope antigen

Anti-HBs: antibody to hepatitis B surface antigen

Antibody: a Y-shaped protein molecule (immunoglobulin) in serum or body fluid that either neutralizes an antigen or tags it for attack by other cells or chemicals; acts by uniting with and firmly binding to an antigen. The prefix *anti-* followed by initials of a virus refers to specific antibody against the virus.

Chronic hepatitis: a condition in which symptoms or signs of hepatitis persist for >6 months

Cirrhosis: irreversible scarring of the liver that may occur after acute or chronic hepatitis

Delta agent: a unique RNA virus that causes acute or chronic hepatitis; requires HBV for replication and infects only patients who are HBsAg-positive; is composed of a delta antigen core and an HBsAg coat; also known as HDV

Endemic: present in a community at all times but occurring in a small number of cases

Enteric route: spread of organisms through the oral-intestinal-fecal cycle

Flavivirus: a family of small RNA viruses; HCV is similar to members of the Flavivirus family

Fulminant hepatitis: the most severe form of hepatitis; may lead to acute liver failure and death

HBcAg: hepatitis B core antigen

HBsAg: hepatitis B surface antigen

Hepatotropic: having an affinity for or exerting a specific effect on the liver

IgG: a form of immunoglobulin that occurs late in an infectious process

IgM: a form of immunoglobulin that occurs early in an infectious process

IgM anti-HAV: M-class immunoglobulin antibody to HAV

IgM anti-HBc: M-class immunoglobulin antibody to HBcAg

Immune globulin: a sterile solution of water-soluble proteins that contains those antibodies normally present in adult human blood; used as a passive immunizing agent against various viruses such as HAV

TABLE 8.5 Summary of Clinical and Epidemiologic Features of Viral Hepatitis Agents

Features	Hepatitis A	Hepatitis B (HBV)	Hepatitis C (HCV)	Hepatitis D	Hepatitis E	Hepatitis G Scan with HBV + HCV
Incubation period	45–50 d	30–150 d	15–110 d	30–150 d	230–240 d	Questionable
Onset	Abrupt	Insidious	Insidious	Abrupt	Insidious	Unknown
Jaundice	Children: 10%; adults: 70%–80%	25%	25%	Varies	Unknown	No
Asymptomatic patients	Most children	Most children; adults: 50%	About 75%	Rare	Rare	Contaminated blood
Routes of transmission						
Fecal-oral	Yes	No	No	No	Yes	No
Parenteral	Rare	Yes	Yes	Yes	No	Blood supply
Sexual	No	Yes	Possible	Yes	No	No
Perinatal	No	Yes	Possible	Possible	No	No
Water/food	Yes	No	No	No	Yes	Yes
Chronic state	No	Adults: 6%–10%; children: 25%–50%; infants: 70%–90%	50%	10%–15%	No	Yes
Case fatality rate	0.6%	1.4% Liver cancer	1%–2% Liver cancer with HBV and HCV	30%	1%–2% Pregnant women: 20%	Unknown

Negative-sense RNA virus: a virus in which the viral proteins are encoded by messenger RNA molecules that are complementary to the viral genome

New viruses—GBV-A, GBV-B, and GBV-C: may be causative agents in non-A through E hepatitis

Non-A, non-B hepatitis: viral hepatitis caused by viruses other than A, B, or D (e.g., C, E)

Parenteral: entering the body subcutaneously, intramuscularly, or intravenously or other means whereby the organisms reach the bloodstream directly

Positive-sense RNA virus: a virus in which the parenteral (or genomic) RNA serves as the messenger RNA for protein synthesis

Recombinant antigen: an antigen that results from the recombination of genetic components, which then are artificially introduced into a cell, leading to synthesis of a new protein

Viral load: the amount or concentration of virus in the circulation

These measurements are used for differential diagnosis of viral hepatitis, viral load. Serodiagnosis of previous exposure and recovery of viral hepatitis is complex because of the number of serum or plasma markers necessary to determine the stage of illness. Testing methods include ELISA, microparticle enzyme immunoassay (MEIA), PCR, and RT-PCR and tests for viral genome (viral load).

Indications for Hepatitis A Vaccine

Pre-exposure Protection

1. Children should be vaccinated between 12 and 23 months of age.
2. Communities with existing vaccination programs for children 2 to 18 years of age should maintain their programs.
3. In areas without vaccination programs, catch-up vaccination of unvaccinated children 2 to 18 years of age can be considered.

Individuals at Increased Risk

1. Persons traveling to or working in countries that have high or intermediate endemicity
2. Users of injection and noninjection illicit drugs
3. Persons with clotting-factor disorders who have received solvent-detergent, treated high-purity factor VIII concentrates
4. Homosexual men
5. Individuals working with nonhuman HAV-infected primates
6. Food handlers
7. Persons employed in child care centers
8. Healthcare workers
9. Susceptible individuals with chronic liver disease

Indications for Hepatitis B Vaccine

1. Family members of adoptees from foreign countries who are HBsAg-positive
2. Healthcare workers and trainees in healthcare fields
3. Hemodialysis patients or patients with early renal failure
4. Household or sexual contacts of persons chronically infected with hepatitis B
5. Immigrants from Africa or Southeast Asia; recommended for children <11 years old and all susceptible household contacts of persons chronically infected with hepatitis B
6. Injection drug users
7. Inmates of long-term correctional facilities
8. Clients and staff of institutions for the developmentally disabled
9. International travelers to countries of high or intermediate HBV endemicity
10. Laboratory workers

11. Public safety workers (e.g., police, fire fighters)
12. Recipients of clotting factors. Use a fine needle (<23 gauge) and firm pressure at injection site for >2 minutes.
13. Persons with STIs or multiple sexual partners in previous 6 months, prostitutes, homosexual and bisexual men
14. Postvaccination blood testing is recommended for sexual contacts of HBsAg-positive persons; healthcare workers, recipients of clotting factors, and those who are HBsAg-positive are at high risk.
15. Persons in nonresidential day care programs should be vaccinated if an HBsAg-positive classmate behaves aggressively or has special medical problems that increase the risk for exposure to blood. Staff in nonresidential day care programs should be vaccinated if a client is HBsAg-positive.
    a. Observe enteric and standard precautions for 7 days after onset of symptoms or jaundice with hepatitis B. Hepatitis A is most contagious before symptoms or jaundice appears.
    b. Use standard blood and body fluid precautions for type B hepatitis and B antigen carriers. Precautions apply until the patient is HBsAg-negative and the anti-HBs appears. Avoid "sharps" (e.g., needles, scalpel blades) injuries. Should accidental injury occur, encourage some bleeding and wash area well with a germicidal soap. Report injury to proper department, and follow up with necessary interventions. Put on gown when blood splattering is anticipated. A private hospital room and bathroom may be indicated.
16. Persons with a history of receiving blood transfusion should not donate blood for 6 months. Transfusion-acquired hepatitis may not show up for 6 months after transfusion. Persons who test positive for HBsAg should *never* donate blood or plasma.
17. Persons who have sexual contact with hepatitis B–infected individuals run a greater risk for acquiring that same infection. HBsAg appears in most body fluids, including saliva, semen, and cervical secretions.
18. Observe standard precautions in all cases of suspected hepatitis until the diagnosis and hepatitis type are confirmed.

Normal Findings

1. Negative (nonreactive) for hepatitis A, B, C, D, or E by ELISA, MEIA, PCR, RIBA, or RT-PCR
2. Negative or undetected viral load (not used for primary infection, only to monitor). PCR requires a separate specimen collection.
3. Hepatitis B viral DNA (HBV-DNA) negative or nonreactive viral load (<0.01 pg/mL) in an infected individual before treatment

Procedure

1. Collect a 7-mL blood serum sample in a red-topped tube or two lavender-topped ethylenediaminetetraacetic acid (EDTA) tubes, 5 mL each, for plasma. Observe standard precautions. Centrifuge promptly and aseptically. Label the specimen with the patient's name, date, and test(s) ordered and place in a biohazard bag for transport to the laboratory. Send specimens frozen on dry ice. Check with your laboratory for protocols and whether plasma or serum is needed.
2. Some specimens need to be split into two plastic vials before freezing and sent frozen on dry ice. Check with your laboratory.

Clinical Implications

1. Individuals with hepatitis may have generalized symptoms resembling the flu and may dismiss their illness as such.

TABLE 8.6 Differential Diagnosis of Viral Hepatitis

Virus	Transmission	Incubation Period	Test for Acute Infection	Social and Clinical History
Hepatitis A	Fecal-oral by person-to-person contact or ingestion of contaminated food	Average, 30 d (range, 15–50 d)	IgM antibody to hepatitis A capsid proteins	Household or sexual contact with an infected person, day care centers, and common source outbreaks from contaminated food
Hepatitis B	Sexual, blood, and other body fluids	Average, 120 d (range, 45–160 d)	HBsAg; the best test for acute or recent infection is IgM antibody to HBcAg	Multiple sexual partners, male-to-male-to-female sexual practices, injection drug use, birth to an infected mother
Hepatitis C	Blood	Commonly 6–9 wk (range, 2 wk–6 mo)	ELISA is the initial test to show if ever infected; it should be confirmed by another test such as PCR	Injection drug use, occupational exposure to blood, hemodialysis, transfusion, possibly sexual transmission
Hepatitis D	Sexual, blood, and other body fluids	2–8 wk (from animal studies)	Total antibody to delta hepatitis shows if ever infected; IgM test is in research laboratories; ELISA	Requires active infection with HBV; injection drug users and persons receiving clotting factor concentrates are at highest risk for infection
Hepatitis E	Fecal-oral	Average, 26–42 d (range, 15–64 d)	Research laboratories	No known cases originated in the United States; international travelers are the only high-risk group to date
Hepatitis G	Blood	Unknown	Occurs with hepatitis B and hepatitis C	Recipient of contaminated blood

ELISA, enzyme-linked immunosorbent assay; HBcAg, hepatitis B core antigen; HBsAg, hepatitis B surface antigen; HBV, hepatitis B; IgM, immunoglobulin M; PCR, polymerase chain reaction.

TABLE 8.7 Viruses for Which Clinical Signs and Symptoms Mimic Hepatitis

Virus	Transmission	Incubation Period	Test for Acute Infection	Social and Clinical History
Epstein-Barr virus (EBV)	Oropharyngeal (saliva)	4–6 wk	IgM antibody to EBV viral capsid	Seroconversion by age 5 yr in 50% of persons in the United States; children with an acutely infected sibling are at greater risk
Cytomegalovirus (CMV, human herpesvirus 5)	Intimate contact with infected fluids; sexual, perinatal, blood transfusion, and infected breast milk	About 3–8 wk for transfusion-acquired CMV	Culture, monoclonal antibody to early antigen	Household sexual contact with an infected person, male-to-male sexual practices, day care centers, perinatal transmission

2. A specific type of hepatitis cannot be differentiated by clinical observations alone. Testing is the only sure method to define the category (see Tables 8.6 and 8.7).
3. Rapid diagnosis of acute hepatitis is essential for the patient so that treatment can be instituted and for those who have close patient contact so that protective measures can be taken to prevent disease spread.
4. Persons at higher risk for acquiring hepatitis A include patients and staff in healthcare and custodial institutions, people in day care centers, intravenous drug abusers, and those who travel to undeveloped countries or regions where food and water supplies may be contaminated.
5. Persons at higher risk for hepatitis B include those with a history of drug abuse, those who have sexual contact with infected persons, those who have household contact with infected persons, and especially those with skin and mucosal surface lesions (e.g., impetigo, saliva from chronic HBV-infected persons on toothbrush racks and coffee cups in their homes); in addition, infants born to infected mothers (during delivery), hemodialysis patients, and healthcare employees are at higher risk for infection. Of all persons with HBV infection, 38% to 40% contract HBV during early childhood.
6. Healthcare workers should be periodically tested for hepatitis exposure and should always observe standard precautions when caring for patients.
7. Persons at risk for hepatitis C include those who have received blood transfusions, engage in intravenous drug abuse, undergo hemodialysis, have had organ transplantation, or have sexual contact with an infected person; hepatitis C can also be transmitted during delivery from mother to neonate. Most people are asymptomatic at the time of diagnosis for hepatitis C. See Table 8.8 for hepatitis markers that appear after infection.
8. Both total (IgG + IgM) and IgM anti-HBc are positive in acute infection, whereas typically only total anti-HBc is present in chronic infection.

TABLE 8.8 Markers That Appear After Infection

Serologic Marker	Time Marker Appears After Infection	Clinical Implications
Hepatitis A Virus (HAV)		
HAV-Ab/IgM	4–6 wk	Positive for acute stage of hepatitis A, develops early in disease course
HAV-Ab/IgG	8–12 wk	Indicates previous exposure and immunity to hepatitis A
Hepatitis B Virus (HBV)		
HBsAg-HBV	12 wk	Positive in acute stage of hepatitis B; earliest indicator of acute antigen infection; also indicates chronic infection
HBeAg	4–12 wk	Positive in acute active stage with viral replication (infectivity factor); highly infective
HBcAb	6–14 wk	This marker may remain in serum for a longer time; together with HBsAb represents convalescent stage; indicates past infection
HBcAb IgM	6–14 wk	Indicates acute infection
HBeAb antibody	8–16 wk	Indicates acute infection resolution
HBsAb antibody	4–10 mo	Indicates previous exposure, clinical recovery, immunity to hepatitis B, not necessarily to other types of hepatitis; marker for permanent immunity to hepatitis B

Ab, antibody; HBcAb, antibody to hepatitis B core antigen; HBeAb, hepatitis B virus e antibody; HBeAg, hepatitis B envelope antigen; HBsAb, hepatitis B surface antibody; HBsAg, hepatitis B surface antigen; IgG, immunoglobulin G; IgM, immunoglobulin M.

Interventions

Pretest Patient Care

1. Assess patient's social and clinical history and knowledge of test. Explain test purpose and procedure.
2. Follow guidelines in Chapter 1 for safe, effective, informed *pretest* care.

Posttest Patient Care

1. Review test results; report and record findings. Modify the nursing care plan as needed. Explain significance of test results and counsel appropriately regarding presence of infection, recovery, and immunity.
2. Counsel healthcare workers and family regarding protective and preventive measures necessary to avoid transmission.
3. Instruct patients to alert healthcare workers and others regarding their hepatitis history in situations in which exposure to body fluids and wastes may occur.
4. Pregnant women may need special counseling.
5. Follow guidelines in Chapter 1 for safe, effective, informed *posttest* care.

CLINICAL ALERT

1. Observe enteric and standard precautions for 7 d after onset of symptoms or jaundice in hepatitis A. Hepatitis A is most contagious before symptoms or jaundice appears.
2. Use standard blood and body fluid precautions with hepatitis B and hepatitis B antigen carriers. Precautions apply until the patient is HBsAg-negative and anti-HBs appears. Avoid "sharps" (e.g., needles, scalpel blades) injuries. Should accidental injury occur, encourage some bleeding, and wash area well with a germicidal soap. Report injury to proper department and follow up with necessary interventions. Put on gown when blood splattering is anticipated. A private hospital room and bathroom may be indicated.
3. If patient has had a blood transfusion, he or she should not donate blood for 6 mo. Transfusion-acquired hepatitis may not show up for 6 mo after transfusion. Persons who test positive for HBsAg should *never* donate blood or plasma.
4. Persons who have sexual contact with hepatitis B–infected individuals run a greater risk for acquiring the infection. HBsAg appears in most body fluids, including saliva, semen, and cervical secretions.
5. Standard precautions must be observed in all cases of suspected hepatitis until the diagnosis and hepatitis type are confirmed.
6. Immunization of persons exposed to the infection should be done as soon as possible. In the case of contact with hepatitis B, both hepatitis B immunoglobulin (HBIG) and HBV vaccine should be administered within 24 hr of skin-break contact and within 14 d of last sexual contact. For hepatitis A, immune globulin (IG) should be given within 2 wk of exposure. In day care centers, IG should be given to all contacts (children and personnel).

● HIV-1/2 Tests

Infection with HIV-1 is most prevalent in the United States and Western Europe. HIV-1 p24 antigen is a viral protein that is present in high amounts in individuals who are newly infected. A combination immunoassay is used to detect HIV-1 and HIV-2 antibodies, as well as HIV-1 p24 antigen (referred to as 4th generation testing). If a specimen is reactive on the initial immunoassay, then additional testing will take place to differentiate between HIV-1 and HIV-2 antibodies. If the results of the additional testing are either nonreactive or indeterminate, then HIV-1 nucleic acid testing (NAT) will be done. This test process provides the foundation for identifying acute and established HIV-1 infections, providing more accurate diagnosis of HIV-2 infection and timely reporting of test results to public health entities. After identification and differentiation of HIV-1 and HIV-2 antibodies, additional tests such as HIV-1 viral load, CD4+T-lymphocyte, and antiretroviral resistance assay are necessary to confirm infection, determine the stage of HIV disease and tailor treatment (Table 8.9). Most cases associated with HIV-2 are reported in West Africa.

Normal Findings

Negative for HIV antibodies and antigens

Procedure

Serum Testing

1. Use a special testing kit such as the FDA-approved commercial Alere Determine HIV-1/2 Ag/Ab Combo. The kit includes a specially treated sample pad, to which a whole blood (from

TABLE 8.9 Diagnostic Testing for HIV

Whom to Test	How to Test	When to Test
Adolescents and adults ages 15–65 yr. Younger adolescents and older adults who are at increased risk (males who have sex with males, IV drug users, recreational drug users, those engaging in unprotected sex, those with signs and symptoms of unusual pneumonia, skin lesions, mononucleosis-like syndrome; persons known to be infected with HIV); all pregnant women, including pregnant women in labor who have not been tested and whose HIV status is unknown.	Screening EIA and confirmatory tests. Combination immunoassay to detect HIV-1/2 antibodies and HIV-1 p24 antigen. Viral RNA and p24 antigen are used along with CD4 count to monitor treatment. Nucleic acid amplification testing (NAT) to monitor "viral load." Rapid testing: single-use diagnostic system (SUDS) results in 1 hr.	Detection should occur as early as possible so that proper treatment, decrease in transmission, and modified behaviors can occur. Mother-to-child (vertical transmission) treated during pregnancy and delivery, and exposed infants within 48 hr of delivery; transmission of HIV can occur in utero, during birth, and by breast-feeding.

EIA, enzyme immunoassay; gp, glycoprotein; IFA, indirect fluorescent antibody; IV, intravenous.

venipuncture or fingerstick), serum or plasma specimen is applied. A Chase Buffer is applied to whole blood samples, and the test results are read between 20 and 30 minutes after application of the Chase Buffer.

2. Interpret the results according to the manufacturer's guidelines and instructions.

Clinical Implications

1. An antibody reactive test is associated with the detection of HIV-1 and/or HIV-2 antibodies in the specimen, and an antigen reactive test is associated with the detection of HIV-1 p24 antigen in the specimen.
2. The presence of HIV-1/2 antibodies or HIV-1 p24 antigen is presumptive for HIV infection.
3. A nonreactive test result does not preclude the possibility of an HIV exposure or infection.
4. Reactive test results should be followed by further confirmatory testing.
5. An HIV infection is described as a continuum of stages that range from the acute, transient, mononucleosis-like syndrome associated with seroconversion to asymptomatic HIV infection to symptomatic HIV infection and, finally, to AIDS. AIDS is end-stage HIV infection.
6. Treatments are more effective and less toxic when begun early in the course of HIV infection.

Interfering Factors

1. Test kits require the use of specific specimens. Refer to test kit instructions to verify that the proper specimen type is being used; otherwise, the kit may produce inaccurate results. Timing of appearance of viral and serologic markers varies (see Fig. 8.1)

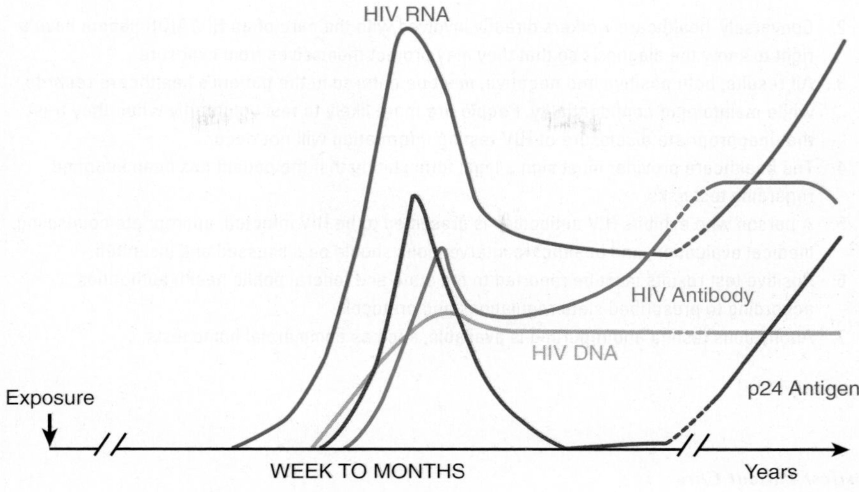

FIGURE 8.1. Time course for appearance of viral and serologic markers during primary HIV infection. (Modified from Busch MP, Satten GA: Time course of viremia and antibody seroconversion following human immunodeficiency virus exposure. Am J Med 102(5B):117–124, 1997. Reproduced with permission of EXCERPTA MEDICA, INC. via Copyright Clearance Center.)

Interventions

Pretest Patient Care

1. An informed, witnessed consent form must be properly signed by any person being tested for HIV/AIDS. This consent form must accompany the patient and the specimen (see Appendix F for sample form).
2. It is essential that counseling precedes and follows the HIV test. This test should not be performed without the subject's informed consent, and persons who need to access results legitimately must be mentioned. Discussion of the clinical and behavioral implications derived from the test results should address the accuracy of the test and should encourage behavioral modifications (e.g., sexual contact, shared needles, blood transfusions).
3. Assess frequency and intensity of symptoms: elevated temperature, anxiety, fear, diarrhea, neuropathy, nausea and vomiting, depression, and fatigue.
4. Infection control measures mandate use of standard precautions (see Appendix A).
5. Follow guidelines in Chapter 1 for safe, effective, informed *pretest* care.

CLINICAL ALERT

1. Issues of confidentiality surround HIV testing. Access to test results should be given judiciously on a need-to-know basis unless the patient specifically expresses otherwise. Interventions to block general computer access to this information are necessary; each healthcare facility must determine how best to accomplish this.

2. Conversely, healthcare workers directly involved with the care of an HIV/AIDS patient have a right to know the diagnosis so that they may protect themselves from exposure.
3. All results, both positive and negative, must be entered in the patient's healthcare records while maintaining confidentiality. People are more likely to test voluntarily when they trust that inappropriate disclosure of HIV testing information will not occur.
4. The healthcare provider must sign a legal form stating that the patient has been informed regarding test risks.
5. A person who exhibits HIV antibodies is presumed to be HIV infected; appropriate counseling, medical evaluation, and healthcare interventions should be discussed and instituted.
6. Positive test results must be reported to the state and federal public health authorities according to prescribed state regulations and protocols.
7. Anonymous testing and reporting is available, such as commercial home tests.

Posttest Patient Care

1. Review test results; report and record findings. Modify the nursing care plan as needed. Counsel the patient regarding abnormal findings; explain the need for possible follow-up testing and treatment. Explain significance of test results along with $CD4^+$ cell counts. Provide options for immediate counseling if necessary. Explain treatment with potent antiviral drugs and protease inhibitors. The International AIDS Society–USA has recommended starting treatment with antiretroviral drugs if the CD4 cell count is $<350/\mu L$ but before it reaches $200/\mu L$.
2. Follow guidelines in Chapter 1 for safe, effective, informed *posttest* care.

VIRAL ANTIBODY TESTS TO ASSESS IMMUNE STATUS

● Rubella Antibody Tests

Rubella, a mild, contagious illness characterized by an erythematous maculopapular rash, is observed primarily in children 5 to 14 years of age and in young adults. The disease, commonly called German or 3-day measles, may be asymptomatic or may involve a 1- to 5-day prodromal period of malaise, headache, cold symptoms, low-grade fever, and suboccipital lymphadenopathy.

Although the illness is mild in children, it may cause the congenital rubella syndrome in the fetus of a mother infected early in pregnancy. As many as 85% of infants infected during the first 8 weeks of gestation have detectable defects by 4 years of age. The classic abnormalities associated with the rubella syndrome include congenital heart disease, cataracts, and neurosensory deafness. After 20 to 24 weeks of gestation, congenital abnormalities are rare.

The quantitative measurement of IgG antibodies to rubella virus aids in the determination of immune status. Assay results of 10 IU/mL of antibody are negative or not immune. Assay results >10 IU/mL are considered positive or immune. A positive result of IgM antibody indicates a congenital or recent infection. The measurement of IgM class antibodies for determination of acute-phase infection is recommended in all age groups. IgM rubella antibody determination is usually not recommended when the patient is >6 months of age. Unlike IgG class antibodies, IgM antibodies are larger molecules and cannot cross the placenta, thus determining that the infant has an active form of the disease.

Normal Findings

Negative for rubella IgG antibodies by ELISA or chemiluminescence (<7 IU/mL: no immunity)
Negative for IgM antibodies by ELISA or chemiluminescence (<0.9 IU/mL: no infection)
Positive for rubella IgG antibodies by ELISA or chemiluminescence (>10 IU/mL; immunity, indicates a current or previous exposure or immunization to rubella)
Positive for rubella IgM antibodies (with or without positive IgG) by ELISA or chemiluminescence (>1.1 IU/mL; indicates a current or recent infection with rubella virus)

Procedure

1. Collect a 7-mL blood serum sample in a red-topped tube. Observe standard precautions. Label the specimen with the patient's name, date, and test(s) ordered and place in a biohazard bag for transport to the laboratory.
2. Follow-up testing may be required.

Clinical Implications

1. When testing for IgG antibody, seroconversion between acute and convalescent sera is considered strong evidence of a current or recent infection. The recommended interval between an acute and convalescent sample is 10 to 14 days.
2. A serum specimen taken very early during the acute stage of infection may contain levels of IgG antibody below 10 IU/mL.
3. Although the presence of IgM antibody suggests current or recent infection, low levels of IgM may occasionally persist for more than 12 months after infection or immunization. Passively acquired rubella antibody levels (IgG) in the infant (which can cross the placenta because of their smaller molecular size) decrease markedly within 2 to 3 months after infection.
4. IgM is detectable soon after clinical symptoms occur and reaches peak levels at 10 days.

Interventions

Pretest Patient Care

1. Assess patient's test knowledge. Explain test purpose and procedure. Advise pregnant women that rubella infection acquired in the first trimester of pregnancy is associated with an increased incidence of miscarriage, stillbirth, and congenital abnormalities.
2. Follow guidelines in Chapter 1 for safe, effective, informed *pretest* care.

Posttest Patient Care

1. Review test results; report and record findings. Modify the nursing care plan as needed. Counsel the patient regarding abnormal findings; explain the need for possible follow-up testing and treatment. Advise women of childbearing age who test negative to be immunized before becoming pregnant. Immunization is contraindicated during pregnancy. Patients who test positive are naturally immune to further rubella infections.
2. Follow guidelines in Chapter 1 for safe, effective, informed *posttest* care.

● Measles (Rubeola) Antibody Tests

Classified as a paramyxovirus, measles produces a highly contagious respiratory infection. The disease is spread during the prodrome phase through direct contact with respiratory secretions in the form of droplets. Clinical infection with measles virus is characterized by high fever, cough, coryza, conjunctivitis, malaise, and Koplik's spots on the buccal mucosa. An erythematous rash then develops behind the ears and over the forehead, spreading to the trunk.

Serology has become increasingly important as a tool for determining the immune status of the young adult population entering college or the military. In addition, the linkage between measles infection and premature delivery or spontaneous abortion supports screening pregnant mothers for susceptibility.

These tests determine susceptibility and immunity to measles virus. Since intensive immunization began in the United States in the 1970s, the incidence of measles infection has been reduced from approximately one half million cases annually (1960s) to fewer than 500 cases in recent years. Many individuals, however, may remain susceptible to measles virus because of vaccine failure or nonimmunization. A positive IgG coupled with a negative IgM result indicates previous exposure to measles virus and immunity to this viral infection. Positive IgM results, with or without positive IgG results, indicate a recent infection with measles virus.

Normal Findings

Negative for measles IgG or IgM antibodies by ELISA: nonimmune
Positive for measles IgG antibody: immune; indicates a current or previous exposure or immunization to measles
Positive for measles IgM antibody (with or without positive IgG): indicates a recent infection with measles virus

Procedure

1. Collect a 7-mL blood serum sample in a red-topped tube. Observe standard precautions. Label the specimen with the patient's name, date, and test(s) ordered and place in a biohazard bag for transport to the laboratory.
2. Follow-up testing may be required.

Clinical Implications

1. When testing for IgG antibody, seroconversion between acute and convalescent sera is considered strong evidence of a current or recent infection. The recommended interval between an acute and convalescent sample is 10 to 14 days.
2. Although the presence of IgM antibody suggests current or recent infection, low levels of IgM may occasionally persist for more than 12 months after infection or immunization.
3. IgM antibody response is detectable 2 to 3 weeks after appearance of the rash.

Interventions

Pretest Patient Care

1. Assess patient's test knowledge. Explain test purpose and procedure. Advise pregnant women that measles poses a high risk for serious complications and may be linked to premature delivery or spontaneous abortion.
2. Follow guidelines in Chapter 1 for safe, effective, informed *pretest* care.

Posttest Patient Care

1. Review test results; report and record findings. Modify the nursing care plan as needed. Counsel the patient regarding abnormal results; explain the need for possible follow-up testing and treatment. Advise women of childbearing age who test negative to be immunized before becoming pregnant. Inform patients who test positive that they are naturally immune to further measles infection.
2. Follow guidelines in Chapter 1 for safe, effective, informed *posttest* care.

● Mumps Antibody Tests

The mumps virus (single-stranded RNA) is a member of the paramyxovirus group (genus *Rubulavirus*) and the etiologic agent of mumps in humans. Mumps is a generalized illness, usually accompanied by parotid (salivary gland) swelling and mild symptoms lasting 2 or more days. Parotitis as a presenting symptom in mumps is usually sufficient to preclude confirmation by serology. However, one third of mumps infections are subclinical and may require viral isolation to confirm mumps infection. Infection with mumps virus, whether symptomatic or subclinical, is generally thought to offer lifelong immunity.

ELISA testing can be both specific and sensitive for the detection and measurement of serum proteins. Current methods for serodiagnosis of mumps include in vitro serum neutralization, hemagglutination inhibition (HAI), IFA, and CF. These test methods, however, lack specificity, which limits their usefulness in establishing immune status.

Normal Findings

Negative for mumps IgG or IgM antibodies by ELISA: nonimmune
Negative for viral antigen by RT-PCR
Positive for mumps IgG antibody: immune; indicates a current or previous exposure or immunization to mumps virus
Positive for mumps IgM antibody: indicates a current or recent infection

NOTE *Serum IgM may be negative in 50% to 60% of vaccinated patients; therefore, a negative IgM cannot rule out mumps in this group.*

Procedure

1. Collect a 7-mL blood serum sample in a red-topped tube. The optimal time to collect serum in unvaccinated persons is 3 to 5 days after they become symptomatic. This is necessary because, in unvaccinated patients, IgM may not be present until 5 days after onset of symptoms, typically peaks in 7 days, and may be present for up to 6 weeks or more. Observe standard precautions. Label the specimen with the patient's name, date, and tests ordered and place in a biohazard bag for transport to the laboratory.
2. The CDC recommends that a blood specimen, buccal/oral swab, and urine be collected from individuals with clinical suspicion of mumps. Buccal/oral and urine specimens should be collected 3 to 5 days after the onset of symptoms. To collect the buccal/oral specimen, massage the parotid gland for 30 seconds and then swab the area between the cheek and gum by sweeping the swab near the upper to lower molar area.
3. Follow-up testing may be required.

Clinical Implications

1. When testing for IgG antibody, seroconversion between acute and convalescent sera is considered strong evidence of a current or recent infection.
2. The recommended interval between an acute and convalescent sample is 10 to 14 days.
3. The clinical case definition of mumps is an acute onset of unilateral or bilateral tender, self-limiting swelling of the parotid gland (or other salivary glands) with or without other apparent cause lasting 2 or more days. A probable case is one that meets the clinical case definition without serologic or virologic testing, whereas a confirmed case meets the clinical definition and is laboratory confirmed.

CLINICAL ALERT

False-positive results by IFA for IgM have been reported.

Interventions

Pretest Patient Care

1. Assess patient's test knowledge. Explain test purpose and procedure.
2. Follow guidelines in Chapter 1 for safe, effective, informed *pretest* care.

Posttest Patient Care

1. Review test results; report and record findings. Modify the nursing care plan as needed. Counsel the patient regarding abnormal findings; explain the need for possible follow-up testing and treatment.
2. If there are no complications, typically, mumps is treated with bed rest and medications to reduce pain and fever, such as acetaminophen or nonsteroidal anti-inflammatory drugs (NSAIDs). Patients younger than 20 years should not be given aspirin because of its link to Reye's syndrome.
3. Follow guidelines in Chapter 1 for safe, effective, informed *posttest* care.

Varicella-Zoster (Chickenpox) Antibody Test

Varicella-zoster virus (VZV) is a herpesvirus and causes chickenpox with primary infection, a highly contagious disease characterized by widely spread vesicular eruptions and fever. The disease is endemic in the United States and most commonly affects children 5 to 8 years of age, although adults and younger children, including infants, may develop chickenpox. VZV infection in a pregnant woman may spread through the placenta to the fetus, causing congenital disease in the infant.

Although a primary infection results in immunity to subsequent chickenpox, the virus remains latent in the body. When it is reactivated, VZV causes shingles (herpes zoster). The incubation period is 10 to 24 days. Fever and painful localized vesicular eruptions of the skin along the distribution of the involved nerves are the most common clinical symptoms.

The sensitivity, specificity, and reproducibility of ELISA immunoassays are comparable to other serologic tests for antibody such as IFA, CF, and HAI. A positive IgG result, coupled with a positive IgM result, indicates a current infection with VZV.

Normal Findings

Negative for varicella-zoster IgG or IgM antibodies by ELISA: nonimmune
Positive for varicella-zoster IgG antibody: indicates a current or previous infection; in the absence of current clinical symptoms, may indicate immunity
Positive for varicella-zoster IgM antibody; indicates a current or recent infection

Procedure

1. Collect a 7-mL blood serum sample in a red-topped tube. Observe standard precautions. Label the specimen with the patient's name, date, and test(s) ordered and place in a biohazard bag for transport to the laboratory.
2. Follow-up testing may be required.

Clinical Implications

1. When testing for IgG antibody, seroconversion between acute and convalescent sera is considered strong evidence of a current or recent infection. The recommended interval between an acute and convalescent sample is 10 to 14 days.

2. Whereas the presence of IgM antibody suggests a current or recent infection, low levels of IgM may occasionally persist for more than 12 months after infection or immunization.
3. Immunosuppressed patients in hospitals may contract severe nosocomial infections from others infected with VZV. Therefore, serologic screening of direct healthcare providers (e.g., physicians, nurses) is necessary to avoid spread of infection.

Interventions

Pretest Patient Care

1. Assess patient's test knowledge. Explain test purpose and procedure. Advise pregnant women that VZV poses a high risk for congenital disease in the infant.
2. Follow guidelines in Chapter 1 for safe, effective, informed *pretest* care.

Posttest Patient Care

1. Review test results; report and record findings. Modify the nursing care plan as needed. Counsel the patient regarding abnormal findings; explain the need for possible follow-up testing and treatment. Inform patients who test positive for VZV IgG that they are naturally immune to chickenpox, but the virus can be reactivated and cause shingles at a later time.
2. Follow guidelines in Chapter 1 for safe, effective, informed *posttest* care.

• Cytomegalovirus (CMV) Antibody Test

Cytomegalovirus (CMV) is a ubiquitous human viral pathogen that belongs to the herpesvirus family. Infection with CMV is usually asymptomatic (up to 60 days) and can persist in the host as a chronic or latent infection. CMV has been linked with STIs. Blood banks routinely screen for CMV antibodies and report these as CMV negative or CMV positive.

This test determines the presence of CMV antibodies and is routinely done in congenitally infected newborns, immunocompromised patients, and sexually active persons who present with mononucleosis-like symptoms. Antibody results must be evaluated in the context of the patient's current clinical symptoms and viral culture results. Tests to detect CMV antigen are available and aid in early detection. Viral culture confirms CMV infection.

Normal Findings

Negative for CMV-specific IgG and IgM by ELISA

Procedure

1. Collect a 7-mL blood serum sample in a red-topped tube. Observe standard precautions. Label the specimen with the patient's name, date, and test(s) ordered and place in a biohazard bag for transport to the laboratory.
2. It is recommended that posttransplantation titers be monitored at weekly intervals, particularly following bone marrow transplantation.

Clinical Implications

1. Infants who acquire CMV during primary infection of the mother are prone to develop severe cytomegalic inclusion disease (CID). CID may be fatal or may cause neurologic sequelae such as mental retardation, deafness, microcephaly, or motor dysfunction.
2. Transfusion of CMV-infected blood products or transplantation of CMV-infected donor organs may produce interstitial pneumonitis in an immunocompromised recipient.
3. When testing for IgG antibody, seroconversion or a significant rise in titer between acute and convalescent sera may indicate presence of a current or recent infection.
4. Although the presence of IgM antibodies suggests current or recent infection, low levels of IgM antibodies may occasionally persist for more than 12 months after infection.

Interventions

Pretest Patient Care

1. Explain test purpose and procedure.
2. Follow guidelines in Chapter 1 for safe, effective, informed *pretest* care.

Posttest Patient Care

1. Review test results; report and record findings. Modify the nursing care plan as needed. Counsel the patient regarding abnormal findings; explain the need for possible follow-up testing and treatment. See Interpreting Results of Immunologic Tests on page 537.
2. Follow guidelines in Chapter 1 for safe, effective, informed *posttest* care.

● Herpes Simplex Virus (HSV) Antibodies (HSV-1 and HSV-2 Tests)

Two types of herpes simplex virus (HSV) exist. HSV type 1 (HSV-1) causes orofacial herpes; type 2 (HSV-2) causes genital and neonatal herpes. Serologic differentiation is difficult; therefore, type-specific antibody tests are required.

These tests identify the herpes simplex infections. Human HSV is found worldwide and is transmitted by close personal contact. The clinical course is variable, and symptoms may be mild enough to go unrecognized. Major signs and symptoms include oral and skin eruptions, genital tract infections and lesions, and neonatal herpes. Herpes simplex is also common in individuals with immune system deficiencies (e.g., cancers, HIV/AIDS, chemotherapy treatment). HSV antibody testing is also widely used for bone marrow recipients and donors.

Normal Findings

Negative for HSV-1 and HSV-2 by ELISA and IFA

Procedure

1. Collect a 7-mL blood serum sample in a red-topped tube. Observe standard precautions.
2. Label the specimen with the patient's name, date, and test(s) ordered and place in a biohazard bag for transport to the laboratory.
3. Follow-up testing is usually required.

Clinical Implications

1. Most persons in the general population have been infected with HSV by 20 years of age. After the primary infection, antibody levels fall and stabilize until a subsequent infection occurs.
2. Diagnosis of current infection is related to determining a significant increase in antibody titers between acute-stage and convalescent-stage blood samples.
3. Serologic tests cannot indicate the presence of active genital tract infections. Instead, direct examination with procurement of lesion cultures should be done.
4. Newborn infections are acquired during delivery through the birth canal and may present as localized skin lesions or more generalized organ system involvement.

Interventions

Pretest Patient Care

1. Assess patient's knowledge regarding the test. Explain test purpose and procedure.
2. Follow guidelines in Chapter 1 for safe, effective, informed *pretest* care.

Posttest Patient Care

1. Review test results; report and record findings. Modify the nursing care plan as needed. Counsel the patient regarding abnormal findings; explain the need for possible follow-up testing and treatment. See Interpreting Results of Immunologic Tests on page 537. Advise pregnant women that the newborn may be infected during birth when active genital area infection is present.
2. Follow guidelines in Chapter 1 for safe, effective, informed *posttest* care.

● Human T-Cell Lymphotropic Virus (HTLV-I/II) Antibody Test

This test detects antibodies to human T-cell lymphotropic virus (HTLV)-I, a retrovirus associated with adult T-cell leukemia (ATL) and demyelinating neurologic disorders. The presence of HTLV-I antibodies in an asymptomatic person excludes that person from donating blood; however, this finding does not mean that leukemia or a neurologic disorder exists or will develop. Specimens with a positive test result by EIA are referred for Western blot. The results of Western blot are for investigational use only at the time of this printing.

Normal Findings

Negative for HTLV-I/II antibodies by EIA and Western blot

Procedure

1. Collect a 7-mL blood serum sample in a red-topped tube. Observe standard precautions.
2. Label the specimen with the patient's name, date, and test(s) ordered and place the specimen in a biohazard bag for transport to the laboratory.

Clinical Implications

1. Positive results (antibodies to HTLV-I) occur in the presence of HTLV-I infection. Infection transmitted to recipients of HTLV-I–infected blood is well documented.
2. The presence of antibodies to HTLV-I bears no relation to the presence of antibodies to HIV-1; its presence does not put a person at risk for HIV/AIDS, but they often occur concurrently because of similar risk factors.
3. HTLV-I is endemic to the Caribbean, Southeastern Japan, and some areas of Africa.
4. In the United States, HTLV-I has been detected in persons with ATL, intravenous drug users, and healthy persons as well as in donated blood products. Transmission can also take place through ingestion of breast milk, sexual contact, and sharing of contaminated intravenous drug paraphernalia.

Interventions

Pretest Patient Care

1. Assess patient's knowledge about test. Explain test purpose and procedure.
2. Follow guidelines in Chapter 1 for safe, effective, informed *pretest* care.

Posttest Patient Care

1. Review test results; report and record findings. Modify the nursing care plan as needed. Counsel the patient regarding abnormal findings; explain the need for possible follow-up testing and treatment. See Interpreting Results of Immunologic Tests on page 537.
2. Follow guidelines in Chapter 1 for safe, effective, informed *posttest* care.

Parvovirus B-19 Antibody Test

These antibody tests detect parvovirus B-19, the only parvovirus known to cause human disease. The B-19 virus destroys red blood cell precursor cells and interferes with normal red blood cell production. In young children, it is associated with erythema infectiosum, a mild, self-limited disease characterized by a low-grade fever and rash. It has also been associated with aplastic crisis in patients with chronic hemolytic anemia and in immunodeficient patients who have bone marrow failure.

Normal Findings

Negative for parvovirus B-19–specific IgG and IgM antibodies by ELISA and IFA

Procedure

1. Collect a 7-mL blood serum sample in a red-topped tube. Observe standard precautions.
2. Label the specimen with the patient's name, date, and test(s) ordered and place in a biohazard bag for transport to the laboratory.

Clinical Implications

1. Positive parvovirus B-19 infection has been implicated in aplastic anemia associated with organ transplantation. It is recommended, therefore, that this test be included in the serologic assessment of prospective organ donors.
2. Immunocompromised patients may have a delayed or absent antibody response. It is recommended that parvovirus DNA detection by PCR be considered.

Interventions

Pretest Patient Care

1. Assess patient's knowledge regarding test. Explain purpose and blood test procedure. Advise any prospective organ donor that this test is part of a panel of tests performed before organ donation to protect the organ recipient from potential infection.
2. Follow guidelines in Chapter 1 for safe, effective, informed *pretest* care.

Posttest Patient Care

1. Review test results; report and record findings. Modify the nursing care plan as needed. Counsel the patient regarding abnormal findings; explain the need for possible follow-up testing and treatment. See Interpreting Results of Immunologic Tests on page 537.
2. Follow guidelines in Chapter 1 for safe, effective, informed *posttest* care.

Rabies Antibody Tests

Rabies, a viral infection, is transmitted in the saliva of infected animals, such as bats, raccoons, skunks, cats, and dogs. Serologic testing is diagnostic for the presence of rabies in animals. It also indicates the degree of antibody responses to rabies immunization (e.g., for people who routinely work with animals).

Normal Findings

IFA <1:16 or DFA examination of the animal brain for presence of the virus

Procedure

Humans

Collect a 7-mL blood serum sample in a red-topped tube. Observe standard precautions. Label the specimen with the patient's name, date, and test(s) ordered and place in a biohazard bag.

Animals

1. If the suspect animal exhibits abnormal behavior, standard procedure is to euthanize the animal and examine its brain for Negri body inclusions in the neurons.
2. Rabies testing is usually performed in a public health laboratory.

Clinical Implications

1. An elevated titer in humans indicates an adequate response after immunization. A rabies titer of 1:16 or greater is considered protective.
2. Pre-exposure vaccination should be offered to individuals in high-risk groups such as veterinarians, animal handlers, or international travelers if they are likely to come in contact with rabid animals and medical care is limited.
3. Postexposure vaccination should be administered to previously vaccinated individuals if exposed to rabies.
4. Postexposure prophylaxis is considered a medical urgency, and each situation should be evaluated by trained medical personnel and in consultation with public health officials. The individual should not be vaccinated unless the animal develops clinical signs of rabies during a 10-day observation period. If the animal is rabid, the person should be vaccinated immediately.

Interventions

Pretest Patient Care

1. Explain test purpose and procedure.
2. Follow guidelines in Chapter 1 for safe, effective, informed *pretest* care.

Posttest Patient Care

1. Review test results; report and record findings. Modify the nursing care plan as needed. Counsel the patient regarding abnormal findings; explain the need for possible follow-up testing and treatment.
2. Follow guidelines in Chapter 1 for safe, effective, informed *posttest* care.

FUNGAL TESTS

● Fungal Antibody Tests: Histoplasmosis, Blastomycosis, Coccidioidomycosis

Certain fungal species are associated with human respiratory diseases acquired by inhaling spores from sources such as dust, soil, and bird droppings. Serologic tests may be used for diagnosis. Fungal diseases are categorized as either superficial or deep. For the most part, superficial mycoses are limited to the skin, mucous membranes, nails, and hair. Deep mycoses involve the deeper tissues and internal organs. Histoplasmosis, coccidioidomycosis, and blastomycosis are caused by deep mycoses.

These tests detect serum precipitin antibodies and CF antibodies present in the fungal diseases of coccidioidomycosis, blastomycosis, and histoplasmosis. Coccidioidomycosis, also known as desert fever, San Joaquin fever, and valley fever, is contracted through inhalation of *Coccidioides immitis* spores found in dust or soil. Blastomycosis is caused by infection with organisms of the genus *Blastomyces*. Histoplasmosis is a granulomatous infection caused by *Histoplasma capsulatum*.

Normal Findings

Negative for fungal antibodies
CF titer: <1:8
Immunodiffusion (ID): negative

Procedure

1. Collect a 7-mL blood serum sample in a red-topped tube. Observe standard precautions.
2. Label the specimen with the patient's name, date, and test(s) ordered and place in a biohazard bag for transport to the laboratory.

Clinical Implications

1. Antibodies to *Coccidioides*, *Blastomyces*, and *Histoplasma* appear early in the course of the disease (weeks 1 to 4) and then disappear.
2. Negative fungal serology does not rule out the possibility of a current infection.
3. CF titers ≥1:8 are considered presumptive of infection.

Interfering Factors

1. Antibodies to fungi may be found in blood samples from apparently healthy people.
2. When testing for blastomycosis, cross-reactions with histoplasmosis may occur.
3. More than 50% of patients having active blastomycosis yield a negative result by CF.
4. Recent histoplasmosis skin tests must be avoided because they cause elevated CF test results, which may be due to the stimulation from the skin test and not the systemic infection.

Interventions

Pretest Patient Care

1. Explain test purpose and procedure.
2. Follow guidelines in Chapter 1 for safe, effective, informed *pretest* care.
3. Specimens for culture of the organism may also be required.

Posttest Patient Care

1. Review test results; report and record findings. Modify the nursing care plan as needed. Counsel the patient regarding abnormal findings; explain the need for possible follow-up testing and treatment. See Interpreting Results of Immunologic Tests on page 537.
2. Follow guidelines in Chapter 1 for safe, effective, informed *posttest* care.

● *Candida* Antibody Test

Candidiasis is usually caused by *Candida albicans* and affects the mucous membranes, skin, and nails (see *Candida* Skin Test, page 490). Compromised individuals with depressed T-cell function are most likely to have invasive disease.

Identifying the *Candida* antibody can be helpful when the diagnosis of systemic candidiasis cannot be shown by culture or tissue sample. Clinical symptomatology must be present for the test to be meaningful. Tests used include ID; counterimmunoelectrophoresis (CIE), which is particularly valuable on CSF and urine specimens; and LA for *Candida* antigen.

Normal Findings

Negative for *Candida* antibodies by ID

Procedure

1. Collect a 7-mL blood serum sample in a red-topped tube. Observe standard precautions.
2. Label the specimen with the patient's name, date, and test(s) ordered and place in a biohazard bag for transfer to the laboratory.

Clinical Implications

1. A titer ≥1:8 by LA or CIE for *Candida* antigen indicates systemic infection.
2. A fourfold rise in titers of paired blood samples 10 to 14 days apart indicates acute infection.
3. Patients on long-term intravenous therapy treated with broad-spectrum antibiotics and diabetic patients commonly have disseminated infections caused by *C. albicans*. The disease also occurs in bottle-fed newborns and in the urinary bladder of catheterized patients.
4. Vulvovaginal candidiasis, common in late pregnancy, can transmit candidiasis to the infant through the birth canal.

Interfering Factors

1. Approximately 25% of the normal population tests positive for the presence of *Candida*.
2. Cross-reaction can occur with LA testing in persons who have cryptococcosis or tuberculosis.
3. Positive results can occur in the presence of mucocutaneous candidiasis or severe vaginitis.

Interventions

Pretest Patient Care

1. Explain test purpose and procedure.
2. Follow guidelines in Chapter 1 for safe, effective, informed *pretest* care.
3. Specimens for culture of the organism may also be required.

Posttest Patient Care

1. Review test results; report and record findings. Modify the nursing care plan as needed. Counsel the patient regarding abnormal findings; explain the need for possible follow-up testing and treatment. See Interpreting Results of Immunologic Tests on page 537.
2. Follow guidelines in Chapter 1 for safe, effective, informed *posttest* care.

● *Aspergillus* Antibody Test

The aspergilli, especially *Aspergillus fumigatus*, *Aspergillus flavus*, and *Aspergillus niger*, are associated with pulmonary infections and invasive fatal disease sequelae in immunosuppressed patients. Manifestations of *Aspergillus* infections include allergic bronchopulmonary disease; lung mycetoma; endophthalmitis; and disseminated brain, kidney, heart, and bone disease.

This test detects antibodies present in aspergillosis, primarily allergic bronchopulmonary disease, or fungus ball.

Normal Findings

Negative for *Aspergillus* antibody by ID
<1:8 by CF

Procedure

1. Collect a 7-mL blood serum sample in a red-topped tube. CSF can also be tested. Observe standard precautions.
2. Label the specimen with the patient's name, date, and tests ordered and place in a biohazard bag for transport to the laboratory.

Clinical Implications

1. Positive test results are associated with pulmonary infections in compromised patients and *Aspergillus* infections of prosthetic heart valves.

2. If blood serum exhibits one to four bands using ID, aspergillosis is strongly suspected. Weak bands suggest an early disease process or hypersensitivity pneumonitis.
3. Best use of the CF test is with paired sera taken 3 weeks apart to detect a rise in titer against a single antigen.

Interventions

Pretest Patient Care

1. Explain test purpose and procedure.
2. Follow guidelines in Chapter 1 for safe, effective, informed *pretest* care.
3. Specimens for culture of the organism may also be required.

Posttest Patient Care

1. Review test results; report and record findings. Modify the nursing care plan as needed. Counsel the patient regarding abnormal findings; explain the need for possible follow-up testing and treatment. See Interpreting Results of Immunologic Tests on page 537.
2. Follow guidelines in Chapter 1 for safe, effective, informed *posttest* care.

● *Cryptococcus* Antibody Test

Cryptococcus neoformans, a yeast-like fungus, causes a lung infection thought to be acquired by inhalation. The organism has been isolated from several natural environments, especially where weathered pigeon droppings accumulate.

This test detects antibodies present in *Cryptococcus* infections. It appears that about 50% of patients who present with antibodies have a predisposing condition such as lymphoma or sarcoidosis or are being treated with steroid therapy. Infection with *C. neoformans* has long been associated with Hodgkin's disease and other malignant lymphomas. In fact, *C. neoformans*, in conjunction with malignancy, occurs to such a degree that some researchers have raised the question regarding the possible etiologic relation between the two diseases. Tests ordered for this disease include LA testing for antigens or antibodies.

Normal Findings

Negative for *Cryptococcus* antibody by IFA or tube agglutination (TA)
IFA test has a specificity of 77%.
TA test has a specificity of 89%.

Procedure

1. Collect a 7-mL blood serum sample in a red-topped tube. A 2-mL spinal fluid sample may also be used. Observe standard precautions.
2. Label the specimen with the patient's name, date, and test(s) ordered and place in a biohazard bag for transport to the laboratory.

Clinical Implications

1. Positive *C. neoformans* tests are associated with infections of the lower respiratory tract through inhalation of aerosols containing *C. neoformans* cells disseminated by the fecal droppings of pigeons.
2. TA titers ≥1.2 are suggestive of infection.

Interventions

Pretest Patient Care

1. Explain test purpose and procedure. Obtain clinical history and assess for exposure.
2. Follow guidelines in Chapter 1 for safe, effective, informed *pretest* care.
3. Specimens for culture of the organism may also be required.

Posttest Patient Care

1. Review test results; report and record findings. Modify the nursing care plan as needed. Counsel the patient regarding abnormal findings; explain the need for possible follow-up testing and treatment. See Interpreting Results of Immunologic Tests on page 537.
2. Follow guidelines in Chapter 1 for safe, effective, informed *posttest* care.

PARASITIC TESTS

● Toxoplasmosis (TPM) Antibody Tests

Toxoplasmosis (TPM) is caused by the sporozoan parasite *Toxoplasma gondii* and is a severe, generalized, granulomatous CNS disease. It may be either congenital or acquired and is found in humans, domestic animals (e.g., cats), and wild animals. Humans may acquire the infection through ingestion of inadequately cooked meat or other contaminated material. Congenital TPM may cause fetal death. Symptoms of subacute infection may appear shortly after birth or much later. Complications of congenital TPM include hydrocephaly, microcephaly, convulsions, and chronic retinitis. It is believed that one fourth to one half of the adult population is asymptomatically infected with TPM. The CDC recommends serologic testing during pregnancy.

The IFA test helps to differentiate TPM from IM. *Toxoplasma* antibodies appear within 1 to 2 weeks of infection and peak at 6 to 8 months. IFA is also a valuable screening test for latent TPM.

Normal Findings

Titer <1:16: no previous infection (except for ocular infection) by IFA
Negative by MEIA
Negative: *T. gondii* DNA not detected by PCR

Procedure

1. Collect a 7-mL blood serum sample in a red-topped tube. Observe standard precautions.
2. Label the specimen with the patient's name, date, and test(s) ordered and place in a biohazard bag for transport to the laboratory.

Clinical Implications

The IFA test is considered positive under any of the following conditions:

1. Titer ≥1:256 indicates recent exposure or current infection; rising titer is of greatest significance.
2. Any titer value is significant in a newborn infant.
3. Titer ≥1:1024 is significant for active disease.
4. Titer ≤1:16 occurs with ocular TPM.

Interventions

Pretest Patient Care

1. Explain test purpose and procedure.
2. Follow guidelines in Chapter 1 for safe, effective, informed *pretest* care.

Posttest Patient Care

1. Review test results; report and record findings. Modify the nursing care plan as needed. Counsel the patient regarding abnormal findings; explain the need for possible follow-up testing and treatment; see Interpreting Results of Immunologic Tests on page 537.
2. Follow guidelines in Chapter 1 for safe, effective, informed *posttest* care.

Amebiasis (*Entamoeba histolytica*) Antibody Test

Entamoeba histolytica, the causative agent of amebiasis, is a pathogenic intestinal parasite. The *E. histolytica* test determines the presence or absence of specific serum antibodies to this parasite. Stool examination is considered the definitive diagnostic tool; however, the absence of detectable stool organisms does not necessarily rule out the disease. Antibiotic therapy, oil enemas, and barium may interfere with the ability to isolate this organism in the stool.

Normal Findings

Negative for *Entamoeba* antibodies by indirect hemagglutination (IHA), latent agglutination, and CIE

Procedure

1. Collect a 7-mL blood serum sample in a red-topped tube. Observe standard precautions.
2. Label the specimen with the patient's name, date, and test(s) ordered and place in a biohazard bag for transport to the laboratory.

Clinical Implications

1. Positive test (titer >1:128) indicates active or recent infection.
2. Amebic liver abscess and amebic dysentery indicate the presence of amebiasis.
3. Titers range from 1:256 to 1:2048 in the presence of current active amebiasis.
4. Titers <1:32 generally exclude amebiasis.

NOTE *A positive test may only reflect past but not current infections.*

Interventions

Pretest Patient Care

1. Explain test purpose and procedure.
2. Follow guidelines in Chapter 1 for safe, effective, informed *pretest* care.

Posttest Patient Care

1. Review test results; report and record findings. Modify the nursing care plan as needed. Counsel the patient regarding abnormal results; explain the need for possible follow-up testing and treatment. See Interpreting Results of Immunologic Tests on page 537.
2. Follow guidelines in Chapter 1 for safe, effective, informed *posttest* care.

TORCH Test

TORCH is an acronym that stands for *Toxoplasma*, rubella, CMV, and HSV. These pathogens are frequently implicated in congenital or neonatal infections that are not clinically apparent but that may result in serious CNS impairment.

Both mothers and newborn infants are tested for exposure to these agents. The test differentiates acute, congenital, and intrapartum infections caused by *T. gondii*, rubella virus, CMV, and herpesvirus. The presence of IgM-associated antibodies in newborns reflects actual fetal antibody production. High levels of IgM at birth indicate fetal in utero response to an antigen. In this instance, an intrauterine infection should be considered. TORCH is more useful in excluding than in establishing etiology.

Normal Findings

Negative for *Toxoplasma*, rubella, CMV, and HSV antibodies

Procedure

1. Collect a 7-mL blood serum sample in a red-topped tube. Observe standard precautions.
2. Label the specimen with the patient's name, date, and test(s) ordered and place in a biohazard bag for transport to the laboratory.

Clinical Implications

1. Persistent rubella antibodies in an infant >6 months of age highly suggests congenital infection. Congenital rubella is characterized by neurosensory deafness, heart anomalies, cataracts, growth retardation, and encephalitic symptoms.
2. A diagnosis of TPM is established through sequential testing rather than by a single positive result. Sequential examination reveals rising antibody titers, changing titers, and the conversion of serologic tests from negative to positive. A titer of 1:256 suggests recent infection. About one third of infants who acquire infection in utero show signs of cerebral calcifications and chorioretinitis at birth; the rest are born without symptoms.
3. A marked and persistent rise in CF antibody titer over time is consistent with a diagnosis of rubella in infants <6 months of age.
4. Presence of herpes antibodies in CSF, together with signs of herpetic encephalitis and persistent HSV-1 or HSV-2 antibody levels in a newborn showing no obvious external lesions, is consistent with a diagnosis of HSV.

Interventions

Pretest Patient Care

1. Explain test purpose and procedure.
2. Follow guidelines in Chapter 1 for safe, effective, informed *pretest* care.

Posttest Patient Care

1. Review test results; report and record findings. Modify the nursing care plan as needed. Counsel the patient regarding abnormal findings; explain the need for possible follow-up testing and treatment for intrauterine and congenital infections. See Interpreting Results of Immunologic Tests on page 537.
2. Follow guidelines in Chapter 1 for safe, effective, informed *posttest* care.

IMMUNOLOGIC TESTS FOR IMMUNE DYSFUNCTION AND RELATED DISORDERS OF THE IMMUNE SYSTEMS

● Quantitative Immunoglobulins: IgA, IgG, IgM

Five classes of immunoglobulins (antibodies)—IgA, IgG (with four subclasses, IgG_1, IgG_2, IgG_3, and IgG_4), IgM, IgD, and IgE—have been isolated. Immunoglobulins function to neutralize toxic substances, support phagocytosis, and destroy microorganism functions. IgA takes two forms: serum and secretory. Serum IgA is present in blood serum; secretory IgA is found in saliva, tears, colostrum, and bronchial, gastrointestinal, and genitourinary secretions, where it can protect against microorganism invasion. IgE is involved in allergic reactions, whereas IgD is involved in humoral immunity.

IgG, the only immunoglobulin that can cross the placenta, is responsible for protection of the newborn during the first months of life. IgM possesses antibody activity against gram-negative organisms and rheumatoid factors and forms natural antibodies such as the ABO blood group. IgM does not cross the placenta and is therefore usually absent in the newborn. It is observed about 5 days after birth.

Quantitative immunoglobulin measurements can monitor the course of a disease and its treatment. If there is a monoclonal protein or M component present on serum protein electrophoresis (SPEP), a quantitative measurement of IgA, IgG, and IgM can identify the specific immunoglobulin. IgD and IgE are present in trace amounts.

Normal Findings

These values are derived from rate nephelometry.

1. *Adults*
   a. IgG: 700 to 1500 mg/dL or 7.0 to 15.0 g/L
   b. IgA: 60 to 400 mg/dL or 600 to 4000 mg/L
   c. IgM: 60 to 300 mg/dL or 600 to 3000 mg/L
   d. IgE: 3 to 423 IU/mL or 3 to 423 kIU/L
   e. IgD: 0 to 14 mg/dL or 0 to 140 mg/L
2. *Children*
   a. IgA (boys and girls)
      (1) 0 to 4 months: 6 to 64 mg/dL or 60 to 640 mg/L
      (2) 5 to 8 months: 10 to 87 mg/dL or 100 to 870 mg/L
      (3) 9 to 14 months: 17 to 94 mg/dL or 170 to 940 mg/L
      (4) 15 to 23 months: 20 to 175 mg/dL or 200 to 1750 mg/L
      (5) 2 to 3 years: 24 to 192 mg/dL or 240 to 1920 mg/L
      (6) 4 to 6 years: 26 to 232 mg/dL or 260 to 2320 mg/L
      (7) 7 to 9 years: 33 to 258 mg/dL or 330 to 2580 mg/L
      (8) 10 to 12 years: 45 to 285 mg/dL or 450 to 2850 mg/L
      (9) 13 to 15 years: 47 to 317 mg/dL or 470 to 3170 mg/L
      (10) 16 to 17 years: 55 to 377 mg/dL or 550 to 3770 mg/L
   b. IgM (boys)
      (1) 0 to 4 months: 14 to 142 mg/dL or 140 to 1420 mg/L
      (2) 5 to 8 months: 24 to 167 mg/dL or 240 to 1670 mg/L
      (3) 9 to 23 months: 35 to 200 mg/dL or 350 to 2000 mg/L
      (4) 2 to 3 years: 41 to 200 mg/dL or 410 to 2000 mg/L
      (5) 4 to 17 years: 55 to 260 mg/dL or 550 to 2600 mg/L
   c. IgM (girls)
      (1) 0 to 4 months: 14 to 142 mg/dL or 140 to 1420 mg/L
      (2) 5 to 8 months: 24 to 167 mg/dL or 240 to 1670 mg/L
      (3) 9 to 23 months: 35 to 242 mg/dL or 350 to 2420 mg/L
      (4) 2 to 3 years: 41 to 250 mg/dL or 410 to 2500 mg/L
      (5) 4 to 17 years: 56 to 260 mg/dL or 560 to 2600 mg/L
   d. IgG (boys and girls)
      (1) 0 to 4 months: 141 to 930 mg/dL or 1.4 to 9.3 g/L
      (2) 5 to 8 months: 250 to 1190 mg/dL or 2.5 to 11.2 g/L
      (3) 9 to 11 months: 320 to 1250 mg/dL or 3.2 to 12.5 g/L
      (4) 1 to 3 years: 400 to 1250 mg/dL or 4.0 to 12.5 g/L
      (5) 4 to 6 years: 560 to 1307 mg/dL or 5.6 to 13.1 g/L
      (6) 7 to 9 years: 598 to 1379 mg/dL or 6.0 to 13.8 g/L
      (7) 10 to 12 years: 638 to 1453 mg/dL or 6.4 to 14.5 g/L
      (8) 13 to 15 years: 680 to 1531 mg/dL or 6.8 to 15.3 g/L
      (9) 16 to 17 years: 724 to 1611 mg/dL or 7.2 to 16.1 g/L

Procedure

1. Collect a 7-mL blood serum sample in a red-topped tube. Observe standard precautions.
2. Label the specimen with the patient's name, date, and test(s) ordered and place in a biohazard bag for transport to the laboratory.

Clinical Implications

1. IgA accounts for 10% to 15% of total immunoglobulin. *Increases* occur in the following conditions or situations:
   a. Chronic, nonalcoholic liver diseases, especially primary biliary cirrhosis (PBC)
   b. Obstructive jaundice
   c. Exercise
   d. Alcoholism
   e. Subacute and chronic infections
2. IgA *decreases* occur in the following conditions or situations:
   a. Ataxia-telangiectasia
   b. Chronic sinopulmonary disease
   c. Congenital deficit
   d. Late pregnancy
   e. Prolonged exposure to benzene immunosuppressive therapy
   f. Abstinence from alcohol after a period of 1 year
   g. In the presence of certain drugs and dextrin
   h. Protein-losing gastroenteropathies
3. IgG constitutes 75% to 80% of total immunoglobulins. *Increases* occur in the following conditions:
   a. Chronic granulomatous infections
   b. Hyperimmunization
   c. Liver disease
   d. Malnutrition (severe)
   e. Dysproteinemia
   f. Disease associated with hypersensitivity granulomas, dermatologic disorders, and IgG myeloma
   g. RA
4. IgG *decreases* occur in the following conditions:
   a. Agammaglobulinemia
   b. Lymphoid aplasia
   c. Selective IgG, IgA deficiency
   d. IgA myeloma
   e. Bence Jones proteinemia
   f. Chronic lymphoblastic leukemia
5. IgM constitutes 5% to 10% of total antibody. *Increases* in adults occur in the following conditions:
   a. Waldenström's macroglobulinemia
   b. Trypanosomiasis
   c. Malaria
   d. IM
   e. Lupus erythematosus
   f. RA
   g. Dysgammaglobulinemia (certain cases)
6. IgM *decreases* occur in the following conditions:
   a. Agammaglobulinemia
   b. Lymphoproliferative disorders (certain cases)

c. Lymphoid aplasia
d. IgG and IgA myeloma
e. Dysgammaglobulinemia
f. Chronic lymphoblastic leukemia

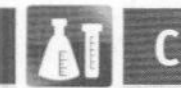

CLINICAL ALERT

Persons with IgA deficiency are predisposed to autoimmune disorders and can develop antibody to IgA, with possible anaphylaxis occurring if transfused with blood containing IgA.

CLINICAL ALERT

In the newborn, a level of IgM >20 mg/dL indicates in utero stimulation of the immune system (e.g., rubella virus, CMV, syphilis, TPM).

Interventions

Pretest Patient Care

1. Explain test purpose and specimen collection procedure.
2. Follow guidelines in Chapter 1 for safe, effective, informed *pretest* care.

Posttest Patient Care

1. See posttest care for protein electrophoresis (PEP).
2. Review test results; report and record findings. Modify the nursing care plan as needed. Counsel the patient regarding abnormal findings; explain the need for possible follow-up testing (such as immunoglobulin and serum viscosity testing, to monitor a patient with monoclonal gammopathy) and treatment.
3. Follow guidelines in Chapter 1 for safe, effective, informed *posttest* care.

• Protein Electrophoresis (PEP), Serum and Urine

Serum proteins represent a diverse microenvironment. They are a source of nutrition and a buffer system. Immunoglobulins and related proteins function as immunologic agents. Carrier proteins (e.g., haptoglobin, prealbumin, transferrin) transport certain ions and molecules to their destinations. Antiproteases (e.g., α_1-antitrypsin [AAT], α_2-macroglobulin) regulate the activity of various proteolytic enzymes, and other classes of proteins regulate oncotic pressure, genetic component pressures (e.g., chromosomal), and metabolic substances (e.g., hormones). Blood serum and urine are commonly screened for the monoclonal immunoglobulin component by means of SPEP. Immunoglobulins are the major component of the serum γ-globulin fraction. In health, the immunoglobulins are polyclonal instead of monoclonal. When a monoclonal band is observed, it frequently signals a neoplastic process such as multiple myeloma or Waldenström's macroglobulinemia. SPEP enhances follow-up procedures such as specific protein quantification of immunoglobulins (IgA, IgG, IgM) and immunofixation. It provides one of the best tools for general screening of the human health state.

These tests can diagnose some inflammatory and neoplastic states, nephrotic syndromes, liver disease, and immune dysfunctions and can evaluate nutritional states and osmotic pressures in edematous and malnourished patients. SPEP produces electrophoretic separation of the five major protein fractions (albumin, α_1-globulin, α_2-globulin, β-globulin, and γ-globulin) in serum and urine specimens so that a more definitive diagnosis can be made. Major components present in each protein fraction or zone exhibit characteristic, unique electrophoretic patterns, and are defined as the albumin zone (albumin); the α_1 zone (α_1-lipoproteins, high-density lipoprotein, AAT); the α_2 zone (α_2-macroglobulin, haptoglobin, β-lipoprotein); the β zone (transferrin, C3 [complement]); and the γ zone (fibrinogen, IgA, IgM, IgG).

Normal Findings

Serum Protein Electrophoresis

Total Protein	SI Units	Albumin	SI Units
Adult: 6.0–8.0 g/dL	60–80 g/L	Adult: 3.8–5.0 g/dL	38–50 g/L
<5 d: 5.4–7.0 g/dL	54–70 g/L	Newborn: 2.6–3.6 g/dL	26–36 g/L
1–3 yr: 5.9–7.0 g/dL	59–70 g/L	1–3 yr: 3.4–4.2 g/dL	34–42 g/L
4–6 yr: 5.9–7.8 g/dL	59–78 g/L	4–6 yr: 3.5–5.2 g/dL	35–52 g/L
7–9 yr: 6.2–8.1 g/dL	62–81 g/L	7–9 yr: 3.7–5.6 g/dL	37–56 g/L
10–19 yr: 6.3–8.6 g/dL	63–86 g/L	10–19 yr: 3.7–5.6 g/dL	37–56 g/L

α_1-Globulin: 0.1 to 0.3 g/dL
α_2-Globulin: 0.6 to 1.0 g/dL
β-Globulin: 0.7 to 1.4 g/dL
γ-Globulin: 0.7 to 1.6 g/dL

Urine Protein Electrophoresis

A descriptive report is prepared by the pathologist.

CLINICAL ALERT

Normally, very little protein is excreted in the urine; however, relatively large amounts may be excreted in certain disease states. In the presence of lipoid nephrosis, selective proteinuria produces excess albumin excretion. With nonselective proteinuria (e.g., glomerulonephritis), all types of serum proteins usually appear in the urine. Urine protein electrophoresis (UPEP) can identify Bence Jones proteins, which migrate in the β-globulin and γ-globulin regions. See Chapter 3 for a complete explanation of urine protein and albumin.

Procedure

1. Collect a 7-mL blood serum sample in a red-topped tube. Observe standard precautions.
2. First voided morning urine specimen or 24-hour timed urine specimen is preferred. A 100-mL sample from a 24-hour urine collection is submitted for Urine protein electrophoresis (UPEP).
3. If blood or urine sample demonstrates the presence of a paraprotein (monoclonal immunoglobin), a follow-up or confirmatory immunofixation electrophoresis (IFE) can be performed on the same specimen submitted for the PEP.
4. To quantify the amount of protein in each fraction, separate proteins are scanned and separated according to net molecular charge by means of a densitometer and are expressed in grams per deciliter (g/dL).

Clinical Implications

The following are the most frequent protein abnormalities in protein quantification and SPE:

1. Total serum protein (the sum of circulating serum proteins) *increases* (hyperproteinemia) in dehydration and hemoconcentration states because of fluid loss (e.g., vomiting, diarrhea, poor kidney function). Increases are also found in the following conditions:
   a. Liver disease
   b. Multiple myeloma and other gammopathies
   c. Waldenström's macroglobulinemia

   d. Tropical disease
   e. Sarcoidosis and other granulomatous diseases
   f. Collagen disorders such as systemic lupus erythematosus (SLE) and RA
   g. Chronic inflammatory states
   h. Chronic infections
2. Total serum protein *decreases* (hypoproteinemia) in the following conditions:
   a. Insufficient nutritional intake (starvation or malabsorption)
   b. Severe liver disease or alcoholism
   c. Renal disease, nephrotic syndrome
   d. Diarrhea (Crohn's disease, ulcerative colitis)
   e. Severe skin diseases or burns
   f. Severe hemorrhage (when plasma volume is replaced more rapidly than protein)
   g. Heart failure
   h. Hypothyroidism
   i. Prolonged immobilization (trauma, orthopedic surgery)
3. Serum albumin *increases* with intravenous infusions and dehydration (elevated hemoglobin and hematocrit indicate higher albumin levels).
4. Serum albumin *decreases* in the following conditions:
   a. Decreased synthesis states such as liver disease, alcoholism, malabsorption syndromes, Crohn's disease, other protein-losing enteropathies, starvation states, and congenital analbuminemia
   b. *Increased* albumin loss (e.g., nephrotic syndrome, third-degree burns)
   c. Poor nutrition states and inadequate iron intake
   d. Low albumin-to-globulin (A/G) ratio (e.g., collagen disease, chronic inflammation, liver diseases, macroglobulinemia, severe infections, cachexia, burns, ulcerative colitis)
5. α_1-Globulin *increases* with infections (acute and chronic) and febrile reactions.
6. α_1-Globulin *decreases* with nephrosis and AAT deficiency.
7. α_2-Globulin *increases* in the following conditions:
   a. Biliary cirrhosis
   b. Obstructive jaundice
   c. Nephrosis
   d. Multiple myeloma (rare)
   e. Ulcerative colitis
8. α_2-Globulin *decreases* in acute hemolytic anemia.
9. β-Globulin *increases* in biliary cirrhosis, obstructive jaundice, and multiple myeloma (occasional).
10. β-Globulin *decreases* in nephrosis.
11. γ-Globulin *increases* in the following conditions:
    a. Chronic infections
    b. Hepatic diseases
    c. Autoimmune diseases
    d. Collagen diseases
    e. Multiple myeloma
    f. Waldenström's macroglobulinemia
    g. Leukemia and other cancers
12. γ-Globulin *decreases* in the following conditions:
    a. Agammaglobulinemia
    b. Hypogammaglobulinemia
    c. Nephrotic syndrome

Interfering Factors

1. Decreased albumin can be seen with rapid intravenous fluid infusions and hydration and during all trimesters of pregnancy.
2. Excessive hemolysis decreases albumin by 0.5 g/mL when patients are in the supine position. Conversely, hemolysis and dehydration elevate the total serum protein.
3. Prolonged bed rest and the last trimester of pregnancy produce lower total protein levels.

Interventions

Pretest Patient Care

1. Explain test purpose and specimen collection procedure.
2. If a 24-hour urine specimen is to be collected, the patient will require specific instructions, an appropriate container, and a receptacle for catching the voided urine (see Chapter 3).
3. Follow guidelines in Chapter 1 for safe, effective, informed *pretest* care.

Posttest Patient Care

1. Review test results; report and record findings. Modify the nursing care plan as needed. Counsel the patient regarding abnormal findings; explain the need for possible follow-up testing and treatment. Very low levels of protein and albumin are associated with edema and hypocalcemia.
2. Assess the patient for signs and symptoms related to these conditions and report and document same. Rarely is any one type of electrophoretic analysis used to diagnose a gammopathy. Follow-up testing may include IFE, quantitative immunoglobulins, and bone marrow studies.
3. Follow guidelines in Chapter 1 for safe, effective, informed *posttest* care.

● Immunofixation Electrophoresis (IFE), Serum and Urine

Monoclonal immunoglobulins consist of heavy and light chains. IFE identifies presence or absence of a monoclonal protein and determines its heavy-chain and light-chain types.

This test measures immune status and competence by identifying monoclonal and particle protein band immunoglobulins involved in the immune response. IFE is a follow-up test performed when monoclonal spike is observed on SPEP or when a monoclonal gammopathy is suspected on the basis of the patient's immunoglobulin concentrations.

Normal Findings

No abnormality present

Procedure

1. Collect a 7-mL blood serum sample in a red-topped tube or a 24-hour urine specimen. Observe standard precautions. Submit 25 mL from a 24-hour urine collection if a urine IFE is to be run simultaneously.
2. If the IFE is a follow-up to a paraprotein being demonstrated by PEP (see Protein Electrophoresis [PEP], Serum and Urine), the same specimen (blood, urine, or both) used for the electrophoresis can be used for this procedure as well.
3. In IFE, high-resolution electrophoresis produces stained bands. By comparing the location of the stained immunofixed band with a band in the same location in the SPEP reference pattern, a particular protein band can be identified.

Clinical Implications

1. *Monoclonal* protein in the serum or urine suggests a neoplastic process; a *polyclonal* increase in immunoglobulins is seen in chronic liver disease, connective tissue disease, and infection.

2. In multiple myeloma, 99% of patients have a monoclonal protein in the serum or urine. Waldenström's macroglobulinemia is characterized by the presence of a serum monoclonal IgM protein in all cases.
3. A monoclonal light chain (K or Bence Jones protein) is found in the urine of about 75% of patients with multiple myeloma. Approximately 75% of patients with Waldenström's macroglobulinemia have a monoclonal light chain in the urine. Heavy-chain fragments as well as free light chains may be seen in the urine of patients with multiple myeloma or amyloidosis.

Interventions

Pretest Patient Care

1. Explain test purpose and specimen collection procedure.
2. Submit the same specimen for the SPEP if a blood sample is needed. If the test is to be performed separately, another 7-mL blood sample collected in a red-topped tube is required. Note patient's age; this procedure is seldom indicated in patients <30 years of age because monoclonal proteins are rarely identified in this age group.
3. A 24-hour urine specimen is preferred. Provide instructions and a 24-hour collection container (see Chapter 3 for protocols).
4. Follow guidelines in Chapter 1 for safe, effective, informed *pretest* care.

Posttest Patient Care

1. Review test results; report and record findings. Modify the nursing care plan as needed. Counsel the patient regarding abnormal findings; explain the need for possible follow-up testing and treatment. Continue to monitor for neoplasms, infection, and liver and connective tissue disease.
2. Follow guidelines in Chapter 1 for safe, effective, informed *posttest* care.

• Cold Agglutinin

This test most commonly diagnoses primary atypical viral pneumonia caused by *Mycoplasma pneumoniae*; it is used to diagnose certain hemolytic anemias (e.g., cold agglutination disease) as well. The diagnosis depends on demonstrating a fourfold or higher increase in antibody titers between an early acute-phase blood serum sample and a blood serum sample taken in the convalescence phase, 7 to 10 days after the first sample. Positive reaction frequency and titer elevation both appear to be directly related to infection severity.

Patient's serum is serially diluted, human red cells are added, and the test is incubated at 4°C (refrigerator, 0° to 10°C). The cold agglutinin antibodies react optimally at 4°C with the I antigen present on human red cells. The reaction is reversed by incubation of the agglutinated serum/cell mixture at 37°C.

Normal Findings

<1:16 by red cell agglutination at 4°C

Procedure

1. Collect a 7-mL blood serum sample in a red-topped tube. Observe standard precautions. Label the specimen with the patient's name, date, and tests ordered and place in a biohazard bag for transport to the laboratory.
2. The sample should be prewarmed to 37°C for at least 15 minutes before the serum is separated from the cells. This allows the cold agglutinating antibodies to be eluted from the red cell membranes so that they can be detected in the agglutination procedure using O-negative indicator cells (pooled group O donors).

Clinical Implications

1. In viral pneumonia, the titer rises 8 to 10 days after onset, peaks in 12 to 25 days, and decreases 30 days after onset. Up to 90% of people with severe illness exhibit positive titers.
2. Chronic increased titer levels are associated with the following conditions:
   a. Cold antibody hemolytic anemia
   b. Chronic cold agglutinin disease
   c. Paroxysmal cold hemoglobinuria
   d. Severe Raynaud's phenomenon (may lead to gangrene)
   e. B-cell chronic lymphocytic leukemia
3. More important than any single high value is the rise in titer during the course of illness. The titer usually decreases by 4 to 6 weeks after the onset of illness.
4. Transient increases in titers are associated with primary atypical viral pneumonia, IM, measles, mumps, CMV, congenital syphilis, hepatic cirrhosis, and trypanosomiasis.

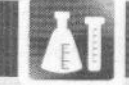
CLINICAL ALERT

A negative test does not rule out infection because only 30%–50% of patients with *M. pneumoniae* infection will develop cold agglutinins.

Interfering Factors

1. A high cold agglutinin titer interferes with blood typing and crossmatching.
2. High titers are sometimes spontaneous in older persons and may persist for years.
3. Antibiotic therapy may interfere with cold agglutinin development.

Interventions

Pretest Patient Care

1. Explain test purpose and procedure.
2. Follow guidelines in Chapter 1 for safe, effective, informed *pretest* care.

Posttest Patient Care

1. Review test results; report and record findings. Modify the nursing care plan as needed. Counsel the patient regarding abnormal findings; explain the need for possible follow-up testing and treatment. See Interpreting Results of Immunologic Tests on page 537. Cold agglutinin titers rise during the second and third week of illness before rapidly returning to baseline levels. The test should be repeated at appropriate intervals.
2. Follow guidelines in Chapter 1 for safe, effective, informed *posttest* care.

● Cryoglobulin Test

Cryoglobulins are proteins that reversibly precipitate or gel at 0° to 4°C. They are classified as follows:

1. Type I (monoclonal)
2. Type II (mixed cryoglobulins, in which a monoclonal is directed against a polyclonal immunoglobulin)
3. Type III (polyclonal, of which no monoclonal protein is found)

Types I and II are associated with monoclonal gammopathies, a group of diseases (see Immunofixation Electrophoresis [IFE], Serum and Urine) in which a monoclonal protein is produced by neoplastic plasma cells or lymphocytes. Types II and III cryoglobulins are circulating immune complexes produced in response to a variety of antigens, including viral, bacterial, and autologous antigens.

The normal proteins of serum do not precipitate in the cold. Blood should be collected, allowed to clot, and centrifuged at 37°C. The serum should be separated at 37°C to ensure that the cryoglobulins will remain in the serum. The serum is then refrigerated and checked each day (up to 7 days) for the presence of a white precipitate or gel. Warming the serum to 37°C will reverse the precipitation.

The amount of cryoglobulin present can be quantified by filling a hematocrit tube with serum, incubating at 1°C, centrifuging at 1°C at 750 g for 30 minutes, and reading the cryocrit.

To characterize the cryoprotein, the precipitate is washed (cold saline) and redissolved (warm saline). IFE will identify the immunoglobulin classes present.

Normal Findings

Negative for cryoglobulin

If positive after 3 to 7 days at 4°C, IFE on the cryoprecipitate is performed to identify the protein complex.

Procedure

1. Collect a 15-mL blood serum sample in a red-topped tube. Observe standard precautions. Keep the specimen at 37°C until the cells are separated.
2. Refrigerate the serum for a minimum of 72 hours, although 7 days is better to determine the presence of a cryoglobulin.

Clinical Implications

The tendency of cryoglobulins to precipitate at low temperatures may occlude blood vessels; symptoms include Raynaud's phenomenon, vascular purpura, bleeding tendencies, cold-induced urticaria, pain, and cyanosis.

Type I cryoglobulinemia is associated with monoclonal gammopathy of undetermined significance (MGUS), macroglobulinemia, or multiple myeloma.

Type II cryoglobulinemia is associated with autoimmune disorders such as vasculitis, glomerulonephritis, SLE, RA, and Sjögren's syndrome. It may also be seen in diseases such as hepatitis, IM, CMV, and TPM.

Type III cryoglobulinemia is usually associated with the same disease spectrum as type II and may take the full 7 days to appear.

A cryoprecipitate in plasma but not serum is caused by *cryofibrinogen*. Cryofibrinogens are rare and can be associated with vasculitis.

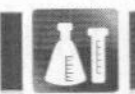

CLINICAL ALERT

The presence of cryoglobulins may cause erroneous results with some automated hematology instruments.

Interventions

Pretest Patient Care

1. Explain test purpose and procedure.
2. Follow guidelines in Chapter 1 for safe, effective, informed *pretest* care.

Posttest Patient Care

1. Review test results; report and record findings. Modify the nursing care plan as needed. Counsel the patient regarding abnormal findings; explain the need for possible follow-up testing and treatment. Continue to monitor for infections, collagen disorders, and malignant blood cell disease.
2. Follow guidelines in Chapter 1 for safe, effective, informed *posttest* care.

● Total Hemolytic Complement (CH_{50})

Complement (C) is a complex sequential cascade system in which inactive proteins become active and interact much like the clotting system. The complement system is important as part of the body's defense mechanism against infection (Fig. 8.2). Activation of complement results in cell lysis, release of histamine from mast cells and platelets, increased vascular permeability, contraction of smooth muscle, and chemotaxis of leukocytes and neutralization of certain viruses. These inactive proteins constitute about 10% of the globulins in normal blood serum. The complement system is also interrelated with

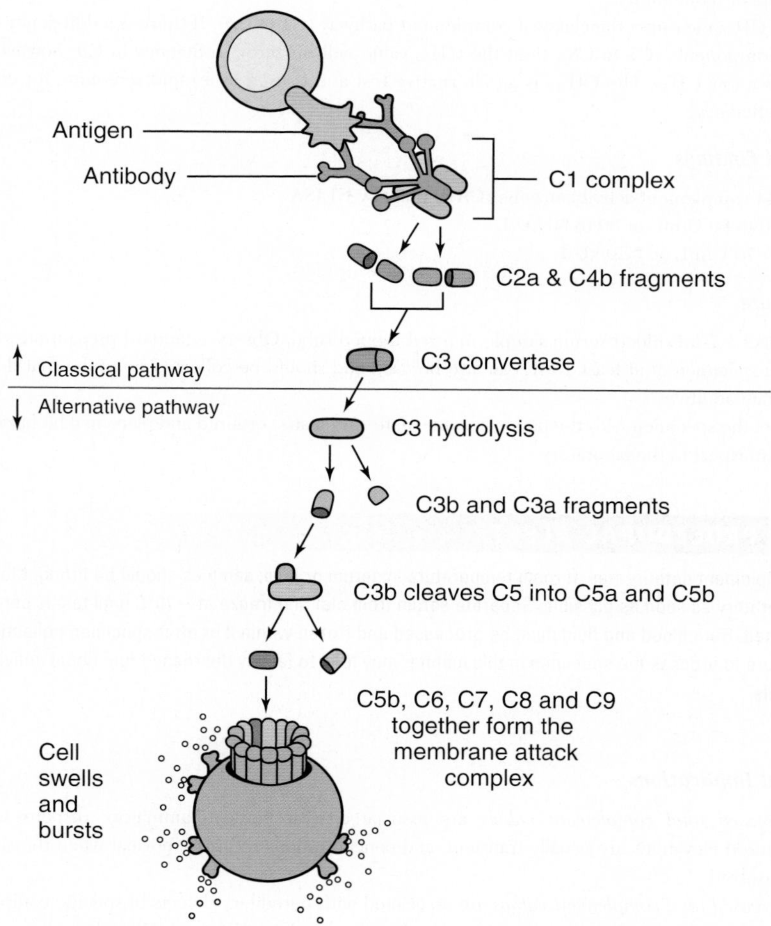

FIGURE 8.2. The complement system is made up of about 25 proteins that work together to "complement" the action of antibodies in destroying bacteria. Complement proteins circulate in the blood in an inactive form. When the first protein in the complement series is activated—typically by antibody that has locked onto an antigen—it sets in motion a domino effect. Each component takes its turn in a precise chain of steps known as the complement cascade. The end product is a cylinder inserted into—and puncturing a hole in—the cell's wall. With fluids and molecules flowing in and out, the cell swells and bursts. (From U.S. Department of Health and Human Services: Understanding the immune system. NIH publication No. 03-5423. Washington, DC, Author, 2003.)

the coagulation, fibrinolytic, and kinin systems. The action of complement, however, is not always beneficial. The potent reactions mediated by this complex system are not always contained. In the presence of gram-negative bacteremia, the complement can escape its built-in control mechanisms, causing severe damage to the body. It is not clear how this happens, but it is known that complement abnormalities develop before shock occurs.

This test screens for certain autoimmune diseases, estimates the extent of immune complex formation, and detects all inherited and most acquired immune deficiencies. Serial measurements monitor disease course and treatment in SLE, RA, and glomerulonephritis. It is a useful adjunct for rheumatoid factor and antinuclear antibody (ANA) testing when immune complexes appear to be the primary mediators of tissue injury.

The CH_{50} measures the classical complement pathway (C1 to C9). If there is a deficiency of one of the components (C1 to C8), then the CH_{50} value will be zero. Deficiency in C9, however, will result in a low CH_{50}. The CH_{100} is an alternative test and is used as a rapid screening for complement deficiency.

Normal Findings

60 to 144 complement activity enzyme (CAE) units by ELISA
CH_{50}: 30 to 60 U/mL or 30 to 60 kU/L
CH_{100}: >70 U/mL or >70 kU/L

Procedure

1. Collect a 7-mL blood serum sample in a red-topped tube. Observe standard precautions. A joint fluid specimen of at least 1 mL can also be used and should be collected in a tube that does not contain additives.
2. Label the specimen with the patient's name, date, and test(s) ordered and place in a biohazard bag for transport to the laboratory.

PROCEDURAL ALERT

Complement deteriorates at room temperature in serum or fluid; samples should be brought to the laboratory as soon as possible. Separate serum from clot and freeze at −70°C until test is performed. Both blood and fluid must be processed and frozen within 2 hr after specimen collection. Failure to process the specimen in this manner may lead to falsely decreased functional activity levels.

Clinical Implications

1. *Increased total complement values* are associated with most inflammatory responses; these acquired elevations are usually transient, and concentrations return to normal when the situation is resolved.
2. *Decreased total complement values* are associated with hereditary defects of specific complement components. In C2 deficiency, autoimmune disorders occur as SLE, and C1q deficiency may cause hereditary angioedema (HAE).
   a. Complement consumption by activation of the alternative pathway, an amplification of the classic pathway not requiring an "immunologic" stimulus, can be seen in the following conditions:
      (1) Gram-negative septicemia
      (2) Subacute bacterial endocarditis
      (3) Acute poststreptococcal glomerulonephritis
      (4) Membranoproliferative glomerulonephritis

b. Complement consumption due to activation of the classic pathway by immune complex formation occurs in the following conditions:
   (1) SLE
   (2) Serum sickness
   (3) Acute vasculitis
   (4) Severe RA
   (5) Hepatitis
   (6) Cryoglobulinemia

Interventions

See Antinuclear Antibody (ANA) Test on pages 591 to 592.

● C3 Complement Component

C3 constitutes 70% of the total protein in the complement system and is essential to the activation of both classic and alternative pathways. Along with the other components of the complement system, C3 may be used up in reactions that occur in some antigen–antibody reactions. C3 is synthesized in the liver, macrophages, fibroblasts, lymphoid cells, and skin.

This test is done when it is suspected that individual complement component concentrations are abnormally reduced. This test and the C1q and C4 tests are the most frequently ordered complement measurements. There is a correlation between most forms of nephritis, the degree of nephritis severity, and C3 levels. C3 is useful for assessing disease activity in SLE.

Normal Findings

75 to 175 mg/dL or 0.75 to 1.75 g/L by rate nephelometry

Procedure

1. Collect a 7-mL blood serum sample in a red-topped tube. Observe standard precautions. This amount is sufficient for both C3 and C4 testing.
2. Label the specimen with the patient's name, date, and test(s) ordered and place in a biohazard bag for transport to the laboratory.

Clinical Implications

1. *Decreased C3 levels* are associated with most active diseases with immune complex formation.
   a. Severe recurrent bacterial infections due to C3 homozygous deficiency
   b. Absence of C3b inactivator factor
   c. Acute poststreptococcal glomerulonephritis
   d. Immune complex disease
   e. Active SLE
   f. Membranoproliferative glomerulonephritis
   g. Nephritis
   h. End-stage liver disease
2. *Increased levels* are found in numerous inflammatory states.

Interventions

See Antinuclear Antibody (ANA) Test.

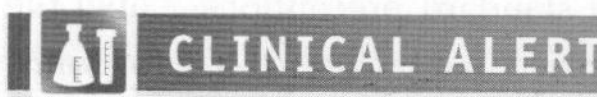

Patients with low C3 levels are in danger of shock leading to death.

• C4 Complement Component

C4 is another of the components of the complement system and is synthesized in bone and lung tissue. C4 may be bypassed in the alternative complement pathway when immune complexes are not involved, or it may be used up in the very complicated series of reactions that follow many antigen–antibody reactions.

This is a follow-up test done when total complement levels are abnormally decreased. It can also be ordered to confirm HAE if the C1 inhibitor result is decreased.

Normal Findings

14 to 40 mg/dL or 140 to 400 mg/L by rate nephelometry.

Procedure

1. Collect a 7-mL blood serum sample in a red-topped tube. Observe standard precautions. This amount is sufficient for both C3 and C4 testing.
2. Label the specimen with the patient's name, date, and tests ordered and place in a biohazard bag for transport to the laboratory.

Clinical Implications

1. *Decreased C4 levels* are associated with the following conditions:
   a. Acute SLE
   b. Early glomerulonephritis
   c. Immune complex disease
   d. Cryoglobulinemia
   e. Inborn C4 deficiency
   f. Hereditary angioneurotic edema
2. *Increased C4 levels* are associated with malignancies.

Interventions

See Antinuclear Antibody (ANA) Test.

• C'1 Esterase Inhibitor (C'1 INH)

C'1 esterase inhibitor is a glycoprotein. It acts as a regulatory brake on the complement activation process. Decreased production of this glycoprotein results in HAE.

This determination is an important tool for diagnosing HAE, a disorder caused by a low concentration of C'1 esterase inhibitor or by an abnormal structure of the protein. Affected persons are apparently heterozygous for the condition. It is also used in the differential diagnosis of the more prevalent but less serious allergic and nonfamilial angioedema.

Normal Findings

18 to 40 mg/dL or 180 to 400 mg/L by an immunoturbidimetric assay

Procedure

1. Collect a 7-mL serum specimen in a red-topped tube. Observe standard precautions. Label the specimen with the patient's name, date, and test(s) ordered and place in a biohazard bag for transport to the laboratory.
2. Spin down, separate from clot, and freeze 1.0 mL of serum at −70°C until testing is performed.

Clinical Implications

1. Decreased values are associated with HAE, a genetic disease characterized by acute edema of subcutaneous tissue, gastrointestinal tract, or upper airway tract.
2. During acute attacks of the disease, C4 and C2 components can be markedly reduced.

Interventions

See Antinuclear Antibody (ANA) Test (next section).

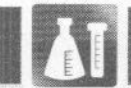

CLINICAL ALERT

Prednisolone and transfusions of fresh-frozen plasma have been successfully used to treat HAE.

TESTS FOR AUTOIMMUNITY AND SYSTEMIC RHEUMATIC DISEASE (SRD)

● Antinuclear Antibody (ANA) Test

Measurement of ANAs in serum is the most commonly performed screening test for autoantibodies in patients suspected of having SRD. SRDs are also called *connective tissue diseases* or *collagen diseases.* Examples of SRDs include SLE, mixed connective tissue disease (MCTD), Sjögren's syndrome, scleroderma, CREST (calcinosis, Raynaud's phenomenon, esophageal dysfunction, sclerodactyly, and telangiectasia) syndrome, RA, and polymyositis dermatomyositis.

The diagnosis of SLE is difficult because clinical signs and symptoms are varied and mimic other SRDs. SLE is characterized by the production of autoantibodies to nuclear antigens; that is, anti–double-stranded DNA (anti-dsDNA). SLE is a multisystem disease that can affect every organ system in the body, especially the kidneys.

Results of tests for ANAs by ELISA show that ELISA and traditional indirect IFA methods for ANA are substantially equivalent; however, ELISAs require less time and technical expertise, whereas IFAs are more sensitive. Many laboratories are using a combination of both methods. ANA samples are screened using an ELISA assay. All samples that screen positive or equivocal are titered using Hep-2 cells, and the titer and pattern are reported. In general, a titer ≥1:160 is considered significantly positive. Low-titer ANAs are common with advancing age. When cell culture substrates (Hep-2 cells) are used, the ANA incidence is 99% in SLE.

Normal Findings

ANA screen: negative by ELISA and IFA methods
If positive by IFA, the specimen is titered and a pattern is reported.
ANA titer: <1:160

Procedure

1. Collect a 7-mL blood serum sample in a red-topped tube. Observe standard precautions.
2. Label the specimen with the patient's name, date, and tests ordered and place in a biohazard bag for transport to the laboratory.

Clinical Implications

1. A positive result does not confirm a disease; low titers of ANAs are present in elderly people and some apparently healthy, normal people.

2. The diagnosis of an SRD is based primarily on the presence of compatible clinical signs and symptoms. The results of tests for autoantibodies, including ANAs and specific autoantibodies (e.g., ribonucleoprotein [RNP], Smith [Sm], SSA, SSB, Scl-70, Jo-1) are ancillary. Additional diagnostic criteria include consistent histopathology or specific radiographic findings.

Interfering Factors

1. Drugs, such as procainamide and hydralazine, may cause a positive ANA result.
2. Positive ANA levels may be found after viral illnesses and with some chronic infections.

Interventions

Pretest Patient Care

1. Explain test purpose and procedure. A strong positive result, that is, >3 on ELISA or ≥1:160 on IFA, may require follow-up testing of specific autoantibodies.
2. Follow guidelines in Chapter 1 for safe, effective, informed *pretest* care.

Posttest Patient Care

1. Review test results; report and record findings. Modify the nursing care plan as needed. Counsel the patient regarding abnormal findings; explain the need for possible follow-up testing and treatment.
2. SRDs, such as SLE, must be dealt with on a continuing basis and may require certain lifestyle changes. Repeat testing evaluates the effectiveness of therapy. Minor symptoms, in the absence of major organ involvement, are frequently treated with NSAIDs such as salicylates. Cutaneous manifestations respond to topical corticosteroid treatments. Short-acting corticosteroids, such as prednisone, are necessary if acute serologic changes and severe clinical manifestations appear.
3. Long-term moderate- to high-dose corticosteroids are central regimens prescribed for diffuse glomerulonephritis as well as RA.
4. Corticosteroid dosage may be reduced and renal disease favorably managed by adding immunosuppressive drugs to the therapy regimen. Infection, secondary to immunosuppressive treatment, is a leading cause of death in patients with SRDs. Patient education plays a major role in prevention of infection.
5. Follow guidelines in Chapter 1 for safe, effective, informed *posttest* care.

● Anticentromere Antibody Test

The variant of scleroderma, the CREST syndrome, is characterized by calcinosis, Raynaud's phenomenon, esophageal dysfunction, sclerodactyly, and telangiectasia. Characteristically, anticentromere antibodies appear in about 90% of these patients. This antibody is detected by using Hep-2 cells in various stages of cell division. The centromere region of the cell chromosomes will stain if an anticentromere antibody is present.

Normal Findings

Negative for anticentromere antibody by IFA or ELISA. If positive by IFA, the serum is titered.

Procedure

1. Collect a 7-mL blood serum sample in a red-topped tube. Observe standard precautions.
2. Label the specimen with the patient's name, date, and test(s) ordered and place in a biohazard bag for transport to the laboratory.

Clinical Implications

Positive results are associated with the CREST syndrome in scleroderma.

Interventions

See Antinuclear Antibody (ANA) Test on pages 591 to 592.

Anti–Double-Stranded DNA (Anti-dsDNA) Antibody Test, IgG

Although not completely understood, the primary mechanism of tissue injury in SLE and related autoimmune disease is the formation of antigen–antibody immune complexes. Not all ANAs are pathogenic. For the few that are harmful, pathogenicity depends on the specific immunoglobulin class, ability to activate complement, size of the immune complex, and site of tissue deposition. For example, studies of immune complex–mediated tissue injury in the kidney have shown a clear relation between deposition of immune complexes and glomerular disease.

The anti-dsDNA test is done specifically to identify or differentiate native (i.e., double stranded) DNA antibodies found in 40% to 60% of patients with SLE during the active phase of their disease from other, nonnative DNA antibodies found in other rheumatic diseases. The presence of antibodies to dsDNA generally correlates with lupus nephritis. An anti-dsDNA test supports a diagnosis, allows monitoring of disease activity and response to therapy, and establishes a prognosis for SLE.

Normal Findings

Negative: <25 IU by ELISA
Borderline: 25 to 30 IU
Positive: 31 to 200 IU
Strongly positive: >200 IU

Procedure

1. Collect a 7-mL blood serum sample in a red-topped tube. Observe standard precautions.
2. Label the specimen with the patient's name, date, and test(s) ordered and place in a biohazard bag for transport to the laboratory.

Clinical Implications

1. Anti-dsDNA concentrations may decrease with successful therapy and may increase with an acute recurrence of SLE.
2. DNA–anti-dsDNA immune complexes play a role in SLE pathogenesis through the deposit of these complexes in the kidney and other tissues.

Interfering Factors

1. The Farr assay, a radioimmunoassay (RIA) method, detects both single-stranded DNA (ssDNA) and dsDNA antibodies.
2. Antibodies to ssDNA are nonspecific but are associated with various other rheumatic diseases.

Interventions

See Antinuclear Antibody (ANA) Test on pages 591 to 592.

Rheumatoid Factor (Rheumatoid Arthritis [RA] Factor) Test

The blood of many persons with RA contains a macroglobulin-type antibody called *rheumatoid factor* (RF). Evidence indicates that rheumatoid factors are anti–γ-globulin antibodies; however, until a specific antigen that produces RF is discovered, the exact nature of RF can only be speculated. Even more uncertain is the role that RF plays in RA. Although RF may cause or perpetuate the destructive changes associated with RA, it may also be incidental to these changes or may even serve some beneficial purpose. RF is sometimes found in blood serum from patients with other diseases, even though RF incidence and values are higher in patients with RA.

This test is useful in the diagnosis of RA. It measures RFs (antibodies directed against the Fc fragment of IgG). These are usually IgM antibodies, but they may also be IgG or IgA. Four of the following clinical criteria must be present to diagnose RA.

Revised American College of Rheumatology Criteria for Rheumatoid Arthritis

1. Morning stiffness for at least 6 weeks
2. Pain on motion or tenderness in at least one joint for at least 6 weeks
3. Swelling in at least one joint for at least 6 weeks
4. Swelling in at least one other joint for at least 6 weeks
5. Symmetrical joint swelling with simultaneous involvement of the same joint on both sides of the body
6. Subcutaneous nodules
7. X-ray changes, including bony decalcification

Normal Findings

0 to 20 U/mL or 0 to 20 kU/L, based on rate nephelometry

Procedure

1. Collect a 7-mL blood serum sample in a red-topped tube. Observe standard precautions.
2. Label the specimen with the patient's name, date, and test(s) ordered and place in a biohazard bag for transport to the laboratory.

Clinical Implications

1. When a patient who tests positive improves, subsequent tests also remain positive unless titers were initially low.
2. A positive RF test result often supports a tentative diagnosis of early-onset RA (e.g., versus rheumatic fever).
3. RFs frequently occur in a variety of other diseases, such as SLE, endocarditis, tuberculosis, syphilis, sarcoidosis, cancer, viral infections, Sjögren's syndrome, and diseases affecting the liver, lung, or kidney as well as in patients who have received skin and renal allografts.
4. Absence of RF does not exclude the diagnosis or existence of RA.

Interfering Factors

The result is normally higher in older patients and in those who have received multiple vaccinations and transfusions.

Interventions

See section on Antinuclear Antibody Test.

● Antibodies to Extractable Nuclear Antigens (ENAs): Anti-Ribonucleoprotein (RNP); Anti-Smith (Sm); Anti-Sjögren's Syndrome (SSA, SSB); Anti-Scleroderma (Scl-70); Anti-Jo-1 (Jo-1)

The extractable nuclear antigens (ENAs), another group of nuclear antigens (nonhistone proteins) to which autoantibodies may develop, are so named because of their presence in saline solution extracts of certain nonhuman cells. The most common ENAs are RNP and Sm.

Anti-RNP is elevated in 35% to 40% of SLE patients and in patients with other connective tissue diseases, notably MCTD. MCTD is characterized by high levels of anti-RNP without autoantibodies to dsDNA or Sm. The disease resembles SLE but is not accompanied by renal involvement.

Anti-Sm is specific for SLE but occurs in only approximately 30% of the patients. The levels of anti-Sm may be related to disease activity in SLE.

Anti-SSA (Ro) has been detected in approximately 25% of patients with SLE and in 40% to 45% of patients with Sjögren's syndrome.

TABLE 8.10 Enzyme-Linked Immunosorbent Assay Screening for Specific Systemic Rheumatic Disease (SRD)

Test	Specific SRD
Anti-RNP	Mixed connective tissue disease (MCTD)
Anti-Sm (with or without RNP)	SLE, MCTD, Sjögren's syndrome
Anti-SSA(Ro) and/or anti-SSB(La)	Sjögren's syndrome
Anti-Scl-70	Scleroderma
Anti-Jo-1	Polymyositis

RNP, ribonucleoprotein; Scl-70, scleroderma; SLE, systemic lupus erythematosus; Sm, Smith; SSA/SSB, Sjögren's syndrome.

Anti-SSB (La) is found in approximately 10% to 15% of patients with SLE and up to 60% of patients with Sjögren's syndrome.

Anti-Scl-70 is considered specific for scleroderma (systemic sclerosis). These autoantibodies are found in up to 60% of scleroderma patients with extensive cutaneous disease and interstitial pulmonary fibrosis.

Anti-Jo-1 (antihistidyl transfer synthase) occurs in approximately 20% of patients with myositis, usually in patients with interstitial pulmonary fibrosis and symmetrical polyarthritis.

The ELISA assay is a screen for several nuclear antibodies. If the ENA screen result is borderline or positive, the following tests (Table 8.10) will be set up to determine the particular SRD.

Normal Findings for ENA and Individual Autoantibody Tests

Negative: <20 U/mL by ELISA
Borderline: 20 to 25 U/mL
Positive: >26 U/mL

Procedure

1. Collect a 7-mL blood serum sample in a red-topped tube. Observe standard precautions.
2. Label the specimen with the patient's name, date, and test(s) ordered and place in a biohazard bag for transport to the laboratory.

Clinical Implications

1. Results of serum tests for autoantibodies should not be relied on extensively to establish the diagnosis of a connective tissue disease. They must always be interpreted in conjunction with clinical findings.
2. Testing for autoantibodies to ENAs is not useful in patients without demonstrable ANAs.

Interventions

See Antinuclear Antibody (ANA) Test.

● Cardiolipin Antibodies, IgA, IgG, IgM

In patients with SLE, antibodies to cardiolipin (a negatively charged phospholipid) have been associated with arterial and venous thrombosis, thrombocytopenia, and recurrent fetal loss. Patients with the anticardiolipin syndrome have one of the aforementioned clinical features and have antibodies to cardiolipin or a positive lupus anticoagulant test.

The antibodies present to cardiolipin may be of the IgA, IgG, or IgM isotype. Testing for the various antibody isotypes to cardiolipin aids in the diagnosis of the antiphospholipid syndrome in patients with SLE or lupus-like disorders. These tests are also useful for the prognostic assessment of pregnant patients with a history of recurrent fetal loss.

Normal Findings

<12 APL (IgA phospholipid units): absent or none detected
<15 GPL (IgG phospholipid units): absent or none detected
<12 MPL (IgM phospholipid units): absent or none detected

Procedure

1. Collect a 7-mL blood serum sample in a red-topped tube. Observe standard precautions.
2. Label the specimen with the patient's name, date, and test(s) ordered and place in a biohazard bag for transport to the laboratory.

Clinical Implications

1. Most patients with antiphospholipid antibody syndrome have moderate or high levels of cardiolipin antibodies and are positive for IgG only or IgG and IgM.
2. Elevated values are seen in spontaneous thrombosis and in patients with connective tissue disease.
3. Patients with current or prior syphilis infection may have a false-positive result without the risk for thrombosis.

Interventions

Pretest Patient Care

1. Explain test purpose and procedure.
2. Follow guidelines in Chapter 1 for safe, effective, informed *pretest* care.

Posttest Patient Care

1. Review test results; report and record findings. Modify the nursing care plan as needed. Counsel the patient regarding abnormal findings in light of the patient's history, physical findings, and other diagnostic procedures and results. Explain the need for possible follow-up testing and treatment. Transiently positive tests do occur for IgG and IgM antibodies, and it is recommended that positive results be confirmed by follow-up assay in 8 weeks.
2. Follow guidelines in Chapter 1 for safe, effective, informed *posttest* care.

● Autoimmune Thyroiditis, Thyroid Antibody Tests: Thyroglobulin Antibody, Thyroid Microsomal Antibody, Thyroperoxidase Antibody

There are several autoantibodies that are organ specific for the thyroid gland, but antithyroglobulin and antithyroperoxidase are ordered most frequently by healthcare providers when evaluating patients for hyperthyroidism, hypothyroidism, and thyroid cancer. In Graves' disease, which is autoimmune hyperthyroidism, and in Hashimoto's thyroiditis, which is autoimmune hypothyroidism, the presence of both antibodies can help confirm the diagnosis.

Thyroglobulin antibodies are directed against the glycoprotein thyroglobulin located in the thyroid follicles; thyroperoxidase (TPO) antibodies are directed against the membrane-bound glycoprotein TPO located in the cytoplasm of the epithelial cells surrounding the follicles.

Along with chemiluminescence technology, highly purified antigens have been used to improve specificity. For the antithyroperoxidase test, instead of using the entire microsomal antigen, this assay uses just the TPO component. TPO is considered the primary autoantigenic component of the microsomal antigen. Test systems that use the purified TPO (in place of the microsomal antigen) have greater specificity for the clinically significant autoantibody. Assays using microsomal antigen are detecting TPO antibody but may also detect antibodies to other parts of the microsomal antigen that have little or no clinical significance.

Normal Findings

Less than 1:100 for thyroglobulin and thyroid microsomal antibodies by CF antibody
Negative for thyroglobulin and thyroid microsomal antibodies by ELISA
Negative for thyroglobulin and TPO antibodies by chemiluminescence

Procedure

1. Collect 7-mL blood serum in a red-topped tube. Observe standard precautions.
2. Label the specimen with the patient's name, date, and test(s) ordered and place in a biohazard bag for transport to the laboratory.

Clinical Implications

1. High titers of thyroglobulin and thyroid microsomal antibodies (>1:400) are found in Hashimoto's disease, but elevations can also be seen in other autoimmune diseases.
2. Increased thyroid antibodies also occur in the following conditions:
   a. Graves' disease
   b. Thyroid carcinoma
   c. Idiopathic myxedema
   d. Pernicious anemia
   e. SLE, RA, Sjögren's syndrome
   f. Subacute thyroiditis
   g. Nontoxic nodular goiter

Interfering Factors

1. About 10% of the normal population may have low levels of thyroid antibodies with no symptoms of the disease. Incidence of low titer is higher in women and increases with age.
2. Antibody production may be confined to lymphocytes within the thyroid, resulting in negative serum test results.

Interventions

Pretest Patient Care

1. Explain test purpose. Thyroid antibody testing is done to confirm diagnosis. It is not to be relied on, however, for management of the disease.
2. Follow guidelines in Chapter 1 for safe, effective, informed *pretest* care.

Posttest Patient Care

1. Review test results; report and record findings. Modify the nursing care plan as needed. Counsel the patient regarding abnormal findings; explain the need for possible follow-up testing. The diagnosis of autoimmune thyroiditis is made on the basis of clinical observations, thyroid function tests (see Chapter 6), and the presence of circulating autoantibodies, such as thyroglobulin and microsomal (TPO).
2. Follow guidelines in Chapter 1 for safe, effective, informed *posttest* care.

AUTOIMMUNE LIVER DISEASE TESTS

● Anti–Smooth Muscle Antibody (ASMA) Test

Anti–smooth muscle antibody (ASMA) is associated with liver and bile duct autoimmune diseases. The immune response itself is believed to be responsible for the disease process.

Sera from patients with autoimmune chronic active hepatitis (CAH) contain antibodies to smooth muscle antigens that are detectable by IFA on tissues that contain smooth muscle, such as mouse stomach. The antibodies are predominantly IgG. This measurement differentiates CAH and PBC from other liver diseases in which ASMAs are seldom present (e.g., SLE). See Table 8.11.

Normal Findings

Negative by IFA
If positive, serum is titered.

Procedure

1. Collect a 7-mL blood serum sample in a red-topped tube. Observe standard precautions. This amount is sufficient for both ASMA and antimitochondrial antibody (AMA) testing.
2. Label the specimen with the patient's name, date, and test(s) ordered and place in a biohazard bag for transport to the laboratory.

Clinical Implications

1. ASMAs are found in CAH, a progressive disease of unknown etiology found predominantly in young women. It has factors characteristic of both acute and chronic hepatitis (80% of patients). If this disease is associated with a positive ANA test, the disease is often called *lupoid hepatitis*.
2. Antibody titers between 80 and 320 occur commonly in patients with CAH.

Interventions

Pretest Patient Care

1. Explain test purpose and procedure.
2. Follow guidelines in Chapter 1 for safe, effective, informed *pretest* care.

TABLE 8.11 Prevalence of Autoantibodies in Liver Disease

Disease	Anti–Smooth Muscle (%)	Antimitochondrial (%)	ANA (%)
Chronic active hepatitis	70–90	30–60	60
Chronic persistent hepatitis	45	15–20	15–30
Acute viral hepatitis	10–30	5–20	20
Acute alcoholic hepatitis	0	0	0
Biliary cirrhosis	30	60–70	5
Cryptogenic cirrhosis	15	30	0
Alcoholic (Laennec's) cirrhosis	0	0	0
Extrahepatic biliary obstruction	5–10	5–10	5

ANA, antinuclear antibody.

Posttest Patient Care

1. Review test results; report and record findings. Modify the nursing care plan if needed. Detection of ASMA by immunofluorescence assists in determining the presence of CAH and need for therapy when used in conjunction with other laboratory tests such as those used to evaluate liver enzymes, ANAs, and IgG levels. All of these are elevated in most patients with CAH.
2. Follow guidelines in Chapter 1 for safe, effective, informed *posttest* care.

● Antimitochondrial Antibody (AMA) Test

AMA is non–organ specific and non–species specific and is directed against a lipoprotein in the inner mitochondrial membrane. AMA is a marker for PBC, a chronic inflammatory liver disease, characterized by the progressive destruction of interlobular bile ducts with development of cholestasis and, eventually, cirrhosis.

The mitochondrial antigens recognized by AMAs in patients' sera have been classified as M1 through M9, with M2 recognized by AMAs in >90% of patients with PBC. The antibodies are predominantly IgG. This measurement aids in the diagnosis of PBC, a progressive disease most commonly seen in women in the second half of their reproductive years. There is also a genetic predisposition.

Normal Findings

Negative: <1.0 U, by IFA
Positive: >1.0 U
If positive, serum is titered.
Reference values are in arbitrary units and will vary with method of testing.

Procedure

1. Collect a 7-mL blood serum sample in a red-topped tube. Observe standard precautions. This amount is sufficient for both AMA and ASMA testing.
2. Label the specimen with the patient's name, date, and test(s) ordered and place in a biohazard bag for transport to the laboratory.

Clinical Implications

1. Elevated concentrations of AMAs are present in >90% of patients with PBC.
2. High titers are also associated with long-standing hepatic obstruction, chronic hepatitis, and cryptogenic cirrhosis.
3. Elevated levels are occasionally present in the following conditions:
   a. SLE
   b. RA
   c. Thyroid disease
   d. Pernicious anemia
   e. Idiopathic Addison's disease

Interventions

Pretest Patient Care

1. Explain test purpose and procedure.
2. Follow guidelines in Chapter 1 for safe, effective, informed *pretest* care.

Posttest Patient Care

1. Review test results; report and record findings. Modify the nursing care plan if needed. Immunofluorescence testing, along with quantitation of IgM and liver enzymes, both of which tend to be elevated in PBC, are reliable follow-up protocols.
2. Follow guidelines in Chapter 1 for safe, effective informed *posttest* care.

● Anti–Liver/Kidney Microsome Type 1 Antibody (LKM) Test

Antibodies to liver/kidney microsome antigens (anti–LKM-1) occur in a subset of patients with chronic autoimmune hepatitis (AIH). The clinical diagnosis of AIH is difficult because there are no particular signs, symptoms, or liver function test abnormalities that are specific enough to be considered diagnostic. Patients with this type of chronic AIH are predominantly children, but some patients are adults.

Different autoantibodies are found in the serum from patients with AIH. The discovery of the LKM-1 antibody led to the establishment of two subtypes of AIH. The percentage of type 2 AIH patients whose serum contains LKM-1 antibodies is 90%.

Patient sera are incubated on slides with mouse kidney and stomach. Anti–LKM-1 antibody produces a characteristic pattern, which allows it to be differentiated from the patterns produced by smooth muscle and mitochondrial antibodies on mouse tissue.

Normal Findings

Negative: <20 U for LKM-1 by IFA
Equivocal: 20 to 25 U
Positive: >25 U
If positive, serum is titered.
Reference values are in arbitrary units and will vary with method of testing.

Procedure

1. Collect a 7-mL blood serum sample in a red-topped tube. Observe standard precautions.
2. Label the specimen with the patient's name, date, and test(s) ordered and place in a biohazard bag for transport to the laboratory.

Interventions

Pretest Patient Care

1. Explain test purpose and procedure.
2. Follow guidelines in Chapter 1 for safe, effective, informed *pretest* care.

Posttest Patient Care

1. Review test results; report and record findings. Modify the nursing care plan if needed. The primary therapy for AIH is administration of corticosteroids. Steroid treatment should lead to rapid reduction in aspartate transaminase (AST) and ALT (liver enzyme) levels.
2. Follow guidelines in Chapter 1 for safe, effective, informed *posttest* care.

● Antiparietal Cell Antibody (APCA) Test

The disruption of normal intrinsic factor production or function due to autoimmune processes can lead to pernicious anemia. Antibodies to two antigens of the gastric parietal cell—antiparietal cell antibodies (APCAs) and intrinsic factor blocking antibodies—are found in patients with pernicious anemia (>80%).

This measurement is helpful in diagnosing chronic gastric disease and differentiating autoimmune pernicious anemia from other megaloblastic anemias. Persons with other anemias do not have detectable APCAs.

Normal Findings

Negative: <1:20 for APCA by IFA
Weakly positive: 1:20 to 1:40
Positive: ≥1:80
If positive, serum is titered.

Procedure

1. Collect a 7-mL blood serum sample in a red-topped tube. Observe standard precautions.
2. Label the specimen with the patient's name, date, and test(s) ordered and place in a biohazard bag for transport to the laboratory.

Clinical Implications

1. APCAs occur in >80% of patients with autoimmune pernicious anemia; 50% have antibodies to intrinsic factor.
2. Occasionally, APCAs are present in the following conditions:
   a. Gastric ulcer
   b. Gastric cancer
   c. Atrophic gastritis
   d. Thyroid disease
   e. Diabetes mellitus
   f. Iron-deficiency anemia

Interfering Factors

APCAs are present in many healthy adults >60 years of age.

Interventions

Pretest Patient Care

1. Explain test purpose and procedure.
2. Follow guidelines in Chapter 1 for safe, effective, informed *pretest* care.

Posttest Patient Care

1. Review test results; report and record findings. Modify the nursing care plan if needed. Detection of APCA may suggest need for more invasive testing, such as gastric biopsy to rule out gastrointestinal disease.
2. Follow guidelines in Chapter 1 for safe, effective, informed *posttest* care.

Antiglomerular Basement Membrane (AGBM) Antibody Test

Antibodies specific for renal structural components such as the glomerular basement membrane of the kidney can bind to respective tissue-fixed antigens to produce an immune response.

This test is primarily used in differentiating glomerular nephritis induced by AGBMs from other types of glomerular nephritis. AGBMs cause about 5% of glomerular nephritis; about two thirds of these patients may also develop pulmonary hemorrhage (Goodpasture's syndrome).

Normal Findings

Negative: <5 EU/mL by ELISA
Borderline: 5.1 to 20.0 EU/mL
Positive: 20.1 to 400 EU/mL
Negative: IgA by IFA
Negative: IgG by IFA
ELISA is about 87% sensitive and 98% specific, whereas the sensitivity of IFA is about 75%.

Procedure

1. Collect a 7-mL blood serum sample in a red-topped tube. Observe standard precautions.
2. Label the specimen with the patient's name, date and time of collection, and test(s) ordered.

Clinical Implications

AGBM antibodies are detected in the following conditions:

1. AGBM glomerular nephritis
2. Tubulointerstitial nephritis
3. AGBM Goodpasture's syndrome
4. Some patients with SLE

Interventions

Pretest Patient Care

1. Explain test purpose and procedure.
2. Follow guidelines in Chapter 1 for safe, effective, informed *pretest* care.

Posttest Patient Care

1. Review test results; report and record findings. Modify the nursing care plan as needed. Counsel the patient regarding abnormal finding; explain the need for possible follow-up testing and treatments that involve immunosuppressants and plasmapheresis, which are effective if started before renal failure is well advanced.
2. Follow guidelines in Chapter 1 for safe, effective, informed *posttest* care.

● Acetylcholine Receptor (AChR) Binding Antibody Test

Acetylcholine receptor antibodies (AChRs) appear in myasthenia gravis (MG). It is believed that this disease involves destruction by the muscle cells of AChRs bound by antibodies at the skeletal muscle motor end plate.

This measurement is considered to be the first-order test for MG in symptomatic patients. It also helps in managing response to immunosuppressive therapy. Second- and third-order tests for modulating and blocking antibodies, respectively, are ordered to confirm the diagnosis of acquired MG; distinguish acquired disease from congenital disease; and monitor the serologic process in the course of MG.

Normal Findings

Negative for AChR or <0.02 nmol/L (SI units are the same) by RIA

Procedure

1. Collect a 7-mL blood serum sample in a red-topped tube. Observe standard precautions.
2. Label the specimen with the patient's name, date, and test(s) ordered and place in a biohazard bag for transport to the laboratory.

Clinical Implications

1. AChR antibodies are found in about 90% of persons with generalized MG, 70% of persons with ocular MG, and 80% of persons in remission. These findings confirm the autoimmune nature of the disease.
2. Patients who have only eye symptoms tend to have lower titers than those with generalized myasthenia symptoms.

Interfering Factors

Positive results can be found in patients with Lambert-Eaton myasthenic syndrome (LES) or autoimmune liver disease.

Interventions

Pretest Patient Care

1. Explain test purpose. Assess for history of immunosuppressive drug treatment. Detection of AChR binding antibody is infrequent in such cases.
2. Follow guidelines in Chapter 1 for safe, effective, informed *pretest* care.

Posttest Patient Care

1. Review test results; report and record findings. Modify the nursing care plan as needed. Counsel the patient regarding abnormal findings; explain the need for possible follow-up testing. Additional tests are available to aid in the serologic diagnosis of MG include AChR blocking antibody, AChR modulating antibody, and striational antibodies. These are ordered according to presentation of neurologic symptoms. All these antibodies are less frequently detected in the early stages of MG (within 1 year of onset) and in patients treated with immunosuppressive drugs. None are found in cases of congenital MG.
2. Follow guidelines in Chapter 1 for safe, effective, informed *posttest* care.

● Anti-Insulin Antibody Test

Patients with diabetes may form antibodies to the insulin they take and require larger doses because insulin is not available for glucose metabolism when it is partially complexed with these antibodies. Insulin antibodies are immunoglobulins called *anti-insulin antibodies*; they act as insulin-transporting proteins. The most common type of anti-insulin antibody is IgG, but it is found in all five classes of immunoglobulins in insulin-treated patients. These immunoglobulins, especially IgE, may be responsible for allergic manifestations; IgM may cause insulin resistance.

This insulin antibody level provides information for determining the most appropriate treatment for certain diabetic patients. It may focus the reason for allergic manifestations. It can identify a state of insulin resistance in which the daily insulin requirement exceeds 200 U for more than 2 days and may be associated with elevated anti-insulin antibody titers and insulin-binding capacity.

Normal Findings

Negative: <3% binding of the patient's serum with labeled beef, human, and pork insulin SI units when performed by RIA

Procedure

1. Collect a 7-mL blood serum sample from a fasting patient. Collect in a red-topped tube. Observe standard precautions.
2. Label the specimen with the patient's name, date, and test(s) ordered and place in a biohazard bag for transport to the laboratory.

Clinical Implications

Anti-insulin antibody elevations are associated with insulin resistance and allergies to insulin.

Interventions

Pretest Patient Care

1. Explain purpose of test. Fasting is required. Check with individual laboratory for time frames.
2. Follow guidelines in Chapter 1 for safe, effective, informed *pretest* care.

Posttest Patient Care

1. Review test results; report and record findings. Modify the nursing care plan if needed. Based on antibody levels present and clinical findings, the dosage of insulin is changed to reduce or prevent further allergic manifestations and insulin resistance.
2. Follow guidelines in Chapter 1 for safe, effective, informed *posttest* care.

● Gliadin Antibodies, IgA and IgG

Antibodies to gliadin (wheat protein) have been shown conclusively to be the toxic agent in celiac disease. Originally, a series of multiple intestinal biopsies was required to diagnose celiac and related intestinal diseases. More recently, serologic testing has been strongly suggested for screening patients with suspected gluten-sensitive enteropathy as well as for monitoring dietary compliance.

Celiac disease usually begins in infancy soon after introduction of cereals to the diet, but symptoms may disappear spontaneously in later childhood despite continued signs of malabsorption. Strict avoidance of gluten in the diet is recommended to control the disease.

Both IgG and IgA gliadin antibodies are detected in sera of patients with gluten-sensitive enteropathy. IgG antigliadin antibodies seem more sensitive but are less specific than the IgA class antibodies. The best strategy for at-risk populations includes testing for both classes of gliadin antibodies.

Normal Findings

Values are given for >2 years of age and are for IgA or IgG.
Negative: <25 U/mL by ELISA
Weakly positive: 25 to 50 U/mL
Positive: >50 U/mL

Procedure

1. Collect a 7-mL blood serum sample in a red-topped tube. Observe standard precautions.
2. Label the specimen with the patient's name, date, and test(s) ordered and place in a biohazard bag for transport to the laboratory.

Clinical Implications

1. The gliadin antibody assay has a sensitivity of 95% for active, untreated celiac disease when both IgG and IgA are used. The test has an overall specificity of 90%.
2. A negative IgA result in an untreated patient does not rule out gluten-sensitive enteropathy, especially when associated with elevated levels of IgG gliadin antibodies.
3. Significant numbers of celiac patients are IgA deficient, which can serve as an explanation for this occurrence.
4. In treated patients known to express IgA antibodies, the IgA gliadin antibody level represents a better indicator of dietary compliance than the IgG level.
5. False-positive results (high antibody levels without the corresponding histologic features) are possible; other gastrointestinal disorders, especially Crohn's disease, postinfection malabsorption, and food protein intolerance (e.g., cow's milk), are known to induce circulating antigliadin antibodies.
6. Results of this assay should be used in conjunction with clinical findings and other serologic tests.

Interventions

Pretest Patient Care

1. Explain test purpose and procedure.
2. Follow guidelines in Chapter 1 for safe, effective informed *pretest* care.

Posttest Patient Care

1. Review test results; report and record findings. Modify the nursing care plan if needed based on the test results in light of the patient's dietary history, including related clinical, laboratory, and histologic data. Positive results are possible in patients with other gastrointestinal disorders.
2. A biopsy of the proximal small bowel is recommended if the test is positive.
3. Often, a diagnosis provides some relief since the patient has been experiencing symptoms for many years and now can be treated appropriately.
4. Follow guidelines in Chapter 1 for safe, effective, informed *posttest* care.

● Antineutrophil Cytoplasmic Antibodies (ANCAs)

There are two types of antineutrophil cytoplasmic antibodies (ANCAs) distinguished by different immunofluorescent staining patterns using human neutrophil substrates:

1. cANCAs produce a diffuse cytoplasmic staining of neutrophils and monocytes and are specific for proteinase 3. cANCA is found in the sera of patients with Wegener's granulomatosis (WG).
2. pANCAs produce a perinuclear staining of neutrophils and are specific for other neutrophil enzymes, including myeloperoxidase (MPO), elastase, and lactoferrin. pANCA specific for MPO is found in the sera of patients with systemic vasculitis, most of whom have renal involvement characterized by pauci-immune necrotizing glomerulonephritis.

Tests for ANCA are performed by an IFA technique. Slides prepared from neutrophils are used as a substrate to bind ANCA so that it can be detected microscopically. Depending on the pattern of staining, as mentioned previously, two types of ANCAs exist: cANCA and pANCA.

Normal Findings

Negative for ANCAs by IFA
If positive for cANCA, results are titered.
If positive for pANCA, MPO testing is performed by ELISA. Not all specimens positive for pANCA are MPO positive.

Procedure

1. Collect a 7-mL blood serum sample in a red-topped tube. Observe standard precautions.
2. Label the specimen with the patient's name, date, and test(s) ordered and place in a biohazard bag for transport to the laboratory.

Clinical Implications

1. In patients with active generalized WG (pulmonary or renal involvement), the frequency of positive cANCA results approaches 85%. A negative test for cANCA does not rule out WG; however, false-positive results are rare.
2. In patients with known WG, rising titers of cANCA suggest relapse, and falling titers suggest successful treatment.
3. In patients with active renal disease, a positive pANCA suggests the presence of antibodies to MPO and pauci-immune necrotizing glomerulonephritis.
4. Results of tests for ANCA should be considered along with other clinical, laboratory, and histopathologic data in establishing the diagnosis of WG or systemic vasculitis.
5. Inflammatory bowel disease (IBD)-associated ANCAs are found in ulcerative colitis and Crohn's disease, specifically pANCA.

Interventions

Pretest Patient Care

1. Explain test purpose and procedure.
2. Follow guidelines in Chapter 1 for safe, effective, informed *pretest* care.

Posttest Patient Care

1. Review test results; report and record findings. Modify the nursing care plan if needed based on the test results in light of the patient's history, including other clinical, laboratory, and histopathologic data. Positive ANCA results (pANCA and, rarely, cANCA) may occur in patients with diseases other than WG or vasculitis, including Goodpasture's syndrome and SLE.
2. Follow guidelines in Chapter 1 for safe, effective, informed *posttest* care.

ALLERGY TESTING

● IgE Antibody, Single Allergen

A large number of substances have been found to have allergic potential. Measurements of IgE antibodies are useful to establish the presence of allergic diseases and to define the allergen specificity of immediate hypersensitivity reactions. Examples of allergic diseases include asthma, allergic rhinitis, dermatitis, anaphylaxis, and urticaria. In 2010, the National Institute of Allergy and Infectious Diseases established guidelines for testing of IgE levels in suspected food allergy cases.

The fluorescent enzyme immunoassay (FEIA) measures the increase and quantity of allergen-specific IgE antibodies and diagnoses an allergy to a specific allergen (e.g., molds, weeds, foods, insects). These measurements are used in people, especially children, with extrinsic asthma, hay fever, and atopic eczema and are an accurate and convenient alternative to skin testing. Although more expensive, they do not cause hypersensitivity reactions.

Additional antigens are continually being added; up-to-date information should be sought. Examples of categories that can be tested for include grasses, trees, molds, venoms, weeds, animal dander, foods, house dust, mites, antibiotics, and insects.

Normal Findings

Based on FEIA, the fluorescence is proportional to the amount of specific IgE present in the patient's sample.
Adult: <100 IU/mL or <100 kIU/L
Child:
<2 years old: <13 IU/mL or <13 kIU/L
<10 years old: <85 IU/mL or <85 kIU/L

Fluorescent Enzyme Immunoassay

Class	Interpretation
0	Negative
1	Equivocal
2	Positive
3	Positive
4	Strongly positive
5	Strongly positive
6	Strongly positive

Procedure

1. Collect a 7-mL blood serum sample in a red-topped tube. Observe standard precautions.
2. Label the specimen with the patient's name, date, and test(s) ordered and place in a biohazard bag for transport to the laboratory.

Clinical Implications

Positive results greater than or equal to class 2 are strongly associated with allergic symptoms on exposure to allergen.

CLINICAL ALERT

Eight foods (eggs, wheat, milk, soy, fish, shellfish, peanuts, tree nuts [e.g., cashews, walnuts]) account for about 90% of food allergies. Approximately 8% of children in the United States have some type of food allergy. Foods are listed below with their associated 95% risk for clinical allergy:
Egg (child): ≥7 IU/mL or ≥7 kIU/L
Milk (child): ≥15 IU/mL or ≥15 kIU/L
Peanuts: ≥14 IU/mL or ≥14 kIU/L
Fish: ≥20 IU/mL or ≥20 kIU/L

(Source: Chapman JA, Berstein IL, Lee RE, et al: Food allergy: A practice parameter. Ann Allergy Asthma Immunol 96:S1–S68, 2006.)

Interventions

Pretest Patient Care

1. Explain test purpose and procedure.
2. Follow guidelines in Chapter 1 for safe, effective, informed *pretest* care.

Posttest Patient Care

1. Review test results; report and record findings. Modify the nursing care plan as needed. Counsel the patient regarding abnormal findings; explain the need for possible follow-up testing and treatment. Negative results effectively rule out allergy induced by that allergen.
2. Follow guidelines in Chapter 1 for safe, effective, informed *posttest* care.

● Latex Allergy Testing (Latex-Specific IgE)

Latex-containing medical devices include gloves, catheters, and bandages, among many others. Millions of people, especially those in the healthcare profession, are susceptible to allergic reactions ranging from mild to severe when exposed to such products. It is recommended that patients at risk for latex allergy be tested before undergoing medical procedures that would expose them to latex. High-risk groups include healthcare workers, workers with industrial exposure to latex, children with spina bifida or urologic abnormalities due to high exposure to latex, and people who have undergone multiple surgeries.

This test measures IgE-mediated latex sensitivity and not irritation or delayed (type IV) reaction to latex. The method for testing is EIA, in which the color reaction measured is directly related to the amount of IgE specific for the test allergen in the sample.

Normal Findings

Negative for latex allergen: <0.35 IU/mL by EIA
Positive for latex allergen: >0.35 IU/mL

Procedure

1. Collect a 7-mL blood serum sample in a red-topped tube. Observe standard precautions.
2. Label the specimen with the patient's name, date, and test(s) ordered and place in a biohazard bag for transport to the laboratory.

Clinical Implications

1. Positive results are strongly associated with a latex allergy.
2. In studies comparing latex-specific IgE results with clinical history, symptoms, and other confirmatory tests, the sensitivity has been >80% and the specificity >90%.

Interventions

Pretest Patient Care

1. Explain test purpose and procedure. Positive history for latex may include the following factors:
   a. Swelling or itching from latex exposure
   b. Hand eczema
   c. Previously unexplained anaphylaxis
   d. Oral itching from cross-reactive foods (e.g., banana, kiwi, avocado, chestnuts)
   e. Multiple surgical procedures in infancy
2. Follow guidelines in Chapter 1 for safe, effective, informed *pretest* care.

Posttest Patient Care

1. Review test results; report and record findings. Modify the nursing care plan as needed. If negative by this test procedure, yet symptomatic, or if positive for this test, refer patient to an allergist.
2. Follow guidelines in Chapter 1 for safe, effective, informed *posttest* care.

PROTEIN CHEMISTRY TESTING/SERUM PROTEINS: ACUTE-PHASE PROTEINS AND CYTOKINES

● Ceruloplasmin

Measurement of ceruloplasmin aids in the diagnosis of copper metabolism disorders—that is, Wilson's disease. Copper bound to ceruloplasmin constitutes the largest amount of Cu^{2+} in the circulation. In Wilson's disease, Cu^{2+} mobilization from the liver is drastically reduced because of the low production of ceruloplasmin.

The test gives a quantitative measurement of the amount of ceruloplasmin in the patient's serum. Values can vary considerably from patient to patient and may be 50% of normal (pointing to some other primary defect). Patients with Wilson's disease are not always extremely low in ceruloplasmin.

Normal Findings

25 to 63 mg/dL or 250 to 630 mg/L by nephelometry

Procedure

1. Collect a 7-mL blood serum sample in a red-topped tube. Observe standard precautions.
2. Label the specimen with the patient's name, date, and test(s) ordered and place in a biohazard bag for transport to the laboratory.

Clinical Implications

1. Values <14 mg/dL are expected in Wilson's disease. Deficient ceruloplasmin, however, is not the primary defect in Wilson's disease and therefore can vary considerably from patient to patient.

Interfering Factors

1. Ceruloplasmin is affected by infections (a late acute-phase reactant) and liver function.
2. Birth control pills and pregnancy will increase ceruloplasmin.

Interventions

Pretest Patient Care

1. Explain test purpose. Measurement of this serum protein aids in diagnosing a copper metabolism disorder known as Wilson's disease.
2. Follow guidelines in Chapter 1 for safe, effective, informed *pretest* care.

Posttest Patient Care

1. Review test results; report and record findings. Modify the nursing care plan as needed. Counsel the patient regarding abnormal findings; explain the need for possible follow-up testing. Values vary from patient to patient and may be 50% or more of normal, pointing to some other defect.
2. Follow guidelines in Chapter 1 for safe, effective, informed *posttest* care.

● α_1-Antitrypsin

AAT is the most abundant serum protease inhibitor and inhibits trypsin and elastin as well as several other proteases. The release of proteolytic enzymes from plasma onto surface organs and into tissue spaces results in tissue damage unless inhibitors are present.

Measurement of AAT aids in the diagnosis of juvenile and adult cirrhosis of the liver. AAT deficiency has been associated with neonatal respiratory distress syndrome, severe protein-losing disorders, and pulmonary emphysema. The test is useful for individuals in whom familial chronic obstructive lung disease is suspected.

Normal Findings

Adults: 100 to 200 mg/dL or 1.0 to 2.0 g/L by nephelometry
Newborns: 145 to 270 mg/dL or 1.45 to 2.70 g/L

Procedure

1. Collect a 7-mL blood serum sample in a red-topped tube. Observe standard precautions.
2. Label the specimen with the patient's name, date, and test(s) ordered and place in a biohazard bag for transport to the laboratory.

Clinical Implications

1. Patients with a serum AAT <70 mg/dL (<0.70 g/L) may have a homozygous deficiency and are at risk for early lung disease. AAT phenotyping should be done to confirm the presence of the homozygous deficiency.
2. If clinically indicated, patients with serum levels <125 mg/dL (<125 g/L) should be phenotyped to identify heterozygous individuals. The latter do not appear to be at increased risk for early emphysema.

Interfering Factors

AAT is an acute-phase reactant, and any inflammatory process will elevate serum AAT levels.

Interventions

Pretest Patient Care

1. Explain test purpose. Follow-up testing, that is, AAT phenotyping, may be necessary if decreased results are obtained.
2. Follow guidelines in Chapter 1 for safe, effective, informed *pretest* care.

Posttest Patient Care

1. Review test results; report and record findings. Modify the nursing care plan as needed. Counsel the patient regarding abnormal findings; explain the need for possible follow-up tests, such as phenotyping, which confirms that the deficiency is homozygous (increased risk of chronic lung disease) or heterozygous (little, if any, risk).
2. Follow guidelines in Chapter 1 for safe, effective, informed *posttest* care.

• C-Reactive Protein (CRP) and High-Sensitivity C-Reactive Protein (hs-CRP)

During an inflammatory process, a specific abnormal protein named C-reactive protein (CRP) appears in the blood in response to inflammatory cytokines such as interleukin-6 (IL-6). This protein is virtually absent from the blood serum of healthy persons. CRP is one of the most sensitive acute-phase reactants. Levels of CRP can increase dramatically (100-fold or more) after severe trauma, bacterial infection, inflammation, surgery, or neoplastic proliferation. Measurement of CRP has been used historically to assess activity of inflammatory disease, to detect infections after surgery, to detect transplant rejection, and to monitor these inflammatory processes.

There are two types of CRP assays. One measures a wide range of CRP levels to include those found in patients with acute infections. The reportable range is typically 0.3 to 20 mg/dL (3 to 200 mg/L). The second is a high-sensitivity CRP (hs-CRP) assay. The latter can detect a lower level of CRP to include those that may be of value in measuring the risk for a cardiac event. The sensitivity is to 0.01 mg/dL (0.10 mg/L). The hs-CRP is useful, therefore, for assessment of risk for developing myocardial infarction in patients presenting with acute coronary syndromes.

Normal Findings

<1.0 mg/dL or <10 mg/L by rate nephelometry for CRP
<0.1 mg/dL or <1 mg/L by immunoturbidimetric assay for hs-CRP

Procedure

1. Collect a 7-mL blood serum sample in a red-topped tube. Observe standard precautions.
2. Label the specimen with the patient's name, date, and test(s) ordered and place in a biohazard bag for transport to the laboratory.

Clinical Implications

1. The traditional test for CRP has added significance over the elevated erythrocyte sedimentation rate (ESR), which may be influenced by altered physiologic states. CRP tends to increase before rises in antibody titers and ESR levels occur. CRP levels also tend to decrease sooner than ESR levels.
2. The traditional test for CRP is elevated in rheumatic fever, RA, myocardial infarction, malignancy, bacterial and viral infections, and postoperatively (declines after fourth postoperative day).
3. A single test for hs-CRP may not reflect an individual patient's basal hs-CRP level; therefore, follow-up tests or serial measurements may be required in patients presenting with increased hs-CRP levels.
4. CRP levels may predict future cardiovascular events and can be used as a screening tool.

CRP Levels

<0.1 mg/dL or <1 mg/L: low risk
0.1 to 0.3 mg/dL or 1 to 3 mg/L: average risk
>0.3 mg/dL or >3 mg/L: high risk
>1.0 mg/dL or >10 mg/L: noncardiovascular cause should be considered

Interventions

Pretest Patient Care

1. Explain the test purpose and procedure. A fasting sample is preferred. Water may be taken.
2. Follow guidelines in Chapter 1 for safe, effective, informed *pretest* care.

Posttest Patient Care

1. Review test results; report and record findings. Modify the nursing care plan as needed. Counsel the patient regarding abnormal findings; explain the need for possible follow-up testing and treatment. Repeat testing is often necessary to establish an individual's basal hs-CRP concentration. A positive test indicates active inflammation but not its cause. CRP is an excellent tool for monitoring disease activity. hs-CRP is a tool for assessing cardiovascular risk.
2. In RA, the traditional test for CRP becomes negative with successful treatment and indicates that the inflammation has subsided.
3. Follow guidelines in Chapter 1 for safe, effective, informed *posttest* care.

● Prion Proteins

Prions are proteins that occur in both heredity forms and infectious disease. Prions do not contain RNA or DNA. No immune response has been detected. This test is done to diagnose prion brain disease, such as Creutzfeldt-Jacob disease and spongiform encephalitis (mad cow disease). The structure and dynamics of proteins become somewhat problematic when developing anti-based diagnostic tests. This is particularly relevant in the case of diagnostic tests for prion diseases. As an example, prion diseases of the CNS are a result of conformational changes in the prion protein. The scrapie prion protein (PrP^{Sc}), which is the lethal form, is chemically indistinguishable from the normal cellular prion protein (PrP^{C}). The conversion from PrP^{C} to the lethal PrP^{Sc} form has been under investigation and several mechanisms have been proposed, such as spontaneous conversion or assisted conversion.

Normal Findings

Negative for PrP^{Sc}

Procedure

1. Brain tissue samples are examined for evidence of the infectious prion or mutated gene in chromosome 20.

NOTE *Researchers continue work on developing diagnostic tests for the detection of prion proteins in blood and urine samples.*

Clinical Implications

1. *Abnormal finding of* PrP^{Sc} protein (disease-causing form) is pathogenic, which affects the cerebral cortex and cerebellum.
2. Gerstmann-Sträussler-Scheinker syndrome, a cause of hereditary dementia, occurs because of mutation in prion gene.
3. Fatal familial insomnia
4. Creutzfeldt-Jakob disease
5. Evidence of prion infectious disease may be transfusion-related

Interventions

Pretest Patient Care

1. Explain test purpose and procedure. Obtain from patient or family signs, symptoms, and history of encephalopathy or dementia (hereditary). Patients are usually very sick, and infectious disease is usually fatal.
2. Behavioral changes include ataxia, peripheral sensory changes, and dementia.

Posttest Patient Care

1. Review test results; report and record findings. Modify the nursing care plan as needed. Counsel the patient regarding abnormal findings; explain the need for possible follow-up testing and treatment. Monitor for encephalitis and dementia.
2. Provide comfort and support and special counseling regarding progression of disease. Death occurs about 12 months after appearance of first signs.

● Cytokines

Cytokines, a diverse group of proteins and peptides secreted by many cells (e.g., lymphocytes, T cells, monocytes, B cells, eosinophils), respond to an immunologic challenge. They are involved in immunity, allergy, and long-term memory (i.e., degenerative aspects of aging) and include interferons, interleukins, chemokines, inflammatory cytokines, and hematopoietic growth factors. Cytokines have been directly implicated in a number of diseases, such as asthma, interstitial cystitis, RA, septic shock, transplant rejection, cirrhosis, and multiple sclerosis. Most interleukins are produced by macrophages and lymphocytes. Interleukins need adequate amounts of fats and pyridoxine to be effective. Some, such as IL-3, are involved in fever, slow-wave sleep, bone resorption, and use of protein by muscles.

These tests are done to evaluate allergy, skin hypersensitivity, asthma, fever, inflammation, and healing. They are also used as tumor markers and to assess immune factors and rheumatic disorders.

Normal Findings

1. IL-1
   a. 3, 5, 7, 9, 11, 12, 13, 14, 15, 16, 17, and 18
   b. Normal: Physiologic levels are normally very low (few pg/mL or ng/L).
2. Interleukin-1a
   a. Plasma: 0.1 ± 1.4 pg/mL or ng/L
   b. Urine median: 1 to 4 pg/µmol creatinine or µg/mol creatinine
3. IL-1b
   a. Blood: 4.60 ± 300 pg/mL or ng/L
   b. Serum: 0.07 ± 0.02 ng/mL or µg/L
4. IL-2
   a. Amniotic fluid (AMF): median, 1.35 ng/mL or 1.35 µg/L
   b. Plasma: 0.3 ± 0.47 pg/mL or 0.3 ± 0.5 ng/L
5. IL-4
   a. Serum: 0.75 ± 0.1 ng/mL or 0.75 ± 0.10 µg/L
   b. See eosinophil count; T cells stimulate eosinophil production.
6. IL-6
   a. Urine: 237 ± 92 ng/L or 237 ± 92 µg/L
   b. Blood: 1609 ± 710 pg/mL or 1.61 ± 0.71 µg/L
   c. Plasma: 2.50 ± 0.35 pg/mL or 2.50 ± 0.55 ng/L
   d. Serum: 0.4 to 2.1 pg/mL or 0.4 to 2.1 ng/L
   e. CSF: 0.04 to 12.5 ng/mL or 0.0 to 12.5 µg/L

7. IL-10
   a. Serum: 0.44 ± 9.5 ng/mL or 44 ± 10 μg/L
   b. AMF: <40 pg/mL or <40 ng/L
8. IL-8
   a. AMF: 237 ± 92 ng/L or same
9. Chemokines
   a. Feces: <22 to 4077 pg/g wet stool or 0.02 to 4.08 ng/g wet stool
   b. Plasma: 3.3 ± 0.3 pg/mL or ng/L
10. Tumor necrosis factors (TNF-α)
    a. ACSF: 22.3 ± 9.5 pg/mL or 1.31 ± 0.56 pmol/L
    b. Feces: <1 to 231 pg/g wet stool or <1 to 231 ng/g wet stool
    c. Plasma: 6.4 ± pg/mL or 6.4 ± 4.6 ng/L
    d. Serum: 0.12 ± 0.02 ng/mL or 7.0 ± 1.2 nmol/L
11. Interferon-γ
    a. Serum (S): 0.7 ± 1.8 pg/mL or 0.7 ± 1.8 ng/L
    b. Plasma (P): 3 ± 1 IU/mL or 3 ± 1 kIU/L

Procedure

1. Collect a stool, urine, or venous blood sample for serum analysis.
2. Cells from synovial fluid, bronchial secretions, AMF, and CSF may also be tested.

PROCEDURAL ALERT

Examine specimens within 5 hr. Avoid a freezing to thawing cycle while stored.

Clinical Implications

1. Pathophysiologic blood levels may indicate inflammation or cancer. Increases are associated with severity of disease.
2. Elevated levels in synovial fluid, CSF, AMF, urine, feces, and bronchoalveolar fluid may indicate immune disorders, SLE, and other pathologic or degenerative conditions.

Interfering Factors

1. Cytokines can continue to be produced after sample collection by the various cells in the fluid, urine, or feces.
2. Collection tubes can become contaminated by microorganisms, a potent stimulus of cytokine production.
3. Cytokines can degrade in the collection container.
4. Cytokines can bind to cell receptors during storage.
5. Circadian rhythms may affect results.

Interventions

Pretest Patient Care

1. Explain the purpose, procedure, benefits, and risks for cytokine tests and the complexities involved. For specimens other than plasma or serum, refer to specific chapters regarding specimen collection and patient care (e.g., urine in Chapter 3, spinal fluid in Chapter 5, amniotic fluid in Chapter 15, and stool [feces] in Chapter 4).
2. Obtain properly signed informed consent when necessary (e.g., spinal fluid sample collection). Explain that a local anesthetic will be injected into the skin. Assess for any previous reactions to any numbing or local anesthetic medicines.
3. Follow guidelines in Chapter 1 for safe, effective, informed *pretest* care.

Intratest Patient Care

Provide psychological support during specimen collection that may require more invasive procedures.

Posttest Patient Care

1. Review test results; report and record findings. Modify the nursing care plan as needed. Counsel the patient regarding abnormal findings; explain the need for possible follow-up testing and treatment. Explain the need for possible identification of chronic disease.
2. Provide the appropriate aftercare if more invasive specimen collection procedures were used (see Chapter 5 for spinal fluid collection aftercare).
3. Follow guidelines in Chapter 1 for safe, effective, informed *posttest* care.

● Tumor Markers

The underlying cause of cancer can be divided into four major classifications: viral, chemical, physical, and genetic. Cancers caused by viruses can be either RNA viruses (e.g., retrovirus HTLV-I, which causes ATL) or DNA viruses (e.g., HBV, which causes hepatocellular carcinoma). Chemical carcinogens can be classified as either genotoxic (targeting the DNA [e.g., nitroso compounds that when heated release toxic fumes or solvents such as trichloroethylene]) or nongenotoxic (targeting cell death directly or hormonal effects [e.g., synthetic pesticides or herbicides]). Physical factors associated with causing cancer include ultraviolet light (sunlight), ionizing radiation (x-rays), and asbestos fibers. Hereditary or genetic cancer can account for up to 30% of some forms of childhood cancers and 5% to 10% of adult cancers.

Cancerous cells differ from normal cells in many respects. Malignant cells grow more rapidly in an uncontrolled fashion and lack normal cell-to-cell interactions, and apoptotic (programmed cell death) mechanisms are disrupted when compared with normal cells. Normal cells, through a series of mutations (referred to as *hits*) and alterations of normal cell growth and cell interactions, can transition into cancerous cells. This unregulated and disorganized increase in cell growth is stimulated by the factors described earlier. Tumors, by definition, are spontaneous growth of abnormal cells leading to a swelling or enlargement of the underlying tissue. This abnormal cell growth, or cancer, can be detected by certain substances (tumor markers) found in the blood.

There are a number of factors that have either a protective effect or promote cancer growth.

Tumor Protectors	Tumor Promoters
Genetic resistance	Genetic susceptibility
Tumor suppressor genes	Age
Immune system	Smoking
Programmed cell death	Asbestos exposure
DNA repair	Resistance to cytotoxicity

Tumor markers include genetic markers (abnormal chromosomes or oncogenes), DNA analysis, oncofetal antigens, enzymes, hormones, placental proteins, steroid receptors, glucoproteins, tumor-associated antigens, tumor-specific antigens, and circulating immune complexes.

Tumor cells differ from normal cells in many ways. Physical examination and standard x-ray techniques can usually detect tumors as small as 1 cm in volume. A tumor mass of this size has completed 30 doublings (two thirds of its growth) and contains 1 billion (10^{-9}) cells. Certain tumor antigens, hormones, oncofetal proteins, and enzymes are secreted into the bloodstream by these tumors.

Malignant tumor cells are produced when DNA is damaged by some form of carcinogen, virus, radiation, or chemical causing the process of mitosis to go out of control. These growing, changed (mutant) cells express oncogenes. These oncogenes are capable of inducing or transforming cells into cancer cells or tumors. Tumor cells capable of forming metastases are likely to invade blood vessel walls; be released into the bloodstream, regional lymphatics, or interstitial stroma; and eventually spread to other organs. Tumor testing has focused on identifying certain tumor-related substances that might allow early detection of malignancy, determination of prognosis, and evaluation of tumor burden (i.e., size, location, and encroachment on other tissues or organs).

Tumor markers are used and developed to obtain greater sensitivity and specificity in determining the presence of cancer and tumor activity. These substances are found in body cells, fluids, and tissue. In general, these markers lack specificity for cancer; none is pathognomonic for any one type of neoplasm. Tumor marker studies do not replace biopsy and pathologic tissue examination and are not ideal for screening for specific cancers, making a diagnosis, or predicting programs for symptomatic patients, but they are effective for tumor staging, monitoring response to therapy, detecting disease recurrence, and early detection of cancer recurrence. Diagnosis still derives from a biopsy and tissue examination, comprehensive patient history, physical examination, and other diagnostic procedures.

The following are diagnostic, prognostic, and predictive markers:

1. Oncofetal antigens (Oncofetal antigens, normally produced in the fetus, are reactivated with cancer cell transformation.)
   a. Carcinoembryonic antigen (CEA)
   b. α-Fetoprotein (AFP)
   c. Proteins
   d. CA 125
   e. CA 19-9
   f. CA 15-3
   g. CA 549
   h. Tissue polypeptide antigen (TPA)
   i. Prostate-specific antigen (PSA)
   j. *hK2* and *hK3* of gene family = kallikreins
   k. Human glandular kallikrein for prostate cancer
2. Placental proteins
   a. Human chorionic gonadotropin (hCG and β-hCG)
   b. Human placental lactogen (HPL)
   c. Placental alkaline phosphatase (PALP)
3. Enzymes and isoenzymes
   a. Prostatic acid phosphatase (PAP)
   b. Creatine kinase (CK)-BB isoenzyme
   c. Alkaline phosphatase (ALP)
   d. Neuron-specific enolase (NSE)
   e. Lactate dehydrogenase isoenzyme (LDI)
   f. Lysozyme (muramidase)
4. Hormones
   a. Hormones, both normally produced by the tissue and ectopic
   b. γ-Glutamyl transpeptidase (GGT)
   c. Luteinizing hormone
   d. Amylase
   e. Terminal deoxynucleotidyl transferase (TDD)
   f. hCG—trophoblastic tumors
   g. Nonseminomatous testicular tumors
   h. Hydroxyindoleacetic acid (HIAA)
   i. Epinephrine and norepinephrine—pheochromocytoma and related malignancies

j. 17-Ketosteroids
k. Gastrin-Zollinger-Ellison syndrome (gastrinoma)
l. Renin—produced by kidney
m. Calcitonin-medullary carcinoma of the thyroid (not normally produced by the tissue)
n. Adrenocorticotropic hormone (ACTH)—small cell carcinoma of the lung
o. Antidiuretic hormone (ADH)
p. Parathyroid-related peptide
q. Erythropoietin
r. Gastrin

5. (Serotonin) immunoglobulins
   a. IgG
   b. IgA
   c. IgM
   d. IgD
   e. IgE
   f. κ and λ light chains
6. Steroid receptors
   a. Estrogen and progesterone receptors (ER and PR)
   b. Epidermal growth factor receptor (EGFR)
   c. HER-2 (human epidermal growth factor receptors)
   d. Androgen receptors
   e. Corticosteroid receptors
7. Immunocomplex typing
   a. Lymphoid cells
   b. Myeloid cells
   c. Cytokines
8. DNA analysis
   a. Ploidy and S-phase fraction
   b. See Chapter 11 for more information.
9. Molecular diagnosis
   a. Oncogene and suppressor genes
   b. Genetic changes
   c. See Chapter 11 for more information.

Normal Findings

See Table 8.12 for the value for each specific tumor marker.

Procedure

1. Be aware that most tumor marker tests involve obtaining either venous plasma or serum, urine or bladder washings, or CSF; some may require fasting.
2. Follow the specific directions from the laboratory or cancer center involved in the testing procedure. Be sure to note factors that interfere with test results.

Clinical Implications

1. Tumor markers, substances produced and secreted by tumor cells and found in serum, urine, or tissue of persons with cancer, are indicative of tumor activity.
2. Table 8.13 includes types of cytokines, their origin and target cells, and clinical implications.

TABLE 8.12 Tumor-Specific and Tumor-Associated Agents

Name of Test Clinical Marker in Current Use and Selected Normal Values[a]	Type of Cancer in Which Tumor Marker May Be Found	Conditions Other Than Cancer Associated With Abnormal Values
Enzymes		
1. Prostatic acid phosphatase (PAP). Major pretreatment tumor marker and used to predict recurrence. Increased values due to increased metabolism and catabolism of cancer cells—levels increase with stage of cancer and age of individual. Prostate-specific antigen (PSA) done to monitor prostate cancer preferred screening marker (<2.7 ng/mL or <2.7 mg/L). Monitor therapy with antineoplastic drugs.	1a. Carcinoma of prostate with the following elevation: carcinoma with no metastasis, 10%–20%; metastasis with one, 20%–40%; metastases with bone involvement, 70%–90% (usually osteoblastic). In three fourths of patients, arises in posterior lobe of prostate. Leukemia (hairy cell) increased. Cancer metastatic to bone (increased osteoblastic lesions). 1b. Is specific for prostate cancer	1. Increased in noncancer prostatic condition, prostate palpation, hyperplasia, infection of prostate following cystostomy, prostate surgery, and chronic prostatitis. Other increases: Gaucher's disease (lipid storage disease), Niemann-Pick disease, Paget's disease, osteoporosis, renal osteopathy, hepatic cirrhosis, pulmonary embolism, and hyperparathyroidism
2. Lactate dehydrogenase (LDH); increased isoenzymes I and II. Total LDH: 166–280 U/L. Detect and monitor testicular cancer.	2. Increased neuroblastomic carcinoma of testis. Elevated in 60% of those with stage III testicular cancer—serial LDH may help to detect recurrence of cancer. Ewing's sarcoma, acute lymphocytic leukemia, non-Hodgkin's lymphoma. LD-1 increased in germ cell tumors; LD-3 increased in leukemia; LD-5 increased in breast, lung, stomach, and colon; elevated in metastatic carcinoma.	2. Increased in cellular injury/hemolysis, early in myocardial infarction (see cardiac marker tests in Chapter 6), hepatic diseases
3. Neuron-specific enolase (NSE) <12.5 mg/mL; normal staining. Produced by neurons and neuroendocrine cells of the central and peripheral nervous system. Used to monitor disease progression, small cell lung cancer and pheochromocytoma, neuroblastoma, medullary thyroid cancer	3. NSE increased in neuroblastomas, amine precursor uptake decarboxylation (APUD) system tumor—small cell lung cancers, pancreatic islet cell, medullary thyroid carcinoma, seminoma (20%) in prostate, breast, and gastrointestinal (GI) tract, also Wilms' tumor and pheochromocytoma	3. Occasionally with benign liver diseases

table continues on pg. 618 >

TABLE 8.12, continued

Name of Test Clinical Marker in Current Use and Selected Normal Values[a]	Type of Cancer in Which Tumor Marker May Be Found	Conditions Other Than Cancer Associated With Abnormal Values
Enzymes		
4. Alkaline phosphatase (ALP) originates in osteoblasts, lining of hepatobiliary tree and intestinal tract, and placenta. Adults (20–60 yr): 35–85 U/L; elderly: slightly higher; children (<2 yr): 85–235 U/L; young persons (2–21 yr): 30–200 U/L. Isoenzymes offer greater specificity.	4. Increased in osteosarcoma, hepatocellular, metastatic to liver, primary or secondary bone tumors, liver and bone leukemia, lymphoma	4. Increased in Paget's disease, nonmalignant liver disease, normal pregnancy, healing fractures, hyperparathyroidism, osteomalacia and rickets, sprue, and malabsorption; decreased in hypoparathyroidism, malnutrition, scurvy, and pernicious anemia
5. Other enzymes: γ-glutamyl transpeptidase (GGT); muramidase, creatinine, phosphokinase isoenzyme BB, β-glucuronidase, terminal deoxynucleotidyl transferase, ribonuclease, histaminase (medullary cancer of thyroid), amylase, and cystine aminopeptidase	5. Creatine phosphokinase (CPK)-BB increased in prostate, lung (small cell), bladder, breast and gastrointestinal (GI) tract cancer; amylase increased in lung and ovarian cancer	5. CPK-BB increased in cardiac muscle and skeletal muscle injury and brain and CNS diseases; Reye's syndrome; hypothyroidism. GGT increased in liver with CPK disease, alcohol abuse, and antiepileptic medications. Amylase increased in pancreatic, diabetic, ketoacidosis, and intestinal obstruction.
6. Squamous cell cancer antigen (SCCA). Used to monitor and detect recurrence of squamous cell cancer of uterus, cervix, head and neck, esophagus, lung, skin, and sinus; also advanced cancer	6. Increased in uterine cancer (89% of stage IV disease). Alert: occurs in saliva, sweat, and respiratory secretions	6. Elevated in pulmonary infection, skin disease, renal failure, and liver disease
Hormones		
1. Human chorionic gonadotropin (hCG) produced by placental syncytiotrophoblast; not usually found in sera of healthy, nonpregnant persons. <2 ng/mL. Useful to monitor testicular tumors and tumors of ovary and to monitor changes	1. Increased in gestational trophoblastic tumors, seminomatous and nonseminomatous testes cancer, ovarian tumors, pancreatic islet-cell cancer, liver (21%), stomach (22%), and less valuable with lung and lymphoproliferative disease	1. Increased in gestational trophoblastic neoplasms (choriocarcinoma); neoplasm of stomach, colon, pancreas, lungs, and liver; multiple pregnancies. Decreased in ectopic pregnancy and abortion; increased in marijuana smokers

2. Calcitonin (CT): malignant C-cell thyroid tumor produces increased CT levels. Calcitonin (see Chapter 6) is a hormone produced by parafollicular C cells of thyroid gland. Ranges vary with method. Serum: adult: <150 pg/mL. Plasma: male, <19 pg/mL; female, <14 pg/mL	2. Increased in metastatic breast (greatly elevated), limited in primary small-tumor-burden breast cancer because levels lower, lung, pancreas, hepatoma, renal cell carcinoid, and skeletal metastases	2. Increased in Zollinger-Ellison syndrome, pernicious anemia, chronic renal failure, pseudohypoparathyroidism, apudomas, alcoholic cirrhosis, Paget's disease, pregnancy, and benign breast or ovarian disease. Decreased with therapy; an increase after therapy suggests progressive disease.
3. Other hormones: adrenocorticotropic hormone (ACTH) (lung—oat cell), parathyroid hormone (PTH) (lung—epidermoid), insulin (lung), glucagon (pancreas), gastrin (stomach and other carcinomas), prostaglandins, and erythropoietin (kidney)	3. Increased in endocrine tumor tissue and nonendocrine tissue (ectopic) tumors	3. See Chapter 6 for specific substance increases.
4. Serotonin (5-hydroxyindoleacetic acid [5-HIAA]). Hydroxyacetic acid: used to detect and monitor carcinoid tumors	4. Increased in carcinoid tumors	4. Increased with many foods (e.g., meats and fruits)
Oncofetal Antigens		
1. α-Fetoprotein (AFP) is a glycoprotein produced by fetal liver, yolk sac, and intestinal epithelium. Disappears from blood soon after birth and is not present in healthy individuals <40 ng/mL. Diagnose and monitor AFP tumors. Follow-up for therapy of testicular, ovarian, and primary liver tumors; used with hCG	1. Increased in primary hepatocellular cancer, embryonal cell (nonseminomatous germ cell) testicular tumors, yolk sac ovarian tumors, teratocarcinoma, gastric, pancreatic, colonic, breast, renal, and lung. >50 ng/mL AFP-producing tumor. Elevations signal recurrence.	1. Increased in fetal distress and death, neural tube defects, viral hepatitis, GI tumors, primary biliary cirrhosis, partial hepatectomy, ataxic telangiectasia, Wiskott-Aldrich syndrome, multiple pregnancy, and abortion
2. Carcinoembryonic antigen (CEA). Initially isolated in endodermally derived adenocarcinoma and fetal gastrointestinal tissue. <2.5–5 ng/mL; up to 5 ng/mL in smokers; <6 ng/mL in spinal fluid. Assess therapy with antineoplastic drugs and following surgery of medullary thyroid cancer, neoplasm of breast, GI tract, lung, and colorectal; monitor cancers of primary colorectal cancer, pancreas, breast, GI, liver, lung, ovaries, prostate.	2. Increased in cancer >3.0 ng/mL (especially metastatic or colon recurrence and germ cell cancer), pancreas, lung, stomach, metastatic breast, ovary, bladder, limbs, neuroblastoma, leukemia, thyroid, and osteogenic carcinoma. >10 ng/mL with CEA-producing tumor. Values <20 ng/mL do *not* rule out recurrent cancer.	2. Increased in pregnancy, inflammatory bowel disease, rectal polyps, active ulcerative colitis, pancreatitis, alcoholic cirrhosis, peptic ulcers, cholecystitis, chronic renal failure, pulmonary emphysema, bronchitis, pulmonary infections, and fibrocystic breast disease; most levels decline with remission of disease. Increase over time suggests recurrent cancer.

table continues on pg.620 >

TABLE 8.12, continued

Name of Test Clinical Marker in Current Use and Selected Normal Values[a]	Type of Cancer in Which Tumor Marker May Be Found	Conditions Other Than Cancer Associated With Abnormal Values
Proteins		
1. CA 15-3 antigen (cancer-associated antigen breast cystic fluid protein [BCFP]; used in conjunction with CEA) is a marker for breast cancer used for serial testing. <30 U/mL males and females encoded by *MUC-l* gene in stage II or III and used with CA 27 and CA 29; most useful to monitor therapy and disease progression in metastatic disease	1. Greatly increased in metastatic breast cancer; limited in small-tumor-burden breast cancer. Decreased with therapy; an increase after therapy suggests progressive disease; increased in pancreas, lung, colorectal, ovarian, and liver cancer	1. Increased in benign breast, ovarian, or liver diseases
2. NMP22 found in urine, used to manage transitional cell cancer of the urinary tract tissue biopsy obtained by cystoscopy	2. Present in transitional cell cancer (TCC) of urinary tract	2. Further study needed
3. Bladder tumor–associated (BTA) analyte found in urine	3. Presence of BTA involves invasion of tumor and/or tumor production associated with recurrence of tumor.	3. Further studies in blood are needed.
4. CA 27–29 (similar to CA 15-3 serum) is a marker for breast carcinoma. Not used for screening. ≤38 U/mL in female and male breast cancer; serial testing for prior stage II or III to detect recurrence	4. Increased in recurrence in stage II or III breast cancer. >38 U/mL indicates recurrence of breast cancer.	4. These antigens are increased by the human *MYC-1* gene; interfering factors: increased levels due to exposure to mouse antigens in environment, treatment, or diagnostic imaging
5. β_2-Microglobulin (b_2-m) (HLA antigen system). 4–12 mg/L	5. Increased in chronic lymphocytic leukemia, multiple myeloma, other B-cell neoplasms, lung cancer, hepatoma, breast cancer	5. Decreased in renal tubular injury; increased in ankylosing spondylitis and Reiter's syndrome, renal failure, AIDS

6. PSA—more sensitive than PAP—correlates with stage of adenocarcinoma and age. Males: 80% <2.0 mg/L; free: total ratio = >0.24 total 2–10 ng/mL = <2.0 ng/mL. Free cascade done. PSA not significantly increased until tumor has grown out of prostate gland. USPSTF recommends against using PSA-based screening for prostate cancer. Medicare provides coverage for an annual PSA test for men over 50 yr.	6. Increased >10.0 ng/mL (in prostate biopsy) in prostate cancer (the higher the level, the greater the tumor burden); successful surgery, chemotherapy, or radiation causes marked reduction in levels. PSA not significantly increased until tumor has grown out of prostate gland.	6. Increase in prostate size and tissue damage, benign prostatic hypertrophy, prostate massage, prostate surgery, and prostatitis. Collect before needle biopsy or resection.
7. CA 19-9 carbohydrate antigen; <37 U/mL. Occurs in serum and tissue; is a marker for colorectal and pancreatic cancer	7. Increased >37 U/mL (very high) in pancreatic cancer, hepatobiliary cancer, lung cancer; primarily mild elevation—gastric and colorectal cancer	7. Increased in pancreatitis (<75 U/mL), cholecystitis, cirrhosis, gallstones, and cystic fibrosis (minimal elevations)
8. CA 125 (ovarian cancer) (glycoprotein antigen) and serum carbohydrate antigen. <35 U/mL. Is a marker for ovarian and endometrial carcinoma; ovarian and endometrial cancer monitoring	8. Greater concentration related to poor survival. Increased in epithelial ovary, fallopian tube, endometrium, endocervix, pancreas, and liver. >35 U/mL indicates residual cancer.	8. Increased in pregnancy (first trimester), endometriosis, pelvic inflammatory disease, menstruation, acute and chronic hepatitis, ascites, peritonitis, pancreatitis, GI disease, Meigs' syndrome, pleural effusion, pulmonary disease, pericarditis, and ovarian cysts
9. CA 50. <17 U/mL. Is a marker for pancreatic and colorectal carcinoma; used to monitor therapy of GI and pancreatic cancer	9. Less increased in colon, breast, lung, and GI cancer	9. None identified
10. CA 72-4 TAG (a micin-like hormone adenocarcinoma associated antigen) <4.0 ng/mL. Is a marker for GI and ovarian cancer; used in gastric carcinoma monitoring	10. Increased in GI and pancreatic cancer and with residual tumor	10. Increased in benign liver and breast disease and in pregnancy
11. C549 (acidic glycoprotein). <15.5 U/mL (results correlate with those using CA 15-3); used in monitoring breast cancer	11. Increased in ovarian and gastric cancer	11. Information not available

table continues on pg. 622 >

TABLE 8.12, continued

Name of Test Clinical Marker in Current Use and Selected Normal Values[a]	Type of Cancer in Which Tumor Marker May Be Found	Conditions Other Than Cancer Associated With Abnormal Values
Proteins		
12. Tissue polypeptide antigen (TPA) 80–100 U/L in serum—may also be detected in urine, washings, and effusions. Is not a specific marker. Monitor GI, genitourinary (GU), breast, lung, and thyroid cancer.	12. Increased in GI, GU tract, breast, lung, thyroid, head and neck, cervix, ovarian, and prostate cancer	12. Increased in hepatitis, cholangitis, cirrhosis, pneumonia, and urinary tract infections
13. Immunoglobulins: monoclonal proteins (M proteins), immunoglobulins produced by B lymphocytes. Normal: absent. Refer to serum protein electrophoresis (SPEP) or urine protein electrophoresis (UPEP).	13. Increased in multiple myeloma, macroglobulinemia, amyloidosis, B-cell lymphoma, multiple solid tumors	13. Increased in cold agglutinin disease, Sjögren's syndrome, Gaucher's disease, lichen myxedematosus, cirrhosis, renal failure, and sarcoidosis
14. Tumor-antigen 4 (TA-4). $\leq$2.6 ng/mL. Diagnose and monitor squamous cancer.	14. Increased in squamous cancer: lung and cervix. Elevations correlate with stage of cancer, especially abnormal high levels. Rising levels after therapy associated with recurrence.	14. Information not available
15. CA 242 is a marker for pancreatic and colorectal cancer	15. Increased in malignant and colorectal cancers	15. Benign colon, gastric, liver, pancreatic, and biliary tract disease
16. Other antigens: colon mucoprotein antigen (CMA), colon-specific antigen (CSA), zinc glycinate marker (ZGM—colon), pancreatic oncofetal antigen (POA), S-100 protein (malignant melanoma), sialoglycoprotein (wide variety of cancers), B protein (wide variety of antigens), and "Tennessee" antigen glycoprotein (wide variety of cancers)	16. Increased levels in colon cancer, malignant melanoma, and a wide variety of cancers	16. Information not available
Cytokines		
1. Interleukin (IL) (also known as interleukin IL-2) T-cell growth factor I; formed from helper T cells and activated B cells; results highly variable. Monitor therapy in leukemia; results highly variable	1. Increased in leukemias (adult T-cell leukemia)	1. HIV infections

Genetic Markers		
Suppressor Genes		
1. *P-53* gene mutation. No mutation; most common genetic mutation in cancer used for prognosis	1. High mutation overexpression in breast, *BRCA*, head and neck, colon, and small cell lung cancer (50%–75%)	1. Increased in colon polyps
2. Retinoblastoma gene	2. Found in ocular tumors arising spontaneously; small portion are hereditary	2. Information not available
3. *BRCA-1* and *BRCA-2* monitor development of breast and ovarian cancer	3. Found in hereditary predisposition to developing breast and ovarian cancer	3. Carriers of *BRCA-1* gene mutation have an 85% risk for developing breast cancer and 45% risk for developing ovarian cancer by age 85 yr.
4. $p21^{WAF1}$ may be clinically useful	4. Uncertain	4. Information not available
5. APC (antigen-presenting cells)	5. Increased in patients with hundreds of polyps; mutations in hereditary colon cancer, also breast and esophageal	5. Premalignant polyps
6. Neurofibromatosis	6. Inactivating mutations in inherited colorectal cancer, melanoma	6. Information not available
7. Wilms' tumor (nephroblastoma)	7. Mutations in Wilms' tumor	7. Information not available
8. NM2, a marker for metastasis	8. Increased in metastatic breast, colon, and prostate cancer	8. Information not available
Oncogenes		
1. *Ras* oncogene; no mutation	1. Oncogene mutations found in leukemia, neuroblastoma, lymphoma, sarcomas, and endotheliomas	1. Information not available
2. *CMYC* gene-defect recurrence	2. Found in B- and T-cell lymphoma and small cell lung cancer	2. Information not available
3. *C-erb B-2, HER-2/Neu* gene, used as prognostic indicator in breast cancer	3. Found in breast, ovarian, and GI carcinomas	3. Information not available
4. *bcl-2* (blocks apoptosis), presence contributes to programmed cell death and survival of cancer cells	4. Found in leukemia and lymphoma. Detection may predict resistance to chemotherapy.	4. Information not available

An inhibitor of apoptosis (programmed cell death), survivin, has been detected in most forms of cancer. Survivin is necessary during mitosis to ensure normal cell division and chromosome distribution. However, in cancerous cells, survivin prolongs their life span, thereby increasing the chances of mutations. Research is being targeted at developing drugs to inhibit survivin expression and thus inhibit tumor growth. Clinical tests are not yet commercially available to measure blood levels of survivin.

[a]Normal values vary greatly; check with your reference laboratory.

TABLE 8.13 Types of Cytokines, Cellular Origin, and Clinical Implications

Cytokine (Synonym)	Cellular Origin	Target Cells	Specific Clinical Implications of Abnormal Results
Interleukin-1			
Also known as B-cell–accelerating factor, catabolin, endogenous pyrogen, epidermal cell–derived thymocyte-activity factor, fibroblast-activity factor, hemoposition-1, hepatogenic stimulatory factor (HSF), leukocyte endogenous mediator, lymphocyte-activating factor, mononuclear cell factor, osteoclast-activating factor, proteolysis-inducing factor, and serum amyloid A inducer	Monocytes, macrophages, antigen-presenting cells (APCs), endothelial cells, T lymphocytes, natural killer (NK) cells	Monocytes, macrophages, hepatocytes, endothelial cells, epithelial cells, fibroblasts, keratinocytes, T lymphocytes, B lymphocytes, NK cells, osteoclasts	Increased in rheumatoid arthritis, septic shock, periodontitis, malignancy, asbestosis, tuberculosis, HIV infection, differential diagnosis; that is, nonallergic bronchial asthma, multisystem organ failure during acute pancreatitis, acute eosinophilic pneumonia, inflammatory intestinal disease. Therapeutically useful in protecting patients against lethal doses of radiation and in stimulation of hematopoiesis.
Interleukin-2			
Also known as T-cell growth factor (TCGF)	T lymphocytes (CD4, T_H0 and T_H1 [CD8]), NK cells, B lymphocytes, mast cells	T lymphocytes (CD4, CD8), B lymphocytes, NK cells	Pregnancy, increased in multiple sclerosis, sarcoidosis, multiple myeloma, acute rheumatic fever, and chronic rheumatic heart disease. Decreased in advanced age, diabetes, Sjögren's syndrome, and AIDS. Therapeutic use in clinical trials for treatment of cancer (kidney, melanoma, and acute myeloid leukemia), AIDS, leprosy, and other immunologic conditions resulting from administration of immunosuppressive agents.
Interleukin-3			
Colony-forming unit (CFU) stimulating activity, colony-stimulating factor (CSF), hematopoietic cell growth factor, mast cell growth factor (MCGF), histamine-producing cell-stimulating factor, multilineage hemopoietic growth factor, P-cell–stimulating factor activity, persisting (P)-cell–stimulating factor, synergistic activity (Thy-1–inducing factor, and WEHI-3 growth factor)	Most interleukins are produced by macrophages or T lymphocytes (CD4, T_H1 and T_H2), NK cells, mast cells, eosinophils.	Hematopoietic stem cells, progenitor cells, B lymphocytes, macrophages, polymorphonuclear leukocytes, mast cells, keratinocytes	Increased production in monocytes and myeloid leukemia and most cell disorders. In blood, only with severe immunization against stimuli such as graft-versus-host disease or parasitic infestations; plays a role in chronic allergic diseases. Therapeutic use in clinical trials to assess the benefit from temperature stimulation, shortening the duration of cytopenia associated with chemotherapy, irradiation, or following bone marrow transplantation.

Interleukin-4			
B-cell differentiating factor (BCDF), B-cell growth factor I (BCGF-I), B-cell–stimulating factor I (BSF-I), MCGF-II, T-cell growth factor II (TCGF-II)	T lymphocytes (CD4, T_H2), basophils, eosinophils, mast cells	T lymphocytes, B lymphocytes, mast cells, myeloid progenitors, erythroid progenitors, NK cells	Regulation of allergic reactions (immediate hypersensitivity). Increased in atopic dermatitis, contact skin sensitivity reactions, T-cell lymphomas (T_H2 subtype). Therapeutic use in humoral immunodeficiency; some effect on solid tumors. Experimental models of vaccination with tumor cells engineered to produce IL-4 have shown release of this cytokine is associated with the immunity that may regress with the development of established cancer.
Interleukin-5			
BCDF for IgM (BCDFu), BCGF-II, eosinophil colony-stimulating factor, eosinophil differentiation factor, IgA-enhancing factor, and T-cell–replacing factor	T lymphocytes (CD4, T_H2), mast cells, eosinophils	Eosinophils, B lymphocytes, basophils, mast cells	Increased in allergic diseases, asthma in late allergen manifestations; patients with acute eosinophilic pneumonia have high bronchoalveolar lavage fluid levels of IL-5, IL-IRA, and soluble type II IL-IR. Production high in severe atopic dermatitis; therapeutic use for hypogammaglobulinemia
Interleukin-6			
26-kd protein, BCDF, B-cell–stimulating factor-2 (BSF-2), cytotoxic T-cell differentiation factor, hybridoma/plasmacytoma growth factor, interferon-β_2 (IFN-β_2) monocytic granulocyte inducer type 2, and thrombopoietin	T lymphocytes, B lymphocytes, monocytes, macrophages, APCs, endothelial cells, epithelial cells, fibroblasts, mast cells	T lymphocytes, B lymphocytes, hepatocytes, endothelial cells, keratinocytes, hematopoietic cells, malignant plasma cells	Increased in gram-negative bacterial infection and inflammatory reactions, bacterial sepsis, acute complications of lung transplantation. IL-6 is produced by macrophages in the periprosthetic membrane surrounding joint replacements, causing osteolysis and prosthetic loosening. Hyperproduction is associated with a variety of malignancies, including plasmacytoma, multiple myeloma, uterine and cervical cancer, and Kaposi's sarcoma. Therapeutic use to support neutrophil and megakaryocyte growth in patients treated with high doses of chemotherapy and to treat patients infected with human T-cell leukemia virus type 1 (HTLV-1).

table continues on pg. 626 >

TABLE 8.13, continued

Cytokine (Synonym)	Cellular Origin	Target Cells	Specific Clinical Implications of Abnormal Results
Interleukin-7			
Lymphopoietin 1, B-cell growth factor, and pre–B-cell growth factor	Stromal cells (bone marrow, thymic), T lymphocytes, spleen cells, epithelial cells, fibroblasts	T lymphocyte progenitors, B lymphocyte progenitors, T lymphocytes (CD4, CD8)	Regulates HIV-1 replication in naturally infected peripheral blood mononuclear cells (ABMCs). Therapeutic use—may be useful in tumor therapy because of its ability to enhance the generation of T lymphocytes and lymphokine-activated killer (LAK) cells, even in the absence of IL-2; helpful for some immunodeficiencies or to accelerate recovery following bone marrow transplantation. May enhance immune system.
Interleukin-8 (see Chemokines)			
Interleukin-9			
B-cell–derived T-cell growth factor, cytokine synthesis-inhibiting factor, MCGF, and thymocyte growth-promoting factor	T lymphocytes (CD4, Th2), lymphoma cells	T lymphocyte progenitor cells	Increased: T-cell tumors, especially of T_H2 lymphocytes. In Hodgkin's lymphoma acts as autoimmune signal for cellular proliferation. No therapeutic applications.
Interleukin-10			
B-cell–derived T-cell growth factor, cytokine synthesis-inhibiting factor, MCGF, and thymocyte growth-promoting factor	T lymphocytes (CD4 T_H0, T_H2) (CD4, T_H1, CD8), B lymphocytes, macrophages, keratinocytes	B lymphocytes, T lymphocytes, NK cells, monocytes, macrophages, mast cells	Increased in virus-induced diseases. IL-10 markedly elevated in acute phase of Kawasaki disease; parasite antigen-induced T-cell hyporesponsiveness in chronic *Schistosoma haematobium* infection. Increased in solid tumors. Therapeutic use—efficient inhibitor of tumor metastasis on experimental level; indicates a possible role in biologic therapy for cancer. As a moderator of cytotoxic cell activity, may ameliorate situations such as septic shock.
Interleukin-11			
Adipogenesis inhibitor factor	Stromal cells (bone marrow), trophoblasts, glial cells, fibroblasts	Hematopoietic progenitors, plasmocytes, adipocytes, neurons	Increased in leukemia myeloid cells, and their proliferation is regulated by this cytokine that acts synergistically as a stimulator of megakaryopoiesis. May be of therapeutic benefit for patients with platelet deficiencies.

Interleukin-12			
Cytotoxic lymphocyte maturation factor, K-cell–stimulating factor, and T-cell–stimulating factor	B lymphocytes, monocytes, macrophages, APCs	T lymphocytes (CD4, CD8), NK cells	Increased or present: A marker for autoimmune type 1 diabetes mellitus, increased in chronic atopic dermatitis, other T_H1-mediated pathologies (e.g., sarcoidosis). Decreased production associated with increased susceptibility to infection (monocytes from HIV-positive individuals secrete decreased IL-12); on experimental level, use for antitumor action and for potential angiogenesis-dependent malignancies. Promotes defense against a variety of pathogens useful for adaptive immunotherapy, especially in immunosuppressed patients (due to cancer or HIV infection).
Interleukin-13			
NC30 (human cDNA) and P6001 mouse cDNA clone	T lymphocytes (CD4, T_H2, T_H0, T_H8), mast cells	B lymphocytes, monocytes, macrophages, endothelial cells	Increased in acute atopic dermatitis skin lesions. Protects vessel wall from monocyte injury leading to atherosclerosis, possible factor in pathogenesis of chronic lymphocytic leukemia. Present in the nasal mucosa in perennial allergic rhinitis. Therapeutic use may be as an agent in toxic shock and type I allergy.
Interleukin-14			
High-molecular-weight BCGF	T lymphocytes, B lymphocytes, dendritic cells, malignant cells	B lymphocytes	Hyperproductive in systemic lupus erythematosus. Therapeutic use in variety of malignant conditions (e.g., lymphoma or leukemia).
Interleukin-15			
	Monocytes, macrophages, epithelial cells, keratinocytes, APCs, many others (tissue)	T lymphocytes, NK cells	UVB-induced downregulation of keratinocytes. IL-15 production may contribute to the relative state of immunosuppression induced by sun exposure. IL-15 triggers the growth of leukemia B cells through IL-2R system subunits, relating to the role of cytokine in regulating neophasic proliferation in chronic lymphoproliferative disorders. Synovial fluid T lymphocytes proliferate in response to IL-15, thereby contributing to rheumatoid arthritis pathogenesis.

table continues on pg. 628 >

TABLE 8.13, continued

Cytokine (Synonym)	Cellular Origin	Target Cells	Specific Clinical Implications of Abnormal Results
Interleukin-16			
Lymphocytic chemoattractant factor	T lymphocytes (CD8), eosinophils, epithelial cells	T lymphocytes (CD4), eosinophils (CD4), monocytes (CD4)	Plays a role in allergic inflammation. Accumulation of CD4-activated lymphocytes in the airways of asthmatic patients is generally attributed to the presence of chemoattractant cytokines. Mast cell histamines may induce the secretion of IL-16 after allergic challenge as in granulomatous inflammatory responses. IL-16 is found in sarcoid granuloma and in granulomas of infective origin, particularly *Mycobacterium tuberculosis*. Possibly effective in treatment of HIV infection.
Interleukin-17			
Cytotoxic T-lymphocyte–associated antigen 8 (CTLA-8)	T lymphocytes (memory CD4)	T lymphocytes, fibroblasts, epithelial cells, endothelial cells	IL-17 may constitute an early initiation of the T-cell–dependent inflammatory reaction and may be an element of the cytokine network that bridges the immune system to hematopoiesis.
Interleukin-18			
IFN-γ–inducing factor	Liver cells	NK cells, T lymphocytes	May play a potential role in immunoregulation or in inflammation by augmenting the function activity of FasL on T_H1 cells
Interferons: IFN-α and IFN-β			
IFN-α: acid-stable IFN, B-cell IFN, buffy coat IFN, leukocyte-derived IFN, lymphoblast IFN, Namoliva IFN, and type I IFN. IFN-β: acid-stable IFN, fibroblast-derived IFN, IFN-β I, and type I IFN	IFN-α: Monocytes, macrophages, lymphocytes. IFN-β: Fibroblasts, epithelial cells. Interferons are produced by virus-infected cells and are the body's first line of defense against many viruses.	T lymphocytes, NK cells, macrophages	IFN-α is detected in plasma of HIV-infected patients during acute uremia and during late-stage disease. Both hyperthyroidism and hypothyroidism have been detected during prolonged recombinant human IFN-α therapy. May have a role in the pathogenesis of atopic dermatitis. Type I IFNs have clinical application in the treatment of viral infections, especially chronic state infections (e.g., hepatitis B and C); also, IFNs have potential as adjuvants in the treatment of HIV infection. Their antitumor effects are significant in lymphoma, multiple myeloma, melanoma, renal cell carcinoma, and Kaposi's sarcoma. IFN-β may be a promising drug for treatment of multiple sclerosis and possibly for gene therapy of malignant glioma.

IFN-γ			
Immune IFN, macrophage-activating factor T-cell IFN, and type II IFN	T lymphocytes (CD4, T_H0, T_H1, CD8), NK cells	T lymphocytes, NK cells, macrophages, endothelial cells, APCs, B lymphocytes	Increased IFN-γ production is associated with food-sensitive atopic dermatitis, Crohn's disease (local mucosal synthesis), rheumatoid arthritis synovial fluid (possible role in the ongoing immunologic reaction of the inflamed joint), and poor antibody-mediated immunity in hypovitaminosis A. Also, IFN-γ is associated with immunodeficiency after allogeneic bone marrow transplantation, the pathophysiology of aplastic anemia, and atherogenesis. Therapeutic use as an antiviral; antiproliferative and immunomodulary effects. Its instability limits its clinical application.
Tumor Necrosis Factor (TNF)			
TFN-α: cachectin, cytotoxin, cytotoxic factor, differentiation-inducing factor, hemorrhagic factor, macrophage cytotoxic factor, and necrosis TNF-β: Cytotoxin, differentiation-inducing factor, and lymphotoxin (LT)	Monocytes, macrophages, T lymphocytes, B lymphocytes, NK cells, mast cells, endothelial cells, APCs, fibroblasts	T lymphocytes, polymorphonuclear leukocytes (PMNs), macrophages, endothelial cells, osteoclasts, fibroblasts, hepatocytes, tumor cells	TNF-α is associated with septic shock and diverse infectious pathology (protective immune response in pulmonary tuberculosis). TNF-α is important in the pathogenesis of allergic respiratory reactions and acute stages of rheumatoid arthritis. Injured patients reveal significantly increased plasma levels of both TNFs compared with healthy persons; severe injury reveals higher levels on day of admission than in patients with minor injury. TNF-α levels higher in peritoneal fluid of women with endometriosis than in healthy women. Increased TNF-α, IL-6, IL-1B levels following transient cerebral ischemia suggest cytokine may be involved in pathophysiologic changes in hippocampus and striatum. TNF-α may play a role in acute pancreatitis and mediate the systemic sequelae of the disease. Increased serum tissue TNF levels observed in alcoholic liver disease; increased plasma levels in nephropathia epidemica. TNF-α involved in pathogenesis of both acute and chronic transplant rejection; those with higher levels of this cytokine are at risk for a number of T-lymphocyte–mediated autoimmune diseases such as type 1 diabetes. TNF-α and IFN-γ are involved in the progression of neurologic disorders such as multiple sclerosis and AIDS complex, anti–TNF-α antibodies, lupus nephritis, inflammatory arthritis, cerebral edema, and neurologic dysfunction.

table continues on pg. 630 >

TABLE 8.13, continued

Cytokine (Synonym)	Cellular Origin	Target Cells	Specific Clinical Implications of Abnormal Results
Chemokines (CKs)			
(Formerly known as intercrines, the scy [small cytokine] family, and small, inducible, secreted cytokines.) A condensation of the term *chemoattractant cytokines.* Now defined as a superfamily of low-molecular-weight proteins (8–10 kD).	Monocytes, macrophages, PMNs, T lymphocytes, B lymphocytes, NK cells, mast cells, endothelial cells, epithelial cells, APCs, stromal cells, fibroblasts, platelets	Monocytes, macrophages, PMNs, T lymphocytes, B lymphocytes, NK cells, mast cells, endothelial cells, epithelial cells, APCs, stromal cells, fibroblasts, megakaryocytes	Regulate the motility and orientation of leukocytes (leukocyte activation/inflammation), lymphocyte activation and diversification, platelet activation, biologic modifier of erythrocyte function, angiogenic activity factors, and cell adhesion. Play an important role as pathogenic mediators in several pathologies, including asthma, allergic diseases, autoimmune diseases, inflammatory/infectious processes (inflammatory bowel disease), rheumatoid arthritis, sarcoidosis, pulmonary fibrosis, AIDS/HIV infections, transplant rejection, kidney pathology and proteinuria, hemolytic decreases/transfusion, and atherosclerosis.

Interventions

Pretest Patient Care

1. Explain purpose and procedure of test.
2. Alleviate fears the patient may have related to cancer test results. Tests for cancer are always anxiety provoking.
3. Follow guidelines in Chapter 1 for safe, effective, informed *pretest* care.

Posttest Patient Care

1. Review test results; report and record findings. Modify the nursing care plan as needed. Counsel the patient regarding abnormal findings; explain the need for possible follow-up testing and treatment.
2. Provide consultation if test results reveal cancer. Tumor drug–resistant assays are performed on tissue obtained in biopsy (see Chapter 11).
3. Provide support through follow-up testing in stages of illness and in forming a therapeutic and diagnostic plan for treating and monitoring the disease.
4. Follow guidelines in Chapter 1 for safe, effective, informed *posttest* care regarding shock, denial, and fear as normal responses to cancer diagnosis.

BLOOD BANKING OR IMMUNOHEMATOLOGY TESTS

These tests are done to select blood components that will have acceptable survival when transfused and to prevent possible transplant and transfusion reactions; to identify potential problems, such as hemolytic disease of newborns and the need for intrauterine transfusion; and to determine parentage. Immunohematology testing identifies highly reactive antigens on blood cells and their antibodies possibly present in serum. See Chart 8.1 for general procedures for blood donation.

CHART 8.1 Procedure for Donating Blood

1. Information for potential blood donors can be obtained at local blood banks or the American Red Cross.
2. The person donating blood must meet certain requirements: age (at least 17 yr), weight (at least 110 pounds or 50 kg), and health history that is negative for cancer and infectious diseases (no fever in past 2 wk). Also, pregnancy, travel to certain parts of the world, and inoculations may require a temporary deferral. A person can typically donate a unit of blood every 56 d. If donating only plasma, the waiting period is only 3 d.
3. A pint of blood (average adult has 10–12 pints) is obtained through a needle inserted into a vein in the arm, filling a bag and four vials. Blood is divided into three parts. Each part (red blood cells, platelets, and plasma) is prepared by spinning and the blood is stored by blood type until the product is used or expired.
4. Blood is shipped to hospitals upon request. Local community blood banks also supply nearby hospitals. The donated pint of blood may also be divided into many products for other uses.
5. The donated blood and products are quarantined until tests show no infection and are checked for antibodies that might cause a transfusion reaction. Unsuitable blood is destroyed.
6. Donated blood in storage that has previously been tested is used to help disaster victims.

Donated Blood Testing and Blood Processing

Pretransfusion testing of blood recipient and donor blood

1. All donated blood, as it is processed, must undergo several measurements. These include tests for the following factors:
   a. ABO groups
   b. Rh type
   c. Antibody screen
   d. HBsAg
   e. HBcAg
   f. HCV (anti-HCV)
   g. Syphilis (VDRL)
   h. HIV-1 and HIV-2
   i. HTLV-I and HTLV-II
   j. HIV antigen (HIV-1-Ag)
   k. NAT (narrow window of infection for HIV and HCV)
   l. Chagas' disease—caused by *Trypanosoma cruzi*
2. Required testing for whole blood or red blood cell recipients includes the following:
   a. ABO group
   b. Rh type
   c. Antibody screen
   d. Crossmatch for compatibility between donor's cells and recipient's serum

Type and screen, when ordered preoperatively, identify ABO and Rh type group and are used for cases that usually do not require transfusion. Even though no crossmatch is needed for plasma administration, compatible ABO typing should be done. Routinely, no crossmatch is needed for platelet administration; compatible ABO and Rh types should be given when possible. If a patient becomes refractory, HLA-matched platelets may be administered. Granulocytes should be tested for HLA compatibility. As a result of previous transfusions or pregnancy, some patients develop antibodies against these antigens and, if given platelets that have these antigens, may have a transfusion reaction. Pretransfusion testing for neonates (<4 months of age) requires determination of ABO group, Rh type, and an antibody screen. The antibody screen may be performed on a specimen obtained from the infant or the mother. If the antibody screen is negative, group O Rh compatible pediatric red blood cells may be used without further crossmatching for the remainder of the neonatal period. If the antibody screen is positive, the antibody is identified, and antigen-negative blood will be crossmatched and provided for transfusion. All infants requiring plasma transfusions will receive group AB pediatric fresh frozen plasma.

A type and screen consists of an ABO group, Rh type, and antibody screen and can be ordered when the need for crossmatched products is unlikely but may be required in an emergency situation. If the patient does have a clinically significant unexpected antibody, at least 2 U of antigen-negative blood will be made available for that patient before surgery. A positive antibody screen will automatically initiate antibody identification to determine the specificity of the antibody detected. If the antibody identified is determined to be clinically significant, antigen-negative blood is required for transfusion.

Procedure

1. Using a 10-mL plain, red-topped tube, collect a venous blood sample for hospital pretransfusion testing.
2. Label with the following information:
   a. Patient's full first and last names
   b. Patient's healthcare record number

c. Date and time of specimen collection
d. Initials (if collected by laboratory personnel) or signature (if collected by nonlaboratory personnel) of phlebotomist
e. Possibly a unique blood bank number (found on special blood bank identification band)

3. Attach a special blood bank band, at the recipient's bedside, at the time of specimen collection. The blood bank band must remain attached to the patient's wrist throughout the transfusion period. The same band may be used throughout one hospital admission as long as the information printed on the band is legible and the band is still securely attached to the patient's wrist.
4. A new blood specimen is required every 3 days if the patient has a history of transfusion or pregnancy during the previous 3 months.

Special Considerations

1. *Autologous donations* are blood products donated by patients for their own use (i.e., blood donor and recipient are the same person). Many patients opt to donate their own blood before scheduled surgery because of the concern regarding transfusion-transmitted diseases. The following are some general guidelines for autologous blood donation.
   a. There is no age limit if donor is healthy.
   b. There are no weight requirements. The volume of blood collected must comply with established weight provisions.
   c. Pregnant women can donate.
   d. Hematocrit should be >33% (or >0.33). If <33% (or <0.33), the patient's healthcare provider must approve the phlebotomy, usually in consultation with the blood bank medical director.
   e. Normally, phlebotomy can be done at 3-day intervals; the final phlebotomy can be done no sooner than 72 hours before the time of the scheduled surgery. Two-unit collections using an automated red cell pheresis machine may also be an option. Iron supplements may be prescribed to maintain adequate hemoglobin levels.
   f. Autologous blood is not "crossed over" into the general (allogeneic) blood supply. It is discarded after its expiration date.
2. *Allogeneic donations* are blood products donated by one individual for use by other individuals (i.e., blood donor and blood recipient are not the same person).
3. *Direct donations* are those in which recipients choose those who donate blood for their transfusions. Laws in several states declare that this request must be honored in nonemergency situations. Standards and testing procedures must be identical to those required for an allogeneic blood donor. (Autologous donors do not need to adhere to the same criteria as do allogeneic blood donors.) Directed donor units can be "crossed over" into the general (allogeneic) blood supply. Each establishment must have a policy describing when this can occur.
4. *CMV testing* is done for patients at risk for transfusion-associated CMV infections. These types of CMV infections include pneumonitis, hepatitis, retinitis, and disseminated infection. They generally occur in immunosuppressed patients, such as premature infants weighing <1200 g at birth, bone marrow and organ transplant recipients, and certain immunocompromised oncology patients. Therefore, to prevent these infections, CMV antibody testing is done. Patients at risk should receive CMV-seronegative blood and blood products. CMV in blood is associated with leukocytes. Leukocyte reduction using highly efficient leukocyte-reduction filters also appears to be an effective way of reducing CMV infection.
5. *Irradiation of blood products* is sometimes done before transfusion for certain immunosuppressed patients. Graft-versus-host disease (GVHD) is a rare complication that follows transfusion in severely immunosuppressed patients. GVHD occurs if donor lymphocytes from blood or blood products engraft and multiply in a severely immunodeficient recipient. The engrafted lymphocytes react against host (recipient) tissues. Clinical symptoms include skin rash, fever, diarrhea, hepatitis, bone marrow suppression, and infection, which frequently leads to death. GVHD can be prevented

by irradiating blood products with a maximum dose (cesium-137) of 2.5 cGy in the center of the container and a minimum dose of 1.5 cGy delivered to all other parts of the component. This practice renders the T lymphocytes in a unit of blood incapable of replication without affecting platelets or granulocytes. Irradiation does affect the red cell membrane, causing it to "leak" potassium. All irradiated red cells are given a 28-day "outdate" or may keep their original outdate of <28 days.

6. *Leukocyte reduction of blood products*: Leukocytes in blood products have long been known to be associated with nonhemolytic febrile transfusion reactions, possibly owing more to cytokines produced by the leukocytes than the leukocytes themselves. Leukocyte reduction may reduce the number of these reactions. It may also decrease the possibility of alloimmunization to the HLA antigens on the leukocytes. Removing leukocytes may effectively reduce the danger of transfusion-transmitted CMV infection.

Interventions

Pretest Patient Care

1. Before transfusion, there is a requirement for healthcare providers to document that all the alternatives to transfusion, risks for transfusion, and transfusion issues were explained to the patient.
2. Discuss with the patient the need for blood or blood components, risks (infection, disease, reactions, alloimmunization), benefits (treatment for active bleeding, anemia, clotting disorders), and alternatives to random allogeneic donation (predeposit autologous donation, intraoperative salvage, directed donor donation). Allow sufficient time for patient to ask questions, resolve concerns, and give voluntary consent.
3. The healthcare provider must document in the health record that the earlier discussions took place and provide documentation, including informed consent (see Appendix F). There must be documentation in the chart before the patient receives the transfusion.
4. Follow guidelines in Chapter 1 for safe, effective, informed *pretest* care.

• Blood Groups (ABO Groups)

Human blood is grouped according to the presence or absence of specific blood group antigens (ABO). These antigens, found on the surface of red blood cells, can induce the body to produce antibodies. More than 300 distinct antigens have been identified. Compatibility of the ABO group is the foundation for all other pretransfusion testing.

All blood donors and potential blood recipients must be tested for blood type to prevent transfusion with incompatible blood products. Specifically linked sugars determine the antigenic activities named A and B. One sugar, *N*-acetylgalactosamine, gives the molecule A activity; another sugar, galactose, determines B activity. The backbone molecule, without galactose or *N*-acetylgalactosamine, has antigenic activity termed H. This H substance, as well as *H* gene activity, is essential for the function of the ABO antigens. Table 8.14 lists the blood groups and their ABO antigens; Table 8.15 shows the relationship between blood antigens and antibodies.

TABLE 8.14 Antigen Values for Blood Types

Blood Group	ABO Antigen
A	A
B	B
AB	A and B
O	Neither

TABLE 8.15 Relationship Between Blood Antigens and Antibodies

Antigen Present on Red Blood Cell	Antibodies Present in Serum	Major Blood Group Designation	Distribution in the United States
None	Anti-A, anti-B	O (universal donor[a] for red blood cells)	O (46%)
A	Anti-B	A	A (41%)
B	Anti-A	B	B (9%)
AB	None	AB (universal recipient for red blood cells)[b] (universal donor for fresh frozen plasma)[c]	AB (4%)

[a]Called universal donor because no antigens are present on red blood cells; therefore, the person is able to donate to all blood groups.

[b]Called universal recipient because no serum antibodies are present; therefore, the person is able to receive blood from all blood groups.

[c]Called universal donor for plasma because no serum antibodies are present; therefore, the plasma can be given to all blood groups.

In general, patients are transfused with blood of their own ABO group because antibodies against the other blood antigens may be present in their blood serum. These antibodies are designated anti-A or anti-B, depending on the antigen they act against. Under normal conditions, a person's blood serum does not contain the antibody specifically able to destroy its antigen. For example, a person with antigen A will not have anti-A antibodies in the serum; however, anti-B antibodies may be present. Therefore, antigen and antibody testing is necessary to confirm ABO grouping.

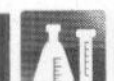 **CLINICAL ALERT**

1. A transfusion reaction can be extremely serious and potentially fatal. Therefore, the blood group must be determined in vitro before any blood is transfused to an individual. Before blood administration, two healthcare professionals (i.e., physicians or nurses) must check the recipient's blood group and type with the donor group and type to ensure compatibility.
2. A blood group change or suppression may be induced by cancer, leukemia, infection, or bone marrow transplant.

Normal Findings

A, B, AB, and O group

Procedure

1. Collect a 7-mL venous clotted blood sample in a red-topped tube. Observe standard precautions.
2. Do not use serum-separating tubes (SSTs) (cell barrier tube).

Interventions

Pretest Patient Care

1. Explain test purpose and procedure. The following are conditions that at some point may require transfusion:
   a. Malignant tumors (leukemias)
   b. Cardiac surgical procedures
   c. Surgical hip procedures
   d. Anemias

e. Certain obstetric or gynecologic procedures or complications
f. Bone and joint diseases
g. Lung disease
h. Kidney disease or genitourinary system surgical procedures
i. Massive trauma
j. Liver disease
k. Certain blood dyscrasias

2. Follow guidelines in Chapter 1 for safe, effective, informed *pretest* care.

Posttest Patient Care

1. Review test results; report and record findings. Modify the nursing care plan as needed. Inform patient of blood group and explain its meaning. Rh type (see next section) may have implications for the pregnant woman and fetus.
2. Follow guidelines in Chapter 1 for safe, effective, informed *posttest* care.

● Rh Typing

Human blood is classified as Rh positive or Rh negative. This relates to the presence or the absence of the D antigen on the red cell membrane. The D antigen (also called Rh_1 [D]) is, after the A and B antigens, the next most important antigen in transfusion practice.

The Rh system is composed of antigens tested for in conjunction with the ABO group. Rh antigens (there are >50) are determined by two closely linked genes on chromosome 1. Investigators (e.g., Dr. Alexander Wiener, Drs. Fisher and Race, and Dr. Tippett) have studied the mechanisms of Rh inheritance, and therefore, different terminology may be used. See Table 8.16. Rh_1 (D) antigen is often the only factor tested for. When this factor is absent, further testing is then done on women of childbearing age to identify if there is Rh_1 (D) antigen present in smaller amounts. This test is called *weak D* (formally known as D testing). Rh-negative individuals may develop antibodies against Rh-positive antigens if they are challenged through a transfusion of Rh-positive blood or through a fetomaternal bleed from an Rh-positive fetus. See Table 8.17.

Normal Findings

1. Caucasian
   a. 85% or 0.85 Rh positive [have the Rh(O) antigen]
   b. 15% or 0.15 Rh negative [lack the Rh(O) antigen]
2. African Americans
   a. 90% or 0.90 Rh positive [have the Rh(O) antigen]
   b. 10% or 0.10 Rh negative [lack the Rh(O) antigen]

TABLE 8.16 Comparison of Terms Used in Rh System Nomenclatures

Wiener	Fisher-Race
Rh1	D
Rh2	C
Rh3	E
Rh4	c
Rh5	e
Rh6	f (ce)
Rh12	G

TABLE 8.17 Incidence and Frequency of Blood Group and Rh Type

Group and Type	Incidence	Frequency of Occurrence (%)
O positive	1 in 3	37.4
O negative	1 in 15	6.6
A positive	1 in 3	35.7
A negative	1 in 16	6.3
B positive	1 in 12	8.5
B negative	1 in 67	1.5
AB positive	1 in 29	3.4
AB negative	1 in 167	0.6

Procedure

1. Blood Rh typing must be done for the following reasons:
   a. Rh-positive blood administered to an Rh-negative person may sensitize the person to form anti-D (Rh_1).
   b. Rh_1 (D)-positive blood administered to a recipient having serum anti-D (Rh_1) could be fatal.
2. Identify Rh immune globulin (RhIG) candidates. RhIG is a concentrated solution of IgG anti-D (Rh_1) derived from human plasma. A 1-mL dose of RhIG contains 300 μg and is sufficient to counteract the immunizing effects of 15 mL of packed red cells or 30 mL of whole blood.
   a. Rh-negative pregnant women with Rh-positive partners may carry Rh-positive fetuses. Fetal cells may cross the placenta to the mother and cause production of antibodies in the maternal blood. The maternal antibody, in turn, may cross through the placenta into the fetal circulation and cause destruction of fetal blood cells. This condition, called *hemolytic disease of the newborn* (formerly called erythroblastosis fetalis), may cause reactions that range from anemia (slight or severe) to fetal death in utero. This condition may be prevented if an Rh-negative pregnant woman receives an RhIG dose antepartum at 28 weeks' gestation and a postpartum injection of RhIG shortly after delivery of an Rh-D (Rh_1)-positive infant. Postpartum Rh immunization can occur despite an injection of RhIG if >30 mL of fetal blood enters the maternal circulation. The American Association of Blood Banks recommends that a postpartum blood specimen of all Rh-D (Rh_1)-negative women (i.e., those at risk for immunization) be examined to detect a fetal maternal hemorrhage of >30 mL.
   b. Rh typing and evaluation for RhIG must also be done for patients who have had abortions, miscarriages, accidents, and amniocentesis.
3. Observe standard precautions.

Clinical Implications

1. The significance of Rh antigens is based on their capacity to immunize as a result of receiving a transfusion or becoming pregnant. The Rh_1 (D) antigen is by far the most antigenic; the other Rh antigens are much less likely to produce isoimmunization. The following general conditions must be met for immunization to Rh antigens to occur:
   a. The Rh blood antigen must be absent in the immunized person.
   b. The Rh blood antigen must be present in the immunizing blood.
   c. The blood antigen must be of sufficient antigenic strength to produce a reaction.
   d. The amount of incompatible blood must be large enough to induce antibody formation.
   e. Factors other than Rh_1 (D) may induce formation of antibodies in Rh-positive persons if the preceding conditions are met.

2. Antibodies for Rh_2 (C) are frequently found together with anti-Rh_1 (D) antibodies in the Rh-negative pregnant woman whose fetus or child is type Rh positive and possesses both antigens.
3. With exceedingly rare exceptions, Rh antibodies do not form unless preceded by antigenic stimulation, as occurs with the following conditions:
   a. Pregnancy and abortions
   b. Blood transfusions
   c. Deliberate immunization, most commonly of repeated intravenous injections of blood for the purpose of harvesting a given Rh antibody

Interventions

Pretest Patient Care

1. Explain purpose and procedure of the typing.
2. Follow guidelines in Chapter 1 for safe, effective, informed *pretest* care.

Posttest Patient Care

1. Review test results; report and record findings. Modify the nursing care plan as needed. Inform and counsel the patient regarding Rh type. Women of childbearing age may need special consideration. See page 637 for incidences of Rh types.
2. Follow Chapter 1 guidelines for safe, effective, informed *posttest* care.

● Rh Antibody Titer Test

This antibody study determines the Rh antibody level in an Rh-negative or pregnant woman whose partner is Rh positive. If the Rh-negative woman is carrying an Rh-positive fetus, the antigen from the fetal blood cells causes antibody production in the mother's serum. The firstborn child usually shows no ill effects; however, with subsequent pregnancies, the mother's serum antibodies increase and eventually destroy the fetal red blood cells, causing hemolytic disease of the newborn.

Normal Findings

Negative is 0 (no antibody detected).

Procedure

1. Obtain a 10-mL venous blood sample (plasma or serum) from the mother using a yellow-topped (ACD) and clotted blood (not SST) tube.
2. Observe standard precautions.

Clinical Implications

Some institutions have established a critical titer for anti-D below which hemolytic disease of the newborn is considered unlikely. No further investigations are undertaken unless the critical titer level is reached.

Interventions

Pretest Patient Care

1. Explain test purpose and procedure.
2. Follow guidelines in Chapter 1 for safe, effective, informed *pretest* care.

Posttest Patient Care

1. Review test results; report and record findings. Modify the nursing care plan as needed. Counsel the patient regarding abnormal findings; explain the need for possible follow-up testing and treatment.
2. Follow guidelines in Chapter 1 for safe, effective, informed *posttest* care.

● Rosette Test, Fetal Red Cells (Fetomaternal Bleed)

This qualitative test detects Rh-positive fetal cells in the Rh-negative maternal circulation. The detection of fetal erythrocytes is important when it is suspected that a severe fetal red cell loss has occurred and when serious risk for the mother becoming immunized against the fetal red cell groups is anticipated. In these instances, the mother's blood sample should be collected immediately after delivery to be examined for fetal cells. This test can be performed only if the mother is Rh negative and the newborn is known to be Rh positive. The rosette test is 97% accurate for detecting a fetomaternal bleed that exceeds 30 mL of whole blood. This test cannot be performed on patients who have had abortions, miscarriages, accidents, or amniocentesis.

Normal Findings

Negative for fetal blood loss
No Rh-positive fetal red blood cells detected in maternal blood

Procedure

1. Obtain a 7-mL venous blood EDTA sample from the mother shortly after delivery.
2. Perform this test and examine results for rosettes or mixed field agglutinates. Following manufacturer's guidelines, the presence of rosettes above a predetermined number indicates a fetal bleed that exceeds 30 mL of whole blood.

Clinical Implications

When the test sample contains few or new Rh_1-positive fetal cells, rosetting or agglutination is absent, and the fetomaternal bleed is <30 mL, one dose of parental RhIG will prevent immunization. If the fetal blood loss into the maternal circulation exceeds 30 mL, a quantitative or semiquantitative test (i.e., Kleihauer-Betke) or quantitative flow cytometry (if available) must be performed to calculate the amount of RhIG to administer.

Interventions

Pretest Patient Care

1. Explain test purpose and procedure.
2. Follow guidelines in Chapter 1 for safe, effective, informed *pretest* care.

Posttest Patient Care

1. Review test results; report and record findings. Modify the nursing care plan as needed. Counsel the patient regarding the findings; explain the need for possible follow-up testing and treatment (RhIG administration).
2. Follow guidelines in Chapter 1 for safe, effective, informed *posttest* care.

● Kleihauer-Betke Test (Fetal Hemoglobin Stain)

The Kleihauer-Betke test is a semiquantitative test to determine the amount of fetomaternal hemorrhage in an Rh_1-negative mother and the amount of RhIG necessary to prevent antibody production. The test is done after full-term delivery if newborn anemia is present or when the mother is Rh negative or weak-negative D. The test is also performed on mothers after invasive procedures (e.g., amniocentesis), miscarriages, or trauma.

Normal Findings

Negative: no fetal cells in maternal circulation (<1% or 0.01)

Procedure

1. A 7-mL maternal venous blood EDTA sample is obtained immediately after delivery, invasive procedure (e.g., amniocentesis), miscarriage, or trauma.
2. Examine the specimen immediately or refrigerate until it can be examined.

Clinical Implications

1. Results indicate moderate to great fetomaternal hemorrhage (50% to 90% of fetal red blood cells contain fetal hemoglobin [HbF]).
2. With full-term delivery, newborn red blood cells must be Rh-D–positive for the Rh-D–negative mother to be a candidate for RhIG.

Interventions

Pretest Patient Care

1. Explain test purpose and procedure.
2. Follow guidelines in Chapter 1 for safe, effective, informed *pretest* care.

Posttest Patient Care

1. Review test results; report and record findings. Modify the nursing care plan as needed. Counsel the patient regarding the findings; explain the need for possible follow-up testing and treatment, including administration of RhIG to suppress the immunization of fetal red cells or whole blood hemorrhage (Table 8.18).

   The calculated dose is as follows:

   $$\text{Vials of RhIG} = \frac{\text{mL of fetal blood}}{30}$$

   Some healthcare providers recommend doubling the calculated dose of RhIG because the method of calculating fetal blood is not precise; the results of undertreatment are serious, but the effects of overtreatment are minor.
2. Follow guidelines in Chapter 1 for safe, effective, informed *posttest* care.

TABLE 8.18 Recommendations for Dose of Rh Immune Globulin in Massive Fetomaternal Blood Based on the Acid Elution Test

	Fetomaternal Hemorrhage Volume (mL Whole Blood)		
Fetal Cells (%)	Average	Range[a]	Vials of RhIG to Inject
0.3–0.5	20	<50	2
0.6–0.8	35	15–80	3
0.9–1.1	50	22–110	4
1.2–1.4	65	30–140	5
1.5–2.0	88	37–200	6
2.1–2.5	115	52–250	6

[a]The range provides for the poor precision of the acid separation elution test. These recommendations are based on one vial needed for each 15 mL of red blood cells or 30 mL of whole blood.

• Crossmatch (Compatibility Test)

The primary purpose of the major crossmatch, or compatibility test, is to prevent a possible transfusion reaction.

Major crossmatch detects antibodies in the recipient's serum that may damage or destroy the cells in the blood donor (Table 8.19). The type and screen determine the ABO and Rh-D type as well as the presence or absence of unexpected antibodies from the recipient. The type and screen is a safe alternative for the routine type and crossmatch ordered preoperatively for cases that may, but usually do not, require transfusion (e.g., hysterectomy, cholecystectomy). If blood is needed, a major crossmatch must be done before transfusion.

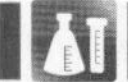

CLINICAL ALERT

Even the most carefully performed crossmatch will not detect all possible incompatible sources.

Normal Findings

No cell clumping or hemolysis and absence of agglutination when serum and cells are appropriately mixed and incubated

The major crossmatch shows compatibility between recipient serum and donor cells.

Procedure

1. Obtain a 10-mL venous blood sample.
2. Observe standard precautions.

Clinical Implications

1. Crossmatch incompatibility implies that the recipient cannot receive the incompatible unit of blood because antibodies are present.
2. A *transfusion reaction* occurs when incompatible blood is transfused, specifically if antibodies in the recipient's serum cause rapid red blood cell destruction in the proposed donor.
   a. Certain antibodies, although not causing immediate red cell destruction and transfusion reaction, may nevertheless reduce the normal life span of transfused incompatible cells; this may necessitate subsequent transfusions.
   b. The patient will derive the most benefit from red cells that survive longest.

CLINICAL ALERT

1. The most common cause of hemolytic transfusion reaction is the administration of incompatible blood to the recipient because of faulty matching in the laboratory, improper patient identification, or incorrect labeling of donor blood. If a transfusion reaction is suspected, discontinue the transfusion and notify the blood bank and attending physician immediately.
2. The probable benefits of each blood transfusion must be weighed against the risks, which include the following:
   a. Hemolytic transfusion reactions due to infusion of incompatible blood (can be fatal)
   b. Febrile or allergic reactions
   c. Transmission of infectious disease (e.g., hepatitis)

TABLE 8.19 Antibodies Found in Crossmatching

Blood Grouping System	Antibody	Description
Rh-hr	Anti-D	Rh1 May cause severe hemolytic disease of newborn
	Anti-C	Rh2 Often found with anti-D, Ce(rh_1), or C^w
	Anti-E	Rh3 Often found with anti-C
	Anti-c	Rh4 Often found with anti-E
	Anti-e	Rh5 Often found with anti-C
	Anti-C^w	Rh8
	Anti-V	Rh10 Alternative antigen names: ce^s, hr^v
Kell	Anti-K	K1 Strongly immunogenic; some non–red cell immune Occasional Kell system antibodies may not react
	Anti-k	K2 Antigen may be depressed by the presence of Kp^a
	Anti-Kp^a	K3 Few non–red cell immune
	Anti-Kp^b	K4
	Anti-Js^a	K6 Few non–red cell immune
	Anti-Js^b	K7
Duffy	Anti-Fy^a	Some antibodies exhibit dosage; quite common and may cause HDN and HTRs
	Anti-Fy^b	Some antibodies may bind complement
Kidd	Anti-Jk^a	Antibodies may exhibit dosage May cause severe delayed hemolytic transfusion reactions
	Anti-Jk^b	Antibody titers may drop rapidly below detectable levels Antibodies may require anti-C3 for detection
Lutheran	Anti-Lu^a	Antibody gives mixed field-like agglutination
	Anti-Lu^b	
MN	Anti-M	Common antibody Seldom clinically significant or implicated in HDN; may be pH-dependent or exhibit dosage
	Anti-N	Rare antibody Formaldehyde-induced anti-N commonly found in dialysis patients
	Anti-S	Antibody may be enhanced if incubated below 37°C before AHG
	Anti-s	—
	Anti-U	Rarely found in S-, s-patients
Lewis	Anti-Le^a	Frequently found in serum of pregnant women
	Anti-Le^b	Neutralized by soluble antigen
	-Le^{bh}	Anti-Le^b often found with anti-Le^a
	-Le^{bL}	Anti-Le^b usually made by Le (a^-b^-) individuals

table continues on pg. 643 >

TABLE 8.19, continued

Blood Grouping System	Antibody	Description
P	Anti-P_1	Antigen strength variable; neutralized by soluble antigen
	Anti-P	Biphasic hemolytic IgG autoantibody in PCH Alloantibody is usually potent IgM hemolysin
	Anti-P^k	Have caused hemolytic transfusion reactions and occasionally HDN
	(Anti-T^{ja})	
Xg	Anti-Xg^a	X-linked
Colton	Anti-Co^a	Rare antibodies
	Anti-Co^b	
Dombrock	Anti-Do^a	Incidence of Do^a lower in African Americans, Native Americans, and Asians
	Anti-Do^b	Infrequently reported antibodies
Diego	Anti-Di^a	Di^a antigen frequently higher in Asians and Native Americans
	Anti-Di^b	
Wright	Anti-Wr^a	IgM and IgG forms of antibody reported Frequently occurring antibody
Vel	Anti-Vel	Antibodies usually IgM; antigen strength variable, binds complement
Sd^a	Anti-Sd^a	Antigen weaker during pregnancy Wide variation of antigen expression Agglutinates have refractile, mixed-field appearance
HLA-associated	Anti-Bg^a	Antigen strength variable
	-Bg^b	Antibodies often found in multitransfused multiparous patients
	-Bg^c	Antibodies characteristically weakly reactive Bg/HLA associations Bg^a/HLA-B7 Bg^b/HLA-B17 Bg^c/HLA-A28
Cartwright	Anti-Yt^a	Antibody not uncommon in Yt (a−) individuals
	Anti-Yt^b	Rare antibody usually found in combination with other antibodies
HTLA	Anti	Antigen strength variable
	-Ch^a	Antibodies characteristically weakly reactive
	-Kn^a	
	-McC^a	
	-Yk^a	
	-Cs^a	
	-Gy^a	
	-Hy	
	-JMH	
	Anti-I	Most frequently detected cold autoagglutination Anti-I in CHD has wide thermal range, high titer Binds complement Seen as alloantibody in adults
	Anti-i	Antibody seen in serum of patients with infectious mononucleosis Rare cause of CHD Antigen very weakly expressed on the cells of most adults

HDN, hemolytic disease of the newborn; CHD, cold hemagglutinin disease; HTR, hemolytic transfusion reaction; AHG, antihuman globulin; Ig, immunoglobulin; PCH, paroxysmal cold hemoglobinuria; HTLA, human T-lymphocyte antigen.

Interventions

Pretest Patient Care

1. Explain purpose and procedure of crossmatching.
2. Follow guidelines in Chapter 1 for safe, effective, informed *pretest* care.

Posttest Patient Care

1. Review test results; report and record findings. Modify the nursing care plan as needed. Counsel the patient regarding potential transfusion reactions.
2. Assess for the following symptoms of transfusion reaction:
   a. Fever
   b. Chills
   c. Chest, abdomen, or flank pain
   d. Hypotension or hypertension
   e. Nausea
   f. Dyspnea
   g. Shock
   h. Oliguria
   i. Back pain
   j. Feeling of heat along vein being transfused
   k. Constricting chest and lumbar back muscles
   l. Facial flushing
   m. Hemoglobinuria
   n. Oozing blood from wounds
   o. Anemia
   p. Allergic reactions such as local erythema, hives, and itching
3. Follow guidelines in Chapter 1 for safe, effective, informed *posttest* care.

● Coombs' Antiglobulin Test

The indirect Coombs' test detects anti-RBC antibodies in the serum, whereas the direct Coombs' test detects antigen–antibody complexes on the red blood cell membrane. Antibody identification is performed when the antibody screen or direct antiglobulin tests produce positive results and unexpected blood group antibodies need to be classified. Antibody identification tests are an important part of pretransfusion testing so that the appropriate antigen-negative blood can be transfused. These tests are also helpful for diagnosing the following conditions:

1. Hemolytic disease of the newborn in which the red cells of the infant are sensitized and exhibit antigen–antibody complexes in vivo
2. Acquired hemolytic anemia in which an antibody is produced that coats the patient's own cells (autosensitization in vivo)
3. Transfusion reaction in which the patient may have received incompatible blood, which in turn has sensitized the donor's and possibly the patient's own red cells
4. Red blood cell sensitization caused by drugs

The indirect Coombs' test detects serum antibodies, reveals maternal anti-Rh antibodies during pregnancy, and can detect incompatibilities not found by other methods.

Normal Findings

Direct Coombs' test: no agglutination
Indirect Coombs' test: no agglutination

Procedure

1. Draw a 7-mL venous blood sample anticoagulated with EDTA and a 20-mL venous blood sample that is allowed to clot.
2. Notify the laboratory of diagnosis, history of recent and past transfusions, pregnancy, and any drug therapy.
3. Observe standard precautions.

Clinical Implications

1. The *direct Coombs' test is positive* (1+ to 4+) in the presence of the following conditions:
   a. Transfusion reactions
   b. Autoimmune hemolytic anemia (most cases)
   c. Cephalothin therapy (75% of cases)
   d. Drugs such as α-methyldopa (Aldomet), penicillin, insulin
   e. Hemolytic disease of newborn
   f. Paroxysmal cold hemoglobinuria
   g. In the presence of specific antibodies, usually from a previous transfusion or pregnancy, or nonspecific antibodies, as in cold agglutinants
2. The *indirect Coombs' test* is positive in the following conditions:
   a. Incompatible blood match
   b. Autoimmune or drug-induced hemolytic anemia
   c. Erythroblastosis fetalis hemolytic disease

Interfering Factors

A number of drugs may cause the direct Coombs' test to be positive, including procainamide, quinidine, and methyldopa.

Interventions

Pretest Patient Care

1. Explain purpose and procedure of test.
2. Follow guidelines in Chapter 1 for safe, effective, informed *pretest* care.

Posttest Patient Care

1. Review test results; report and record findings. Modify the nursing care plan as needed. Counsel the patient regarding abnormal findings; explain the need for possible follow-up testing and treatment. Hemolytic disease of the newborn can occur when the mother is Rh negative and the fetus is Rh positive. Diagnosis is derived from the following information: Mother is Rh negative, newborn is Rh positive, and the direct Coombs' test is positive. Newborn jaundice results from Rh incompatibility, but more often, the jaundice results from an ABO incompatibility.
2. Follow guidelines in Chapter 1 for safe, effective, informed *posttest* care.

TYPES OF TRANSFUSION REACTIONS

Acute Hemolytic Transfusion Reaction (HTR)

Hemolytic transfusion reaction (HTR) is triggered by an antigen–antibody reaction and activates the complement and coagulation systems. These are most always due to ABO incompatibility because of misidentification resulting in the patient receiving incompatible blood. Symptoms include fever, chills, backache, vague uneasiness, and red urine. HTR is potentially fatal.

Bacterial Contamination

Bacteria may enter the blood during phlebotomy. These microbes will multiply faster in components stored at room temperature than in refrigerated components. Although rare, bacteria in blood or its components can cause a septic transfusion reaction. Symptoms include high fever, shock, hemoglobinuria, disseminated intravascular coagulation, and renal failure. Such reactions can be fatal.

Cutaneous Hypersensitivity Reactions

Urticarial reactions are very common, second in frequency only to febrile nonhemolytic (FNH) reactions, and are usually characterized by erythema, hives, and itching. Allergy to some soluble substance in donor plasma is suspected.

Noncardiogenic Pulmonary Reactions (NPR)

Transfusion-related acute lung injury (TRALI) should be considered whenever a transfusion recipient experiences acute respiratory insufficiency or x-ray films show findings consistent with pulmonary edema without evidence of cardiac failure. These are possibly reactions between the donor's leukocyte antibodies and the recipient's leukocytes. TRALI produces white cell aggregates that become trapped in the pulmonary microcirculation. The findings on chest x-ray films are typical of acute pulmonary edema. If subsequent transfusions are needed, leukocyte-reduced red cells may prevent NPR reactions.

The diagnosis of TRALI includes the following:

- Acute onset of respiratory distress
- Hypoxemia
- Bilateral lung infiltration on x-ray
- No evidence of circulatory overload

Febrile Nonhemolytic (FNH) Reactions

FNH reactions are defined as a temperature increase of >1°C. They are seldom dangerous and may be caused by an antibody–antigen reaction.

Anaphylactic Reactions

Anaphylactic reactions occur after infusion of as little as a few milliliters of blood or plasma. Anaphylaxis is characterized by coughing, bronchospasm, respiratory distress, vascular instability, nausea, abdominal cramps, vomiting, diarrhea, shock, and loss of consciousness. Some reactions occur in IgA-deficient patients who have developed anti-IgA antibodies after immunization through previous transfusion or pregnancy.

Circulatory Overload

Rapid increases in blood volume are not tolerated well by patients with compromised cardiac or pulmonary function. Symptoms of circulatory overload include coughing, cyanosis, orthopnea, difficulty breathing, and a rapid increase in systolic blood pressure.

● Leukoagglutinin Test

Leukoagglutinins are antibodies that react with white blood cells and sometimes cause febrile, non-HTRs. Patients who exhibit this type of transfusion reaction should receive leukocyte-poor blood for any subsequent transfusions.

This study is done when a blood reaction occurs even though compatible blood has been given. The donor plasma contains an antibody that reacts with recipient white cells to produce an acute clinical syndrome of fever, dyspnea, cough, pulmonary infiltrates, and, in more severe cases, cyanosis and hypertension. Patients immunized by previous transfusions, by pregnancy, or during allografts often experience these febrile, non-HTRs because of incompatible transfused leukocytes. This type of reaction must be confirmed (as compared with hemolytic reactions) before additional transfusions can be safely administered.

Normal Findings

Negative for leukoagglutinins

Procedure

1. Obtain a 10-mL venous blood sample.
2. Observe standard precautions.

Clinical Implications

1. Agglutinating antibodies may appear in the donor's plasma.
2. When the agglutinating antibody appears in the recipient's plasma, febrile reactions are common; however, pulmonary manifestations do not occur.
3. Febrile reactions are more common in pregnant women and in individuals with a history of multiple transfusions.

CLINICAL ALERT

1. Febrile reactions can be prevented by separating out white cells from the donor blood before transfusion.
2. Patients whose blood contains leukoagglutinins should be instructed that they generally need to be transfused with leukocyte-reduced blood to minimize these reactions.

Interventions

Pretest Patient Care

1. Explain test purpose and procedure.
2. Follow guidelines in Chapter 1 for safe, effective, informed *pretest* care.

Posttest Patient Care

1. Review test results; report and record findings. Modify the nursing care plan as needed. Counsel the patient regarding future transfusion precautions.
2. Follow guidelines in Chapter 1 for safe, effective, informed *posttest* care.

● Platelet Antibody Detection Test

Platelet antibody detection studies are used to diagnose posttransfusion purpura, alloimmune neonatal thrombocytopenic purpura, idiopathic thrombocytopenic purpura, paroxysmal hemoglobinuria, and drug-induced immunologic thrombocytopenia.

Normal Findings

PLAI (negative platelet hyperlysibility): negative
ALTP (negative drug-dependent platelet antibodies): negative
PAIgG (platelet-associated IgG antibody): negative

Procedure

1. Obtain a 10-mL to 30-mL venous blood sample. Obtain 30 mL of venous blood when platelet count is 50,000 to 100,000/mm^3; 20 mL of venous blood when platelet count is 100,000 to 150,000 mm^3; and 10 mL of venous blood when platelet count is >150,000/mm^3.
2. Use standard precautions.

Interfering Factors

1. Alloantibodies formed in response to previous blood transfusions during pregnancies may produce positive reactions. Such antibodies are usually specific for HLAs found in platelets and other cells.
2. Whenever possible, obtain samples for platelet antibody testing before transfusion.

Clinical Implications

1. Antibodies to platelet antigens are of two types: Autoantibodies develop in response to one's own platelets as in idiopathic thrombocytopenic purpura, and alloantibodies develop following exposure to foreign platelets during transfusion.
2. Antiplatelet antibody, usually having anti-PLAI specificity, occurs in posttransfusion purpura.
3. A persistent or rising antibody titer during pregnancy is associated with neonatal thrombocytopenia.
4. PLAI incompatibility between mother and fetus appears to account for >60% of alloimmune neonatal thrombocytopenic purpura. A finding of a PLAI-negative mother and a PLAI-positive father provides presumptive diagnostic evidence.
5. PAIgG is present in 95% of both acute and chronic cases of idiopathic (autoimmune) thrombocytopenic purpura. Patients responding to steroid therapy or undergoing spontaneous remission show increased circulatory times that correlate with decreased PAIgG levels.
6. The platelet hyperlysibility assay measures the sensitivity of platelets to lysis. This test is positive in and specific for paroxysmal hemoglobinuria.
7. In drug-induced immunologic thrombocytopenia, antibodies that react only in the presence of the inciting drug can be detected. Quinidine, quinine, chlordiazepoxide, sulfa drugs, and diphenylhydantoin most commonly cause this type of thrombocytopenia. Gold-dependent antibodies and heparin-dependent platelet IgG antibodies can be detected by direct assay. Approximately 1% of persons receiving gold therapy develop thrombocytopenia as a side effect. Thrombocytopenia is also a well-known side effect of heparin.

NOTE *Platelet compatibility typing is done to ensure that hemostatically stable platelets can be transfused (e.g., for aplastic anemia and malignant disorders). This is important because most patients repeatedly transfused with platelets from random donors become partially or totally refractory to further platelet transfusion because of alloimmunization. Platelet typing also provides diagnostic evidence of posttransfusion purpura. Platelets are routinely typed for PLAI, HLH-A2, and PLEI. Those matched for HLA antigens generally produce satisfactory posttransfusion improvement. A standard platelet count performed 1 hour after the end of a fresh platelet concentrate transfusion is a sensitive indicator for the presence or absence of clinically important antibodies against HLA antigens.*

Interventions

Pretest Patient Care

1. Explain test purpose and procedure.
2. Follow guidelines in Chapter 1 for safe, effective, informed *pretest* care.

Posttest Patient Care

1. Review test results; report and record findings. Modify the nursing care plan as needed. Counsel the patient regarding abnormal findings; explain the need to assess and monitor the patient for bleeding tendencies. Assess for prescribed medications as cause of purpura.
2. Follow guidelines in Chapter 1 for safe, effective, informed *posttest* care.

● Human Leukocyte Antigen (HLA) Test

The major histocompatibility antigens of humans belong to the HLA system. They are present on all nucleated cells but can be detected most easily on lymphocytes. Each antigen results from a gene that shares a locus on the chromosome with another gene, one paternal and one maternal (two alleles). More than 27 of these antigens have been identified. The HLA complex, located in the short arm of chromosome 6, is a major histocompatibility complex that is responsible for many important immune functions in humans.

This test determines the leukocyte antigens present on human cell surfaces. When tissue or organ transplantation is contemplated, HLA typing identifies the degree of histocompatibility between donor and recipient. By matching donors and potential recipients with compatible lymphocytes and similar HLA types, it is possible to prolong transplant survival and to reduce rejection episodes. The HLA also aids in diagnosis of parentage as well as correlation with certain disease syndromes and rheumatoid diseases, particularly ankylosing spondylitis. HLA-B27, one of the HLA antigens, is found in 90% of patients with ankylosing spondylitis. Generally, the presence of a certain HLA antigen may be associated with increased susceptibility to a specific disease; however, it does not mandate that that person will develop the disease. This test is also done before HLA-matched platelet transfusion.

Normal Findings

Requires clinical correlation

Procedure

1. Obtain a 10- to 24-mL (two green-topped tubes) heparinized venous blood sample in three lavender-topped EDTA tubes (14 mL) or two plain red-topped tubes, 10 mL minimum, or 5 mL of clotted blood or two yellow-topped (ACD) tubes.
2. Observe standard precautions.
3. Determine the patient's HLA type by testing the patient's lymphocytes against a panel of defined HLA antisera directed against the currently recognized HLA antigens. The HLA antigens are identified by letter and number. When viable human lymphocytes are incubated with a known HLA cytotoxic antibody, an antigen–antibody complex is formed on a cell surface. The addition of serum that contains complement kills the cells, which are then recognized as possessing a defined HLA antigen.
4. Label carefully with patient's name, date, and special laboratory number. Include diagnosis and history.

Clinical Implications

1. Particular HLA antigens are associated with certain disease states:
   a. Ankylosing spondylitis (HLA-B27)
   b. Multiple sclerosis (HLA-B27 + Dw2 + A3 + B18)
   c. Sarcoidosis (HLA-B8)
   d. Psoriasis (HLA-A13 + B17)
   e. Reiter's syndrome (B27)

f. Juvenile type 1 diabetes (Bw15 + B8)
g. Acute anterior uveitis (B27)
h. Graves' disease (B27)
i. Juvenile RA (B27)
j. Celiac disease (B8)
k. Autoimmune CAH (B8)

2. Four groups of cell surface antigens (HLA-A, HLA-B, HLA-C, and HLA-D) constitute the strongest barriers to tissue transplantation.
3. In parentage determination, if a reputed father presents a phenotype (genotype completely determined by heredity; two haplotypes or gene clusters: one from father and one from mother) with no haplotype or antigen pair identical with one of the child's, he is excluded as the supposed father. If one of the reputed father's haplotypes (gene clusters) is the same as one of the child's, he *may* be the father. The chances of his being accurately identified as the father increase in direct proportion to the rarity of the presenting haplotype in the general population. Put another way, if the haplotype is very common, there is an increased probability that another man with the same haplotype also could be the father. When the frequency of the haplotype is known, the probability that the nonexcluded man is the father can be calculated. However, the degree of certainty diminishes as the incidence of the haplotype increases.

Interventions

Pretest Patient Care

1. Explain HLA test purposes and procedure. It is also used for postmortem testing before a renal transplantation.
2. Follow guidelines in Chapter 1 for safe, effective, informed *pretest* care.

Posttest Patient Care

1. Review test results; report and record findings. Modify the nursing care plan as needed. Counsel the patient regarding abnormal findings; explain the need for possible follow-up testing and treatment. HLA testing is best used as a diagnostic adjunct and should not be considered as diagnostic by itself.
2. Follow guidelines in Chapter 1 for safe, effective, informed *posttest* care.

BIBLIOGRAPHY

Abbas AK, Lichtman AH, Pillai S: Basic Immunology: Functions & Disorders of the Immune System, 5th ed. Philadelphia, Elsevier Health Sciences, 2015

Alere: Alere Determine™ HIV-1/2 Ag/Ab Combo. Available at: http://www.alere.com

American Association of Blood Banks: Standards for Blood Banks and Transfusion Services, 30th ed. Bethesda, MD, Author, 2016

Bartlett JG: 2005–2006 Pocket Book of Infectious Disease Therapy, 13th ed. Philadelphia, Lippincott Williams & Wilkins, 2005

Centers for Disease Control and Prevention: Human rabies prevention—United States, 2008: Recommendations of the Advisory Committee on Immunization Practices (ACIP). MMWR Recomm Rep 57(RR-3):1–28, 2008; updated by MMWR Recomm Rep 59(RR-2), 2010

Centers for Disease Control and Prevention: Laboratory testing for the diagnosis of HIV infection: Updated recommendations. Available at: http://stacks.cdc.gov/view/cdc/23447/cdc_23447_DS1.pdf; published June 27, 2014

Centers for Disease Control and Prevention: Prevention of hepatitis A through active or passive immunization. MMWR Recomm Rep 55(RR-7):1–23, 2006

Centers for Disease Control and Prevention: Screening recommendations and considerations referenced in treatment guidelines and original sources; STD & HIV screening recommendations. Available at: https://www.cdc.gov/std/tg2015/screening-recommendations.htm; last updated April 27, 2017

Centers for Disease Control and Prevention: Updated U.S. Public Health Service guidelines for the management of occupational exposures to HIV and recommendations for postexposure prophylaxis. MMWR Recomm Rep 54(RR-9):1–17, 2005; updated September 25, 2013

Chapman JA, Berstein IL, Lee RE, et al: Food allergy: A practice parameter. Ann Allergy Asthma Immunol 96:S1–S68, 2006

Detrick B, Schmitz, JL, Hamilton RG: Manual of Molecular and Clinical Immunology, 8th ed. Washington, DC, ASM Press, 2016

DeVita VT, Lawrence TS, Rosenberg SA: Cancer: Principles and Practice of Oncology, 10th ed. Philadelphia, Lippincott Williams & Wilkins, 2014

Diamandis EP, Bruns DE: Cancer diagnostics: Discovery and clinical applications—Introduction. Clin Chem 48(8):1145–1146, 2002

Doan T, Melvold R, Waltenbaugh C: Concise Medical Immunology. Philadelphia, Lippincott Williams & Wilkins, 2005

International AIDS Society-USA Panel: Treatment for adult HIV infection: 2006 recommendations. JAMA 296(7): 827–843, 2006

International Antiviral Society-USA: Practice Guidelines for HIV Prevention in Clinical Care Settings; 2014. Available at: https://www.iasusa.org/guidelines

Lukan A, Vranac T, Serbec VC: TSE Diagnostics: Recent Advances in Immunoassaying Prions. J Immunol Res 2013(2013):360304, 2013

Microplate Allergen-Specific IgE Standard Scoring: Product Insert from DPC's AlaSTAT Test Kit. Los Angeles, Diagnostic Products Corp, 2000

Myers JW, Moorman JP, Salgado CD: Gantz's Manual of Clinical Problems in Infectious Disease, 6th ed. Philadelphia, Lippincott Williams & Wilkins, 2012

National Cancer Institute: Prostate-Specific Antigen Test. Available at: https://www.cancer.gov/types/prostate/psa-fact-sheet#q2

Papp JR, Schachter J, Gaydos CA, et al: Recommendations for the laboratory-based detection of Chlamydia trachomatis and Neisseria gonorrhoeae—2014, MMWR Recomm Rep 63:1–19, 2014

Popovsky MA: Transfusion Reactions, 4th ed. Bethesda, MD, American Association of Blood Banks, 2012

Seage GR, Losina E, Goldie SJ, et al: The relationship of preventable opportunistic infections, HIV-1 RNA, and CD4 cell counts to chronic mortality. J Acquir Immune Defic Syndr 30:421–428, 2002

Stowel C, Dzik W: Emerging Technologies in Transfusion Medicine. Bethesda, MD, American Association of Blood Banks, 2003

Urban A: Laboratory monitoring in the management of HIV infection. Lab Med 33(3):193–202, 2002

U.S. Department of Health and Human Services: Exposure to Blood: What Health Care Workers Need to Know. Bethesda, MD, Centers for Disease Control and Prevention, 2003

U.S. Preventive Services Task Force: Prostate Cancer Screening Recommendations; release date May 2012

U.S. Preventive Services Task Force: Screening for HIV: Recommendation statement. Ann Intern Med 159(1): 1–36, 2013; Final Update Summary; available at: https://www.uspreventiveservicestaskforce.org/Page/Document/UpdateSummaryFinal/human-immunodeficiency-virus-hiv-infection-screening

Willis MS, Latimer MJ: Autoimmune hepatitis type 2. ASCP Lab Med 33(4):273–277, 2002

Woodhouse S: C-reactive protein: From acute phase reactant to cardiovascular disease risk factor. Med Lab Observ 34(3):2–21, 2002

Nuclear Medicine Studies

9

OVERVIEW OF NUCLEAR MEDICINE STUDIES

Nuclear medicine is a diagnostic modality that studies the *physiology* or *function* of any organ system in the body. Other diagnostic imaging modalities, such as ultrasound, magnetic resonance imaging (MRI), computed tomography (CT), and x-ray, generally visualize anatomic structures.

A pharmaceutical is labeled with a radioactive isotope to form a *radiopharmaceutical*. The radioisotope emits gamma and positron rays. Radioisotopes are reactor produced (iodine-131 [^{131}I]), cyclotron produced (fluorine-18 [^{18}F] for positron emission tomography [PET]), or generator produced (technetium-99m [^{99m}Tc]).

To visualize the function of an organ system, a radiopharmaceutical is administered. A time delay (in some cases, up to several hours) may be required for the radiopharmaceutical to reach its target site, and then the organ of interest is imaged with a gamma camera. Image formation technology involves the detection with very great density of a signal (gamma rays) emanating from the radioactive isotope. There is very little signal in the image that does not come from the radiopharmaceutical. The normal background level of radiation within the human body is minimal, with small amounts of radioactive potassium and some cesium. Routes of radiopharmaceutical administration vary with the specific study. Most commonly, a radiopharmaceutical is injected through a vein in the arm or hand. Other routes of administration include the oral, intramuscular, inhalation, intrathecal, subcutaneous, and intraperitoneal routes. See Table 9.1 for possible side effects of or adverse reactions to the administration of radiopharmaceuticals.

Nuclear medicine studies are performed by certified nuclear medicine technologists, interpreted by radiologists or nuclear medicine physicians, and performed in a hospital or clinic-based nuclear medicine department. The collaborative approach to care is evidenced by interventions from pharmacists, laboratory personnel, and nurses, among others.

Principles of Nuclear Medicine

The radiopharmaceutical is generally made up of two parts: the pharmaceutical, which is targeted to a specific organ, and the radionuclide, which emits gamma rays (high-energy electromagnetic radiation; short wavelength) and allows the organ to be visualized by the gamma camera. Nuclear medicine imaging can yield quantitative as well as qualitative data. A measurement of the ejection fraction of the heart is an example of quantitative data derived from a multigated acquisition (MUGA) or a myocardial stress procedure.

In general, nuclear medicine images visualize the distribution of a particular radiopharmaceutical, with hot, warm, or cold spots of activity indicating an abnormality. In a *hot spot*, there is an increased area of uptake of the radiopharmaceutical in diseased tissue compared with the distribution in normal tissue. Examples of this type of uptake can be seen on bone images. An example of a *warm spot* would be in a thyroid nodule. In a *cold spot*, there is an area of decreased uptake of the radiopharmaceutical compared with the distribution in normal tissue. Liver and lung imaging are examples of this

TABLE 9.1 Potential Side Effects in the Administration of Radiopharmaceuticals

Radiopharmaceutical (Trade Name)	Possible Side Effects
Iodine-131 [^{131}I]	Chills, nausea, vomiting, headache, dizziness, diffuse rash, tachycardia
Fluorine-18 [^{18}F]	None have been reported
Thallium-201 [^{201}Tl]	Fever, flushing, diffuse rash, hypotension
Technetium-99m [^{99m}Tc] ^{99m}Tc pertechnetate (Minitec, UltratecKow)	Chills, nausea, vomiting, headache, dizziness, diffuse rash, hypertension
^{99m}Tc tetrofosmin (Myoview)	Angina, hypertension, hypotension, vomiting, dyspnea, dizziness, metallic taste, abdominal discomfort
^{99m}Tc pyrophosphate [^{99m}Tc-PYP] (Pyrolite, TechneScan PYP, Phosphotec)	Chills, fever, nausea, vomiting, dizziness, diffuse rash, flushing, chest pain, syncope
^{99m}Tc disofenin (Hepatolite)	None have been reported
^{99m}Tc mebrofenin (Choletec)	Hives, urticaria
^{99m}Tc sulfur colloid (AN-Sulfur Colloid, TechneColl, Tesuloid)	Chills, fever, nausea, vomiting, headache, dizziness, diffuse rash, flushing, chest pain, vertigo, hypertension, hypotension, dyspnea
^{99m}Tc bicisate dihydrochloride (Neurolite)	Nausea, diffuse rash, dizziness, chest pain, seizures, syncope, vertigo
^{99m}Tc methylenediphosphonate (MDP) (Osteolite, TechneScan)	Chills, fever, nausea, vomiting, headache, dizziness, diffuse rash, flushing, chest pain, vertigo, hypertension, hypotension, syncope
^{99m}Tc pentetate (diethylenetriaminepentaacetate [DTPA]) (TechneScan DTPA, Techneplex)	Chills, fever, nausea, flushing, vomiting, headache, dizziness, diffuse rash, syncope, hypertension, hypotension, dyspnea
^{99m}Tc exametazime (Ceretec)	Fever, flushing, diffuse rash, hypertension, hypotension, seizures, dyspnea
^{111}In capromab pendetide (ProstaScint)	Increase in bilirubin, hypotension, hypertension, injection site reactions, fever, rash, headache, production of human antimouse antibody (HAMA)
Indium-111 [^{111}In] DTPA (MPI-DTPA)	Fever, nausea, vomiting, flushing, headache, hypertension
Indium oxine (^{111}In)	Fever
^{123}I metaiodobenzylguanidine (MIBG)	Nausea, flushing, hypertension, dizziness, vertigo, tachypnea
Gallium citrate (^{67}Ga) (Neoscan)	Nausea, vomiting, flushing, diffuse rash, tachycardia, dizziness, vertigo, metallic or salty taste
Cobalt (^{57}Co)	None has been reported
Chromium-51 (^{51}Cr)	Flushing, hypertension, tachycardia

Note: Most adverse drug reactions (ADRs) include such symptoms as nausea, vomiting, hypotension, rash, dyspnea, tachycardia, fever, and headaches; however, it is difficult to determine whether these are due to administration of the radiopharmaceutical or other medications the patient is taking. The ADR rate has been estimated at about 0.003% (3 per 100,000). The half-life of radiopharmaceuticals ranges from a couple of minutes to several days.

Adapted from Silberstein EB, Ryan J, Pharmacopeia Committee of the Society of Nuclear Medicine: Prevalence of adverse reactions in nuclear medicine. J Nucl Med 37:185–192, 1996.

type of uptake. Prompt uptake in transplanted organs correlates with (1) adequate perfusion, such as reperfusion of the transplanted lungs or pancreas; (2) excretory function, such as in kidney transplants; and (3) evidence of cardiac viability and reinnervation. Poor uptake and nonvisualization of the transplanted organ are evidence of rejection.

NOTE *Units of measure: curie (Ci) or becquerel (Bq) = radiation emitted by a radioactive material (1 Ci = 3.7×10^{10} Bq) rad or gray (Gy) = radiation dose absorbed by a person (1 rad = 0.01 Gy) rem or sievert (Sv) = biologic risk of exposure to radiation (1 rem = 0.01 Sv)*

Principles of Imaging

All gamma cameras have the same basic components. The camera may have one, two, or three heads, with the capability of imaging in multiple configurations. The camera is networked with a multitasking computer capable of acquiring and processing the data.

Several methods of imaging are used: dynamic, static, whole-body, and single photon emission computed tomography (SPECT). These imaging capabilities are available on all camera systems.

Dynamic imaging allows serial display of multiple frames of data, each frame lasting 1 to 3 seconds, to visualize the blood flow associated with a particular organ. Static imaging is also known as *planar* imaging. The camera acquires one image at a time, covering the field of view. This image is two-dimensional. Whole-body imaging acquires both anterior and posterior sweeps of the patient's body. This type of imaging also gives two-dimensional information.

SPECT imaging has revolutionized the field of nuclear medicine. SPECT imaging provides three dimensions of data. SPECT imaging increased the specificity and sensitivity of nuclear imaging through improved resolution and is often combined with CT scans. A combined gamma camera and CT scanner allows both procedures to be performed without patient transfer. Therefore, positioning is not compromised, and both abnormal and normal areas are visualized without position change.

General Procedure

1. Alert the patient that he or she may be required to follow a study-specific preparation regimen before imaging determined by the type of nuclear medicine procedure (e.g., nothing by mouth [NPO], no caffeine for 24 hours, hydration, bowel preparation).
2. Administer a radiopharmaceutical through the ordered route: oral, inhalation, intravenous, intramuscular, intrathecal, or intraperitoneal. On occasion, additional pharmaceuticals may be administered to enhance the function of the organ of interest.
3. A time delay may be necessary for the radiopharmaceutical to reach the organ of interest.
4. Imaging time depends on:
    a. Specific study radiopharmaceutical used and the time that must be allowed for concentration in tissues
    b. Type of imaging equipment used
    c. Patient cooperation
    d. Additional views based on patient history and nuclear medicine protocol
    e. Patient's physical size

PROCEDURAL ALERT

The nuclear medicine department should be notified if the patient may be pregnant or is breastfeeding or is younger than 18 yr of age.

Benefits and Risks

Benefits and risks should be explained before testing. Patients retain the radioisotope for a relatively short period. The radioactivity decays over time. Some of the radioisotope is eliminated in urine, feces, and other body fluids.

^{99m}Tc, the most commonly used radiopharmaceutical, has a radioactive half-life of 6 hours. This means that half of the dose decays in 6 hours. Other radioisotopes, such as iodine, indium, thallium, and gallium, take 13 hours to 8 days for half of the dose to decay.

1. Benefits
    a. Nuclear medicine yields functional data that are not provided by other modalities.
    b. Nuclear imaging is relatively safe, painless (except for intravenous administration), and noninvasive.
2. Risks
    a. Radiation exposure is minimal.
    b. Hematoma at intravenous injection site
    c. Reactions to the radiopharmaceutical (hives, rash, itching, constriction of throat, dyspnea, bronchospasm, anaphylaxis [rare])

Clinical Considerations

The following information should be obtained before diagnostic nuclear imaging:

1. Pregnancy (confirmed or suspected): Pregnancy is a contraindication for most nuclear imaging.
2. Lactating women may be advised to stop nursing for a set period (e.g., 2 to 3 days with ^{99m}Tc). Most radiopharmaceuticals are excreted in the mother's milk.
3. Radiopharmaceutical uptake from a recent nuclear medicine examination could interfere with interpretation of the current study.
4. The presence of any prostheses in the body must be recorded on the patient's history because certain devices can shield the gamma rays from imaging.
5. Current medications, treatments, and diagnostic measures (e.g., telemetry, oxygen, urine collection, intravenous lines)
6. Age and current weight: This information is used to calculate the radiopharmaceutical dose to be administered. If the patient is younger than 18 years of age, notify the examining department before testing. The amount of radioactive substance administered is adjusted downward for anyone younger than 18 years of age.
7. Allergies: Past history of allergies, especially to contrast substances (e.g., iodine) used in diagnostic procedures.

Interventions

Pretest Patient Care and Standard Precautions for Nuclear Medicine Procedures

1. Explain the purpose, procedure, benefits, and risks of the nuclear medicine procedure.
2. Assess for allergies to substances such as iodine.
3. Reassure the patient that the procedure is safe and painless.
4. Inform the patient that the procedure is performed in the nuclear medicine department. Contact the department to determine the expected time and length of the procedure.
5. Have the patient appropriately dressed.
6. Obtain an accurate weight because the radiopharmaceutical dose may be calculated by weight.
7. If a female patient is premenopausal, determine whether she may be pregnant. Pregnancy is a contraindication to most nuclear imaging to avoid irradiation of the fetus.

CLINICAL ALERT

1. Nuclear medicine procedures are usually contraindicated in pregnant women. Lactating women may need to discard their breast milk for several days following the procedure.
2. These precautions should also be followed for the radionuclide laboratory procedures and PET imaging.

Posttest Patient Care and Standard Precautions for Nuclear Medicine Procedures

1. Use routine disposal procedures for body fluids and excretions unless directed otherwise by the nuclear medicine department. Special considerations for disposal must be followed for therapeutic procedures.
2. Record any problems that may have occurred during the procedure.
3. Monitor the injection site for signs of bruising, hematoma, infection, discomfort, or irritation.
4. Assess for side effects of radiopharmaceuticals.

Pediatric Nuclear Medicine Considerations

Many of the nuclear medicine procedures that are performed on adults may be indicated in children.

Interventions

Pediatric Pretest Care

1. Verify that the female patient is not pregnant.
2. Be aware that depending on hospital policy, a valid consent form may be requested to be signed by the parents or legal guardians of the patient.
3. Explain the procedure and its purpose, benefits, and risks to the parents or legal guardians and to the patient. Reassure the patient that the test is safe and painless.
4. Assess for allergy to medications.
5. Have the patient appropriately dressed, ensuring that there are no metal objects on the patient during the procedure.
6. Obtain an accurate weight; the dose is calculated based on the patient's weight. Because pediatric patients have a different body metabolism than adults, a lower dose is given. Use of a body surface area (BSA) formula is recommended. The most commonly used is the DuBois formula:

$$BSA = 0.007184 \times W^{0.425} \times H^{0.725}$$

(W = weight in kg and H = height in cm)

7. Remember that immobilization techniques are often used during the imaging of pediatric patients. Wrapping an infant or small child is often necessary. Head clamps, arm boards, or sandbags may be used for patient immobilization.
8. Administer sedative drugs to reduce patient motion during the examination. Disadvantages of sedation may include nausea and vomiting.
9. Start an intravenous line for administration of radiopharmaceuticals.
10. Do not leave patients unattended during the procedure.
11. Pediatric patients need constant reassurance and emotional support.
12. Patient urination is often difficult to control. A urinary catheter may be required.

Pediatric Posttest Care

1. Follow *posttest* guidelines for adults.
2. Observe pediatric patients for adverse reactions to radiopharmaceuticals. Infants are more at risk for reactions.

CARDIAC STUDIES

Myocardial Perfusion: Rest and Stress (Sestamibi/Tetrofosmin/Thallium Stress Test)

^{99m}Tc sestamibi, thallium-201 (^{201}Tl), and ^{99m}Tc tetrofosmin are the radioactive imaging agents available for myocardial perfusion imaging to diagnose ischemic heart disease and allow differentiation of ischemia and infarction. This test reveals myocardial wall defects and heart pump performance during increased oxygen demands. Nuclear medicine imaging may also be done before and after streptokinase treatment for coronary artery thrombosis, after surgery for great vessel translocation, and after transplantation to detect organ rejection and myocardial viability. Pediatric indications include evaluation for ventricular septal defects and congenital heart disease and postsurgical evaluation of congenital heart disease. Studies have shown the efficacy of performing SPECT imaging with ^{99m}Tc sestamibi when triaging patients with diabetes who arrive in the emergency department with symptoms suggestive of acute cardiac ischemia.

^{201}Tl is a physiologic analogue of potassium. The myocardial cells extract potassium, as do other muscle cells. ^{99m}Tc sestamibi is taken up by the myocardium through passive diffusion, followed by active uptake within the mitochondria. Unlike thallium, technetium does not undergo significant redistribution. Therefore, there are some procedural differences. Myocardial activity also depends on blood flow. Consequently, when the patient is injected during peak exercise, the normal myocardium has much greater activity than the abnormal myocardium. Cold spots indicate a decrease or absence of flow.

A completely normal myocardial perfusion study may eliminate the need for cardiac catheterization in the evaluation of chest pain and nonspecific abnormalities of the electrocardiogram (ECG). SPECT imaging can accurately localize regions of ischemia.

Administration of dipyridamole (Persantine) or regadenoson (Lexiscan) is indicated in adults and children who are unable to exercise to achieve the desired cardiac stress level and maximum cardiac vasodilation. These medications have an effect similar to that of exercise on the heart. Physical stress testing may be initiated in children beginning at 4 to 5 years. Candidates for drug-induced stress testing are those with lung disease, peripheral vascular disease with claudication, amputation, spinal cord injury, multiple sclerosis, or morbid obesity. Dipyridamole stress testing is also valuable as a significant predictor of cardiovascular death, reinfarction, and risk for postoperative ischemic events and to reevaluate unstable angina.

Ejection fraction and wall motion can be assessed by computer analysis.

Reference Values

Normal

Normal stress test: ECG and blood pressure normal

Normal myocardial perfusion under both rest and stress conditions

Procedure

1. Myocardial perfusion general imaging
   a. There are two phases to this procedure: the rest imaging and the stress imaging. Either ^{201}Tl, ^{99m}Tc sestamibi, or ^{99m}Tc tetrofosmin may be used.
      (1) Rest imaging
         (a) Perform an intravenous injection of the radioisotope. Allow a 30- to 60-minute delay for the radioisotope to localize in the heart.
         (b) Perform SPECT imaging.

(2) Stress imaging
   (a) The patient undergoes an exercise or a pharmacologic cardiac stress test. At the peak level of stress, inject the patient with the radioisotope.
   (b) SPECT imaging may begin 30 minutes after injection.

b. Pharmacologic stress tests may be performed with any of three routine stressing agents:
   (1) Infuse dipyridamole over 4 to 6 minutes. Inject the radiopharmaceutical. Two minutes later, administer aminophylline, an antidote to the dipyridamole, at the nuclear medicine physician or cardiologist's discretion. Patient monitoring may last 20 minutes. Contraindication: caffeine.
   (2) Infuse regadenoson over 20 seconds. Inject the radiopharmaceutical 3 minutes after the infusion.
   (3) Infuse dobutamine until the predicted heart rate is achieved. The infusion protocol lasts 3 minutes at each dose increment.

2. ^{201}Tl
   a. During the cardiac stress test, the patient is monitored by a nuclear medicine physician, cardiologist, a registered nurse, an electrophysiologist, or an ECG technician.
   b. Have the patient begin walking on the treadmill.
   c. When the patient has reached 85% to 95% of maximum heart rate, inject radioactive thallium. Take the patient for immediate imaging.
   d. SPECT imaging begins within 5 minutes of injection.
   e. Acquire a second image approximately 3 to 4 hours later, with the patient at rest, to determine redistribution of the thallium.
   f. See Chapter 1 guidelines for safe, effective, informed *intratest* care.
3. ^{99m}Tc sestamibi and ^{99m}Tc tetrofosmin
   a. Follow myocardial perfusion general imaging procedures.
   b. Observe standard precautions.

PROCEDURAL ALERT

Myocardial perfusion imaging protocols vary among nuclear medicine departments. Some departments use a rest–stress, stress–rest, dual-isotope, or 2-d protocol, separating the phases into 2 different days.

NOTE *Regadenoson has an extremely short half-life: Once the infusion has stopped, any symptoms will subside. Contraindications: caffeine and theophylline-based drugs.*

PROCEDURAL ALERT

Some nuclear medicine protocols may require the patient to return 24 hr later for delayed imaging.

Clinical Implications

1. Imaging that is abnormal during exercise but remains normal at rest indicates transient ischemia.
2. Nuclear cardiac imaging that is abnormal both at rest and under stress indicates a past infarction.
3. Hypertrophy produces an increase in uptake.
4. The progress of disease can be estimated.
5. The location and extent of myocardial disease can be assessed.
6. Specific and significant abnormalities in the stress ECG usually are indications for cardiac catheterization or further studies.

Interfering Factors

1. Inadequate cardiac stress
2. Caffeine intake
3. Injection of dipyridamole in the upright or standing position or with isometric handgrip may increase myocardial uptake.

Interventions

Pretest Patient Care for Stress Testing

1. Explain test purpose and procedure, benefits, and risks. See standard nuclear medicine imaging *pretest* precautions.
2. Before the stress test has begun, start an intravenous line and prepare the patient. Perform a resting 12-lead ECG and blood pressure measurement.
3. Advise the patient that the exercise stress period will be continued for 1 to 2 minutes after injection to allow the radiopharmaceutical to be cleared during a period of maximum blood flow.
4. The patient should experience no discomfort during the imaging.
5. Alert the patient that fasting may be recommended for at least 2 hours before the stress test. Caffeine intake must be eliminated for 24 hours before the stress test.
6. For dipyridamole administration:
   a. Fasting may be required before the stress test, and avoidance of any caffeine products for at least 24 hours before the test is necessary.
   b. Blood pressure, heart rate, and ECG results are monitored for any changes during the infusion. Aminophylline may be given to reverse the effects of the dipyridamole.
7. Follow guidelines in Chapter 1 for safe, effective, informed *pretest* care.

CLINICAL ALERT

1. The stress study is contraindicated in patients who:
   a. Have a combination of right and left bundle branch block
   b. Have left ventricular hypertrophy
   c. Are taking digitalis or quinidine
   d. Are hypokalemic
2. Adverse short-term effects of dipyridamole may include nausea, headache, dizziness, facial flush, angina, ST-segment depression, and ventricular arrhythmia.

Posttest Patient Care

1. Observe the patient for possible effects of dipyridamole infusion.
2. Review test results; report and record findings. Modify the nursing care plan as needed.
3. Refer to nuclear scan *posttest* precautions.
4. Follow guidelines in Chapter 1 for safe, effective, informed *posttest* care.

• Myocardial Infarction Pyrophosphate (PYP) Imaging

^{99m}Tc pyrophosphate (^{99m}Tc-PYP) is the radioactive imaging agent used to evaluate the general location, size, and extent of myocardial infarction 24 to 96 hours after suspected myocardial infarction and as an indication of myocardial necrosis to differentiate between old and new infarcts. In some instances, the test is sensitive enough to detect an infarction 12 hours to 7 days after its occurrence. Acute infarction is associated with an area of increased radioactivity (hot spot) on the myocardial image. This test is useful when ECG and enzyme studies are not definitive.

Reference Values

Normal

Normal distribution of the radiopharmaceutical in sternum, ribs, and other bone structures
No myocardial uptake

Procedure

1. Myocardial imaging involves a 4-hour delay before imaging after the intravenous injection of the radionuclide. During this waiting period, the radioactive material accumulates in the damaged heart muscle.
2. Alert the patient that imaging takes 30 to 45 minutes, during which time the patient must lie still on an imaging table.
3. See Chapter 1 guidelines for safe, effective, informed *intratest* care.

Clinical Implications

1. Imaging that is entirely normal indicates that an acute infarction is not present and the myocardium is viable.
2. Myocardial uptake of the PYP is compared with the ribs (2+) and sternum (4+). Higher uptake levels (4+) reflect greater myocardial damage.
3. Larger defects have a poorer prognosis than small defects.

Interfering Factors

False-positive infarct-avid PYP can occur in cases of chest wall trauma, recent cardioversion, and unstable angina.

Interventions

Pretest Patient Care

1. Imaging can be performed at the bedside in the acute phase of infarction if the nuclear medicine department has a mobile gamma camera.
2. Explain the purpose, procedure, benefits, and risks of the nuclear medicine study. See standard *pretest* precautions.
3. Remember that imaging must occur within a period of 12 hours to 7 days after the onset of symptoms of infarction. Otherwise, false-negative results may be reported.
4. Follow guidelines in Chapter 1 for safe, effective, informed *pretest* care.

Posttest Patient Care

1. Review test results; report and record findings. Modify the nursing care plan as needed. If heart surgery is needed, counsel the patient concerning follow-up testing after surgery.
2. Refer to standard precautions and *posttest* care.
3. Follow additional guidelines in Chapter 1 for safe, effective, informed *posttest* care.

● Multigated Acquisition (MUGA) Imaging: Rest and Stress

The term *gated* refers to the synchronization of the imaging equipment and computer with the patient's ECG to evaluate left ventricular function. The primary purpose of this test is to provide an ejection fraction (the amount of blood ejected from the ventricle during the cardiac cycle).

Once injected, the distribution of radiolabeled red blood cells (RBCs) is imaged by synchronization of the recording of cardiac images with the ECG. This technique provides a means of obtaining information about cardiac output, end-systolic volume, end-diastolic volume, ejection fraction, ejection velocity, and regional wall motion of the ventricles. Computer-aided imaging of wall motion of the ventricles can be portrayed in the cinematic mode to visualize contraction and relaxation. This procedure may also be performed as a stress test. MUGA images are not often performed on children.

Reference Values

Normal

Normal myocardial wall motion and ejection fractions under conditions of stress and rest

Procedure

1. This procedure may be performed with or without stress. A MUGA with the patient at rest could be performed at the bedside if necessary, if the nuclear medicine department has a mobile gamma camera.
2. Label the patient's own RBCs with ^{99m}Tc-PYP by any of several methods. Inject the blood once it is labeled. In children and adults, administer the ^{99m}Tc-labeled RBCs slowly through an intravenous line. For children younger than 3 years of age, sedation may be required for the injection and to allow the pediatric patient to hold still for the required 20 to 30 minutes. Alternatively, perform a cardiac flow study.
3. During an ECG, the patient's R wave signals the computer and camera to take several image frames for each cardiac cycle.
4. Image the patient immediately after injection of the labeled RBCs.
5. See Chapter 1 guidelines for safe, effective, informed *intratest* care.

Clinical Implications

Abnormal MUGA procedures as associated with:

1. Congestive cardiac failure
2. Change in ventricular function due to infarction
3. Persistent arrhythmias from poor ventricular function
4. Regurgitation due to valvular disease
5. Ventricular aneurysm formation

Interfering Factors

If a reliable ECG cannot be obtained because of arrhythmias, the test cannot be performed.

Interventions

Pretest Patient Care

1. Explain the purpose, procedure, benefits, and risks.
2. Follow standard nuclear medicine imaging *pretest* precautions.
3. Follow guidelines in Chapter 1 for safe, effective, informed *pretest* care.

Posttest Patient Care

1. Review test results; report and record findings. Modify the nursing care plan as needed. Review MUGA outcomes and monitor appropriately for cardiac disease.
2. Refer to standard nuclear scan *posttest* precautions.
3. Follow guidelines in Chapter 1 for safe, effective, informed *posttest* care.

● Cardiac Flow Study (First-Pass Study; Shunt Imaging)

The cardiac flow study is performed to check for blood flow through the great vessels and after vessel surgery; it is useful in the determination of both right and left ventricular ejection fractions. Immediately after the injection, the camera traces the flow of the radiopharmaceutical in its "first pass" through the cardiac chambers in multiple rapid images. The first-pass study uses a jugular or antecubital vein injection of the radiopharmaceutical. A large-bore needle is used.

This study is useful in examining heart chamber disorders, especially left-to-right and right-to-left shunts. Children are commonly candidates for this procedure. Indications for pediatric patients include evaluation for congenital heart disease, transposition of the great vessels, and atrial or ventricular septal defects and quantitative assessment of valvular regurgitation. In neonates, the cardiac flow study can be used in conjunction with computer software for quantitative assessments. These quantitative values are useful in determining the degree of cardiac shunting with septal defects in the atria or ventricles.

Reference Values

Normal

Normal wall motion and ejection fraction
Normal pulmonary transit times and normal sequence of chamber filling

Procedure

1. Use a three-way stopcock with saline flush for radionuclide injection into the jugular vein or the antecubital fossa. For a shunt evaluation, inject the radionuclide into the external jugular vein to ensure a compact bolus.
2. Have the patient lie supine with the head slightly raised.
3. Although the total patient time is approximately 20 to 30 minutes; the actual imaging time is only 5 minutes.
4. Perform resting MUGA imaging with a shunt study.
5. See Chapter 1 guidelines for safe, effective, informed *intratest* care.

NOTE *With pediatric patients, it is important that the child not cry because this disrupts the flow of the radiopharmaceutical and negates the results of the test.*

Clinical Implications

1. Abnormal first-pass ejection fraction values are associated with:
   a. Congestive heart failure
   b. Change in ventricular function due to infarction
   c. Persistent arrhythmias from poor ventricular function
   d. Regurgitation due to valvular disease
   e. Ventricular aneurysm formation
2. Abnormal heart shunts reveal:
   a. Left-to-right shunt
   b. Right-to-left shunt
   c. Mean pulmonary transit time
   d. Tetralogy of Fallot

Interfering Factors

Inability to obtain intravenous access to the jugular vein or large-bore antecubital access

Interventions

Pretest Patient Care

1. Explain the purpose, procedure, benefits, and risks. An intravenous line is required.
2. Follow guidelines in Chapter 1 for safe, effective, informed *pretest* care.
3. Refer to standard nuclear scan *pretest* precautions.
4. Obtain a signed, witnessed consent form if stress testing is to be done.

Posttest Patient Care

1. Review test results; report and record findings. Modify the nursing care plan as needed. Monitor injection site and counsel patient appropriately.
2. Refer to standard nuclear scan *posttest* precautions.
3. Follow guidelines in Chapter 1 guidelines for safe, effective, informed *posttest* care.

ENDOCRINE STUDIES

● Thyroid Imaging

The thyroid imaging test systematically measures the update of radioactive iodine (either ^{131}I or ^{123}I) by the thyroid. Iodine (and, consequently, radioiodine) is actively transported to the thyroid gland and is incorporated into the production of thyroid hormones. The test is required for the evaluation of thyroid size, position, and function. It is used in the differential diagnosis of masses in the neck, base of the tongue, or mediastinum. Thyroid tissue can be found in each of these three locations.

Benign adenomas may appear as nodules of increased uptake of iodine ("hot" nodules), or they may appear as nodules of decreased uptake ("cold" nodules). Malignant areas generally take the form of cold nodules. The most important use of thyroid imaging is the functional assessment of these thyroid nodules. Pediatric indications include evaluation of neonatal hypothyroidism or thyrocarcinoma.

Thyroid imaging performed with iodine is usually acquired in conjunction with a radioactive iodine uptake study, which is performed 4 to 6 hours and 24 hours after dosing. For a complete thyroid workup, in both adults and children, thyroid hormone blood levels are usually measured. A thyroid ultrasound examination also may be performed.

Reference Values

Normal

Normal or evenly distributed concentration of radioactive iodine
Normal size, position, shape, site, weight, and function of the thyroid gland
Absence of nodules

Procedure

1. Have the patient swallow radioactive iodine in a capsule or liquid form.
2. Determine an uptake 4 to 6 hours and 24 hours after dosing. Four hours after dosing, the thyroid (neck area) is imaged if ^{123}I is used for both the uptake and the image.
3. Normal scan time is about 45 minutes.
4. See Chapter 1 guidelines for safe, effective, informed *intratest* care.

Clinical Implications

1. Cancer of the thyroid most often manifests as a nonfunctioning cold nodule, indicated by a focal area of decreased uptake.
2. Some abnormal results are:
    a. Hyperthyroidism, represented by an area of diffuse increased uptake
    b. Hypothyroidism, represented by an area of diffuse decreased uptake
    c. Graves' disease, represented by an area of diffuse increased uptake
    d. Autonomous nodules, represented by focal area of increased uptake
    e. Hashimoto's disease (chronic lymphocytic thyroiditis, an autoimmune disease), represented by mottled areas of decreased uptake
3. Imaging alone cannot definitively determine the diagnosis; uptake information is essential for a definitive diagnosis.

Interfering Factors

1. Thyroid imaging needs to be completed before radiographic examinations using contrast media (e.g., intravenous pyelogram, cardiac catheterization, CT with contrast, myelogram) are performed.
2. Any medication containing iodine should not be given until the nuclear medicine thyroid procedures are concluded. Notify the attending healthcare provider if thyroid studies have been ordered or if there are interfering radiographs or medications.

Interventions

Pretest Patient Care

1. Instruct the patient about nuclear medicine imaging purpose, procedure, and special restrictions. Refer to standard nuclear medicine imaging *pretest* precautions.
2. Because the thyroid gland responds to small amounts of iodine, the patient may be requested to refrain from iodine intake for at least 1 week before the test. Patients should consult with a healthcare provider. Restricted items include the following:
   a. Certain thyroid drugs
   b. Weight-control medicines
   c. Multiple vitamins
   d. Some oral contraceptives
   e. X-ray contrast materials containing iodine
   f. Cough medicine
   g. Iodine-containing foods, especially kelp and other natural foods
3. Alleviate any fears the patient may have about radionuclide procedures.
4. Follow guidelines in Chapter 1 for safe, effective, informed *pretest* care.

CLINICAL ALERT

1. Nuclear medicine thyroid imaging is contraindicated in pregnancy. Thyroid testing in pregnancy is routinely limited to blood testing.
2. This study should be completed before thyroid-blocking radiographic contrast agents are administered and before thyroid or iodine drugs are given.
3. Occasionally, tests are performed purposely with iodine or some thyroid drug in the body. In these cases, the healthcare provider is testing the response of the thyroid to these drugs. These stimulation and suppression tests are usually done to determine the nature of a particular nodule and whether the tissue is functioning or nonfunctioning.

Posttest Patient Care

1. If iodine has been administered, observe the patient for signs and symptoms of allergic reaction.
2. Explain test outcomes and possible treatment.
3. Refer to standard nuclear medicine imaging *posttest* precautions.
4. Follow guidelines in Chapter 1 for safe, effective, informed *posttest* care.

● Radioactive Iodine (RAI) Uptake Test

This direct test of the function of the thyroid gland measures the ability of the gland to concentrate and retain iodine. When radioactive iodine is administered, it is rapidly absorbed into the bloodstream. This procedure measures the rate of accumulation, incorporation, and release of iodine by the thyroid. The rate of absorption of the radioactive iodine, which is determined by the increase in radioactivity of the thyroid gland, is a measure of the ability of the thyroid to concentrate iodine from blood plasma. The radioactive isotopes of iodine used are ^{131}I and ^{123}I.

This procedure is indicated in the evaluation of hypothyroidism, hyperthyroidism, thyroiditis, goiter, and pituitary failure and for posttreatment evaluation. The patient who is a candidate for this test may have a lumpy or swollen neck or complain of pain in the neck; the patient may be jittery and ultrasensitive to heat or sluggish and ultrasensitive to cold. The test is more useful in the diagnosis of hyperthyroidism than hypothyroidism.

Reference Values

Normal

Absorption (uptake) by the thyroid gland:
1% to 13% after 2 hours
5% to 20% after 6 hours
15% to 40% after 24 hours
Values are laboratory dependent.

Procedure

NOTE *The test usually is done in conjunction with thyroid imaging and assessment of thyroid hormone blood levels.*

1. A fasting state is preferred. A complete history and listing of all medications is a must for this test. This history should include over-the-counter medications, as well as herbal supplements, vitamins, and patient dietary habits.
2. Administer a liquid form or a tasteless capsule of radioactive iodine orally.
3. Measure the amount of radioactivity by an uptake calculation of the thyroid gland 2, 4, 6, and 24 hours later. There is no pain or discomfort involved.
4. Have the patient return to the laboratory at the designated time because the exact time of measurement is crucial in determining the uptake.

Clinical Implications

1. Increased uptake (e.g., 20% in 1 hour, 25% in 6 hours, 45% in 24 hours) suggests hyperthyroidism but is not diagnostic for it.
2. Decreased uptake (e.g., 0% in 2 hours, 3% in 6 hours, 10% in 24 hours) may be caused by hypothyroidism but is not diagnostic for it.
   a. If the administered iodine is not absorbed, as in severe diarrhea or intestinal malabsorption syndromes, the uptake may be low even though the gland is functioning normally.
   b. Rapid diuresis during the test period may deplete the supply of iodine, causing an apparently low percentage of iodine uptake.
   c. In renal failure, the uptake may be high even though the gland is functioning normally.

CLINICAL ALERT

1. This test is contraindicated in pregnant or lactating women, in children, in infants, and in persons with iodine allergies.
2. Whenever possible, this test should be performed before any other radionuclide procedures are done, before any iodine medications are given, and before any radiographs using iodine contrast media are taken.

Interfering Factors

1. The chemicals, drugs, and foods that interfere with the test by *lowering* the uptake are:
   a. Iodized food and iodine-containing drugs such as Lugol's solution, expectorants, cough medications, saturated solutions of potassium iodide, and vitamin preparations that contain minerals: The duration of the effects of these substances in the body is 1 to 3 weeks.
   b. Radiographic contrast media such as iodopyracet (Diodrast), sodium diatrizoate (Hypaque, Renografin), poppy-seed oil (Lipiodol), ethiodized oil (Ethiodol), iophendylate (Pantopaque), and iopanoic acid (Telepaque): The duration of the effects of these substances is 1 week to 1 year or more; consult with the nuclear medicine laboratory for specific times.
   c. Antithyroid drugs such as propylthiouracil (PTU) and related compounds: The duration of the effects of these drugs may last 2 to 10 days.
   d. Thyroid medications such as liothyronine sodium (Cytomel), desiccated thyroid, thyroxine (Synthroid, levothyroxine sodium): The duration of the effects of these medications is 1 to 2 weeks.
   e. Miscellaneous drugs such as thiocyanate, perchlorate, nitrates, sulfonamides, tolbutamide (Orinase), corticosteroids, para-aminosalicylate, isoniazid, phenylbutazone (Butazolidin), thiopental (Pentothal), antihistamines, adrenocorticotropic hormone, aminosalicylic acid, cobalt, and warfarin sodium (Coumadin) anticoagulants: Consult with the nuclear medicine department for duration of effects of these drugs as they vary widely.
2. The compounds and conditions that interfere by *enhancing* the uptake are:
   a. Thyroid-stimulating hormone (TSH) (thyrotropin)
   b. Pregnancy
   c. Cirrhosis
   d. Barbiturates
   e. Lithium carbonate
   f. Phenothiazines (duration, 1 week)
   g. Iodine-deficient diet
   h. Renal failure

Interventions

Pretest Patient Care

1. Explain test purpose and procedure; the test takes 24 hours to complete. Assess and record pertinent dietary and medication history.
2. Advise that iodine intake is restricted for at least 1 week before testing.
3. Refer to standard nuclear medicine imaging *pretest* precautions.
4. Follow guidelines in Chapter 1 for safe, effective, informed *pretest* care.

Posttest Patient Care

1. Explain test outcomes and possible treatment.
2. Refer to standard nuclear medicine imaging *posttest* precautions.
3. Review test results; report and record findings. Modify the nursing care plan as needed. Counsel the patient appropriately.
4. Follow guidelines in Chapter 1 for safe, effective, informed *posttest* care.

● Adrenal Gland Metaiodobenzylguanidine (MIBG) Imaging

The adrenal gland is divided into two different components: cortex and medulla. The scope of adrenal imaging is limited to the medulla. Testing can be performed in both adults and children.

The purpose of adrenal medulla imaging is to identify sites of certain tumors that produce excessive amounts of catecholamines. Pheochromocytomas develop in cells that make up the adrenergic portion of the autonomic nervous system. A large number of these well-differentiated cells are found in adrenal medullas. Adrenergic tumors have been called *paragangliomas* when they are found outside the adrenal medulla, but many practitioners refer to all neoplasms that secrete norepinephrine and epinephrine as *pheochromocytomas*. Because the only definite and effective therapy is surgery to remove the tumor, identification of the site using adrenal gland imaging, CT, and ultrasound is an essential goal of treatment.

Reference Values

Normal

No evidence of tumors or hypersecreting hormone sites

Normal salivary glands, urinary bladder, and vague shape of liver and spleen can be seen.

Procedure

1. Inject intravenously the radionuclide ^{131}I- or ^{123}I-metaiodobenzylguanidine (MIBG).
2. Take images at the healthcare provider's discretion, usually 4 and 24 hours after injection.
3. Advise the patient that imaging may take 2 hours.
4. See Chapter 1 guidelines for safe, effective, informed *intratest* care.

Clinical Implications

1. More than 90% of primary pheochromocytomas occur in the abdomen.
2. Pheochromocytomas in children often represent a familial disorder.
3. Bilateral adrenal tumors often indicate a familial disease.
4. Multiple extrarenal pheochromocytomas are often malignant.
5. The presence of two or more pheochromocytomas strongly indicates malignant disease.

Interfering Factors

Barium interferes with the test.

Interventions

Pretest Patient Care

1. Explain nuclear medicine imaging purpose, procedure, benefits, and risks.
2. Give Lugol's solution (potassium iodine) 1 day prior to the injection, the day of the injection, and 4 days postinjection to prevent uptake of radioactive iodine by the thyroid.
3. Refer to standard nuclear medicine imaging *pretest* precautions.
4. Follow guidelines in Chapter 1 for safe, effective, informed *pretest* care.

Posttest Patient Care

1. Review test results; report and record findings. Modify the nursing care plan as needed. Counsel appropriately about the need for possible follow-up tests. Follow-up tests include:
   a. Kidney and bone imaging to give further orientation to abnormalities discovered by MIBG scan
   b. CT procedure if MIBG imaging failed to locate the tumor
   c. Ultrasound of the pelvis if the tumor produces urinary symptoms
2. Refer to standard nuclear medicine imaging *posttest* precautions.
3. Follow guidelines in Chapter 1 for safe, effective, informed *posttest* care.

Parathyroid Imaging

Parathyroid imaging is done to localize parathyroid adenomas in clinically proven cases of primary hyperparathyroidism. It is helpful in demonstrating intrinsic or extrinsic parathyroid adenoma. ^{99m}Tc sestamibi, ^{123}I capsules, or ^{201}Tl, or a combination of these three, can be used for imaging. In children, nuclear medicine imaging is done to verify presence of the parathyroid gland after thyroidectomy.

Reference Values

Normal

No areas of increased perfusion or uptake in parathyroid or thyroid

Procedure

1. Administer ^{123}I. Four hours later, image the neck.
2. Inject ^{99m}Tc sestamibi without moving the patient; after 10 minutes, acquire additional images. Computer processing involves subtracting the technetium-visualized thyroid structures from the ^{123}I accumulation in a parathyroid adenoma.
3. Alert patient that total examination time is 1 hour.
4. See Chapter 1 guidelines for safe, effective, informed *intratest* care.

Clinical Implications

Abnormal concentrations of the radiopharmaceuticals reveal parathyroid adenoma, both intrinsic and extrinsic, but cannot differentiate between benign and malignant adenomas.

Interfering Factors

Recent ingestion of iodine in food or medication and recent tests with iodine contrast are contraindications and reduce the effectiveness of the study.

Clinical Considerations

Pregnancy is a relative contraindication. However, if primary hyperparathyroidism is suspected and surgical exploration is essential before delivery, the study may be performed.

Interventions

Pretest Patient Care

1. Explain the purpose, procedure, benefits, and risks of parathyroid imaging.
2. Assess for the recent intake of iodine. However, this finding is not a specific contraindication to performing the study.
3. Palpate the thyroid carefully.
4. Refer to standard nuclear scan *pretest* precautions.
5. Follow guidelines in Chapter 1 for safe, effective, informed *pretest* care.

Posttest Patient Care

1. Refer to standard nuclear medicine imaging *posttest* precautions.
2. Review test results; report and record findings. Modify the nursing care plan as needed.
3. Follow guidelines in Chapter 1 for safe, effective, informed *posttest* care.

GENITOURINARY STUDIES

● Renogram: Kidney Function and Renal Blood Flow Imaging (With Furosemide or Captopril/Enalapril)

The renogram is performed in both adult and pediatric patients to study the function of the kidneys and to detect renal parenchymal or vascular disease or defects in excretion. The radiopharmaceutical of choice, ^{99m}Tc mertiatide (MAG-3), permits visualization of renal clearance. In pediatric patients, this procedure is done to evaluate hydronephrosis, obstruction, reduced renal function (premature neonates), renal trauma, and urinary tract infections. The renogram is ideal for pediatric evaluation because of the nontoxic nature of the radiopharmaceuticals, compared with the contrast media used in radiology procedures. Post–kidney transplantation scans, which assess perfusion and excretory function as a reflection of glomerular filtration rate (GFR), are done when the serum creatinine level increases and determine kidney damage leading to acute tubular necrosis (ATN).

Reference Values

Normal

Equal blood flow in right and left kidneys
In 10 minutes, 50% of the radiopharmaceutical should be excreted.

Indications

1. To detect the presence or absence of unilateral kidney disease
2. For long-term follow-up of hydroureteronephrosis
3. To study the hypertensive patient to evaluate for renal artery stenosis. The captopril test is a first-line study to determine a renal basis for hypertension.
4. To study the azotemic patient when urethral catheterization is contraindicated or impossible
5. To evaluate upper urinary tract obstruction
6. To assess renal transplant efficacy

Procedure

1. Place the patient in either an upright sitting or supine position for imaging; the supine position is preferred for pediatric patients.
2. Inject the radiopharmaceutical intravenously. An intravenous diuretic (furosemide [Lasix]) or angiotensin-converting enzyme (ACE) inhibitor (enalapril/captopril) may also be administered during a second phase of the renogram.
3. Start imaging immediately after injection.
4. Alert patient that total examination time is approximately 45 minutes for a routine, one-phase renogram.
5. See Chapter 1 guidelines for safe, effective, informed *intratest* care.

PROCEDURAL ALERT

1. The test should be performed before an intravenous pyelogram.
2. A renogram may be performed in a pregnant woman if it is imperative to assess renal function.

Clinical Implications

Abnormal distribution patterns may indicate:

1. Hypertension
2. Obstruction due to stones or tumors
3. Renal failure
4. Decreased renal function
5. Diminished blood supply
6. Renal transplant rejection
7. In pediatric patients, urinary tract infections in male neonates; the finding shifts to females after 3 months of age.

Interfering Factors

Diuretics, ACE inhibitors, and beta blockers are medications that may interfere with the test results.

Interventions

Pretest Patient Care

1. Explain the purpose, procedure, benefits, and risks of the procedure. Pediatric patients have a detectible GFR after 6 months of age. In the neonate, ultrasound is used in combination with nuclear medicine procedures for a more complete renal assessment. Refer to standard nuclear medicine imaging *pretest* precautions. An intravenous line is placed before imaging. Check for history of previous transplantation.
2. Unless contraindicated, ensure that the patient is well hydrated with two to three glasses of water (10 mL/kg of body weight) before undergoing the test.
3. Follow guidelines in Chapter 1 for safe, effective, informed *pretest* care.

Posttest Patient Care

1. Encourage fluids and frequent bladder emptying to promote excretion of radioactivity.
2. Review test results; report and record findings. Modify the nursing care plan as needed. Counsel the patient appropriately.
3. Refer to standard nuclear medicine imaging *posttest* precautions.
4. Follow guidelines in Chapter 1 for safe, effective, informed *posttest* care.

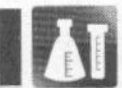

CLINICAL ALERT

Some renal transplant recipients may have more than two kidneys—for example, the transplanted kidney, their native kidney or kidneys, and an older, failing transplant. Sometimes, two pediatric kidneys will both be transplanted.

● Testicular (Scrotal) Imaging

This test is performed on an emergency basis to evaluate acute, painful testicular swelling. It also is used in the differential diagnosis of torsion or acute epididymitis and in evaluation of injury, trauma, tumors, and masses. The radiopharmaceutical ^{99m}Tc pertechnetate is injected intravenously. The images obtained differentiate lesions associated with increased perfusion from those that are primarily ischemic. In pediatric patients, the procedure is done to diagnose acute or latent testicular torsion, epididymitis, or testicular hydrocele and for evaluation of testicular masses such as abscesses and tumors.

Reference Values

Normal

Normal blood flow to scrotal structures, with even distribution and concentration of the radiopharmaceutical

Procedure

1. Have the patient lie supine under the gamma camera. Tape the penis gently to the lower abdominal wall. For proper positioning, use towels to support the scrotum. Place lead shielding in the perineal area to reduce any background activity.
2. Inject the radionuclide intravenously. In pediatric patients, do not inject the radiopharmaceutical through veins in the legs because this interferes with the study.
3. Perform imaging in two phases: first as a dynamic blood flow study of the scrotum and second as an assessment of distribution of the radiopharmaceutical in the scrotum.
4. Advise the patient that total examining time is 30 to 45 minutes.
5. See Chapter 1 guidelines for safe, effective, informed *intratest* care.

Clinical Implications

1. Abnormal concentrations reveal:
   a. Tumors
   b. Hematomas
   c. Infection
   d. Torsion (with reduced blood flow): In the neonatal patient, torsion is caused primarily by developmental anomalies.
   e. Acute epididymitis
2. The nuclear medicine imaging is most specific soon after the onset of pain.

Interventions

Pretest Patient Care

1. Explain the purpose, procedure, benefits, and risks of the test. There is no discomfort involved in testing.
2. If the patient is a child, a parent should accompany the child to the department.
3. Tape the penis to the lower abdominal wall.
4. Refer to standard nuclear medicine imaging *pretest* precautions.
5. Follow guidelines in Chapter 1 for safe, effective, informed *pretest* care.

Posttest Patient Care

1. Refer to standard nuclear imaging *posttest* precautions.
2. Review test results; report and record findings. Modify the nursing care plan as needed.
3. Follow guidelines in Chapter 1 for safe, effective, informed *posttest* care.

● ProstaScint Imaging

This test is done to determine whether curative therapy and radiotherapy are treatment options in patients with prostate cancer who are at high risk for metastasis or have a rising prostate-specific antigen (PSA) following a prostatectomy. ProstaScint (^{111}In capromab pendetide) uses a murine monoclonal antibody (MAB) that attaches to prostate-specific membrane antigen (PSMA) located on prostate cancer cells.

Reference Values

Normal

No areas of uptake or ProstaScint activity

Procedure

1. The patient is injected with 5.5 to 6.5 mCi of ^{111}In capromab pendetide intravenously over a 5-minute period.
2. The patient then drinks 8 to 12 oz of water and undergoes the first imaging session.
3. On day 3 (48 hours before second imaging session) and day 4 (24 hours before second imaging session), the patient is instructed to take an oral laxative. Also, a cleansing enema should be performed just before arrival for the second imaging session, which is 5 days after injection.
4. Depending on the results of the imaging sessions, a third imaging session on day 6 or 7 may be necessary.

CLINICAL ALERT

ProstaScint is contraindicated in patients who are hypersensitive to murine-origin products.

Clinical Implications

Increased activity or uptake in the lymph nodes indicates the likelihood of metastatic disease.

Interventions

Pretest Patient Care

1. Explain the purpose, procedure, benefits, and risks of the test.
2. Refer to standard nuclear imaging *pretest* precautions.
3. Follow guidelines in Chapter 1 for safe, effective, informed *pretest* care.

Posttest Patient Care

1. Refer to standard nuclear medicine imaging *posttest* precautions.
2. Review test results; report and record findings. Modify the nursing care plan as needed.
3. Follow guidelines in Chapter 1 for safe, effective, informed *posttest* care.

● Vesicoureteric Reflux (Bladder and Ureters) Imaging

Vesicoureteric reflux imaging usually is done on pediatric patients to assess abnormal bladder filling and possible reflux into the ureter. ^{99m}Tc pentetate (diethylenetriaminepentaacetate [DTPA] used as a chelating vehicle) is administered through a urinary catheter, followed by sufficient saline until the patient has an urge to urinate. The ureters and kidneys are scanned by the camera during administration to detect the reflux.

Reference Values

Normal

Normal bladder filling without any reflux into the ureters

Procedure

1. Place the patient in the supine position. Use a special urinary catheter kit and insert a urinary catheter.
2. Start the camera immediately for dynamic acquisition while the radiopharmaceutical and saline are administered until the bladder is full or there is patient discomfort.
3. Remove the catheter once the imaging is complete.

Clinical Implications

Abnormal vesicoureteric reflux may be either congenital (immature development of the urinary tract) or caused by infection.

Interventions

Pretest Patient Care

1. See standard *pretest* care for nuclear imaging of pediatric patients.
2. Place a urinary catheter with sterile saline. Place an absorbent, plastic-backed pad under the patient to absorb any leakage of radioactive material. If a urinary catheter is contraindicated for the patient, use an alternative indirect renogram method.

Posttest Patient Care

1. Refer to standard nuclear imaging *posttest* precautions for adults.
2. Depending on cause and severity, antibiotic therapy or surgery is used to treat the condition.
3. Remember that special handling of the patient's urine (gloves and handwashing before donning gloves and after gloves are removed) is necessary for 24 hours after completion of the test.

GASTROINTESTINAL STUDIES

● Hepatobiliary (Gallbladder, Biliary) Imaging with Cholecystokinin

This study, using ^{99m}Tc disofenin or mebrofenin, is performed to visualize the gallbladder and determine patency of the biliary system. In pediatric patients, this test is done to differentiate biliary atresia from neonatal hepatitis and to assess liver trauma, right upper quadrant pain, and congenital malformations.

A series of images traces the excretion of the radionuclide. Through computer analysis, the activity in the gallbladder is quantitated, and the amount ejected (ejection fraction) is calculated.

Indications for the Test

1. To evaluate cholecystitis
2. To differentiate between obstructive and nonobstructive jaundice
3. To investigate upper abdominal pain
4. For biliary assessment after surgery
5. For evaluation of biliary atresia

Reference Values

Normal

Rapid transit of the radionuclide through the liver cells to the biliary tract (15 to 30 minutes) with significant uptake in the normal gallbladder

Normal distribution patterns in the biliary system, from the liver, through the gallbladder, to the small intestines

Procedure

1. Inject the radionuclide intravenously. In adults and older children, give cholecystokinin (CCK) to stimulate gallbladder contraction. In infants, give phenobarbital to distinguish between biliary atresia and neonatal jaundice.
2. Start imaging immediately after injection. Take a series of images at 5-minute intervals for as long as it takes to visualize the gallbladder and small intestine.
3. In the event of biliary obstruction, obtain delayed views (2 to 24 hours).
4. Remember that if CCK is administered, computer-assisted quantitative measurements can determine an ejection fraction.
5. See Chapter 1 guidelines for safe, effective, informed *intratest* care.

Clinical Implications

1. Abnormal concentration patterns reveal unusual bile communications.
2. Gallbladder visualization excludes the diagnosis of acute cholecystitis with a high degree of certainty.

Interfering Factors

1. Patients with high serum bilirubin levels (>10 mg/dL or >171 mmol/L) have less reliable test results.
2. Patients receiving total parenteral nutrition or with long-term fasting may not have gallbladder visualization.

Interventions

Pretest Patient Care

1. Explain the purpose, procedure, benefits, and risks of the procedure.
2. Ensure that the patient is NPO for at least 4 hours (3 to 4 hours for pediatric patients) before testing. In case of prolonged fasting (>24 hours), notify the nuclear medicine department. Fasting does not apply when the indication is for biliary atresia or jaundice.
3. Discontinue opiate- or morphine-based pain medications 2 to 6 hours before the test to avoid interference with transit of the radiopharmaceutical.
4. Refer to standard nuclear medicine imaging *pretest* precautions.
5. Follow guidelines in Chapter 1 for safe, effective, informed *pretest* care.

Posttest Patient Care

1. Review test results; report and record findings. Modify the nursing care plan as needed.
2. Refer to standard nuclear imaging *posttest* precautions.
3. Follow guidelines in Chapter 1 for safe, effective, informed *posttest* care.

● Gastroesophageal Reflux Imaging

This test is indicated for both adult and pediatric patients to evaluate esophageal disorders such as regurgitation and to identify the cause of persistent nausea and vomiting. In infants, the study is used to distinguish between vomiting and reflux (for those with more severe symptoms). A certain amount of reflux occurs naturally in infants. If timely diagnosis and treatment of gastrointestinal reflux do not occur, additional complications may result, such as recurrent respiratory infections, apnea, or sudden infant death syndrome (SIDS).

After oral administration of the radioisotope ^{99m}Tc sulfur colloid in orange juice or scrambled eggs, the patient is immediately imaged to verify that the dose is in the stomach. Images are acquired in 2 hours. A computer analysis is used to calculate the percentage of reflux into the esophagus for each image.

Reference Values

Normal

<40% gastric reflux across the esophageal sphincter

Procedure

1. Have the patient ingest the radionuclide in orange juice or in scrambled eggs. For infants, perform the test at the normal infant feeding time to determine esophageal transit. Have the infant drink ^{99m}Tc-labeled sulfur colloid mixed with milk. Give a portion of the milk containing the radioisotope and burp the infant before the remainder is given. Give some unlabeled milk to clear the esophagus of the radioactive material. If a nasogastric tube is required for radiopharmaceutical administration, remove it before the imaging occurs to avoid a false-positive result.
2. Images are obtained in 2 hours.
3. Remember that a computer analysis generates a time–activity curve to calculate the reflux.
4. See Chapter 1 guidelines for safe, effective, informed *intratest* care.

PROCEDURAL ALERT

Patients who have esophageal motor disorders, hiatal hernias, or swallowing difficulties should have an endogastric tube inserted for the procedure.

Clinical Implications

More than 40% reflux is abnormal. The percentage of reflux is used to evaluate patients before and after surgery for gastroesophageal reflux.

Interfering Factors

1. Previous upper gastrointestinal radiographic procedures may interfere with this test.
2. Previous gastric banding (bariatric procedure for morbid obesity) may interfere with esophageal motility and gastroesophageal reflux.

Interventions

Pretest Patient Care

1. Explain the purpose, procedure, benefits, and risks. See standard nuclear medicine *pretest* precautions.
2. Perform imaging with the patient in a supine position.
3. Ensure that the patient is fasting for the appropriate amount of time before the examination.
4. Monitor oral intake of the orange juice or scrambled eggs containing ^{99m}Tc sulfur colloid.
5. Follow guidelines in Chapter 1 for safe, effective, informed *pretest* care.

Posttest Patient Care

1. Remove endogastric tubes, if placed for the examination, after the radiopharmaceutical is administered.
2. Refer to standard nuclear medicine *posttest* precautions.
3. Review test results; report and record findings. Modify the nursing care plan as needed.
4. Follow guidelines in Chapter 1 for safe, effective, informed *posttest* care.

● Gastric Emptying Imaging

Gastric emptying imaging is used in both adult and pediatric patients to assess gastric motility disorders and in patients with unexplained nausea, vomiting, diarrhea, and abdominal cramping. The emptying of food by the stomach is a complex process that is controlled by food composition (fats, carbohydrates), food form (liquid, solid), hormone secretion (gastrin, CCK), and innervation. Because clearance of liquids and clearance of solids vary, the imaging procedure traces both food forms. Indications for imaging include both mechanical and nonmechanical gastric motility disorders. Mechanical disorders include peptic ulcerations, gastric surgery, trauma, and cancer. Nonmechanical disorders include diabetes, uremia, anorexia nervosa, certain drugs (opiates), and neurologic disorders. Clearance of liquids, solids, or a combination (dual-phase examination) may be studied.

Reference Values

Normal

Normal half-time clearance ranges:
45 to 110 minutes for solids
10 to 65 minutes for liquids

Procedure

1. Have the fasting patient consume the solid phase (^{99m}Tc sulfur colloid, usually in scrambled eggs or oatmeal or chicken livers) followed by the liquid phase (indium-111 [^{111}In] DTPA in 300 mL of water). For infants, perform the test at the normal feeding time. Have the infant drink ^{99m}Tc sulfur colloid mixed with milk. Provide older children solids such as scrambled eggs mixed with ^{99m}Tc sulfur colloid.
2. Perform imaging immediately, with the patient in the supine position.

3. Obtain subsequent images over the next 2 hours.
4. Use computer processing to determine the half-time clearance for both liquid and solid phases of gastric emptying.
5. See Chapter 1 guidelines for safe, effective, informed *intratest* care.

Clinical Implications

1. *Slow or delayed* emptying is usually seen in the following conditions:
   a. Peptic ulceration
   b. Diabetes
   c. Smooth muscle disorders
   d. After radiation therapy
   e. In pediatric patients, hypomotility of the antrum portion of the stomach is the primary cause of delayed gastric emptying. However, all abnormal functions of the stomach do contribute to the delay.
2. *Accelerated* emptying is often seen in the following conditions:
   a. Zollinger-Ellison syndrome (triad of peptic ulceration, pancreatic non–beta cell islet tumors, and hypersecretion of gastric acid)
   b. Certain malabsorption syndromes
   c. After gastric or duodenal surgery

Interfering Factors

Administration of certain medications (e.g., gastrin, CCK) interferes with gastric emptying.

Interventions

Pretest Patient Care

1. Explain the purpose, procedure, benefits, and risks of the procedure.
2. Have the adult patient fast for 8 hours before the test.
3. Refer to standard nuclear medicine procedures *pretest* precautions.
4. Follow guidelines in Chapter 1 for safe, effective, informed *pretest* care.

Posttest Patient Care

1. The patient may eat and drink normally.
2. Review test results; report and record findings. Modify the nursing care plan as needed.
3. Refer to standard nuclear medicine procedures *posttest* precautions.
4. Follow guidelines in Chapter 1 for safe, effective, informed *posttest* care.

● Gastrointestinal Bleeding Imaging

This test is very sensitive in the detection and location of acute gastrointestinal bleeding that occurs distal to the ligament of Treitz (suspensory ligament of the duodenum). (Gastroscopy is the procedure of choice for diagnosis of upper gastrointestinal bleeding.) Before this diagnostic technique was refined, barium enemas were used to identify lesions reflecting sites of bleeding, but that test was not specific and frequently missed small sites of bleeding. This procedure is also indicated for detection and localization of recent hemorrhage, both peritoneal and retroperitoneal. The radiopharmaceutical of choice for suspected active bleeding is ^{99m}Tc-labeled RBCs.

Reference Values

Normal

No sites of active bleeding

Procedure

1. Inject ^{99m}Tc-labeled RBCs intravenously.
2. Begin imaging immediately after injection and continue every few minutes. Obtain anterior images over the abdomen at 5-minute intervals for 60 minutes or until a bleeding site is located. If the study is negative after 1 hour, obtain delayed images 2, 6, and sometimes 24 hours later, when necessary, to identify the location of difficult-to-determine bleeding sites.
3. Total examining time varies.
4. See Chapter 1 guidelines for safe, effective, informed *intratest* care.

CLINICAL ALERT

1. This test is contraindicated in patients who are hemodynamically unstable. In these instances, angiography or surgery should be the procedure of choice.
2. Assess the patient for signs of active bleeding during the examining period.
3. Recent blood transfusion may be a contraindication for this study.

Clinical Implications

Abnormal concentrations of RBCs (hot spots) are associated with active gastrointestinal bleeding sites, both peritoneal and retroperitoneal.

Interfering Factors

Presence of barium in the gastrointestinal tract may obscure the site of bleeding because of the high density of barium and the inability of the technetium to penetrate the barium.

Interventions

Pretest Patient Care

1. Explain the purpose, procedure, benefits, and risks of the gastrointestinal blood loss imaging.
2. Determine whether the patient has received barium as a diagnostic agent within the past 24 hours. If the presence of barium in the gastrointestinal tract is questionable, an abdominal radiograph may be ordered.
3. Advise the patient that delayed images may be necessary. Also, if active bleeding is not seen on initial imaging, additional images must be obtained for up to 24 hours after injection in a patient with clinical signs of active bleeding.
4. Refer to standard nuclear medicine procedures *pretest* precautions.
5. Follow guidelines in Chapter 1 for safe, effective, informed *pretest* care.

Posttest Patient Care

1. Refer to standard nuclear medicine procedures *posttest* precautions.
2. Review test results; report and record findings. Modify the nursing care plan as needed.
3. Follow guidelines in Chapter 1 for safe, effective, informed *posttest* care.

• Parotid (Salivary) Gland Imaging

This study is helpful in the evaluation of swelling or masses in the parotid region. This imaging is done to detect blocked tumors of parotid or salivary glands and to diagnose Sjögren's syndrome (a systemic autoimmune disease). The radionuclide injected intravenously is ^{99m}Tc pertechnetate. One of the limitations of the test is that it cannot furnish an exact preoperative diagnosis.

Reference Values

Normal

No evidence of tumor-type activity or blockage of ducts
Normal size, shape, and position of the glands

Procedure

1. Inject the radionuclide pertechnetate intravenously. Perform imaging immediately. There are three phases to imaging: blood flow, uptake or trapping mechanism, and secreting capability.
2. Take images of the gland every minute for 30 minutes.
3. If a secretory function test is being performed to detect blockage of the salivary duct, three quarters of the way through the test, ask the patient to suck on a lemon slice. If the salivary duct is normal, this causes the gland to empty. This is not done in studies undertaken for tumor detection.
4. Alert patient that total test time is 45 to 60 minutes.
5. See Chapter 1 guidelines for safe, effective, informed *intratest* care.

Clinical Implications

1. The reporting of a hot nodule amidst normal tissue that accumulates the radionuclide is associated with tumors of the ducts, as in:
   a. Warthin's tumor
   b. Oncocytoma
   c. Mucoepidermoid tumor
2. The reporting of a cold nodule amidst normal tissue that does not accumulate the radionuclide is associated with:
   a. Benign tumors, abscesses, or cysts, which are indicated by smooth, sharply defined outlines
   b. Adenocarcinomas, which are indicated by ragged, irregular outlines
3. Diffuse decreased activity occurs in obstruction, chronic sialadenitis, or Sjögren's syndrome.
4. Diffuse increased activity occurs in acute parotitis.

Interventions

Pretest Patient Care

1. Explain the purpose, procedure, benefits, and risks.
2. No pain or discomfort is involved.
3. Lemon may be given to the patient to stimulate parotid secretion.
4. Refer to standard nuclear scan *pretest* precautions.
5. Follow guidelines in Chapter 1 for safe, effective, informed *pretest* care.

Posttest Patient Care

1. Review test results; report and record findings. Modify the nursing care plan as needed.
2. Refer to standard nuclear scan *posttest* precautions.
3. Follow guidelines in Chapter 1 for safe, effective, informed *posttest* care.

● Liver/Spleen Imaging and Liver RBC Imaging

This test is used to demonstrate the anatomy and size of the liver and spleen. It is helpful in determining the cause of right upper quadrant pain and in the detection of metastatic disease, cirrhosis, ascites, infarction due to trauma, and liver damage due to radiation therapy. Most liver and spleen imaging evaluates for metastatic disease and for the differential diagnosis of jaundice. Post–liver transplantation scans detect bile and anastomotic leaks and rule out abnormal perfusion as a sign of rejection.

The radioactive material, ^{99m}Tc-labeled sulfur colloid, is injected intravenously. Liver/spleen SPECT imaging provides three-dimensional images of radiopharmaceutical uptake. The radiopharmaceutical most specific for detection of hemangioma in the liver is ^{99m}Tc labeled to a patient's own RBCs. In many instances, ultrasound imaging replaces this test.

Reference Values

Normal

Normal liver size, shape, and position within the abdomen
Normal spleen size, cell function, and blood flow
Normally functioning liver and spleen reticuloendothelial system

NOTE *The amount of uptake in the spleen should always be less than in the liver.*

Procedure

1. Inject the radiopharmaceutical intravenously.
2. Perform a SPECT study and planar images.
3. The entire study usually takes 60 minutes from injection to completion.
4. See Chapter 1 guidelines for safe, effective, informed *intratest* care.

Clinical Implications

1. Abnormal liver and spleen scan patterns occur in:
   a. Cirrhosis
   b. Hepatitis
   c. Trauma
   d. Hepatomas
   e. Sarcoidosis
   f. Metastasis
   g. Cysts
   h. Perihepatic abscesses
   i. Hemangiomas
   j. Adenomas
   k. Ascites
2. Abnormal splenic concentrations reveal:
   a. Unusual splenic size
   b. Infarction
   c. Ruptured spleen
   d. Accessory spleen
   e. Tumors
   f. Metastatic spread
   g. Leukemia
   h. Hodgkin's disease
3. Spleens larger than 14 cm are abnormally enlarged; those smaller than 7 cm are abnormally small. Areas of absent radioactivity or holes in the spleen images are associated with abnormalities that displace or destroy normal splenic pulp.
4. About 30% of persons with Hodgkin's disease (lymphoma, cancer of lymph tissue) with splenic involvement have a normal splenic image.

Interventions

Pretest Patient Care

1. Explain the purpose, procedure, benefits, and risks.
2. This test can be performed in cases of trauma or suspected ruptured spleen, at the bedside or in the emergency room.

3. Refer to standard nuclear medicine procedures *pretest* precautions.
4. Follow guidelines in Chapter 1 for safe, effective, informed *pretest* care.

Posttest Patient Care

1. Refer to standard nuclear medicine procedures *posttest* precautions.
2. Review test results; report and record findings. Modify the nursing care plan as needed. Explain need for medical treatment or surgery.
3. Follow guidelines in Chapter 1 for safe, effective, informed *posttest* care.

● Meckel's Diverticulum Imaging

The test for Meckel's diverticulum, a congenital abnormality of the small intestine, usually is done in pediatric patients diagnosed with congenital abnormality of the ileum, which sometimes continues to the umbilicus with fistula formation. The uptake of ^{99m}Tc pertechnetate occurs in the parietal cells of the gastric mucosa and is detected by the gamma camera. Meckel's diverticulum shows uptake in the distal portion of the ileum. This anomaly contains secretory cells similar to those of gastric mucosa. An alternative radiopharmaceutical, ^{99m}Tc-labeled RBCs, may be considered in cases of suspected bleeding sites associated with the diverticulum.

Reference Values

Normal

Normal blood pool distribution and clearance of the radioactive tracer into the duodenum and jejunum

Procedure

1. Have the patient lie supine and inject with the radiopharmaceutical.
2. Start the camera immediately with a series of static images obtained at 5-minute intervals for 30 minutes.
3. Extra spot views may be requested by the healthcare provider.
4. See Chapter 1 guidelines for safe, effective, informed *intratest* care.

Clinical Implications

1. Abnormal results reveal rectal bleeding, the most common symptom of Meckel's diverticulum. Meckel's diverticulum can occur with or without abdominal symptoms.
2. If it is left undetected and untreated, ulceration of the ileum may occur, and strangulation may cause intestinal obstruction.

Interventions

Pretest Patient Care

1. See standard *pretest* care for nuclear imaging of pediatric patients. Explain the purpose and procedures of the examination. Patients should be fasting. Other diagnostic procedures involving the gastrointestinal tract and medications affecting the intestines should be avoided for 2 to 3 days before the examination. This is especially true of lower and upper gastrointestinal radiographic procedures.
2. Have patients void immediately before the examination.

Posttest Patient Care

1. Refer to standard *posttest* precautions, the same as for adults. Special handling of the patient's urine (gloves and handwashing before donning gloves and after glove removal) is necessary for 24 hours after test completion.
2. Review test results; report and record findings. Modify the nursing care plan as needed.
3. Follow guidelines in Chapter 1 for safe, effective, informed *posttest* care.

NEUROLOGIC STUDIES

● Brain Imaging and Cerebral Blood Flow Imaging

Brain imaging provides information about regional perfusion and brain function, whereas CT and MRI show structural changes. Developments in radiopharmaceuticals and SPECT have rejuvenated brain imaging. Technetium complexes, such as ^{99m}Tc bicisate (ethyl cysteinate dimer [ECD]) and ^{99m}Tc exametazime, are radiopharmaceuticals that cross the blood–brain barrier. The blood–brain barrier is not an anatomic structure but a complex system of select mechanisms that oppose the passage of most ions and high-molecular-weight compounds from the blood to the brain tissue. This complex system includes capillary endothelium with closed intracellular clefts, a small or absent extravascular fluid space between endothelium and glial sheaths, and the membrane of the neurons themselves. SPECT technology allows for three-dimensional slices, providing depth resolution from different angles. Although PET imaging is more effective in functional diagnosis, SPECT is less expensive and more readily available. This test is indicated in both adults and children to determine brain death or the presence of encephalitis; it is also used in children with hydrocephalus, to localize epileptic foci, to assess metabolic activity, to evaluate brain tumors, and for the assessment of childhood development disorders.

Reference Values

Normal

Normal extracranial and intracranial blood flow

Normal distribution, with highest uptake in the gray matter, basal ganglia, thalamus, and peripheral cortex and less activity in the central white matter and ventricles

Procedure

1. Inject the radionuclide intravenously. During the injection, have the patient in a relaxed, controlled environment to minimize anxiety. In uncooperative children, do not use sedation until after the injection because it may affect brain activity. Secure the patient's head during the examination.
2. Begin imaging immediately after administration of the radiopharmaceutical or after a 1-hour delay. The test takes about 1 hour to complete.
3. With the patient in the supine position, obtain SPECT images around the circumference of the head.
4. With administration of iodoamphetamines, some departments require a dark and quiet environment.
5. See Chapter 1 guidelines for safe, effective, informed *intratest* care.

PROCEDURAL ALERT

In children, for localization of the area in the brain where a seizure originates, the radiopharmaceutical is injected at the time of the seizure (20-s window), and the patient is immediately transported to the nuclear medicine department to obtain SPECT images. This procedure is done under a controlled environment in which the patient has been previously weaned from medication and under continuous observation by healthcare professionals.

Clinical Implications

1. Abnormal radionuclide distribution patterns indicate:
   a. Alzheimer's disease
   b. Stroke

   c. Dementia
   d. Seizure disorders
   e. Epilepsy
   f. Systemic lupus erythematosus
   g. Huntington's disease
   h. Parkinson's disease
   i. Psychiatric disorder (schizophrenia)
2. The cerebral blood flow in a patient with brain death shows a very distinct image: There is a lack of tracer uptake in the anterior and middle cerebral arteries and in the cerebral hemisphere, but perfusion is present in the scalp veins.

Interfering Factors

1. Any patient motion (e.g., coughing, leg movement) can alter cerebral alignment.
2. Sudden distractions or loud noises can alter the distribution of the radionuclide.

Interventions

Pretest Patient Care

1. Explain the purpose, procedure, benefits, and risk.
2. Refer to standard nuclear medicine imaging *pretest* precautions.
3. Because precise head alignment is crucial, advise the patient to remain quiet and still.
4. Obtain a careful neurologic history before testing.
5. Follow guidelines in Chapter 1 for safe, effective, informed *pretest* care.

Posttest Patient Care

1. Refer to standard nuclear medicine procedures *posttest* precautions.
2. Review test results; report and record findings. Modify the nursing care plan as needed. Monitor patient appropriately, especially if sedation is used.
3. Follow guidelines in Chapter 1 for safe, effective, informed *posttest* care.

● Cisternography (Cerebrospinal Fluid [CSF] Flow Imaging)

This study, in which the radiopharmaceutical ^{111}In DTPA is injected intrathecally during a lumbar puncture, is a sensitive indicator of altered flow and reabsorption of cerebrospinal fluid (CSF). Congenital malformations are the most common causes of hydrocephalus in the neonate. In older patients and in cases of trauma, CT or MRI is often used to identify anatomic origins of obstructive hydrocephalus. In the treatment of hydrocephalus, this test aids in selection of the type of shunt and pathway and in determining the prognosis of both shunting and hydrocephalus.

Reference Values

Normal

Unobstructed flow of CSF and normal reabsorption

Procedure

1. Perform a sterile lumbar puncture after the patient has been positioned and prepared (see Chapter 5 for lumbar puncture procedure). Inject the radionuclide into the cerebrospinal circulation.
2. Have the patient lie flat after the puncture; the length of time depends on the physician's order.
3. Perform imaging 2 to 6 hours after injection and repeat after 24 hours, 48 hours, and 72 hours if the healthcare provider so directs.
4. Advise the patient that exam time is about 1 hour for each imaging.
5. See Chapter 1 guidelines for safe, effective, informed *intratest* care.

Clinical Implications

Abnormal filling patterns reveal:

1. Cause of hydrocephalus (e.g., trauma, inflammation, bleeding, intracranial tumor)
2. Subdural hematoma
3. Spinal mass lesions
4. Posterior fossa cysts
5. Parencephalic and subarachnoid cysts
6. Communicating versus noncommunicating hydrocephalus
7. Shunt patency
8. Diagnosis and localization of rhinorrhea and otorrhea

Interventions

Pretest Patient Care

1. Explain the purpose, procedure, benefits, and risks of both lumbar puncture and cisternography.
2. Refer to standard nuclear medicine imaging *pretest* precautions.
3. Advise the patient that it may take as long as 1 hour for each imaging session.
4. Because of the lumbar puncture, transport the patient by cart to the nuclear medicine department for the first imaging session.
5. Follow guidelines in Chapter 1 for safe, effective, informed *pretest* care.

Posttest Patient Care

1. Follow instructions for lumbar puncture (see Chapter 5) and standard nuclear medicine imaging *posttest* precautions.
2. Be alert to complications of lumbar puncture, such as meningitis, allergic reaction to anesthetic, bleeding into spinal canal, herniation of brain tissue, and mild to severe headache.
3. Review test results; report and record findings. Modify the nursing care plan as needed.
4. Follow guidelines in Chapter 1 for safe, effective, informed *posttest* care.

● DaTscan Imaging

DaTscan (radiopharmaceutical, ^{123}I-ioflupane) is used to differentiate essential tremor from tremor due to Parkinson's syndromes (idiopathic Parkinson's disease, multiple system atrophy, and progressive supranuclear palsy). ^{123}I-ioflupane is injected into the bloodstream and will bind with healthy dopamine-containing neurons.

Reference Values

Normal

Normal images reveal two symmetrical, comma- or crescent-shaped regions in the striata (subcortical part of the forebrain).

Procedure

1. Patient will need to lie still for 40 to 60 minutes.
2. Patient should be given potassium perchlorate (400 mg) to block ^{123}I thyroid uptake 1 hour before DaTscan dose.
3. The patient will be injected with DaTscan via an intravenous line.
4. Imaging will take place 3 to 6 hours later, typically at 4 hours postinjection. To avoid movement artifact, a strip of tape may be placed across the forehead.

Contraindications

1. DaTscan is contraindicated in patients with known hypersensitivity to the active substance or to any of the excipients, or to iodine.
2. DaTscan is contraindicated in pregnancy, nursing mothers, and in pediatric patients.
3. DaTscan is excreted by the kidneys, and patients with severe renal impairment may have altered DaTscan images.

Interfering Factors

Drugs that bind to the dopamine transporter with high affinity may interfere with the image obtained.

Interventions

Pretest Patient Care

1. Explain purpose, procedure, benefits, and risks of test.
2. Patient should wear comfortable clothes.
3. Assess for contraindications.
4. Follow guidelines in Chapter 1 for safe, effective, informed *pretest* care.

Posttest Patient Care

1. Instruct the patient to drink plenty of fluids for at least 2 days following the test.
2. Follow guidelines in Chapter 1 for safe, effective, informed *posttest* care.

PULMONARY STUDIES

● Lung Scan (Ventilation and Perfusion Imaging)

Lung imaging is performed for three major purposes:

1. To diagnose and locate pulmonary emboli
2. To detect the percentage of the lung that is functioning normally
3. To assess the pulmonary vascular supply by providing an estimate of regional pulmonary blood flow

Lung imaging in both adults and children is done to assess pneumonia, cystic fibrosis, cyanosis, asthma, airway obstruction, infection, inflammation, and AIDS-related pulmonary diseases. It is a simple method for monitoring the course of embolic disease because an area of ischemia persists after apparent resolution on chest radiographs. In the case of pulmonary embolus, the blood supply beyond an embolus is restricted. Imaging results in poor or no visualization of the affected area. Assessment of the adequacy of pulmonary artery perfusion in areas of known disease can also be done reliably as well as after lung transplantation to detect reperfusion of lung and bronchiolitis obliterans.

There are two parts to the lung imaging: the ventilation ($\dot{V}$) imaging and the perfusion ($\dot{Q}$) imaging. The ventilation imaging reveals the movement or lack of air in the lungs. An aerosol of ^{99m}Tc DTPA or xenon-133 (^{133}Xe) gas demonstrates the ventilation properties of the patient's lungs. The perfusion imaging demonstrates the blood supply to the tissues in the lungs.

When inhaled, the radioactive gas or aerosol follows the same pathway as the air in normal breathing. In some pathologic conditions affecting ventilation, there is significant alteration in the normal ventilation process. The $\dot{V}/\dot{Q}$ is significant in the diagnosis of pulmonary emboli. It is also helpful in diagnosing bronchitis, asthma, inflammatory fibrosis, pneumonia, chronic obstructive pulmonary disease, and lung cancer.

The lung perfusion study can be performed after the ventilation test. A macroaggregated albumin (MAA) labeled with technetium is injected intravenously, and assessment of the pulmonary vascular supply is achieved by imaging.

Certain limitations exist with these tests. With a positive chest film and a positive $\dot{V}/\dot{Q}$, the differential possibilities are multiple: pneumonia, abscess, bullae, atelectasis, and carcinoma, among others. A pulmonary arteriogram is still necessary before an embolectomy can be attempted. Pulmonary embolism (PE) is determined by a mismatch between the ventilation and perfusion images. In other words, a normal ventilation image and an abnormal perfusion image with segmental defects indicate PE.

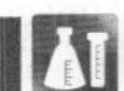

CLINICAL ALERT

Pulmonary perfusion imaging is contraindicated in patients with primary pulmonary hypertension unless reduced MAA particles are used in the preparation of the imaging agent ^{99m}Tc MAA.

Reference Values

Normal

Normal functioning lung
Normal pulmonary vascular supply
Normal gas exchange

Procedure

1. Ask the patient to breathe for approximately 4 minutes through a closed, nonpressurized ventilation system. During this time, administer a small amount of radioactive gas or aerosol. It is important that the patient not swallow the radioactive aerosol during the ventilation portion of the lung imaging. Doing so causes radioactive interference with the lower lobes of the lung and makes an accurate diagnostic interpretation difficult. Also, take care that the patient does not aspirate the aerosol.
2. Alert the patient that breath holding will be required for a brief period at some time during the imaging.
3. The imaging time is 10 to 15 minutes. When the ventilation imaging is performed with lung perfusion imaging (e.g., in differential diagnosis of PE), the testing time is 30 to 45 minutes.
4. Perform the perfusion imaging immediately after the ventilation study.
5. In the pediatric patient, reduce the number of particles given in the MAA dose because of the smaller size of the capillary beds. Use caution with MAA in patients with atrial and ventricular septal defects.
6. See Chapter 1 guidelines for safe, effective, informed *intratest* care.

Clinical Implications

1. Abnormal ventilation and perfusion patterns indicate possible:
   a. Tumors
   b. Emboli
   c. Pneumonia
   d. Atelectasis
   e. Bronchitis
   f. Asthma
   g. Inflammatory fibrosis
   h. Chronic obstructive pulmonary disease
   i. Lung cancer
2. In pediatric patients, there is an increased incidence of an airway obstruction caused by mucus plugs or foreign bodies. However, pulmonary emboli do not occur in children as often as in adults.

Interfering Factors

1. False-positive images occur in vasculitis, mitral stenosis, and pulmonary hypertension and when tumors obstruct a pulmonary artery with airway involvement.
2. During the injection of MAA, care must be taken that the patient's blood does not mix with the radiopharmaceutical in the syringe. Otherwise, hot spots may be seen in the lungs.

Interventions

Pretest Patient Care

1. Explain the purpose, procedure, benefits, and risks of the test.
2. Alleviate any fears the patient may have concerning nuclear medicine procedures.
3. It is important that a recent chest radiograph be available.
4. Remember that the patient must be able to follow directions for breathing and holding the breath, including breathing through a mouthpiece or into a facemask.
5. Refer to standard nuclear medicine imaging *pretest* precautions.
6. Follow guidelines in Chapter 1 for safe, effective, informed *pretest* care.

Posttest Patient Care

1. Refer to standard nuclear medicine imaging *posttest* precautions.
2. Review test results; report and record findings. Modify the nursing care plan as needed. Monitor appropriately for post-procedural signs of aspiration.
3. Follow guidelines in Chapter 1 for safe, effective, informed *posttest* care.

ORTHOPEDIC STUDIES

● Bone Imaging

This test is used primarily to evaluate and monitor persons with known or suspected metastatic disease. Breast cancer, prostate cancer, lung cancer, and lymphoma tend to metastasize to bone. Bone images visualize lesions 6 to 12 months before they appear on radiographs. Bone imaging may also be performed to evaluate patients with unexplained bone pain, primary bone tumors, arthritis, osteomyelitis, abnormal healing of fractures, fractures, shin splints, or compression fractures of the vertebral column; to evaluate pediatric patients with hip pain (Legg-Calvé-Perthes disease); and to assess child abuse, bone growth plates, sports injuries, and stress fractures. It is also performed to determine the age and metabolic activity of traumatic injuries and infections.

Other indications are evaluation of candidates for knee and hip prostheses, diagnosis of aseptic necrosis and vascularity of the femoral head, presurgical and postsurgical assessment of viable bone tissue, and evaluation of prosthetic joints and internal fixation devices to rule out loosening of prosthesis or infection.

Bone imaging has greater sensitivity in the pediatric patient than in the adult and is used for early detection of trauma. Normally, there is increased activity in the growth plates of the long bones. The child's history is significant for correlation and diagnostic differentiation. In older children with unexplained pain who participate in sports, stress fractures are often found on bone imaging.

A bone-seeking radiopharmaceutical is used to image the skeletal system. An example is ^{99m}Tc-labeled phosphate injected intravenously. Imaging usually begins 2 to 3 hours after injection. Abnormal pathology, such as increased blood flow to bone or increased osteocytic activity, concentrates the radiopharmaceutical at a higher or lower rate than the normal bone does. The radiopharmaceutical mimics calcium physiologically; therefore, it concentrates more heavily in areas of increased metabolic activity.

Reference Values

Normal

Homogeneous distribution of radiopharmaceutical

Procedure

1. Inject radioactive ^{99m}Tc methylenediphosphonate (MDP) intravenously.
2. A 2- to 3-hour waiting period is necessary for the radiopharmaceutical to concentrate in the bone. During this time, the patient may be asked to drink 4 to 6 glasses of water.
3. Before the imaging begins, ask the patient to void because a full bladder masks the pelvic bones.
4. Imaging takes about 30 to 60 minutes to complete. The patient must be able to lie still during the imaging.
5. Additional spot views of a specific area or three-dimensional SPECT imaging may be requested by the healthcare provider.
6. See Chapter 1 guidelines for safe, effective, informed *intratest* care.

PROCEDURAL ALERT

For osteomyelitis, images are acquired during the injection of the radiopharmaceutical, thus giving the image of the blood flow to the bone.

Clinical Implications

Abnormal concentrations indicate the following:

1. Very early bone disease and healing are detected by nuclear medicine bone images long before they are visible on radiographs. Radiographs are positive for bone lesions only after 30% to 50% decalcification (decrease in bone calcium) has occurred.
2. Many disorders can be detected but not differentiated by this test (e.g., cancer, arthritis, benign bone tumors, fractures, osteomyelitis, Paget's disease, aseptic necrosis). The findings must be interpreted in light of the whole clinical picture because any process inducing an increased calcium excretion rate will be reflected by an increased uptake in the bone.
3. In patients with breast cancer, the likelihood of a positive bone image finding in the preoperative period depends on the staging of the disease, and imaging tests are recommended before initial therapy. *Stages 1 and 2*: 40% have a positive bone image. *Stage 3*: 19% have a positive bone image. Yearly nuclear medicine bone imaging is recommended for follow up.
4. Multiple myeloma is the only tumor that shows better detectability with a plain radiograph than a radionuclide bone procedure.
5. Multiple focal areas of increased activity in the axial skeleton are commonly associated with metastatic bone disease. The reported percentage of solitary lesions due to metastasis varies on a site-by-site basis. With a single lesion in the spine or pelvis, the cause is more likely to be metastatic disease than with a single lesion occurring in the extremities or ribs.

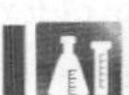

CLINICAL ALERT

The "flare phenomenon" occurs in patients with metastatic disease who are receiving a new treatment. The bone imaging may show increased activity or new lesions in patients with clinical improvement. This is caused by a healing response in patients with prostate or breast cancer within the first few months of starting a new treatment. These lesions should show marked improvement on imaging taken 3 to 4 months later. Radiographic correlation is necessary to rule out a benign process when solitary areas of increased or decreased uptake occur.

Interfering Factors

1. False-negative bone images occur in multiple myeloma of the bone. When this condition is known or suspected, the bone image is an unreliable indicator of skeletal involvement.
2. Patients with follicular thyroid cancer may harbor metastatic bone marrow disease, but these lesions are often missed by bone scans.

Interventions

Pretest Patient Care

1. Instruct the patient about the purpose and procedure of the test. Alleviate any fears concerning the procedure. Advise the patient that frequent drinking of fluids and activity during the first 6 hours help to reduce excess radiation to the bladder and gonads.
2. The patient can be mobile and active during the waiting period. There are no restrictions during the day before imaging.
3. Remind the patient to void before the imaging. If the patient is in pain or debilitated, offer assistance to the restroom.
4. Order and administer a sedative to any patient who will have difficulty lying quietly during the imaging period.
5. Refer to standard nuclear medicine imaging *pretest* precautions. Follow guidelines in Chapter 1 for safe, effective, informed *pretest* care.

Posttest Patient Care

1. Advise the patient to empty the bladder when imaging is completed, to decrease radiation exposure time.
2. Refer to standard nuclear medicine imaging *posttest* precautions.
3. Review test results; report and record findings. Modify the nursing care plan as needed.
4. Follow guidelines in Chapter 1 for safe, effective, informed *posttest* care.

● Bone Mineral Density (Bone Densitometry; Osteoporosis Imaging)

Bone densitometry enables the clinician to obtain a diagnosis of osteoporosis or osteopenia, often before fractures occur, by measuring bone mineral density. No radiopharmaceuticals are used in this procedure, but special imaging techniques are used. X-ray absorptiometry for measuring bone mineral density includes these special modalities:

1. Dual-energy absorptiometry (DEXA or DXA) to measure spine, hip, and forearm density
2. Peripheral dual-energy absorptiometry (pDXA) to measure forearm density
3. Single-energy x-ray absorptiometry (SXA) to measure the heel and forearm density
4. Radiographic absorptiometry (RA) to measure the density of the phalanges

DEXA is the most common and preferred method of measuring bone mineral density because of its precision and low radiation exposure. With the use of laser x-ray imaging and specific computer software, DEXA can assess fracture risk with relative ease and patient comfort. Fracture risk is measured in standard deviations (SDs) by comparing the patient's bone mass to that of healthy 25- to 35-year-olds. Test scores are printed out and reported with a T-score and a Z-score. The T-score is the number of SDs for the patient compared with normal young adults with mean peak bone mass. Fracture risk increases about 1.5 to 2.5 times for every SD. According to the World Health Organization, T-scores of <2.5 SDs may confirm a diagnosis of osteoporosis; scores of 2.5 to 1.0 SDs are associated with osteopenia; and scores of 1.0 SD or greater are considered normal. The Z-score is defined as the number of SDs for the patient compared with normal persons in the same age category. The T-score is the score most commonly reported and is the preferred reference point for diagnosing osteoporosis.

Reference Values

Normal

Absence of osteoporosis or osteopenia
T-score: <1.0 SD below normal (>−1.0)
Osteopenia: 1.0 to 2.5 SD below normal (−1.0 to −2.5)
Osteoporosis: >2.5 SD below normal (<−2.5)

Procedure

1. Position the patient so the area being imaged is immobile.
2. Place a foam block under both knees during the spine imaging. Use a leg brace immobilizer during the femur imaging and use an arm brace when imaging the forearm.
3. DEXA images of the spine and hip take approximately 20 minutes to complete. An additional 15 minutes is needed to image the forearm.
4. See Chapter 1 guidelines for safe, effective, informed *intratest* care.

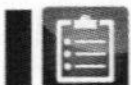

PROCEDURAL ALERT

Additional means of measuring bone mineral density include:

1. Quantitative computed tomography (QCT) to measure spine density
2. Peripheral quantitative computed tomography (pQCT) to measure forearm density

Clinical Implications

Abnormal imaging may be associated with the following:

1. Estrogen deficiency in postmenopausal women
2. Vertebral abnormalities
3. Patients with radiographic osteopenia
4. Hyperparathyroidism
5. Patients receiving long-term corticosteroid therapy

Interfering Factors

False readings may occur with the following:

1. Nuclear medicine imaging within the previous 72 hours (longer for gallium or indium imaging) may cause residual emission that can be misinterpreted.
2. Barium studies within the previous 7 to 10 days may interfere with the spine imaging.
3. Prosthetic devices or metallic objects surgically implanted in areas of interest may interfere with the image.

Interventions

Pretest Patient Care

1. Explain the purpose and procedure for measuring bone density of spine, hip, forearm, heel, and phalanges. No radiopharmaceuticals are administered.
2. Encourage patients to wear cotton garments that are free of metal or plastic zippers or buttons.
3. Follow guidelines in Chapter 1 for safe, effective, informed *pretest* care.

Posttest Patient Care

1. Review test results; report and record findings. Modify the nursing care plan as needed. If needed, serial studies may be ordered to measure the effectiveness of treatment.
2. Follow guidelines in Chapter 1 for safe, effective, informed *posttest* care.

TUMOR IMAGING STUDIES

● Gallium (^{67}Ga) Imaging

This image is used to detect the presence, location, and size of lymphoma; to detect chronic infections and abscesses; to differentiate malignant from benign lesions; and to determine the extent of invasion of known malignancies. The entire body is imaged looking for lymph node involvement. In both adult and pediatric patients, these studies are used to help stage bronchogenic cancer, Hodgkin's lymphomas, and non-Hodgkin's lymphomas. Gallium images may also be used to record tumor regression after radiation or chemotherapy. The radionuclide used in this study is gallium citrate (^{67}Ga).

The underlying mechanism for the uptake of ^{67}Ga is not well understood. Uptake in some neoplasms may depend on the presence of transferrin receptors in tumor cells, but this is only speculation. Once gallium enters a tissue, it remains there until radioactive decay dissipates the isotope. Medical centers that have PET/CT scanners have seen a major reduction in gallium imaging procedures because of PET/CT superior tumor imaging ability.

Reference Values

Normal

No evidence of tumor-type activity or infection

Procedure

1. Laxatives, suppositories, or tap water enemas are often ordered before imaging. The patient may eat breakfast on the day of imaging.
2. Inject the radionuclide 24 to 96 hours before imaging.
3. Have the patient lie quietly without moving during the imaging procedure. Take anterior and posterior views of the entire body.
4. Additional imaging may be done at 24-hour intervals to differentiate normal bowel activity from pathologic concentrations.
5. See Chapter 1 guidelines for safe, effective, informed *intratest* care.

Clinical Implications

1. Abnormal gallium concentration usually implies the existence of underlying pathology:
   a. Malignancy, especially lung and testes
   b. Mesothelioma
   c. Stages of lymphoma, Hodgkin's disease, melanoma, hepatoma, soft tissue sarcoma, primary tumor of bone or cartilage, neuroblastoma, and leukemia
   d. Abscesses
   e. Tuberculosis
   f. Thrombosis
   g. Abscessed sarcoidosis
   h. Chronic infection
   i. Interstitial pulmonary fibrosis
2. Further diagnostic studies usually are performed to distinguish benign from malignant lesions.
3. Tumor uptake of ^{67}Ga varies with tumor type, among persons with tumors of the same histologic type, and even among tumor sites of a given patient.
4. Tumor uptake of ^{67}Ga may be significantly reduced after effective treatment.
5. Although ^{111}In-labeled leukocyte imaging is more specific for acute abscess localization, gallium imaging may be used as a multipurpose screening procedure for chronic infection.

Interfering Factors

1. A negative study cannot be definitely interpreted as ruling out the presence of disease. (The rate of false-negative results in gallium studies is 40%.)
2. It is difficult to detect a single, solitary nodule (e.g., adenocarcinoma). Lesions smaller than 2 cm can be detected. Tumors near the liver are difficult to detect, and interpretation of iliac nodes is difficult.
3. Because gallium does collect in the bowel, there may be an abnormal concentration in the lower abdomen. For this reason, laxatives and enemas may be ordered.
4. Degeneration or necrosis of tumor and use of antineoplastic drugs immediately before imaging cause false-negative results.

Interventions

Pretest Patient Care

1. Explain the purpose, procedure, benefits, and risks of gallium imaging.
2. Usually no change in eating habits is required before testing. However, some departments request that patients eat a low-residue lunch and a clear-liquid supper the day before the examination.
3. See standard nuclear medicine procedures *pretest* precautions.
4. The usual preparation includes oral laxatives taken on the night before the first imaging session and again on the night before each imaging session. Enemas or suppositories may also be given. These preparations clear normal gallium activity from the bowel.
5. Actual imaging time is 45 to 90 minutes per imaging session.
6. Follow guidelines in Chapter 1 for safe, effective, informed *pretest* care.

Posttest Patient Care

1. Refer to standard nuclear medicine procedures *posttest* precautions.
2. Review test results; report and record findings. Modify the nursing care plan as needed.
3. Follow guidelines in Chapter 1 for safe, effective, informed *posttest* care.

CLINICAL ALERT

Breastfeeding should be discontinued for at least 4 wk after testing.

OVERVIEW OF MONOCLONAL ANTIBODY TUMOR IMAGING (ONCOSCINT, PROSTASCINT, OCTREOTIDE, AND OTHER PEPTIDES)

These classes of tumor imaging have revolutionized the foundation of radiopharmaceutical production. Like other radiopharmaceuticals, MABs and peptides have two parts: a radioisotope linked to a substance specific to a target organ. In the case of MABs, that substance is an antibody that has been cloned and mass produced. Because all the daughter antibodies are identical, a high yield of very specific antibodies can be produced.

1. OncoScint MAB. This was the first MAB radiopharmaceutical to be approved by the U.S. Food and Drug Administration and mass-marketed. OncoScint was approved for the detection of ovarian and colon cancer. OncoScint is an antibody linked to ^{111}In.
2. ProstaScint MAB. ProstaScint is a MAB approved for the detection of lymph node metastasis from prostate cancer.
3. Octreotide-peptide. This radiopharmaceutical peptide is used for localizing neuroendocrine tumors.

● Antibody and Peptide Tumor Imaging

Antibody and peptide tumor imaging is used to detect the location and size of known extrahepatic malignancies. These procedures are not screening techniques.

Reference Values

Normal

Distribution occurs in the normal liver, spleen, bone marrow, and bowel.

Procedure

1. Inject the patient with the radioisotope over a period of 5 minutes. Observe the patient for any reaction to the radiopharmaceutical.
2. Optimal whole-body images are obtained between 2 and 4 days after injection; additional images may be obtained at 24 hours and at 5 days.
3. Perform SPECT imaging if necessary.
4. See Chapter 1 guidelines for safe, effective, informed *intratest* care.

Clinical Implications

1. Abnormal distributions are found in tumors. Any change in the distribution provides information regarding the effectiveness of surgery or therapy.
2. Abnormal results have been observed in nonspecific areas such as inflammatory bowel disease, colostomy sites, and postoperative bowel adhesions.
3. The patient's medical history should be reviewed carefully.

Interfering Factors

Radioactivity in the bowel may interfere with colorectal assessment. Follow-up imaging is useful after administration of a cathartic to clarify equivocal findings.

During the ProstaScint procedure, the close proximity of the prostate to the bladder requires that a urinary catheter be placed during the delayed imaging. The catheter allows for the bladder to remain empty during the entire imaging session of the prostate and the surrounding body area. The catheter is removed immediately after the 1- to 2-hour imaging session.

Interventions

Pretest Patient Care

1. Explain the purpose, procedure, benefits, and risks.
2. Refer to standard nuclear medicine procedures *pretest* precautions.
3. Establish an intravenous line before injecting the radiopharmaceutical.
4. Advise the patient that a cathartic is required to differentiate bowel activity from abnormal pathology.
5. Follow guidelines in Chapter 1 for safe, effective, informed *pretest* care.

Posttest Patient Care

1. Refer to standard nuclear medicine procedures *posttest* precautions.
2. Review test results; report and record findings. Modify the nursing care plan as needed.
3. Observe the patient for 1 hour after injection of OncoScint for antibody reactions (e.g., chills, fever, nausea).
4. Realize that some patients develop human antimouse antibody (HAMA) titers after OncoScint injection.
5. Follow guidelines in Chapter 1 for safe, effective, informed *posttest* care.

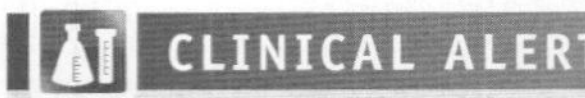

CLINICAL ALERT

Following OncoScint imaging, HAMA titers may result in falsely elevated immunoassay levels for CA 125.

Iodine-131 Whole-Body (Total-Body) Imaging

Whole-body imaging using ^{131}I can identify functioning thyroid tissue throughout the body. It is useful to determine the presence of metastatic thyroid cancer and the amount and location of residual tissue after thyroidectomy. The procedure is routinely performed in conjunction with thyroid therapy using ^{131}I for thyrocarcinoma.

Reference Values

Normal

No functioning thyroid tissues outside of the thyroid gland

Procedure

1. Administer radionuclide orally in a capsule form.
2. Perform imaging 24 to 72 hours after administration of the radiopharmaceutical. Imaging may take as long as 2 hours to perform.
3. Sometimes thyrotropin (TSH) is administered intravenously before the radionuclide is given. This stimulates any residual thyroid tissue and enhances ^{131}I uptake.
4. See Chapter 1 guidelines for safe, effective, informed *intratest* care.

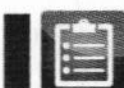

PROCEDURAL ALERT

1. If possible, this test should be performed before any other radionuclide procedures and before use of anti-iodine contrast medium, surgical preparation, or other form of iodine.
2. The test is most effective when endogenous TSH levels are high, so as to stimulate radionuclide uptake by metastatic neoplasms.

Clinical Implications

Abnormal uptake of iodine reveals:

1. Areas of extrathyroid tissue such as:
   a. Struma ovarii
   b. Substernal thyroid
   c. Sublingual thyroid
2. Residual tissue after thyroidectomy
3. Metastatic thyroid cancer

Interventions

Pretest Patient Care

1. Explain the purpose, procedure, benefits, and risks.
2. Advise the patient that the imaging process may take several hours. If iodine allergies are suspected, observe the patient for possible reactions.

3. Refer to standard nuclear medicine procedures *pretest* precautions.
4. Follow guidelines in Chapter 1 for safe, effective, informed *pretest* care.

Posttest Patient Care

1. Refer to standard nuclear medicine procedures *posttest* precautions.
2. Review test results; report and record findings. Modify the nursing care plan as needed.
3. Follow guidelines in Chapter 1 for safe, effective, informed *posttest* care.

● Breast Imaging (Scintimammography); Lymph Node Imaging (Lymphoscintigraphy)

Although x-ray mammography is the preferred examination for routine breast screening, scintimammography is often used in cases of indeterminate mammography. Other indications for performing breast imaging include follow-up to surgery, biopsy, radiation therapy, or chemotherapy. The test is more specific than x-ray mammography and may differentiate between benign and malignant lesions. The test is also used to detect any axillary lymph node involvement from breast cancer and decreases the number of unnecessary breast biopsies. Sentinel and satellite node identification and staging in early breast cancer using lymphoscintigraphy and intraoperative gamma node and tissue biopsy show micrometastasis more frequently than standard dissection. Lymphoscintigraphy assesses the lymphatic drainage of tumors.

Reference Values

Normal Breast

Uniform distribution of radiopharmaceutical uptake in the breasts without focal points of concentration

No focal uptake in lymphatic tissue

Normal Lymph Node

No abnormal nodes (indicated by obstruction to tracer)

(The first node the tracer goes to is identified.)

Procedure

Breast Imaging

1. Inject the radiopharmaceutical intravenously in the arm opposite from the breast of concern.
2. Have the patient lie prone on a special table with a cut out section that allows the breasts to hang through the table unobstructed.
3. Place the patient in the supine position with the arms raised for obtaining images of the axillary lymph nodes.
4. Although the total patient time is approximately 45 to 60 minutes, the actual scan time is only 25 to 30 minutes.
5. For sentinel node identification, see Chapter 11 for a complete discussion of the procedure.
6. Remember that an optional SPECT examination may be requested by the nuclear medicine physician. This examination may take an additional 30 to 40 minutes.
7. See Chapter 1 guidelines for safe, effective, informed *intratest* care.

Lymph Node Imaging

1. Special positioning is required. (See sentinel node evaluation in Chapter 11.)
2. The tracer is injected by intradermal method for melanoma evaluation or subcutaneously for breast cancer evaluation. Massage after injection for at least 30 seconds, moving the breast to optimally clear the overlying soft tissue.

3. Images are obtained immediately and 2 to 4 hours after injection.
4. Sentinel lymph node (SLN) identification may also be performed to evaluate metastatic spread of cancer to penis, vulva, uterus, head, and neck.

Clinical Implications

Breast Imaging

1. Abnormal increased focal uptake is found in cases of a fibroadenoma and adenocarcinoma.
2. Nonuniform increased diffuse uptake of activity is associated with fibrous dysplasia, which may be unilateral or bilateral.
3. Several areas of increased focal uptake are often seen in cases of multifocal breast cancer.
4. In patients with a breast prosthesis, a focal decrease in activity is observed in relation to the size and shape of the prosthesis.
5. Axillary metastasis is detected as focal areas of increased uptake in the axillary nodes.
6. This scan is used to evaluate radiation therapy and chemotherapy.

Lymph Node Imaging

1. Abnormal nodes show leaks into adjacent tissue, a blush around the affected node, and unusual collateral lymph drainage pathways.
2. The first lymph node to drain the tumor invariably contains the tumor.
3. It has been found that there are more than one lymphatic channels draining the tumor, and that there are one, two, or three SLNs as well as satellite nodes.
4. Micrometastasis of biopsied tissue is found more frequently than standard axillary node dissection.

Interfering Factors

1. There should not be any other detectable amount of radioactivity in the patient.
2. The patient should be lying supine for the injection of the radiopharmaceutical (for breast imaging) to prevent a "streaking" artifact found on the resulting image in the breast region, which corresponds to the arm that received the injection.
3. To eliminate a false-positive appearance, the patient should be injected on the side opposite of a known lymphatic lesion. If the patient is known to have bilateral breast cancer, a foot vein may be used for injection.
4. Extravasation of the radiopharmaceutical can result in hot spots of radioactivity in the location of the axillary lymph nodes.

Interventions

Pretest Patient Care

1. Explain the purpose, procedure, benefits, and risks of the nuclear image. See Chapter 11 for more information on sentinel node biopsy.
2. Have the patient remove all clothing and jewelry from the waist up. The patient wears a hospital gown with the opening of the gown in the front. There are no dietary or medication restrictions.
3. Follow guidelines in Chapter 1 for safe, effective, informed *pretest* care.
4. See standard nuclear medicine procedures *pretest* precautions.

Posttest Patient Care

1. Review test results; report and record findings. Modify the nursing care plan as needed. Counsel appropriately about need for further tests (e.g., biopsy and possible immediate surgery).
2. Refer to standard nuclear medicine procedures *posttest* precautions.
3. Follow guidelines in Chapter 1 for safe, effective, informed *posttest* care.

INFLAMMATORY PROCESS IMAGING

● Leukocyte (WBC) Imaging (Indium- or Ceretec-Labeled WBCs)

The leukocyte imaging test—in which a sample of the patient's own white blood cells (WBCs) are isolated, labeled with indium oxine (^{111}In) or ^{99m}Tc exametazime, and reinjected—is used for localization of acute abscess formation. The study is indicated in both adults and children with signs and symptoms of a septic process, fever of unknown origin, osteomyelitis, or suspected intra-abdominal abscess. It is also helpful in determining the cause of complications of surgery, injury, or inflammation of the gastrointestinal tract and pelvis. The test results are based on the fact that any collection of labeled WBCs outside the liver, spleen, and functioning bone marrow indicates an abnormal area to which the cells localize. This procedure is 90% sensitive and 90% specific for acute inflammatory disease or acute abscess formation.

Reference Values

Normal

Normal leukocyte concentration and radiopharmaceutical distribution in liver, spleen, and bone marrow

No signs of leukocyte localization outside of the reticuloendothelial system

Procedure

1. Obtain a venous blood sample (lavender-topped tube) of 60 mL for the purpose of isolating and labeling the WBCs. The laboratory process takes about 2 hours to complete. The patient's WBC count needs to be at least 4.0 so that there are enough cells to label for this procedure.
2. Label the WBCs with radioactive ^{111}In, oxine, or ^{99m}Tc exametazime and inject intravenously.
3. Have the patient return for imaging after 4 hours with Ceretec (exametazime) and after 24 or 48 hours with indium.
4. Imaging time is about 1 hour per session.
5. See Chapter 1 guidelines for safe, effective, informed *intratest* care.

Clinical Implications

Abnormal concentrations indicate:

1. Acute abscess formation
2. Acute osteomyelitis and infection of orthopedic prostheses
3. Active inflammatory bowel disease
4. Postsurgical abscess sites and wound infections

Interfering Factors

1. False-negative reactions are known to occur when the chemotactic function of the WBC has been altered, as in hemodialysis, hyperglycemia, hyperalimentation, steroid therapy, and long-term antibiotic therapy.
2. Gallium scans up to 1 month before the test can interfere.
3. False-positive scans occur in the presence of gastrointestinal bleeding and in upper respiratory infections and pneumonitis when patients swallow purulent sputum.

NOTE *See Clinical Considerations, Pretest Patient Care, and Posttest Patient Care for nuclear medicine imaging.*

CLINICAL ALERT

If the patient does not have an adequate number of WBCs, additional blood may have to be drawn. Gallium imaging may be necessary if too few WBCs are present, or donor cells can be used.

OVERVIEW OF RADIONUCLIDE (NON-RADIOIMMUNOASSAY) LABORATORY STUDIES

Very small amounts of radioactive substances may be administered to patients, and subsequently, their body fluids and glands may be examined in the laboratory for concentrations of radioactivity. Minute quantities of radioactive materials may be detected in blood, feces, urine, other body fluids, and glands.

Some procedures check the ability of the body to absorb the administered radioactive compound. Others, such as blood volume determinations, test the ability of the body to localize or dilute the administered radioactive substance.

● Total Blood Volume; Plasma Volume; Erythrocyte (RBC) Volume

The purposes of the blood volume test are to determine circulating blood volume, to help evaluate the bleeding or debilitated patient, and to determine the origin of hypotension in the presence of anuria or oliguria when dehydration may be the cause. This determination is one way to monitor blood loss during surgery; it is used as a guide in replacement therapy after blood or body fluid loss and in the determination of whole-body hematocrit. The results are useful in choosing the most appropriate blood component for replacement therapy (whole blood, plasma, or packed RBCs).

Total blood volume determinations are of value in the following situations:

1. To evaluate gastrointestinal and uterine bleeding
2. To aid in the diagnosis of hypovolemic shock
3. To aid in the diagnosis of polycythemia vera
4. To determine the required blood component for replacement therapy, as in persons undergoing surgery

These tests reveal an increased or decreased volume of RBC mass. A sample of the patient's blood is mixed with a radioactive substance, incubated at room temperature, and reinjected. Another blood sample is obtained 15 minutes later. The most commonly used tracers in blood volume determinations are serum albumin tagged with ^{131}I or ^{125}I and patient or donor RBCs tagged with chromium-51 (^{51}Cr). The combination of procedures (total blood volume) is the only true blood volume. Other volume studies are plasma volume and RBC volume, which may be done separately. Serum albumin tagged with ^{131}I or ^{125}I may not always be available from the manufacturer.

The plasma volume is used to establish a vascular baseline, to determine changes in plasma volume before and after surgery, and to evaluate fluid and blood replacement in patients with gastrointestinal bleeding, burns, or trauma. The ^{51}Cr RBC volume study is done to see what percentage of the circulating blood is composed of RBCs. This procedure is performed in connection with evaluation of RBC survival or gastrointestinal blood loss and in ferrokinetic (turnover or clearance rate of iron in the body) studies. These tests can be done simultaneously.

Reference Values

Normal

Total blood volume: 55 to 80 mL/kg or 0.055 to 0.080 L/kg
Erythrocyte volume: 20 to 35 mL/kg or 0.020 to 0.035 L/kg (greater in men than in women)
Plasma volume: 30 to 45 mL/kg or 0.030 to 0.045 L/kg

NOTE *Because adipose tissue has a sparser blood supply than lean tissue, the patient's body type can affect the proportion of blood volume to body weight; for this reason, test findings should always be reported in milliliters per kilogram of body weight.*

Procedure

1. Record the patient's height and current weight.
2. Obtain venous blood samples and mix one blood sample with a radionuclide.
3. Fifteen to 30 minutes later, reinject the blood radiopharmaceutical.
4. About 15 minutes later, obtain another venous blood sample and have it examined in the laboratory.
5. See Chapter 1 guidelines for safe, effective, informed *intratest* care.

Clinical Implications

1. A normal total blood volume with a decreased RBC content indicates the need for a transfusion of packed red cells.
2. Polycythemia vera may be differentiated from secondary polycythemia.
   a. Increased total blood volume due to an increased RBC mass suggests polycythemia vera. The plasma volume most often is normal.
   b. Normal or decreased total blood volume due to a decreased plasma volume suggests secondary polycythemia. The RBC most often is normal.

CLINICAL ALERT

If intravenous blood component therapy is ordered for the same day, the blood volume determination should be done before the intravenous line is started.

Interventions

Pretest Patient Care

1. Explain the purpose, procedure, benefits, and risks of the test. Blood samples and intravenous injection are part of this test. No imaging takes place.
2. Weigh the patient just before the test if possible.
3. Refer to standard nuclear medicine *pretest* precautions.
4. Follow guidelines in Chapter 1 for safe, effective, informed *pretest* care.

Posttest Patient Care

1. Refer to standard nuclear medicine *posttest* precautions.
2. Review test results; report and record findings. Modify the nursing care plan as needed.
3. Follow guidelines in Chapter 1 for safe, effective, informed *posttest* care.

● Red Blood Cell (RBC) Survival Time Test

The RBC survival time test has its greatest use in the evaluation of known or suspected hemolytic anemia and is also indicated when the cause for anemia is obscure (abnormal sequestration of RBCs in the spleen), to identify accessory spleens, and to determine abnormal RBC production or destruction. Typically, the normal RBC survives about 110 to 120 days in a normal healthy adult. Under normal circumstances, RBCs are eliminated due to the aging of the RBC (senescence) and random hemolysis.

Scanning of the spleen is often done as part of this test. The RBC survival test usually is ordered in conjunction with a blood volume determination and radionuclide iron uptake and clearance tests. When stool specimens are collected for 3 days, the test is often referred to as the "gastrointestinal blood loss test."

Reference Values

Normal

Normal half-time for survival of ^{51}Cr-labeled RBCs is approximately 25 to 35 days.
^{51}Cr in stool: <3 mL/24 hours or <3 mL/day

Procedure

1. Obtain a venous blood sample of 20 mL.
2. Ten to 30 minutes later, reinject the blood after being tagged with a radionuclide, ^{51}Cr.
3. Blood samples are usually obtained on the first day; again after 24, 48, 72, and 96 hours; and then at weekly intervals for 3 weeks. Time may be shortened depending on the outcome of the test. After counting the specimens, the results are plotted, and the RBC survival time is calculated. Results are based on the fact that disappearance of radioactivity from the circulation corresponds to disappearance of the RBCs, thereby determining overall erythrocyte survival. As part of this procedure, a radioactive detector may be used over the spleen, sternum, and liver to assess the relative concentrations of radioactivity in these areas. This external counting helps to determine whether the spleen is taking part in excessive sequestration of RBCs as a causative factor in anemia.
4. In some instances, a 72-hour stool collection may be ordered to detect gastrointestinal blood loss. Obtain special collection containers labeled for radiation hazard. At the end of each 24-hour collection period, the total stool is to be collected by the department of nuclear medicine. This test can be completed in 3 days.
5. See Chapter 1 guidelines for safe, effective, informed *intratest* care.

Clinical Implications

1. Shortened RBC survival may result from blood loss, hemolysis, or removal of RBCs by the spleen, as in:
   a. Chronic granulocytic leukemia
   b. Hemolytic anemia
   c. Hemoglobin C disease
   d. Hereditary spherocytosis
   e. Pernicious anemia
   f. Megaloblastic anemia of pregnancy
   g. Sickle cell anemia
   h. Uremia
2. Prolonged RBC survival time may result from an abnormality in RBC production, as in thalassemia minor, and false-negative results when transfusion is given during the procedure.
3. If hemolytic anemia is diagnosed, further studies are needed to establish whether the RBCs have intrinsic abnormalities or whether anemia results from immunologic effects of the patient's plasma.
4. Results are normal in:
   a. Hemoglobin C trait
   b. Sickle cell trait
5. Half of the radioactivity in the plasma may not disappear for 7 to 8 hours.

Interfering Factors

1. Dehydration or blood loss can affect the RBC volume.
2. Blood transfusion during the testing period

Interventions

Pretest Patient Care

1. Explain the purpose and procedure of the test. Emphasize that this test requires a minimum of 2 weeks of the patient's time, with trips to the diagnostic facility for venipunctures.
2. If stool collection is required, advise the patient of the importance of saving all stool and that stool must be free of urine contamination.
3. Refer to standard nuclear medicine *pretest* precautions.
4. Follow guidelines in Chapter 1 for safe, effective, informed *pretest* care.

CLINICAL ALERT

1. The test usually is contraindicated in a patient who is actively bleeding.
2. Record and report signs of active bleeding.
3. Transfusions should not be given while the test is in progress. If it is necessary to do so, notify the nuclear medicine department to terminate the test.

Posttest Patient Care

1. Refer to standard nuclear medicine *posttest* precautions.
2. Review test results; report and record findings. Modify the nursing care plan as needed. Explain need for further testing and possible treatment (splenectomy).
3. Follow guidelines in Chapter 1 for safe, effective, informed *posttest* care.

OVERVIEW OF POSITRON EMISSION TOMOGRAPHY (PET) IMAGING STUDIES

PET imaging involves the combined use of positron-emitting radionuclides and emission CT. PET technology generates high-resolution images of body function and metabolism. PET uses radiopharmaceuticals that are the basic elements of biologic substances. In this way, normal and abnormal biologic function of cells and organs can be determined. It produces images of molecular-level physiologic function, including glucose metabolism, oxygen utilization, blood flow, and tissue perfusion. The radiopharmaceutical dose is injected and emits radioactivity in the form of positrons, which are detected and transformed into a visual display by computer.

A broad spectrum of radiopharmaceuticals is used in PET imaging. A main advantage of PET derives from the positron-emitting isotopes themselves: carbon-11 (^{11}Ca), nitrogen-13 (^{13}N), and oxygen-15 (^{15}O), which are present in organic molecules, and ^{18}F, which can be substituted for hydrogen. Typically, radionuclides used in PET imaging have very short half-lives (2 minutes to 2 hours).

^{18}F is used for several purposes. Its half-life is long enough to trace biochemical reactions. It can be used to label a glucose compound, permitting imaging of a variety of tissues. ^{18}F is administered primarily in a glucose form called fluorodeoxyglucose (FDG). FDG is highly sensitive. Neoplastic cells are hypermetabolic and appear to have an FDG affinity that results in high contrast. FDG has >90% specificity for myocardial viability, neoplastic processes, and infection. FDG is an outstanding tracer that can be used in many areas of the body. It is a glucose analogue and has a broad application because every cell uses glucose as fuel.

Indications for the Test

Clinical PET is a useful tool aiding diagnosis of many disease states, primarily in oncology, neurology, and cardiology. However, the technique is applicable to all parts of the body for diagnosis, disease staging, and monitoring of therapy. Unlike MRI or CT, PET provides physiologic, anatomic, and biochemical data.

Although PET is more sensitive than gamma SPECT, it is considerably more expensive. The use of FDG imaging with specially equipped gamma cameras has been an alternative to exclusive PET imaging systems. The patient preparation for nuclear medicine use of FDG in gamma SPECT imaging is similar to that for PET imaging of FDG. Because of the physics of ^{18}F, only multiheaded cameras can be used for gamma SPECT acquisitions. Currently, there are certain limitations with gamma SPECT imaging when compared with true PET imaging.

In oncology, FDG-PET has proved useful in several areas, including the diagnosis of pulmonary nodules, the differentiation of pancreatic cancer from mass-forming pancreatitis, and the diagnosis of breast cancer in selected cases of mammography and biopsy failure. PET imaging is used for the initial preoperative staging of cancer involving the lung, liver, colon, breast, head, and neck as well as in melanomas and lymphomas. For example, in lung cancer, PET is useful in determining the degree of operability. With extensive metastasis in the mediastinum, surgery is contraindicated. Staging, detection of recurrence, and response to therapy also can be determined.

In cardiology, PET has demonstrated excellent utility for measuring myocardial blood flow and perfusion and for detecting coronary artery disease. The high-energy photons of PET tracers produce high-quality images even in obese patients. In these cases, PET can provide important information for determining which patients will benefit from the more invasive procedures.

In neurology, FDG-PET imaging is a noninvasive aid in predicting prognosis and for surgical planning in epilepsy. By revealing areas of increased and decreased glucose utilization, PET helps surgeons pinpoint the surgical site. PET is being used to diagnose a wide variety of dementias, including Alzheimer's disease, which shows a distinct pattern of glucose consumption in the temporal and parietal regions of the brain. Also, distinct brain patterns can be seen in the involuntary movement disorders, such as Parkinson's disease, Huntington's disease, and Tourette's syndrome.

Reference Values

Normal

Normal patterns of tissue metabolism based on oxygen, glucose, and fatty acid utilization and protein synthesis

Normal blood flow and tissue perfusion

Procedure

1. Although the actual imaging time required for a single image is 30 minutes to 45 minutes, the actual time involved with the patient may be several hours and occurs before and during radiopharmaceutical injection. Delayed imaging may produce different results than early imaging after injection (after 45 minutes for body tumor and 30 minutes for brain tumor).
2. Position the patient on a table and then within the scanner. Before administration of the radiopharmaceutical, perform a background transmission scan. In certain procedures, this preliminary scan is optional. A number of positions are assumed, 2 to 6 minutes at each position.
3. Administer the radioactive drug intravenously. The patient waits 30 to 45 minutes in the department.
4. Patients undergoing PET procedures for colon cancer, suspected pelvic pathology, or kidney studies may require a urinary catheter or Lasix and oral contrast.
5. All patients require fasting, and glucose monitoring may be part of the patient preparation before the scan. Elevated glucose results in decreased FDG uptake in cancer cells. Hydrate patient before and after FDG injection to minimize bladder uptake.

6. Combined PET and CT images result in more sensitive, improved images.
7. See Chapter 1 guidelines for safe, effective, informed *intratest* care.

Interventions

Patient preparation for FDG-PET imaging varies among institutions. However, some generalizations can be made.

Pretest Patient Care

1. Explain test purpose and procedure. Fasting is required for all tests. Sometimes, fasting blood glucose levels are obtained. Caution must be taken if insulin is given because it suppresses glucose tissue uptake. Insulin also suppresses FDG tissue uptake, which affects the quality of the resulting scan. Insulin should not be given within 4 hours of the FDG injection.
2. Administer the FDG radiopharmaceutical intravenously. Blood pressure is monitored.
3. Follow guidelines in Chapter 1 for safe, effective, informed *pretest* care.

Posttest Patient Care

1. Review test results; report and record findings. Modify the nursing care plan as needed.
2. Refer to standard nuclear medicine procedures *posttest* precautions.
3. Follow guidelines in Chapter 1 for safe, effective, informed *posttest* care.

● Brain Imaging

Clinical Implications

1. *Epilepsy.* Focal areas with increased metabolism have been seen during actual episodes of epilepsy, with decreased oxygen utilization and blood flow during interictal episodes. (PET/CT becomes an alternative to depth electrode implants.)
2. *Stroke.* An extremely complex pathophysiologic picture is revealed, including anaerobic glycolysis, depressed oxygen utilization, and decreased blood flow.
3. *Coronary artery disease.* Excellent images of decreased myocardial blood flow and perfusion are observed.
4. *Dementia.* Decreased glucose consumption (hypometabolic activity) is revealed by PET/CT imaging. PET/CT is used to differentiate Alzheimer's disease from other types of dementia.
5. *Schizophrenia.* Some studies using labeled glucose indicate reduced metabolic activity in the frontal region.
6. *Brain tumors.* Data have been collected concerning oxygen use and blood flow relations for these tumors. The PET/CT images can also distinguish the developmental stages of cranial tumors and give information about the operability of such tumors. Gliomas have relatively good perfusion compared with their decreased oxygen utilization. The high uptake of radiopharmaceutical in gliomas is reported to correlate with the tumor's histologic grade.

Interfering Factors

Excessive anxiety can alter the test results when brain function is being tested. Tranquilizers cannot be given before the test because they alter glucose metabolism.

Interventions

Pretest Patient Care

1. Instruct the patient about the purpose, procedure, and special requirements of PET/CT imaging. Refer to standard nuclear medicine procedures *pretest* precautions.
2. Advise the patient that lying as still as possible during the imaging is necessary. However, the patient is not to fall asleep.

3. Maintain a quiet environment.
4. Follow guidelines in Chapter 1 for safe, effective, informed *pretest* care.

Posttest Patient Care

1. Review test results; report and record findings. Modify the nursing care plan as needed.
2. Refer to standard nuclear medicine procedures *posttest* precautions.
3. Follow guidelines in Chapter 1 for safe, effective, informed *posttest* care.

• Cardiac Imaging

Clinical Implications

1. In cardiology, PET/CT imaging provides measurements of blood flow, myocardial perfusion, and myocardial viability. These measurements are used to detect:
   a. Coronary artery disease, which is characterized by areas of decreased blood flow, decreased perfusion, or both
   b. Transient ischemia (both stress and rest images are performed)
2. A high rate of glucose consumption is required to meet the energy needs of the heart. Low glucose metabolism in areas of decreased blood flow indicates nonviable myocardial tissue.

Interventions

Pretest Patient Care

1. Instruct the patient about the purpose, procedure, and special requirements of PET/CT imaging. Refer to standard nuclear medicine procedures *pretest* precautions.
2. An intravenous line may be necessary. Cardiac viability patients require fasting and may be given glucose and/or insulin as part of patient preparation. Smoking and medication restrictions may be required before imaging. Consult with the referring healthcare provider or the nuclear imaging department.
3. It may be necessary to place ECG leads on the patient.
4. Follow guidelines in Chapter 1 for safe, effective, informed *pretest* care.

Posttest Patient Care

1. Review test results; report and record findings. Modify the nursing care plan as needed.
2. Refer to standard nuclear medicine procedures *posttest* precautions.
3. Follow guidelines in Chapter 1 for safe, effective, informed *posttest* care.

• Tumor Imaging

Clinical Implications

1. Measurements of glucose (FDG) metabolism are used to determine tumor growth. Because small amounts of FDG can be visualized, early tumor detection is possible before structural changes detectable by MRI or CT occur. Tumor grading can be assessed by the rate of increase in glucose metabolism. In cases of suspected tumor recurrence after therapy, PET differentiates any new growth from necrotic tissue.
2. PET/CT is used to distinguish between recurrent, active tumor growth and necrotic masses in soft tissue; this differentiation is difficult to make by MRI or CT.

Interventions

Pretest Patient Care

1. Explain the purpose, procedure, and special requirements of PET/CT imaging. Refer to standard nuclear medicine procedures *pretest* precautions.

2. Usually, no special preparation is needed. Sometimes, a urinary catheter, Lasix (furosemide), and contrast may be used for abdominal tumors.
3. Follow guidelines in Chapter 1 for safe, effective, informed *pretest* care.

Posttest Patient Care

1. Review test results; report and record findings. Modify the nursing care plan as needed.
2. Refer to standard nuclear medicine procedures *posttest* precautions.
3. Follow guidelines in Chapter 1 for safe, effective, informed *posttest* care.

BIBLIOGRAPHY

Adam A, Dixon AK: Grainger & Allison's Diagnostic Radiology, 6th ed. Philadelphia, Elsevier Saunders, 2014

Alazraki N, Styblo T, Grant S, et al: Sentinel node staging of early breast cancer using lymphoscintigraphy and intraoperative gamma-detecting probe. Semin Nucl Med 30:56–64, 2000

Christian PE, Waterstram-Rich KM: Nuclear Medicine and PET/CT, 7th ed. Philadelphia, Elsevier Mosby, 2012

DePuey EG, Garcia EV, Berman DS: Cardiac SPECT Imaging, 2nd ed. Philadelphia, Lippincott Williams & Wilkins, 2001

Elgazzar A: The Pathophysiologic Basis of Nuclear Medicine, 3rd ed. New York, Springer, 2015

Gore RM, Levine MS: Textbook of Gastrointestinal Radiology, 4th ed. Philadelphia, Elsevier Saunders, 2014

Iskandrian AE, Garcia EV: Nuclear Cardiac Imaging, 5th ed. Oxford University Press, 2015

Kapetanopoulos A, Heller GV, Selker HP, et al: Acute resting myocardial perfusion imaging in patients with diabetes mellitus: results from the Emergency Room Assessment of Sestamibi for Evaluation of Chest Pain (ERASE Chest Pain) trial. J Nucl Cardiol 11(5):570–577, 2004

Mettler FA, Guiberteau MJ: Essentials of Nuclear Medicine Imaging, 6th ed. Philadelphia, Elsevier Saunders, 2012

Morton KA, Clark PB, Christensen CR, et al: Diagnostic Imaging: Nuclear Medicine. Philadelphia, Elsevier, 2007

Pickhardt P, Arluk G: Atlas of Gastrointestinal Imaging: Radiologic-Endoscopic Correlation. Philadelphia, Elsevier Saunders, 2007

Saha GB: Fundamentals of Nuclear Pharmacy, 6th ed. New York, Springer 2010

Sandler MP, Coleman RE, Patton JA, et al: Diagnostic Nuclear Medicine, 4th ed. Philadelphia, Lippincott Williams & Wilkins, 2003

Taylor A, Schuster D, Alazraki N: A Clinician's Guide to Nuclear Medicine, 2nd ed. Reston, VA, Society of Nuclear Medicine, 2000

Treves ST: Pediatric Nuclear Medicine/PET, 4th ed. New York, Springer, 2014

X-Ray and Computed Tomography (CT) Studies

10

OVERVIEW OF X-RAY STUDIES

X-ray studies, also known as *radiographs*, are used to examine soft and bony tissues of the body. X-rays are short-wavelength electromagnetic waves produced when fast-moving electrons collide with substances in their pathways. X-rays travel in straight lines at the speed of light (186,000 miles/second). When an x-ray beam passes through matter, some of its intensity is absorbed—the more dense the matter, the greater the degree of x-ray absorption. The composite image produced represents these varying degrees of tissue density in shades of black, white, and gray. Images may be captured on photographic film, displayed on a video screen, or recorded on digital media. The basic principle of radiography is that differences in density among various body structures produce images of varying light or dark intensity, much like the negative print of a photograph. Dense structures appear white, whereas air-filled areas are black. Fluoroscopy is an imaging technique that uses x-rays to demonstrate movement of body organs and/or contrast agents.

USE OF CONTRAST AGENTS

Many radiographic techniques use the natural contrasts and varying densities that exist in body tissues representing air, water (in soft tissue), fat, and bone. The lungs and gastrointestinal (GI) tract normally contain air or gases. Other body structures are encased in a fatty envelope. Bone contains naturally occurring mineral salts. However, diagnosis of certain pathologic conditions requires visualization of details that cannot be revealed through plain x-rays. In these cases, details can be highlighted by the presence of *contrast media* in the area. These contrast substances can be administered through oral, rectal, or injection routes.

The ideal contrast agent should be relatively harmless (low toxicity, nonantigenic, nonallergenic, and inert), should not interfere with any physiologic functions, and should allow high and repeated dosing at a moderate cost. A contrast medium may be classified as either *radiopaque* (not permitting the transmission of x-rays) or *radiolucent* (permitting partial transmission of x-rays). The adverse pharmacodynamics of contrast media causes death in an estimated 1 of every 20,000 to 40,000 administrations. The most commonly used contrast agents are *water-soluble* non-iodine agents for GI examinations and intravascular procedures. Ultimately, one must always be alert to the possibility of an adverse reaction to contrast media. Consequently, emergency supplies and equipment should be readily available when using these agents.

The following contrast agents are used routinely in x-ray studies:

1. Alimentary canal contrast agents
   a. Water-soluble agents (e.g., Gastrografin [Bracco Diagnostics], Gastroview [Guerbet Inc.], Hypaque [GE Healthcare] sodium oral powder)
   b. Water-insoluble agents (e.g., $BaSO_4$, Polibar Plus [Bracco Diagnostics], Anatrast [Mallinckrodt Inc.])
   c. Gases (CO_2 gas, gas-producing calcium citrate and magnesium citrate)
2. Injectable contrast agents
   a. Nonionic iodinated contrast (low osmolar agents; e.g., Omnipaque [GE Healthcare], Optiray [Mallinckrodt Inc.])
   b. Ionic iodinated contrast (high osmolar agents; e.g., Hypaque, Conray [Guerbet])
3. Specific-use agents
   a. Bile agents (e.g., Conray)
   b. Iodized oil contrast agents

ADVERSE REACTIONS TO CONTRAST AGENTS

All contrast agents have the potential for causing allergic reactions that can range from mild (e.g., nausea and vomiting) to severe anaphylaxis (e.g., cardiovascular collapse and central nervous system depression leading to death if untreated). Table 10.1 lists the range of possible adverse reactions to iodine contrast media. Reactions happen quickly and usually occur within minutes of administration of the contrast agent. Such reactions can occur in anyone.

TABLE 10.1 Signs, Symptoms, and Incidence of Reactions to Iodine Contrast Media

Cardiovascular	Respiratory	Cutaneous	Gastrointestinal	Neurologic	Genitourinary
Pallor	Sneezing	Erythema	Nausea	Anxiety	Flank pain
Diaphoresis	Coughing	Feeling of warmth	Vomiting	Headache	Hematuria
Tachycardia	Rhinorrhea	Parotitis	Metallic taste	Dizziness	Oliguria
Bradycardia	Wheezing	Urticaria	Abdominal cramps	Agitation	Albuminuria
Palpitations	Acute asthma attack	Pruritus	Diarrhea	Vertigo	WBCs in blood
Arrhythmia	Laryngospasm	Pain at the injection site	Paralytic ileus	Slurred speech	Acute renal failure
Acute pulmonary edema	Cyanosis	Angioneurotic edema		Disorientation	Uterine cramps
Shock	Laryngeal edema	Swelling of eyes		Stupor	Urgency to urinate
Congestive heart failure	Apnea			Coma	
Cardiac arrest	Respiratory arrest			Convulsions	
	Dyspnea				

All Iodine Contrast Reactions	Incidence (%)
Minor reactions requiring no treatment: sensation of heat, nausea, vomiting, local urticaria, rash, dizziness, light-headedness, transient arrhythmia, pain at injection site, mild pallor, pruritus, facial swelling	1:20 (5)
Intermediate reactions that require treatment but no hospitalization and are not life-threatening: vomiting, extensive urticaria, bronchospasm, faintness, dyspnea, mild chest pain, headache, chills, and fever	1:100 (1)
Severe reactions that require hospitalization and are life-threatening: syncope, laryngeal and pulmonary edema, hypotension, convulsions, circulatory collapse, pulmonary edema, severe angina, myocardial infarction, cardiac arrhythmia, coma, respiratory arrest	1:2000 (0.05)
Cardiac arrest	1:6000 (0.017)
Death	1:40,000 (0.0025)

Clinical Considerations When Iodine Contrast Agents Are Used

1. Know the patient's age and health status. Children and elderly people, especially those with medical problems, may be especially sensitive to contrast agents. This sensitivity may increase the chance for side effects.
2. The presence of other medical problems may increase the risk for side effects.
   a. Individuals with asthma or hay fever are at a greater risk for having an allergic reaction to the contrast agent.
   b. Diabetic patients have a greater risk for developing kidney problems.
   c. Patients with severe hypertension may experience a dangerous rise in blood pressure and tachycardia.
   d. Patients with kidney and liver disease may experience exacerbation of their disease.
   e. Individuals with multiple myeloma may develop severe kidney problems.
   f. Patients with overactive thyroid may experience a sudden increase in symptoms or thyroid storm.
   g. Patients with sickle cell disease may experience the formation of abnormal blood cells.
   h. Patients using beta blockers may have a higher risk for developing anaphylactoid reactions.
   i. Patients with chronic obstructive pulmonary disease (COPD) have an increased risk for postinjection dyspnea.
3. Patients who are allergic to iodine contrast media must have this information documented in their healthcare records. The risk for subsequent reactions increases 3 to 4 times after the first reaction; however, subsequent reactions will not necessarily be more severe than the first. The patient must be made aware of the implications of the situation. Assess for and document allergies to iodine-containing substances (e.g., seafood, cabbage, kale, raw leafy vegetables, turnips, iodized salt). Also, determine each person's reaction to penicillin or skin test for allergies because these patients have a greater chance of having a reaction.
4. Check the patient's fasting status before the x-ray procedure has begun. Except in an extreme emergency, iodine contrast media should never be administered intravenously sooner than 90 minutes after the patient has eaten. In most instances, the patient should fast the night before undergoing any x-ray procedure using an iodine contrast agent.
5. Death from an allergic reaction can occur if severe symptoms go untreated. Staff in attendance must be qualified to administer cardiopulmonary resuscitation should it be necessary. Emergency equipment and supplies must be readily available.
6. Promptly administer antihistamines per healthcare provider's order if mild to moderate reactions to iodine contrast substances occur (see Table 10.1).
7. When coordinating x-ray testing with a contrast agent, keep in mind that studies using iodine and those using barium should be scheduled at different times.
8. Some physiologic change can be expected when an iodine contrast substance is injected, as during an intravenous pyelogram (IVP). Physiologic responses to iodine given intravenously include hypotension, tachycardia, and arrhythmias. For this reason, always check blood pressure, pulse, and respirations before and after these tests are performed.
9. If appropriate for the patient, encourage intake of large amounts of oral fluids after the test to promote frequent urination. This flushes the iodine out of the body.
10. Possible contraindications to the administration of iodine contrast substances include the following conditions:
    a. Hypersensitivity to iodine
    b. Sickle cell anemia (iodine use may increase sickling effect)
    c. Syphilis (iodine use may lead to nephrotic syndrome)
    d. Long-term steroid therapy (iodine substances may render part of the drug inactive)
    e. Pheochromocytoma (iodine use may produce sudden, potentially fatal rise in blood pressure)

f. Hyperthyroidism
g. COPD
h. Multiple myeloma
i. Acute asthma
j. History of renal failure
k. Pregnancy
l. Diabetes mellitus
m. Severe dehydration
n. Congestive heart failure
o. Drug therapy known to be nephrotoxic (e.g., cisplatin)

11. Nonionic contrast agents tend to produce fewer side effects than do ionic materials.
12. Patients with renal failure may develop acidosis when iodine contrast is administered.

CLINICAL ALERT

1. Careful patient preparation considers patient safety, prevents complications, and can avoid the necessity of repeat procedures. Assess for the following risk factors associated with a higher incidence of undesirable contrast agent reactions:
   a. Allergy
   b. Asthma
   c. Previous reactions to contrast media
   d. Repeat and high dosages administered
   e. Diabetes mellitus
   f. Renal failure (preexisting); many laboratories require preprocedural assessment of creatinine levels in older adults
   g. Liver insufficiency
   h. Multiple myeloma
   i. Dehydration
   j. Older adult (>65 yr)
   k. Newborns
   l. History of seizures
   m. Pheochromocytoma
2. No contrast agent is without risk for causing reactions. Benefit versus risk must be considered. For example, in a workup to detect cancer, the benefits of early detection far outweigh the dangers of cumulative radiation exposure. The patient must be informed of the risk-to-benefit ratio; the patient has a legal right to this knowledge. In instances in which contrast must be delivered to high-risk patients, prophylactic premedication with prednisone may be ordered. Consult the radiology department for further information.
3. Never inject iodized oils or barium into the bloodstream.
4. Contrast agent–induced acute renal insufficiency is a rare and dangerous complication that occurs 1–5 d following intravenous (IV) injection of a contrast medium. Dehydrated patients and those with serum creatinine levels >1.4 mg/dL (>123.8 μmol/L) are at greatest risk.
5. Intravascular iodinated contrast may interact with certain IV medications. These interactions produce insoluble precipitates that may lead to embolism. For that reason, an existing IV line should be flushed with saline before using this line as the mechanism for delivering contrast.
6. Special attention is necessary for patients with diabetes because of their increased potential for renal failure and development of lactic acidosis. Diabetic persons taking oral hypoglycemic metformin (Glucophage) should have this drug withheld the day of and 48 hr following

the injection of iodinated contrast. In addition, advise the patient that his or her serum creatinine level should be rechecked 24–48 hr after he or she has received parenteral contrast. Examinations requiring extremely small volumes of contrast (myelography, arthrography) may not require such stringent precautions. Check with the radiology department for specific instructions.

7. Tests for thyroid function (serum tests as well as nuclear medicine studies) are adversely affected for several weeks to months following iodinated contrast injection.
8. Late reactions (2–3 d after procedure) most often occur with the use of agents such as iotrolan and iodohexane for intravascular procedures such as angiography.

Clinical Considerations When Barium Contrast Is Used

There is always some risk when introducing barium sulfate or a similar contrast agent into the GI tract.

1. Barium radiography may interfere with many other abdominal examinations. A number of studies—including other x-rays, tests using iodine, ultrasound procedures, radioisotope studies, tomograms, computed tomography (CT), and proctoscopy—must be scheduled before or several days following barium studies. Consult with the radiography department for the proper sequencing of studies.
2. Increased consumption of fluids will help to clear the bowel of barium.
3. Elderly, inactive persons should be checked for stool impaction if they fail to defecate within a reasonable length of time after a barium procedure. The first sign of impaction in an elderly person is fainting.
4. Observe and record findings regarding stool color and consistency for at least 2 days to determine whether barium has been evacuated. Stools will be light in color until all barium has been expelled. Outpatients should be given a written reminder to observe their stools for at least 2 days following barium administration.
5. If possible, avoid giving narcotics, especially codeine, when barium x-rays are ordered because these drugs can cause decreased bowel motility that can compound possible barium-associated constipation.

CLINICAL ALERT

1. Rare instances of severe allergic reactions to barium sulfate have been reported. All patients should be questioned regarding their allergic history before administration of any type of contrast agent. A history of hay fever, asthma, and other allergies places the patient at higher risk for reactions to all types of contrast agents.
2. The risk for postprocedure constipation or blockage of the bowel is increased in patients with the following conditions:
   a. Cystic fibrosis
   b. Dehydration
   c. Acute ulcerative colitis
3. Barium should *not* be used for intestinal study in the following circumstances:
   a. When a bowel perforation is suspected
   b. Following sigmoidoscopy or colonoscopy, especially if a biopsy was performed, because leakage of barium from the alimentary canal can cause peritonitis. Iodinated contrast should be used in these cases.

There are special clinical considerations for ostomy patients undergoing bowel preparation for GI studies; exam preparation and procedure should be tailored by the primary care provider and the radiology department to achieve the most optimal outcomes. In most cases, standard dietary and medication restrictions apply, but modifications involving mechanical bowel cleansing with enemas and physiologic cleansing with laxatives may be necessary.

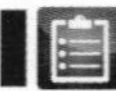

PROCEDURAL ALERT

1. Enemas and laxatives should not be given to a person with an ileostomy in preparation for x-rays or endoscopy (see Chapter 12) because this puts the person at risk for dehydration and electrolyte imbalance. The person with a sigmoid colostomy requires irrigation of the stoma the night before and the morning of the study. Consequently, it is important to identify the type of surgical procedure the patient has undergone. Moreover, not all colostomies need irrigation. For example, a person with an ascending right-sided colostomy will usually pass a liquid, pasty stool high in water content and digestive enzymes—such a patient may only require laxatives.
2. Notify the radiology department that the person has an ostomy.
3. Advise all patients to bring extra ostomy supplies and pouches for use after the procedure is completed.

RISKS OF RADIATION

Exposure of the human body to radiation carries certain risks. The biologic effects of ionizing radiation change the chemical makeup of cells, causing cell damage and mutation and promoting carcinogenesis. However, not all forms of radiation are equal in the potential for causing damage, and often no perceptible or long-lasting damage occurs. As a general rule, the higher the dose, as determined by the "strength" of the radiation and the duration of the exposure, the greater the risk.

Deterministic effects, such as erythema, nausea, fatigue, depressed sperm count, and temporary sterility, occur due to significant cell damage or death that occurs after a threshold amount of radiation has been exceeded. The severity of deterministic effects increases as the exposure dose increases. Stochastic effects, such as cancer, are associated with long-term low-level exposure to radiation. Low doses of radiation received over a period of time can lead to radiation-induced malignancy and genetic effects and are of most concern in diagnostic radiology. Because the embryo is most radiosensitive during the first trimester of pregnancy, special precautions must be taken to prevent or minimize radiation exposure to the pregnant uterus (Tables 10.2 through 10.5).

TABLE 10.2 Principal Early Effects of Radiation Exposure on Humans and Approximate Threshold Dose

Effect	Anatomic Site	Minimum Dose (Gray)
Death	Whole body	2
Hematologic depression	Whole body	0.25
Skin erythema	Small field	3
Epilation	Small field	3
Chromosome aberration	Whole body	0.05
Gonadal dysfunction	Local tissue	0.1

Reprinted with permission from Bushong SC: Radiologic Science for Technologists, 9th ed. Philadelphia, Elsevier Saunders, 2008.

TABLE 10.3 Relative Risk for Childhood Leukemia After Irradiation in Utero by Trimester

Time of X-Ray Examination	Relative Risk
First trimester	8.3
Second trimester	1.5
Third trimester	1.4
Total	1.5

Reprinted with permission from Bushong SC: Radiologic Science for Technologists, 9th ed. St. Louis, CV Mosby, 2008.

TABLE 10.4 Summary of Effects After 10 Radians in Utero

Time of Exposure	Type of Response	Natural Occurrence	Radiation Response
0–2 wk	Spontaneous abortion	25%	0.1%
2–10 wk	Congenital abnormalities	5%	1%
2–15 wk	Mental retardation	6%	0.5%
0–9 mo	Malignant disease	8/10,000	12/10,000
0–9 mo	Impaired growth and development	1%	Nil
0–9 mo	Genetic mutations	10%	Nil

Reprinted with permission from Bushong SC: Radiologic Science for Technologists, 9th ed. St. Louis, CV Mosby, 2008.

TABLE 10.5 Representative Radiation Quantities From Various Diagnostic X-Ray Procedures

Examination	Technique (kVp/mAs)	Entrance Skin Exposure (mrad)	Mean Marrow Dose (mrad)	Gonad Dose (mrad)
Skull	76/50	200	10	<1
Chest	110/3	10	2	<1
Cervical spine	70/40	150	10	<1
Lumbar spine	72/60	300	60	225
Abdomen	74/60	400	30	125
Pelvis	70/50	150	20	150
Extremity	60/5	50	2	<1
CT (head)	125/300	4000	20	50
CT (pelvis)	124/400	2000	50	2000

CT, computed tomography; kVp, kilovoltage potential; mAs, milliamperage second; mrad, milliradian.

Reprinted with permission from Bushong SC: Radiologic Science for Technologists, 9th ed. St. Louis, CV Mosby, 2008.

Safety Measures

Certain precautions must be taken to protect patients, visitors, and staff from unnecessary exposure to radiation.

General Precautions

1. The patient's medical records should be reviewed for previous radiologic studies in order to minimize the potential for unwarranted repeat studies.
2. The size or area irradiated must be carefully adjusted so that no extra tissue than necessary is exposed to the x-irradiation. Collimators (shutters), cones, or lead diaphragms can ensure proper sizing and x-ray exposure area.
3. Fluoroscopy yields a higher dose of radiation than radiographs or CT studies. Significant dose reduction is achieved by employing pulsed digital fluoroscopy.
4. The gonads should be shielded in both female and male patients of childbearing age unless the examination involves the abdomen or gonad areas.
5. The primary x-ray beam should pass through layers of aluminum adequate to filter out low-energy radiation while still providing detailed images.
6. Staff in the radiology department should wear lead aprons (and gloves if indicated) when not within a shielded booth during x-ray exposures. Patients should be shielded appropriately insofar as the procedure allows.
7. The x-ray tube housing should be checked periodically to detect radiation leakage and to indicate when repairs or adjustments are necessary.

Precautions to Be Used with Pregnant Patients

1. Women of childbearing age who could possibly be in the first trimester of pregnancy should *not* have x-ray examinations involving the trunk or pelvic regions. A brief menstrual history should be obtained to determine whether a possible pregnancy exists. If pregnancy is possible, a pregnancy test should be done before proceeding with x-ray examination.
2. All pregnant patients, regardless of trimester, should avoid radiographic, fluoroscopic, and serial film studies of the pelvic region, lumbar spine, and abdomen if at all possible.
3. Should x-ray studies be necessary for obstetric regions, repeat images should be avoided.
4. If x-ray studies of nonreproductive tissues are necessary (e.g., dental x-rays), the abdominal and pelvic region should be shielded with a lead apron.

Responsibilities in Ordering, Scheduling, and Sequencing X-Ray Examinations

Correct and complete information should be entered into the computer or on the x-ray requisition. An appropriate order will include the name of the exam, the ordering healthcare provider's name, and the clinical indication for the exam. Explain to the patient the purpose and procedure of the x-ray examination. Written patient instructions may be helpful.

When a complete genitourinary (GU) and GI workup is scheduled, the sequence of x-ray procedures should follow a definite order:

1. First day: IVP and barium enema
2. Second day (or subsequent day): upper GI (UGI) series

Barium studies should be scheduled after the following procedures:

1. Abdominal or pelvic ultrasound examination
2. Lumbar-sacral spine x-rays

3. Pelvic x-rays
4. Hysterosalpingogram
5. IVP

As a general rule, examinations that *do not* require contrast should *precede* examinations that *do* require contrast. All examinations that require contrast agents should be completed before those that require barium contrast. In addition, examinations that require contrast agents must precede nuclear medicine examinations that require radioactive iodine administrations (e.g., thyroid scans). Other x-ray examinations that do not require preparation can be performed at any time. Such examinations include the following:

1. X-rays of the head, spine, and extremities
2. Noncontrast abdominal x-rays (e.g., kidney, ureters, bladder [KUB], abdomen series)
3. Mammograms

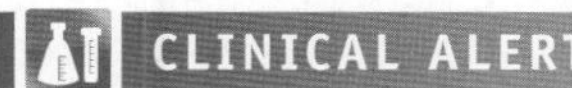

Nursing home patients should be accompanied by an adult to the x-ray testing site. If a nonfasting patient will be in the x-ray department during mealtime, the nursing facility should send food or money for food with the patient.

PLAIN (CONVENTIONAL) X-RAYS/RADIOGRAPHY

● Chest X-Ray

The chest x-ray is the most frequently requested radiograph. It is used to diagnose cancer, tuberculosis and other pulmonary diseases, and disorders of the mediastinum and bony thorax. The chest x-ray provides a record of the sequential progress or development of a disease. It can also provide valuable information about the condition of the heart, lungs, GI tract, and thyroid gland. A chest x-ray must be done after the insertion of chest tubes or subclavian catheters to determine their anatomic position as well as to detect possible pneumothorax related to the insertion procedure. A postbronchoscopy chest x-ray is done to ensure there is no pneumothorax following a biopsy.

Reference Values

Normal

Normal-appearing and normally positioned chest, bony thorax (all bones present, aligned, symmetrical, and normally shaped), soft tissues, mediastinum, lungs, pleura, heart, and aortic arch

Procedure

1. Routine chest radiography consists of two images: a frontal view (posterior to anterior [PA]) and a left lateral view. Upright chest radiographs (digital images) are preferred and are of utmost importance because images taken in the supine position do not demonstrate fluid levels. This observation is especially important when testing patients on bed rest.
2. Street clothing that is covering the chest is removed to the waist. Allow only cloth or paper hospital gowns free of buttons and snaps to be worn during the x-ray. Remove jewelry on or adjacent to the chest.
3. Ensure that monitoring cables and patches do not obscure the chest area, if possible.
4. Instruct the patient to take a deep breath and to exhale and then to take another deep breath and to hold it while the x-ray image is taken. After the x-ray is completed, the patient may breathe normally.
5. The actual procedure takes only a few minutes.
6. Follow guidelines in Chapter 1 for safe, effective, informed *intratest* care.

Clinical Implications

1. Abnormal chest x-ray results may indicate the following lung conditions:
   a. Presence of foreign bodies
   b. Aplasia
   c. Hypoplasia
   d. Cysts
   e. Lobar pneumonia
   f. Bronchopneumonia
   g. Aspiration pneumonia
   h. Viral pneumonia
   i. Lung abscess
   j. Middle lobe syndrome
   k. Pneumothorax
   l. Pleural effusion
   m. Atelectasis
   n. Pneumonitis
   o. Congenital pulmonary cysts
   p. Pulmonary tuberculosis
   q. Sarcoidosis
   r. Pneumoconiosis (e.g., asbestosis)
   s. Coccidioidomycosis
2. Abnormal conditions of the bony thorax include the following:
   a. Scoliosis
   b. Hemivertebrae
   c. Kyphosis
   d. Trauma
   e. Bone destruction or degeneration
   f. Osteoarthritis
   g. Osteomyelitis
3. Cardiac enlargement

Interfering Factors

An important consideration in interpreting chest radiographs is to ask whether the film was taken in full inspiration. Certain disease states do not allow the patient to inhale fully. The following conditions may alter the patient's ability to breathe properly and should be considered when evaluating radiographs:

1. Obesity
2. Severe pain
3. Congestive heart failure
4. Scarring of lung tissues

Interventions

Pretest Patient Care

1. No special preparation is required. However, the patient should be given a brief explanation of the purpose of and procedure for the test and assured that there will be no discomfort. Screen for pregnancy status of female patients. If positive, advise the radiology department.
2. Remove all jewelry and other ornamentation in the chest area before the x-ray.
3. Remind the patient of the need to remain motionless and to follow all breathing instructions during the procedure.
4. Follow guidelines in Chapter 1 for safe, effective, informed *pretest* care.

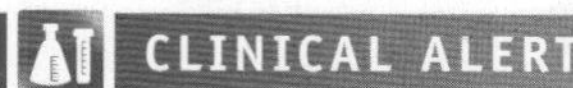

A portable x-ray machine may be brought to the nursing unit if the patient cannot be transported. The nurse may need to assist x-ray personnel in positioning the patient and image receptor (IR). It is the x-ray technologist's responsibility to clear all unnecessary personnel from the radiation field before x-ray exposure.

Posttest Patient Care

1. Review test results; report and record findings. Modify the nursing care plan as needed. Monitor for pulmonary disease and chest disorders. Explain changes in therapy based on chest x-ray results (e.g., diuretics for pulmonary edema, endotracheal tube repositioning, starting or stopping mechanical ventilation) per the healthcare provider's orders.
2. Follow guidelines in Chapter 1 for safe, effective, informed *posttest* care.

● Mammography (Breast X-Ray)

Soft tissue mammography visualizes the breast to detect small abnormalities that could suggest a malignancy or benign disease. Its primary use is to screen for and discover cancers that escape detection by other means such as palpation. Typically, lesions <1 cm cannot be detected by routine clinical or self-examinations. Although the average breast cancer has likely been present for some time before it reaches the clinically palpable 1-cm size, the prognosis for cure is excellent if detected in this preclinical or presymptomatic phase.

The low-energy x-ray beam used for this procedure is applied to a tightly restricted area and consequently does not produce significant radiation exposure to other areas of the body. Therefore, it is quite acceptable from a radiation safety standpoint to recommend routine screenings. Diagnosis by mammography is based on the radiographic appearance of gross anatomic structures. Benign lesions tend to push breast tissue aside as they expand, whereas malignant lesions may invade surrounding breast tissue. Although false-negative and false-positive readings can occur, mammography is highly accurate.

Most breast lumps are not malignant; many are benign cysts. For women >40 years of age, the benefits of using low-dose mammography to find early, curable cancers outweigh possible risks from radiation exposure (Table 10.6).

The American College of Radiology (ACR) accredits mammography machines, and the U.S. Food and Drug Administration (FDA) certifies mammographic facilities. To earn accreditation, mammograms must be performed by specially trained and credentialed radiographers, and the resulting images must be interpreted by radiologists who meet criteria for continuing education in mammography. Additionally, the ACR has stringent standards for equipment, image quality, and radiation dose. Health insurers, including Medicare, require mammographic services to be performed at an accredited institution. The FDA has approved certain digital systems to record breast anatomy electronically.

TABLE 10.6 Likelihood of Diagnosis of Breast Cancer in Next 10 Years

Starting at Age (yr)	Odds
30	1 in 227
40	1 in 68
50	1 in 42
60	1 in 28
70	1 in 26

Source: National Cancer Institute, 2016.

Indications for Mammography

1. To detect clinically nonpalpable breast cancer in women >45 years of age, younger women at high risk, or those with a history of breast cancer
2. When signs and symptoms of breast cancer are present
   a. Skin changes (e.g., "orange peel" skin associated with inflammatory-type cancer)
   b. Nipple or skin retraction
   c. Nipple discharge or erosion
3. Breast pain
4. "Lumpy" breast; multiple masses or nodules
5. Pendulous breasts that are difficult to examine manually
6. Survey of opposite breast after mastectomy
7. Patients at risk for having breast cancer (e.g., family history of breast cancer)
8. Adenocarcinoma of undetermined origin
9. Previous breast biopsy
10. Tissue samples removed from the breast may be imaged using detailed mammography techniques
11. Follow-up studies for questionable mammographic images

NOTE *The American Cancer Society recommends that women between 40 and 44 years of age should have the choice to start annual mammography if they wish, that women 45 to 54 years of age have annual mammograms, and that women 55 and over have mammograms every 2 years or continue annually.*

Reference Values

Normal

Essentially normal breast tissue: calcification, if present, should be evenly distributed; normal ducts with gradual narrowing ductal system branches

Procedure

1. Mammogram
   a. Perform mammograms with the person in an upright position, preferably standing. Make accommodations for patients using wheelchairs.
   b. Expose the breast. Elevate the inframammary fold to its maximum height. Lift onto a cassette or digital plate to the level of the inferior surface of the patient's breast. Adjust the breast tissue by hand, smoothing out all skin folds and wrinkles. Lower a movable paddle onto the breast, rigorously compressing the breast tissue.
   c. Make an x-ray exposure quickly and immediately lift the compression.
   d. Take two views (craniocaudal [CC] and mediolateral oblique [MLO]) of each breast.
   e. Before the x-ray examination, the technologist visually observes and manually palpates the breasts.
   f. Tell the patient that the complete examination takes about 30 minutes.
   g. Follow guidelines in Chapter 1 for safe, effective, informed *intratest* care.
2. X-ray–guided biopsy (stereotactic technique)
   a. Administer a local anesthetic.
   b. Have the patient lie on her abdomen, allowing her breast to protrude through an opening in a special table.
   c. Take two stereo-view mammograms, allowing precise positioning of the biopsy needle.
   d. Insert the needle into the breast at precise locations using sterile lacerations. Take multiple core tissue samples because tumors have both benign and malignant areas. In vacuum-assisted biopsy procedure, a probe is inserted directly into the suspicious area, and tissue is gently vacuumed out for subsequent analysis. See Chart 10.1 for comparison of these two methods.
   e. Cleanse the breast and apply a sterile dressing.

CHART 10.1 Comparisons of Core Needle and Vacuum-Assisted Biopsy

Core Needle Biopsy	Technique	Disadvantages	Advantages
Advanced breast biopsy instrumentation (ABBI)	Automated gun	Requires multiple passes into tissue	Excellent for dense lesions
SiteSelect (SiteSelect Medical Technologies) Centrica (Scion Medical Technologies)	Large-core needle		Relatively inexpensive equipment
Vacuum-Assisted Biopsy (VAB)			
Minimally invasive breast biopsy (MIBB)	Dual-lumen needle/probe with rotating cutter	Increased potential for postprocedural bleeding	Single pass into tissue yields multiple samples
Mammotome (Devicor Medical Products) ATEC (Hologic)		Expensive equipment	Larger tissue sample

3. Needle x-ray localization and surgical biopsy
   a. Administer a local anesthetic.
   b. Insert a needle that holds a fine wire, clip, or biodegradable marker into the breast tissue, using stereotactic or sonographic guidance. When the needle point is at the tip of the lesion, the device is released. It stays there until the surgeon, guided by the wire, removes a specimen of the abnormal tissue.

NOTE *Rigorous compression is a brief and uncomfortable but critical step in ensuring a high-quality mammogram. It lowers dose and improves image quality.*

CLINICAL ALERT

1. Computer software (computer-assisted diagnosis [CAD]) scans the image and notes suspicious areas that a radiologist could miss, thus acting as a second opinion.
2. Many radiologists double-read all mammograms.
3. Comparison with prior mammograms is very important. Consequently, patients are advised to have all mammograms performed at the same facility or retrieve prior mammograms and bring them along when having a new study performed.
4. Mammographic examination of augmented breasts requires additional views that add to procedure time. The presence of implants should be communicated to the radiology department when scheduling the procedure.

Clinical Implications

Abnormal mammogram findings reveal the following conditions:

1. Breast mass
   a. Benign breast masses (e.g., cysts, fibroadenomas) are usually round and well demarcated.
   b. Malignant breast masses are often irregularly shaped with extensions into adjacent tissue, generally with an increased number of blood vessels (Fig. 10.1).

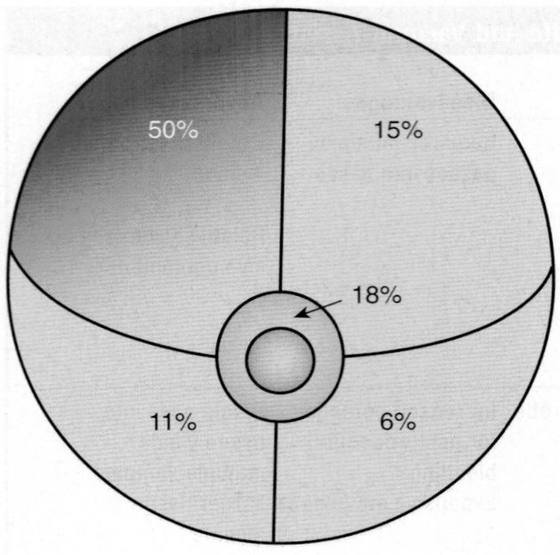

FIGURE 10.1. Half of all breast cancers develop in the upper outer section. (Courtesy of Department of Health and Human Services, 1994.)

c. When a mass is detected, additional studies are performed to help differentiate the nature of the mass. These studies may include the following:
   (1) Special x-ray magnification views of the area in question
   (2) Spot compression views performed using a paddle that isolates the suspicious tissue (Fig. 10.2)
   (3) Ultrasound of the area to help differentiate a cystic (fluid-filled) mass from a solid lesion
2. Calcifications present in the malignant mass (duct carcinoma) or in adjacent tissue (lobular carcinoma) are described as innumerable punctuate calcifications resembling fine grains of salt or rod-like calcifications that appear thin, branching, and curvilinear. Macrocalcifications (large mineral deposits) generally represent benign degenerative processes. Microcalcifications ($<1/50$ inch) are of more concern and require close examination.
3. The likelihood of malignancy increases with a greater number of calcifications in a cluster. However, a cluster with as few as three calcifications, particularly if they are irregular in shape or size, can occur in cancer.
4. Typical parenchymal patterns are as follows:
   a. N1: normal
   b. P1: mild duct prominence on less than one fourth of the breast
   c. P2: marked duct prominence
   d. DY: dysplasia (some diagnosticians believe that the person who exhibits dysplasia is 22 times more likely to develop breast cancer than the person with normal results)
5. Findings of breast cancer when contrast is injected are associated with extravasation of contrast, filling defects, obstruction, or irregular narrowing of ducts (Chart 10.2).

Interventions

Pretest Patient Care

1. Explain the purpose, procedure, benefits, and risks of mammograms. Mammography is the single best method for detecting breast cancer while it is still in a curable stage (Fig. 10.3). Some discomfort is to be expected when the breast is compressed.
2. Assess pregnancy status of female patients. If positive, advise radiology department.
3. Instruct the patient not to apply deodorant, perfume, powders, or ointment to the underarm or chest area on the day of the examination. Residue from these preparations can obscure optimal visualization.

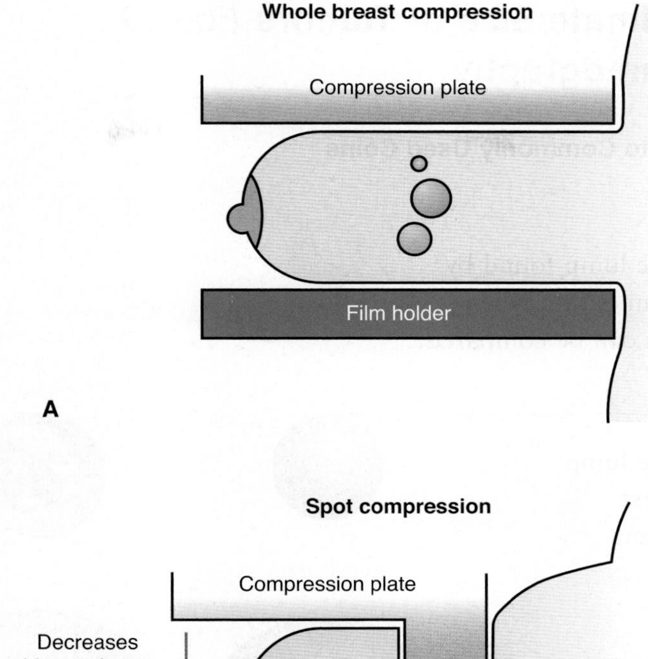

FIGURE 10.2. Examples of whole breast compression (**A**) and spot compression (**B**).

CHART 10.2 Clinical Note

1. *Contrast mammography* (ductogram, galactogram) is a valuable aid for diagnosing intraductal papillomas. Mammary duct injection is used when cytologic examination of breast fluid or discharge is abnormal. In contrast mammography, after careful cannulation of a discharging duct, about 1 mL of a radiopaque substance (e.g., 50% sodium diatrizoate) is injected into the breast duct with a blunt 25-gauge needle.
2. *Ductal lavage* is a technique in which the milk ducts are cannulated. Saline is injected and, when withdrawn, will "wash out" ductal cells. These cells are examined in the laboratory, in much the same way as a Pap test is reviewed. (See Chapter 11 for additional information.)

Approximate Size of Tumors Found by Mammography

Compared to Commonly Used Coins

Average-size lump found by yearly mammogram when past images can be compared.

Average-size lump found by first mammogram.

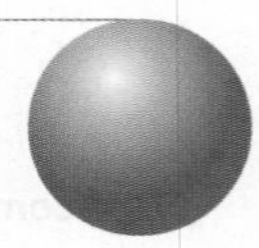

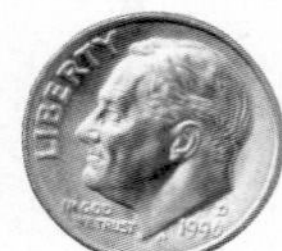

Average-size lump found by accident.

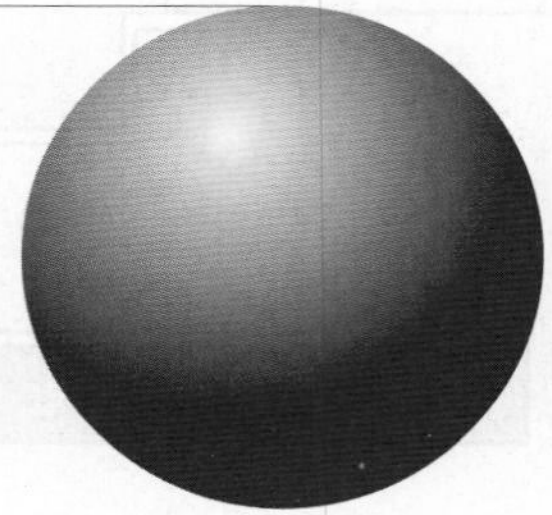

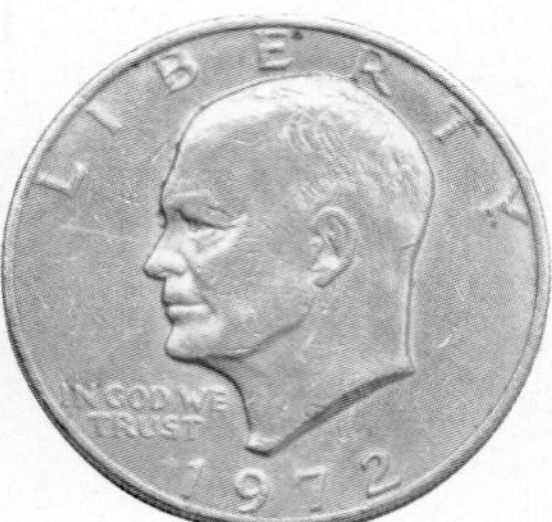

FIGURE 10.3. Approximate size of tumors found by mammography compared to commonly used coins. (Reprinted with permission of Susan G. Komen®. All images are copyrighted. © 2013, Susan G. Komen®. Adapted from Item No. KOMEED007100 Mammography Card 5/13.)

4. Advise the patient to wear separates rather than a dress because clothing must be removed from the upper body.
5. Suggest that patients who have painful breasts refrain from caffeinated foods and beverages (e.g., coffee, tea, cola, chocolate, some over-the-counter medications, and most antiasthmatic medication) for up to 2 weeks before testing.
6. Follow guidelines in Chapter 1 for safe, effective, informed *pretest* care.

NOTE *Patients in the reproductive age group are advised to have mammograms performed in the 2 weeks that follow their last menstrual period.*

Posttest Patient Care

1. Review test results; report and record findings. Modify the nursing care plan as needed. If a biopsy is necessary, see procedures for biopsy using x-ray technology.
2. Follow guidelines in Chapter 1 for safe, effective, informed *posttest* care.

CLINICAL ALERT

1. A mammogram detects abnormalities that could warn of cancer. The actual diagnosis of cancer is made by biopsy. Only 1 in 5 biopsies tests positive for cancer.
2. Several methods can be used to provide a breast tissue sample necessary for cancer diagnosis. These include core needle biopsy, surgical biopsy, and vacuum-assisted biopsy. Any of these methods can utilize either x-ray mammography or ultrasound for image guidance.

● Orthopedic X-Ray: Bones, Joints, and Supporting Structures

Orthopedic radiography examines a particular bone, group of bones, or joint. The bony or osseous system presents five functions of radiologic significance: structure support of the body, locomotion, red marrow storage, calcium storage, and protection of underlying soft tissue and organ structures. Orthopedic radiography is performed on the following structures:

1. The extremities (e.g., hand, wrist, shoulder, foot, knee, hip)
2. The bony thorax (e.g., ribs, sternum, clavicle)
3. The spine (e.g., cervical, thoracic, lumbar, sacrum, coccyx)
4. The head and skull (e.g., facial bones, mastoids, sinuses)

Optimal results from orthopedic x-ray examinations depend on proper immobilization of the area being studied. To produce a thorough image of the body part, at least two projections are required. These are taken at angles of 90 degrees to one another (e.g., anteroposterior and lateral views).

To examine more complex structures such as the spine and skull, or to examine a structure in greater detail, several projections from various angles may be required.

Reference Values

Normal

Normal osseous (bone) and supporting tissue structures

Procedure

1. Inform the patient that dietary restrictions are not necessary.
2. Have the patient assume the positions most favorable to capturing the best images. However, the degree of patient mobility and physical condition may also need to be considered. Typically, the anatomic structures being studied are examined from several angles and positions. This may require the technologist to manipulate the body area physically into a position that will allow optimal visualization.
3. Jewelry, zippers, snaps, monitoring cables, and so forth interfere with proper visualization. These objects must be removed from the visual field if possible. Skull x-rays require removal of dentures and partials.
4. Removal of any surgical-type hardware used to stabilize a traumatized area should be done only under the direction of the attending physician.
5. Follow guidelines in Chapter 1 for safe, effective, informed *intratest* care.

Clinical Implications

Abnormal orthopedic x-ray results may reveal the following conditions:

1. Fractures
2. Dislocations
3. Arthritis
4. Osteoporosis
5. Osteomyelitis
6. Degenerative joint disease
7. Hydrocephalus

8. Sarcoma
9. Abscess and aseptic necrosis
10. Paget's disease
11. Gout
12. Acromegaly
13. Metastatic processes
14. Myeloma
15. Osteochondrosis
    a. Legg-Calvé-Perthes disease
    b. Osgood-Schlatter disease
16. Bone infarcts
17. Bone tumors (benign and malignant)
18. Foreign bodies

Interfering Factors

Images of the lumbosacral spine, coccyx, or pelvis must be completed before barium studies because residual barium may interfere with proper visualization. Jewelry and accessories, heavy clothing, metallic objects, zippers, buttons, snaps, cables, and monitoring equipment and supplies can interfere with optimal views and need to be removed before the examination.

Interventions

Pretest Patient Care

1. Explain the purpose and procedure of the test. No preparation or dietary restrictions are necessary. Screen for pregnancy status of female patients. If positive, advise the radiology department.
2. Assure the patient that the procedure in and of itself causes no pain. However, necessary manipulation of the body may cause discomfort. If appropriate, pain medication may be administered before the procedure.
3. Advise the patient that all dentures, partials, jewelry, and other ornamentation worn in the anatomic area being examined must be removed before the study. If possible, simple clothing should be worn, and the previously mentioned items should be left at home or locked in the patient's room.
4. Emphasize the importance of not moving during the procedure unless specifically instructed otherwise. Movement distorts or "blurs" the image and often requires repeat exposures.
5. Follow guidelines in Chapter 1 for safe, effective, informed *pretest* care.

Posttest Patient Care

1. Review test results; report and record findings. Modify the nursing care plan as needed. Advise the patient to monitor for and report signs and symptoms of fractures, dislocations, and other orthopedic disorders. Counsel the patient about need for follow-up procedures and treatment.
2. Follow guidelines in Chapter 1 for safe, effective, informed *posttest* care.

CLINICAL ALERT

1. Orthopedic radiography also can provide information about soft tissue structures, such as swelling or calcifications. However, radiography alone cannot provide data about the condition of cartilage, tendons, or ligaments.
2. Portable x-ray machines can be taken to the nursing unit if the patient cannot be transported to the radiology department. Nursing personnel may need to assist in the process. The x-ray technologist is responsible for clearing all unnecessary personnel from the immediate radiation field before activating the exposure.

Abdominal X-Ray: Plain Film or KUB (Kidney, Ureters, Bladder); Scout Film; Abdominal Series

This radiographic study does *not* use contrast media. It is done to aid in the diagnosis of intra-abdominal diseases such as nephrolithiasis, intestinal obstruction, soft tissue mass, or ruptured viscus. It may be the preliminary step in evaluating the GI tract, the gallbladder, or the urinary tract, and it is done before IVP or other renal studies. Abdominal images may provide information on the size, shape, and position of the liver, spleen, and kidneys.

Reference Values

Normal

Normal abdominal structures

Procedure

1. Have the patient wear a hospital gown. All metallic objects must be removed from the abdominal area.
2. Have the patient lie in a supine position on the x-ray table.
3. Take multiple images (including upright or left decubitus) for an abdominal series to assess air–fluid levels.
4. Follow guidelines in Chapter 1 for safe, effective, informed *intratest* care.

Clinical Implications

Abnormal abdominal x-ray results reveal the following conditions:

1. Calcium deposits in blood vessels and lymph nodes; cysts, tumors, or stones
2. Ureters are not clearly defined, although calculi may be visualized within the ureters.
3. The urinary bladder can often be identified by the shadow it casts, especially in the presence of urine with high specific gravity.
4. Abnormal kidney size, shape, and position
5. Appendicolithiasis
6. Foreign bodies
7. Abnormal fluid; ascites
8. Large tumors and masses (e.g., bladder, ovarian, or uterine), if they displace normal bowel configurations
9. Abnormal gas distribution associated with bowel perforation or obstruction
10. Fusion anomalies
11. Horseshoe-shaped kidneys

Interfering Factors

1. Barium may interfere with optimal visualization. Therefore, this examination should be done before barium studies.
2. The supine position of the abdomen does not detect free air.

Interventions

Pretest Patient Care

1. Explain the purpose and procedure of the test. Normal diet is allowed unless contraindicated. Assure the patient that the procedure in itself is not painful.
2. Remove belts, zippers, jewelry, and other ornamentation from the abdominal area.
3. Instruct the patient to remain still and to follow breathing instructions.
4. Follow guidelines in Chapter 1 for safe, effective, informed *pretest* care.

CLINICAL ALERT

1. Abdominal plain images are not diagnostic for certain conditions, such as esophageal varices or bleeding peptic ulcer.
2. A portable x-ray machine may be brought to the nursing unit if the patient cannot be moved. Assist with positioning as necessary. The x-ray technologist is responsible for clearing all unnecessary personnel from the radiation field before the x-ray is taken.

Posttest Patient Care

1. Review test results; report and record findings. Modify the nursing care plan as needed. Monitor for intra-abdominal disease.
2. Follow guidelines in Chapter 1 for safe, effective, informed *posttest* care.

CONTRAST X-RAYS/RADIOGRAPHY

To visualize hollow internal viscera, contrast media are administered to highlight the structure. Refer to pages 729–733 for special care when using contrast media. Careful sequencing of multiple examinations is necessary. As a general rule, the following instructions for sequencing should be followed:

1. Perform abdominal pelvic plain images, CT, ultrasound, and nuclear medicine studies before contrast studies of the intestines.
2. Perform examinations of the lower intestine (barium enema) 1 or 2 days before UGI examinations.
3. Perform examinations requiring an injection of iodinated contrast, such as an IVP, before any barium studies (e.g., barium enema, UGI).
4. Consult the radiology department for specific sequencing information.
5. Take special caution when administering contrast agents to diabetic persons and persons with kidney problems.
6. See cautions on effects of concurrent use of codeine and barium contrast agents.
7. Use fluoroscopy for imaging of diagnostic (moving) structures such as those of the alimentary canal. Use fluoroscopy to localize tumors for biopsy and drainage, guide catheter placement, aid filter stent placement, and monitor vascular filling for both diagnostic and therapeutic purposes (angioplasty).

The radiation dose received from a fluoroscopic exam is higher than that of conventional x-rays. Dose is directly related to length of exposure. The use of digital fluorography tends to reduce dose by pulsing the x-ray beam.

● Contrast X-Ray of the Stomach: Gastric X-Ray Including Upper Gastrointestinal Examination (Upper GI [UGI] Series, Barium Swallow, Esophagram)

Gastric radiography visualizes the form, position, mucosal folds, peristaltic activity, and motility of the stomach and UGI tract. A UGI series includes the esophagus, stomach, duodenum, and upper portion of the jejunum.

Preliminary images without the use of a contrast medium are useful in detecting perforation, presence of radiopaque foreign substances, gastric wall thickening, and displacement of the gastric air bubble, which may indicate a mass external to the stomach.

Oral contrast substances, such as barium sulfate or diatrizoate meglumine (Gastrografin), highlight conditions such as hiatal hernia, pyloric stenosis, gastric diverticulitis, presence of undigested food, gastritis, congenital anomalies (e.g., dextroposition, duplication), or diseases of the stomach (e.g., gastric ulcer, cancer, stomach polyps).

Reference Values

Normal

Normal stomach size, contour, motility, and peristaltic activity
Normal esophagus

NOTE *A swallow study is typically performed to evaluate swallowing disorders, particularly in poststroke patients and after head and neck surgery with plastic repair. This examination generally includes evaluation by a speech pathologist.*

Procedure

1. Have patient change from street clothing into a hospital gown. Neck and torso jewelry and other ornamentation must be removed.
2. Instruct the patient to swallow the barium after the patient is properly positioned in front of the fluoroscopy machine. Some changes in position may be necessary during the procedure. A motorized tabletop shifts the patient from an upright to a supine position when appropriate. Fluoroscopy allows visualization and imaging of actual activity taking place in real time.
3. Take several conventional x-ray images following fluoroscopic examination. The patient will need to hold his or her breath during each exposure.
4. Inform the patient that examination time may be 20 to 45 minutes.
5. Follow guidelines in Chapter 1 for safe, effective, informed *intratest* care.

PROCEDURAL ALERT

1. If the patient has diabetes, alert the radiology department and schedule examination for early morning. If a patient with diabetes is taking metformin (Glucophage), special considerations may be necessary. Consult with radiology department to determine whether this medication regimen must be suspended for the day of and several days after the study.
2. Determine whether the patient is allergic to barium. Although rare, presence of this allergy must be communicated to the radiology department so that alternate contrast can be used.
3. All female patients of reproductive age must be screened for pregnancy before performing this study.

Clinical Implications

Abnormal UGI x-ray results reveal the following conditions:

1. Congenital anomalies
2. Gastric ulcer
3. Carcinoma of stomach
4. Gastric polyps
5. Gastritis
6. Foreign bodies
7. Gastric diverticula
8. Pyloric stenosis
9. Reflux and hiatal hernia
10. Volvulus of the stomach

NOTE *Normal contours may be deformed by intrinsic tumors or consistent filling defects as well as by stenosis in conjunction with dilation.*

Interfering Factors

1. If the patient is debilitated, proper examination may be difficult; it may be impossible to visualize the stomach adequately.
2. Retained food and fluids interfere with optimal image clarity.

Interventions

Pretest Patient Care

1. Explain purpose and procedure (consult barium contrast test precautions on pages 711–712. Written instructions on pretest preparation are helpful for the patient. Screen female patients for pregnancy status. If positive, inform the radiology department.
2. Inform patient that complete fasting from food and fluids is required for a minimum of 8 hours before the procedure. Necessary oral medications (other than metformin) may be taken with a small sip of water. Inform radiology department because pills may be visualized during the study.
3. Instruct the patient to hold still and follow breathing instructions during the procedure.
4. Follow guidelines in Chapter 1 for safe, effective, informed *pretest* care.

Posttest Patient Care

1. Review test results; report and record findings. Modify the nursing care plan as needed.
2. Diet and activity may be resumed. Provide food and ample fluids.
3. Observe and record stools for color and consistency. Monitor evacuation of barium. Counsel that follow-up procedures may be necessary.
4. Follow guidelines in Chapter 1 for safe, effective, informed *posttest* care.

● Small Bowel X-Ray: Intestinal Radiography and Fluoroscopy

These small intestine studies, usually scheduled in conjunction with UGI series, are done to diagnose small bowel diseases (e.g., ulcerative colitis, tumors, active bleeding, obstruction). In fluoroscopy imaging, the x-rays are transmitted to a computer monitor allowing visualization of movement, whether of an organ or contrast agent, to be viewed in detail. The contrast material, such as barium sulfate or Gastrografin, highlights Meckel's diverticulum, congenital atresia, obstruction, filling defects, regional enteritis, lymphoid hyperplasia, tuberculosis of the small intestine (malabsorption syndrome), sprue, Whipple's disease (infectious disease caused by *Tropheryma whipplei* leading to malabsorption), intussusception, and edema.

The mesenteric small intestine begins at the duodenojejunal valve and ends at the ileocecal valve. The mesenteric small intestine is not routinely included as part of a UGI study.

Reference Values

Normal

Normal small intestine contour, position, and motility

Procedure

1. Have the patient change into a hospital gown after removing street clothes and accessories. Perform a preliminary radiograph with the patient on the examining table.
2. Have the patient swallow the prescribed amount of contrast media while the patient is standing in front of the fluoroscopy machine.
3. Take timed images after contrast material is swallowed, usually every 30 minutes.

4. Remember that the examination is not complete until the ileocecal valve has filled with contrast material. This may take several minutes (for those patients with a gastric bypass) to several hours.
5. Follow guidelines in Chapter 1 for safe, effective, informed *intratest* care.

PROCEDURAL ALERT

1. If the patient has diabetes, alert the radiology department and schedule examination for early morning. If the diabetic patient is taking metformin, special considerations may be necessary. Consult with the radiology department to determine whether this medication regimen must be suspended during and for several days after study.
2. Determine whether the patient is hypersensitive to barium. Although rare, presence of this allergy must be communicated to the radiology department so alternate contrast can be used.
3. All female patients of reproductive age must be screened for pregnancy before performing this study.

Clinical Implications

Abnormal small bowel x-ray results indicate the following conditions:

1. Anomalies of small intestine
2. Errors of rotation
3. Meckel's diverticulum
4. Atresia
5. Neoplasms
6. Regional enteritis
7. Tuberculosis
8. Malabsorption syndrome
9. Intussusception
10. Roundworms (ascariasis)
11. Intra-abdominal hernias

Interfering Factors

1. Delays in small intestine motility can be due to the following circumstances:
   a. Morphine use
   b. Severe or poorly controlled diabetes
2. Increases in motility in the small intestine can be due to the following circumstances:
   a. Fear or anxiety
   b. Excitement
   c. Nausea
   d. Pathogens
   e. Viruses
   f. Diet (e.g., very high fiber)

Interventions

Pretest Patient Care

1. Explain the purpose and procedure of the test. Refer to barium contrast test precautions on pages 711–712. Written reminders for pretest instructions are helpful, especially for diet limitations. Screen female patients for pregnancy status. If positive, advise the radiology department.
2. Maintain total fast for at least 8 hours prior to the examination.
3. Do not administer laxatives or enemas to a patient with an ileostomy.

4. Instruct the patient regarding the need to hold still and to follow breathing instructions during the procedure.
5. Follow guidelines in Chapter 1 for safe, effective, informed *pretest* care.

Posttest Patient Care

1. Review test results; report and record findings. Modify the nursing care plan as needed.
2. Diet and activity may be resumed. Assist the patient if necessary.
3. Monitor stools for color and consistency.
4. Counsel the patient about motility disorders and other small intestine abnormalities. Follow-up procedures may be necessary.
5. Follow guidelines in Chapter 1 for safe, effective, informed *posttest* care.

• Colon X-Ray: Defecography; Barium Enema; Air Contrast Study

This fluoroscopic and filmed examination of the large intestine (colon) allows visualization of the position, filling, and movement of contrast medium through the colon. It can reveal the presence or absence of diseases such as diverticulitis, mass lesions, polyps, colitis, obstruction, or active bleeding. High-density barium sulfate is instilled into the large intestine through a rectal tube inserted into the colon. The radiologist, with the aid of a fluoroscope, observes the barium as it flows through the large intestine. X-ray images are taken concurrently.

If polyps are suspected, an air contrast colon examination may be done. The procedure is basically the same as that for the barium enema; however, more complex radiographs need to be taken with the patient in several different positions. A double contrast mixture of air and barium is instilled into the colon under fluoroscopic visualization.

Reference Values

Normal

Normal colon position, contour, filling, movement time, and patency

Procedure

1. Have the patient lie on his or her back while a preliminary x-ray film is made; this step may be omitted at some institutions.
2. Have the patient lie on his or her side while barium is administered by rectal enema (i.e., through the rectum and up through the sigmoid, descending, transverse, and ascending colon to the ileocecal valve).
3. Take conventional x-ray images following fluoroscopy, which includes several spot films. After these are completed, the patient is free to expel the barium. After evacuation, another film is made.
4. Defecography is a contrast-enhanced study of anus and rectum function during evacuation. Often used in young patients to evaluate rectoceles, rectal prolapse, or rectal intussusception, this examination requires the patient to evacuate into a specially designed commode while being evaluated fluoroscopically.
5. Follow guidelines in Chapter 1 for safe, effective, informed *intratest* care.

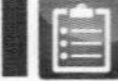

PROCEDURAL ALERT

A pretest preparation is vital for this exam. For a satisfactory examination, the colon must be thoroughly cleansed of fecal matter. Accurate identification of small polyps is possible only in a clean bowel. The presence of stool can also make the search for bleeding sources much more difficult.

Colonic Transit Time

This examination is performed on patients with suspected colonic motility disorder. The patient must *not* take any laxatives, enemas, or suppositories before beginning this test or during the 4 to 7 days it takes to perform this test.

1. The patient receives several pills that contain radiopaque markers (sitz markers).
2. A KUB or series of KUBs are performed at fixed times several days later.
3. The passage of or retention of these markers is noted and recorded.
4. Retention of a significant portion of markers 5 days after administration is considered abnormal and is evidence of dysmotility or an outlet obstruction.

Clinical Implications

1. Abnormal colon x-ray results indicate the following conditions:
   a. Lesions or tumors (benign)
   b. Obstructions
   c. Megacolon
   d. Fistulas
   e. Inflammatory changes
   f. Diverticula
   g. Chronic ulcerative colitis
   h. Stenosis
   i. Right-sided colitis
   j. Hernias
   k. Polyps
   l. Intussusception
   m. Carcinoma
2. Appendix size, position, and motility can also be evaluated; however, a diagnosis of acute or chronic appendicitis *cannot* be made from x-ray findings. Instead, typical signs and symptoms of appendicitis provide the most accurate data for this diagnosis.

Interfering Factors

A poorly cleansed bowel is the most common interfering factor. Fecal matter interferes with accurate and complete visualization. Therefore, it is imperative that proper bowel cleansing be conscientiously carried out, or the procedure may need to be repeated.

Special Considerations

1. For children or elderly patients receiving barium enemas
   a. Because a successful examination of the large intestine depends on the ability of the bowel to retain contrast medium during visualization and filming, special techniques are used for infants and young children and the infirm or uncooperative adult patient.
   b. After inserting a small enema tip into the rectum, the infant's buttocks are gently taped together to prevent leakage of contrast material during the study.
   c. For the older patient, a special retention enema tip may be used. This device resembles a regular enema tip, but it can be inflated, much like an indwelling urinary catheter, after insertion into the rectum. When the examination is done, the retention balloon is deflated and the tip removed.
2. Barium enema in the presence of a colostomy
   a. See page 712 for assessment criteria.
   b. Laxatives can be taken.
   c. Suppositories are of no value.

   d. Follow the healthcare provider's diet orders.
   e. If irrigation is necessary, a preassembled colostomy irrigation kit or a soft, standard-tip Foley catheter attached to a disposable enema bag may be used.
   f. Advise the patient that a Foley catheter is used to introduce the barium into the stoma.
   g. The patient should bring additional colostomy supplies to the radiology department for *posttest* use.
3. Patients with stomas
   a. Patients with descending or sigmoid colostomies may need a normal saline or tap-water irrigation to wash out the barium.
   b. Advise those who normally irrigate their colostomy to wear a disposable pouch for several days until all the barium has passed.

Interventions

Pretest Patient Care

Preparation involves a three-step process over a 1- to 2-day period and includes diet restrictions and a bowel cleaning regimen. Follow institutional protocols.

1. Explain the purpose and procedure of the test. Patients may be apprehensive or embarrassed. If the patient consents, also include a family member in the patient education process if it appears likely that the patient will need assistance with preparation. Explain the need to cooperate to expedite the procedure. Emphasize that the actual time frame when the colon is full is quite brief. Screen female patients for pregnancy status. If positive, advise the radiology department.
2. A written reminder about the following may be helpful to the patient:
   a. Only a clear liquid diet should be taken before testing (according to protocols).
   b. Stool softeners, laxatives, and enemas need to be taken to ensure bowel cleanliness necessary for optimal visualization. Agents such as X-Prep or citrate of magnesia assist in emptying the ascending and right to mid-transverse colon (proximal large bowel). Enemas cleanse the left transverse, descending, and sigmoid colon and the rectum. Suppositories also empty the rectum.
   c. Fasting from food and fluids is prescribed before the test. Nothing should be eaten or drunk from midnight until the test is completed. Oral medications should also be temporarily discontinued unless specifically ordered otherwise. Check with the clinician who orders the test.
3. Refer to barium contrast test precautions.
4. Follow guidelines in Chapter 1 for safe, effective, informed *pretest* care.

CLINICAL ALERT

1. Determine whether the patient is allergic or hypersensitive to barium. Although rare, the presence of this allergy must be communicated to the radiology department so that alternate contrast media can be used.
2. Determine whether the patient is allergic to latex. Latex products are typically used to administer the contrast agent; alternate materials must be used if the patient is allergic or hypersensitive. Inform the radiology department of any known or suspected latex allergies.
3. Inform the radiology department if this procedure is to follow a sigmoidoscopy or colonoscopy, particularly if a biopsy was performed. In the case of biopsy, an iodinated contrast agent, rather than barium, is used.

Posttest Patient Care

1. Review test results; report and record findings. Modify the nursing care plan as needed. Diet and activity may be resumed. Assist the patient if necessary. This bowel examination can be very exhausting. Patients may be weak, thirsty, hungry, and tired. Provide a calm, restful environment to promote return to normal status.
2. Follow guidelines in Chapter 1 for safe, effective, informed *posttest* care.

CLINICAL ALERT

1. Multiple enemas given before the procedure, especially to a person at risk for electrolyte imbalances, could induce a rather rapid hypokalemia. Enema fluid, if not expelled within a reasonable time, can be absorbed through the bowel wall and deposited into the intestinal spaces and eventually within extracellular spaces.
2. Caution should dictate administration of cathartics or enemas in the presence of acute abdominal pain, active bleeding, ulcerative colitis, or obstruction. Consult with the healthcare provider or radiology department and consider the following points:
   a. Introducing large quantities of water into the bowel of a patient with megacolon should be avoided because of the potential danger of water intoxication. In general, patients with toxic megacolon should *not* receive enemas.
   b. In the presence of colon obstruction, large volumes of water from enemas may be reabsorbed and impaction may occur.
   c. Rectal obstruction makes it difficult or impossible to give cleansing enemas because the solution will not be able to enter the colon. Consult the healthcare provider or radiology department.
3. Strong cathartics administered in the presence of obstructive lesions or acute ulcerative colitis can present hazardous or life-threatening situations.
4. Be aware of complications that can occur when barium sulfate or other contrast media are introduced into the GI tract. For example, barium may aggravate acute ulcerative colitis or cause a progression from partial to complete obstruction. Barium also should not be given as contrast for intestinal studies when a bowel perforation is suspected because leakage of barium through the perforation may cause peritonitis. Iodinated contrast substances should be used if perforation is suspected.
5. Fasting orders include oral medications except when specified otherwise.
6. If the patient has diabetes, alert the radiology department and schedule examination for early morning. If a patient with diabetes is taking metformin, special consideration may be necessary. Consult with the radiology department to determine whether this medication regimen must be suspended the day of and several days after the study.

● Bile Duct X-Ray (Cholangiography), T-Tube Cholangiogram, Operative Cholangiogram, Percutaneous Transhepatic Cholangiogram

A cholangiogram visualizes the bile ducts by enhancing them with an iodinated contrast agent. Often performed on the postcholecystectomy patient, the cholangiogram is used to identify intraductal mass lesions and calculi. A number of approaches may be used to opacify and image the bile ducts:

1. *T-tube cholangiogram*: Following cholecystectomy, a self-retaining T-shaped drainage tube may be surgically inserted into the common bile duct. Before removal, patency is verified by injecting iodinated contrast into the T-tube to fill the biliary tree.

2. *Cholangiogram with stone removal*: This study combines diagnostic visualization of the bile ducts with therapeutic capture and removal of ductal calculi.
3. *Intravenous cholangiography*: This study allows radiographic visualization of the large hepatic ducts and the common ducts by means of IV injection of a contrast medium. It is rarely performed.
4. *Operative cholangiography*: Cannulation and injection of contrast medium into the exposed cystic duct or common bile duct is performed during surgery.
5. *Percutaneous transhepatic cholangiography*: A Chiba (thin, 22-gauge) needle is percutaneously introduced into the liver and the bile duct. Following injection of the contrast agent, the hepatic and common ducts should be visualized. The dilated biliary tree can be shown up to the point of obstruction, which is usually in the common duct. This procedure is frequently done for patients with jaundice whose liver cells are unable to transport oral or IV contrast agents properly.
6. *Intravenous cholecystography*: Radiographic visualization of the gallbladder is performed after IV injection of a contrast agent.
7. *Oral cholecystography*: Radiographic visualization of the gallbladder is performed after oral administration of an opaque medium. This test is often combined with or replaced by gallbladder sonography.
8. *Endoscopic retrograde cholangiopancreatography (ERCP)*: This endoscopic procedure uses an injection of a contrast agent to evaluate the patency of pancreatic and common bile ducts, the duodenal papilla, and the normalcy of the gallbladder (see Chapter 12). Often, the ERCP is performed therapeutically, involving stone extraction, stent placement, or other treatments.

Reference Values

Normal

Patent bile ducts

Procedure: T-Tube Cholangiogram

1. Have the patient lie on the x-ray table as an iodine contrast medium is injected into the T-tube.
2. Alert the patient that typically no pain or discomfort should be felt; however, some persons may feel pressure during the injection.
3. Unclamp the T-tube after the procedure and allow it to drain freely unless otherwise ordered. This minimizes prolonged, irritating contact of residual contrast in the bile duct.
4. Follow guidelines in Chapter 1 for safe, effective, informed *intratest* care.

Clinical Implications

Abnormal duct and gallbladder x-ray results reveal stenosis, obstruction, or choledocholithiasis (calculi of the common bile duct).

Interventions

Pretest Patient Care

1. Explain the purpose and procedure of the test. Assure the patient that the procedure is not painful, but some discomfort or pressure may be felt when the contrast is injected. If the patient has diabetes, special precautions may be necessary.
2. Instruct the patient to remove street clothing and accessories such as jewelry before the study. Provide a gown for patient use.
3. Stress the importance of remaining still and following breathing instructions during the procedure.
4. Refer to iodine test precautions. Assess female patients for pregnancy status. If positive, advise the radiology department.
5. Omit food and fluid before the examination. Check institutional protocols for specific dietary and fluid restrictions. A laxative may be ordered the evening before the examination.
6. Follow guidelines in Chapter 1 for safe, effective, informed *pretest* care.

CLINICAL ALERT

1. If the patient has diabetes, assess whether he or she is taking metformin. Because of an increased risk for renal failure, this medication regimen must be discontinued the day of and several days after administration of contrast media. Consult the radiology department for specific instructions.
2. Assess the patient for allergies to all substances, specifically latex, and inform the radiology department of any known or suspected sensitivities before study.
3. Assess whether the patient is allergic to iodine. If iodine contrast sensitivities are known or suspected, inform the radiology department before study.

Posttest Patient Care

1. Review test results; report and record findings. Modify the nursing care plan as needed.
2. Nausea, vomiting, and transient elevated temperature may occur as a reaction to the iodine contrast.
3. Document observations and notify the healthcare provider if necessary.
4. Follow guidelines in Chapter 1 for safe, effective, informed *posttest* care.

CLINICAL ALERT

1. Persistent fever, especially if associated with chills, may indicate bile duct inflammation.
2. Monitor for hemorrhage, pneumothorax, or peritonitis after percutaneous transhepatic cholangiography. Unusual pain or tenderness, difficulty breathing, or change in vital signs may signal these complications. If these side effects occur, take immediate action to treat.

● Intravenous Urography (IVU); Excretory Urography or Intravenous Pyelography (IVP)

Intravenous urography (IVU) is one of the most frequently ordered tests in cases of suspected renal disease or urinary tract dysfunction.

NOTE *IVU is indicated during the initial investigation of any suspected urologic problem, especially to diagnose kidney and ureter lesions and impaired renal function.*

An IV radiopaque iodine contrast substance is injected and concentrates in the urine. Following this injection, a series of x-ray images is made at predetermined intervals over 20 to 30 minutes. A final postvoid film is taken after the patient empties the bladder.

These images demonstrate the size, shape, and structure of the kidneys, ureters, and bladder and the degree to which the bladder can empty. Renal function is reflected by the length of time it takes the contrast material first to appear and then to be excreted by each kidney. Kidney disease, ureteral and bladder stones, and tumors can be detected with IVU.

CT also may be done in conjunction with IVU to obtain better visualization of renal lesions. This increases examination time. If kidney tomography or nephrotomograms are ordered separately, the procedure and preparation are the same as for IVU.

Reference Values

Normal

1. Normal size, shape, and position of the kidneys, ureters, and bladder. Normal kidneys measure approximately 4.5 inches in length and 2 to 3 inches in width. Therefore, kidney size is estimated in relation to this rule of thumb.

2. Normal renal function
   a. Two to 8 minutes after the injection of contrast material, the kidney outline appears on an x-ray film. Threadlike strands of contrast material appear in the calyces.
   b. When the second film is taken several minutes after contrast injection, the entire renal pelvis can be visualized.
   c. Later films show the ureters and bladder as the contrast material makes its way into the lower urinary tract.
   d. No evidence of residual urine should be found on the postvoid film.

Procedure

1. Take a preliminary x-ray (KUB) with the patient in a supine position to ensure that the bowel is empty and the kidney location can be visualized.
2. Inject the IV contrast material, usually into the antecubital vein.
3. Alert the patient that during and following the IV contrast injection, he or she may experience warmth, flushing of the face, salty taste, and nausea.
   a. Instruct the patient to take slow, deep breaths should these sensations occur. Have an emesis basin and tissue wipes available. Use standard precautions when handling secretions.
   b. Assess for other untoward signs, such as respiratory difficulty, diaphoresis, numbness, palpitations, or urticaria. Be prepared to respond with emergency drugs, equipment, and supplies. These items should be readily available whenever this procedure is performed.
4. Take at least three x-ray images at predetermined intervals following injection of the contrast material.
5. After these three images are taken, instruct the patient to void before the final image is made to determine the ability of the bladder to empty.
6. Follow guidelines in Chapter 1 for safe, effective, informed *intratest* care.

Clinical Implications

1. Abnormal IVU findings may reveal the following conditions:
   a. Altered size, form, and position of the kidneys, ureters, and bladder
   b. Duplication of the pelvis or ureter
   c. Presence of only one kidney
   d. Hydronephrosis
   e. Supernumerary kidney
   f. Renal or ureteral calculi
   g. Tuberculosis of the urinary tract
   h. Cystic disease
   i. Tumors
   j. Degree of renal injury subsequent to trauma
   k. Prostate enlargement
   l. Enlarged kidneys suggesting obstruction or polycystic disease kidney
   m. Evidence of renal failure in the presence of normal-sized kidneys suggesting an acute rather than chronic disease process
   n. Irregular scarring of the renal outlines, suggesting chronic pyelonephritis
2. A time delay in radiopaque contrast visualization is indicative of renal dysfunction. No contrast visualization may indicate very poor or no renal function.

Interfering Factors

1. Feces or intestinal gas will obscure urinary tract visualization.
2. Retained barium can obscure optimal views of the kidneys. For this reason, barium tests should be scheduled after IVU when possible.

Interventions

Pretest Patient Care

1. Explain the purpose and procedure of the test. A written reminder may be helpful to the patient. Screen female patients for pregnancy status. If positive, advise the radiology department. If the patient has diabetes or takes metformin, special precautions may be necessary.
2. Observe iodine contrast test precautions. Assess for all allergies and determine prior allergic reaction to contrast substances. Many radiology departments require a recent creatinine level for all patients >40 years of age before performing this procedure in order to ensure the absence of renal insufficiency.
3. Because a relative state of dehydration is necessary for contrast material to concentrate in the urinary tract, instruct the patient to abstain from *all* food, liquid, and medication (if possible) for 12 hours before examination. Fasting after the evening meal the day before the test will meet this criterion.
4. Do not give children <7 years of age pretest cathartics or enemas. Should the preliminary radiographs show intestinal gas obscuring the kidneys, a few ounces of carbonated beverage may relieve the concentration of gas at that particular location.
5. Evaluate stool and check for abdominal distention to evaluate for possible barium retention if it has been used in previous studies. Additional bowel preparation may be necessary.
6. Follow guidelines in Chapter 1 for safe, effective, informed *pretest* care.

NOTE *Elderly or debilitated patients with poor renal reserves may not tolerate these dehydration protocols (fasting, laxatives, enemas). In such instances, consult with the radiologist or the patient's healthcare provider to ascertain the proper procedure. For infants and small children, fasting time usually varies from 6 to 8 hours pretest. If in doubt, verify protocols with the radiologist or attending physician.*

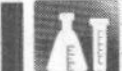

CLINICAL ALERT

Assess for latex allergy and inform the radiology department of any known or suspected sensitivities before study.

Posttest Patient Care

1. Review test results; report and record findings. Modify the nursing care plan as needed.
2. Resume prescribed diet and activity after the examination.
3. Teach and encourage the patient to drink sufficient fluids to replace those lost during the *pretest* phase.
4. Encourage rest, as needed, following the examination.
5. Observe and document mild reactions to the iodine material, which may include hives, skin rashes, nausea, or swelling of the parotid glands. Notify the healthcare provider if the signs and symptoms persist. Oral antihistamines may relieve more severe symptoms.
6. Follow guidelines in Chapter 1 for safe, effective, informed *posttest* care.

CLINICAL ALERT

1. Contraindications to IVU or IVP include the following conditions:
   a. Hypersensitivity or allergy to iodine preparations
   b. Combined renal and hepatic disease
   c. Oliguria or anuria

   d. Renal failure: Most radiology departments require recent creatinine test levels to determine whether to administer contrast materials. Generally, creatinine levels >1.5 mg/dL (>133 μmol/L) raise suspicion and signal the need for repeat laboratory work. A blood urea nitrogen (BUN) level >25 mg/100 mL also may contraindicate the use of iodine contrast.
   e. Multiple myeloma, unless the patient can be adequately hydrated during and after the study
   f. Advanced pulmonary tuberculosis
   g. Patients receiving drug therapy for chronic bronchitis, emphysema, or asthma
   h. Congestive heart failure
   i. Pheochromocytoma
   j. Sickle cell anemia
   k. Diabetes, especially diabetes mellitus
2. If the patient has diabetes, assess whether he or she is taking metformin. Because of an increased risk for renal failure and lactic acidosis, this medication regimen must be discontinued the day of and several days after administration of contrast media. Consult the radiology department for specific instructions.
3. Some physiologic changes can be expected after radiopaque iodine injections. Hypertension, hypotension, tachycardia, arrhythmias, or other electrocardiographic (ECG) changes may occur.
4. An iodine-based contrast medium is given with caution in the presence of hyperthyroidism, asthma, and hay fever or other allergies.
5. Observe for anaphylaxis or severe reactions to iodine, as evidenced by shock, respiratory distress, precipitous hypotension, fainting, convulsions, or actual cardiopulmonary arrest. Resuscitation supplies and equipment should be readily available.
6. In all cases except emergencies, a contrast medium should not be injected sooner than 90 minutes after eating.
7. IV iodine can be highly irritating to the intimal layer of the veins and may cause painful vascular spasm. If this occurs, a 1% procaine IV injection may relieve vascular spasm and pain. Sometimes, local vascular irritation is severe enough to induce thrombophlebitis. Warm or cold compresses to the area may relieve pain; however, these do not prevent sloughing. The attending physician should be notified. Anticoagulant therapy may need to be instituted.
8. Local reactions to iodine may be evidenced by extensive redness, swelling, and pain at the injection site. Even a small amount of iodine contrast entering subcutaneous tissues can cause tissue sloughing, which may require skin grafting. Radiographic evidence of iodine contrast leakage within soft tissues surrounding the injection site confirms extravasation.

• Retrograde Pyelography

Retrograde pyelography generally confirms IVU findings and is indicated when IVU yields insufficient results because of kidney nonvisualization (congenital kidney absence), decreased renal blood flow that impairs renal function, obstruction, kidney dysfunction, presence of calculi, or patient allergy to IV contrast material. This x-ray examination of the upper urinary tract begins with cystoscopy to introduce ureteral catheters up to the level of the renal pelvis. Following this, iodine contrast is injected into the ureteral catheter, and x-ray images are then taken. The chief advantage of retrograde pyelography lies in the fact that the contrast substance can be indirectly injected under controlled pressure so that optimal visualization is achieved. Renal function impairment does not influence the degree of visualization. See Chart 10.3 for additional tests that are used to examine the urinary system.

Reference Values

Normal

Normal contour and size of ureters and kidneys

CHART 10.3 Tests Used to Examine the Urinary System

1. *Excretory urography or intravenous pyelography*: After injection of an IV contrast agent, the collecting system (i.e., calyces, pelvis, and ureter) of each kidney is progressively opacified. Radiographs are made at 5- to 15-min intervals until the urinary bladder is visualized.
2. *Drip infusion pyelography*: This is a modification of conventional pyelography. An increased volume of contrast agent is administered by continuous IV infusion.
3. *Cystography*: The urinary bladder is opacified by means of a contrast agent instilled through a urethral catheter. After the patient voids, air may be introduced into the bladder to obtain a double-contrast study.
4. *Retrograde cystourethrography*: After catheterization, the bladder is filled to capacity with a contrast agent, and radiography is used to visualize the bladder and urethra.
5. *Voiding cystourethrography*: After contrast material has been instilled into the urinary bladder, images are taken of the bladder and urethra during the process of voiding.

Procedure

1. This examination is usually done in the surgical department in conjunction with cystoscopy (see Chapter 12).
2. Sedation and analgesia may precede insertion of a local anesthetic into the urethra (see Sedation and Analgesia in Chapter 1). General anesthesia may be required if the patient is not able to cooperate fully with the procedure.
3. Follow guidelines in Chapter 1 for safe, effective, informed *intratest* care.

PROCEDURAL ALERT

1. Renal function tests of blood and urine must be completed before this examination is done.
2. Assess whether the patient is allergic to iodine. If iodine contrast sensitivities are known or suspected, inform the radiology department before study.
3. Refer to Clinical Alerts for Cystoscopy in Chapter 12.

Clinical Implications

Urinary system x-ray results may reveal the following conditions:

1. Intrinsic abnormality of ureters and kidney pelvis (e.g., congenital defects)
2. Extrinsic abnormality of the ureters (e.g., obstructive tumor or stones)

Interfering Factors

Because barium may interfere with test results, these studies must be done before barium x-rays are performed.

Interventions

Pretest Patient Care

1. Explain the purpose and procedure of the test. Screen female patients for pregnancy status. If positive, advise the radiology department.
2. The patient or other authorized person must sign and have witnessed a legal consent form before examination in the operating room.

3. Follow iodine contrast test precautions. A recent creatinine level may be required by the radiology department to evaluate the kidney's ability to clear the contrast.
4. Have the patient fast from food and fluids after midnight before the test.
5. Administer cathartics, suppositories, or enemas as ordered.
6. Follow guidelines in Chapter 1 for safe, effective, informed *pretest* care.

Posttest Patient Care

1. Review test results; report and record findings. Modify the nursing care plan as needed.
2. Observe the patient for signs of allergic reaction to iodine contrast.
3. Check vital signs frequently for the first 24 hours following the test. Follow institutional protocols if general anesthetics were administered.
4. Record accurate urine output and appearance for 24 hours following the procedure. Hematuria or dysuria may be common after the examination. If hematuria does not clear and dysuria persists or worsens, notify the healthcare provider. Instruct the patient to do the same.
5. Administer analgesics as necessary. Discomfort may be present immediately following the examination and may require a prescription analgesic (e.g., codeine).
6. Follow guidelines in Chapter 1 for safe, effective, informed *posttest* care.

• Arthrography (Joint X-Ray)

Arthrography involves multiple x-ray examinations of encapsulated joint structures following injection of contrast agents into the joint capsular space. Arthrography is done in cases of persistent, unexplained joint discomfort. Although the knee is the most frequently studied joint, the shoulder, hip, elbow, wrist, and other joints may also be examined. Local anesthetics are used, and aseptic conditions are observed.

Reference Values

Normal

Normal filling of encapsulated joint structures, joint space, bursae, menisci, ligaments, and articular cartilage

Procedure

1. Position the patient on the examining table.
2. Surgically prepare and drape the skin around the joint.
3. Inject a local anesthetic into tissues around the joint. It is usually unnecessary to anesthetize the actual joint space.
4. Aspirate any effusion fluids present in the joint. Inject the contrast agents (e.g., gaseous medium and water-soluble iodinated medium). Remove the needle and manipulate the joint to ensure even distribution of the contrast material. In some cases, ask the patient to walk or exercise the joint for a few minutes.
5. During the examination, several positions are assumed so as to obtain various x-ray views of the joint.
6. Pillows and sandbags also may be used to position the joint properly.
7. Follow guidelines in Chapter 1 for safe, effective, informed *intratest* care.

PROCEDURAL ALERT

If a patient with diabetes is taking metformin, special considerations may be necessary. Consult with the radiology department to determine whether this medication regimen must be discontinued the day of and several days after the study.

Clinical Implications

Abnormal joint x-ray results reveal the following conditions:

1. Arthritis
2. Dislocation
3. Ligament tears
4. Rotator cuff rupture
5. Synovial abnormalities
6. Narrowing of joint space
7. Cysts

Interventions

Pretest Patient Care

1. Explain the purpose and procedure of the test. Advise the patient that some discomfort is normal during contrast injection and joint manipulation.
2. Obtain a properly signed and witnessed consent form.
3. Refer to iodine test precautions. Check for known allergies to iodine, other contrast substances, and latex.
4. Advise the patient to bring any prior x-ray images of the joint in question to the arthrogram appointment.
5. Follow guidelines in Chapter 1 for safe, effective, informed *pretest* care.

Posttest Patient Care

1. Review test results; report and record findings. Modify the nursing care plan as needed.
2. The joint should be rested for 12 hours.
3. Ice can be applied to the area if swelling occurs. Pain can usually be controlled with a mild analgesic.
4. Cracking or clicking noises in the joint may be heard for 1 or 2 days following the test. This is normal. Notify the healthcare provider if crepitant noises persist or if increased pain, swelling, or restlessness occurs.
5. Follow guidelines in Chapter 1 for safe, effective, informed *posttest* care.

● Myelogram

Myelography is a radiographic study of the spinal subarachnoid space in which non-iodine, water-soluble contrast medium is introduced into the subarachnoid space so that the spinal cord and nerve roots are outlined and dura mater distortions can be detected.

This study is done to detect neoplasms, ruptured intervertebral disks, ankylosing spondyloses, and bone fragments. This examination is also indicated when compression of the spinal cord or posterior fossa neural structure or nerve roots is suspected. The test is frequently done before surgical treatment for a ruptured vertebral disk or release of stenosis. Symptoms may include unrelieved back pain, pain radiating down the leg, absent or abnormal ankle and knee reflexes, claudication of neurospinal origin, or past history of cancer with loss of mobility or bladder control.

Nonionic, water-soluble contrast is the most commonly used medium for myelograms and is often followed by CT scanning to improve visualization.

Reference Values

Normal

Normal lumbar, cervical, or thoracic myelogram

Procedure

1. The test is usually done in the radiography department with the patient positioned on his or her abdomen.
2. Prepare and drape the puncture area.
3. The procedure is the same as those for lumbar puncture (see Chapter 5), except for the injection of the contrast substance and fluoroscopic x-ray images. With the use of nonionic water-soluble contrast, a narrow-bore needle (22-gauge) may be used. A lumbar puncture is done when a lumbar defect is suspected; a cervical puncture is done for a suspected cervical lesion. In children, the level at which the lumbar puncture is performed is much lower than the level in adults to avoid puncturing the spinal cord.
4. Tilt the table during the procedure to achieve optimal visualization. Use shoulder and foot braces to maintain correct position.
5. Follow guidelines in Chapter 1 for safe, effective, informed *intratest* care.

Clinical Implications

Abnormal myelogram results reveal distorted outlines of the subarachnoid space that indicate the following conditions:

1. Ruptured intervertebral disk
2. Compression and stenosis of spinal cord
3. The exact level of intravertebral tumors
4. Spinal canal obstruction
5. Avulsion of nerve roots

Interventions

Pretest Patient Care

1. Explain the purpose, procedure, benefits, and risks of the test. Explain that some discomfort may be felt during the procedure. Disadvantages of water-soluble and air contrast include poor visualization and painful headache (with air contrast) because of the difficulty in controlling the gas introduced into the area. Refer to iodine contrast test precautions if iodine is used (see pages 709–711).
2. A legal consent form must be properly signed and witnessed before the test.
3. Assess pregnancy status of female patients. Alert the radiology department if positive.
4. Explain that the examination table may be tilted during the test but that the patient will be securely fastened and will not fall off the table.
5. Most diagnostic departments require the patient to refrain from eating for approximately 4 hours before testing. Clear liquids may be permitted and even encouraged to lower the incidence of headaches after the test. Check with the radiology department and healthcare provider for specific orders.
6. Inform the patient that a myelogram usually produces some discomfort. If the patient has trouble moving, a pain reliever may be necessary to allow easier positioning and movement during the test.
7. Follow guidelines in Chapter 1 for safe, effective, informed *pretest* care.

CLINICAL ALERT

1. This test is to be avoided unless there is a reason to suspect a lesion. Multiple sclerosis, for example, may be worsened by this procedure.
2. Assess whether the patient is allergic to latex or iodine and inform the radiology department of any known or suspected sensitivities before study.

3. If the patient has diabetes, assess whether he or she is taking metformin. Because of an increased risk for renal failure and lactic acidosis, this medication regimen may need to be discontinued the day of and several days after administration of contrast media. Consult the radiology department for specific instructions.
4. Many radiology departments require the discontinuation of warfarin sodium (Coumadin) therapy for several days before performance of a myelogram. Often, a prothrombin time is required before beginning the examination.

Posttest Patient Care

1. Review test results; report and record findings. Modify the nursing care plan as needed.
2. Bed rest is necessary for 4 to 24 hours after testing. If a water-soluble contrast is used, the head of the bed should be elevated at 45 degrees for 8 to 24 hours after the procedure. The patient is also advised to lie still and quietly. This position reduces upward dispersion of the contrast medium and keeps it out of the head, where it may cause headache. If oil contrast dye is used, the patient usually must lie prone for 2 to 4 hours and then remain on his or her back for another 2 to 4 hours. If the entire amount of oil contrast is not withdrawn at the end of the procedure, the head must be elevated to prevent the oil from flowing into the brain.
3. Encourage fluid intake to hasten absorption of residual contrast material, to replace cerebrospinal fluid, and to reduce risk for headache and unusual or metallic taste.
4. Check for bladder distention and adequate voiding, especially if metrizamide has been used.
5. Check vital signs frequently (at least every 4 hours) for the first 24 hours after the examination.
6. Follow guidelines in Chapter 1 for safe, effective, informed *posttest* care.

CLINICAL ALERT

1. Observe the patient for possible complications such as nausea and vomiting, headache, fever, seizure, paralysis of one side of the body or both arms or legs (rare), arachnoiditis (inflammation of the spinal cord coverings), change in level of consciousness, hallucinations, drowsiness, stupor, neck stiffness, and sterile meningitis reaction (severe headache, symptoms of arachnoiditis, slow-wave patterns on electroencephalogram).
2. Alteration of cerebrospinal fluid pressure may cause an acute exacerbation of symptoms that may require immediate surgical intervention. Lumbar punctures should not be done unless absolutely necessary.
3. Determine whether water-soluble, oil, or air contrast was used for the procedure because *posttest* interventions differ.
4. If nausea or vomiting occur after the procedure and a water-soluble contrast has been used, do not administer phenothiazine antiemetics such as prochlorperazine (Compazine).

● Hysterosalpingography (Uterine and Fallopian Tube X-Rays)

Hysterosalpingography involves radiographic visualization of the uterine cavity and the fallopian tubes to detect abnormalities that may be the cause of infertility or other problems. Normally, a contrast agent introduced into the uterine cavity will travel through the fallopian tubes and "spill" into the peritoneal cavity, where it will be naturally reabsorbed.

Reference Values

Normal

Normal intrauterine cavity
Patent fallopian tubes

Procedure

1. Have the patient remove all clothing and put on a hospital gown. The bladder should be emptied before the study begins.
2. Have the patient lie supine on the x-ray table in a lithotomy position. Preliminary pelvic x-ray images may be taken.
3. The radiologist or gynecologist introduces a speculum into the patient's vagina and inserts a cannula through the cervical canal. Administer the iodinated contrast agent into the uterus through this cannula.
4. Remove the speculum (unless it is radiolucent) and perform both fluoroscopic and conventional images.
5. Follow guidelines in Chapter 1 for safe, effective, informed *intratest* care.

Clinical Implications

Abnormal uterine and fallopian tube x-ray findings include the following conditions:

1. Bicornuate uterus or other uterine cavity anomalies
2. Tubal tortuosity
3. Tubal obstruction evidenced by failure of the contrast dye to spill into the peritoneal cavity on one or both sides (bilateral tubal obstruction causes infertility)
4. Scarring and evidence of past pelvic inflammatory disease

Interventions

Pretest Patient Care

1. Explain test purpose and procedure. Some institutions require a properly signed and witnessed informed consent.
2. Refer to iodine contrast test precautions.
3. Verify date of last menstrual period to ensure that the patient is not pregnant.
4. Advise the patient that some discomfort may be experienced but subsides quickly.
5. Provide sanitary napkins to wear because some spotting and contrast agent discharge may occur.
6. Follow guidelines in Chapter 1 for safe, effective, informed *pretest* care.

CLINICAL ALERT

1. Pregnancy, active vaginal bleeding, and active pelvic inflammatory disease are contraindications to hysterosalpingography. It is best to perform this test 7–10 d after the onset of menses.
2. If the patient has diabetes and is taking metformin, special considerations may be necessary. Consult with the radiology department to determine whether this medication regimen must be discontinued the day of and for several days after the study.
3. Assess whether the patient is allergic to latex and inform the radiology department of any known or suspected allergies or sensitivities before study.
4. Assess whether the patient is allergic to iodine. If iodine contrast allergies or sensitivities are known or suspected, inform the radiology department before the study.

Posttest Patient Care

1. Review test results; report and record findings. Modify the nursing care plan as needed.
2. Monitor the patient for discomfort and administer analgesics as ordered.
3. Instruct the patient to report heavy vaginal bleeding, abnormal discharge, unusual pain, or fever to the referring healthcare provider.
4. Review test outcomes and counsel about infertility problems.
5. Follow guidelines in Chapter 1 for safe, effective, informed *posttest* care.

Angiography (Digital Subtraction Angiography, Transvenous Digital Subtraction, Vascular X-Ray)

Digital angiography is a computer-based method of performing vascular imaging studies that require catheterization of certain venous or arterial vessels. Vasculature studies include the carotid vessels; intracranial vessels; those vessels originating from the aortic arch; abdominal vessels, including the celiac, renal, and mesenteric branches; and other, peripheral vessels. Digital subtraction angiography began as an IV technique, but because of its limitations, other methods of iodine contrast administration may be employed. Although carrying a greater complication risk, intra-arterial injection can be used for detailed visceral studies. The presence of the contrast material blocks the path of x-rays and makes blood vessels visible. An image taken just before contrast injection is subtracted from that taken when the contrast material is actually within the vascular system. The resulting image shows only the distribution of the contrast substance. Digital subtraction is used to isolate a clinically relevant subset of information and is particularly useful in preoperative and postoperative evaluations for anomalies, vascular, and tumor surgery.

Visualization of the carotid and vertebral vasculature is possible in patients with a history of stroke, transient ischemic attacks, bruit, or subarachnoid hemorrhage. The procedure may be used as an adjunct to CT or magnetic resonance scanning and may be performed just before these studies in persons who have evidence of an aneurysm, vascular malformation, or hypervascular tumor. A bi-plane imaging device is used, producing simultaneous images 90 degrees apart.

The study names are derived from the vascular structure studied and the study method used. *Arteriography* refers to contrast agent studies of arterial vessels. Venous structures may also be visualized as these procedures progress. *Venography* is the contrast agent study of peripheral or central veins. *Lymphography* studies lymph vessels and nodes. *Angiocardiography* investigates the interior of the heart and adjacent great vessels such as the pulmonary arteries. *Aortography* refers to a contrast study of aortic segments such as the thoracic aorta (*thoracic aortography*), the abdominal aorta (*abdominal aortography*), or the lumbar aorta (*lumbar aortography*).

Angiographic examinations also can be named for the route used to inject the contrast substance. For example, *renal arteriography* is performed by inserting a catheter into the abdominal aorta and then directing it into the renal artery. During *peripheral arteriography*, the contrast is injected directly into the vessel being studied (e.g., femoral artery). If done through the venous route, a large bolus of contrast medium is directly injected into a peripheral vein (e.g., venous aortography). X-ray images are taken to track the flow of contrast through the right side of the heart, the lungs, and the left side of the heart.

Reference Values

Normal

Normal carotid arteries, vertebral arteries, abdominal aorta and its branches, renal arteries, and peripheral arteries

Procedure

1. Cleanse, prepare, and inject the vascular access area with a local anesthetic, using the sterile technique. Depending on the type of study and patient factors, this is commonly the femoral, brachial, or axillary artery.
2. Follow standard procedure for the Seldinger technique:
   a. Puncture occurs in the femoral artery just below the inguinal ligament.
   b. A beveled compound needle containing an inner cannula pierces the artery.
   c. The needle is withdrawn slowly until there is blood flow.
   d. The needle's inner cannula is removed, and a flexible guidewire is inserted.

e. The needle is removed; pressure fixes the wire and reduces hemorrhage.
f. The catheter is slipped over the wire and into the artery.
g. The guidewire is removed, leaving the catheter in the artery.

3. Remove the catheter after the procedure is terminated.
4. Place a dressing over the insertion site and apply manual pressure to the puncture site for about 5 minutes (vein) and 15 minutes (artery) or until bleeding stops. Tape a more permanent pressure dressing in place; this usually can be removed in 24 hours.
5. Monitor the patient frequently for hemorrhage or hematoma formation.
6. Follow guidelines in Chapter 1 for safe, effective, informed *intratest* care.

Clinical Implications

Abnormal digital subtraction angiography results reveal the following conditions:

1. Arterial stenosis
2. Large aneurysms
3. Intravascular or extravascular tumors or other masses
4. Total occlusion of arteries
5. Thoracic outlet syndrome
6. Large or central pulmonary emboli
7. Ulcerative plaque
8. Tumor circulation

Interfering Factors

1. Because this examination is very sensitive to physical movement, motion artifact will produce poor images. Consequently, uncooperative or agitated patients cannot be studied. Even the act of swallowing results in unsatisfactory images. Measures to reduce swallowing, such as breath holding, do not always yield satisfactory results.
2. Vessel overlap of external and internal carotid arteries makes it almost impossible to obtain a select view of a specific carotid artery because contrast fills both arteries almost simultaneously.

Interventions

Pretest Patient Care

1. Explain test purpose and procedure. Reinforce explanation of test benefits and risks.
2. Ensure that the patient is coherent and cooperative and is able to hold his or her breath and remain absolutely still when so instructed.
3. A legal consent form must be properly signed and witnessed.
4. Refer to iodine contrast test precautions.
5. Determine whether the patient has any known allergies, especially those to iodine, contrast media, or latex.
6. Assess pregnancy status of female patients. If positive, advise the radiology department.
7. Ensure that preprocedure laboratory work is performed in accordance with departmental standards. This generally will include the following tests:
    a. Prothrombin time drawn on day of procedure for any patients on anticoagulation therapy (e.g., warfarin sodium [Coumadin])
    b. Creatinine levels for all patients
    c. Recent prothrombin time and partial thromboplastin time (PT/PTT) and platelet count (generally within 30 days)
8. In many instances, administer glucagon intravenously just before abdominal examinations. This serves to reduce motion artifacts by stopping peristalsis.
9. Be alert to the risk of venous thrombosis and infection. When contrast is administered through the venous route, the arteries—which are normally under higher pressure than the veins—can

clear the contrast agent through the process of normal circulation. For the same reason, there is less risk for loosening plaques.

10. Advise the patient that no food (6 hours) or clear fluids (2 hours) should be taken before the study to minimize vomiting if an iodine contrast reaction occurs.
11. Arteries in a specific area can be visualized during one series of exposures. This overview gives the advantage of being able to evaluate the entire blood supply to a given area at one time. In contrast, during routine angiography, only one specific artery at a time can be visualized.
12. Follow guidelines in Chapter 1 for safe, effective, informed *pretest* care.

CLINICAL ALERT

1. These tests should be used cautiously in patients with renal insufficiency or unstable cardiac disease. Assess for contraindications to iodinated contrast drugs listed on pages 709–711.
2. In the presence of diabetes, assess whether the patient is taking metformin. Because of an increased risk for renal failure and lactic acidosis, this medication regimen must be discontinued the day of and several days after administration of contrast media. Consult the radiology department for specific instructions.

Posttest Patient Care

1. Review test results; report and record findings. Modify the nursing care plan as needed.
2. Check vital signs frequently and report unstable signs to the healthcare provider.
3. Observe the catheter insertion site for signs of infection, hemorrhage, or hematoma. Use sterile aseptic technique at all times. Monitor neurovascular status of the extremity. Report problems to the healthcare provider promptly.
4. Observe for allergic reactions to iodine. Mild side effects include nausea, vomiting, dizziness, and urticaria. Assess for other complications such as abdominal pain, hypertension, congestive heart failure, angina, myocardial infarction, and anaphylaxis. In susceptible persons, renal failure may occur because higher doses of contrast materials are given compared with conventional arteriograms. Resuscitation equipment and emergency supplies should be readily available. Immediately report these conditions to the healthcare provider.
5. Instruct the patient to increase fluid intake to at least 2000 mL (2 L) during the 24 hours following the procedure to facilitate excretion of the iodine contrast substance.
6. Review test outcomes and monitor appropriately.
7. Follow guidelines in Chapter 1 for safe, effective, informed *posttest* care.

CLINICAL ALERT

1. The catheter puncture site must be observed frequently and closely for hemorrhage, pseudoaneurysm, or hematoma formation. These can be serious complications and require immediate attention should they occur.
2. Vital sign assessment, puncture site assessment, and neurovascular assessments may need to be done as frequently as every 15 min for the first few hours after the procedure. Neurovascular assessments include evaluation of color, motion, sensation, capillary refill time, pulse quality, and temperature (warm or cool) of the affected extremity. Compare the affected extremity with the nonaffected extremity.
3. Review the chart or question the patient or healthcare provider regarding deficits that were present before the procedure to establish baseline levels of circulatory function. Report post-procedure changes immediately.

4. If an arterial puncture was performed, the affected extremity must *not* be bent for several hours, and the patient must lie flat other than a pillow under the head. Do not raise the head of the bed or cart because this can put a strain on a femoral puncture site. The patient may turn if the affected extremity is maintained in a straight position without putting strain on the femoral puncture site. If needed, a fracture bedpan can lessen strain on a groin puncture site.
5. If bleeding or hematoma occurs, apply pressure to the site. Sometimes, sandbags may be applied to the puncture site as a routine part of postprocedure protocols.
6. Maintain a functional IV access site. Usually, the patient will return to the nursing unit with an IV line in place.
7. A Doppler device may reveal audible pulse sounds if pulses are nonpalpable.
8. Sudden onset of pain, numbness or tingling, greater degree of coolness, decreased or absent pulses, and blanching of extremities are always cues to notify the healthcare provider immediately. These signs can indicate arterial occlusion, which may require rapid surgical intervention.

Lymphangiography (X-Rays of Lymph Nodes and Vessels)

Lymphangiography examines the lymphatic channels and lymph nodes by means of radiopaque iodine contrast injected into the small lymphatics of the foot. This test is commonly ordered for patients with Hodgkin's disease or cancer of the prostate to check for nodal involvement. Lymphangiography is also indicated to evaluate edema of an extremity without known cause, to determine the extent of adenopathy, to stage lymphomas, and to localize affected nodes as part of surgical or radiotherapeutic treatment.

Reference Values

Normal

Normal lymphatic vessels and nodes

Procedure

1. Place the patient in the supine position on the x-ray table.
2. After injection of a local anesthetic, inject a blue contrast subcutaneously between each of the first three toes of each foot to stain the lymphatic vessels 15 minutes before the start of the examination.
3. Make a 1- to 2-inch incision on the dorsum of each foot after the site is infiltrated with local anesthetic.
4. Identify and cannulate the lymphatic vessel to facilitate extremely low-pressure injection of the iodine contrast medium over a 30-minute period.
5. Discontinue the injection when the contrast medium reaches the level of the third and fourth lumbar vertebrae as seen on fluoroscopy.
6. Observe that abdominal, pelvic, and upper body images demonstrate the lymphatic vessels filling.
7. Obtain a second set of images 12 to 24 hours later to demonstrate filling of the lymph nodes.
8. View the nodes in the inguinal, external iliac, common iliac, and periaortic areas, as well as the thoracic duct and supraclavicular nodes, using this procedure.
9. When a lymphatic of the hand is injected, the axillary and supraclavicular nodes should be visible.
10. Because the contrast dye remains present in the nodes for several months after lymphangiography, repeat studies can be done to track disease activity and to monitor treatment

without the need to repeat contrast injection. The patient may need to have additional images taken.

11. Follow guidelines in Chapter 1 for safe, effective, informed *intratest* care.

Clinical Implications

Abnormal lymph node and vessel x-ray results indicate the following conditions:

1. Retroperitoneal lymphomas associated with Hodgkin's disease
2. Metastasis to lymph nodes
3. Abnormal lymphatic vessels

Interventions

Pretest Patient Care

1. Explain test purpose and procedure. Obtain a signed, witnessed consent form.
2. See iodine contrast test precautions.
3. Assess pregnancy status of female patients. If positive, advise the radiology department.
4. Tell the patient that no fasting is necessary. Usual medications can be taken.
5. Instruct the patient that he or she may feel some discomfort when the local anesthetic is injected into the feet.
6. Administer oral antihistamines per healthcare provider orders if allergy to the iodized contrast agents is suspected.
7. Follow guidelines in Chapter 1 for safe, effective, informed *pretest* care.

CLINICAL ALERT

1. Lymphangiography is usually contraindicated in the following conditions:
   a. Known iodine hypersensitivity
   b. Severe pulmonary insufficiency
   c. Cardiac disease
   d. Advanced renal or hepatic disease
2. The major complication of this procedure relates to contrast media embolization into the lungs. This will diminish pulmonary function temporarily and, in some patients, may produce lipid pneumonia. The patient may require aggressive respiratory management if this complication is life threatening.
3. If the patient has diabetes and is taking metformin, special considerations may be necessary. Consult with the radiology department to determine whether this medication regimen must be discontinued the day of and several days after the study.
4. Assess whether the patient is allergic to latex and inform the radiology department of any known or suspected sensitivities before study.
5. Assess whether the patient is allergic to iodine. If iodine contrast sensitivities are known or suspected, inform the radiology department before study.

Posttest Patient Care

1. Review test results; report and record findings. Modify the nursing care plan as needed.
2. Check and record the patient's temperature every 4 hours for 48 hours after the examination.
3. Provide a restful environment.
4. If ordered, elevate the legs to prevent swelling.
5. Watch for complications such as delayed wound healing, infection, extremity edema, allergic dermatitis, headache, sore mouth and throat, skin rashes, transient fever, lymphangitis, and oil embolism.
6. Follow guidelines in Chapter 1 for safe, effective, informed *posttest* care.

COMPUTED TOMOGRAPHY (CT)

CT, also called CT scanning or computerized tomography, produces images similar to those used in conventional radiography; however, CT scans are taken with a special scanner system. Conventional x-rays pass though the body and produce an image of bone, soft tissues, and air. With CT scans, a computer provides rapid complex calculations that determine the extent to which tissues absorb multiple x-ray beams. CT is unique because it can produce cross-sectional images (i.e., "slices") of anatomic structures without superimposing tissues on each other. Additionally, CT can discern the different characteristics of tissue structures within solid organs. Agents may be used for delineation of blood vessels, the opacification of certain tissue (e.g., kidneys), demonstration of bowel, and blood flow patterns.

The patient lies on a motorized table positioned inside a doughnut-shaped frame called the *gantry* (Fig. 10.4). The gantry contains the x-ray tubes, which rotate around the patient during the scan. By rotating the narrow-beamed x-ray source around the patient's body, multiple attenuation readings are gathered and processed by the computer. The display, similar to a conventional radiograph, demonstrates varying densities that correspond to the absorption of x-rays by the patient's anatomy. As with traditional x-ray techniques, bones appear white, and gas and fat appear black. However, with CT, discrete differences in attenuation can be *quantified*. This means a CT scan can demonstrate minor differences in density and composition in shades of gray. A CT scan can differentiate tumors from soft tissues, air space from cerebrospinal fluid, and normal blood from clotted blood.

By interpreting the scan, structures are identified by appearance, shape, size, symmetry, and position. Usually, space-occupying lesions show characteristic displacement of surrounding viscera. Scans can be performed at different levels and planes and in different slice thicknesses to isolate small lesions. Often, hollow viscera (e.g., intestines) and blood vessels need to be accentuated with the use of contrast media.

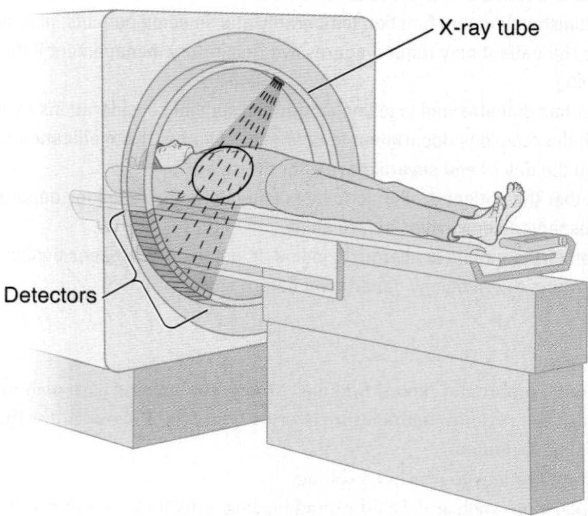

FIGURE 10.4. Computed tomography (CT) scanner showing patient position, x-ray tube, and detectors. (From Moore KL, Dalley AF, Agur AMR: Clinically Oriented Anatomy, 7th ed. Philadelphia, Wolters Kluwer, 2014.)

Spiral CT scanners, also known as helical CT scanners, are a modification of the conventional CT technique. A spiral scan employs a continuous corkscrew pattern that produces a three-dimensional raw data set. This allows for three-dimensional reconstruction and CT angiography. Multirow scanners are capable of producing up to 64 image slices simultaneously. Following image acquisition on a multirow or spiral CT scanner, several postprocessing techniques can be applied to the data sets. This computer manipulation allows for:

1. *CT angiography*, which allows the vascular system to be viewed in three dimensions without the visualization of overlying structures. Considered a complement to true angiography, the CT angiography technique has the advantage of requiring only an IV needle puncture rather than an arterial puncture.
2. *Shaded surface display*, which is a computer-generated surface rendering. The resultant images have the perception of depth, which may be of particular value to surgeons, especially during reconstruction (e.g., posttrauma) procedures.

CT scans can be performed on virtually any body part and can isolate virtually any abdominal organ. Typical CT applications include the following studies:

1. Abdominal: to include liver, pancreas, gallbladder, kidneys, adrenals, spleen, retroperitoneum, and abdominal blood vessels
2. Pelvic: to include urinary bladder, uterus, ovaries, distal colon, and prostate
3. Spine
4. Head: to include sinuses, orbits, mastoids, internal auditory canals, facial bones, neck
5. Chest: to include lungs, mediastinum, and heart
6. Joints and specific bones
7. CT-guided biopsy
8. Fee-for-service screening test may be available to evaluate the heart, lungs, colon, or the entire body

• Computed Tomography (CT) of the Head and Neck; Brain, Eyes, and Sinus

CT of the head is a relatively simple x-ray examination done by means of a special scanning machine to evaluate for suspected intracranial lesions. The results form a cross-sectional picture of the anatomic structure of the head that includes the internal cranial structure, brain tissue, and surrounding cerebrospinal fluid. This axial image of the head is similar to a view looking down through the top of the head.

Reference Values

Normal

No evidence of tumor, other pathology, or fracture

Typically, low-density tissue areas appear black, whereas higher density tissues appear as shades of gray; the lighter the shading, the higher the density of the tissue or structure.

Procedure

1. During the test, have the patient lie completely still on a motorized table with his or her head comfortably immobilized. The table is moved into a doughnut-shaped frame called a *gantry*. X-ray tubes situated within the gantry move around the patient in a circular fashion.
2. Inject an iodinated radiopaque contrast substance if tissue density enhancement is desired because a questionable area needs further clarification. Some patients experience nausea and vomiting after receiving this contrast agent.

3. Take additional images during contrast injection.
4. During and after the IV injection, the patient may experience warmth, flushing of the face, salty taste, or nausea. Encourage the patient to breathe deeply. An emesis basin should be readily available.
5. Watch for other untoward signs such as respiratory difficulty, diaphoresis, numbness, or palpitations.
6. Follow guidelines in Chapter 1 for safe, effective, informed *intratest* care.

Clinical Implications

Abnormal CT head and neck scan results reveal the following conditions:

1. Bony and soft tissue tumor masses such as meningiomas, astrocytomas, angiomas, and cysts
2. Intracranial bleeding or hematoma
3. Aneurysm
4. Infarction
5. Infection
6. Sinusitis
7. Foreign bodies

Interfering Factors

1. A false-negative CT scan can occur in the presence of hemorrhage. As hematomas age, their appearance on CT scans changes from high-intensity to low-intensity levels partly because older hematomas become more transparent to x-rays.
2. Patient movements negatively affect image quality and accuracy.

Interventions

Pretest Patient Care

1. Explain test purpose and procedure. Provide written instructions. Reinforce knowledge regarding possible adverse effects such as radiation exposure or allergy to iodine contrast media.
2. Assess pregnancy status of female patients. If positive, advise the radiology department.
3. Refer to iodine contrast test precautions. A creatinine level may be required before the study.
4. Generally, the patient should fast 2 to 3 hours before the test if a contrast study is planned. In most cases, prescribed medications can be taken before CT studies.
5. Check for patient allergies. Nausea and vomiting, warmth, and flushing of the face may signal a possible iodine allergy.
6. Reassure the patient who is prone to claustrophobia that claustrophobic fear of the scanner is common. Pictures of the scanner or introduction to the scanner may alleviate these fears.
7. Administer analgesics and sedatives, especially to minimize pain and unnecessary movement.
8. Follow guidelines in Chapter 1 for safe, effective, informed *pretest* care.

CLINICAL ALERT

1. If the patient has diabetes and is taking metformin, special considerations may be necessary. Consult with the radiology department to determine whether this medication regimen must be discontinued the day of and several days after the study.
2. Assess whether the patient is allergic to iodine or latex. If iodine contrast or latex allergies or sensitivities are known or suspected, inform the radiology department before study.

Posttest Patient Care

1. Review test results; report and record findings. Modify the nursing care plan as needed.
2. Determine whether an iodine contrast substance was used. If used, observe and record information about reactions if they occurred. Reactions may include hives, skin rashes, nausea, swelling of parotid glands, or, most serious of all, anaphylaxis.
3. Notify the healthcare provider immediately if allergic reactions occur. Antihistamines may be necessary to treat symptoms.
4. Documentation should include assessment of information needs, instructions given, time examination was completed, patient response to the procedure, and any allergic reactions.
5. Follow guidelines in Chapter 1 for safe, effective, informed *posttest* care.

● Computed Tomography (CT) of the Body; Chest, Spine, Extremities, Abdomen, and Pelvis

Body CT imaging provides detailed cross-sectional images of the chest, abdomen, pelvis, spine, and extremities. When used to evaluate neoplastic and inflammatory disease, CT data acquisition can be rapidly sequenced to evaluate blood flow and to determine vascularity of a mass. This technique, known as *dynamic CT scanning*, requires the administration of IV contrast. In addition, CT can be used to detect intervertebral disk disease, herniation, and soft tissue damage to ligaments within joint spaces.

Conventional x-ray machines produce a flat picture, with organs in the front of the body appearing to be superimposed over organs toward the back of the body. The result is a two-dimensional image of the three-dimensional body part. CT imaging produces many cross-sectional anatomic views without superimposing structures. Spiral scanners allow CT angiography and three-dimensional reconstruction techniques.

Reference Values

Normal

No apparent tumor or pathology

On CT scans, air appears black, bone appears white, and soft tissue appears in various shades of gray. Shade patterns and their correlation to different tissue densities, together with the added dimensions of depth, allow identification of normal body structures and organs.

Procedure

1. Have the patient drink a special contrast preparation several minutes before the CT abdominal examination. This contrast material outlines the bowel so that it can be more readily differentiated from other structures.
2. Have the patient lie supine on a motorized couch that moves into a doughnut-shaped frame called a *gantry*. X-ray tubes within the gantry move around the patient as the pictures are taken. These images are concurrently projected onto a monitor screen.
3. Have the patient lie motionless and give breathing instructions.
4. Inject iodine contrast substance and take more pictures if a questionable area requires further clarification. Patients having pelvic CT scans are given a barium contrast enema. Furthermore, female patients undergoing pelvic CT scans may require insertion of a contrast-enhanced vaginal tampon to delineate the vaginal wall. Another indication for contrast is blood vessel delineation, the opacification of well-vascularized tissue, and evaluation of blood flow patterns (as for differential diagnosis of hemangioma).
5. The patient may experience warmth, flushing of the face, salty taste, and nausea with IV injection of the contrast material. Slow, deep breaths may alleviate these symptoms. Have an emesis basin

readily available. Watch for other untoward signs such as respiratory difficulty, heavy sweating, numbness, palpitations, or progression to an anaphylactic reaction. Resuscitation equipment and drugs should be readily available. Notify the healthcare provider immediately should any of these side effects occur.

6. Follow guidelines in Chapter 1 for safe, effective, informed *intratest* care.

Clinical Implications

Abnormal body CT scan findings reveal the following conditions:

1. Tumors, nodules, and cysts
2. Ascites
3. Fatty liver
4. Aneurysm of abdominal aorta
5. Lymphoma
6. Enlarged lymph nodes
7. Pleural effusion
8. Cancer of pancreas
9. Retroperitoneal lymphadenopathy
10. Abnormal collection of blood, fluid, or fat
11. Skeletal bone metastasis
12. Cirrhosis of liver
13. Fractures
14. Soft tissue or ligament damage
15. Abscess

Interfering Factors

1. Retained barium can obscure organs in the upper and lower abdomen. Barium tests should be scheduled after CT scans when possible.
2. Inability of the patient to lie quietly produces less-than-optimal pictures.

Interventions

Pretest Patient Care

1. Explain test purpose and procedure. Written explanations may be helpful. Benefits and risks of the test should be explained to the patient before the procedure.
2. Assess pregnancy status of female patients. If positive, advise the radiology department.
3. Refer to iodine and barium contrast test precautions.
4. In most cases, allow the patient to take usual prescribed medications before CT studies.
5. Inform the patient that an iodine contrast substance may be administered before and during the examination. Determine whether the patient is allergic to iodine. Pelvic CT examinations usually require both IV and rectal administration of contrast material. A creatinine level may be required before the study.
6. Abdominal cramping and diarrhea may occur; therefore, drugs such as glucagon, or Donnatal (atropine, hyoscyamine, phenobarbital, and scopolamine) may be ordered to decrease these side effects.
7. Inform the patient that solid foods are usually withheld on the day of the examination until after test completion. Clear liquids may be taken up to 2 hours before examination. If in doubt, check with the diagnostic department for specific protocols. A patient with diabetes may need to adjust his or her insulin dose and diet before the test. For CT of the abdomen, the patient usually can take nothing by mouth.
8. Instruct the patient that he or she may experience warmth, flushing of the face, a salty metallic taste, and nausea or vomiting if IV iodine is administered.

9. Claustrophobic sensations while in the CT scanner are common. Show the patient a picture of the scanner before the procedure to alleviate anxiety.
10. Remember that sedation and analgesics may help the patient lie quietly during the test to achieve optimal results.
11. Follow guidelines in Chapter 1 for safe, effective, informed *pretest* care.

CLINICAL ALERT

1. If the patient has diabetes and is taking metformin, special considerations may be necessary. Consult with the radiology department to determine whether this medication regimen must be discontinued the day of and several days after the study.
2. Assess whether the patient is allergic to iodine. If iodine contrast allergies or sensitivities are known or suspected, inform the radiology department before study.

Posttest Patient Care

1. Review test results; report and record findings. Modify the nursing care plan as needed.
2. Observe and document reactions to iodine contrast material such as hives, skin rashes, nausea, swelling of parotid glands, iodine poisoning, or anaphylactic reaction.
3. Notify the healthcare provider immediately if symptoms are serious.
4. Administer antihistamines.
5. Document preparation and instructions given to the patient or significant others, the time the procedure was completed, the patient's response to the procedure, any allergic reactions, and subsequent treatment.
6. Follow guidelines in Chapter 1 for safe, effective, informed *posttest* care.

BIBLIOGRAPHY

Adam A, Dixon AK: Grainger & Allison's Diagnostic Radiology, 6th ed. Philadelphia, Elsevier Saunders, 2014

Adler AM, Carlton RR: Introduction to Radiographic Sciences and Patient Care, 5th ed. Philadelphia, Elsevier Saunders, 2012

American Cancer Society: American Cancer Society guidelines for the early detection of cancer, 2006. CA Cancer J Clin 56:11–25, 2006; last medical review, March 11, 2015

Ballinger PW, Frank ED: Merrill's Atlas of Radiographic Positions and Radiologic Procedures, Vols. 1–3, 12th ed. Philadelphia, Elsevier Saunders, 2012

Bontrager KL, Lampignano J: Textbook of Radiographic Positioning and Related Anatomy, 8th ed. Philadelphia, Elsevier Saunders, 2013

Brant WE, Helms C: Fundamentals of Diagnostic Radiology, 4th ed. Philadelphia, Lippincott Williams & Wilkins, 2012

Bushong SC: Radiologic Science for Technologists: Physics, Biology, and Protection, 11th ed. Philadelphia, Elsevier Saunders, 2016

Carlton RR, Adler AM: Principles of Radiographic Imaging, an Art and a Science, 5th ed. Albany, NY, Delmar Thomson, 2012

Cochran ST: Determination of serum creatinine levels prior to administration of radiographic contrast media. JAMA 277(7):517–518, 1997

Daffner RH: Clinical Radiology: The Essentials, 4th ed. Philadelphia, Lippincott Williams & Wilkins, 2013

Food & Drug Administration: Fluoroscopy. Available at: https://www.fda.gov/Radiation-EmittingProducts, 2017

Jensen SC, Peppers MP: Pharmacology and Drug Administration for Imaging Technologists, 2nd ed. Philadelphia, Elsevier Saunders, 2005

Lin, EC: Radiation Risk from Medical Imaging. Mayo Clin Proc 85(12):1142–1146, 2010

Smith RA, Brooks D, Cokkinides V, et al: Cancer screening in the United States 2013: A review of current American Cancer Society guidelines, current issues in cancer screening, new guidance on cervical cancer screening and lung cancer screening. CA Cancer J Clin 63(2):87–105, 2013

Statkiewicz-Sherer MA, Visconti PJ, Ritenour ER: Radiation Protection in Medical Radiography, 7th ed. Philadelphia, Elsevier Saunders, 2013

INTERNET SITES

http://acr.org
http://auntminnie.com
http://breastcancer.org
http://cancernews.com
http://diabetesmonitor.com
http://emedicine.com
http://epa.gov/radiation
http://imaginis.com
http://intelihealth.com
http://postgradmed.com

Cytologic, Histologic, and Genetic Studies

11

OVERVIEW OF CYTOLOGIC (CELLS) AND HISTOLOGIC (TISSUE) STUDIES

Cytologic Studies

Exfoliated cells in body tissues and fluid are studied to determine the types of cells present and to diagnose malignant and premalignant conditions. The staining technique developed by Dr. George N. Papanicolaou has been especially useful in diagnosis of malignancy and is now used routinely in the cytologic study of the female genital tract as well as in many types of nongynecologic specimens.

Some cytologic specimens (e.g., smears of the mouth, genital tract, nipple discharge) are relatively easy to obtain for study. Other samples (e.g., amniotic fluid, pleural effusions, cerebrospinal fluid [CSF]) are from less accessible sources, and special techniques, such as fine-needle aspiration (FNA), are required for collection. Histologic samples may be obtained by biopsy during surgery or during outpatient diagnostic procedures such as endoscopy. In all studies, the source of the sample and its method of collection must be documented so that the evaluation can be based on complete information.

Specimens for cytologic and histologic study usually consist of many different cells. Some are normally present, whereas others indicate pathologic conditions. Cells normally observed in one sample may, under certain conditions, be indicative of an abnormal state when observed elsewhere. All specimens are examined for the number of cells, cell distribution, surface modifications, size, shape, appearance and staining properties, functional adaptations, and inclusions. The cell nucleus is also examined. Any increases or decreases from normal values are noted.

Gynecologic specimens may be smeared and fixed in 95% alcohol. Some types of spray fixative are also available. (Gynecologic specimens collected using the liquid-based technique are collected in special [e.g., PreservCyt, Hologic Inc., Marlborough, MA] solution.) Nongynecologic specimens are generally collected without preservative. They may be placed in saline, and they must be handled carefully to prevent drying or degeneration. Check with your individual laboratory for collection requirements. It is important that all cytology specimens be sent to the laboratory as soon as they are obtained to prevent disintegration of cells or any other process that could cause alteration of the material for study (Table 11.1).

CLINICAL ALERT

1. Test analysis and results depend on the quality of the specimen obtained.
2. Specimens collected from patients in isolation should be clearly labeled on the specimen container (patient's name, date, and test[s] ordered) and requisition form with appropriate warning stickers. The specimen container should then be placed inside two sealed, protective biohazard bags before it is transported to the laboratory.
3. The U.S. Occupational Safety and Health Administration (OSHA) requires that all specimens be placed in a secondary container before transportation to the laboratory. Most laboratories prefer plastic biohazard bags. Requisitions should be kept on the outside of the bag or in a separate compartment in the biohazard bag, if available.

Results of cytologic studies are commonly reported as:

1. Inflammatory
2. Benign
3. Atypical
4. Suspicious for malignancy
5. Positive for malignancy (in situ vs. invasive)

TABLE 11.1 Nucleic Acid Testing Performed in Gynecologic Cytology

Organism	Sample	Method
Human papillomavirus low and high risk	Liquid-based Pap; PreservCYT	Hybrid Capture II (Digene)
Chlamydia trachomatis	Liquid-based Pap; PreservCYT	Cervical cytology plus Hybrid Capture II
Neisseria gonorrhoeae	Liquid-based Pap; PreservCYT	Polymerase chain reaction
Herpes simplex virus types 1 and 2	Liquid-based Pap; PreservCYT	Polymerase chain reaction

Pap, Papanicolaou.

Modified from Bentz JS: Molecular testing in cytopathology: Where are we, where do we go from here? Northfield, IL, CAP Today, *College of American Pathologists*, 20:2, 2006.

Histologic Studies

Material submitted for tissue examination may be classified according to its histologic or cellular characteristics. A basic method for classifying cancers according to the histologic or cellular characteristics of the tumor is Broder's classification of malignancy:

1. Grade I: tumors showing a marked tendency to differentiate; 75% or more of cells differentiated
2. Grade II: 75% to 50% of cells differentiated, slight to moderate dysplasia and metaplasia
3. Grade III: 50% to 25% of cells differentiated, marked dysplasia, marked atypical features, and cancer in situ
4. Grade IV: 25% to 0% of cells differentiated

The tumor-node-metastasis (TNM) system is a method of identifying tumor stage according to spread of the disease. This system evolved from the work of the International Union Against Cancer and the American Joint Committee on Cancer. In addition, the TNM system further defines each specific type of cancer (e.g., breast, head, neck). This staging system is used for previously untreated and treated cancers and classifies the primary site of cancer and its extent and involvement, such as lymphatic and venous invasion.

CYTOLOGIC AND HISTOLOGIC STUDIES

● Fine-Needle Aspirates: Cytologic (Cell) and Histologic (Tissue) Study

FNA is a method of obtaining diagnostic material for cytologic (cell) and histologic (tissue) study that causes a minimal amount of trauma to the patient. Aspirates may be obtained from all parts of the body, including the mouth, breast, liver, genital tract, respiratory tract, urine, CSF, and thyroid. Bacteriologic studies may also be done on material obtained during FNA. Unfixed material, left in the syringe or on a needle rinsed in sterile saline, may be taken to the microbiology department for study.

Reference Values

Normal

Benign or negative: no abnormal cells or abnormal tissue present

No pathogenic organisms

Procedure

1. Use local anesthesia in most cases. Aspirate superficial or palpable lesions without radiologic aid but aspirate nonpalpable lesions using radiographic imaging as an aid for needle placement. Use sterile technique.
2. Insert the needle with syringe attached. Vacuum pressure inside the syringe causes fluid to be drawn up through the needle into the syringe.
3. Express material obtained onto glass slides, which must either be fixed immediately in 95% alcohol, spray-fixed, or air-dried, depending on the staining procedure used by the laboratory. The remaining material may be placed in a preservative solution, such as 50% alcohol. Check with your laboratory for recommended fixation requirements. Material may also be sent to the laboratory in the syringe.
4. Record the source of the sample and method of collection so that evaluation can be based on complete information.
5. Clearly label specimens collected from patients in isolation on the specimen container (patient's name, date, and test[s] ordered) and on the requisition form with an appropriate warning sticker. Place the specimen container inside two sealed, protective biohazard bags before transport.
6. See Chapter 1 guidelines for *intratest* care.

Clinical Implications

Abnormal results reported as atypical, suspicious for malignancy, and positive for malignancy (in situ vs. invasive) are helpful in identifying:

1. *Infectious processes*. The infectious agent may be seen, or characteristic cellular changes may indicate the infectious agent that is present.
2. *Benign conditions*. Some characteristic cellular changes may be present, indicating the presence of a benign process.
3. *Malignant conditions, either primary or metastatic*. If the disease is metastatic, the findings may be reported as consistent with the primary malignancy.

Interventions

Pretest Patient Care

1. Explain the purpose, procedure, benefits, and risks of the test. Even though a local anesthetic is used, the procedure causes some discomfort, and this should not be minimized. If the approach involves passing near a rib, the pain may be greater because of the sensitivity of the bone; this is not a cause for alarm. Unexpected pain may induce a vasovagal or other undesirable response. Other risks include infection and hematoma or hemorrhage, depending on the site aspirated.
2. See guidelines in Chapter 1 for safe, effective, informed *pretest* care.

Posttest Patient Care

1. Review test results; report and record findings. Modify the nursing care plan as needed. Monitor for signs of inflammation and use site care infection control measures. Treat pain, which may be common in sensitive areas such as the breast, nipple, prostate, and scrotum. Monitor for specific problems, which vary depending on the site aspirated (e.g., hemoptysis after a lung aspiration).
2. Counsel about follow-up procedures for infections and malignant conditions.
3. Follow guidelines in Chapter 1 for safe, effective, informed *posttest* care.

● Sentinel Node Location Before Biopsy (Breast, Melanoma); Special Prebiopsy Study

The concept of identifying and localizing the sentinel node or nodes before biopsy is that these nodes receive initial lymphatic drainage and are the first filter to remove metastatic cells; thus, if this sentinel node is free of disease, the rest of the nodes in the patient will also be free of disease. Three methods (along with marking of the skin) are used: (1) lymphoscintigraphy (preoperative), (2) nuclear probe localization (intraoperative), and (3) blue dye injection (intraoperative). Often, all three techniques are used together, the lymph nuclear scan being the most common (see Procedures).

These special prebiopsy procedures are done before biopsies to diagnose cancer of breast or melanoma. Indications for lymph nuclear scan lymphoscintigraphy include detection of metastasis, mapping of all sentinel nodes, and staging and monitoring cancers such as melanoma, breast, head, neck, and skin. Indications for using the nuclear gamma-radiation probe include detecting the most sentinel nodes and providing auditory confirmation. See Chapter 9 for more information on nuclear scans. Indications for blue dye staining include to provide visual confirmation of nodes and to map tumor route (urine will turn blue and skin will stain).

Reference Values

Normal

No evidence of tumor activity

No blocked lymphatic drainage

Procedure

1. *Lymph nuclear scan (lymphoscintigraphy)*
    a. For the breast, inject the radiopharmaceutical (large volume) subcutaneously into the breast and adjacent to suspected breast tumor; for lymphedema, inject into webs of fingers and toes.
    b. For melanoma, make four to six intradermal injections around the tumor or excision site, avoiding scar tissue.
    c. Perform immediate imaging with the patient in the position expected during surgery.
2. *Nuclear radiation (gamma) probe*
    a. A previously administered radiopharmaceutical and the sound radiation detector permit node detection and localization to determine where the initial operative incisions can be made.
    b. Use the sound-radiation gamma probe to locate the area of radioactivity not associated with the injection sites. Of the three procedures, the probe is the most sensitive.
3. *Blue dye*
    a. In order to identify the nodes to undergo biopsy, inject the feet in the web between the toes and the hands between the second and third fingers (allergic reaction to the dye may occur).
    b. Operative biopsy procedure may follow this test.

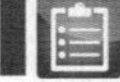

PROCEDURAL ALERT

Only when the sentinel node is positive is a complete nodal dissection performed.

Clinical Implications

1. Abnormal findings reveal metastatic nodes and routes of spread.
2. Asymmetry may indicate lymph flow obstruction.

Interventions

Pretest Patient Care

1. Explain purpose of sentinel node identification procedures.
2. Inform the patient that if the results are positive, surgery usually follows soon after.

Intratest Patient Care

1. Be aware that sedation or analgesia is not usually ordered.
2. Mark the site of lymph nodes with indelible marker.
3. Provide support, assist with positioning, and provide reassurance to the patient that testing is proceeding as expected.

Posttest Patient Care

1. Review test results; report and record findings. Modify the nursing care plan as needed. Monitor injection site (breast, toes, fingers, or around tumor excision site). Check for signs of inflammation or bleeding.
2. If surgery is planned, prepare according to established protocol. Also, see Biopsy Studies Overview section (pages 762 to 764).
3. When surgery is scheduled, take images just before transfer to the operating room.
4. Counsel about outcomes and possible need for further testing or treatment.

● Histologic (Tissue) Biopsy Studies: Overview; Prognostic and Predictive Markers

Tissue biopsies from body sites (e.g., breast, liver, kidney, lymph nodes, skin, bone, muscle, lung, bladder, prostate, thyroid, cervix) may be examined for the presence of benign, toxic, or malignant cells and conditions. The amount of tissue obtained and submitted to the laboratory depends on the specimen site and disease process (e.g., in liver biopsy, at least two to three liver cores >2 cm in length). These procedures may be performed in outpatient or inpatient settings. Some specimens should be collected early in the day. For ultrasound-guided prostate specimens (i.e., transrectal ultrasound [TRUS]), 6 to 12 threadlike sections of tissue are obtained, ranging from 0.5 to 1.5 cm in length. Pain and bloody urine are common afterward. Depending on the body site sampled, anesthetic (i.e., local or general) or conscious sedation and analgesia may be indicated.

Tissue obtained for routine histologic and pathologic examination requires special handling (e.g., place in 10% formalin or send fresh and intact). Tissue needed for frozen-section examination must be delivered to the laboratory immediately with no fixative added. Tissue needed for special studies (e.g., special stains for microorganisms, hormonal studies, DNA ploidy, bone biopsies) may need special handling. A frozen section is done upon the pathologist's recommendation. In some cases, tissue freezing (frozen section) may be contraindicated because it is not in the patient's best interest. Contact your individual laboratory for specific instructions.

After the biopsy specimen is sent to the laboratory, various tests are done to identify the unique characteristics of the patient's tumor cells and to select correct chemotherapy based on resistance to specific drugs. Multiple and complex genetic changes result from loss of control over normal cell growth, and these alterations may influence the tumor's response to chemotherapy. To measure these changes, four major testing groups are used and include the following:

1. *Extreme drug resistance (EDR) assay* tests solid tumors and malignant fluids (blood, bone marrow effusions), which determine the probability of a tumor's resistance to specific chemotherapeutic drugs. If the tumor cells grow in the presence of extreme exposures to a specific drug, this indicates the presence of significant drug resistance and, by identifying inactive agents, avoids exposing patients to the toxicity of drugs that are likely to be ineffective, saves valuable treatment time, and decreases the possibility of cross-resistance to other effective agents.
2. *Differential staining and cytotoxicity (DiSC) assay* uses special stains and techniques to detect drug resistance in leukemia, lymphoma, blood, and bone marrow specimens.
3. *Prognostic markers* measure the tumor's growth potential or ability to invade other tissues (metastasis). Tumor cells release proteases and angiogenic factors to break down basement membranes

and induce new vascularization of the tumor, which delivers oxygen and nutrients to the tumor and allows micrometastasis to distant sites.

4. *Predictive markers* identify specific mechanisms of drug resistance and provide information on how effective clinically indicated chemotherapy agents will be in treating the patient's tumor cells. Prognostic and predictive markers use molecular probes to determine the genetic characteristics, amount of protein, proliferation index, resistance mechanisms, receptor status, and other defining factors of the patient's malignant tumor. To obtain the most comprehensive analysis of the patient's unique tumor biology, drug resistance testing is done in combination with oncoprofiles and prognostic and predictive markers for the specific cancer type. A *radiation resistance assay* can also be done before the treatment actually begins.

These combined studies identify cervical cancer resistive to internal and external radiation plus chemotherapy (the standard treatment is prognostic indicators of progression-free survival). Also included are p53, thrombospondin-1 (Tsp-1), CD31, and angiogenesis index. Prognostic and predictive markers are as follows:

1. *Androgen receptor*. This receptor predicts prostate cancer's response to hormone therapy.
2. *Angiogenesis index* (AI) (p53, Tsp-1, CD31). The AI defines a patient's risk for occult metastatic disease and is composed of factors that characterize the capacity for new blood vessel formation: *p53*, Tsp-1, and CD31 (vessel count). The *p53* gene contributes to tumor growth suppression by slowing cell cycle progression and promoting apoptosis in damaged tumor cells. It also suppresses tumor angiogenesis. Tsp-1 levels have been found to decrease after the tumor sustains mutations in *p53*. CD31 is expressed on the membrane of endothelial cells, allowing for microvessel count in the tumor.
3. *BAX*. Increased levels of BAX, a 21-kD protein and amino acid, indicate accelerated programmed cell death induced by apoptotic stimulus.
4. *Proto-oncoprotein bcl2 (apoptosis regulator)*. The translocation of the *bcl2* gene, occurring in follicular lymphomas, is brought under control of the immunoglobulin gene promoter, resulting in increased intracellular levels of bcl2 protein. This protein suppresses programmed cell death (apoptosis). Induction of cell death is an important mechanism for many chemotherapeutic agents. An abnormal expression of bcl2 protein can render tumor cells resistant to chemotherapeutic agents.
5. *Cathepsin D (invasion potential)*. Cathepsin D, a lysosomal acid protease, has been associated with metastatic potential. Elevated levels of cathepsin D are predictors of early recurrence and death in node-negative cancer and breast cancer.
6. *CD31 (component of tumor angiogenesis index)*. CD31 stains microvessels, allowing for counting, and helps to predict more aggressive disease, metastases, poor survival, and new vascularization of the tumor mass.
7. *DNA ploidy and S-phase (flow cytometry)*. DNA ploidy and proliferative index are independent indicators of prognosis. Patients with aneuploid tumors or high S-phase fractions have poor disease-free survival compared with patients with diploid or low S-phase fraction tumors. DNA ploidy (image analysis) (Feulgen stain) is an indicator of prognosis in selected tumor types in fresh specimens.
8. *Epidermal growth factor receptor (EGF-R)*. This growth factor receptor is a glycoprotein tyrosine kinase, either EGF or transforming growth factor-α (TGF-α). When high levels occur in breast, prostate, ovarian, lung, and squamous cell carcinomas, there is an association with poorer prognosis and poor disease-free survival.
9. *Endoglin (CD105)*. Endoglin normally occurs in vascular endothelial cells of capillaries, arterioles, small arteries, and venules. Increased levels are found in tumor vessels and proliferating endothelial cells. Endoglin has been found in non-T/non-B and pre-B acute lymphoblastic leukemia (ALL) and acute myelocytic and myelomonocytic leukemia cells.
10. *Estrogen receptor (ER) and progesterone receptor (PR)*. ER and PR positivity is associated with a 70% response rate to antihormonal therapy. In contrast, the response rate is <10% among

patients whose tumors are ER and PR negative. Patients whose tumors are ER and PR positive generally achieve superior disease-free survival.

11. *Glutathione S-transferase (GST) (alkylator resistance).* GST is an enzyme that inactivates certain anticancer agents by linking glutathione to the drug. Increased GST levels are associated with tumor resistance to chlorambucil and melphalan.
12. *HER2/neu c-erbB2 oncoproteins.* The presence of HER2/neu, a protein that functions as an oncogene, is associated with poorer prognosis. HER2/neu detection also provides information on the potential treatment response to trastuzumab (Herceptin).
13. *Ki-67 (proliferative index).* This is a staining technique. Monoclonal antibody Ki-67 is associated with increased cell proliferative activity in tumors and with more aggressive tumors and poor disease-free survival.
14. *MDR-1 (P170 glycoprotein: multidrug resistance).* The presence of MDR-1 cancer cells is associated with resistance to naturally produced chemotherapeutic agents such as paclitaxel (Taxol), doxorubicin, and etoposide and plays a critical role in the selection of a treatment regimen.
15. *O(6)-methylguanine-DNA-methyltransferase (MGMT) (nitrosourea resistance).* MGMT, a repair protein, occurs after DNA damage caused by nitrosoureas, such as bis-chloroethylnitrosourea (BCNU). Brain cancer patients with high levels of the *MGMT* gene and alkyltransferase (AT) have shorter disease-free and overall survival.
16. *Multidrug resistance protein (MRP).* This protein is similar to, but distinct from, MDR-1 and is strongly associated with resistance to cisplatin drugs in ovarian cancer.
17. *p21.* A protein-like tumor suppressor like p53, p21 controls when and how the cell replicates. Low levels of p21 are associated with increased risk for tumor occurrence, and the absence of p21 contributes to aggressive growth in some tumors.
18. *p53 (cell cycle and Tsp-1 regulator).* The tumor suppressor gene *p53* regulates cell cycle progression, cellular proliferation, DNA repair, apoptosis, and angiogenesis. Increased levels of mutated p53 protein in tumor cell nuclei are associated with tumor progression and a poorer prognosis.
19. *Proliferating cell nuclear antigen (PCNA) (proliferative index).* Presence of PCNA protein is associated with cell proliferation, and increased levels occur with more aggressive tumors and are associated with poor disease-free survival.
20. *Thymidylate synthase (TS; 5-fluorouracil [5-FU] resistance).* Drug resistance tests of TS, a cellular enzyme essential for DNA biosynthesis and cell proliferation that is a target for 5-FU, is an important component of some breast cancer and colon cancer treatment regimens. Increased TS expression correlates with poorer response rates to 5-FU and with shorter survival in breast and colon cancer.
21. *Thrombospondin-1 (Tsp-1).* This extracellular matrix protein is involved in wound healing. Low value is associated with increased tumor neovascularity and mutant *p53* expression.
22. *UIC2 (MDR-1) shift assay.* This staining technique can be performed on solid tumors. The UIC2 shift assay can be performed on blood and bone marrow specimens from patients with acute myelogenous leukemia (AML), multiple myeloma, or lymphoma and, if the sample contains an adequate amount of viable tumor cells, on solid tumors.
23. *Vascular endothelial growth factor (VEGF).* VEGF, or vascular permeability factor (VPF), plays an important role in angiogenesis, which promotes tumor progression and metastasis.

Oncoprofiles provide the maximum useful information from a single biopsy specimen. These disease-specific marker studies include tests that have been associated with clinical outcomes for each cancer type. Oncoprofiles identify relative risk for relapse and assist in planning therapy for each patient's specific tumor. Table 11.2 shows an example of oncoprofiles offered by Oncotech, Inc. (Irvine, CA).

TABLE 11.2 Useful Information from a Single Biopsy Specimen[a]

Oncoprofile	Basic Profile	Comprehensive Profile
Bladder cancer	DNA, p53, HER2/neu	DNA, p53, HER2/neu, CD31
Brain cancer	DNA, p53, HER2/neu	DNA, p53, HER2/neu, CD31
Breast cancer	DNA, ER/PR, HER2/neu	DNA, ER/PR, HER2/neu, p53, CD31
Colon cancer	DNA, p53	DNA, p53, TS, MDR-1, CD31
Endometrial cancer	DNA, ER/PR, Ki-67	DNA, ER/PR, Ki-67, CD31, MDR-1, p53
Kidney cancer	DNA, MDR-1	DNA, MDR-1, p53, CD31
Leukemia/non-Hodgkin's lymphoma	DNA, Ki-67	DNA, Ki-67, bc12, p53, MDR-1
Lung cancer	DNA, p53	DNA, p53, MDR-1, bc12
Melanoma	DNA, MDR-1	DNA, MDR-1, p53, CD31
Ovarian cancer	DNA, ER/PR, HER2/neu, EGF-R	DNA, ER/PR, HER2/neu, EGF-R, p53, MDR-1
Prostate cancer	DNA, AR	DNA, AR, p53, CD31
Sarcoma	DNA, p53	DNA, p53, MDR-1
Unknown primary site	DNA, p53, HER2/neu	DNA, p53, HER2/neu, MDR-1

[a]The laboratory report from these tumor studies should provide answers to questions such as "Is the tumor malignant?" "Is type of cancer identified?" "How aggressive is the cancer?" "Is the cancer likely to recur?" and "To which drugs is the tumor resistant?"

Interventions

Pretest Patient Care

1. Explain the purpose and biopsy procedure and obtain a signed, witnessed consent form.
2. Remember that patient preparation depends on the predetermined biopsy site. Complete blood count (CBC), prothrombin time (PT), and other bleeding time determinants may be required. Obtain a pertinent history (e.g., prior radiation therapy, other cancer, current medications, pregnancy).
3. Follow Chapter 1 guidelines for safe, effective, and informed *pretest* care.

CLINICAL ALERT

Contraindications to tissue biopsy depend on the body site sampled: bleeding diathesis, anticoagulant therapy, highly vascular lesions, sepsis, seriously impaired lung function, an uncooperative patient, or local infection near the biopsy site.

Posttest Patient Care

1. Review test results; report and record findings. Modify the nursing care plan as needed.
2. Monitor for signs of bleeding, inflammation, infection, laceration of tissue and organs, and perforation. Treat pain, which may be experienced to various degrees depending on the body site sampled.
3. Counsel the patient about follow-up procedures and treatment for infections and malignant conditions.
4. Follow the guidelines in Chapter 1 for safe, effective, and informed *posttest* care.

Breast Biopsy: Cytologic (Cell) and Histologic (Tissue) Study and Prognostic Markers

Breast biopsies are among the most common type of biopsy done. The cells and tissue obtained by breast biopsy establish the presence of breast disease, diagnose histopathology, and classify the process. They also confirm and characterize calcifications noted in prebiopsy mammograms. The breast tissue is examined to determine surgical margins, presence or absence of vesicular invasion, tumor type, staging, and grading. Secondary studies relevant to survival may include imaging procedures, along with the following prognostic markers. (Also see Tumor Markers in Chapter 8 for more information.)

1. *ER and PR.* These hormone receptors are indicators of prognosis and are used to manage hormonal therapy in breast and endometrial cancer. Immunohistochemical (IHC) staining aids recognition of metastatic breast cancer.
2. *DNA ploidy.* This test measures cell turnover or replication; it is used to predict prognosis and shorter survival times by the presence of aneuploid (rapidly replicating cells) for certain tumor types, such as breast, prostate, and colon; it is less clear for ovarian, lung, kidney, and bladder (urine) tumors (66% of breast cancers are aneuploid).
3. *S-phase fraction (SPF).* This test is done to predict survival and reduced chance of relapse. Low levels of SPF appear to have longer survival and reduced chance of relapse. SPF is the DNA synthesis phase obtained by a statistical method.
4. *Cathepsin D.* This test is done to determine prognosis. The presence of this lysosomal protease is estrogen related and may promote tumor spread. Prognostic significance remains ambiguous.
5. *EGF reception.* This test is done to predict survival time. Presence is correlated with ER negativity, aneuploidy, increased S-phase factors, and lymph node metastases. Increased EGF reception may be associated with worse relapse-free and survival time.
6. *p53 gene.* This test is used to predict prognosis. This tumor suppressor gene regulates cell cycles. Some healthcare providers believe that the prognostic value of the *p53* gene is second only to lymph node status.
7. *c-erbB2 (HER2) oncogene.* This test determines which patients are most likely to benefit from high doses of chemotherapy. High levels of this oncogene receptor are associated with poor response to conventional chemotherapy and may be a marker for patients likely to benefit from high doses of chemotherapy. HER2/neu levels may also be determined in a blood specimen.

Gene profiling technologies have also allowed identification of different types of breast cancer, such as *luminal* A and *luminal B* (hormone receptor–positive tumors that arise from luminal cells), HER2 (hormone receptor–negative tumors), BRCA (tumors due to gene mutations), and *basal* (negative for PR and ER).

Reference Values

Normal

Negative for malignant or other abnormal cells and tissue
Prognostic markers: of no significance or negative
No vascular invasion
DNA index: 0.8 to 1.2 on the diploid scale
Proliferative antigen index of 10% S phase: 7% = amount of cells on the S phase

Procedure

1. See Chapter 10 for image-guided tumor localization study before biopsy.
2. Breast tissue specimens may be obtained by open surgical technique, x-ray–guided core biopsy, needle biopsy, or magnetic resonance imaging (MRI)-guided biopsy.
3. MRI-guided breast biopsy is performed by positioning the patient with both breasts in a dedicated surface breast coil. The breast to be biopsied is positioned in a compression device, and a

marker is taped over the suspected area of the lesion. Subsequently, an intravenous injection of gadopentetate dimeglumine is given, and images are acquired after contrast injection. This process is used to determine the depth and location of the lesion for insertion of a probe. A needle can now be introduced and a small, cylindrical tissue sample obtained. The procedure generally takes <60 minutes.

4. Label specimen with the patient's name, date, and test(s) ordered and place these specimens in a biohazard bag, take directly to the laboratory, and give to the pathologist or histotechnologist. The breast tissue is examined and the extent of the tumor determined. Reaction margins and the grade and stage of disease are identified.
5. See Chapter 1 guidelines for *intratest* care.

PROCEDURAL ALERT

MRI-guided breast biopsy is indicated when ultrasound-guided or stereotactic-guided biopsy cannot clearly define the area of concern.

Clinical Implications

1. After breast tissue is examined, the extent of the tumor is determined. Resection margins are evaluated, and grade and stage of disease are identified. The further dedifferentiated a tumor becomes, the further it deviates from the normal diploid state. This may be expressed as a tetraploid or aneuploid state according to the amount of DNA on the stained tissue (DNA index of between 1.0 and 2.0). The more cells in the S or DNA phase, the more aggressive the tumor.
2. Favorable prognostic indicators include tumor size <1 cm, a low histologic grade, negative axillary lymph nodes, and positive ER and PR.
3. Fibroplasia and fibroadenoplasia are benign conditions.

Interventions

Pretest Patient Care

1. Explain biopsy purpose and procedure. Obtain and record relevant family or personal history of prior biopsy, trauma, recent or current pregnancy, nipple discharge, location of lump, and how lesion was detected. Obtain signed, witnessed consent form.
2. Be aware that open breast biopsies are performed under local or general anesthesia. Sedation may be used with local anesthetics. Nothing by mouth (NPO) is required when general anesthesia is used.
3. Provide information and support, recognizing the fear the patient experiences about the procedure.
4. Follow guidelines in Chapter 1 for safe, effective, informed *pretest* care.

Posttest Patient Care

1. If general anesthesia is used, follow the recovery protocols.
2. Review test results; report and record findings. Modify the nursing care plan as needed. Counsel the patient appropriately about possible further testing and treatment (surgery, radiation, and medication [chemotherapy]).
3. Follow guidelines in Chapter 1 for safe, effective, informed *posttest* care.

● Ductal Lavage of Breast Cells (Cytologic) Study; Gail Index Score of Breast Cancer Risk

Ductal lavage collects cells from the milk ducts of the nipple, where most breast cancers begin. If cytologic study shows abnormal cells, this is an indication of increased risk for breast cancer development. Ductal lavage is used to assess breast cancer risk and for ongoing surveillance. A statistical model computes a Gail index score in a woman of a given age and with the presence of certain factors that indicate risk for developing breast cancer over a specified interval. The Gail index score is based on risk factors (e.g., late age at menarche, late age at first live birth, number of previous biopsies, and number of first-degree relatives with breast cancer).

Reference Values

Normal

No atypical or abnormal cells

Gail index of breast cancer risk = odds ratio ≤1.7. For more information, see Gail et al. (1989).

Procedure

1. Apply a local anesthetic cream to the nipple area using a special kit; use a suction device to draw tiny amounts of fluid droplets from the milk ducts to the nipple surface. These droplets locate the milk ducts' natural opening on the surface of the nipple.
2. Insert a very fine (hair-thin) catheter (Fig. 11.1) into the periareolar duct. Administer local anesthetic into the duct. Use a saline wash to separate the cells. Place the specimen in a special collector vial; label with the patient's name, date, and test(s) ordered; and send for examination in a biohazard bag.

Clinical Implications

1. Abnormal findings include atypical hyperplasia and evidence of proliferative breast disease. The presence of atypical cells increases the risk for breast cancer by 4 to 5 times compared with women who do not have atypical cells.
2. Relative risk is increased even further in the presence of a family history of breast cancer (mother, daughter, sister, or two or more close relatives with history of breast cancer), specific genetic change (*BRCA-1* and *BRCA-2* mutations), and a Gail index score of at least 1.7.
3. The age-specific composite evidence rate of the Gail model increases rapidly with age, although the conversion model changes little with age.
4. Later relative risk (percentage) or estimate of developing breast cancer within 10, 20, or 30 years of follow-up is based on projected probability.

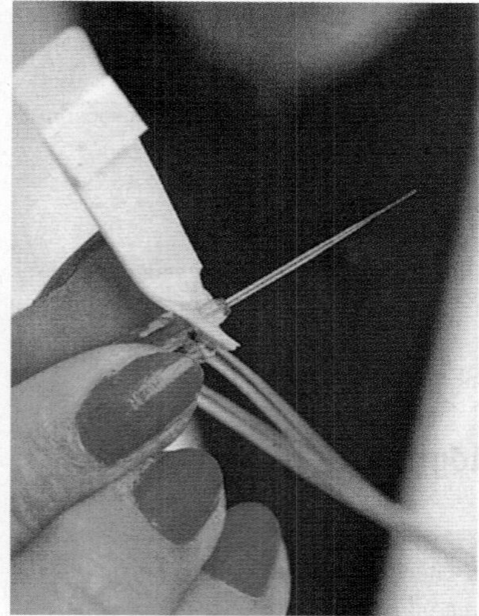

FIGURE 11.1. A ductal lavage microcatheter. (From Titus K: Breast specimens: FNA, core, more. CAP Today 16[2], 2002. Copyright Bob Self.)

Interventions

Pretest Patient Care

1. Explain the lavage purpose, procedure, benefits, and risks.
2. Be aware that high-risk women of any age may be good candidates for ductal lavage. Obtain and document history and risk factors.
3. Describe sensations that might be felt: feelings of fullness, pinching, and gentle tugging on the breast, which is uncomfortable but not usually painful.
4. Follow guidelines in Chapter 1 for safe, effective, informed *pretest* care.

Posttest Patient Care

1. Review test results; report and record findings. Modify the nursing care plan as needed. Counsel the patient appropriately about the chance of breast cancer development, follow-up, close monitoring (yearly examinations), and preventive drug treatment (e.g., tamoxifen) or surgery (oophorectomy or bilateral mastectomy).
2. Remember that test outcomes are interpreted in conjunction with mammogram and physical examination findings.
3. Follow guidelines in Chapter 1 for safe, effective, informed *posttest* care.

● Liver Biopsy: Cytologic (Cell) and Histologic (Tissue) Study

Liver needle biopsy is an invasive procedure that is done to confirm diagnosis of chronic hepatitis and liver cirrhosis, evaluate disease severity, and establish etiology. Cellular material from the liver may be useful in evaluating the status of the liver in diffuse disorders of the parenchyma and in the diagnosis of space-occupying lesions. Liver biopsy is especially useful when the clinical findings and laboratory test results are not diagnostic (e.g., an aspartate aminotransferase [AST] level 10 to 20 times less than the upper defined limit with an alkaline phosphatase [ALP] level <3 times the limit) and when the diagnosis or cause cannot be established by other means (enlarged liver of unknown cause or systemic disease affecting the liver, such as miliary tuberculosis). Other indications for liver biopsy include evaluation of chronic hepatitis, portal hypertension, and fever of unknown origin (tuberculosis and brucellosis) and to confirm alcoholic liver disease.

Reference Values

Normal

Negative for malignant or other abnormal cells and abnormal tissue
No evidence of local or diffuse liver disease
No evidence of toxic reaction to drugs or inflammatory reactions
No pathogenic organisms present

Procedure

1. See Fine-Needle Aspirates: Cytologic (Cell) and Histologic (Tissue) Study.
2. Be aware that in most cases, this is an outpatient procedure.
3. Remember that the test may be done at the bedside in a designated area, usually under local anesthesia. Obtain specimens with ultrasound or computed tomography (CT) x-ray guidance and a tissue core biopsy needle, such as the Menghini needle, that provides histologic and cytologic material; or use an FNA needle, which obtains cytologic material only and is useful for cancer diagnosis but not diagnosis of other liver diseases.
4. Place tissue specimens in 10% formalin for fixation. Do not place specimens for culture in a fixative. Check with your laboratory for specific instructions for handling special cases (e.g., liver biopsies for copper levels).

5. Express cytology specimens on glass slides and fix immediately in 95% alcohol. Needle rinses may provide helpful diagnostic material as well.
6. See Chapter 1 for safe, effective, informed *intratest* care. See Chapter 12 on endoscopic examination and liver biopsy.

Clinical Implications

Abnormalities in test results of liver biopsies may be helpful in detecting the following liver diseases:

1. Benign disorders, such as those causing liver cirrhosis, and presence of pathogenic organisms in liver abscess
2. Metabolic disorders
   a. Fatty metamorphosis
   b. Hemosiderosis
   c. Accumulation of bile (due to hepatitis, obstructive jaundice, malignancy)
   d. Diabetic pathology and Wilson's disease
   e. Hepatic cysts (congenital or hydatid)
   f. Malignant processes, such as end-stage lymphoma

Interfering Factors

Reported effectiveness of liver aspirates or biopsies varies. Because a very small fragment of tissue, often partially destroyed, is taken in a random manner from a large organ, localized disease may be missed.

1. False-negative results may be caused by:
   a. Sampling error. Detection rate of liver metastases is approximately 50% to 70% with blind biopsy and about 85% (range, 67% to 96%) with the use of ultrasound guidance. Also, many diseases produce nonspecific changes that may be spotty, healing, or minimal.
   b. Degeneration or distortion caused by faulty preparation of specimen.
2. False-positive results may be caused by misinterpretation of markedly reactive hepatocytes.

Interventions

Pretest Patient Care

1. Explain the purpose, procedure, benefits, and risks of the test. Obtain signed, witnessed consent form. The procedure usually causes minimal discomfort but only for a short while. Explain that a local anesthetic will be injected into the skin. Remember to ask whether the patient has ever had a reaction to any numbing medicines. Discontinue all aspirin and nonsteroidal anti-inflammatory drugs (NSAIDs) for at least 7 days before the procedure. PT, partial thromboplastin time (PTT), blood urea nitrogen (BUN), bleeding time, and type L screen cross-match for possible transfusion are usually ordered before biopsy.
2. Ensure that the patient takes NPO for 4 to 6 hours before the procedure. Ask the patient to lie supine with the right arm above the head. During the biopsy, the patient should take a deep breath in, blow the air out, and then hold the breath.
3. Be aware that risks include a small but definite risk for intra-abdominal bleeding and bile peritonitis. Percutaneous liver biopsy results in complications in ~1% of cases.
4. Follow guidelines in Chapter 1 for safe, effective, informed *pretest* care.

CLINICAL ALERT

Contraindications include:

1. Bleeding diathesis (anticoagulant therapy)
2. Highly vascular lesions
3. Uncooperative patient

4. PT in the anticoagulant range; PTT >20 s over control
5. Severe anemia (hemoglobin <9.5 g/dL or <95 g/L) or marked prolonged bleeding time
6. Infection
7. Platelet count >50,000/mm^3 (50 × 10^9/L)
8. Marked or tense ascites (risk for leakage)
9. Septic cholangitis

Posttest Patient Care

1. Strict bed rest for at least 6 hours is usually ordered, with observation for 24 hours.
2. Review test results; report and record findings. Modify the nursing care plan as needed. Monitor in a recovery area. Assess pulse, blood pressure, and respiration every 15 minutes for the first hour, every 30 minutes for the next 2 hours, once in each of the next 4 hours, and then every 4 hours until the patient's condition is stable.
3. Notify the surgeon if the blood pressure differs markedly from baseline or if the patient is in severe pain.
4. Maintain NPO status for 2 hours; previous diet can then be resumed. Take action immediately if a bleeding episode occurs. Assess for pain and treat as ordered.
5. After 6 hours, a blood specimen for hematocrit testing is usually ordered to rule out internal bleeding. A small number of patients need transfusion for intraperitoneal bleeding.
6. Warn the patient not to cough hard or strain for 2 to 4 hours after the procedure. Heavy lifting and strenuous activities should be avoided for about 1 week.
7. The most common complications include uncontrolled pain, hemorrhage, peritonitis, bile leakage, lacerations of other organs, sepsis, and bacteremia.
8. Follow the guidelines in Chapter 1 for safe, effective, informed *posttest* care.

● Kidney Biopsy: Cytologic (Cell) and Histologic (Tissue) Study

Kidney biopsy is used to establish a diagnosis in the presence of renal dysfunction, evaluate severity and extent of disease, guide therapy, and identify candidates for kidney transplantation.

Reference Values

Normal

No patterns of abnormality or abnormal glomeruli
No evidence of drug toxicity, infection, or inflammation

Procedure

1. Obtain a specimen of kidney tissue (containing 8 to 10 glomeruli) by needle biopsy or open surgical technique using x-ray or ultrasound as a guide.
2. Place in normal saline until frozen or place in a fixative or saline and send immediately to the laboratory. Check with your laboratory for specific handling instructions. Proper handling is critical to ensure that the specimen is properly preserved for necessary testing.
3. See Fine-Needle Aspirates: Cytologic (Cell) and Histologic (Tissue) Study for information regarding obtaining kidney material for cytologic study.

Clinical Implications

Abnormal patterns reveal interstitial fibroses and scleroses, diabetic nephrotic pathology syndrome, chronic renal failure, kidney transplant reactions, rejection or failure, past infections, glomerulonephritis, and renal pathology in systemic diseases.

Interventions

Pretest Patient Care

1. Explain purpose, procedure, benefits, and risks of kidney biopsy.
2. Use sedation and local or general anesthesia if necessary.
3. Obtain signed, witnessed consent form.
4. Be aware that contraindications include uncontrolled bleeding, cancer, large cysts, abscess, pregnancy, acute pyelonephritis, aneurysm, and renal artery.
5. Follow guidelines in Chapter 1 for safe, effective, informed *pretest* care.

Posttest Patient Care

1. Review test results; report and record findings. Modify the nursing care plan as needed. Counsel the patient appropriately.
2. Monitor for complications, which include hematuria (more common in uncontrolled hypertension and uremia), hematomas (presence of a local mass), infection, and laceration of other organs.
3. Follow guidelines in Chapter 1 for safe, effective, informed *posttest* care.

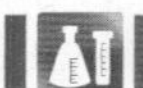

CLINICAL ALERT

Death (although very rare) has occurred in 0.12% of patients.

● Respiratory Tract: Cytologic (Cell) and Histologic (Tissue) Study

The lungs and the passages that conduct air to and from the lungs form the respiratory tract, which is divided into the upper and lower respiratory tracts. The upper respiratory tract consists of the nasal cavities, the nasopharynx, and the larynx; the lower respiratory tract consists of the trachea and the lungs.

Sputum is composed of mucus and cells. It is the secretion of the bronchi, lungs, and trachea and is therefore obtained from the lower respiratory tract (bronchi and lungs). Sputum is ejected through the mouth but originates in the lower respiratory tract. Saliva produced by the salivary glands in the mouth is not sputum. A specimen can be correctly identified as sputum in microscopic examination by the presence of dust cells (carbon dust–laden macrophages). Although the glands and secretory cells in the mucous lining of the lower respiratory tract produce up to 100 mL of fluid daily, a healthy person normally does not cough up sputum.

Cytologic studies of sputum and bronchial specimens are important as diagnostic aids because of the frequency of cancer of the lung and the relative inaccessibility of this organ. Also detectable are cell changes that may be related to the future development of malignant conditions and to inflammatory conditions.

Reference Values

Normal

Negative for abnormal cells or tissue
No pathogenic organisms

Procedures

1. Procedure for obtaining sputum
   a. Be aware that the preferred material is an early-morning specimen. Usually, three specimens are collected on 3 separate days.
   b. Have the patient inhale air to the full capacity of the lungs and then exhale the air with an expulsive deep cough.
   c. Have the patient cough the specimen directly into a wide-mouthed, clean container containing 50% alcohol. (Some cytology laboratories prefer the specimen to be fresh if it will be delivered

to the laboratory immediately.) If microbiologic studies are also ordered, the container must be sterile, and no fixative should be added.

d. Cover the specimen with a tight-fitting, clean lid.

e. Label the specimen with the patient's name, date and time of collection, test(s) ordered, and sequence of specimen (one, two, or three) and send immediately to the laboratory.

2. Procedure for obtaining bronchial secretions
   a. Obtain bronchial secretions during bronchoscopy (see Chapter 12). Diagnostic bronchoscopy involves removal of bronchial secretions and tissue for cytologic and microbiologic studies.
   b. Collect secretions obtained in a clean container and take to the cytology laboratory. If microbiologic studies are ordered, the container must be sterile.
3. Procedure for obtaining bronchial brushings
   a. Obtain bronchial brushings during bronchoscopy.
   b. Smear the material collected directly on all-frosted slides and immediately fix, or place the actual brush in a container of 50% ethyl alcohol or saline and deliver to the cytology laboratory.
4. Procedures for bronchopulmonary lavage
   a. Use bronchopulmonary lavage to evaluate patients with interstitial lung disease.
   b. Inject saline into the distal portions of the lung and aspirate back through the bronchoscope into a specimen container. This essentially "washes out" the alveoli.
   c. Take the fresh specimen directly to the laboratory. A total cell count and a differential cell count are performed to determine the relative numbers of macrophages, neutrophils, and lymphocytes.

For all procedures, see Chapter 1 guidelines for *intratest* care.

Clinical Implications

Abnormalities in sputum and bronchial specimens may sometimes be helpful in detecting the following:

1. Benign atypical changes in sputum, as in:
   a. Inflammatory diseases
   b. Asthma (Curschmann's spirals and eosinophils may be found, but they are not diagnostic of the disease.)
   c. Lipid pneumonia (Lipophages may be found, but they are not diagnostic of the disease.)
   d. Asbestosis (ferruginous or asbestos bodies)
   e. Viral diseases
   f. Benign diseases of lung, such as bronchiectasis, atelectasis, emphysema, and pulmonary infarcts
2. Metaplasia (the substitution of one adult cell type for another); severe metaplastic changes are found in patients with:
   a. History of chronic cigarette smoking
   b. Pneumonitis
   c. Pulmonary infarcts
   d. Bronchiectasis
   e. Healing abscess
   f. Tuberculosis
   g. Emphysema
3. Viral changes and the presence of virocytes (viral inclusions) may be seen in:
   a. Viral pneumonia
   b. Acute respiratory disease caused by adenovirus
   c. Herpes simplex
   d. Measles
   e. Cytomegalic inclusion disease
   f. Varicella

4. Degenerative changes, as seen in viral diseases of the lung
5. Fungal and parasitic diseases (in parasitic diseases, ova or parasite may be seen)
6. Tumors (benign and malignant)

Interfering Factors

1. False-negative results may be caused by:
   a. Delays in preparation of the specimen, causing a deterioration of tumor cells
   b. Sampling error (diagnostic cells may not have exfoliated into the material examined)
2. The frequency of false-negative results is about 15%, in contrast to about 1% in studies for cervical cancer. This high incidence occurs even with careful examination of multiple deep cough specimens.

Selection of Medications and Media for All Respiratory Cell and Tissue Procedures

1. Mild sedative and analgesia and/or local anesthetic may be used during bronchoscopy. Analgesia is indicated for pain after bronchoscopy. See Chapter 12 for bronchoscopy care.
2. Sputum specimens are collected in a wide-mouthed container; 50% alcohol may be added if transportation to the laboratory will be delayed.
3. Bronchial washings may be collected in a trap tube or wide-mouthed container.
4. Bronchial brushes may be smeared directly on glass slides, which are then fixed immediately in 95% alcohol or spray fixative. Brushes may be placed in a fixative solution such as 50% alcohol.

Interventions

Pretest Patient Care

1. Explain the purpose and procedure of the test. Tell the patient *not* to drink fixative liquid in specimen container.
2. Emphasize that sputum is not saliva. If a patient is having difficulty producing sputum, a hot shower before obtaining a specimen may improve the yield.
3. Advise the patient to brush the teeth and rinse the mouth well before obtaining the sputum specimen to avoid introduction of saliva into the specimen. The specimen should be collected before the patient eats breakfast.
4. If bronchoscopy is performed, maintain NPO for 6 hours before the procedure.
5. Manage pain with sedation as indicated.
6. Provide emotional support.
7. Instruct the patient to breathe in and out of the nose with the mouth open during the procedure. The fiber optic bronchoscope is inserted through the nose or mouth; the rigid bronchoscope is inserted through the mouth.
8. Follow guidelines in Chapter 1 for safe, effective, informed *pretest* care.

Posttest Patient Care

1. If the specimen is obtained by bronchoscopy, check the patient's blood pressure and respirations every 15 minutes for 1 hour, then every 2 hours for 4 hours, and then as ordered.
2. Assist and teach the patient to not eat or drink until the gag reflex returns.
3. Maintain bed rest and elevate the head of the bed 45 degrees.
4. Manage pain as indicated.
5. Auscultate the chest for breath sounds every 2 to 4 hours and then as ordered.
6. Perform postural drainage and oropharyngeal suctioning as ordered. (Refer to bronchoscopy care in Chapter 12.)
7. Review test results; report and record findings. Modify the nursing care plan as needed. Provide support for abnormal outcomes.
8. Follow guidelines in Chapter 1 for safe, effective, informed *posttest* care.

Gastrointestinal Tract: Cytologic (Cell) and Histologic (Tissue) Study

Exfoliative cytology of the gastrointestinal tract is useful in the diagnosis of benign and malignant diseases. It is not, however, a specific test for these diseases. Many benign diseases, such as leukoplakia of the esophagus, esophagitis, gastritis, pernicious anemia, and granulomatous diseases, may be recognized because of their characteristic cellular changes. Response to radiation may also be noted from cytologic studies.

Reference Values

Normal
Negative for abnormal cells
Squamous epithelial cells of the esophagus may be present.

Procedure

1. Give a sedative before the procedure. For esophageal studies, pass a nasogastric Levin tube ~40 cm (to the cardioesophageal junction) with the patient in a sitting position.
2. For stomach studies, pass a Levin tube into the stomach (~60 cm) with the patient in a sitting position.
3. For pancreatic and gallbladder drainage, pass a double-lumen gastric tube orally 45 cm, with the patient in a sitting position. Then, place the patient on his or her side and pass the tube slowly 8.5 cm. It takes about 20 minutes for the tube to reach this distance. Confirm the tube location by biopsy. Lavage with physiologic salt solution is done during all upper gastrointestinal cytology procedures.
4. Be aware that specimens can also be obtained during endoscopy procedures.
5. Material obtained with the use of brushes may be smeared directly on glass slides, which are fixed immediately in 95% alcohol or spray fixative. Brushes may also be placed in a fixative such as 50% alcohol. See Chapter 12 for endoscopic biopsy procedures. Washings must be delivered immediately to the laboratory and may need to be placed on ice. Check with your individual laboratory for specific instructions on handling of washings from the gastrointestinal tract.

Clinical Implications

1. The characteristics of benign and malignant cells of the gastrointestinal tract are the same as for cells of the rest of the body.
2. Abnormal results in cytologic studies of the esophagus may be a nonspecific aid in the diagnosis of:
   a. Acute esophagitis, characterized by increased exfoliation of basal cells with inflammatory cells and polymorphonuclear leukocytes in the cytoplasm of the benign squamous cells
   b. Vitamin B_{12} and folic acid deficiencies, characterized by giant epithelial cells
   c. Malignant diseases, characterized by typical cells of esophageal malignancy
3. Abnormal results in studies of the stomach may be a nonspecific aid in the diagnosis of:
   a. Pernicious anemia, characterized by giant epithelial cells. An injection of vitamin B_{12} causes these cells to disappear within 24 hours.
   b. Granulomatous inflammations seen in chronic gastritis and sarcoidosis of the stomach, which is characterized by granulomatous cells
   c. Gastritis, characterized by degenerative changes and an increase in the exfoliation of clusters of surface epithelial cells

d. Malignant diseases, most of which are gastric adenocarcinomas. Lymphoma cells can be differentiated from adenocarcinoma. The Reed-Sternberg cell, a multinucleated giant cell, is the characteristic cell found along with abnormal lymphocytes in Hodgkin's disease.

4. Abnormal results in studies of the pancreas, gallbladder, and duodenum may reveal malignant cells (usually adenocarcinoma), but it is sometimes difficult to determine the exact site of the tumor.
5. Abnormal results in examination of the colon may reveal:
   a. Ileitis, characterized by large, multinucleated histocytes
   b. Ulcerative colitis, characterized by hyperchromatic nuclei surrounded by a thin cytoplasmic rim
   c. Malignant cells (usually adenocarcinoma)

Interfering Factors

The barium and lubricant used in Levin tubes interfere with results because they distort the cells and prevent accurate evaluation.

Interventions

Pretest Patient Care

1. Tell the patient the purpose of this test, the nature of the procedure, and to anticipate some discomfort.
2. A liquid diet usually is ordered for the 24 hours before testing. Encourage the patient to take fluids throughout the night and in the morning before the procedure.
3. Do not administer oral barium for the preceding 24 hours.
4. Laxatives and enemas are ordered for colon cytologic studies.
5. Because insertion of the nasogastric tube can cause considerable discomfort, devise a system (e.g., raising a hand) with the patient to indicate discomfort. (See gastric analysis procedure in Chapter 16.)
6. Inform the patient that panting, mouth breathing, or swallowing can help to ease insertion of the tube.
7. Tell the patient that sucking on ice chips or sipping through a straw also makes insertion of the tube easier.
8. Ballottement and massage of the abdomen are needed to release cells when a gastric wash technique is used.
9. Follow guidelines in Chapter 1 for safe, effective, informed *pretest* care.

CLINICAL ALERT

1. The uncooperative patient is a contraindication.
2. Immediately remove the tube if the patient shows signs of distress: coughing, gasping, or cyanosis.

Posttest Patient Care

1. Review test results; report and record findings. Modify the nursing care plan as needed. The patient may be given food and fluids after the tests are completed.
2. Provide rest. Patients having colon studies will feel quite tired.
3. Potential complications of endoscopy include respiratory distress and esophageal, gastric, or duodenal perforation. Complications of proctosigmoidoscopy include possible bowel perforation. Decreased blood pressure, pallor, diaphoresis, and bradycardia are signs of vasovagal stimulation and require immediate notification of the healthcare provider.
4. Follow Chapter 1 guidelines for safe, effective, informed *posttest* care.

Papanicolaou (Pap) Smear: Cytologic (Cell) Study of the Female Genital Tract, Vulva, Vagina, and Cervix; DNA Test for Human Papillomavirus (HPV)

Characteristic physiologic cellular changes occur in the genital tract from birth through the postmenopausal years. Three major cell types occur in a characteristic pattern in normal vaginal smears:

1. Superficial squamous cells are mature squamous, usually polygonal, containing a pyknotic (thick, compact, dense) nucleus.
2. Intermediate squamous cells are mature squamous, usually polygonal, containing a clearly structured vesicular nucleus, which may be either well preserved or changed as a result of bacterial cytolysis.
3. Parabasal cells are immature squamous, usually round or oval.

Findings indicate that presence of human papillomavirus (HPV) may be associated with the development of cervical cancer.

The Papanicolaou (Pap) cytologic smear is used principally for early detection of cervical cancer and diagnosis of precancerous and cancerous conditions of the vulva and vagina. In the United States, 50 million Pap smears are performed annually. The U.S. Preventive Services Task Force recommends conventional Pap tests every 3 years for women ages 21 to 65 years. Women ages 30 to 65 years may choose co-testing (Pap test plus HPV testing) every 5 years. After age 65 years with prior normal tests, she may choose to stop cervical screening (Table 11.3). This test is also used for diagnosis of inflammatory and infectious diseases. HPV testing is recommended for all women with a Pap cytologic diagnosis of atypical squamous cells of undetermined significance (ASCUS).

The value of the Pap smear depends on the fact that cells readily exfoliate (or can be easily stripped) from genital cancers. Cytologic study can also be used for assessing response to administered sex hormones. The microbiologic examination on cytology samples is not as accurate as bacterial culture, but it can provide valuable information.

Specimens for cytologic examination of the genital tract are usually obtained by vaginal speculum examination or by colposcopy with biopsy. Material from the cervix, endocervix, and posterior fornix is obtained for most smears. Smears for hormonal evaluation are obtained from the vagina.

CLINICAL ALERT

1. Cytologic findings alone do not form the basis for a diagnosis of cancer or other diseases. Often, they are used to justify further procedures, such as biopsy.
2. The Pap smear has been approved by the U.S. Food and Drug Administration (FDA) for diagnosis of cancer and HPV.

In an effort to standardize reporting of cervical-vaginal cytology specimens, the Bethesda System for reporting cervical-vaginal diagnoses was developed by a 1977 National Cancer Institute workshop and slightly modified after a second workshop in 1991 and revised in 2001. This reporting system has been adapted by many laboratories nationwide. The terminology of this reporting system appears in Chart 11.1. The Bethesda System 2001 recommends deleting hormonal evaluation. Hormonal evaluation is a crude measure of estrogen-like effects on squamous cells.

The AutoPap System received preliminary approval from the FDA in early 1998 and is the first device of its kind to receive a recommended approval for automated initial Pap smear screening. With the AutoPap system (NeoPath, Inc., Redmond, WA), ~25% of submitted Pap smears would receive AutoPap review only and would not need to be seen by a technologist.

TABLE 11.3 Cervical Cancer Screening Guidelines for Average-Risk Women[a]

		American Cancer Society (ACS), American Society for Colposcopy and Cervical Pathology (ASCCP), and American Society for Clinical Pathology (ASCP)[b] 2012	U.S. Preventive Services Task Force (USPSTF)[c] 2012	American Congress of Obstetricians and Gynecologists (ACOG)[d] 2012
When to start screening[e]		Age 21. Women age <21 yr should not be screened regardless of the age of sexual initiation or other risk factors. *(Strong recommendation)*	Age 21. *(A recommendation)* Recommend against screening women age <21 yr. *(D recommendation)*	Age 21 regardless of the age of onset of sexual activity. Women age <21 yr should not be screened regardless of age at sexual initiation and other behavior-related risk factors. *(Level A evidence)*
Statement about annual screening		Women of any age should not be screened annually by any screening method. *(Strong recommendation)*	Individuals and healthcare providers can use the annual Pap test screening visit as an opportunity to discuss other health problems and preventive measures. Individuals, healthcare providers, and health systems should seek effective ways to facilitate the receipt of recommended preventive services at intervals that are beneficial to the patient. Efforts also should be made to ensure that individuals are able to seek care for additional health concerns as they present.	In women ages 30–65 yr, annual cervical cancer screening should not be performed. (*Level A evidence*) Patients should be counseled that annual well-patient visits are recommended even if cervical cancer screening is not performed at each visit.
Screening method and intervals[f]				
Cytology (conventional or liquid based)	21–29 yr of age	Every 3 yr.[g] *(Strong recommendation)*	Every 3 yr. *(A recommendation)*	Every 3 yr. *(Level A evidence)*
	30–65 yr of age	Every 3 yr.[g] *(Strong recommendation)*	Every 3 yr. *(A recommendation)*	Every 3 yr. *(Level A evidence)*

HPV co-test (cytology + HPV test administered together)	21–29 yr of age	HPV co-testing should not be used for women age <30 yr.	Recommend against HPV co-testing women age <30 yr. *(D recommendation)*	HPV co-testing[h] should not be performed in women age <30 yr. *(Level A evidence)*
	30–65 yr of age	Every 5 yr *(Strong recommendation)*; this is the preferred method *(Weak recommendation)*.	For women who want to extend their screening interval, HPV co-testing every 5 yr is an option. *(A recommendation)*	Every 5 yr; this is the preferred method. *(Level A evidence)*
Primary HPV testing[i]		For women age 30–65 yr, screening by HPV testing alone is not recommended in most clinical settings. *(Weak recommendation)*[j]	Recommend against screening for cervical cancer with HPV testing (alone or in combination with cytology) in women age <30 yr. *(D recommendation)*	Not addressed.
When to stop screening		Age >65 yr with adequate screening history.[k,l]	Age >65 yr with adequate screening history. *(D recommendation)*[k]	Age >65 yr with adequate screening history.[k,m] *(Level A evidence)*
Screening post-hysterectomy		Women who have had a total hysterectomy (removal of the uterus and cervix) should stop screening.[n] Women who have had a supracervical hysterectomy (cervix intact) should continue screening according to guidelines. *(Strong recommendation)*	Recommend against screening in women who have had a hysterectomy (removal of the cervix).[m] *(D recommendation)*	Women who have had a hysterectomy (removal of the cervix) should stop screening and not restart for any reason.[m] *(Level A evidence)*[o]

table continues on pg. 780 >

TABLE 11.3, continued

	American Cancer Society (ACS), American Society for Colposcopy and Cervical Pathology (ASCCP), and American Society for Clinical Pathology (ASCP)[b] 2012	U.S. Preventive Services Task Force (USPSTF)[c] 2012	American Congress of Obstetricians and Gynecologists (ACOG)[d] 2012
The need for a bimanual pelvic exam	Not addressed in 2012 guidelines but was addressed in 2002 ACS guidelines.[p]	Addressed in USPSTF ovarian cancer screening recommendations (draft).[q]	Addressed in 2012 well-patient visit recommendations.[r] **Age <21 yr**, no evidence supports the routine internal examination of the healthy, asymptomatic patient. An "external-only" genital examination is acceptable. **Age ≥21 yr**, no evidence supports or refutes the annual pelvic examination or speculum and bimanual examination. The decision whether or not to perform a complete pelvic examination should be a shared decision after a discussion between the patient and her healthcare provider. Annual examination of the external genitalia should continue.[s]
Screening among those immunized against HPV 16/18	Women at any age with a history of HPV vaccination should be screened according to the age-specific recommendations for the general population.	The possibility that vaccination might reduce the need for screening with cytology alone or in combination with HPV testing is not established. Given these uncertainties, women who have been vaccinated should continue to be screened.	Women who have received the HPV vaccine should be screened according to the same guidelines as women who have not been vaccinated. *(Level C evidence)*

HPV, human papillomavirus; CIN, cervical intraepithelial neoplasia; Pap, Papanicolaou.

[a]These recommendations do not apply to women who have received a diagnosis of a high-grade precancerous cervical lesion (CIN 2 or 3) or cervical cancer, women with in utero exposure to diethylstilbestrol, or women who are immunocompromised or are HIV positive.

[b]Saslow D, Solomon D, Lawson HW, et al. American Cancer Society, American Society for Colposcopy and Cervical Pathology, and American Society for Clinical Pathology screening guidelines for the prevention and early detection of cervical cancer. CA Cancer J Clin 62(3):147–172, 2012. doi:10.3322/caac.21139. Available at: http://www.cancer.org/Cancer/CervicalCancer/DetailedGuide/cervical-cancer-prevention

[c]USPSTF. Screening for Cervical Cancer. 2012. Available at: http://www.uspreventiveservicestaskforce.org/uspstf11/cervcancer/cervcancerrs.htm. These recommendations apply to women who have a cervix, regardless of sexual history.

[d]ACOG Practice Bulletin No. 131: Screening for Cervical Cancer. ACOG Committee on Practice Bulletins—gynecology. Obstet Gynecol 120(5):1222–1238, 2012. doi:10.1097/AOG.0b013e318277c92a

[e]Because cervical cancer is believed to be caused by sexually transmissible HPV infections, women who have not had sexual exposures (e.g., virgins) are likely at low risk. Women age >21 years who have not engaged in sexual intercourse may not need a Pap test depending on circumstances. The decision should be made at the discretion of the woman and her healthcare provider. Women who have had sex with women are still at risk of cervical cancer. Providers should also be aware of instances of nonconsensual sex among their patients.

[f]Conventional cytology and liquid-based cytology are equivalent regarding screening guidelines, and no distinction should be made by test when recommending next screening.

[g]There is insufficient evidence to support longer intervals in women ages 30–65 years, even with a screening history of consecutive negative cytology tests.

[h]All ACOG references to HPV testing are for high-risk HPV testing only. Tests for low-risk HPV should not be performed.

[i]Primary HPV testing (HPV testing alone) is defined as conducting the HPV test as the first screening test. It may be followed by other tests (like a Pap) for triage.

[j]No further explanation of which clinical settings HPV testing should be used to screen women ages 30–65 years as a stand-alone test.

[k]Current guidelines define adequate screening as three consecutive negative cytology results or two consecutive negative co-tests within 10 years before cessation of screening, with the most recent test performed within 5 years, and are the same for ACS, ACOG, and USPSTF.

[l]Women age >65 years with a history of CIN2, CIN3, or AIS should continue screening for at least 20 years after spontaneous regression or appropriate management. (Weak recommendation)

[m]And no history of CIN 2 or higher.

[n]Unless the hysterectomy was done as a treatment for cervical pre-cancer or cancer.

[o]Women should continue to be screened if they have had a total hysterectomy and have a history of CIN 2 or higher in the past 20 years or cervical cancer ever. Continued screening for 20 years is recommended in women who still have a cervix and a history of CIN 2 or higher. Therefore, screening with cytology alone every 3 years for 20 years after the initial posttreatment surveillance for women with a hysterectomy is reasonable. (Level B evidence)

[p]2002 guidelines statement: The ACS and others should educate women, particularly teens and young women, that a pelvic exam does not equate to a cytology test and that women who may not need a cytology test still need regular healthcare visits including gynecologic care. Women should discuss the need for pelvic exams with their providers. Saslow D, Runowicz CD, Solomon D, et al: American Cancer Society Guideline for the Early Detection of Cervical Neoplasia and Cancer. CA Cancer J Clin 52:342–362, 2002.

[q]The bimanual pelvic examination is usually conducted annually in part to screen for ovarian cancer, although its effectiveness and harms are not well known and were not a focus of this review. No randomized trial has assessed the role of the bimanual pelvic examination for cancer screening. In the PLCO Trial, bimanual examination was discontinued as a screening strategy in the intervention arm because no cases of ovarian cancer were detected solely by this method and a high proportion of women underwent bimanual examination with ovarian palpation in the usual care arm.

[r]ACOG Committee Opinion No. 534: Well-Woman Visit. Committee on Gynecologic Practice. Obstet Gynecol 120(2):421–424, 2012. doi:10.1097/AOG.0b013e3182680517

[s]For women age ≥21 years, annual pelvic examination is a routine part of preventive care even if they do not need cervical cytology screening; but data are lacking to support a specific time frame or frequency of such examinations. The decision to receive an internal examination can be left to the patient if she is asymptomatic and has undergone a total hysterectomy and bilateral salpingo-oophorectomy for benign indications and is of average risk.

Source: http://www.cdc.gov/cancer/cervical/pdf/guidelines.pdf

CHART 11.1 Bethesda System for Reporting Cervical-Vaginal Diagnoses

Bethesda System—2001 (Specimen type: Conventional [Pap] vs. liquid vs. other)

SPECIMEN ADEQUACY

Satisfactory for evaluation (describe presence or absence of endocervical/transformation zone component and any other quality indicators)

Unsatisfactory for evaluation (specify reason):

1. Specimen rejected but processed (specify reason)
2. Specimen processed and examined but unsatisfactory for evaluation of epithelial abnormality because of (specify reason)

GENERAL CATEGORIZATION

Negative for intraepithelial lesion or malignancy

Epithelial cell abnormality (followed by interpretation)

Other: see interpretation/result

INTERPRETATION/RESULT

Negative for intraepithelial lesion or malignancy

Organisms

1. *Trichomonas vaginalis*
2. Fungal organisms morphologically consistent with *Candida* species
3. Shift in flora suggestive of bacterial vaginosis (coccobacillus)
4. Bacteria morphologically consistent with *Actinomyces* species
5. Cellular changes consistent with herpes simplex virus

Other nonneoplastic findings

1. Reactive changes associated with inflammation (includes repair), radiation, intrauterine device (IUD), atrophy, glandular cell status after hysterectomy, or endometrial cells (in women >40 yr of age)

EPITHELIAL CELL ABNORMALITIES

SQUAMOUS CELL TYPE

Squamous cell

Atypical squamous cells of undetermined significance (ASCUS) , cannot exclude high-grade squamous intraepithelial lesion (HSIL) (ASC-H)

LSIL encompassing human papillomavirus (HPV), mild dysplasia, cervical intraepithelial neoplasm (CIN) grade 1 (low-grade precursor)

HSIL encompassing moderate, severe, CIS/ CIN 2 and CIN 3 (grades 2 and 3 are high-grade precursors)

Squamous cell carcinoma

GLANDULAR CELL LESIONS

Atypical

1. Endocervical cells (not otherwise specified [NOS] or specify in comments)
2. Endometrial cells (NOS or specify in comments)
3. Glandular cells (NOS or specify in comments)
4. Endocervical cells, favor neoplastic
5. Glandular cells, favor neoplastic

Endocervical adenocarcinoma in situ

Adenocarcinoma

1. Endocervical
2. Endometrial
3. Extrauterine
4. NOS

ThinPrep Pap Test (Hologic, Marlborough, MA) is a liquid-based cytology method for HPV testing. The Pap smear collection device for ThinPrep is rinsed in a special solution (i.e., PreservCyt) and sent to the lab. A special machine prepares a uniform monolayer Pap smear. These slides are then manually screened in the usual manner. Studies have shown that these ThinPrep smears have a higher rate of detection of biopsy-proven high-grade lesions and a lower rate of false-negative results than conventional Pap smears.

HPV has been identified as the primary causal factor in cervical cancer. Although there are more than 100 types of HPV, types 16 and 18 have been implicated in 70% of cervical cancers and types 6 and 11 in about 90% of genital warts. The Digene HPV Test (Qiagen, Germantown, MD), also known as the hc2 High-Risk HPV DNA Test, is approved in the United States for HPV DNA detection. This test can identify 13 of the high-risk types of HPV in cervical specimens: types 16, 18, 31, 33, 35, 39, 45, 51, 52, 56, 58, 59, and 68 (Fig. 11.2).

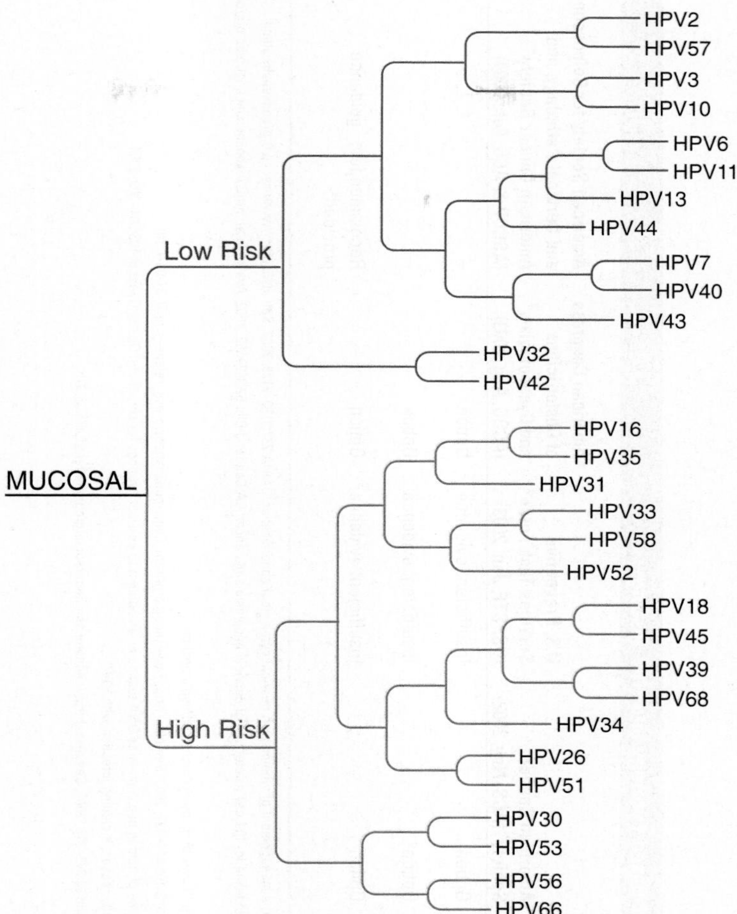

FIGURE 11.2. The human papillomavirus (HPV) DNA high-risk and low-risk subtypes and their relationship. (From Levenson D: A new era in cervical cancer screening. Clin Lab News 33(6), 2007. Reprinted with permission from Mark H. Stoler, MD.)

Primarily, this test is useful to triage or manage women with an ASCUS or equivocal cytology result. It is an efficient, rapid test that is able to differentiate patients with high-risk versus low-risk HPV and can be performed from the same patient specimen when the ThinPrep Pap Test is used. In addition, the FDA has approved testing for *Chlamydia trachomatis* and *Neisseria gonorrhoeae* directly from the ThinPrep sample vial. If the ThinPrep Pap Test is not used, a collection kit is available from Qiagen. Clinicians should check with their laboratories for ordering and collection instructions for any of these tests (Table 11.4).

Reference Values

Normal Pap

No abnormal or atypical cells

No inflammation, no infection, no partially obscuring blood

TABLE 11.4 Recommendations for Liquid-Based Cytology and HPV Testing

	American Society for Colposcopy and Cervical Pathology[a] (ASCCP, Apr. 2002)	American Cancer Society[b] (ACS, Nov. 2002)	U.S. Preventive Services Task Force[c] (USPSTF, Jan. 2003)	American Congress of Obstetricians and Gynecologists[d] (ACOG, Aug. 2003)	American Society for Colposcopy and Cervical Pathology, and American Cancer Society[e] (ASCCP & ACS, Feb. 2004)
Liquid-based cytology	—	Option	Insufficient evidence	Option	—
HPV testing					
Women with ASC-US (reflex testing)	Recommended,[f] guidance provided[a]	Option[g]	Insufficient evidence	Option	—
Women ≥30 years (adjunct to Pap test)	—	Option	Insufficient evidence	Option	Recommended,[f] guidance provided[e]

[a]Wright TC Jr, Cox JT, Massad LS, et al: 2001 consensus guidelines for the management of women with cervical cytological abnormalities. JAMA 287:2120–2129, 2002. See also: http://www.asccp.org/consensus.shtml

[b]Saslow D, Runowicz CD, Solomon D, et al: American Cancer Society guideline for the early detection of cervical neoplasia and cancer. CA Cancer J Clin 52:342–362, 2002. Available at: http://caonline.amcancersoc.org/cgi/content/full/52/6/342

[c]USPSTF: Screening for Cervical Cancer. January 2003. Available at: http://www.ahcpr.gov/clinic/uspstf/uspscerv.htm

[d]ACOG: Cervical Cytology Screening. ACOG Practice Bulletin No. 45. ACOG 102:417–427, 2003. See also: http://www.acog.org/from_home/publications/press_releases/nr07-31-03-1.cfm

[e]Wright TC Jr, Schiffman M, Solomon D, et al: Interim guidance for the use of human papillomavirus DNA testing as an adjunct to cervical cytology for screening. Obstet Gynecol 103:304–309, 2004.

[f]Some exceptions apply (e.g., women who are immunosuppressed for any reason, including infection with HIV).

[g]ACS. Patient Pages: Early Detection of Cervical Cancer. CA Cancer J Clin 52:375–376, 2002. See also: http://caonline.amcancersoc.org/cgi/content/full/52/6/375

Major cell types within normal limits
Negative for intraepithelial cell abnormality of malignancy
Negative for HPV

Procedure

1. Ask the patient to remove clothing from the waist down.
2. Place the patient in a lithotomy position on an examining table.
3. Gently insert an appropriately sized bivalve speculum, lubricated and warmed only with water, into the vagina to expose the cervix (Fig. 11.3).
4. Observe standard precautions (see Appendix A).
5. If a conventional Pap smear, as opposed to liquid base, is being taken, scrape the posterior fornix and the external os of the cervix with a wooden spatula, a cytobrush, or a cytobroom. Smear material obtained on glass slides and place immediately in 95% alcohol or spray fixative before air-drying occurs.
6. If a ThinPrep Pap smear is being taken, use a broom-like collection device. Insert the central bristles of the broom into the endocervical canal deep enough to allow the short bristles to contact the ectocervix fully. Push gently and rotate the broom in a clockwise direction five times. Rinse the broom with a PreservCyt solution vial by pushing the broom into the bottom of the vial 10 times, forcing the bristles apart. As a final step, swirl the broom vigorously to release material. Discard the collection device. Tighten the cap on the solution container so that the torque line on the cap passes the torque line on the vial.
7. Label the specimen with the patient's name, date and time of collection, test(s) ordered, and the area from which the specimen was obtained. Send the specimen to the laboratory with a properly completed information sheet, including date of collection, patient's date of birth, date of last menstrual period, and pertinent clinical history.
8. Examination takes about 5 minutes.
9. See Chapter 1 guidelines for *intratest* care.

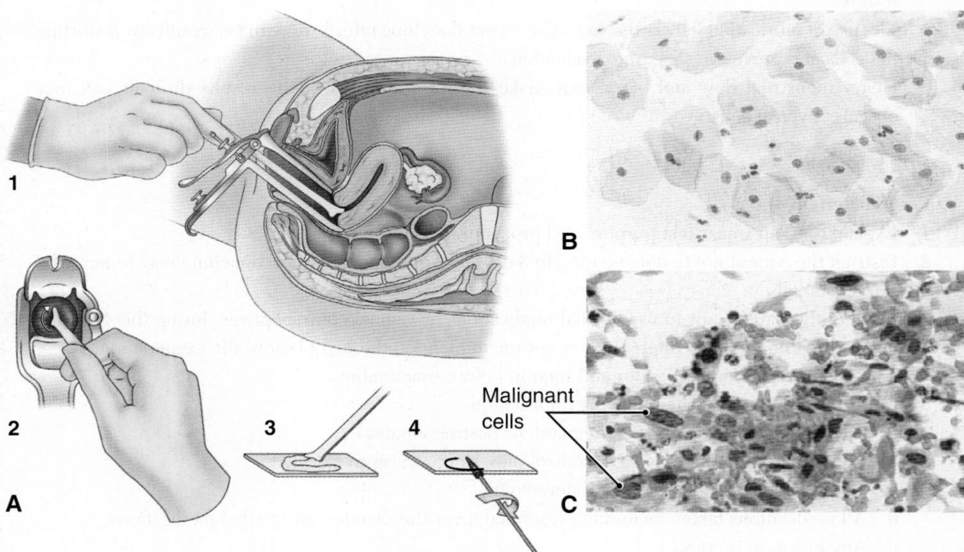

FIGURE 11.3. Papanicolaou (Pap) smear procedure **(A)**; normal cells **(B)**; and malignant cells **(C)**. (A, Reprinted with permission from Timby BK, Smith NE: Introductory Medical-Surgical Nursing, 10th ed. Philadelphia, Lippincott Williams & Wilkins, 2009; B and C, Reprinted with permission from McConnell TH: The Nature of Disease, 2nd ed. Philadelphia, Lippincott Williams & Wilkins, 2013.)

PROCEDURAL ALERT

1. The best time to take a Pap smear is 2 wk after the first day of the last menstrual period, not when the patient is menstruating or bleeding, unless bleeding is a continuous condition.
2. Cytologic specimens should be considered infectious until fixed with a germicidal fixative. Observe standard precautions when handling specimens from all patients.
3. A cytobrush should not be used to obtain a cervical specimen from a pregnant patient.
4. Some nonpregnant patients experience heavy bleeding after a cytobrush is used.

Clinical Implications

1. Abnormal Pap cytologic responses include ASCUS and can be classified as protective, destructive, reparative (regenerative), or neoplastic.
2. Inflammatory reactions and microbes (*Trichomonas vaginalis* and *Monilia, Coccobacillus, Candida,* and *Actinomyces* species, cells indicative of herpes simplex virus [HSV]) can be identified to help in the diagnosis of vaginal diseases and evidence of *Chlamydia trachomatis* and *N. gonorrhoeae.*
3. Reactive cells associated with inflammation, typical surgical repair, radiation, intrauterine contraception devices (IUDs), post-hysterectomy glandular cells, atrophy, and endometrial cells in a woman 40 years of age or older
4. Positive DNA test for HPV
5. Precancerous and cancerous lesions of the cervix can be identified.
6. Deviation from normal physiologic cell patterns may be indicative of a pathologic condition. See Figure 11.4 for a sample cytopathology report.

Interfering Factors

1. Medications such as tetracycline and digitalis, which affect the squamous epithelium, alter test results.
2. The use of lubricating jelly in the vagina or recent douching interferes with test results by distorting the cells and preventing accurate evaluation.
3. Heavy menstrual flow and blood may make the interpretation of the results difficult and may obscure atypical cells.

Interventions

Pretest Patient Care

1. Explain the Pap smear test purpose and procedure.
2. Instruct the patient not to douche for 2 to 3 days before the test because douching may remove the exfoliated cells.
3. Instruct the patient not to use vaginal medications or vaginal contraceptives during the 48 hours before the examination. Intercourse is not recommended the night before the examination.
4. Have the patient empty bladder and rectum before examination.
5. Ask the patient to give the following information:
   a. Age—indicate if adolescent, pregnant, or postmenopausal
   b. Use of hormone therapy, birth control pills, or contraceptive devices
   c. Past vaginal surgical repair or hysterectomy
   d. All medications taken, including prescribed, over-the-counter, and herbal medications
   e. Any radiation therapy
   f. Any other pertinent clinical history (e.g., previous abnormal Pap smear, signs of inflammation or bleeding)
6. Follow Chapter 1 guidelines for safe, effective, informed *pretest* care.

Community Hospital
CYTOPATHOLOGY REPORT

Name: **SMITH, JANE M.** Cytology ID: **C02-4133**
DOB: 9/30/55 (Age: 48) MRN#:
000000000
SS#: 999-99-9999 Collected:
Location: Community Clinic Received:
Provider: Mark Simpson MD

Specimen Source: ThinPrep Pap Test, Cervix/Endocervix
Last Menstrual Period: 2/27/03
Previous Gynecologic Pathology: ASCUS: one time
Treatment History: Colposcopy: 02/02

Specimen Adequacy
Satisfactory for Evaluation
-transformation zone component present

General Categorization
Epithelial cell abnormality

Interpretation
Squamous Cell Abnormality—Atypical squamous cells, undetermined significance.

Educational Notes/Recommendations
Community Hospital recommends following the "2001 Consensus Guidelines for the Management of Women with Cervical Cytological Abnormalities" (JAMA,2002;287:2120–9). Management algorithms have been distributed by Community Hospital and are available online at www.ASCCP.org.

Document reviewed and electronically signed by:
John M. Smith MD
Report Date: 03/15/03

James Doe, M.D. Director 25 Maple Street Burlington, VT 05401 802-999-9999

Note: A disclaimer may appear on cytology reports:
The Pap smear is a screening test for cervical cancer and its precursors. Since its introduction, it has reduced the death rate from cervical cancer by more than 70%. However, the smear is not perfect. As a screening test is has an inherent false negative and false positive rate. Regular Pap smear testing should be used in conjunction with other established clinical practices in evaluating patients for cervical disease. If the results of this Pap test do not correlate with the clinical impression, or do not explain the patient's clinical signs/symptoms, additional studies would be warranted. The Pap test is not a screening test for detecting endometrial pathology.

FIGURE 11.4. Sample cytopathology report.

TABLE 11.5 Further Testing After Abnormal Results of Pap Testing[a]

Adolescents—LSIL	Postmenopausal Women—ASCUS	Women With HSIL
Repeat Pap at 6 and 12 months.	Intravaginal estrogen therapy	Colposcopy with endocervical assessment
Colposcopy if repeat Pap is ASC or above, or HPV DNA at 12 months	After treatment, repeat Pap cytology in 1 week.	If no CIN, review cytology, colposcopy, and histology. If necessary, a revised report is issued.
If positive for high-risk HPV, refer for colposcopy. If positive, perform another colposcopy.	If Pap is negative, repeat at 4–6 months. If repeat is negative, return to regular screening schedule; if either Pap is ASC or above, refer for colposcopy.	If no change found upon review, biopsy to confirm CIN Manage and treat per ASCCP.

[a]For complete recommendations, refer to 2001 ASCCP Consensus Guidelines.

Pap, Papanicolaou; LSIL, low-grade squamous intraepithelial lesions; ASCUS, atypical squamous cells of undetermined significance; HSIL, high-grade squamous intraepithelial lesions; ASC, atypical squamous cell; HPV, human papillomavirus; CIN, cervical intraepithelial neoplasm; ASCCP, American Society for Colposcopy and Cervical Pathology.

2001 Consensus guidelines for the management of women with cervical cytological abnormalities. JAMA 287:2120–2129, 2002.

Posttest Patient Care

1. Give the patient a perineal pad after the procedure to absorb any bleeding or drainage.
2. Review test results; report and record findings. Modify the nursing care plan as needed. Counsel the patient appropriately regarding repeat cytology testing if atypical or abnormal cells are present (Table 11.5).
3. Explain that monitoring and management of women with atypical or abnormal cells follows American Society for Colposcopy and Cervical Pathology (ASCCP) consensus guidelines. Repeat HPV DNA tests and repeat cytology Pap smears are standard.
4. Counsel the patient that treatment may include intravaginal estrogen therapy, diagnostic excisional procedures, or referral to an expert. Management options may vary if the woman is an adolescent, pregnant, or postmenopausal (see Table 11.4 and Chapter 12 for typical procedures). The FDA approved Gardasil in 2006 (cervical cancer vaccine; Merck & Co., Inc., Whitehouse Station, NJ) for girls and women ages 9 to 26 years who have not been exposed to HPV. Gardasil (quadrivalent HPV types 6, 11, 16, and 18, recombinant vaccine) is approved for the prevention of cervical cancer, cervical precancers, vaginal precancers, and genital warts. Topotecan HCl (Hycamtin, GlaxoSmithKline, Philadelphia, PA) has been approved for treatment of stage 4B recurrent or persistent cervical cancer.
5. Follow guidelines in Chapter 1 for safe, effective, informed *posttest* care.

● Anal Smears: Cytologic (Cell) Study

The incidence of anal squamous neoplasms has been increasing, especially in homosexual and bisexual men and in women with multicentric genital tract squamous lesions. When evaluating high-risk populations, the rate of anal cancer has been reported to be as high as 70 cases per 100,000. The etiology and pathogenesis of anal squamous neoplasia are similar to that of cervical squamous neoplasia, including an association with HPV, which has been identified in 90% of anal squamous cancers in reported studies.

Although there are no official guidelines regarding anal cytology screening for anal squamous intraepithelial lesions, smears of the anorectal junction are being done with increasing frequency on high-risk patients. Taking an anal "Pap" is a fairly simple procedure, and samples are handled in a similar fashion to cervical-vaginal Pap smears. Healthcare providers should check with their laboratories for specific handling instructions.

Reference Values

Normal

Negative for intraepithelial cell abnormality or malignancy
Negative for HPV

Procedure

1. Ask the patient to remove clothing from the waist down.
2. Place the patient on the side with the knees drawn up to the chest.
3. Gently insert a Dacron swab or cytobrush into the anus to a distance of 2 to 3 cm, ensuring sampling of the anorectal junction by passing and including the dentate line.
4. Rotate the swab or cytobrush 360 degrees while gently pulling back and forth.
5. Transfer the sample by inserting the swab or brush into a vial of fixative fluid and gently agitate or, if the laboratory prefers, directly apply the sample to a glass slide, which is then placed in 95% alcohol or spray-fixed.
6. Label specimen with the patient's name, date, and test(s) ordered; seal the sample vial in a biohazard bag; and forward to the laboratory with a properly completed requisition.
7. See Chapter 1 guidelines for *intratest* care.

Clinical Implications

1. Abnormal results are indicative of abnormal cytology, anal squamous intraepithelial lesions, or malignancy.
2. Anoscopic and histologic assessment of anal lesions is critical to classify lesions accurately. Any cytologic abnormality should be followed with high-resolution anoscopy, and any lesion should be biopsied to confirm the grade of dysplasia.

Interventions

Pretest Patient Preparation

1. Explain the purpose of the test and the collection procedure. No rectal suppositories should be used before the day of obtaining the smear.
2. Advise that there may be a slight discomfort (e.g., pressure sensation) during insertion and rotation of swab.
3. Follow guidelines in Chapter 1 for safe, effective, and informed *pretest* care.

Posttest Patient Care

1. Give the patient a perineal pad after the procedure to absorb any bleeding or drainage.
2. Review test results; report and record findings. Modify the nursing care plan as needed. Counsel the patient appropriately regarding subsequent testing (anoscopy and biopsy) if an abnormal result is received and there is a possible need for treatment (i.e., excisional procedures).
3. Follow Chapter 1 guidelines for safe, effective, informed *posttest* care.

● Aspirated Breast Cysts and Nipple Discharge: Cytologic (Cell) Study, Fine-Needle Aspiration (FNA) and Cytologic Study of Breast Aspirate and Biomarkers of Cancer Risk

Nipple discharge usually is normal only during the lactation period. Any other nipple discharge is abnormal, and when it occurs, the breasts should be examined for mastitis, duct papilloma, and intraductal cancer. (However, certain situations increase the possibility of finding a normal nipple discharge, such as pregnancy, perimenopausal state, and use of birth control pills.) About 3% of breast cancers and 10% of benign lesions of the breast are associated with abnormal nipple discharge. The contents of the identified breast cyst are obtained by FNA biopsy and are examined to detect malignant cells. Fine-needle periareolar breast aspiration, along with the Gail risk model and certain biomarkers, is used to predict cancer development in high-risk individuals.

Reference Values

Normal

Negative for neoplasia or hyperplasia with atypia
No evidence of high-risk results
No expression of select biomarkers as predictors of future cancer development

Procedure

Nipple Discharge

1. Limit this procedure to patients who have no palpable masses in the breast or other evidence of breast cancer.
2. Wash the nipple with a cotton pledget and pat dry.
3. Gently strip, or milk, the nipple to obtain a discharge. Express fluid until a pea-sized drop appears. The patient may assist by holding a bottle of fixative beneath the breast so that the slide may be dropped in immediately.
4. Spread the nipple discharge directly on glass slides and then drop into the fixative bottle containing 95% alcohol, or spray-fix the slide.
5. Identify the specimen with pertinent data, including from which breast it was obtained, and send it without delay to the laboratory.
6. For all procedures, see Chapter 1 guidelines for *intratest* care.

Fine-Needle Aspiration

1. Administer buffered lidocaine (1%) as a local anesthetic. Use a 1.5-inch, 21-gauge needle with attached 10- to 12-mL syringe prewetted with tissue culture medium. Position needle directly adjacent to areola, avoiding superficial blood vessels. A number of aspirations may be performed in the upper, outer, and inner quadrants of the breast.
2. All cells, if from multiple aspirations, may be pooled in 5 mL of an ice-cold medium in an ice bath and fixed in acetone, methanol, or formalin until stained. Part of the specimen is used for cytologic study, and the rest is used for expression of biomarkers.
3. Use sterile measures and standard precautions.

Clinical Implications

Abnormal results are helpful in identifying:

1. Benign breast conditions, such as mastitis or intraductal papilloma
2. Malignant breast conditions, such as intraductal cancer or intracystic infiltrating cancer
3. FNA results of hyperplasia with atypia are associated with a greater risk for future development of breast cancer.
4. Expression of DNA aneuploidy (≥2+ intensity), p53 expression (≥2+ intensity), HER2/neu expression (≥2+ intensity), nER expression (≥1+ intensity), and EGF-R expression (≥2+ intensity)
5. Also, see breast biopsy prognostic markers and ER, PR, and DNA ploidy.

Interfering Factors

Use of drugs that alter hormone balance (e.g., phenothiazines, digitalis, diuretics, steroids) often results in a clear nipple discharge.

Interventions

Pretest Patient Care

1. Explain the purpose and procedure of the nipple discharge procedure. Oral lorazepam may be given for anxiety.
2. The nipple should be washed with a cotton pledget and patted dry.
3. Follow guidelines in Chapter 1 for safe, effective, informed *pretest* care.

CLINICAL ALERT

The only contraindication is an uncooperative patient.

Posttest Patient Care

1. No special instructions are needed for nipple discharge aftercare because this is not an invasive procedure.
2. Review test results; report and record findings. Modify the nursing care plan as needed. Counsel the patient appropriately about possible further testing (e.g., biopsy) and treatment (e.g., tamoxifen, which reduces breast cancer risk, or antibiotics for infection).
3. After FNA, monitor for hematoma formation and infection. Apply cold packs for approximately 10 minutes, bind breast and chest wall with gauze, and instruct patient to wear a tight-fitting sports bra.
4. Follow guidelines in Chapter 1 for safe, effective, informed *posttest* care.

CLINICAL ALERT

1. Any nipple discharge, regardless of color, should be reported and examined. A bloody or blood-tinged discharge is especially significant.
2. After FNA, a large hematoma may require surgery, and infection may require antibiotics.

• Urine: Cytologic (Cell) Study

Cells from the epithelial lining of the urinary tract exfoliate readily into the urine. Urine cytology is most useful in the diagnosis of cancer and inflammatory diseases of the bladder, the renal pelvis, the ureters, and the urethra. This study is also valuable in detecting cytomegalic inclusion disease and other viral diseases and in detecting bladder cancer in high-risk populations, such as workers exposed to aniline dyes, smokers, and patients previously treated for bladder cancer. A Pap stain of smears prepared from the urinary sediment, filter preparations, or cytocentrifuged smears is useful to identify abnormalities.

Reference Values

Normal

Negative

Epithelial and squamous cells are normally present in urine.

(See also Chapter 3, especially Microscopic Examination of Urine Sediment.)

Procedure

1. Obtain a clean-voided urine specimen of at least 180 mL for an adult or 10 mL for a child.
2. Obtain a catheterized specimen, if possible, if cancer is suspected.
3. Deliver the specimen immediately to the cytology laboratory. Urine should be as fresh as possible when it is examined. If a delay is expected, an equal volume of 50% alcohol may be added as a preservative.

4. Collect urine specimens or bladder washings in wide-mouthed containers; add 50% alcohol if laboratory transport will be delayed. Check with your laboratory for specific instructions.
5. See Chapter 1 guidelines for *intratest* care.

Clinical Implications

1. Findings possibly indicative of inflammatory conditions of the lower urinary tract include:
   a. Epithelial hyperplasia
   b. Atypical cells
   c. Abundance of red blood cells
   d. Leukocytes
2. Findings indicative of viral disease include the following:
   a. Cytomegalic inclusion disease: large intranuclear inclusions
      (1) Cytomegaloviruses or salivary gland viruses are related to the herpes varicella agents.
      (2) Infected people may excrete virus in the urine or saliva for months.
      (3) About 60% to 90% of adults have experienced infection.
      (4) In closed populations (e.g., institutionalized mentally disabled persons, household contacts), high infection rates may occur at an early age.
   b. *Measles*: Characteristic cytoplasmic inclusion bodies may be found in the urine before the appearance of Koplik's spots.
3. Findings possibly indicative of malacoplakia and granulomatous disease of the bladder or upper urinary tract include:
   a. Histocytes with multiple granules in an abundant, foamy cytoplasm
   b. Michaelis-Gutmann bodies in malacoplakia
4. Cytologic findings possibly indicative of malignancy. If the specimen shows evidence of any of the changes associated with malignancy, cancer of the bladder, renal pelvis, ureters, kidney, or urethra may be suspected. Metastatic tumor should be ruled out as well.

NOTE *Inflammatory conditions could be caused by benign prostatic hyperplasia, adenocarcinoma of the prostate, kidney stones, diverticula of bladder, strictures, or malformations.*

NOTE *Cytomegalic inclusion disease is a viral infection that usually occurs in childhood but is also seen in cancer patients treated with chemotherapy and in transplantation patients treated with immunosuppressive drugs. The renal tubular epithelium is usually involved.*

Interventions

Pretest Patient Care

1. Patient preparation depends on the type of procedure being done. Explain the purpose, procedure, benefits, and risks to the patient.
2. If cystoscopy is done, give the patient anesthesia (general, spinal, or local). Refer to Chapter 12 for cystoscopy care.
3. If voided urine is required, instruct the patient in the procedure for collection of a clean-catch specimen.
4. Follow guidelines in Chapter 1 for safe, effective, informed *pretest* care.

CLINICAL ALERT

The only contraindication is an uncooperative patient.

Posttest Patient Care

1. Review test results; report and record findings. Modify the nursing care plan as needed. If cystoscopy is performed gently and with adequate lubrication, the patient should experience only minimal discomfort after the procedure.
2. Be aware that aftereffects may include mild dysuria and transient hematuria, but these should disappear within 48 hours after the procedure. The patient should be able to void normally after a routine cystoscopic examination. Refer to Chapter 12 for cystoscopy care.
3. Follow Chapter 1 guidelines for safe, effective, informed *posttest* care.

● Cerebrospinal Fluid (CSF): Cytologic (Cell) Study

CSF obtained by lumbar puncture is examined for the presence of abnormal cells and for an increase or decrease in the normally present cell population. Most laboratory procedures for study of CSF involve an examination of the leukocytes and a leukocyte count; chemical and microbiologic studies are also done. Cell studies of the CSF also have been used to identify neoplastic cells. These studies have been especially helpful in diagnosis and treatment of the different phases of leukemia. The nature of neoplasia is such that for tumor cells to exfoliate, they must actually invade the CSF circulation and enter such areas as the ventricle wall, the choroid plexus, or the subarachnoid space.

Reference Values

Normal

Total cell count, adult: 0 to 10/mm^3 or 0 to 10 $\times$ 10^9 cells/L (all mononuclear cells)
Total cell count, infant: 0 to 20/mm^3 or 0 to 20 $\times$ 10^9 cells/L
Negative for neoplasia
A variety of normal cells may be seen. Large lymphocytes are most common. Small lymphocytes are also seen, as are elements of the monocytomacrophage series.
The CSF of a healthy person should be free of all pathogens.
Negative for blood

Procedure

1. Obtain four specimens of at least 1 to 3 mL each by lumbar puncture (see Chapter 5).
2. Generally, only one specimen of 1 to 3 mL goes to the cytology laboratory. Other tubes are sent to different laboratories for examination.
3. Label the specimen with the patient's name, date and time of collection, and test(s) ordered.
4. Send the sample immediately to the cytology laboratory for processing.

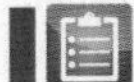

PROCEDURAL ALERT

The laboratory should be given adequate warning that a CSF specimen is being delivered. Time is a crucial factor; cells begin to disintegrate if the sample is kept at room temperature for >1 hr.

Clinical Implications

1. CSF abnormalities may indicate:
   a. Malignant gliomas that have invaded the ventricles or cortex of the brain: leukocytes, 150/mm^3 or 150 $\times$ 10^9 cells/L
   b. Ependymoma (neoplasm of differentiated ependymal cells) and medulloblastoma (a cerebellar tumor) in children
   c. Seminoma and pineoblastoma (tumors of the pineal gland)

d. Secondary carcinomas
   (1) Secondary carcinomas metastasizing to the central nervous system have multiple avenues to the subarachnoid space through the bloodstream.
   (2) The breast and lung are common sources of metastatic cells exfoliated in the CSF. Infiltration of acute leukemia is also common.
e. Central nervous system leukemia
f. Fungal forms
   (1) Congenital toxoplasmosis: leukocytes, 50 to 500/mm^3 or 50 to 500 $\times$ 10^9 cells/L (mostly monocytes present)
   (2) Coccidioidomycosis: leukocytes, 200/mm^3 (200 $\times$ 10^9 cells/L)
g. Various forms of meningitis
   (1) Cryptococcal meningitis: leukocytes, 800/mm^3 or 800 $\times$ 10^9 cells/L (lymphocytes are more abundant than polynuclear neutrophilic leukocytes)
   (2) Tuberculous meningitis: leukocytes, 25 to 1000/mm^3 or 25 to 1000 $\times$ 10^9 cells/L (mostly lymphocytes present)
   (3) Acute pyogenic meningitis: leukocytes, 25 to 1000/mm^3 or 25 to 1000 $\times$ 10^9 cells/L (mostly polynuclear neutrophilic leukocytes present)
h. Meningoencephalitis (primary amebic meningoencephalitis)
   (1) Leukocytes, 400 to 21,000/mm^3 or 400 to 21,000 $\times$ 10^9 cells/L
   (2) Red blood cells are also found.
   (3) Wright's stain may reveal amebas.
i. Hemosiderin-laden macrophages, as in subarachnoid hemorrhage
j. Lipophages from central nervous system destructive processes

2. Characteristics of neoplastic cells
   a. Marked increase in size (usually sarcoma and carcinoma)
   b. Exfoliated cells tend to be more polymorphic as the neoplasm becomes increasingly malignant.

Interfering Factors

The lumbar puncture can occasionally cause contamination of the specimen with squamous epithelial cells or spindly fibroblasts.

Interventions

Pretest Patient Care

1. Explain the procedure to the patient (see Chapter 5). A local anesthetic will be used. Ask whether the patient has a history of reacting to local anesthetic. CSF is collected in tubes and delivered immediately to the laboratory. No fixative is added to the specimen. Instruct the patient that the procedure may be uncomfortable and that immobilization is extremely important. The patient should be instructed to breathe normally and not to hold the breath. Provide the patient with physical and emotional support during the procedure.
2. Follow guidelines in Chapter 1 for safe, effective, informed *pretest* care.

CLINICAL ALERT

The only contraindication is an uncooperative patient.

Posttest Patient Care

1. Place the patient in a supine position. Keep the head of the bed flat for 4 to 8 hours as ordered; if headache occurs, elevate the feet 10 to 15 degrees above the head. Assist and teach the patient to turn and deep breathe every 2 to 4 hours. Blood pressure, pulse, and respiration should be checked

every 15 minutes four times, then every hour four times, and then as ordered. Control pain as ordered and observe the site of puncture for redness, swelling, or drainage; report any symptoms to the healthcare provider.

2. Review test results; report and record findings. Modify the nursing care plan as needed.
3. Follow guidelines in Chapter 1 for safe, effective, and informed *posttest* care.

● Effusions (Thoracentesis and Paracentesis): Cytologic (Cell) Study

Effusions are accumulations of fluids. They may be exudates, which generally accumulate as a result of inflammation (tuberculosis, abscess, pancreatitis), lung infarct or embolus, trauma, or systemic lupus erythematosus (SLE), or transudates, which are fluids not associated with inflammation (i.e., cirrhosis, congestive heart failure, and nephrotic syndromes). Table 11.6 compares these two effusions.

Fluid contained in the pleural, pericardial, peritoneal, or abdominal cavity is a serous fluid. Accumulation of fluid in the peritoneal cavity is called ascites.

Cytologic studies of effusions (exudates or transudates) are helpful in determining the cause of these abnormal collections of fluids. The effusions are found in the pericardial sac, the pleural cavities, and the abdominal cavities. The chief problem in diagnosis is in differentiating malignant cells from reactive mesothelial cells.

Reference Values

Normal

Negative for abnormal cells

Procedure

1. General procedure
   a. Obtain material for cytologic examination of effusions by either thoracentesis or paracentesis.
   b. Remember that both of these procedures involve surgical puncture or a cavity aspiration of a fluid.
   c. Fluid may be obtained in syringes, vacuum bottles, or other containers, depending on the volume of accumulated fluid. Heparin may be added to prevent clotting. Check with your laboratory for specific instructions.

TABLE 11.6 Comparison of Exudate and Transudate Effusions

Exudate	Transudate
1. Accumulates in body cavities and tissues because of malignancy or inflammation	1. Accumulates in body cavities from impaired circulation
2. Associated with an inflammatory process	2. Not associated with an inflammatory process
3. Viscous; opaque to purulent	3. Highly fluid
4. High content of protein, cells, and solid materials derived from cells	4. Low content of protein (<2.5–3.0 g/dL or <25–30 g/L), cells, or solid materials derived from cells
5. May have high white blood cell content	5. Has low white blood cell content
6. Clots spontaneously (contains high concentration of fibrinogen)	6. Will not clot
7. Malignant cells as well as bacteria may be detected	7. Malignant cells may be present
8. Specific gravity >1.016	8. Specific gravity <1.016

2. Thoracentesis procedure
   a. Ensure that chest x-rays are available at the patient's bedside so that the location of fluid may be determined.
   b. Give the patient a sedative if necessary.
   c. Expose the chest. The healthcare provider inserts a long thoracentesis needle with a syringe attached.
   d. Withdraw at least 40 mL of fluid. It is preferable to withdraw 300 to 1000 mL of fluid.
   e. Collect the specimen in a clean container and add heparin if necessary, particularly if the specimen is very bloody (5 to 10 U of heparin per milliliter of fluid). Do *not* add alcohol.
   f. Label the specimen with the patient's name, date and time of collection, and test(s) ordered; the source of the fluid; and the diagnosis.
   g. Send the covered specimen immediately to the laboratory. (If the specimen cannot be sent at once, it may be refrigerated.)
3. Paracentesis (abdominal) procedure
   a. Ask the patient to void.
   b. Place the patient in Fowler's position.
   c. Give a local anesthetic.
   d. Introduce a no. 20 needle into the patient's abdomen and withdraw fluid, 50 mL at a time, until 300 to 1000 mL has been withdrawn.
   e. Follow the same procedure for collection and transport of the specimen as for thoracentesis.
   f. For all procedures, see Chapter 1 guidelines for *intratest* care.

CLINICAL ALERT

Paracentesis can precipitate hepatic coma in a patient with chronic liver disease. The patient must be continually assessed for indications of shock: pallor, cyanosis, or dizziness. Emergency stimulants should be ready.

Clinical Implications

1. All effusions contain some mesothelial cells. (Mesothelial cells make up the epithelial layer covering the surface of all serous membranes.) The more chronic and irritating the condition, the more numerous and atypical are the mesothelial cells. Histiocytes and lymphocytes are common.
2. Evidence of abnormalities in serous fluids is characterized by:
   a. Degenerating red blood cells, granular red cell fragments, and histiocytes containing blood. Presence of these structures means that injury to a vessel or vessels is part of the condition causing fluid to accumulate.
   b. Mucin, which is suggestive of adenocarcinoma
   c. Large numbers of polymorphonuclear leukocytes, which is indicative of an acute inflammatory process such as peritonitis
   d. Prevalence of plasma cells, which suggests parasitic infestation, Hodgkin's disease, or hypersensitive state
   e. Presence of many reactive mesothelial cells together with hemosiderin histiocytes, which may indicate:
      (1) Leaking aneurysm
      (2) Rheumatoid arthritis
      (3) Lupus erythematosus
   f. Malignant cells

3. Abnormal cells may be indicative of:
   a. Malignancy
   b. Inflammatory conditions

Interfering Factors

Vigorous shaking and stirring of specimens causes altered results.

Interventions

Pretest Patient Care

1. Explain the purpose of the test and the procedure. The procedure varies depending on the site of fluid accumulation. General patient preparation includes measuring blood pressure, temperature, pulse, and respiration; administering sedation as ordered; preparing local anesthetic as ordered; providing emotional support; and obtaining a signed consent form.
2. Be aware that local anesthetic and sedative may be ordered to achieve a state of conscious sedation.
3. Follow guidelines in Chapter 1 for safe, effective, informed *pretest* care.

CLINICAL ALERT

The only contraindication is an uncooperative patient.

Posttest Patient Care

1. Review test results; report and record findings. Modify the nursing care plan as needed. Monitor according to agency protocols.
2. Check blood pressure, pulse, and respirations every 15 minutes for 1 hour, then every 2 hours for 4 hours, and as ordered. Check temperature every 4 hours for 24 hours. Apply adhesive bandage or dressing to site of puncture. Check dressing every 15 to 30 minutes. Turn patient onto the unaffected side for 1 hour and then to a position of comfort. Manage pain as indicated. Measure and record the total amount of fluid removed; note its color and character.
3. See guidelines in Chapter 1 for safe, effective, informed *posttest* care.

● Skin/Cutaneous Immunofluorescence Biopsy: Cytologic (Cell) Study and Histologic (Tissue) Study

Biopsy of the skin for direct epidermal fluorescent studies is indicated in the investigation of certain disorders such as lupus erythematosus, blistering disease, and vasculitis. Skin biopsies are also used to confirm the histopathology of skin lesions, to rule out other diagnoses (e.g., herpes simplex and psoriasis), and to monitor the results of treatment.

Reference Values

Normal

A descriptive interpretative report of the skin biopsy is made.

Procedure

1. Obtain a 3- to 6-mm punch biopsy or shave biopsy, excisional biopsy, or incisional biopsy specimen of involved or uninvolved skin. Scraping smears and/or aspirates also may be obtained. Take care not to crush the specimen.
2. Check with your laboratory for specific guidelines for specimen handling.
3. See Chapter 1 guidelines for *intratest* care.

Clinical Implications

1. Biopsy of skin shows the lesions of discoid lupus erythematosus as a band-like immunofluorescence of immunoglobulins and complement components. Similar findings in a biopsy of normal skin are consistent with SLE and may be used to monitor the results of treatment.
2. In blistering diseases such as pemphigus and pemphigoid, in which circulating antibodies may not be present, a lesion may show intercellular epidermal antibody of pemphigus or basement membrane antibody of pemphigoid.

Interventions

Pretest Patient Care

1. Explain the purpose and procedure of the skin biopsy. Local anesthesia will be used.
2. Follow guidelines in Chapter 1 for safe, effective, informed *pretest* care.

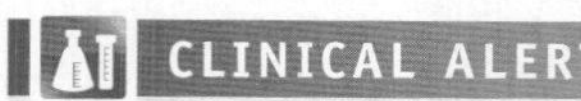

Contraindications include:

1. An uncooperative patient
2. Bleeding diathesis—anticoagulant therapy

Posttest Patient Care

1. Review test results; report and record findings. Modify the nursing care plan as needed. Monitor biopsy site for infection or bleeding.
2. See Chapter 1 for safe, effective, informed *posttest* care.

● Estrogen/Estradiol Receptor (ER), Progesterone Receptor (PR) Histologic (Tissue) Study and DNA Ploidy (Tumor Aneuploidy)

Cancers have abnormal amounts of nuclear DNA. The higher the grade of tumor cells, the more likely the DNA content will be abnormal. The determination of tumor ploidy (the number of chromosome sets in a cell; i.e., diploid, two sets; triploid, three sets) is made by various methods: Flow cytometry, histograms, and image analysis divide cells into triploid/diploid (slowly replicating cells) or aneuploid (rapidly replicating cells).

ER and PR in the cells of breast and endometrial cancer tissues are measured to determine whether the cancer is likely to respond to endocrine therapy or to removal of the ovaries. DNA ploidy measures cell turnover in a specimen identified as cancer and predicts progress, shorter survival, and relapse in some patients with cancer of the bladder, breast, colon, endometrial, prostate, kidney, or thyroid. The predictive value is greater for breast, prostate, and colon.

Reference Values

Normal

ER: negative; <3 femtomole (fmol)/mg (<3.0 nmol/kg) of protein

PR: negative; <5 fmol/mg (<5.0 nmol/kg) of protein

DNA index (DI): 0.9 to 1.0 is normal DNA ploidy (content) or the diploid state.

An interpretive histogram by flow cytometry classifies the stained nucleic as DNA diploid, DNA aneuploid, DNA tetraploid, or DNA uninterpretable.

Procedure

1. Obtain a fresh specimen by biopsy, keep on ice, and deliver immediately to the histology laboratory.
2. Examine a 1-g specimen of quickly frozen tumor for saturation and express in a Scatchard plot. Do not place the specimen in formalin. Some laboratories can perform estrogen receptor assay (ERA)/progesterone receptor assay (PRA) studies on paraffin-embedded tissue. Check with your laboratory for specific instructions.
3. Classify specimens for DNA ploidy on the basis of the percentage of epithelial cells that contain diploid (2n) DNA content and nondiploid DNA (aneuploid). DNA content is calculated as the DNA index.
4. See Chapter 1 guidelines for *intratest* care.

Clinical Implications

1. A positive test for ER occurs at levels of 10 fmol/mg (10 nmol/kg) and for PR binding at levels of 10 fmol/mg (10 nmol/kg). The frequency of positive ER and PR is higher in postmenopausal women.
2. Approximately 50% of ER-*positive* tumors respond to antiestrogen therapy, and 60% to 70% respond in patients with both ER- and PR-positive tumors.
3. ER-*negative* tumors rarely respond to antiestrogen therapy.
4. The finding of positive progesterone increases the predictive value of selecting patients for hormonal therapy.
5. The presence of aneuploid peaks in the replicative activity of neoplastic cells may be prognostically significant, independent of tumor grade and stage.
6. The greater the amount of cells in S phase (DNA synthesis) of the cell cycle, the more aggressive the tumor.
7. Positive aneuploidy points to a favorable prognosis in some conditions, such as acute lymphoblastic lymphoma and neuroblastoma and perhaps transitional cell bladder cancer.

Interventions

Pretest Patient Care

1. Explain purpose and procedure of testing. See Histologic (Tissue) Biopsy Studies: Overview; Prognostic and Predictive Markers and Breast Biopsy: Cytologic (Cell) and Histologic (Tissue) Study and Prognostic Markers. Obtain appropriate clinical history so that this information can be provided with the specimen.
2. Be aware that positive ER and PR means that antiestrogen drug therapy may be beneficial.
3. Follow guidelines in Chapter 1 for safe, effective, informed *pretest* care.

CLINICAL ALERT

Contraindications include:

1. An uncooperative patient
2. Bleeding diathesis tendency—anticoagulant therapy

Posttest Patient Care

1. Review test results; report and record findings. Modify the nursing care plan as needed. Counsel the patient appropriately about possible treatment.
2. Follow Chapter 1 guidelines for safe, effective, informed *posttest* care.

OVERVIEW OF GENETIC STUDIES

Genetics is concerned with the components and function of biologic inheritance. Genetic testing investigates the presence, absence, or activity of genes through direct and indirect means and by chemical analysis, microscopic methods, submicroscopic techniques, and molecular biology studies. Cytogenetics is the part of genetics concerned with the structure and functions of cells, especially chromosomes. Genetic tests are done to identify inborn errors of metabolism, to determine sex when ambiguous genitalia are present, and to detect chromosome aberrations such as Down syndrome. As genetics moves toward genomics, the thrust expands from considering the effects of single genes to the interactions and subsequent functions of genes within the genome.

Insight into causes of developmental problems, birth defects, and heritable disorders often involves genetic studies. Basic technology counts the chromosomes in a person's cells or measures the amount of specific proteins and enzymes. At the other end of the spectrum, cellular DNA can be assayed with molecular probes designed to identify a unique genetic sequence. Genetic testing is a rapidly evolving field that has shown expanding possibilities, an ever-increasing number of tests, and a unique set of limitations and dilemmas. The challenge includes the interactions of maternal, paternal, and fetal genomes.

Many disease states reflect hereditary components even though general clinical studies usually focus on the disorder itself rather than on its genetic components. This section addresses circumstances that may require biochemical analysis (enzymes, organic acids, amino acids) and DNA tests or cytogenetic (chromosome) studies for proper diagnosis and management.

Testing may be done before birth, neonatally, during childhood or adult life, or postmortem.

Biochemical analysis and tests to detect carrier status of inborn errors of metabolism are done, primarily through detection of abnormal accumulation in body fluids and tissue. Advances in the study of molecular genetics have been affected by the completion of the Human Genome Project. Tests in this category include diagnosis of neoplastic disease (e.g., Philadelphia chromosome in chronic myelocytic leukemia and *N-MYC* gene in neuroblastoma) and inherited disorders (e.g., cystic fibrosis, spinal cerebellar ataxia). Along with genetic testing, a thorough clinical assessment and family history are integral components when diagnosing genetic disorders.

In 2004, the FDA approved Roche Diagnostics' (Indianapolis, IN) DNA technology to aid health-care providers in assessing treatment strategy and dose. The Roche AmpliChip CYP450 Test is used to identify a patient's CYP2D6 and CYP2C19 (cytochrome P-450 isoenzymes) genotype from genomic DNA. These isoenzymes are involved in the metabolism of several antidepressants, antipsychotics, and antiarrhythmics. Identification of the patient's genotype can be predictive of drug metabolism, thereby improving outcome by reducing adverse drug reactions and improving efficacy.

When considering whether or not a patient is a candidate for genetic testing, the following should be taken into consideration: a comprehensive history of the patient's health and lifestyle, family history (tracing back two or three generations if possible), reasons for requesting testing, and available support system. A support system is crucial should the results of testing be positive.

Indications for Testing

1. Prenatal care: Medical management of potentially problematic pregnancies identified through abnormal maternal screening, ultrasound, or family history may include specific genetic testing and realistic information about fetal abnormalities to allow parents to make informed decisions about pregnancy continuation.
2. Newborn screening to detect preventable, common, or treatable disease
3. Investigation of fetal death, stillbirth, or miscarriage
4. Decisive diagnosis: Diagnostic and presymptomatic studies may be done to investigate certain syndromes or diseases related to chromosomal or single gene disorders, for gene status in the diagnosis of cancer, for inherited diseases in carrier status, and to test asymptomatic relatives at risk for

developing significant medical or reproductive problems. As a general rule, presymptomatic testing is *not* offered to minors.

5. Cytogenetic analysis or DNA probes are used to study bone marrow and to check for diagnostic translocations, particularly in leukemias (cells with genetic changes).
6. Assignment of gender in the presence of ambiguous genitalia
7. Genetic counseling: to address prognosis and diagnosis as well as causes and recurrence risks in the context of the family as well as individuals. Genetic counseling often depends on precise testing or chromosomal analysis.

CLINICAL ALERT

1. Tests are not performed purely for information's sake; instead, they are ordered for diagnostic purposes in symptomatic individuals after testing implications are explained for conditions for which treatment is available or in situations in which treatment would be useless.
2. Genetic counseling ideally should be available before and after testing and linked to management (proper medications, diets, hormone replacement) and to educational and age-appropriate therapy programs.
3. Patients should be able to use test results to make their own informed decisions about issues such as childbearing and medical treatment. Privacy is an issue in genetic testing.
4. Everyone carries genes that are potentially harmful or defective to some degree; genetic counseling can put these risks into perspective.
5. Family history along with the medical and personal health records are major tools in identifying genetic disorders.
6. Recognize and document signs of possible genetic disorders:
   a. Birth defects: cleft palate, congenital heart disease
   b. Dysmorphic features: abnormally shaped or low-set ears, extra fingers or toes, large tongue, upward slanting of eyes, flattened face, characteristic features of Down syndrome, hypopigmentation of skin, abnormal color of urine, brittle hair
   c. Growth problems: short stature (found in Down syndrome and Turner's syndrome); tall stature (found in Marfan's syndrome)
   d. Developmental delay: failure to thrive, late achievement of walking or talking, hypotonia
   e. Sensory deficits: early-onset hearing loss or visual impairment; vomiting with hypoglycemia (suggests galactosemia); also, many metabolic disorders only become apparent during recurrent fever and infections
   f. Adult retardation: fragile X syndrome; long face; prominent ears, jaw, and forehead in persons (usually male) with undiagnosed mental retardation

Inheritance in Human Disorders

Genetic information is coded within DNA. This information is packaged into chromosomes that are present in cell nuclei. In humans, 46 chromosomes contain an estimated 30,000 to 50,000 gene pairs. DNA contains four distinct molecules (base pairs). These four base pairs code the information that controls growth, development, and function by providing a template for message molecules called RNA. RNA molecules are involved in the process of transcription (changing a DNA message into a protein) as well as in providing molecules that regulate expression, make the hardware within the cell for building proteins (ribosomes), and also perform many housekeeping functions.

With the exception of red blood cells and egg/sperm cells, there are 23 pairs of chromosomes in human cell nuclei. One of each pair comes from each parent. Twenty-two of these pairs match up and contain copies of the same genes (although the copies may not be identical). These chromosomes are assigned numbers, and they are called *autosomes*. Then, there are two sex chromosomes: X and Y. Females have two X chromosomes; males have one X and one Y chromosome. The Y chromosome is unique to males and contains genes that determine male structure and function and also affect fertility. The Y chromosome contains very few genes, but its presence or absence determines male or female development. Genes, like chromosomes, come in pairs, except for genes on the sex chromosomes.

1. *Autosomal dominant inheritance*. Within one gene pair, an abnormality in a single copy of the gene may produce a disorder. A person with such a gene combination would have a theoretical 50–50 chance of passing this gene on to any offspring. Dominant disorders may therefore be inherited from a parent, or they may arise as a new mutation in an egg or sperm cell that participates in fertilization. For many dominantly inherited conditions, manifestations of the disorder are not consistent. This observation is known as *variable expression*. Examples of dominantly inherited disorders include Huntington's disease, neurofibromatosis, familial hypercholesterolemia, and hereditary colon cancer (Chart 11.2).

   One form of diabetes mellitus (DM), type 2, is an example of autosomal dominant inheritance, although not all cases are hereditary. DM, a disorder of carbohydrate metabolism, can be divided into two categories: type 1 (juvenile onset or insulin dependent) and type 2 (adult onset or non–insulin dependent). The cause of DM is deficient insulin action (insulin action is equal to the product of insulin concentration [B-cell control] and insulin sensitivity [target cell function]). Deficient insulin action leads to disordered carbohydrate, lipid, and protein metabolism. DM type 1 results from insulin deficiency; DM type 2 results from a combination of insulin resistance and relative insulin deficiency.

   About 7% to 10% of breast cancers show an autosomal dominant inheritance pattern. Mutations of the *BRCA-1* (breast cancer 1) and *BRCA-2* (breast cancer 2) genes, found on chromosomes 17 and 13, respectively, account for most breast cancers. Individuals who test positive for mutations should be monitored closely (monthly self-breast examinations and annual or semiannual clinic follow-up), consider chemoprevention (e.g., tamoxifen), and possibly undergo prophylactic surgery (controversial).

   DM type 1: Autoimmune diabetes may result from an interaction of genetics and the environment and results in an absolute insulin deficiency. Type 1 diabetes resulting from autoimmune destruction of pancreatic B cells is not inherited, but susceptibility to type 1 disease is. The major genetic loci indicative of susceptibility to type 1 are located in the HLA complex: DRBI, DQAI, and DQBI.

   DM type 2: Patients with type 2 diabetes (due to insulin resistance and B-cell failure) often have a first-degree relative with the disease and a genetic predisposition to type 2 resulting in a restricted ability of the B cells to secrete insulin. Type 2 DM is inherited as a dominant gene, although not all cases are hereditary. Persons at risk include those with a family history and those who develop gestational diabetes. Type 2 diabetes has been associated with metabolic syndrome. *Metabolic syndrome* is defined as having at least three of the following conditions: hypertension, obesity, hyperglycemia, hypertriglyceridemia, and low high-density lipoprotein (HDL) cholesterol.

CHART 11.2 Types of Genetic Disorders

Autosomal Dominant	Autosomal Recessive	X-Linked Recessive
Familial breast cancer	Sickle cell anemia	Hemophilia A and B
Huntington's disease	Thalassemia β and α	Duchenne's and Becker's muscular dystrophy
Adult polycystic disease (some types)	Cystic fibrosis	Fragile X syndrome
Myotonic dystrophy	α_1-Antitrypsin deficiency	Ornithine transcarbamylase deficiency
	Tay-Sachs disease	

2. *Autosomal-recessive inheritance.* Both copies of the gene pair must not function correctly for a problem to be apparent. If both parents carry the same nonfunctional gene, there is a 1-in-4 chance that any child could inherit two nonfunctional copies, leading to possible disease. Examples of autosomal recessively inherited diseases include cystic fibrosis, sickle cell disease, Tay-Sachs disease, some nonsyndromic early-onset hearing loss, and recurrent pyogenic infections. Primary hemochromatosis, an example of an inherited autosomal recessive disease, is caused by a mutation of the *HFE* gene. This disorder is characterized by excessive absorption and accumulation of iron resulting in tissue damage and subsequently organ damage, such as liver dysfunction. This disorder, treated by phlebotomy at regular intervals (about 500 mL of blood per week, which equates to about 250 mg of iron), is fatal if not diagnosed early. Genotyping is done of the *HFE* gene to include the C2824 and H63D mutations.
3. *X-linked recessive inheritance.* Males have only one X chromosome, so that abnormal genes on the X chromosome can cause problems. Females have a second X chromosome, which usually masks the effects of an abnormal gene, although not always completely. A woman with a disease-causing gene on one X chromosome would have a 50–50 chance of passing this gene to any child, and this is independent of her 50–50 chance of having a son. Examples of X-linked disorders include hemophilia and Duchenne's muscular dystrophy.
4. *Multifactorial inheritance.* Some developmental processes, as well as some adult disease states, are influenced by the interactions of many genes associated with environmental factors. Examples of multifactorial disorders include pyloric stenosis, cleft lip and palate, spina bifida, and schizophrenia.
5. *Cytogenic inheritance.* Chromosomal abnormalities may include abnormal numbers of chromosomes (e.g., Down syndrome is caused by three copies of chromosome 21). Chromosomal rearrangements, called *translocations*, can be unbalanced, causing multiple congenital abnormalities. A molecular abnormality within a single gene can cause structural differences like fragile X mental retardation syndrome. Submicroscopic deletions of chromosomes can be studied using fluorescent in situ hybridization. Examples of human syndromes caused by microdeletions include Williams syndrome and DiGeorge syndrome.
6. *Mitochondrial inheritance.* Separate from the nucleus of the cell are the energy-processing organelles called *mitochondria*. These organelles possess a unique set of genes on a single chromosome. Mutations in these genes can cause a wide variety of disorders, including neuromuscular disorders. Examples include Kearns-Sayre syndrome and Leber's hereditary optic neuropathy. Mitochondria are inherited exclusively from the mother.
7. *Nontraditional inheritance.* Some human genes are sensitive to modification (known as *imprinting* or *methylation*) that alters gene expression, depending on the gender of the parent in which the gene originates. Some human syndromes are caused by the presence of two copies of a gene or chromosome originating from one parent and none from the other (called *uniparental disomy*, or UPD). Examples include Beckwith-Wiedemann syndrome and Prader-Willi syndrome.

Genetic Counseling

Genetic counseling is the process of providing individuals and families with information on the nature, inheritance, and implications of genetic disorders in order to help them make informed medical and personal decisions. Risk assessment, family history, and genetic testing to clarify genetic status of family members may be part of the genetic counseling process.

Genetic counselors are healthcare professionals with specialized education, training, and experience in medical genetics. They frequently work as part of a team that includes physicians and other specialists in biochemistry and genetics, and they coordinate activities with many medical specialties, including prenatal care, pediatric specialties, neurology, hematology, and laboratory testing.

Genetic counseling services are available at or through most major medical centers in the United States and serve the medical and lay communities as sources of information, clinical evaluation, management of genetic conditions and birth defects, and coordination with appropriate testing services. Geographic listings of genetic clinics and genetic counselors can be found online at http://www.genetests.org and http://www.nsgc.org.

When testing for genetic disease is being considered, pretest counseling may include additional attention to issues of realistic usefulness of currently available tests and consideration of personal, family, privacy, and insurance implications of testing. Just because a test is available does not mean it is appropriate—unwanted information can be generated by genetic testing, tests may cost thousands of dollars, and ambiguous results are possible.

Posttest counseling not only presents test results but also reviews medical and psychological implications for the family and potentially may be expanded to include other family members for counseling and testing. Once identified, experience with rare genetic diseases will add to the direction of specific medical care and therapy, and patient education and counseling can assist with the process of identifying options and resources.

The number of specific genetic tests is increasing rapidly, although availability may be limited and the cost may not be covered by health insurance. An additional dilemma is the lack of usefulness of testing in many disorders to rule out a specific diagnosis. (For example, a tall, thin individual with some cardiac findings like mitral valve prolapse may be thought to have Marfan's syndrome. Currently, testing for the gene that causes Marfan's syndrome can be done, but it does not find many mutations, even in individuals who are known to have the syndrome.)

Often, it is necessary to study an affected family member to determine what gene mutation is present in a family. This can be problematic in diseases like breast cancer because the affected person may be deceased, unavailable, or uncooperative because of family dynamics. If a family wishes to be studied but no gene mutation is identified, linkage studies might be considered to estimate risks within a family.

Because the possibility of identifying gene changes associated with human disease now exists, so does the expectation and challenge of improving treatment and understanding of both rare and common diseases.

GENETIC STUDIES

Direct Detection of Abnormal Genes by DNA Testing

Many genetic diseases continue to be detected by the effects they produce in body structure, function, or chemistry. With the elucidation of gene structure and the cataloging of human gene mutations, direct detection of hundreds of mutations is possible. For known genetic disorders for which specific mutational analysis is not available, indirect analysis using varied techniques, including protein expression, may be applicable.

Genetic testing for diagnostic purposes requires patient education and consent, healthcare provider request, and coordination of sample collections. Diagnostic tests must be done in a Clinical Laboratory Improvement Act (CLIA)–approved laboratory. Research labs cannot provide this service and should not be contacted for clinical testing.

Sensitivity of testing in genetic disease needs to be addressed because many diseases may have different causes, and many genetic tests are not capable of finding all mutations in complex genes. For example, nearly 1000 gene mutations have been linked to cystic fibrosis, but still, an estimated 3% to 10% of mutations cannot be found. Interpretation of results can be a challenge also, especially in situations in which a gene change can be demonstrated, but it is not known whether it is a harmless change. An example of this is polymorphism in the *BRCA-1* gene. In such situations, interpretation may rely on comparison to gene changes found in known affected relatives.

A variety of morbid genetic changes have been discovered, including gain or loss of a single base pair or larger group of base pairs as well as repetitive sequences that get copied over and over so many times that they disable the function of the gene. Detection strategies are tailored to the type of mutation present or suspected.

Procedure

1. Establish availability and sensitivity of clinical testing and inform the patient of the benefits, limitations, and consequences of testing (see Genetic Counseling). Informed consent may be required. Prepayment may be required. Test results may take weeks or months.
2. Obtain samples or specimens of body fluids or tissues as specified by the receiving CLIA-approved laboratory. Overnight shipment must usually be arranged.

Clinical Implications

1. Improved diagnosis of types of cancer may have therapeutic implications.
2. Discovery of hereditary disease or cancer may have implications for other family members.
3. Precise DNA tests can be done for some inherited diseases (e.g., cystic fibrosis, Duchenne's and Becker's muscular dystrophy, some polycystic kidney diseases).
4. Paternity identity testing and forensic testing
5. Identification of microbes in infectious diseases (e.g., *Chlamydia*, cytomegalovirus)
6. Prediction of progression in neuromuscular disorders (e.g., Huntington's disease, myotonic dystrophy, cerebellar ataxia)
7. Identification of comorbid disease risks (e.g., progressive kidney failure in some hearing loss syndromes)
8. Identification of reproductive risks
9. Explanation of miscarriage and stillbirth
10. Potential associations with common diseases of aging (e.g., cardiovascular disease, Alzheimer's disease)

CYTOGENETICS

● Chromosomal Analysis

The karyotype, a study of chromosome distribution for an individual, determines chromosome numbers and chromosome structure (Chart 11.3); alterations in either of these can produce problems. The standard karyotype can be a diagnostic precursor to genetic counseling. Additional or missing pieces of most chromosomal material cause developmental problems. Despite much speculation, it is not known exactly how these abnormalities translate into structural or functional anomalies. Predictions almost always depend on comparisons with clinical findings from other similar cases that present the same evidence.

Standard chromosome studies can be helpful in evaluation of the following clinical situations:

1. Multiple malformations of structure and function
2. Failure to thrive
3. Mental retardation
4. Ambiguous genitalia or hypogonadism
5. Recurrent miscarriages
6. Infertility
7. Primary amenorrhea or oligomenorrhea
8. Delayed onset of puberty
9. Stillbirths or miscarriages (particularly with associated malformations)

CHART 11.3 Definition and Nomenclature of Karyotype

Background

The karyotype is an arrangement of the chromosomes on a cell in a specific order, from the largest size to the smallest, so that their number and structure can be analyzed. This is routinely done through banding, a technique that permits detection of the differences in structure between the different pairs. Before banding, it was often impossible to pair chromosomes correctly; instead, they were arranged in groups according to size and structure and labeled A through G. The X chromosomes were part of group C, and the Y chromosomes belonged to group E. Now, they are usually placed with each other, apart from the other pairs.

The pairs of chromosomes are differentiated according to the following characteristics:

1. Their length
2. The location of the centromere, the constriction that divides chromosomes into long (q) and short (p) arms
3. Ratio of the long and short arms to each other
4. Secondary constrictions
5. Satellites, which are small, variable pieces of DNA seen at the ends of the arms of some chromosomes
6. Staining or banding patterns. A variety of different stains and techniques can be used. The most common is Giemsa banding. Most of the other methods, such as centromeric or fluorescent staining, are restricted to specific situations.

Nomenclature of the Karyotype

The standard conventions for listing karyotypes are as follows:

1. The first number denotes the total number of chromosomes.
2. The sex chromosome complement follows (usually XX for normal females and XY for normal males).
3. The missing, extra, or abnormal chromosomes are identified.
4. The letter "p" refers to the short arm, "q" to the long arm.
5. Bands are numbered from the centromere out. As techniques evolve, these are further subdivided. For example, in the two-digit number 32, the first number (3) is the band and the second number (2) is the subdivision of that band (band 32). Decimal points indicate further division under the same system; for example (working backward), 32.41 is the first subdivision (1) of the fourth subdivision (4) of the second subdivision of the third band.
6. A three-letter code at the end designates the banding technique. The first letter is the type of banding; the second letter denotes the general technique; the third letter indicates the stain. Probably the most common code is GTG: band type G, banding by trypsin, using Giemsa stain. Special or unusual techniques are used only in selected circumstances.

More than 80 other abbreviations can be used to label other structural findings. Some of the more common ones are mentioned in clinical implications of chromosome analyses.

10. Prenatal diagnosis of potential or actual abnormalities related to chromosome disorders (e.g., Down syndrome, especially in offspring of mothers >35 years of age)
11. Detection of parents with chromosomal mosaicism or translocations, who may be at high risk for transmitting genetic abnormalities to their children
12. Selected cancers and leukemias in which abnormalities of the chromosomes may reveal prognosis or disease stage

Reference Values

Normal

46 chromosomes

Women: 44 autosomes + 2 X chromosomes (karyotype 46,XX)

Men: 44 autosomes + 1 X and 1 Y chromosome (karyotype 46,XY)

A photograph of representative karyotype is included with report.

Procedure

Specimens for chromosome analyses are generally obtained as follows, using aseptic procedures and special kits and containers:

1. Heparinized venous blood leukocytes from peripheral vascular blood samples are used most frequently because they are the most easily obtained. Preparation of the cells takes at least 3 days. The time required is directly proportional to the complexity of the analytic process.
2. Collect bone marrow in a green-topped tube, at least 5 mL in a heparinized syringe (20 to 25 units of heparin). Biopsies can sometimes be completed within 24 hours. Bone marrow analysis is often done to diagnosis certain categories of leukemias.
3. Fibroblasts from skin or other surgical specimens can be grown and preserved in long-term culture mediums for future studies. Growth of a sufficient amount of the specimen for studies usually requires at least 1 week. These specimens are especially helpful in detecting mosaicism (different chromosome constitutions in different tissues) and in the study of stillbirths, neonatal death, and spontaneous abortion.
4. Amniotic fluid in the prenatal period obtained through amniocentesis and stored in a sterile container requires at least 1 week to produce a sufficient amount of cell growth for analysis. These studies are often done for prenatal detection of chromosomal abnormalities (see Chapter 15).
5. Chorionic villus sampling (CVS) can be done at earlier stages of pregnancy (~9 weeks) than can amniocentesis. Some initial CVS studies can be done almost immediately after conception. Occasional false-positive results represent mosaicism of the placenta (the presence of several cell lines, some of which may not be found in the fetus). These studies need confirmation of findings through long-term culture (see Chapter 15).
6. Grow cells from fetal tissue or from early-trimester products of conception to determine causes of spontaneous abortion. Cells from the fetal surface of the placenta may be easiest to grow and are the most likely to be successful.
7. Take the buccal smear, for detecting sex chromosomes, from the inner cheek and use fluorescent in situ hybridization with probes specific for the X or Y chromosome.
8. Take dried blood spot from heel of newborn.
9. Place specimens of lymph nodes or solid tumors in sterile containers.
10. Chromosome analysis is often performed using other specimens, such as skin, fascia, lung tissue, kidney, or the placenta. At least 2 mm of volume is needed for an adequate specimen.
11. See Chapter 1 guidelines for *intratest* care.

Clinical Implications

Many chromosomal abnormalities can be placed into one of two classes (abnormalities of number and abnormalities of structure).

1. Abnormalities of number
   a. Autosomal
      (1) Trisomy 21 (Down syndrome)
      (2) Trisomy 18 (Edwards' syndrome)
      (3) Trisomy 13 (Patau's syndrome)

b. Sex chromosome syndromes
   (1) Ullrich-Turner syndrome (45, single X)—short stature, webbed neck, and renal and C anomalies
   (2) Klinefelter's syndrome (47,XXXY)—hypogonadism, infertility, learning disabilities, undeveloped secondary characteristics
   (3) XXY; 47,XXY—tall, increased risk for behavior problems
   (4) Triple XXX—increased risk for infertility and behavior problems

2. Abnormalities of structure
   a. Deletions
      (1) Cri du chat (cat's cry syndrome): The distal part of the chromosome 5 short arm is deleted.
      (2) Missing short arm of chromosome 18: 18p– is deleted.
      (3) Prader-Willi syndrome: 15q is deleted in some cases.
   b. Duplications: extra material from the second band in the long arm of the third chromosome: 3q2 trisomy (Cornelia de Lange's syndrome resemblance)
   c. Translocations: translocation of chromosomes 11 and 22: t(11;22) or 14 and 21
   d. Isochromosomes: a single chromosome with duplication of the long arm of the X chromosome: i(Xq) (a variant of Turner's syndrome)
   e. Ring chromosomes: a chromosome 13 with the ends of the long and short arms joined together, as in a ring: r(13)
   f. Mosaicism: two cell lines, one normal female and the other for Turner's syndrome: 46,X; 45,X

Interventions

Pretest Patient Care

1. Provide information and referrals for appropriate genetic counseling and treatment if necessary.
2. Explain the purpose, procedure, and limitations of the genetic test together with the known risks and benefits. This education process should be done by a genetic counselor.
3. Obtain a signed, witnessed consent form. This is required for most genetic tests.
4. Follow Chapter 1 guidelines for safe, effective, informed *pretest* care.

Posttest Patient Care

1. If an amniotic fluid specimen or CVS is obtained for analysis, follow the same precautions as listed in Chapter 15.
2. Provide timely information and compassionate support and guidance for parents, children, and significant others.
3. Follow guidelines in Chapter 1 for safe, effective, informed *posttest* care.

CLINICAL ALERT

1. Occasionally, it is possible to line up a certain chromosomal pattern with specific genes and to then understand the clinical picture from analyzing these results. However, for the most part, the association between specific chromosomal abnormalities and specific sets of findings is not yet well understood. Interpretations from karyotype studies usually come from correlations with similar cases rather than from any theoretical considerations. Therefore, because many variables exist, predictions must be made cautiously and judiciously.
2. Most laboratories provide interpretations of results. However, it may be necessary to talk directly with laboratory personnel to fully understand the meaning of an unusual karyotype.

Special Chromosomal Studies

Fragile X syndrome is one of the most common genetic causes of mental retardation. An X-linked trait, it is more commonly seen in males. Females may carry this gene without exhibiting any of its characteristics; however, they can also be as severely affected as males. This syndrome takes its name from the small area on the long arm of the X chromosome that looks like a break in the arm (although it actually is not). The cells need to be grown in a special medium to reveal this pattern; a regular karyotype will miss it. Even with the special medium, not all cells show the characteristic. In female carriers of this trait, the syndrome becomes harder to detect as the woman ages. Accurate detection of fragile X syndrome at a molecular level is now available.

Rare conditions such as excess chromosome breakage (Fanconi's anemia) or abnormal centromeres (Roberts' syndrome) merit special analytic processes and procedures. Chromosome and molecular analyses are done using a venous blood sample (5 mL with ethylenediaminetetraacetic acid tube) to identify the fragile X mental retardation syndrome and possible carrier status.

Newborn Screening for Congenital Disorders

Most industrialized countries of the world require screening of newborns to detect congenital and metabolic disorders within the first week of life. In the United States, only three disorders—phenylketonuria (PKU), congenital hypothyroidism (CH), and galactosemia (GAL)—are screened in all states. Some states have expanded screening using tandem mass spectrometry (MS/MS) technology to screen for >20 genetic metabolic disorders. Providing and performing the testing and following up on all abnormal results are the responsibility of state health departments. For those babies with a confirmed congenital disorder, genetic counseling, treatment, and long-term care are also provided in most states (e.g., special dietary formula for PKU children). Recently, pilot programs have been undertaken to develop protocols to screen for severe combined immune deficiency (SCID), which affects 1 in 100,000 newborns. SCID is often fatal, characterized by no immune response because of a defect of the white blood cell. If identified within a few weeks of birth, 95% of cases can be cured by bone marrow transplantation.

Screening for congenital hearing loss has become a standard of care for all newborns in the United States. The prevalence of permanent hearing loss is about 1 to 3 of every 1000 live births. Before implementation of newborn hearing screening, most children were typically older than 2 years before congenital hearing loss was detected. Unfortunately, by this age, children have difficulty developing speech and language skills. However, when identified at a much earlier age and with intervention, by 6 months, these children can develop language skills equal to children with normal hearing.

Procedure

1. Newborn blood is sampled using a heel-stick procedure in the first week of life (see Chapter 2).
2. Apply the blood drops (<0.5 mL in total) to a piece of special filter paper, which usually contains three to five printed circles.
3. Fill all the printed circles with blood, which in most cases can be done with one drop of blood per circle.
4. Be sure the attached coverslip does not come into contact with the blood until completely dry. Do not permit the blood-soaked portion of the collection kit to come in contact with another surface (e.g., desktop, absorbent paper). Proper collection procedures are based on the National Committee on Clinical Laboratory Standards (NCCLS) document LA4-A5: Blood Collection on Filter Paper for Newborn Screening Programs; Approved Standard.
5. In addition to the filter paper, the collection kit also contains a multipart form requesting information regarding the baby's name, mother's name, birth date and time, specimen collection

data and time, birth weight, and so forth. It is important that this form be filled out completely because the information is critical for the laboratory staff in the interpretation of test results. For example, differentiating normal from abnormal thyroid-stimulating hormone (TSH) results for potential hypothyroidism may be dependent on the age (in hours) of the infant at the time of specimen collection.

6. After the specimen is collected, allow the blood card to air-dry in a horizontal position for a minimum of 3 hours at room temperature. After the blood is dried, the specimen should be forwarded (mail or courier) to the screening laboratory within 24 hours.
7. Although the process may vary among newborn screening laboratories, most testing begins by punching a ⅛-inch blood spot into a 96-well microplate (or some other vessel such as a test tube or dimple tray).
   a. Basic chemistry procedures are completed, such as measurement of phenylalanine or galactose metabolites.
   b. Electrophoresis technology or liquid chromatography is used to separate hemoglobin fractions.
   c. Immunochemistry (e.g., antigen-antibody reactions) is used to measure thyroid hormones (hypothyroidism), 17-hydroxyprogesterone (congenital adrenal hyperplasia), and immunoreactive trypsinogen enzyme (cystic fibrosis).
   d. Gene mutation analysis is used to detect the genetic mutation causing the disorder (e.g., cystic fibrosis, abnormal hemoglobin). Mutation analysis is used as a second-tier assay to improve the specificity of the primary assay.
   e. MS/MS technology has allowed newborn screening programs to expand significantly the number of disorders screened. The disorders fall into four groups: fatty acid oxidation (FAO), organic acidemia (OA), urea cycle (UC), and aminoacidopathies (AA). The FAO and OA disorders are detected by measuring acylcarnitine (an intermediate compound containing fatty acids or organic acids combined with carnitine that occurs from blocked metabolic pathways), and the UC and AA disorders are determined by measuring a specific set of amino acids. At least 30 different disorders can be detected by this technology.
8. Urine samples can also be collected using dried urine filter paper strips. Because the collection of liquid urine from neonates is difficult and transportation of frozen urine is expensive, the use of filter paper strips is more convenient.
9. Hearing can be tested using otoacoustic emissions (OAEs) or automated auditory brainstem responses (ABR). With OAEs, an earphone is placed in the infant's ear canal and emits certain tones or clicks. Sounds subsequently produced by the inner ear are recorded. Alternatively, ABR also requires an earphone being placed in the ear canal; however, three electrodes on the head, neck, and shoulder record neural activity in response to tapping noises emitted from the earphone. The infant is asleep during these procedures.

Chart 11.4 is a list of disorders that currently can be detected through newborn screening. It should be noted that the information provided is generally not considered all-inclusive, and results are considered presumptive (requiring confirmation before a formal diagnosis is made and treatment implemented). The State Public Health Laboratory or Health Department in specific states or regions can provide information about the status of newborn screening in a particular state or region. Most screening programs have two levels of abnormal results. The first level are those abnormal results considered borderline. The likelihood of such results being indicative of a disorder is low, and most are resolved by repeating the newborn screen. The second level of abnormal results are those considered urgent. These results are highly indicative of a disorder and require immediate follow-up and confirmation, usually at a clinic specializing in the disorder. Abnormal values represent the absence of expected enzyme activity, elevated or decreased hormone values, presence of abnormal or variant hemoglobins, abnormal levels of amino acids, or presence of a genetic mutation.

CHART 11.4 Disorders Currently Detectable Through Newborn Screening

Biotinidase

Prevalence:	1:100,000
Substance measured:	Biotinidase enzyme activity
Determined by:	Basic chemistry
Abnormal:	No enzyme activity
Interfering factors:	Transfusions may cause a false-negative result
Additional diagnostic testing:	Serum/plasma enzyme quantification
Treatment:	Biotin—daily supplements
Clinical symptoms (not treated):	Seizures, dermatitis, hair loss

Congenital Adrenal Hyperplasia (CAH)

Prevalence	1:10,000
Substance measured:	17-Hydroxyprogesterone (17-OHP)
Determined by:	Immunochemistry
Abnormal (cutoff):	Elevated 17-OHP: typical cutoff range: >90 ng/dL (>2.7 nmol/L) is considered critical in full-term babies. Cutoffs will vary by program in low-birth-weight babies.
Interfering factors:	False positives can be expected in low-birth-weight babies and early sample collections (<24 hr).
Diagnostic testing:	Refer to a pediatric endocrinologist for CAH workup
Treatment:	Glucocorticoid replacement, 9-α-fluorohydrocortisone
Clinical symptoms (not treated):	Salt-losing crisis in males that often results in death Virilization (ambiguous genitalia) in females

Congenital Hypothyroidism

Prevalence:	1:3000
Substance measured:	Thyroid-stimulating hormone (TSH) and/or thyroxine (T_4)
Determined by:	Immunochemistry
Abnormal (cutoff):	Elevated TSH: typical cutoff range: 20–50 μIU/mL (258–645 nmol/L) (program dependent) Decreased T_4: typical cutoff range: 6–8 μg/dL (77–103 nmol/L) (program dependent)
Interfering factors:	False positives can be expected in early (<24 hr) discharges. False negatives can occur in very-low-birth-weight babies.
Additional diagnostic testing:	Serum T_4 and TSH measurements Thyroid scan (warranted in some cases)
Treatment:	Synthroid—daily supplements
Clinical symptoms (not treated):	Mental retardation, cretinism, liver failure

Cystic Fibrosis (CF)

Prevalence:	1:4000 (Caucasians)
Substance measured:	Immunoreactive trypsinogen (IRT) Mutant alleles
Determined by:	Immunochemistry Polymerase chain reaction (PCR)
Interfering factors:	False negatives can occur because some CF mutations may not cause an IRT elevation.
Abnormal (cutoff):	Elevated IRT: typical cutoff range: 140–180 ng/mL (program dependent) Mutation analysis: detection of one or two mutant alleles

continues on pg. 812 >

CHART 11.4, continued

Additional diagnostic testing:	Pilocarpine iontophoresis sweat chloride test
Treatment:	Care at a CF foundation–approved center
Clinical symptoms (not treated):	Persistent diarrhea, malnutrition, chronic cough, respiratory diseases (infections)
Hemoglobinopathies (Sickle Cell Disease)	
Prevalence:	1:400 (African Americans)
Substance measured:	Hemoglobin fractions (e.g., fetal, sickle, adult, hemoglobin C)
Determined by:	Electrophoresis and/or high performance liquid chromatography (HPLC)
Abnormal:	Detection of hemoglobin(s) other than fetal and adult
Interfering factors:	Transfusions will invalidate testing for up to 60 days
Additional diagnostic testing:	Hemoglobin detection and quantification on whole blood
Treatment:	Penicillin—daily supplements
Clinical symptoms (not treated):	Sepsis, pain crisis, death (25% of babies)

Fatty Acid Oxidation (FAO) Disorders

	Prevalence:
Medium-chain acyl-CoA dehydrogenase (MCAD)	1:20,000
Short-chain acyl-CoA dehydrogenase (SCAD)	1:10,000
Long-chain 3-hydroxyacyl-CoA dehydrogenase (LCHAD)	1:50,000
Very-long-chain acyl-CoA dehydrogenase (VLCAD)	1:50,000
Glutaric acidemia type II (GAII)	1:100,000
Carnitine palmitoyltransferase deficiency type II (CPT-II)	Unknown
2,4-Dienoyl-CoA reductase deficiency	Unknown
Carnitine/acylcarnitines translocase (CAT)	Unknown
Carnitine uptake defect (CUD)	Unknown
Medium/short-chain hydroxyacyl-CoA dehydrogenase (M/SCHAD)	Unknown
Medium-chain 3-ketoacyl-CoA thiolase (MCKT)	Unknown
Trifunctional protein (TFP) deficiency	Unknown

Substance measured:	Acylcarnitines
Determined by:	Tandem mass spectrometry
Abnormal:	Each FAO disorder has a distinctive acylcarnitine profile. The exact profile is program dependent.
Interfering factors:	False negatives may occur if specimen collection is delayed (>14 d).
Diagnostic testing:	Consult with a certified biochemical geneticist. Urine organic acids; mutation analysis
Treatment:	Diet restrictions that are disorder dependent
Clinical symptoms (not treated):	Vomiting, lethargy, hypoglycemia, hypotonia; sudden death or permanent neurologic damage can occur
Galactosemia	
Prevalence:	1:50,000
Substance measured:	Total metabolites (galactose and galactose-1-phosphate) and/or galactose-1-phosphate uridyltransferase (GALT)
Determined by:	Basic chemistry
Abnormal (cutoff)	Elevated metabolites
	Typical cutoff range: 10–15 mg/dL or 555–832 µmol/L (program dependent)
	No GALT activity

continues on pg. 813 >

CHART 11.4, continued

Interfering factors:	False negatives may occur if there has not been a lactose load before specimen collection. Transfusions may cause false negatives also.
Additional diagnostic testing:	Serum/plasma metabolite levels, GALT activity quantification Mutation analysis
Treatment:	Lactose restriction diet
Clinical symptoms (not treated):	Sepsis, milk intolerance; mental retardation, sudden death can occur.

Organic Acidemia (OA) disorders

	Prevalence:
Glutaric acidemia type I (GAI)	1:100,000
Isovaleric acidemia (IVA)	1:100,000
2-Methylbutyryl-CoA-dehydrogenase (2MBCD)	1:45,000
3-Methylcrotonyl-CoA carboxylase (3MCC)	1:30,000
Methylmalonic acidemia (Mutase, Cbl A and Cbl B, Cbl C and Cbl D)	1:50,000
Mitochondrial acetoacetyl-CoA thiolase (β-KT)	1:150,000
Propionic acidemia (PA)	1:150,000
3-Hydroxy-3-methylglutaryl-CoA lyase (HMG)	Unknown
Isobutyryl-CoA dehydrogenase (IBD)	Unknown
Malonyl-CoA decarboxylase (MA)	Unknown
3-Methylglutaconyl-CoA hydratase (3MGA)	Unknown
2-Methyl-3-hydroxybutyryl-CoA dehydrogenase (MHBD)	Unknown
Multiple CoA carboxylase (MCD)	Unknown

Substance measured:	Acylcarnitines
Determined by:	Tandem mass spectrometry
Abnormal:	Each OA disorder has a distinctive acylcarnitine profile. The exact profile is program dependent.
Interfering factors:	False negatives may occur if specimen collection is delayed (>14 days).
Diagnostic testing:	Consult with a certified biochemical geneticist. Urine organic acids; mutation analysis
Treatment:	Diet restrictions that are disorder dependent
Clinical symptoms (not treated):	Vomiting, lethargy, hypoglycemia, hypotonia, sudden death, or permanent neurologic damage can occur.

Phenylketonuria (PKU)

Prevalence:	1:15,000
Substance measured:	Phenylalanine
Determined by:	Basic chemistry or tandem mass spectrometry
Abnormal (cutoff):	Elevated phenylalanine: typical cutoff range: 2.0–4.0 mg/dL or 121.1–242.2 μmol/L (program dependent)
Interfering factors:	False negatives may occur due to lack of protein.
Diagnostic testing:	Serum/plasma amino acid quantification
Treatment:	Dietary restriction of phenylalanine
Clinical symptoms (not treated):	Mental retardation

Maple Syrup Urine Disease (MSUD)

Prevalence:	1:100,000
Substance measured:	Leucine, isoleucine, valine
Determined by:	Basic chemistry or tandem mass spectrometry

continues on pg. 814 >

CHART 11.4, continued

Abnormal (cutoff):	Elevated leucine/isoleucine/valine. Typical cutoff range: 4.0–6.0 mg/dL or 304.9–457.4 μmol/L (program dependent) Elevated valine: Typical cutoff 2.0 mg/dL (250 μmol/L)
Interfering factors:	False negatives may occur because of lack of protein.
Diagnostic testing:	Serum/plasma amino acid quantification
Treatment:	Dietary restrictions of branched-chain amino acids
Clinical symptoms (not treated):	Lethargy, vomiting, coma, mental retardation
Homocystinuria	
Prevalence:	1:150,000
Substance measured:	Methionine
Determined by:	Basic chemistry or tandem mass spectrometry
Abnormal (cutoff):	Elevated methionine. Typical cutoff range: 1.0–2.0 mg/dL or 67–134 μmol/L (program dependent)
Interfering factors	False negatives may occur because of lack of protein.
Diagnostic testing:	Serum/plasma amino acid quantification
Treatment:	Dietary restrictions of methionine. Cystine supplementation, folic acid, betaine
Clinical symptoms (not treated):	Dislocated lenses, cataracts, muscle weakness, arterial and venous thrombosis, developmental delay
Tyrosinemia	
Prevalence:	1:150,000
Substance measured:	Tyrosine
Determined by:	Basic chemistry or tandem mass spectrometry
Abnormal (cutoff):	Elevated tyrosine: typical cutoff range: 4.0–6.0 mg/dL or 220.8–331.0 μmol/L (program dependent)
Interfering factors	False negatives may occur because of lack of protein.
Additional diagnostic testing:	Serum/plasma amino acid quantification
Treatment:	Dietary restrictions of phenylalanine and tyrosine; liver transplantation
Clinical symptoms (not treated):	Vomiting, diarrhea, renal dysfunction, chronic liver disease, speech delays
Citrullinemia	
Prevalence:	1:150,000
Substance measured:	Citrulline
Determined by:	Tandem mass spectrometry
Abnormal (cutoff):	Elevated citrulline: typical cutoff range: 1.0–2.0 mg/dL or 57.1–114.2 μmol/L (program dependent)
Interfering factors:	False negatives may occur because of lack of protein.
Additional diagnostic testing:	Serum/plasma amino acid quantification Urine—normal levels of argininosuccinic acid
Treatment:	Dietary protein restriction of arginine
Clinical symptoms (not treated):	Vomiting, lethargy, coma, seizures, anorexia, death
Argininosuccinic Acidemia	
Prevalence:	1:150,000
Substance measured:	Citrulline
Determined by:	Tandem mass spectrometry

continues on pg. 815 >

CHART 11.4, continued

Abnormal (cutoff):	Elevated citrulline: typical cutoff range: 1.0–2.0 mg/dL or 57.1–114.2 μmol/L (program dependent)
Interfering factors:	False negatives may occur because of lack of protein.
Additional diagnostic testing:	Serum/plasma amino acid quantification Urine elevations of argininosuccinic acid
Treatment:	Dietary restriction of protein; arginine supplement
Clinical symptoms (not treated):	Lethargy, coma, progressive neurologic deterioration, ataxia

Clinical Implications

1. Most of the congenital disorders are autosomal recessive genetic disorders (the exception being hypothyroidism). This means that for the baby to have one of these disorders, both the mother and father have to carry the abnormal gene that causes the disorder. If the mother and father are carriers, there is a 1-in-4 chance that with each pregnancy, the couple will have an affected baby.
2. Although the disorders can be quite varied in clinical expression, there are common issues. All the disorders are relatively rare. The most frequently detected disorder is hypothyroidism, which occurs in 1 of 3000 births in most states or regions. Some disorders have a frequency rate of 1 in 100,000 or less.
3. All of the disorders, if not detected early and treated promptly, will cause severe medical complications. These complications include mental retardation, neurologic problems, or death.
4. All of the disorders can be detected by laboratory tests in the first few days of life before there are any clinical symptoms.
5. If a disorder is detected early and promptly treated, the baby's quality of life can be significantly improved.
6. The treatments are relatively simple and inexpensive when compared against a lifetime of medical care. For example, several of the metabolic disorders are treated by changes in diet and vitamin supplements.

Interventions

Pretest Patient Care

1. Parents should be informed about the timing and importance of newborn screening. The state newborn screening programs provide, free of charge, educational brochures regarding newborn screening. Be sure the parents receive this material.
2. Most states do not require informed consent to perform newborn screening and have limited reasons for parental refusals. If the parent refuses to have the baby screened and the reason is valid under specific state criteria, have the parents sign a waiver for the baby's healthcare record.
3. Complete the form associated with the newborn screening blood collection kit. Be sure the name on the blood collection card matches the baby whose blood is being drawn.
4. Collect the newborn screening specimen before discharge from the hospital. If the initial specimen was collected before 24 hours of age, obtain a repeat in about 14 days as recommended by the American Academy of Pediatrics.
5. For premature and sick infants, collect an initial specimen as soon as medically possible but no later than the first week of life. Be familiar with your local newborn screening laboratory procedures and policies regarding initial and repeat testing.
6. Collect initial specimen before transfusion, if possible. Be familiar with your local newborn screening laboratory procedures and policies regarding repeat testing when a baby has been transfused.
7. Record the date the specimen was sent to the screening laboratory.

Posttest Patient Care

1. After the testing is complete, the screening laboratory will send a report back to the hospital. Record the receipt and review of the report. The newborn screening laboratory should be contacted if a report is unreasonably delayed (within 10 days of specimen being sent). All reports should be added to the baby's healthcare records as soon as possible after receipt.
2. Most newborn screening programs report two types of abnormal results. One type is considered borderline or possible, if the test results are equivocal or only marginally indicative of a disorder. In most cases, the recommendation is to repeat the newborn screening testing. If the repeat test results are normal, no further action is necessary. Care must be taken to neither alarm the parents nor trivialize the importance of repeat testing. The second type of report issued is when the screening test result is highly indicative of a particular disorder. In this case, the screening laboratory will contact the healthcare provider directly, provide recommendations, and often refer the baby and parents to a specialty clinic for evaluation.
3. Do not institute disorder-specific intervention (e.g., diet changes, antibiotics) until directed by a healthcare provider after consultation with a specialist. The state newborn screening program can provide contact for appropriate specialty clinics or experts in the disorders.
4. Ensure that genetic counseling is provided for those parents whose baby has a confirmed disorder.

CLINICAL ALERT

1. If there is a family history of one of the disorders screened for, notify the newborn screening laboratory so that the specialist can be alerted.
2. The most frequent reason for a retest is that the first specimen was unsatisfactory (inadequate amount of blood or improper use of capillary collection tubes).
3. Be sure the baby gets the newborn screen before hospital discharge or by the seventh day of life for extended hospital stays.
4. Ensure there is a positive correlation between the name written on the blood collection card and the name of the baby being screened.
5. Ensure there is a newborn screening test report in the medical report.
6. Check newborn screening results (including calling the newborn screening laboratory) on babies being readmitted to hospital with severe jaundice, anemia, failure to thrive, seizures, and so forth.
7. Follow-up:
   a. Determine whether family of affected children is compliant with appropriate care.
   b. Additional newborn testing may be done (e.g., electroencephalogram procedure for evoked auditory response).

SPECIAL TYPES OF GENETIC STUDIES

Biochemical Genetics

Testing for hereditary metabolic disorders identifies inborn errors of metabolism (IEMs) and enzyme disorders. Included are amino acids, carbohydrates, cholesterol, cofactors and vitamins, lysosomal shortage, lactic acids, fatty acids, carnitines, organic acids, porphyrins, purines and pyrimidine, and urea.

Molecular genetics includes the diagnosis of neoplastic disorders (e.g., Philadelphia chromosome and neuroblastoma) and the carrier identification and prenatal diagnosis of various inherited disorders (e.g., thalassemia, cystic fibrosis, hemophilia A). In general, it is the mature protein product of a gene that carries out its function.

Population Genetics

Population genetics is the study of genes in populations and of factors that maintain or change the frequency of genes and genotypes from generation to generation. Multifactorial inherited disease deals with traits or diseases not inherited in factors believed to play an important role in causation; examples of these disorders are hypertension, schizophrenia, DM, and common birth defects such as cleft lip, cleft palate, and neural tube defects.

Pharmacogenomics

Pharmacogenomics studies genetic variations and drug metabolism to match the best drug for phenotype (in specific diseases) before beginning therapy. Matching effective drugs to DNA-based diagnostic and predictive markers is expected to be at the forefront of treatment. Examples of tests and collaborating drug and diagnostic test companies include diagnostic tests, genetic markers, and drug targets for schizophrenia, hematochromatosis, peripheral arterial occlusive disease, rheumatoid arthritis, obesity, severe anxiety, stroke, type 2 diabetes (Roche and deCode Genetics Co.), progression of advanced heart disease (Pharmacia and deCode Genetic Companies), and obesity and diabetes (Bayer Corp. and CuraGen Corp.), and markers for colon, breast, and ovarian cancer.

BIBLIOGRAPHY

Abraham J, Gulley JL, Allegra CJ: The Bethesda Handbook of Clinical Oncology, 4th ed. Philadelphia, Lippincott Williams & Wilkins, 2014

American Cancer Society: American Cancer Society guidelines for the early detection of cancer, 2006. CA Cancer J Clin 56:11–25, 2006; last medical review March 11, 2015; last updated July 26, 2016

American Society of Cytopathology Cervical Cytology Practice Guidelines. November 2000. (Online.) Available at: http://www.cytopathology.org/guidelines/guide_cervical_cytology.php

Bertrand J, Floyd RL, Weber MK: Guidelines for identifying and referring persons with fetal alcohol syndrome. MMWR Recomm Rep 54(RR-11):1–14, 2005

Burke W, Atkins D, Gwinn M: Genetic test evaluation: Information needs of clinicians, policy makers, and the public. Am J Epidemiol 156(4):311–318, 2002

DeMay RM: The Art & Science of Cytopathology, 2nd ed. Chicago, ASCP Press, 2012

DeMay RM: Practical Principles of Cytopathology, revised edition. Chicago, ASCP Press, 2009

DeVita VT, Hellman S, Rosenberg SA: Cancer: Principles and Practice of Oncology, 10th ed. Philadelphia, Lippincott Williams & Wilkins, 2014

Dolan S, Biermann J, Damus K: Genomics for health in preconception and prenatal periods. J Nursing Scholarship 39(1):4–9, 2007

Ducatman BS: A tale of two tests: Cytology gyn screening and mammography. Northfield, IL, CAP Today, College of American Pathologists 20(9):67–68, 2006

Hologic, Inc.: The ThinPrep Pap Test. Copyright 2017. (Online.) Available at: http://www.thinprep.com

Gail MH, Brinton LA, Byar DP, et al. Projecting individualized probabilities of developing breast cancer for white females who are being examined annually. J Natl Cancer Inst 81(24):1879–1886, 1989

Kaye CI, Committee on Genetics: Newborn screening fact sheets. Pediatrics 118:934–963, 2006

Kaz AM, Brentnall TA: Genetic testing for colon cancer. Nat Clin Pract Gastroenterol Hepatol 3(12):670–679, 2006

Kuppermann M, Nease RF, Gates E, et al: How do women of diverse backgrounds value prenatal testing outcomes? Prenatal Diagnosis 24:424–429, 2004

Lea DH, Williams JK, Cooksey JA, et al: U.S. genetics nurses in advanced practice. J Nurs Scholarship 38(3):213–218, 2006

Lehman CD, DePeri ER, Peacock S, et al: Clinical experience with MRI-guided vacuum-assisted breast biopsy. Am J Roentgenol 184:1782–1787, 2005

Pasacreta JV, Jacobs L, Cataldo JK: Genetic testing for breast and ovarian cancer risk: The psychological issues. Am J Nursing 102(12):40–47, 2002

Prows CA, Glass M, Nicol MJ, et al: Genomics in nursing education. J Nurs Scholarsh 37(3):196–202, 2005

Salem-Schatz S, Peterson LE, Palmer RH, et al: Barriers to first-week follow-up of newborns: Findings from parents and clinician focus groups. Joint Commission Journal on Quality and Safety 30(11):593–601, 2004

Saslow D, Solomon D, Lawson HW, et al: American Cancer Society, American Society for Colposcopy and Cervical Pathology, and American Society for Clinical Pathology screening guidelines for the prevention and early detection of cervical cancer. CA Cancer J Clin 62(3):147–172, 2012; updated July 26, 2016

Solomon D, Nayar R, Davey DD, et al: The Bethesda System for Reporting Cervical Cytology: Definitions, Criteria and Explanatory Notes, 3rd ed. New York, Springer, 2015

Titus K: Breast specimens: FNA, core, more. CAP Today 16(2), 2002

Tripath Care Technologies: U.S. Products. January 2003. (Online.) Available at: http://www.tripathimaging.com/usproducts/index.htm

U.S. Preventive Services Task Force: Screening for cervical cancer: Clinical summary of U.S. Preventive Services Task Force recommendation, AHRQ Publication No. 11-05156-EF-3, March 2012

U.S. Preventive Services Task Force: Screening for ovarian cancer. Ann Fam Med 2:260–262, 2004; recommendations updated September 2012

Watson MS, Mann MY, Lloyd-Puryear MA, et al: Newborn screening: Toward a uniform screening panel and system. Genetics Med 8(5):15–115, 2006

Wolff AC, Hammond EH, Schwartz JN, et al: American Society of Clinical Oncology/College of American Pathologists: Guideline recommendations for human epidermal growth factor receptor 2 testing in breast cancer. J Clin Oncol 25(1):115–145, 2007

Wright TC Jr, Massad LS, Dunton CJ, et al: 2006 Consensus guidelines for the management of women with abnormal cervical cancer screening tests. Am J Obstet Gynecol 197(4):346–355, 2007

12 Endoscopic Studies

OVERVIEW OF ENDOSCOPIC STUDIES

Endoscopy is the general term given to all examination and inspection of body organs or cavities using endoscopes. Endoscopes can also provide access for certain kinds of surgical procedures or treatments. Endoscopes, known generally as *fiberoptic instruments*, are used for direct visual examination of certain internal body structures by means of a lighted lens system attached to either a rigid or flexible tube. Fiberoptic instruments transmit signals from the tip of the scope via glass or plastic threads to a monitor. Light travels through an optic fiber by means of multiple reflections. Fiberoptic instruments, composed of fiber bundle systems, redirect and transmit light around twists and bends in cavities and hollow organs of the body. An image fiber and a light fiber allow visualization at the distal tip of the scope. Separate ports allow instillation of drugs, lavage, suction, and insertion of a laser, brushes, forceps, or other instruments used for excision, sampling, or other diagnostic and therapeutic procedures. The flexible scope can be inserted into orifices or other areas of the body not easily accessed or directly visualized by rigid scopes or other means. Procedures are done for health screening, diagnosis of pathologic conditions, or therapy, such as removal of tissue (polyps) or foreign objects. Sedatives or analgesia (to achieve a state of conscious sedation) or local or general anesthetics may be used. The use of video documentation and endoscopic sonography (diagnostic imaging for visualizing subcutaneous body structures) also aids in cancer diagnosis, staging of cancer, and determining operability. Biopsy tissue is submitted to the laboratory for histologic examination (see Chapter 11).

● Mediastinoscopy

Mediastinoscopy, performed under general anesthesia, requires insertion of a lighted mirror-lens instrument, similar to a bronchoscope, through an incision at the base of the anterior neck, to examine and biopsy mediastinal lymph nodes. Because these nodes receive lymphatic drainage from the lungs, mediastinal biopsy specimens can allow identification of diseases such as carcinoma, granulomatous infection, sarcoidosis, coccidioidomycosis, and histoplasmosis. Mediastinoscopy is used to stage lung tumors, diagnose sarcoidosis, biopsy and remove mediastinal lymph nodes directly, and assess hilar adenopathy of unknown origin. It has virtually replaced scalene fat pad biopsy for examining suspicious nodes on the right side of the mediastinum. It is the routine method of establishing tissue diagnosis and staging of lung cancer and for evaluating the extent of lung tumor metastasis, done just before thoracotomy. Nodes on the left side of the chest are usually resected through left anterior thoracotomy (mediastinoscopy). This procedure is performed by a thoracic surgeon.

Reference Values

Normal

No evidence of disease
Normal lymph glands

Procedure

1. Mediastinoscopy is considered a surgical procedure and is usually performed under general anesthesia in a hospital.
2. Biopsy is performed through a suprasternal incision in the neck (2 to 3 cm or 3 to 4 cm). When the Chamberlain procedure is performed, a small transverse incision is done in the second intercostal space or over the second or third costal cartilage.
3. Follow guidelines in Chapter 1 for safe, effective, informed *intratest* care.

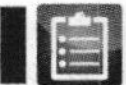

PROCEDURAL ALERT

1. Observe standard precautions and latex precautions for all endoscopic procedures.
2. Endoscopically related bacteremia infections may result from tissue manipulations, bloodstream invasion by pathogens, or a contaminated endoscope, usually due to improper cleansing and disinfection. It is important that strict infection control guidelines be followed by persons who clean and disinfect the endoscopes. Hospitals and clinics should follow the infection control policies for their institution, which should include documentation of all endoscopic procedures, including name of patient, type of procedure, date and time of procedure, and serial number of the endoscope used in each procedure. A log documenting the time, date, and serial number of each endoscope cleaned and disinfected should also be maintained. These records allow for tracing an infection back to a specific instrument. Any infections suspected to have been caused by a contaminated instrument should be reported immediately to the appropriate infection control and risk management departments for investigation.

Clinical Implications

1. Abnormal findings may include the following conditions:
   a. Sarcoidosis (chronic inflammatory cell accumulation in multiple organs)
   b. Tuberculosis
   c. Histoplasmosis (disease caused by the fungus *Histoplasma capsulatum*)
   d. Hodgkin's disease (cancer of the lymphatic system)
   e. Granulomatous infections and inflammatory processes
   f. Carcinomatous lesions
   g. Coccidioidomycosis
   h. *Pneumocystis carinii* infection
2. Results assist in defining the extent of metastatic process, staging of cancer (N2 and N3, IIIa and IIIb), and possibility of successful surgical resectability.

Interventions

Pretest Patient Care

1. Explain the purpose, procedure, benefits, and risks of the test. It is usually used after computed tomography (CT) scan has indicated enlarged mediastinal nodes (>1 cm).
2. A legal surgical consent form must be appropriately signed and witnessed preoperatively (see Chapter 1).
3. Remember that preoperative care is the same as that for any patient undergoing general anesthesia and surgery.
4. Have the patient fast for 8 or more hours before the test.
5. Follow guidelines in Chapter 1 for safe, effective, informed *pretest* care.

Posttest Patient Care

Care is the same as for any patient who has had surgery under general anesthesia.

1. Evaluate breath and lung sounds; check wound for bleeding and hematoma.
2. At time of discharge, monitor for complications (e.g., breathing difficulties, coughing up blood). Instruct the patient to call healthcare provider if problems occur.
3. After endoscopic procedures, assess for fever, elevated white blood cells, signs of bloodstream infection, and signs of sepsis (rigors and hypotension, hypothermia, or hyperthermia).

4. Review test results; report and record findings. Modify the nursing care plan as needed. Monitor patient appropriately and explain any need for follow-up tests or treatment (e.g., medication for tuberculosis, antibiotics).
5. Follow guidelines in Chapter 1 for safe, effective, informed *posttest* care.

CLINICAL ALERT

1. Previous mediastinoscopy contraindicates repeat examination because adhesions make satisfactory dissection of nodes extremely difficult or impossible.
2. Complications can result from the risks associated with general anesthesia and from preexisting conditions, pneumothorax, and subcutaneous emphysema.
3. Damage to major vessels can occur during this procedure.

● Bronchoscopy

Bronchoscopy permits visualization of the trachea, bronchi, and select bronchioles. There are two types of bronchoscopy: flexible (Fig. 12.1), which is almost always used for diagnostic purposes, and rigid, which is less frequently used. This procedure is done to diagnose tumors, coin lesions, or granulomatous lesions; to find hemorrhage sites; to evaluate trauma or nerve paralysis; to obtain biopsy specimens; to take brushings for cytologic examinations; to improve drainage of secretions; to identify inflammatory infiltrates; to lavage; and to remove foreign bodies. Bronchoscopy can determine resectability of a lesion as well as provide the means to diagnose bronchogenic carcinoma. A transbronchial needle biopsy may be performed during this procedure, thus obviating the need for diagnostic open-lung biopsy. A flexible needle is passed through the trachea or bronchus and is used to aspirate cells from the lung. This procedure is performed on patients with suspected sarcoidosis or pulmonary infection.

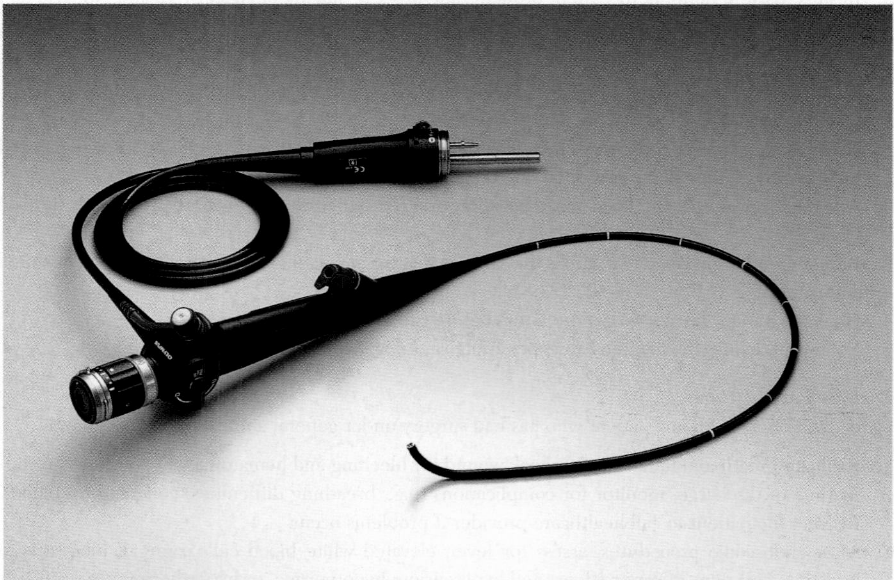

FIGURE 12.1. Fiberoptic bronchoscope (Olympus BF Type P60). (Image courtesy of Olympus America Inc.)

Indications for the Test

1. Diagnostic
   a. Staging of bronchogenic carcinoma
   b. Differential diagnosis in recurrent unresolved pneumonia
   c. Evaluation of cavitary lesions, mediastinal masses, and interstitial lung disease
   d. Localization of bleeding and occult sites of cancer
   e. Evaluate immunocompromised patients (e.g., HIV-positive patients, bone marrow or lung transplant recipients)
   f. Differentiate rejection from infection in lung transplantation
   g. Assess airway damage in thoracic trauma
   h. Evaluate underlying etiology of nonspecific symptoms of pulmonary disease such as chronic cough (>6 months), hemoptysis, or unilateral wheezing
2. Therapeutic
   a. Removal of mucus plugs and polyps
   b. Removal of an aspirated foreign body and to relieve endobronchial obstruction
   c. Brachytherapy (radioactive treatment of malignant endobronchial tumors)
   d. Placement of a stent to maintain airway patency
   e. Drainage of lung abscess
   f. Decompression of bronchogenic cysts
   g. Laser photoresection of endotracheal lesions
   h. Bronchoalveolar lavage (BAL) to remove intra-alveolar proteinaceous material
   i. Alternative to difficult endotracheal intubations
   j. Control bleeding and airway hemorrhage in the presence of massive hemoptysis

The examination is usually done under local anesthesia combined with some form of sedation in an outpatient setting, diagnostic center, or operating room. It also can be done in a critical care unit, in which case the patient may be unresponsive or ventilator dependent.

Reference Values

Normal

Normal trachea, bronchi, nasopharynx, pharynx, and select bronchioles (conventional bronchoscopy cannot visualize alveolar structures)

Procedure

1. Spray and swab topical anesthetic (e.g., 4% lidocaine) onto the back of the nose, the tongue, the pharynx, and the epiglottis. Give an antisialagogue (e.g., atropine) to reduce secretions. If the patient has a history of bronchospasms, administer a bronchodilator (e.g., albuterol) through a handheld nebulizer. Morphine sulfate is contraindicated in patients who have problems with bronchospasm or asthma because it can cause bronchospasm. Analgesics, barbiturates, tranquilizer-sedatives, and atropine may be ordered and administered 30 minutes to 1 hour before bronchoscopy. The patient should be as relaxed as possible before and during the procedure but also needs to know that anxiety is normal.
2. Insert the flexible or rigid bronchoscope carefully through the mouth or nose into the pharynx and the trachea (Fig. 12.2). The scope also can be inserted through an endotracheal tube or tracheostomy. Suctioning, oxygen delivery, and biopsies are accomplished through bronchoscope ports designed for these purposes.
3. Be advised that because of sedation, usually with diazepam (Valium) or midazolam (Versed), the patient is usually comfortable when a state of conscious sedation is achieved. However, when the bronchoscope is advanced, some patients may feel as if they cannot breathe or are suffocating.

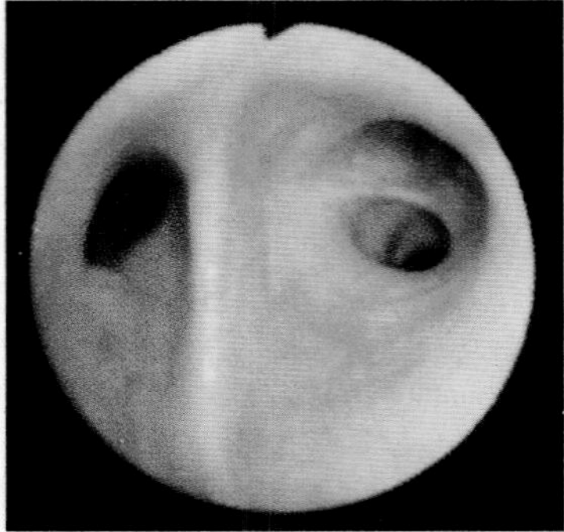
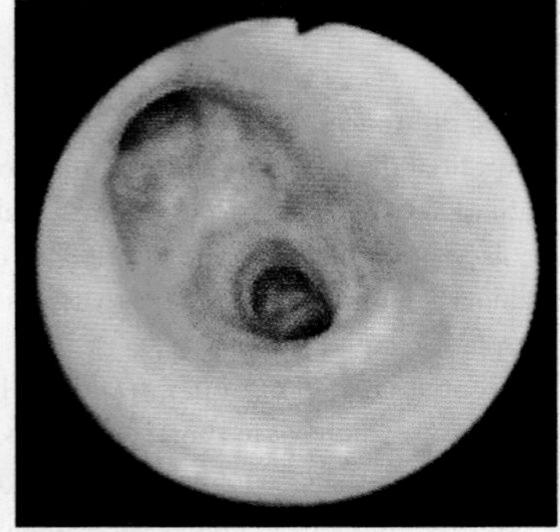

FIGURE 12.2. View of the airway through a bronchoscope. (Image courtesy of Olympus America Inc.)

4. Arterial blood gas measurement during and after bronchoscopy may be ordered, and arterial blood oxygen may remain altered for several hours after the procedure (see Chapter 14). Sputum specimens taken during and after bronchoscopy may be sent for cytologic examination or culture and sensitivity testing. These specimens must be handled and preserved according to institutional protocols (see Chapter 16).
5. Continuous monitoring of electrocardiogram (ECG), blood pressure, pulse oximetry, and respirations is routinely performed. Monitoring of pulse oximetry is especially important to indicate levels of oxygen saturation before, during, and after the procedure.
6. The right lung is usually examined before the left lung.
7. Bronchoscopic procedures include any one or a combination of the following:
   a. Bronchial washings for cytology and staining for fungi and mycobacteria
   b. BAL for infectious diseases (e.g., alveolar proteinosis, eosinophilic granuloma)
   c. Bronchial brushings of both visible and peripheral (under fluoroscopy) endobronchial lesions or transbronchial biopsies, both visible and peripheral
8. Follow guidelines in Chapter 1 for safe, effective, informed *intratest* care.

PROCEDURAL ALERT

Bronchoscopy instruments can decrease an already small airway lumen even more by causing inflammation and edema. Consequently, a child can rapidly become hypoxic and desaturate oxygen very quickly. Resuscitation, oxygen administration equipment, and drugs must be readily accessible when this procedure is performed on a child. Close monitoring of respiratory and cardiac status is imperative during and after the procedure. The same precautions and treatment apply to children and adults. When cardiac arrest occurs in children, it is usually because of respiratory problems, not cardiac problems.

Clinical Implications

Abnormalities revealed through bronchoscopy include the following conditions:

1. Abscesses
2. Bronchitis
3. Carcinoma of the bronchial tree (occurs in the right lung more often than the left)
4. Tumors (usually appear more often in larger bronchi)

5. Tuberculosis
6. Alveolitis
7. Evidence of surgical nonresectability (e.g., involvement of tracheal wall by tumor growth, immobility of a main-stem bronchus, widening and fixation of the carina)
8. *P. carinii* infection
9. Inflammatory processes
10. Cytomegalovirus infection
11. Aspergillosis
12. Idiopathic nonspecific pulmonary fibrosis
13. *Cryptococcus neoformans* infection
14. Coccidioidomycosis
15. Histoplasmosis (disease caused by the fungus *H. capsulatum*)
16. Blastomycosis (fungal infection caused by inhalation of *Blastomyces dermatitidis*)
17. Phycomycosis (group of fungal diseases caused by *Phycomycetes*)

Clinical Considerations

The following data must be available before the procedure: history and physical examination, recent chest x-ray film, recent arterial blood gas values, and if the patient is >40 years of age or has heart disease, ECG. Appropriate blood work (coagulation), urinalysis, pulmonary function tests, and sputum studies (especially for acid-fast bacilli) must be done as well. Bronchoscopy is often done as an ambulatory surgical procedure.

Interventions

Pretest Patient Care

1. Reinforce information related to the purpose, procedure, benefits, and risks of the test. Record signs and symptoms (e.g., dyspnea, bloody sputum, coughing, hoarseness).
2. Emphasize that pain is not usually experienced because lungs do not have pain fibers.
3. Explain that the local anesthetic may taste bitter, but numbness will occur in a few minutes. Feelings of a thickened tongue and the sensation of something in the back of the throat that cannot be coughed out or swallowed are not unusual. These sensations will pass within a few hours following the procedure as the anesthetic wears off.
4. Informed consent form must be properly signed and witnessed (see Chapter 1).
5. Have the patient fast for at least 6 hours before the procedure to reduce the risk for aspiration. Gag, cough, and swallowing reflexes will be blocked during and for a few hours after surgery.
6. Ensure that the patient removes wigs, nail polish, makeup, dentures, jewelry, and contact lenses before the examination.
7. Use techniques to help the patient relax and breathe more normally during the procedure. The more relaxed the patient is, the easier it is to complete the procedure.
8. Follow guidelines in Chapter 1 for safe, effective, informed *pretest* care.

CLINICAL ALERT

Contraindications to bronchoscopy include the following conditions:

1. Severe hypoxemia
2. Severe hypercapnia (carbon dioxide retention)
3. Certain cardiac arrhythmias, cardiac states
4. History of being hepatitis B carrier
5. Bleeding or coagulation disorders
6. Severe tracheal stenosis

Posttest Patient Care

1. Swallowing, gagging, and coughing reflexes should be present before allowing food or liquids to be ingested orally. Usually, the patient has fasted for at least 2 to 6 hours before the procedure.
2. Provide gargles to relieve mild pharyngitis. Monitor ECG, blood pressure, temperature, pulse, pulse oximeter readings, skin and nail bed color, lung sounds, and respiratory rate and patterns according to institution protocols. Document observations.
3. The following may be ordered:
   a. Oxygen by mask or nasal cannula: Humidified oxygen at specific concentrations up to 100% by mask may be necessary.
   b. A chest x-ray film: This will check for pneumothorax or to evaluate the lungs.
   c. Sputum specimen: These must be preserved in the proper medium or solution.
4. Elevate the head of the bed for comfort.
5. Review test results; report and record findings. Modify the nursing care plan as needed. Monitor patient appropriately and explain need for other tests or treatment. Follow-up procedures may be necessary. CT-guided fine-needle cytology aspiration may be done when bronchoscopy is not diagnostic.
6. Do not allow the patient to drive or sign legal documents for 24 hours because of the effects of anesthetics and sedation.
7. Refer to intravenous sedation precautions in Chapter 1.
8. Follow guidelines in Chapter 1 for safe, effective, informed *posttest* care.

CLINICAL ALERT

1. Observe for possible complications of traditional bronchoscopy, which may include the following conditions:
   a. Shock
   b. Bleeding following biopsy (rare, but can occur if there is excessive friability of airways or massive lesions, or if patient is uremic or has a hematologic disorder)
   c. Hypoxemia
   d. Partial or complete laryngospasm (inspiratory stridor) that produces a "crowing" sound; may be necessary to intubate
   e. Bronchospasm (pallor and increasing dyspnea are signs)
   f. Infection or gram-negative bacterial sepsis
   g. Pneumothorax
   h. Respiratory failure
   i. Cardiac arrhythmias
   j. Anaphylactic reactions to drugs
   k. Seizures
   l. Febrile state
   m. Hypoxia, respiratory distress
   n. Empyema (accumulation of pus in the lung pleura)
   o. Aspiration
2. Virtual noninvasive bronchoscopy using spiral CT technology requires no sedation or analgesics. Indications include pulmonary embolism and staging of lung cancer.

• Thoracoscopy

Thoracoscopy is an examination of the thoracic cavity using an endoscope. Video-assisted thoracoscopy (VAT) is available for diagnosing intrathoracic diseases. This procedure can be used as a diagnostic device when other methods of diagnosis fail to present adequate and accurate findings.

Moreover, the discomfort and many of the risks associated with traditional diagnostic thoracotomy procedures are reduced with thoracoscopy. Thoracoscopy allows visualization of the parietal and visceral pleura, pleural spaces, thoracic walls, mediastinum, and pericardium without the need for more extensive procedures. It is used most frequently to investigate pleural effusion and can be used to perform laser procedures; diagnose and stage lung disease; assess tumor growth, pleural effusion, emphysema, inflammatory processes, and conditions predisposing to pneumothorax; and perform biopsies of pleura, mediastinal lymph nodes, and lungs.

Reference Values

Normal

Thoracic cavity and tissues normal and free of disease

Procedure

1. Thoracoscopy is considered an operative procedure. The patient's state of health, the particular positioning needed, and the procedure itself determine the need for either local or general anesthesia. The incision is usually made at the midaxillary line and the sixth intercostal space.
2. Many patients are discharged the following day, provided the lung has reexpanded properly and chest tubes have been removed.
3. Follow guidelines in Chapter 1 for safe, effective, informed *intratest* care.

Clinical Implications

Abnormal findings can include the following conditions:

1. Carcinoma or metastasis of carcinoma
2. Empyema (accumulation of pus in the lung pleura)
3. Pleural effusion
4. Conditions predisposing to pneumothorax or ulcers
5. Inflammatory processes
6. Bleeding sites
7. Tuberculosis, coccidioidomycosis, or histoplasmosis

Interventions

Pretest Patient Care

1. Reinforce and explain the purpose, procedure, benefits, and risks of the examination and describe what the patient will experience. Record preprocedure signs and symptoms.
2. A surgical consent form must be appropriately signed and witnessed before the procedure begins (see Chapter 1).
3. Complete and review required blood tests, urinalysis, recent chest x-ray film, and ECG (for certain individuals) before the procedure.
4. Have the patient fast for 8 hours before the procedure.
5. Insert an intravenous line for the administration of intraoperative intravenous fluids and intravenous medication.
6. Perform skin preparation and correct positioning in the operating room.
7. Place a chest tube and connect to negative suction or sometimes to gravity drainage after the thoracoscopy is completed.
8. Follow guidelines in Chapter 1 for safe, effective, informed *pretest* care.

Posttest Patient Care

1. Take a postoperative chest x-ray film to check for abnormal air or fluid in the chest cavity.
2. Monitor vital signs, amount and color of chest tube drainage, fluctuation of fluid in the chest tube, bubbling in the chest drainage system, and respiratory status, including arterial blood gases. Promptly report abnormalities to the healthcare provider.

3. Administer pain medication as necessary. Encourage relaxation exercises as a means to lessen the perception of pain. Monitor quality and rate of respirations. Be alert to the possibility of respiratory depression related to narcotic administration or intrathecal narcotics.
4. Encourage frequent coughing and deep breathing. Assist the patient in splinting the incision during coughing and deep breathing to lessen discomfort. Promote leg exercises while in bed and assist with frequent ambulation if permitted.
5. Use open-ended questions to provide the patient with an opportunity to express concerns.
6. Document care accurately.
7. Review test results; report and record findings. Modify the nursing care plan as needed.
8. Follow guidelines in Chapter 1 for safe, effective, informed *posttest* care. Provide written discharge instructions.

CLINICAL ALERT

1. *Do not clamp chest tubes unless specifically ordered to do so.* Clamping chest tubes may cause tension pneumothorax. Sudden onset of sharp pain, dyspnea, uneven chest wall movement, tachycardia, anxiety, and cyanosis may indicate pneumothorax. Notify the healthcare provider immediately.
2. Possible wound and pulmonary complications include the following:
   a. Acute respiratory distress, hypoxia
   b. Infection
   c. Hemorrhage (watch for unusually large outputs of blood in a relatively short period of time into the chest drainage system and notify healthcare provider immediately)
   d. Empyema (accumulation of pus in the lung pleura)
   e. Atelectasis
   f. Aspiration
3. Nerve damage may occur during the procedure.

● Esophagogastroduodenoscopy (EGD); Upper Gastrointestinal (UGI) Study; Endoscopy; Gastroscopy

Endoscopy is a general term for visual inspection of any body cavity with an endoscope. Endoscopic examination of the upper gastrointestinal (UGI) tract (mouth to upper jejunum) is referred to when the following examinations are ordered: panendoscopy, esophagoscopy, gastroscopy, duodenoscopy, esophagogastroscopy, or esophagogastroduodenoscopy (EGD).

EGD allows direct visualization of the interior lumen of the UGI tract with a fiberoptic instrument designed for that purpose. EGD is indicated for patients with dysphagia; reflux symptoms; weight loss; hematemesis; melena; persistent nausea and vomiting; persistent epigastric, abdominal, or chest pain; and persistent anemia. EGD can confirm suspicious x-ray findings and establish a diagnosis in symptomatic patients with negative x-ray reports. EGD can be used to diagnose and treat many abnormalities of the UGI tract, including hernias, gastroesophageal reflux disease (GERD), esophagitis, gastritis, strictures, varices, ulcers, polyps, and tumors. It can be used to remove swallowed foreign objects (e.g., a swallowed coin in a small child) and for placement of a percutaneous gastric or duodenal feeding tube. For patients who require some form of UGI surgery, it provides a safe way to perform presurgical screening and postsurgical surveillance.

Reference Values

Normal

UGI tract within normal limits

Procedure

1. Remember that this examination is usually performed in an outpatient setting of a hospital or ambulatory clinic. It also may be performed in the operating room or in a critical care setting.
2. Use a topical spray to anesthetize the patient's throat.
3. Start an intravenous line and use for administration of sedation alone or in combination with analgesics. These medications are given to achieve a state of conscious sedation. Resuscitation equipment must be available.
4. Perform continuous monitoring of the patient's vital signs, ECG, and oxygen saturation (pulse oximetry).
5. Remove partial dental plates or dentures. Insert a mouthpiece to prevent the patient from biting the endoscope and to prevent injury to the patient's teeth, tongue, or other oral structures.
6. Lubricate the endoscope well. Gently insert through the mouthpiece into the esophagus and advance slowly into the stomach and duodenum. Insufflate air through the scope to distend the area being examined so that optimal visualization of the mucosa is possible. Obtain tissue biopsy specimens and brushings for cytology. Take photos to provide a permanent record of observations.
7. Inform the patient that he or she may have an initial gagging sensation that quickly subsides. During the procedure, the patient may belch frequently. Sensations of abdominal pressure or bloating are normal, but the patient should not experience actual pain.
8. Immediately after the examination is completed, ask the patient to remain on his or her left side until fully awake.

Clinical Implications

Abnormal results may indicate the following conditions:

1. Hemorrhagic areas or erosion of an artery or vein
2. Hiatal hernia
3. Esophagitis, gastritis, duodenitis
4. Neoplastic tissue
5. Gastric ulcers (benign or malignant)
6. Esophageal or gastric varices
7. Esophageal, pyloric, or duodenal strictures

Interventions

Pretest Patient Care

1. Explain the purpose and procedure of the examination, the sensations that may be experienced, and the benefits and risks of the test. Refer to intravenous conscious sedation precautions in Chapter 1. Reassure the patient that the endoscope is thinner than most food swallowed. Inform the patient that he or she may be quite sleepy during the EGD and may not recall much or any of the experience. Record preprocedure signs and symptoms (e.g., vomiting, melena [black, tarry feces], dysphagia, and persistent upper gastrointestinal [GI] pain).
2. Patients should be instructed to fast before the procedure, according to the hospital or clinic policy. Generally, adult patients should fast 6 to 8 hours before the examination, and children may have clear liquids up until 2 hours before the procedure; however, each patient should be assessed on an individual basis, according to age, size, and general health status. Inpatients may have intravenous fluids to prevent dehydration. Outpatients need education about potential risks for aspiration and possible cancellation of the procedure if fasting is not maintained.
3. Confirm informed consent. A legal consent must be signed and witnessed before the procedure.
4. Encourage the patient to urinate and defecate if possible before the examination.
5. Follow guidelines in Chapter 1 for safe, effective, informed *pretest* care.

Posttest Patient Care

1. Do not permit food or liquids until the patient's gag reflex returns.
2. Monitor blood pressure, pulse, respirations, and oxygen saturation according to the hospital or clinic policy, usually every 15 to 30 minutes, until the patient is fully awake.
3. Ask the patient to remain on his or her left side with side rails raised until fully awake. This position usually prevents aspiration.
4. Encourage the patient to belch or expel air inserted into the stomach during the examination.
5. Remember that the patient should not experience discomfort or side effects once the sedative has worn off. Occasionally, the patient may complain of a slight sore throat.
6. Review test results; report and record findings. Modify the nursing care plan as needed.
7. Follow guidelines in Chapter 1 for safe, effective, informed *posttest* care.

CLINICAL ALERT

Complications are rare; however, the following complications can occur:

1. Perforation
2. Bleeding or hemorrhage
3. Aspiration
4. Infection
5. Complications from drug reaction (leading to hypotension, respiratory depression or arrest, allergic or anaphylactic response)
6. Complications from unrelated diseases (e.g., myocardial infarction, cerebrovascular accident)
7. Death (very rare)

● Esophageal Manometry

Esophageal manometry measures the movement, coordination, and strength of esophageal peristalsis as well as the function of the upper and lower esophageal sphincters. The test consists of recording intraluminal pressures at various levels in the esophagus and at the upper and lower esophageal sphincters. Intraluminal pressures can be measured with the use of a manometric catheter, which is passed intranasally and then attached to an infusion pump, transducer, and recorder. The intraluminal pressures produce waveform readings (somewhat similar to ECG readings), which can be used to assess esophageal function.

Indications for the Test

1. Abnormal esophageal muscle function
2. Difficulty swallowing (dysphagia)
3. Heartburn
4. Noncardiac chest pain
5. Regurgitation
6. Vomiting
7. Esophagitis

Another test, often done in conjunction with manometry, is the *Bernstein test* (discussed in the following Procedure section, item 6). The Bernstein test is useful for evaluating heartburn, esophagitis, and noncardiac chest pain.

Reference Values

Normal

Normal esophageal and stomach pressure readings
Normal contractions
No acid reflux

Procedure

1. The examination is usually performed in an outpatient setting, such as an ambulatory clinic or healthcare provider's office.
2. Attach the manometric catheter to the infusion pump. Set up the transducer and recording equipment and calibrate according to manufacturer's recommendations.
3. Assess the patient's nasal passage for adequate size and patency. Generously apply a topical anesthetic to the selected nostril.
4. Lubricate the manometric catheter and pass it through the nostril, down the esophagus, and just below the lower esophageal sphincter with the patient in a sitting position. Facilitate this with the patient drinking sips of water through a straw.
5. Begin recording. Pull the catheter through the lower esophageal sphincter, then the esophageal body, and finally the upper esophageal sphincter. Different techniques may be used to obtain recordings. The patient may be asked to swallow, not swallow, take sips of water, or hold his or her breath while the catheter is pulled through.
6. The Bernstein test evaluates for acid reflux by means of a nasogastric tube passed to a point 5 cm above the gastroesophageal junction. Concentration of hydrochloric acid (0.1 N HCl) is infused for 10 minutes into the esophagus to reproduce symptoms of heartburn or chest discomfort. In the first 5 minutes of testing, 0.9% sodium chloride (NaCl) is infused as a control. Testing takes about 15 minutes. The patient may lie down or sit up.
7. Follow guidelines in Chapter 1 for safe, effective, informed *intratest* care.

Clinical Implications

Abnormal recordings reveal the following conditions:

1. Primary esophageal motility disorders, such as achalasia, nutcracker esophagus, or diffuse esophageal spasm
2. Hypertensive lower esophageal sphincter
3. Acid reflux

Interventions

Pretest Patient Care

1. Explain the purpose, procedure, benefits, and risks of the test.
2. Obtain an informed consent that is properly signed and witnessed.
3. Confirm that the patient has fasted for 6 hours before testing.
4. Instruct the patient on the techniques of swallowing, sipping water, and so forth to facilitate accurate recordings.
5. Follow guidelines in Chapter 1 for safe, effective, informed *pretest* care.

Posttest Patient Care

1. Advise the patient that a sore throat and nasal passage irritation are common for 24 hours after the examination. Sensations of heartburn may also persist. Administer antacids if ordered.
2. Observe for or instruct patient to watch for nasal bleeding, signs and symptoms of GI bleeding, or unusual pain.
3. Review test results; report and record findings. Modify the nursing care plan as needed.
4. Follow guidelines in Chapter 1 for safe, effective, informed *posttest* care. Provide written discharge instructions.

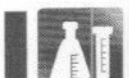

CLINICAL ALERT

Complications are rare; however, the following can occur: aspiration; perforation of nasopharynx, esophagus, or stomach; epistaxis.

Endoscopic Retrograde Cholangiopancreatography (ERCP) and Manometry

This examination of the hepatobiliary system is done through a side-viewing flexible fiberoptic endoscope by instillation of contrast medium into the duodenal papilla, or ampulla of Vater. This allows for radiologic visualization of the biliary and pancreatic ducts. It is used to evaluate jaundice, pancreatitis, persistent abdominal pain, pancreatic tumors, common duct stones, extrahepatic and intrahepatic biliary tract disease, malformation, and strictures and as a follow-up study in confirmed or suspected cases of pancreatic disease.

ERCP manometry can be done to obtain pressure readings in the bile duct, pancreatic duct, and sphincter of Oddi at the papilla. Measurements are obtained using a catheter that is inserted into the endoscope and placed within the sphincter zone.

Reference Values

Normal

Normal appearance and patent pancreatic ducts, hepatic ducts, common bile ducts, duodenal papilla (ampulla of Vater), and gallbladder

Manometry: Normal pressure readings of bile and pancreatic ducts and sphincter of Oddi

Procedure

1. This examination is usually performed in a hospital or outpatient setting where fluoroscopy and x-ray equipment are available.
2. Have the patient gargle, or spray his or her throat with, a topical anesthetic.
3. Start an intravenous line and use for administration of sedatives and analgesics. These medications are given to achieve a state of conscious sedation. In some situations, general anesthesia may be used. Resuscitation equipment must be available.
4. Perform continuous monitoring of the patient's vital signs, ECG, and oxygen saturation (pulse oximetry).
5. Remove partial dental plates or dentures. Insert a mouthpiece to prevent the patient from biting the endoscope and to prevent injury to the patient's teeth, tongue, or other oral structures.
6. Have the patient assume a left lateral position with the knees flexed. The endoscope is well lubricated and inserted via the mouthpiece, down the esophagus and stomach, and into the duodenum. At this point, have the patient assume a prone position.
7. Instill simethicone to reduce bubbles from bile secretions. Give glucagon or anticholinergic agents intravenously to relax the duodenum so that the papilla can be cannulated. (Atropine increases the heart rate.)
8. Pass a catheter into the ampulla of Vater and instill a contrast agent through the cannula to outline the pancreatic and common bile ducts. Perform fluoroscopy and x-rays at this time.
9. Take biopsy specimens or cytology brushings before the endoscope is removed.
10. Monitor for side effects and drug allergy reactions (e.g., diaphoresis, pallor, restlessness, hypotension).
11. Follow guidelines in Chapter 1 for safe, effective, informed *intratest* care.

Clinical Implications

Abnormal results reveal stones, stenosis, and other abnormalities that are indicative of the following conditions:

1. Biliary cirrhosis
2. Primary sclerosing cholangitis
3. Cancer of bile ducts, gallstones

4. Pancreatic cysts
5. Pseudocysts
6. Pancreatic tumors
7. Cancer of the head of the pancreas
8. Chronic pancreatitis
9. Pancreatic fibrosis
10. Cancer of duodenal papilla
11. Papillary stenosis
12. Peptic ulcer disease

CLINICAL ALERT

Contraindications include:

1. Acute pancreatitis, pancreatic pseudocysts, and cholangitis
2. Obstructions or strictures within the esophagus or duodenum
3. Acute infections
4. Recent myocardial or severe pulmonary disease
5. Coagulopathy
6. Recent barium x-rays of the GI tract (barium obscures views during ERCP)

Interventions

Pretest Patient Care

1. Explain the purpose, procedure, benefits, and risks of the test. If done as an outpatient procedure, the patient should arrange for a ride home and should leave all valuables at home. Blood work, urinalysis, x-ray films, and scans should be reviewed and charted before the procedure. Record baseline vital signs and preprocedure signs and symptoms (e.g., jaundice, persistent abdominal pain, and signs of pancreatic cancer).
2. An informed consent form must be properly signed and witnessed.
3. Have the patient fast for 8 to 12 hours before ERCP.
4. Inform the patient to expect the following:
   a. The patient may be quite sleepy during ERCP and may not recall much of the experience.
   b. The patient should swallow when requested to do so and should not attempt to talk (to prevent damage to the oral pharynx).
   c. Initially, the patient may experience a gagging or choking sensation that quickly subsides. Slow, deep breathing may help with this feeling. Sensations of abdominal pressure or bloating are normal.
   d. The patient will have to lie still while x-rays are being taken.
   e. Encourage the patient to urinate and defecate before the procedure.
5. Refer to conscious sedation precautions in Chapter 1.
6. Follow guidelines in Chapter 1 for safe, effective, informed *pretest* care.

Posttest Patient Care

1. Do not permit food or liquids until the patient's gag reflex returns.
2. Monitor the blood pressure, pulse, respirations, oxygen saturation, and temperature according to institutional policy.
3. Observe the patient for signs of complications such as infection, urinary retention, cholangitis, or pancreatitis. Check for temperature elevation, which may be the first sign of inflammation. Monitor the white blood cell count and assess for signs of sepsis.
4. Infection may result from obstructed and infected biliary systems or contaminated endoscopes used during the procedure.

5. Monitor for respiratory and central nervous system depression from narcotics (naloxone may be used to reverse narcotic effects, and flumazenil is used for reversing benzodiazepines).
6. Explain that some abdominal discomfort may be experienced for several hours after the procedure.
7. Advise patient that drowsiness may last up to 24 hours. During this time, the patient should not perform any tasks that require mental alertness, and legal documents should not be signed.
8. Tell patient that a sore throat can be relieved by gargles, ice chips, fluids, or lozenges if permitted.
9. Notify healthcare provider of any of the following signs or symptoms:
   a. Prolonged, sharp abdominal pain; abnormal weakness; faintness
   b. Fever
   c. Nausea or vomiting
10. Review test results; report and record findings. Modify the nursing care plan as needed.
11. Follow guidelines in Chapter 1 for safe, effective, informed *posttest* care. Provide written instructions to outpatients. Outpatients should be discharged to the care of a responsible adult.

CLINICAL ALERT

Observe for possible complications:

1. Pancreatitis (most common complication)
2. Sepsis
3. Hemorrhage
4. Perforation
5. Aspiration
6. Respiratory depression or arrest
7. Medication reaction

● Enteroscopy, Virtual Enteroscopy

Enteroscopy is the examination of the small bowel with a fiberoptic endoscope. The endoscope is about 250 to 300 cm long, depending on the manufacturer. This long instrument is passed down the esophagus, through the stomach, through the distal duodenum, and then into the jejunum. Once in the jejunum, the endoscopist uses a series of movements to advance the endoscope as far as possible. A device known as an *overtube* may be applied to the endoscope to prevent it from looping in the stomach and inhibiting deep intubation of the small intestine. Fluoroscopy may also be useful in determining the position of the endoscope in the small bowel.

Virtual enteroscopy uses a video capsule to aid in the diagnosis of small bowel abnormalities. The video capsule is a wireless virtual endoscope that transmits video images as it travels through the bowel.

The main indication for enteroscopy is unexplained GI bleeding. It may also be used to help diagnose patients with unexplained chronic diarrhea or suspicious x-ray findings. It is very useful in diagnosing a small bowel abnormality out of reach of a standard endoscope that might otherwise be done surgically.

Reference Values

Normal

Small intestinal tract within normal limits

Procedure

1. This examination is usually performed in an outpatient setting of a hospital or ambulatory clinic. It also may be performed in the operating room or in a critical care setting.
2. Use a topical spray to anesthetize the patient's throat.

3. Start an intravenous line and use for administration of sedation alone or in combination with analgesics. These medications are given to achieve a state of conscious sedation. Resuscitation equipment must be available.
4. Perform continuous monitoring of the patient's vital signs, ECG, and oxygen saturation (via pulse oximetry).
5. Remove partial dental plates or dentures. Insert a mouthpiece to prevent the patient from biting the endoscope and to prevent injury to the patient's teeth, tongue, or other oral structures.
6. Depending on the endoscopist's preference, an overtube may be back-loaded onto the endoscope. The endoscope is well lubricated and gently inserted through the mouthpiece into the esophagus and advanced into the stomach and duodenum. To advance into the distal duodenum and jejunum, the endoscopist may use a series of pushing and pulling movements that serve to pleat the small bowel onto the endoscope, allowing deeper intubation. Fluoroscopy is useful to determine location in the small bowel.
7. Obtain biopsy specimens and brushing for cytology. Take photos to provide a permanent record of observations.
8. Inform the patient that he or she may initially have a strong gagging or choking sensation. During the procedure, the patient may belch frequently and have a sensation of abdominal pressure and bloating.
9. Immediately after the procedure, have the patient remain on his or her left side until fully awake.
10. If virtual enteroscopy is being performed, the patient will swallow a small video capsule (size of a large pill). As the video capsule travels through the GI tract, due to normal peristalsis, images are transmitted to a recorder and subsequently reviewed.

Clinical Implications

Abnormal results indicate the following:

1. Vascular abnormalities, such as angiodysplasia or varices
2. Ulcerative lesions, such as in Crohn's disease
3. Diverticula such as Meckel's diverticulum (congenital defect in the lower part of the small intestine resulting in an outpocketing of tissue)
4. Tumors

Interventions

Pretest Patient Care

1. Explain the purpose and procedure of the examination, the sensations that may be experienced, and the benefits and risks of the test. Refer to the conscious sedation and analgesia precautions in Chapter 1.
2. Inform the patient that the procedure may be several hours long, depending on the ease of passing the endoscope, diagnosis, and treatment.
3. Inform the patient that he or she might be quite sleepy during the test and may not recall much of the experience.
4. Instruct the patient to fast for 10 to 12 hours before the procedure to avoid the risks for aspiration and possible cancellation of the procedure.
5. Confirm informed consent. A legal consent form must be signed and witnessed before the procedure.
6. Encourage the patient to urinate and defecate if possible before the examination.
7. Follow guidelines in Chapter 1 for safe, effective, informed *pretest* care.

Posttest Patient Care

1. No food or liquids are permitted until the patient's gag reflex returns. Sucking on ice chips or throat lozenges, if permitted, may be helpful to relieve a sore throat.
2. Monitor blood pressure, pulse, respirations, and oxygen saturation according to the hospital or clinic policy, until the patient is fully awake.
3. The patient should remain on his or her left side with side-rails raised until fully awake.

4. Encourage the patient to belch or expel air inserted during the procedure.
5. Review test results; report and record findings. Modify the nursing care plan as needed.
6. Follow guidelines in Chapter 1 for safe, effective, and informed *posttest* care. Provide written discharge instructions to outpatients. Outpatients should be discharged to the care of a responsible adult.

CLINICAL ALERT

Potential complications include:

1. Shearing or stripping of gastric mucosa (which may arise from use of the overtube)
2. Pancreatitis
3. Hemorrhage
4. Perforation

Colposcopy

Colposcopy permits examination of the vagina and cervix with the colposcope, an instrument with a magnifying lens. The colposcope is also used to examine male genital lesions suspected in sexually transmitted diseases, condylomas, or human papillomavirus. Indications for this procedure in women include abnormal Papanicolaou (Pap) smear results or other cervical lesions, leukoplakia, and other cancerous lesions. Biopsy specimens and cell scrapings are obtained under direct visualization. Colposcopy can be used to assess women with a history of exposure to diethylstilbestrol (DES) *in utero*, born between 1938 and 1971 (referred to as DES Daughters) who are at an increased risk of developing a rare form of vaginal and cervical cancer called clear cell adenocarcinoma. Advantages of colposcopy include the following:

1. Lesions can be localized and their extent determined.
2. Inflammatory processes can be differentiated from neoplasia.
3. Invasive or noninvasive disease processes can be differentiated.

Colposcopy *cannot* readily detect endocervical lesions. Cervicitis and other changes can produce abnormal findings. When combined with findings from Pap smears, colposcopy can be a means of enhancing diagnostic accuracy. Tables 12.1 and 12.2 present correlation of findings and advantages and disadvantages of Pap smears and colposcopy. See Chapter 11 for Pap smear procedure.

Whitish areas of epithelium (squamous cell hyperplasia, formerly called leukoplakia), mosaic staining patterns, irregular blood vasculature, hyperkeratosis, and other abnormal-appearing tissues can be seen using colposcopy. The colposcope has a definite advantage for detecting atypical epithelium, designated in the literature as *basal cell activity*. Atypical epithelium cannot be called benign and yet does not fulfill all criteria for carcinoma in situ. Its early detection promotes cancer prophylaxis.

Patients receiving colposcopy may often be spared having to undergo surgical conization (the removal of a cone of tissue from the cervix).

Another gynecology procedure, a hysteroscopy, can be done to determine the cause of abnormal uterine bleeding, size and shape of the uterine cavity, location of a misplaced intrauterine device (IUD), and uterine abnormalities. A hysteroscopy is performed in a healthcare provider's office early in the menstrual cycle. A local anesthetic is usually administered into the cervix and paracervical area before insertion of the hysteroscope.

Reference Values

Normal

Normal vagina, cervix, vulva, and genital areas
Normal pink squamous epithelium and capillaries
Normal color, tone, and surface contours

TABLE 12.1. Correlation of Colposcopic and Histologic (Tissue) Findings

Colposcopic Term	Colposcopic Appearance	Histologic Correlate
Original squamous epithelium	Smooth, pink; indefinitely outlined vessels; no change after application of acetic acid	Squamous epithelium
Columnar epithelium	Grape-like structures after application of acetic acid	Columnar epithelium
Transformation zone	Tongues of squamous metaplasia; gland openings; nabothian cysts	Metaplastic squamous epithelium
White epithelium	White, sharp-bordered lesion visible only after application of acetic acid; no vessels visible	From minimal dysplasia to carcinoma in situ
Punctation	Sharp-bordered lesion; red stippling; epithelium whiter after application of acetic acid	From minimal dysplasia to carcinoma in situ
Mosaic	Sharp-bordered lesion, mosaic pattern; epithelium whiter after application of acetic acid	Usually hyperkeratosis or parakeratosis; seldom carcinoma in situ or invasive disease
Hyperkeratosis	White patch; rough surface; already visible before application of acetic acid	Usually hyperkeratosis or parakeratosis; seldom carcinoma in situ or invasive disease
Atypical vessel	Horizontal vessels running parallel to surface; constrictions and dilations of vessels; atypical branching, winding course	From carcinoma in situ to invasive carcinoma

TABLE 12.2. Pros and Cons of Colposcopy and Cytology (Examination of Cells)

Advantages	Disadvantages
Colposcopy	
Localizes lesion	Inadequate for detection of endocervical lesions
Diagnostic biopsy reveals cause of cancer	
Evaluates extent of lesion	More intensive training is necessary
Differentiates between inflammatory atypia and neoplasia	Cervicitis and regenerative changes may produce abnormal findings
Differentiates between invasive and noninvasive cervical lesions	
Enables follow-up	
Cytology	
Ideal for mass screening	Cannot localize lesion
Economical	Inflammation, atrophic changes, or folic acid deficiency may produce suspicious changes
Detection of human papilloma virus (HPV) by DNA for cervical cancer	
Specimen can be obtained by most healthcare personnel	Many steps between patient and cytopathologist allow misdiagnosis
Detects lesion in endocervical canal	Value of single smear is limited
Detects endocervical and endometrial carcinoma	False-negative rate is 5%–10%
High correlation with biopsy material (>90%)	

See Chapter 11 for more information on cytology and histology.

Procedure

1. Place the patient in the modified lithotomy position. Expose the vagina and cervix with a speculum after the internal and external genitalia have been carefully examined. Do not insert any part of the colposcope into the vagina.
2. Swab the cervix, vagina, or male genital areas with 3% acetic acid as needed during the procedure to improve visibility of epithelial tissues (it precipitates nuclear proteins within the cells). Remove the cervical mucus completely. Do not use cotton-wool swabs because fibers left on the cervix interfere with proper visualization.
3. Begin actual visualization with the colposcope with a field of white light and decreased magnification to focus on sites of white epithelium or irregular cervical contours. The light is then switched to a green filter for magnification of vascular changes.
   a. Diagram suspicious lesions and take photographs for the permanent healthcare record.
   b. The transformation zone and squamocolumnar junction (where the squamous epithelium meets the columnar epithelium of the cervix) are areas where many women exhibit atypical cells. It is imperative that these zones be visualized completely, especially in older women, because of changes associated with aging.
4. Obtain biopsy specimens of the lesions using a fine biopsy forceps. Some patients note discomfort at this time.
5. Place specimen in proper preservative, label accurately, and route to the appropriate department.
   a. Endocervical curettage *must* be performed before colposcope-directed biopsy so that epithelial fragments dislodged during colposcopy do not cause false-positive results in the endocervical curettage. The endocervical smear (curettage biopsy samples) should be placed on a slide in formalin.
   b. Sterile saline or sterile water should be used to cleanse and rinse acetic acid from the vaginal area to prevent burning or irritation. Bleeding can be stopped by applying toughened silver nitrate cautery sticks or ferric subsulfate (Monsel's solution).
6. Inform the patient that a small amount of vaginal bleeding or cramping for a few hours is not abnormal.
7. A paracervical block (e.g., with lidocaine) may be necessary in patients who are extremely anxious.
8. Follow guidelines in Chapter 1 regarding safe, effective, informed *intratest* care.

Clinical Implications

1. Abnormal lesions or unusual epithelial patterns include the following:
   a. Leukoplakia (white patches appear on mucous membranes of the urinary tract and genitals)
   b. Abnormal vasculature
   c. Slight, moderate, or marked dysplasia
   d. Abnormal-appearing tissue is classified by punctation (i.e., sharp borders, red stippling, epithelium whiter with acetic acid), mosaic pattern (i.e., sharp borders, mosaic pattern, epithelium whiter with acetic acid), or hyperkeratosis (i.e., white epithelium, rough, visible without acetic acid)
2. Extent of abnormal epithelium (with acetic acid) and extent of nonstaining with iodine
3. Clinical cervical cancer, cervical exfetation pain (fetus developing outside of the uterus)
4. Acute inflammation with human papillomavirus or bacterial infections (e.g., chlamydia), bacterial vaginosis, and gonorrhea

Interventions

Pretest Patient Care

1. Explain test purpose and procedure. Record preprocedure signs and symptoms (e.g., abnormal Pap, cervical or vaginal drainage or bleeding).
2. Obtain a urine specimen and a pertinent gynecologic history.
3. Follow guidelines in Chapter 1 for safe, effective, informed *pretest* care.

Posttest Patient Care

1. Patients may experience a vasovagal response. Watch for bradycardia and hypotension and treat accordingly. Have the patient sit for a short while before standing.
2. Monitor for complications, including heavy bleeding, infection, or pelvic inflammatory disease.
3. Instruct the patient to abstain from sexual intercourse and to not insert anything into the vagina for 2 to 7 days (per healthcare provider's orders) after the procedure.
4. If specimens are taken, slight vaginal bleeding may occur. Excessive bleeding, pain, fever, or abnormal vaginal discharge should be reported immediately. Ibuprofen may relieve cramps.
5. Review test results; report and record findings. Modify the nursing care plan as needed. Note that cervical scars from previous events may prevent satisfactory visualization and counsel appropriately regarding follow-up treatment such as cone biopsy and loop electrosurgical excision procedure (LEEP). If radiation treatment is prescribed, cervical tumor tissue may be tested for the presence of glutathione as a possible indicator of radiation resistance.
6. Follow guidelines in Chapter 1 for safe, effective, informed *posttest* care. Provide written discharge instructions.

● Loop Electrosurgical Excision Procedure (LEEP), Cone Biopsy, Cervical Conization

These procedures are done as a follow-up for an abnormal Pap smear and colposcopy findings, to enhance accuracy of colposcopy, and to investigate squamous intraepithelial lesions (SILs). They are done to exclude invasive cancer, determine extent of noninvasive lesions, and treat (LEEP and cone biopsy) and remove abnormal cervical dysplasia, based on lesion size, distribution, and grade, when there is lack of correlation between Pap smear, previous biopsy, and colposcopy.

Reference Values

Normal

Normal cervix cells, which flatten as they grow

Procedure

1. Place the patient's feet in stirrups and insert a speculum, as with a Pap test and colposcopy.
2. Apply a local anesthetic to the cervix and a mild vinegar (acetic acid) or iodine, depending on the procedure type. For LEEP procedures, a grounding pad is placed on or under the patient's thigh and a fine wire loop with a special high-frequency current is used to remove a small piece of cervical tissue.
3. Apply a paste to the cervix to reduce bleeding. This may cause a dark vaginal discharge.
4. A laser or a cone biopsy may also be one of the procedures.

CLINICAL ALERT

Complications may include heavy bleeding, severe cramping, infection, and accidental cutting or burning of normal tissue. Cervical stenosis may be an untoward effect of this procedure.

Clinical Implications

Abnormal findings include dysplasia and invasive cancer into deeper parts of the cervix.

Interventions

Pretest Patient Care

1. Explain purpose, procedure, and equipment used.
2. Provide support and take measures to relieve fear and anxiety about possible diagnosis of cervical cancer.
3. Follow guidelines in Chapter 1 for safe, effective, informed *pretest* care.

Posttest Patient Care

1. Instruct patient to call healthcare provider if heavy or bright-red bleeding or clots, chills, aching, severe abdominal pain (not relieved by pain medication), foul-smelling discharge, or unusual swelling occurs.
2. Watery discharge and white, dark, and light spotting may last approximately 4 weeks. The heaviest discharge occurs for about 1 week after treatment. Do not use tampons.
3. No douching or bubble baths. Delay sexual intercourse for approximately 4 weeks. Check with healthcare provider.
4. Be sure to stress the importance of returning for follow-up appointment to evaluate satisfactory healing.
5. Follow Chapter 1 guidelines for safe, effective, informed *posttest* care.

● Flexible Proctoscopy; Sigmoidoscopy; Proctosigmoidoscopy

These tests involve the examination of the rectum, anal canal, and sigmoid colon, up to 65 cm, with a proctosigmoidoscope. Rigid scopes are not as commonly used since the advent of flexible fiberoptic instruments, which are more comfortable for patients. Their main use is for the investigation of rectal bleeding, evaluation of colonic symptoms, and detection and diagnosis of cancers and other abnormalities such as diverticula in this area of the GI tract. Because the risk for developing colorectal cancer increases with age, the American Society of Colon and Rectal Surgeons has recommended screening guidelines for individuals >50 years of age. These guidelines include annual fecal occult blood testing (FOBT), annual FOBT in conjunction with flexible sigmoidoscopy every 5 years, or colonoscopy every 10 years, or double contrast barium enema every 5 years. Most colorectal cancers develop from a malignant change in a polyp that has been in the lining of the bowel for 10 to 15 years. These tests can also evaluate hemorrhoids, polyps, blood or mucus in the stool, unexplained anemia, and other bowel conditions. Sigmoidoscopy is used along with air-contrast barium studies.

Reference Values

Normal

Normal anal, rectal, and sigmoid colon mucosa

Procedure

1. Have the patient assume the knee-to-chest position for rigid proctoscopy (inserted 25 cm). When the flexible proctoscope is used, the patient must be in the left lateral position. Carefully insert the proctoscope (inserted 35 to 60 cm) or sigmoidoscope into the rectum.
2. The examination can be done with the patient in bed or positioned on a special tilt-table.
3. Inform the patient that he or she may feel a very strong urge to defecate or pass gas. The patient may also experience a feeling of bloating or cramping, which is normal.
4. Follow guidelines in Chapter 1 for safe, effective, informed *intratest* care.

Clinical Implications

Examination may reveal the following: edematous, red, or denuded mucosa; granularity; friability; ulcers; polyps; cysts; thickened areas; changes in vascular pattern; pseudomembranes;

spontaneous bleeding; or normal mucosa. These findings may help to confirm or to rule out the following conditions:

1. Inflammatory bowel disease
   a. Chronic ulcerative colitis
   b. Crohn's disease
   c. Proctitis (acute and chronic)
   d. Pseudomembranous colitis
   e. Antibiotic-associated colitis
2. Polyps
   a. Adenomatous
   b. Familial
   c. Diminutive
3. Cancer and tumors
   a. Adenocarcinoma
   b. Carcinoids
   c. Other tumors, such as lipomas
4. Anal and perianal conditions
   a. Hemorrhoids
   b. Abscesses and fistulas
   c. Strictures and stenoses
   d. Rectal prolapse
   e. Fissures
   f. Contractures

Interventions

Pretest Patient Care

1. Explain the test purpose, procedure, and benefits. Record pertinent preprocedure signs and symptoms (e.g., rectal bleeding). Obtain a signed, witnessed informed consent form, if required.
2. There is no need for the patient to fast. However, a restricted diet such as clear liquids the evening before the test may be prescribed.
3. Remind patient that laxatives and enemas may be taken the night before the examination. Enemas or a rectal laxative suppository may be administered the morning of the procedure. For patients of all ages, one or two phosphate (Fleet) enemas are frequently ordered to be performed about 1 to 2 hours before the examination. This is considered ample preparation by many endoscopy departments.
4. Follow guidelines in Chapter 1 for safe, effective, informed *pretest* care.

CLINICAL ALERT

1. Patients with acute symptoms, particularly those with suspected ulcerative or granulomatous colitis, should be examined *without* any preparation (i.e., without enemas, laxatives, or suppositories).
2. Perforation of the intestinal wall can be an infrequent complication of these tests.
3. Notify the patient's healthcare provider before administering laxatives or enemas to a pregnant woman.
4. Notify healthcare provider immediately of any instance of decreased blood pressure, diaphoresis, or bradycardia.

Posttest Patient Care

1. Review test results; report and record findings. Modify the nursing care plan as needed. Monitor the patient and counsel appropriately about possible further testing (colonoscopy).
2. Colon cancer is highly treatable and, if detected at an early stage, often curable. Typically stage 0 and I colon cancer is treated with surgery, stage II with surgery and possible chemotherapy or radiation therapy, stage III with surgery and possible chemotherapy or radiation therapy or immunotherapy, and stage IV (denotes metastatic disease) with surgery and palliative care.
3. Rectal cancer is also highly treatable and curable if localized. In stage 0 (limited to mucosa) rectal cancer, the main treatment is surgical excision followed by local radiation therapy. Stage I treatment includes surgical excision followed by external-beam radiation and fluorouracil (5-FU). Stage II treatment combines chemotherapy and radiation followed by surgery. In stages III and IV, surgery is accompanied by intraoperative external-beam radiation, chemotherapy (5-FU), or both. In stage IV (metastatic disease), the treatment includes surgery and palliative care.
4. Follow guidelines in Chapter 1 for safe, effective, informed *posttest* care. Provide written discharge instructions.

• Colonoscopy, Virtual Colonoscopy (VC), Optical Colonoscopy

Colonoscopy visualizes, examines, and photographs the large intestine with a flexible fiberoptic or video-colonoscope inserted through the anus and advanced to the ileocecal valve. Air introduced through an accessory channel of the colonoscope distends the intestinal walls to enhance visualization. Virtual colonoscopy (VC) uses CT generating both two-dimensional and three-dimensional views of the rectum and colon. VC may be indicated in those patients who cannot undergo optical colonoscopy because of an occlusive mass or excessive spasms within the colon. An added benefit of VC is that it also allows for extracolonic findings, such as bronchogenic, ovarian, and renal carcinomas. Colonoscopy can differentiate inflammatory disease from neoplastic disease and can evaluate polypoid lesions that are beyond the reach of the sigmoidoscope. Polyps, foreign bodies, and biopsy specimens can be removed through the colonoscope. Photographs of the large intestine lumen can also be taken. Before colonoscopy was available, major abdominal surgery was the only way to remove polyps or suspicious tissue to determine malignancy or nonmalignancy. Periodic colonoscopy is a valuable adjunct to the follow-up of persons with previous polyps, colon cancer, family history of colon cancer, or high risk factors. It is also helpful in locating the source of lower GI bleeding. It provides a safe way to perform presurgical screening and postsurgical surveillance of anastomotic suture lines. Colonoscopy is recommended as the primary screening tool for individuals of higher-than-average risk for colon cancer.

Reference Values

Normal

Normal large intestine mucosa

Procedure

1. A clear liquid diet is usually ordered for 48 to 72 hours before examination. Have the patient fast for 8 hours before the procedure. Laxatives may be ordered to be taken for 1 to 3 days before the test; enemas may be ordered to be given the night before the test.
2. For an oral saline iso-osmotic and isotonic laxative, have the patient drink 3 to 6 L of the prescribed solution over a 2- to 3.5-hour period. The typical volume taken is 1 gallon (~4 L), and this volume of fluid can be administered by nasogastric tube if necessary. Expect initial results in 30 minutes to 1 hour. Ingestion of the washout solution continues until feces expelled are nothing but clear liquid. Notify the healthcare provider before administering >6 L of this solution. Patients with congestive heart failure or renal failure may be at risk for fluid volume overload if this preparation is used.

3. An alternative bowel preparation method is a combination of sodium phosphate tablets (OsmoPrep), and clear liquids, which should be taken according to the prescribed schedule and dosage. Large, watery bowel movements usually begin within one hour of taking the first dose of pills and clear liquids. This bowel-cleansing preparation works by drawing large amounts of water into the colon, and is contraindicated in patients with acute phosphate nephropathy, bowel obstruction or perforation, gastric bypass or stomach stapling, and used with extreme caution in patients with chronic kidney disease, electrolyte disorders, cardiac arrhythmias, seizures, inflammatory bowel disease or swallowing problems.
4. Start an intravenous line and use for administration of sedatives and narcotics. These medications are given to achieve a state of conscious sedation (see Chapter 1). Ensure that the patient is responsive enough to inform the doctor of any subjective reactions during the examination. Ensure that resuscitation equipment is available.
5. Perform continuous monitoring of the patient's vital signs, ECG, and oxygen saturation (pulse oximetry).
6. On occasion, intravenous anticholinergic agents and glucagon may be used to relax bowel spasms.
7. Have the patient assume the left-sided or Sims' position and drape properly. Insert a well-lubricated colonoscope about 12 cm into the bowel. Ask the patient to take deep breaths through the mouth during this time. Introduce air into the bowel through a special port on the colonoscope to aid viewing. As the colonoscope advances, the patient may need to be repositioned several times to aid in proper visualization of the colon. Sensations of pressure, mild pain, or cramping are not unusual.
8. Remember that the best views are obtained during withdrawal of the colonoscope. Therefore, a more detailed examination is usually performed during withdrawal than during advancement.
9. If the patient is undergoing VC, the process takes about 15 minutes and, in most cases, does not require sedation.
10. Follow guidelines in Chapter 1 for safe, effective, informed *intratest* care.

PROCEDURAL ALERT

Four-dimensional elastic light-scanning fingerprinting (4D-ELF) is a less invasive optical scan that allows probing at the nanoscale/microscale level of living cells in the detection of colon cancer from measurements made within the rectum. This technique makes use of light scattering properties on the cells lining the colon in predicting cancer without the need for a biopsy.

Clinical Implications

Abnormal findings may reveal the following conditions:

1. Polyps
2. Tumors (benign or malignant)
3. Areas of ulceration
4. Inflammation
5. Colitis, diverticula
6. Bleeding sites
7. Strictures
8. Foreign bodies

Clinical Considerations

1. Keep colon electrolyte lavage preparations refrigerated; however, the patient may drink the solution at room temperature. Use within 48 hours of preparation and discard unused portions.
2. Before testing, the complete blood count, prothrombin time, platelet count, and thromboplastin time results should be reviewed and charted.

3. Persons with known heart disease may receive prophylactic antibiotics before testing.
4. Patients should not mix or drink anything with the colonic washout preparation. Do not add ice or glucose to the solution.
5. Diabetic persons are usually advised not to take insulin before the procedure but to bring insulin with them to the clinic.

Interventions

Pretest Patient Care

1. Explain the purpose, procedure, benefits, and risks of the test. Record preprocedure signs and symptoms (e.g., GI bleeding). If done as an outpatient procedure, the patient should arrange for a ride home and should leave valuables at home. Blood work, urinalysis, x-ray films, and scans should be reviewed and charted before the procedure. Record baseline vital signs.
2. When ordered, have the patient take one 12-oz glass of liquid preparation every 10 minutes before the examination. (Each gallon holds approximately eleven 12-oz [360 mL] glasses.) The entire gallon should be taken in 2 hours, if possible. Timing is important. Slower drinking does not clean the colon properly. Some patients will receive another type of preparation when ordered (e.g., liquid Fleet laxatives and enemas).
3. Some patients will be on a clear liquid diet for 72 hours before the test, and then fasting, except for medications, after a clear-liquid supper the evening before the test. No solid food, milk, or milk products are permitted. Strained fruit juices without pulp (e.g., apple, white grape), lemonade, Hi-C drink, water, clear liquid, Gatorade, Kool-Aid, Jell-O, Popsicles, and hard candy are permitted, but no red or purple fluids are allowed.
4. To be effective, a purgative must produce fluid diarrhea. This shows that unaltered small intestinal contents are emerging and colonic residue has been cleared. Enemas must be repeated until solid matter is no longer expelled (clear liquid returns). Soapsuds enemas are contraindicated because they cause increased mucus secretion as a result of irritant stimulation. Preparation is complete when fecal discharge is clear. If returns are not clear after 4 L of solution have been ingested, continue until returns are clear, up to 6 L total.
5. A legal consent form must be signed and properly witnessed (see Chapter 1) after patient has received proper instruction about the test.
6. Discontinue iron preparations 3 or 4 days before examination because iron residues produce an inky, black, sticky stool that interferes with visualization, and the stool can be viscous and difficult to clear. Aspirin and aspirin-containing products should also be discontinued 1 week before the examination because they may cause bleeding problems or localized hemorrhages.
7. Inform the patient to expect the following:
   a. The patient may feel quite sleepy during the test and may not recall much of the procedure.
   b. The patient may experience abdominal pressure, mild pain, or cramping.
   c. The patient may pass gas (expel flatus) or have the urge to defecate, which is normal.
   d. The patient may be asked to assume various positions to aid with passing the colonoscope.
8. Follow guidelines in Chapter 1 for safe, effective, informed *pretest* care.

CLINICAL ALERT

1. Solid food should never be taken within 2 hr before the oral cleansing regimen is begun.
2. Orally administered colon lavage is contraindicated in the following conditions:
   a. Actual or suspected ulcers
   b. Gastric outlet obstruction
   c. Weight <20 kg
   d. Toxic colitis
   e. Megacolon

3. Relative contraindications for colonoscopy include the following conditions:
   a. Perforating disease of the colon
   b. Peritonitis
   c. Radiation enteritis
   d. Recent abdominal or bowel surgery
   e. Acute conditions of the anus and rectum
   f. Serious cardiac or respiratory problems (e.g., recent myocardial infarction)
   g. Situations in which the bowel cannot be adequately prepared for the procedure (i.e., fulminant granulomatous or irradiation colitis)
4. No barium studies should be done during the preparation phase for colonoscopy.
5. Bloating, nausea, and occasional vomiting after oral laxatives are common. Advise patient to adhere to instructions if at all possible.

Posttest Patient Care

1. The patient may have liquids or a light meal when fully awake.
2. Stools should be observed for visible blood. The patient should be instructed to report abdominal pain or other unusual symptoms because perforation and hemorrhage are possible complications.
3. Monitor the blood pressure, pulse, respirations, and oxygen saturation, according to institutional policy, until the patient is fully awake.
4. The most frequent adverse reactions to oral purgatives include nausea, vomiting, bloating, rectal irritation, chills, and feelings of weakness.
5. The patient may expel large amounts of gas/flatus after the procedure.
6. Review test results; report and record findings. Modify the nursing care plan as needed. Monitor for complications.
7. Follow guidelines in Chapter 1 for safe, effective, informed *posttest* care. Provide written discharge instructions to outpatients. Outpatients should be discharged to the care of a responsible adult.

CLINICAL ALERT

1. Observe for the following possible complications:
   a. Perforations of the bowel
   b. Hypotensive episodes
   c. Cardiac or respiratory arrest, which can be provoked by the combination of oversedation and intense vagal stimulus from instrumentation
   d. Hemorrhage, especially if polypectomy has been performed
2. If colon preparations are administered by lavage to an unconscious patient or to a patient with impaired gag reflexes, observe for aspiration or regurgitation, especially if a nasogastric tube is in place. Keep the head of the bed elevated. If this is not possible, position the patient on his or her side. Have continuous suction equipment and supplies readily available.
3. Signs of bowel perforation include malaise, rectal bleeding, abdominal pain, distention, and fever.

● Peritoneoscopy; Laparoscopy; Pelviscopy; Fertiloscopy

These examinations of the intra-abdominal and pelvic cavities are performed using a laparoscope or pelviscope inserted through a slit in the anterior abdominal wall. The pelvic organs, as well as abdominal organs such as the greater curvature of the stomach or the liver, can be viewed. The use of a laparoscopic intracorporeal ultrasound (LICU) probe in the evaluation of GI malignancies is an important technology. The different types of examinations include peritoneoscopy, laparoscopy (intra-abdominal), pelviscopy (gynecologic), and fertiloscopy (gynecologic). These procedures are frequently performed under general anesthesia in a surgical setting; however, many are also done with local anesthesia.

Peritoneoscopy is most commonly done to evaluate liver disease and to obtain biopsy specimens when the liver is too small, when previous liver biopsy proves inadequate, when contraindications to percutaneous liver biopsy exist (e.g., ascites), when there is unexplained portal hypertension or liver function abnormalities, and when the liver cannot be properly palpated for a conventional liver biopsy. It does away with the need for a blind liver biopsy. Other indications for peritoneoscopy include unexplained ascites, staging of lymphomas, or staging and follow-up of ovarian cancer or abdominal masses. Sometimes, patients with advanced chest, gastric, pancreatic, endometrial, or rectal tumors are evaluated by peritoneoscopy before surgical intervention is attempted.

Indications for laparoscopy include diagnosis and staging of cancer, evaluating cause of ascites, and examination of the abdomen with ultrasound probes. Biopsies of abdominal and lymph node masses and hepatic lesions can also be done using a core needle biopsy, wedge biopsy using electrocautery, or cup forceps biopsy.

Gynecologic laparoscopy and pelviscopy are used to diagnose cysts, adhesions, fibroids, malignancies, inflammatory processes, or infections in persons with pelvic and abdominal pain. Evaluation of the fallopian tubes can be done for infertile patients. These procedures also provide a means to release adhesions, to obtain biopsy specimens, to do select operative procedures such as tubal ligations, or to perform laser treatments for endometriosis. Gynecologic laparoscopy or pelviscopy is commonly performed under general anesthesia as a same-day surgical procedure.

These techniques can frequently replace laparotomy. They are less stressful to the patient; require only small incisions; can be done in shorter periods of time; can be done using local, spinal, or general anesthetics; reduce potential for formation of adhesions; and hasten healing and recovery time.

Pelviscopy differs from laparoscopy in two major respects—*endocoagulation* as a method for controlling bleeding and *endoligation* as a technique that permits suturing using extracorporeal (outside the body) or intracorporeal (inside the body) ligating and suturing methods by means of special instruments.

The pelviscope is angled at 30° for better visualization. A video camera attachment offers the healthcare provider a choice of viewing the process on a video screen instead of through the scope. Printouts and video recordings of the pelviscopy can be produced. Thus, pelviscopy is both a diagnostic and an operative modality.

Fertiloscopy, using an instrument called a *fertiloscope*, is used to examine the entire female reproductive system. It is used to diagnose infertility and replaces laparoscopic tests done to diagnose infertility. Local anesthetics are used. Future applications include testing to rule out ovarian cancer, biopsy of the ovary, and drainage of cysts.

Reference Values

Normal

Gynecologic examination: normal size, shape, and appearance of uterus, fallopian tubes, and ovaries.

Intra-abdominal examination: normal liver, gallbladder, spleen, and greater curvature of the stomach

Procedure

1. The patient will lie supine or be placed in a lithotomy position depending on the procedure.
2. Cleanse the skin and, if the procedure is to be performed under local anesthesia, inject a local anesthetic into areas where the scope will be introduced. Otherwise, prep the patient as for an abdominal procedure under general anesthesia. Maintain a sterile field.
3. Place an intravenous line so that medications may be given intravenously as needed.
4. Place an indwelling catheter into the bladder to reduce the risk for bladder perforation.
5. Make a small incision near the umbilicus through which a trocar is introduced, followed by passage of the pelviscope or laparoscope. Sometimes, more than one puncture site will be made so that accessory

instruments can be used during the procedure. Carbon dioxide introduced into the peritoneal cavity causes the omentum to rise away from the organs and allows for better visualization. A few stitches or Steri-Strips are usually needed to close the incisions. Apply adhesive bandages as dressings.

6. Follow guidelines in Chapter 1 for safe, effective, informed *intratest* care.

Clinical Implications

Abnormal findings can reveal the following conditions:

1. Endometriosis
2. Ovarian cysts
3. Pelvic inflammatory disease
4. Metastasis stage of cancer
5. Uterine fibroids
6. Abscesses
7. Tumors (benign and malignant)
8. Enlarged fallopian tubes (hydrosalpinx)
9. Ectopic pregnancy
10. Infection
11. Adhesions or scar tissue
12. Ascites
13. Cirrhosis
14. Liver nodules (often an indication of cancer)
15. Engorged peritoneal vasculature (correlates with portal hypertension)

CLINICAL ALERT

1. These procedures may be contraindicated in persons known to have the following conditions:
   a. Advanced abdominal wall cancer
   b. Severe respiratory or cardiovascular disease
   c. Intestinal obstruction, dilated bowel loops
   d. Palpable abdominal mass
   e. Large abdominal hernia
   f. Chronic tuberculosis
   g. History of peritonitis
   h. Noncorrectable coagulation disorders
2. Possible complications include the following:
   a. Bleeding from the puncture injury or from liver biopsy
   b. Misplacement of gas
   c. Thermal burns
3. The endoscopy should be aborted in favor of a laparotomy in the event of uncontrolled bleeding or suspected malignancy.

Interventions

Pretest Patient Care

1. Complete laboratory tests and other appropriate diagnostic modalities before these endoscopies.
2. Bowel preparation may include an enema or suppository.
3. Explain the test purpose and procedure and the type of anesthesia chosen (general, spinal, or local) as well as postoperative expectations such as activity, deep breathing, and shoulder pain.
4. Ensure that a properly signed and witnessed consent form is obtained (see Chapter 1).

5. Maintain sensitivity to cultural, sexual, and modesty issues as an important part of psychological support.
6. Follow guidelines in Chapter 1 for safe, effective, informed *pretest* care.

Posttest Patient Care

1. Check blood pressure frequently according to institutional policies.
2. Observe for infection, hemorrhage, and bowel or bladder perforation.
3. Advise the patient that shoulder and abdominal discomfort may be present for 1 to 2 days because of residual carbon dioxide gas in the abdominal cavity. This can be controlled with mild oral analgesics. Sitting or resting in a semi-Fowler's (lying flat with head of the bed elevated to 30° to 45°) position can also alleviate discomfort.
4. If the patient has had a general or spinal anesthetic, follow the usual cautions and protocols for the care of any person having undergone those types of anesthesia.
5. Review test results; report and record findings. Modify the nursing care plan as needed. Counsel the patient appropriately.
6. Follow guidelines in Chapter 1 for safe, effective, informed *posttest* care. Provide written discharge instructions.

● Cystoscopy (Cystourethroscopy)

Cystoscopy and cystourethroscopy are used to diagnose and treat disorders of the lower urinary tract. They provide views of the interior bladder, urethra, prostatic urethra, and ureteral orifices by means of tubular, lighted, telescopic lens instruments called cystoscopes or cystourethroscopes. These scopes come in many sizes and variations as well as in flexible fiberoptic instruments. Urethroscopy is an important part of this examination because it allows visualization of the prostate gland.

Cystoscopy is the most common of all urologic diagnostic procedures. It may be indicated in the following conditions:

1. Unexplained hematuria (gross or microscopic)
2. Recurrent or chronic urinary tract infection
3. Infection resistant to medical treatment
4. Unexplained urinary symptoms such as dysuria, frequency, urgency, hesitancy, intermittency, straining, incontinence, enuresis, or retention
5. Bladder tumors (benign and malignant)
6. Pediatric considerations include the above and the following:
   a. Posterior urethral valves, ureteroceles in females, and other congenital anomalies
   b. Complete workup of children with daytime incontinence usually done in conjunction with urodynamic studies
   c. Removal of foreign objects and stents placed in previous surgeries

Because intravenous pyelography (IVP) does not allow proper visualization of the area from the neck of the bladder to the end of the urethra, cystoscopy makes it possible to diagnose and to treat abnormalities in this area.

Cystoscopy may be used to perform meatotomy and to crush and retrieve small stones and other foreign bodies from the urethra, ureter, and bladder. Biopsy specimens can be obtained. Bladder tumors can be fulgurated, and strictures can be dilated through the cystoscope. In conjunction with cystoscopy, ureteroscopy can be done to determine the cause of hematuria, to detect tumors and stones, and to manipulate stones.

Reference Values

Normal

Normal structure and function of the interior bladder, urethra, ureteral orifices, and prostatic urethra

Procedure

1. The examination can be performed in a special operating room designed for this purpose, in a clinic, or in the urologist's office. The patient's age, state of health, and extent of surgical procedure necessary determine the setting. Pediatric cystoscopy is done in the operating room under general anesthesia.
2. The external genitalia are prepped with an antiseptic solution such as povidone-iodine after the patient is properly grounded, padded, and draped.
3. Local anesthetic jelly is instilled into the urethra. For males, the anesthetic is retained in the urethra by a clamp applied near the end of the penis. For best results, the local anesthetic should be administered 5 to 10 minutes before passage of the cystoscope.
4. The scope is connected to an irrigation system, and fluid is infused into the bladder throughout the procedure. Solutions used are nonconductive and retain clarity during the procedure (e.g., glycine, sterile water). The solution also distends the bladder to allow better visualization. The infusion is stopped and the bladder drained when it becomes filled with 300 to 500 mL of fluid.
5. Should blood or other matter be present in the bladder, the fiberoptic cystoscope will not provide as clear a view as a rigid cystoscope because it is more difficult to flush.
6. During transurethral resection procedures, venous sinuses may be opened, and irrigation fluid may enter the circulatory system, causing water intoxication. Therefore, isotonic solutions such as sorbitol, mannitol, or glycine must be used.
7. Institutional policies dictate general perioperative care and procedures. Follow guidelines in Chapter 1 regarding safe, effective, informed *intratest* care.

Clinical Implications

Abnormal conditions revealed by cystoscopy include the following:

1. Prostatic hyperplasia or hypertrophy
2. Cancer of the bladder
3. Bladder stones
4. Urethral strictures or abnormalities
5. Prostatitis
6. Ureteral reflux (shown on cystogram)
7. Vesicle neck stenosis
8. Urinary fistulas
9. Ureterocele
10. Diverticula
11. Abnormally small or large bladder capacity
12. Polyps

Interventions

Pretest Patient Care

1. Explain the purpose and procedure of the test. Special sensitivity to concern for cultural, sexual, and modesty issues is an important part of psychological support. Emphasize that there is little pain or discomfort from cystoscopy; however, a strong desire to void may be experienced.
2. Facilitate bowel preparation and other laboratory and diagnostic tests if extensive procedures are planned.
3. Obtain a properly signed and witnessed consent form (see Chapter 1).
4. Liquids may be encouraged until the time of the examination to promote urine formation if the procedure is a simple cystoscopy done under local anesthesia. Fasting guidelines are followed when spinal or general anesthesia is planned.

5. Start an intravenous line for the administration of drugs to achieve a state of conscious sedation. Medications such as diazepam (Valium) or midazolam (Versed) are used to relax the patient. Amnesia may be a side effect. Younger men may experience more pain and discomfort than older men. Women usually require less sedation because the female urethra is shorter. The patient should be instructed to relax the abdominal muscles to lessen discomfort. See Chapter 1 regarding sedation and analgesia precautions.
6. Follow guidelines in Chapter 1 regarding safe, effective, informed *pretest* care.

Posttest Patient Care

1. After cystoscopy, voiding patterns and bladder emptying should be monitored. Check vital signs as necessary.
2. The intake of fluids should be encouraged.
3. Clots may form and may cause difficulty in voiding.
4. Report unusual bleeding or difficult urination to the healthcare provider promptly.
5. Urinary frequency, dysuria, pink to light-red urine, urethral burning, and posttest bladder spasms are common after cystoscopy.
6. Antibiotics may be prescribed before and after cystoscopy to prevent infection. Rectal opioid suppositories may also be administered.
7. The potential for gram-negative shock is always present with urologic procedures because the urethra is so vascular that any break in the tissues can allow bacteria to enter the bloodstream directly. Onset of symptoms can be rapid and may actually begin during the procedure if it is fairly lengthy. Observe for and *promptly* report chills, fever, increasing tachycardia, hypotension, and back pain to the healthcare provider. Blood cultures are usually ordered, followed by an aggressive regimen of antibiotic therapy.
8. Urethral catheters may be left in place to facilitate urinary drainage, especially if there is concern about edema.
9. Routine catheter care is necessary for retention of urethral catheters. Follow institutional protocols. The patient may need instructions if discharged with catheter in place.
10. Review test results; report and record findings. Modify the nursing care plan as needed. Counsel the patient appropriately.
11. Follow guidelines in Chapter 1 for safe, effective, informed *posttest* care. Provide written discharge instructions.

CLINICAL ALERT

1. If urethral dilation has been part of the procedure, the patient is advised to rest and to increase fluid intake.
2. Monitor patient's voiding patterns and bladder emptying (or instruct to self-monitor).
3. Evaluate and instruct the patient to watch for edema. Edema may cause urinary retention, hesitancy, weak urinary stream, or urinary dribbling any time within several days after the procedure. Warm sitz baths and mild analgesics may be helpful; however, an indwelling catheter may sometimes be necessary for relief.

● Urodynamic Studies: Cystometrogram (CMG); Urethral Pressure Profile (UPP); Rectal Electromyogram (EMG); Cystourethrogram

These tests evaluate bladder, urethral, and sphincter function; identify abnormal voiding patterns; check status of neuroanatomic connectives between brain, spinal cord, and bladder; and consist of two main components: the cystometrogram (CMG) and the rectal electromyogram (EMG).

The combined measurement of the CMG and the EMG provides information about how the bladder adapts to being filled as well as how it reacts to the filling itself. These studies are indicated in an incontinent person and when there is evidence of neurologic disease (neurogenic bladder), spinal cord injury, dysuria, enuresis, infection, or specific neuropathies such as those found in multiple sclerosis, diabetes, and tabes dorsalis (degeneration of the sensory neurons to the brain).

Reference Values

Normal

Normal bladder sensations of fullness, heat, and cold

Adult: Normal bladder capacity of 400 to 500 mL, residual urine <30 mL, desire to void is at 175 to 250 mL; sensation of fullness felt at 350 to 450 mL; stream is strong and uninterrupted

Normal voiding pressures and muscle coordination

Normal rectal EMG readings; urethral pressure profile readings normal

Pediatric: Bladder capacity varies with age. Compliant bladder: stretches to capacity without pressure increase. Bladder stability: no involuntary contractions

Procedures

1. CMG
   a. Have the patient void and record urine flow rate, voiding pressure, and amount of urine voided.
   b. Insert a nonlatex double-lumen catheter into the bladder. Place adhesive patch electrodes parallel on each side of the anus and attach a ground to the thigh. Measure the residual urine. Connect the catheter to the cystometer. (A cystometer evaluates the neuromuscular mechanism of the bladder by measuring bladder capacity and pressure.) The bladder is gradually filled with sterile saline or sterile water or carbon dioxide gas in predetermined increments, and pressure readings are taken at these increments. Water or saline offers a more physiologic result and is less irritating.
   c. Make observations during the CMG about the patient's perception of heat and cold, bladder fullness, urge to void, and ability to inhibit voiding when bladder contractions occur.
   d. Remove the catheter and patch electrodes when the bladder is completely emptied of fluid.
   e. Inject cholinergic and/or anticholinergic drugs to determine their effects on bladder function (after CMG procedure).
   f. Perform the cystometric study as a control, followed by repeat study 20 to 30 minutes after injection of the drugs.
   g. Be aware that a change in posture from supine to standing or walking may be required during the examination.
   h. Remember that sleep studies may be performed in conjunction with an electroencephalogram (EEG) to evaluate persons having nocturnal incontinence (see Chapter 16 for EEG study).
   i. Pediatric CMG: The bladder is filled until the pressures reach 40 to 60 cm of water, the child voids around the catheter, or the child seems very uncomfortable. In older children, ask questions about bladder fullness, when they would normally void, and ask them to hold urine until extreme urgency ensues. Patients may void on the table with the catheter in place, or they may void in a special container that measures urine flow, voiding pressure, and length of time to void. These pressures are depicted on a graph.
2. Rectal EMG—monitors the pelvic floor muscles responsible for holding urine in the bladder.
   a. Apply electrodes next to the anus, and attach a ground to the thigh, or introduce a needle electrode into the periurethral striated muscle. These electrodes record electromyographic activity during voiding and produce a simultaneous recording of urine flow rate. (See Chapter 16 for EMG study.)
   b. Pediatric rectal EMG: Patch electrodes record the coordination of the external sphincter and the pelvic floor muscle response to filling and the ability to inhibit bladder contractions. If the child voids on the table, the sphincter relaxes during voiding (which is normal).

3. UPP
   a. Use a specially designed catheter, coupled to a transducer, to record pressures along the urethra as it is slowly withdrawn.
   b. Pediatric UPP: This profile assesses the functional urethral length as well as general competency of the urethra and sphincter. The same double-lumen catheter is used, which has premarked lines on it for both the CMG and the UPP. Slowly withdraw the catheter and note the pressures at the premarked spots.
4. Cystourethrogram—evaluates bladder wall and urethral abnormalities and tumors. It can be used to assess reflux and stress incontinence in women and to identify posttraumatic urine extravasation.
   a. Instill an x-ray contrast medium into the bladder through a catheter until the bladder fills. Clamp the catheter and take x-rays with the patient assuming several different positions.
   b. Remove the catheter and take more x-rays as the patient voids and the contrast material passes through the urethra (voiding cystourethrogram [VCUG]).
   c. Pediatric cystourethrogram: Rarely are VCUGs done at the same time as EMGs. VCUGs are done in children to assess vesicourethral reflux, to identify structural abnormalities, and to evaluate for voiding dysfunction, and they are usually done as part of the workup before considering EMG.
5. See Chapter 1 guidelines for safe, effective, informed *intratest* care for all procedures.

PROCEDURAL ALERT

In children, the bladder is filled at 10% of what the bladder is expected to hold at a specific age.

Clinical Implications

Abnormal results reveal motor and sensory defects, altered pressures or bladder capacity, and inappropriate or absent contractions of the pelvic floor muscles and internal sphincter during voiding.

1. Bladder noncompliance: During filling, the bladder is stiff, does not stretch as expected, and can possibly compromise kidney function over time. A large-capacity low-pressure bladder (high compliance) may indicate chronic overdistention from infrequent voiding habits or disturbed muscle coordination.
2. Bladder instability (hyperreflexia): During filling, the bladder contracts involuntarily; this occurs when the pressures go up and down in a wavelike pattern during filling due to overactivity of involuntary contractions. The unstable bladder may be asymptomatic; many times, no contractions are felt, but commonly, patients have frequency, urgency, and incontinence.
3. The most common cause of incontinence is a vesicle–sphincter dyssynergia (disturbance of muscular coordination). This dyssynergia is thought to be responsible for incomplete emptying of the bladder, inappropriate voiding, perineal dampness, and predisposition to urinary tract infections.
4. Detrusor hyperreflexia: The patient cannot suppress voiding on command owing to upper or lower motor neuron lesions, as in cerebrovascular aneurysm, Parkinson's disease, multiple sclerosis, cervical spondylosis, and spinal cord injury above the conus medullaris.
5. Detrusor areflexia occurs when the detrusor reflex cannot be evoked because the peripheral innervation of the detrusor muscle has been interrupted, resulting in difficulty in initiating voiding without a residual volume being present in the bladder. The cause may be associated with trauma, spinal arachnoiditis, spinal cord birth defects, diabetic neuropathy, or anticholinergic effects of phenothiazines. In postmenopausal women, the urethral pressure profile may be altered because the mucosal sphincter is deprived of estrogen.
6. Urethrovesical hyperreflexia is caused by benign prostatic hypertrophy and stress urge incontinence.

Interfering Factors

Disorientation or inability of the patient to cooperate affects the test results.

Interventions

Pretest Patient Care

1. Explain the purpose and procedure of the bladder function test, often done before and after certain types of spinal surgery. Sensitivity to the patient's potential anxiety or modesty concerns is important. Record signs and symptoms of incontinence and voiding problems.
2. Ensure that the patient is relaxed and cooperative for accurate results. For children, a favorite toy or book may provide security. Sedation is not given because patient participation is necessary to verify sensations and perceptions. However, the patient must avoid movement during the examination unless instructed otherwise.
3. Allow the test and filling of the bladder to continue until the patient either leaks or voids around the catheter.
4. Follow guidelines in Chapter 1 for safe, effective, informed *pretest* care.

Posttest Patient Care

1. Encourage the patient to increase oral fluid intake to dilute the urine and to minimize bladder sensitivity.
2. Explain that some minor discomfort or burning may be noted, especially if carbon dioxide is used, but it will lessen and disappear with time.
3. Review test results; report and record findings. Modify the nursing care plan as needed. Counsel the patient appropriately (bladder capacity varies with age). Explain possible treatments (medication).
4. Follow Chapter 1 guidelines for safe, effective, informed *posttest* care. Provide written discharge instructions.

CLINICAL ALERT

1. Certain patients with cervical cord lesions may exhibit an autonomic reflex that produces an elevated blood pressure, severe headache, lower pulse rate, flushing, and diaphoresis. Propantheline bromide (Pro-Banthine) alleviates these symptoms.
2. Careful use of sterile technique reduces the incidence of urinary tract infections. Preprocedural urinary tract infections can lead to sepsis as a result of bacterial spread into the bloodstream.

● Arthroscopy

Arthroscopy is the direct visual examination of the interior of a joint by means of a specially designed fiberoptic endoscope and is frequently associated with a surgical procedure. It is most commonly done for the diagnosis of athletic injuries (meniscus, patella, condyle, extrasynovial area, and synovium) and for the differential diagnosis of acute or chronic joint disorders. For example, degenerative processes can be accurately differentiated from injuries. Postoperative rehabilitation programs can be initiated to shorten recovery periods. Arthroscopy can also assess response to treatment or identify whether other corrective procedures are indicated.

Although the knee is the joint most frequently examined, the shoulder, ankle, hip, elbow, wrist, and metacarpophalangeal joints can also be explored. Calcium deposits, biopsy specimens, loose bodies, bone spurs, torn meniscus or cartilage, and scar tissue can be removed during the procedure. These procedures are often performed in an ambulatory surgical setting.

Reference Values

Normal

Normal joint: normal vasculature and color of the synovium, capsule, menisci, ligaments, and articular cartilage

Procedure

1. The examination is usually performed under general or spinal anesthesia for the following reasons:
   a. The joint is very painful.
   b. Definitive treatment or surgical intervention can be done at the same time if within the realm of arthroscopic surgery.
   c. An inflated tourniquet may be used during part of the procedure to minimize bleeding at the site.
   d. Complete muscle relaxation permits a thorough examination and eliminates the risk for inadvertent patient movement while the arthroscope is in the joint.
2. Start an intravenous line. Drape and prep the surgical site according to institutional protocols. Attach proper monitoring equipment to the patient.
3. Apply a tourniquet to the appropriate area (by use of an elastic bandage or elevation) and then insert an arthroscope into the joint through a small insertion. Some surgeons choose not to inflate the tourniquet unless bleeding cannot be controlled by irrigation.
4. Aspirate the joint and subsequently perform continuous irrigation and flushing throughout the procedure.
5. Collect joint washings and examine for loose bodies or cartilage fragments.
6. Examine all parts of the joint carefully. Take photographs or video record of the procedure. The healthcare provider may choose to perform surgical interventions for problems that can be corrected using arthroscopy.
7. As the arthroscope is slowly withdrawn, compress the joint to squeeze out excess irrigation fluid.
8. Inject steroids or local anesthetics into the joint for postoperative pain control and reduction of inflammation. Close the wounds with sutures or adhesive strips and apply small dressings to the wound or wounds (e.g., two to three small incisions for the knee joint). Apply compressive dressings and splints or immobilizers.
9. Follow guidelines in Chapter 1 for safe, effective, informed *intratest* care.

Clinical Implications

Abnormal results reveal the following conditions:

1. Torn or displaced meniscus or cartilage (symptoms relate to clicking, locking, and/or swelling of the joint)
2. Trapped synovium
3. Loose fragments of joint contents
4. Torn or ruptured ligaments
5. Necrosis
6. Nerve entrapment
7. Fractures or nonunion of fractures
8. Ganglions
9. Infections
10. Degenerative disease
11. Osteochondritis dissecans
12. Chronic inflammatory arthritis
13. Secondary osteoarthritis caused by injury, metabolic disorders, and wearing away of weight-bearing joints
14. Chondromalacia of femoral condyle

Interfering Factors

Ankylosis, fibrosis, sepsis, or presence of contrast agent from previous arthrogram may affect results.

Interventions

Pretest Patient Care

1. Ensure that the history and physical examination, requisite laboratory work, x-ray films, and other preoperative requirements are completed, reviewed, and documented in the patient's record.
2. Explain the purpose and procedure of the test. The patient should fast from midnight before the examination unless otherwise ordered (e.g., if scheduled late in the day, a liquid breakfast may be permitted).
3. A properly signed and witnessed consent form must be completed (see Chapter 1).
4. Check peripheral pulses in the operative area. The surgical site is prepped, positioned, and draped according to institutional protocols. An intravenous line is started.
5. Teach crutch-walking before the procedure if its necessity is anticipated postoperatively.
6. Follow guidelines in Chapter 1 for safe, effective, informed *pretest* care.

CLINICAL ALERT

1. Arthroscopy is usually contraindicated if ankylosis or fibrosis is present because it is very difficult to maneuver the examining instrument in this type of joint.
2. For knee arthroscopy, the posterior approach is not used because of the neurovascular structures present in that area.
3. Do not place pillows under the knee; flexion contractures can occur as a result. If the patient's leg is ordered to be elevated, make sure the entire leg is elevated in a straight position. The knee is not flexed because a flexion contracture may result. Pad pressure points such as the heel.
4. If there is risk for sepsis or if sepsis is present in any part of the body, the procedure should not be done.
5. Arthroscopy is usually not done less than 7–10 d after arthrography because chemical synovitis caused by a contrast medium can adversely affect the visual examination. However, it may be necessary to perform arthroscopy if the patient is experiencing severe pain. In this case, the joint must be thoroughly irrigated to remove contrast medium.

Posttest Patient Care

1. Assess vital signs, bleeding, neurologic status, and circulatory status of the affected extremity (e.g., color, pulse, temperature, capillary refill times, sensation, and motion).
2. Apply cold pack and, if ordered, elevate the extremity to minimize swelling and pain. Dressing changes and suture removal are performed at the healthcare provider's discretion. The dressing must be kept clean and dry. Notify the healthcare provider of unusual bleeding or swelling.
3. Administer appropriate pain medication.
4. The patient can usually be ambulatory after recovery from the anesthetic. Crutches may be used. Degree of weight-bearing and joint motion is at the discretion of the healthcare provider; however, patient should be cautioned to avoid excessive joint use for at least 24 to 48 hours.
5. Exercise and physical therapy may be ordered postoperatively. These are designed to strengthen and maximize use of the joint.
6. Make arrangements preoperatively for transportation by another person if the patient is discharged the same day as the procedure. The patient should not drive for at least 24 hours.
7. Advise the patient to consume no alcohol for 24 hours after the procedure. Progress diet from fluid to solid foods as tolerated.

8. Instruct the patient to report fever, altered sensation, numbness, tingling, coldness, duskiness (i.e., bluish color), swelling, bleeding, or abnormal pain to the healthcare provider immediately. Mild soreness and a mild grinding sensation for a few days are normal.
9. Review test results; report and record findings. Modify the nursing care plan as needed. Counsel the patient appropriately.
10. Follow guidelines in Chapter 1 for safe, effective, informed *posttest* care. Provide written discharge instructions.

CLINICAL ALERT

1. Watch for signs of thrombophlebitis postoperatively. Instruct patient to watch for calf tenderness, pain, and heat and to report these symptoms to the healthcare provider immediately. *Warn the patient not to massage the affected area.*
2. Other complications may include hemarthrosis, adhesions, neurovascular injury, pulmonary embolus, effusion, scarring, and compartmental syndrome as a result of swelling. Compartmental syndrome is a musculoskeletal complication that occurs most commonly in the forearm or leg. The compartment of fascia surrounding muscles does not expand when bleeding or edema occurs. Consequently, the neurovascular status of the extremity may be severely compromised. This presents an emergency situation that usually requires surgical intervention to release pressure. Assess the neurovascular status of an affected extremity frequently for 24 hr after the procedure.

Sinus Endoscopy

Sinus endoscopy visualizes the anterior ethmoid, middle turbinate region, and middle meatus sinus areas. Although the purposes of sinus endoscopy are primarily to relieve infection and other symptoms of inflammation and to alter structural abnormalities in these areas, it can also be a valuable diagnostic tool. Retained secretions may contribute to chronic recurrent sinus infections, which may lead to systemic infections, cyst formation, or mucoceles that can erode sinus walls into areas of the eyeball, eye orbit, or brain.

Patients having recurrent episodes of acute or chronic sinusitis that are not responsive to antibiotic or allergy therapy are candidates for sinus endoscopy as both a diagnostic and therapeutic modality.

Reference Values

Normal

Normal sinuses or resolution of sinus disease

Procedure

Sinus endoscopy may be performed as an outpatient or office procedure. More extensive examination and operative procedures may require admission to a healthcare facility or special diagnostic center.

1. Spray or instruct the patient to inhale ordered medication to produce local anesthesia. Introduce the endoscope to permit visualization of the nasal interior; the sinus cavities are *not* opened.
2. Sinus computed axial tomography (CAT) scans and magnetic resonance imaging (MRI) may be necessary adjuncts to this procedure to permit visualization of areas not accessible through endoscopy.
3. Perform treatment for underlying disease or malformations using local or general anesthesia and medications to achieve a state of conscious sedation. Diagnostic and surgical techniques vary according to preoperative findings.

4. Endoscopes using a fiberoptic light delivery system are the mainstay of visualization for diagnosis and treatment.
5. Follow guidelines in Chapter 1 for safe, effective, informed *intratest* care.

Clinical Implications

Abnormalities that may be revealed include the following conditions:

1. Chronic sinusitis (edematous or polypoid mucosa)
2. Cysts
3. Mucocele
4. Sinus erosion
5. Anatomic deformities or obstructions
6. Pathologic sinus discharge (infectious process)
7. Enlarged middle turbinates

Interventions

Pretest Patient Care

1. Explain the test purpose, benefits, risks, and procedure.
2. Obtain and record a properly signed and witnessed consent form (see Chapter 1), appropriate laboratory and diagnostic test results, history and physical examination, current drug therapies, and allergies before the procedure.
3. Preprocedure preparation may require the patient to:
   a. Be processed through preadmission testing if procedure will be done in a hospital surgical setting.
   b. Fast from midnight the day of the procedure.
   c. Remove facial prostheses, dentures, hairpieces, and jewelry before the procedure.
   d. Have an intravenous line placed.
   e. Arrange transportation home when discharged.
4. Have the patient assume a supine position in the surgical suite. Prep the face and throat according to established protocols and properly drape the area. Tape eye pads in place to protect the eyes from injury. Perform other positioning and pressure-point padding as necessary.
5. Administer intravenous sedation as needed. Spray the nose with a topical anesthetic, and inject a small amount of 1% lidocaine with 1:200,000 aqueous epinephrine into the appropriate areas (unless contraindicated because of allergy or for other reasons) to provide anesthesia and control of bleeding. Refer to Chapter 1 for intravenous conscious sedation precautions.
6. Follow guidelines in Chapter 1 for safe, effective, informed *pretest* care.

Posttest Patient Care

1. Fill a 10-mL syringe with antibiotic ointment at the end of the procedure. Use a small catheter attached to the syringe tip to direct ointment to the appropriate areas. Insert nasal packing into the nares. Tape a small (2 × 2 inches) "mustache dressing" to the end of the nose to collect secretions and blood. Usually, this dressing can be changed as needed.
2. Encourage oral fluids after nausea or vomiting has resolved; the patient may experience nausea or vomiting if blood is swallowed because blood is irritating to the GI system.
3. Postprocedural instructions may include the following:
   a. Take prescribed medications as ordered (usually a broad-spectrum antibiotic and pain medication). Soothing gargles may be ordered.
   b. Report excessive bleeding or sinus discharge, unusual pain, fever, nausea or vomiting, or visual problems immediately.
   c. Do not allow the patient to drive or sign legal documents for 24 hours because of the effects of anesthetics and sedation.

4. Follow the usual precautions involved in the care of any person having received sedation and analgesia. The patient who has received drugs to achieve conscious sedation may require closer monitoring, positioning on the side to prevent aspiration, and a longer recovery time than those who receive local anesthesia.
5. Review test results; report and record findings. Modify the nursing care plan as needed. Counsel the patient appropriately about possible treatment (medications [e.g., steroids, antibiotics]). Numbness of the face may continue for several weeks.
6. Follow guidelines in Chapter 1 for safe, effective, informed *posttest* care. Provide written discharge instructions.

CLINICAL ALERT

1. **Sinuses are poorly visualized through routine sinus x-ray films.**
2. **If sinus problems appear to be related to dental problems, the patient should see a dentist or oral surgeon before sinus endoscopy is performed.**
3. **Severe nasal septal deviation must be corrected before endoscopy.**
4. **Potential complications include periorbital bleeding, cerebrospinal fluid leak, cellulitis, visual disturbances, and subcutaneous orbital emphysema.**
5. **Direct trauma to the nasofrontal duct is associated with increased risk for postoperative stenosis.**

BIBLIOGRAPHY

American Cancer Society: Treatment of Rectal Cancer, by Stage. Available at: https://www.cancer.org/cancer/colon-rectal-cancer/treating/by-stage-rectum.html. Last medical review: January 15, 2017; last revised: March 2, 2017

American Society of Anesthesiologists, Inc., Task Force on Sedation and Analgesia by Non-Anesthesiologists: Practice guidelines for sedation and analgesia by non-anesthesiologists. Anesthesiology 96(4):1004–1017, 2002

Centers for Disease Control: Known health effects for DES daughters. Available at: www.cdc.gov/DES/consumers/about/effects_daughters.html

DeVita VT, Hellman S, Rosenberg SA: Cancer Principles and Practice of Oncology, 10th ed. Philadelphia, Lippincott Williams & Wilkins, 2014

Finkelmeier BA: Cardiothoracic Surgical Nursing, 2nd ed. Philadelphia, Lippincott Williams & Wilkins, 2000

Goroll AH, Mulley AG: Primary Care Medicine: Office Evaluation and Management of the Adult Patient, 7th ed. Philadelphia, Lippincott Williams & Wilkins, 2014

Hatchett R, Thompson DR: Cardiac Nursing: A Comprehensive Guide, 2nd ed. Philadelphia, Churchill Livingstone, 2008

Hutchisson B, Phippen ML, Wells MP: Review of Perioperative Nursing. Philadelphia, Elsevier Mosby Saunders, 2000

Jamieson E, McCall JM, Whyte LA: Clinical Nursing Practice, 5th ed. Philadelphia, Elsevier Mosby Saunders, 2007

Nagelhout JJ, Plaus KL: Nurse Anesthesia, 5th ed. Philadelphia, Elsevier Mosby Saunders, 2013

Nettina SM: Lippincott Manual of Nursing Practice, 10th ed. Philadelphia, Lippincott Williams & Wilkins, 2013

Society of Gastroenterology Nurses and Associates, Core Curriculum Committee: Gastroenterology Nursing: A Core Curriculum, 5th ed. Chicago, SGNA, 2013

Thompson JM, McFarland GK, Hirsch JE, et al: Clinical Nursing, 5th ed. St. Louis, Mosby, 2002

U.S. Food and Drug Administration: Medication guide: OsmoPrep® tablets. Available at: https://www.fda.gov/downloads/drugs/drugsafety/ucm135936

INTERNET SITES

http://www.sgna.org

13 Ultrasound Studies

OVERVIEW OF ULTRASOUND STUDIES

Ultrasound (ultrasonography) is a noninvasive procedure for visualizing soft tissue structures of the body by recording the reflection of inaudible sound waves directed into the tissues. The image produced by the ultrasound is called a sonogram. The diagnostic procedure, which requires very little patient preparation, is used in many branches of medicine for accurate diagnosis of certain pathologic conditions (Chart 13.1). It may be used diagnostically with the obstetric, gynecologic, or cardiac

CHART 13.1 Uses of Ultrasound

Obstetric ultrasound: commonly performed to evaluate fetal health, size, and number of fetuses; level of amniotic fluid; and maternal and placental anatomy

Abdominal ultrasound: used to characterize soft tissue organs, including:

- Hepatobiliary: to evaluate organ size and presence of masses, calculi, or diffuse parenchymal conditions. Doppler ultrasound is helpful in demonstrating signs of portal hypertension.
- Pancreas: to detect pathologic states such as tumor involvement, pseudocysts, and inflammatory processes
- Kidneys, ureters, and bladder: to diagnose cysts, masses, hydronephrosis, and certain diffuse conditions. Doppler evaluation of the renal vessels and parenchyma is commonly used to evaluate transplanted kidneys and in the staging of known renal cell carcinoma.
- Aorta and other large abdominal vessels: to detect aneurysms, the presence of clots or tumors, and other defects
- Spleen and lymph nodes: to evaluate organ size and pathologic states such as lymphoma and metastatic spread of known cancers
- Additional structures: to demonstrate suspected ascites, abscesses, retroperitoneal tumors, and signs of appendicitis

Pelvic ultrasound: Gynecologic scan is done to evaluate the urinary bladder, uterus, and ovaries; is used to monitor follicle development during infertility treatments and also as a guide for oocyte retrieval.

Male reproductive organs ultrasound: used to evaluate scrotal masses and swelling and combined with Doppler examination of the penis to detect physiologic causes for male impotence. Transrectal ultrasound is an accepted method of screening for prostatic disease.

Head and neck ultrasound: used to evaluate pathologies in the following structures:

- Thyroid and parathyroid: for differentiating cysts from solid tumors
- Carotid and vertebral arteries: to demonstrate vessel patency and flow patterns
- Eye: to assist ophthalmologist in the removal of foreign bodies and in the evaluation of the eye's structure
- Neonatal brain: to diagnose cerebral hemorrhage and other intracranial pathologies
- Adult cerebral blood flow: By using a method known as transcranial Doppler, the larger blood vessels within the brain may be interrogated to rule out vascular disturbance.

Breast ultrasound: performed to differentiate cysts from solid lesions and to guide cyst aspirations and needle biopsies

Extremities ultrasound: used to evaluate arterial and venous blood flow and to characterize soft tissue masses such as Baker's cysts. Sonography is often used to evaluate the pediatric hip for dislocations or other structural deformities. Certain adult joint anatomy can be visualized, such as the wrist in the evaluation of carpal tunnel syndrome.

Invasive procedures: serve as a guide for diagnostic procedures, such as paracentesis, amniocentesis, thoracentesis, and biopsy

Cardiac ultrasound: performed to evaluate the cardiac structure and blood flow through chambers and valves

patients and in patients with abnormal conditions of the kidney, pancreas, gallbladder (GB), lymph nodes, liver, spleen, abdominal aorta, bile ducts, ureters, bladder, thyroid, or peripheral blood vessels. Frequently, it is used in conjunction with radiology or nuclear medicine scans. The procedure is relatively quick (often requiring only a few minutes to an hour) and causes little discomfort. No harmful effects have yet been established at the low intensities that are used (<100 mW/cm^2). However, as with any diagnostic procedure, ultrasound should not be used frivolously.

Principles and Techniques

Ultrasound uses high-frequency sound waves to produce an "echo map" that characterizes the position, size, form, and nature of soft tissue organs. Echoes of varying strength are produced by different types of tissues and are displayed as a visual pattern after computer processing of the echo information. The capability of acquiring real-time images means that ultrasound can readily demonstrate motion, as in the fetus or the heart. Ultrasound, however, cannot appropriately image air-filled structures such as the lungs.

Doppler Method

A phenomenon that accompanies movement, the *Doppler effect*, can be combined with diagnostic ultrasound imaging to produce duplex scans. Duplex scans provide anatomic visualization of blood vessels and a graphic representation of blood flow characteristics. Flow direction, velocity, and the presence of flow disturbances can readily be assessed. Certain equipment is capable of advanced Doppler imaging techniques, such as:

1. *Color Doppler* imaging provides a color-coded depiction of selected blood flow parameters.
2. *Doppler energy, power Doppler,* or *color angio* is sensitive to very low blood velocity states and is often used to evaluate blood flow through solid organs.
3. *B-flow Doppler* images the blood itself, producing images that resemble an angiogram.

These techniques establish the patency of a given blood vessel and are useful in investigating perfusion to an organ or mass. They are also helpful in evaluating complications in transplanted organs.

General Procedure

1. A couplant is a nontoxic gel, paste, or liquid that is used to transmit sound energy between the body and the transducer. The couplant is applied to the skin over the area to be examined in order to conduct the sound waves.
2. An operator, known as an ultrasonographer or *sonographer,* holds a microphone-like device called a *transducer.* The transducer is moved over a specific body part, producing a display that is viewed on the monitor.
3. Sonography of structures in the abdominal region often requires that the patient control breathing patterns. Deep inspiration and exhalation may be used.
4. Selected images are recorded for documentation purposes.
5. The examination causes no physical pain. However, in certain applications, pressure may be applied to the transducer, causing some degree of discomfort. Long examinations may leave the patient feeling tired.
6. Tests usually take 20 to 45 minutes. This is the actual procedure time and does not include waiting and preparation times.
7. Some examinations require the patient to fast or to have a filled urinary bladder. Each examining department determines its own guidelines for patient preparation.

Advances in technology have allowed the development of very small high-resolution transducers. Catheter-sized transducers are used to visualize blood vessels "from the inside out" during angiographic procedures. Endoscopic ultrasound is used to evaluate gastrointestinal lesions and may be used to visualize pancreatic biliary structures. Small transducers passed through the esophagus permit exquisite visualization of the heart during transesophageal echocardiography (TEE). Slim transducers are introduced into the vagina to visualize gynecologic anatomy. Transrectal visualization of the prostate gland is an accepted method of screening for disease in the organ.

Implications of Ultrasound Studies

Benefits and Risks

1. Ultrasound is a noninvasive procedure with no radiation risk to patient or examiner.
2. It requires little, if any, patient preparation and aftercare.
3. The examination can be repeated as often as necessary without being injurious to the patient. No harmful cumulative effect has been seen.
4. Ultrasound is useful in the detection and examination of moving parts, such as the heart.
5. It does not require the injection of contrast materials or isotopes or ingestion of opaque materials.

Disadvantages

1. An extremely skilled examiner is required to operate the transducer. The scans should be read immediately and interpreted for adequacy. If the scans are not satisfactory, the examination must be repeated.
2. Air-filled structures (e.g., the lungs) cannot be studied by ultrasonography.
3. Certain patients (e.g., restless children, extremely obese patients) cannot be studied adequately unless they are specially prepared.

Difficult-to-Study Patients

The following general categories of patients may provide some difficulties in ultrasound studies:

1. *Postoperative patients and those with abdominal scars*: The area surrounding an incision is to be avoided whenever possible. If a scan must be performed over an incision, the dressing must be removed and a sterile coupling agent and probe must be used.
2. *Children and agitated adults*: Because the procedure requires the patient to remain still, some patients may need to be sedated so that their movements do not cause artifacts.
3. *Obese patients*: Certain patients cannot be studied adequately in any case. For example, it may be difficult to obtain an accurate scan on a very obese patient, owing to alteration of the sound beam by fatty tissue.

Interfering Factors

1. Barium has an adverse effect on the quality of abdominal studies, so sonograms should be scheduled before barium studies are done.
2. If the patient has a large amount of gas in the bowel, the examination may be rescheduled because air (bowel gas) is a very strong reflector of sound and does not permit accurate visualization.

OBSTETRIC AND GYNECOLOGIC ULTRASOUNDS

● Obstetric Sonogram

Ultrasound studies of the obstetric patient are valuable in (1) confirming pregnancy; (2) facilitating amniocentesis by locating a suitable pool of amniotic fluid; (3) determining fetal age; (4) confirming multiple pregnancy; (5) ascertaining whether fetal growth is normal, through sequential studies;

(6) determining fetal viability; (7) localizing placenta; (8) confirming masses associated with pregnancy; (9) identifying postmature pregnancy (increased amount of amniotic fluid and degree of placental calcification); (10) serving as a guidance method for chorionic villus sampling (CVS), embryo transfer, intrauterine device (IUD) extraction, and percutaneous umbilical vein sampling (PUVS); and (11) determining fetal nuchal translucency (FNT). A pregnancy can be dated with considerable accuracy if an ultrasound is done at 20 weeks' gestation and a follow-up scan is done at 32 weeks' gestation. This validation is most important when early delivery is anticipated and prematurity is to be avoided. Conditions in which determination of pregnancy duration is useful include maternal diabetes, Rh immunization, and preterm labor (Chart 13.2).

The pregnant uterus is ideal for echographic evaluation because the amniotic fluid–filled uterus provides strong transmitting interfaces between the fluid, placenta, and fetus. Ultrasonography has become the method of choice for evaluating the fetus and placenta, eliminating the need for the potentially injurious radiographic studies that were used previously.

Reference Values

Normal Obstetric Sonogram

Normal image of placental position, size, and structure

Normal fetal position and size with evidence of fetal movement, cardiac activity, and breathing activity

Adequate amniotic fluid volume

Normal fetal intracranial, thoracic, and abdominopelvic anatomy; four limbs visualized

Procedure

1. Most laboratories use a transvaginal (endovaginal) approach during the first trimester of pregnancy. No patient preparation is required for this method. Contact the laboratory performing the study to determine the method to be used.
2. Most laboratories use a transabdominal approach in the second trimester of pregnancy. Exceptions are made when the scan is performed to locate the placenta before amniocentesis, for evaluation of an incompetent cervix, or during labor and delivery. With this approach, the patient will need to have a full bladder. The patient is asked to drink five to six glasses of fluid (water or juice) about 1 to 2 hours before the examination. If she is unable to do so, intravenous fluids may be administered. She is asked to refrain from voiding until the examination is complete. Tell the patient that she will have a strong urge to void during the examination. Discomfort caused by pressure applied over a full bladder may be experienced. If the bladder is not sufficiently filled, three to four 8-oz glasses of water should be ingested, with rescanning done 30 to 45 minutes later. A full bladder allows the examiner to assess the true position of the placenta, repositions the uterus, and acts as a sonic window to the pelvic organs.
3. Have the pregnant woman lie on her back with her abdomen exposed during the test. This may cause some shortness of breath and supine hypotensive syndrome, which can be relieved by elevating the upper body or turning the patient onto her side.
4. In the transvaginal (endovaginal) procedure, a slim transducer, properly covered and lubricated, is gently introduced into the vagina. Because the sound waves do not need to traverse abdominal tissue, exquisite image detail is produced.
5. In the transabdominal approach, a coupling agent (special transmission gel, lotion, or mineral oil) is liberally applied to the skin to prevent air from absorbing sound waves. The sonographer slowly moves the transducer over the entire abdomen to obtain a picture of the uterine contents.
6. Check with your laboratory to determine the approach to be used.
7. Tell the patient that the examining time is about 30 to 60 minutes.
8. See Chapter 1 guidelines for *intratest* care.

CHART 13.2 Major Uses of Obstetric Ultrasound—Levels I and II[a]

Indications During First Trimester

Confirm pregnancy.
Confirm viability.
Rule out ectopic pregnancy in the first trimester.
Confirm gestational age.[b]
- Birth control pill use
- Irregular menses
- No dates
- Postpartum pregnancy

Previous complicated pregnancy
- Cesarean delivery
- Rh incompatibility
- Diabetes mellitus
- Fetal growth retardation

Clarify discrepancy between dates and size.
- If large for dates, rule out:
  - Leiomyomas
  - Bicornuate uterus
  - Adnexal mass
  - Multiple gestation
  - Poor estimate of dates
  - Missed abortion
  - Blighted ovum

As guidance method for:
- Chorionic villus sampling
- Amniocentesis
- Embryo transfer

Indications During Second Trimester

Establish or confirm dates.[b]
- If no fetal heart tones:
  - Clarify discrepancy between dates and size.
- If large for dates, rule out:
  - Poor estimate of dates
  - Molar pregnancy
  - Multiple gestation
  - Leiomyomas
  - Polyhydramnios
  - Congenital anomalies
- If small for dates, rule out:
  - Poor estimate of dates
  - Fetal growth retardation
  - Congenital anomalies
  - Oligohydramnios

If history of bleeding, rule out total placenta previa
If Rh incompatibility, rule out fetal hydrops
Evaluation and follow-up of suspected fetal anomalies

Indications During Third Trimester

If no fetal heart tones:
- Clarify discrepancy between dates and size.
- If large for dates, rule out:
  - Macrosomia (diabetes mellitus)
  - Multiple gestation
  - Polyhydramnios
  - Congenital anomalies
  - Poor estimate of dates[a]
- If small for dates, rule out:
  - Fetal growth retardation
  - Oligohydramnios
  - Congenital anomalies
  - Poor estimate of dates[c]

Determine fetal position, rule out:
- Breech
- Transverse lie

If history of bleeding, rule out:
- Placenta previa
- Abruptio placentae

Determine fetal maturity
- Amniocentesis for lecithin/sphingomyelin ratio
- Placental maturity (grades 0–3)

Evaluation and follow-up of suspected fetal anomalies
Estimation of fetal weight

[a]Ultrasound is a diagnostic tool for assessment of fetal age, health, and growth. Level I ultrasound is performed to assess gestational age, number of fetuses, fetal viability, and the placenta. Level II ultrasound is used for assessment of specific congenital anomalies or abnormalities. (See also Fetal Echocardiography, p. 884.)
[b]Accuracy ±3 days.
[c]Accuracy ±1 to 1.5 days.

Clinical Implications

1. During the first trimester, the following information can be obtained:
   a. Number, size, and location of gestational sacs
   b. Presence or absence of fetal cardiac activity and body movement
   c. Presence or absence of uterine abnormalities (e.g., bicornuate uterus, fibroids) or adnexal masses (e.g., ovarian cyst, ectopic pregnancy)
   d. Pregnancy dating (e.g., biparietal diameter, crown–rump length)
2. During the second and third trimesters, ultrasound can be performed to obtain the following information:
   a. Fetal viability, number, position, gestational age, growth pattern, and structural abnormalities
   b. Amniotic fluid volume
   c. Placental location, maturity, and abnormalities
   d. Uterine fibroids and anomalies
   e. Adnexal masses
   f. Early diagnosis of fetal structural abnormalities
3. ***Fetal viability***: Fetal heart activity can be demonstrated at 5 weeks' gestation in most cases. This information is helpful in establishing dates and in the management of vaginal bleeding. Molar pregnancies (a nonviable fertilized egg implants into the uterus; the pregnancy will not come to term) and incomplete, complete, and missed abortions can be differentiated.
4. ***Gestational age***: Indications for gestational age evaluation include uncertain dates for the last menstrual period, recent discontinuation of oral hormonal suppression of ovulation, bleeding episode during the first trimester, amenorrhea of at least 3 months' duration, uterine size that does not agree with dates, previous cesarean birth, and other high-risk conditions.
5. ***Fetal growth***: The conditions that serve as indicators for ultrasound assessment of fetal growth include poor maternal weight gain or pattern of weight gain, previous intrauterine growth retardation (IUGR), chronic infection, ingestion of drugs such as anticonvulsants or heroin, maternal diabetes, pregnancy-induced or other hypertension, multiple pregnancy, and other medical or surgical complications. Serial evaluation of biparietal diameter and limb length can help differentiate between wrong dates and IUGR. Doppler evaluation of the umbilical artery, uterine artery, and fetal aorta can also assist in the detection of IUGR. IUGR can be symmetric (the fetus is small in all measurements) or asymmetric (head and body growth vary). Symmetric IUGR may be caused by low genetic growth potential, intrauterine infection, maternal undernutrition, heavy smoking by the mother, or chromosomal anomaly. Asymmetric IUGR may reflect placental insufficiency secondary to hypertension, cardiovascular disease, or renal disease. Depending on the probable cause, the therapy varies.
6. ***Fetal anatomy***: Depending on the gestational age, the following structures may be identified: intracranial anatomy, neck, spine, heart, stomach, small bowel, liver, kidneys, bladder, and extremities. Structural defects may be identified before delivery. The following are examples of structural defects that may be diagnosed by ultrasound: Hydrocephaly, anencephaly, and myelomeningocele are often associated with polyhydramnios (excessive accumulation of amniotic fluid; occurs in <1% of pregnancies). Potter's syndrome (renal agenesis) is associated with oligohydramnios defects (dwarfism, achondroplasia, osteogenesis imperfecta) and diaphragmatic hernias. Other structural anomalies that can be diagnosed by ultrasound are pleural effusion (after 20 weeks), intestinal atresias or obstruction (early pregnancy to second trimester), hydronephrosis, and bladder outlet obstruction (second trimester to term with fetal surgery available). Two-dimensional (2D) studies of the heart, together with echocardiography, allow diagnosis of congenital cardiac lesions and prenatal treatment of cardiac arrhythmias.
7. ***Detection of fetal death***: Inability to visualize the fetal heart beating, lack of fetal movement, and overlapping of skull bones (Spalding sign) are signs of death.

8. ***Placental position and function***: The site of implantation (e.g., anterior, posterior, fundal, in lower segment) can be described, as can location of the placenta on the other side of midline. The pattern of uterine and placental growth and the fullness of the bladder influence the apparent location of the placenta. For example, when ultrasound scanning is done in the second trimester, the placenta seems to be overlying the os in 15% to 20% of all pregnancies. At term, however, the evidence of placenta previa (placenta is partially in lower uterine segment) is only 0.5%. Therefore, the diagnosis of placenta previa can seldom be confirmed until the third trimester. Placenta abruptio (premature separation of placenta) can also be identified. A transverse scan through the umbilical cord confirms the number of vessels. Doppler of the cord detects flow abnormalities.
9. ***Fetal well-being***: Ultrasound findings are a major component of the biophysical profiles. The following physiologic measurements can be accomplished with ultrasound: heart rate and regularity, fetal breathing movements, urine production (after serial measurements of bladder volume), fetal limb and head movements, and analysis of vascular wave forms from fetal circulation. Fetal breathing movements are decreased with maternal smoking and alcohol use and increased with hyperglycemia. Fetal limb and head movements serve as an index of neurologic development. Identification of amniotic fluid measuring at least 1 cm is associated with normal fetal status. The presence of one pocket measuring <1 cm or the absence of a pocket is abnormal; it is associated with increased risk of perinatal death.
10. ***Assessment of multiple pregnancy***: Two or more gestational sacs, each containing an embryo, may be seen after 6 weeks. Of twin pregnancies diagnosed in the first trimester, only about 30% will deliver twins, owing to loss or absorption of one fetus. Of value is assessment of the relative fetal growth of twins when IUGR or twin-to-twin transfusion is suspected. One cannot unequivocally diagnose whether twins are monozygotes (identical; develop from one zygote) or heterozygotes (fraternal; two eggs are fertilized) with ultrasound alone unless fetuses of opposite sex are evident.
11. If the fetal position and amniotic fluid volumes are favorable, fetal sex can be determined by visualization of the genitalia. It must be cautioned, however, that sex determination is not the purpose of obstetric sonography.

Interfering Factors

1. Artifacts may be produced when the transducer is moved out of contact with the skin. This can be resolved by adding more coupling agent to the skin and repeating the scan.
2. Artifacts (reverberation) may be produced by echoes emanating from the same surface several times. This can be avoided by careful positioning of the transducer.
3. A posterior placental site may be difficult to identify because of the angulation of the reflecting surface or insufficient penetration of the sound beam owing to the patient's size.

Interventions

Pretest Patient Care

1. A brief explanation of the procedure to be performed is given, emphasizing that it is not uncomfortable or painful and does not involve ionizing radiation that might be harmful to the mother or fetus. The studies can be repeated without harm, but the procedure is being studied carefully to determine whether there are any long-term adverse side effects. Benefits of the procedure should be explained.
2. Explain that a liberal coating of coupling agent must be applied to the skin so that there is no air between the skin and the transducer and to allow for easy movement of the transducer over the skin. A sensation of warmth or wetness may be felt. The couplant (ultrasound gel) does not stain or discolor clothing, but the patient may prefer to don a gown.
3. The woman may face the screen, and the sonographer may explain the images in basic terms. A photograph or video recording may be provided (per institutional policy).
4. Follow guidelines in Chapter 1 for safe, effective, informed *pretest* care.

CLINICAL ALERT

1. A full bladder may not be needed or desired for patients in the late stages of pregnancy or active labor. However, if a full bladder is required and the woman has not been instructed to report with a full bladder, at least another hour of waiting time may be needed before the examination can begin.
2. Endovaginal studies typically involve the use of a latex condom to sheath the transducer before it is inserted into the vagina. Contact the laboratory if the patient has known or suspected latex sensitivity.
3. Fetal age determinations are most accurate during the crown–rump stage in the first trimester. The next most accurate time for age estimation is during the second trimester. Sonographic dating during the third trimester has a large margin of error (up to ±3 wk).

Posttest Patient Care

1. Review test results; report and record findings. Modify the nursing care plan as needed. Counsel the patient appropriately. Explain the possible need for follow-up testing (e.g., fetal echocardiography) and/or treatment: medical (to stimulate early onset of labor) or surgical (fetal surgery or immediate surgery for ectopic pregnancy).
2. If fetal death is suspected, careful and considerate counseling and support are offered to parents.
3. Follow guidelines in Chapter 1 for safe, effective, informed *posttest* care.

● Fetal Echocardiography (Fetal Doppler)

Fetal echocardiography is performed after the detection of a potential cardiac abnormality during an obstetric sonogram or in patients with a strong history of congenital cardiovascular disease. Additionally, women exposed to cardiac teratogens are usually advised to have this study. Not a screening procedure, fetal echocardiograms are most commonly performed in specialized laboratories or teaching hospitals. The heart is imaged in numerous planes, using pulsed Doppler and M-mode tracings, similar to an electrocardiogram (see Cardiac Ultrasound, page 892). Valves and other cardiac structures are measured, and blood velocities and volumes are calculated. Optimal fetal echocardiographic studies are performed between 18 and 22 gestational weeks. Before 18 weeks, the fetal heart is too small, and after 22 weeks, image quality may be degraded by overlying structures.

Reference Values

Normal Sonogram

Normal structure of heart and great vessels

Normal heart rate and rhythm, with proper hemodynamic flow through heart and great valves

Procedure

1. Perform the fetal echocardiogram in the same manner as a routine obstetric scan, which also requires similar patient preparation, although a full bladder is not necessary. The pregnant patient lies on her back with the abdomen exposed. A couplant (ultrasound gel) is applied to the skin, and a transducer is moved across the abdomen.
2. Although the fetal echocardiogram does not require the patient to have a full bladder, if combined with an obstetric sonogram, the mother is then required to have a full bladder. The patient is asked to drink five to six glasses of fluid (water or juice) about 1 to 2 hours before the examination. If she is unable to do so, intravenous fluids may be administered. She is asked to refrain from voiding until the examination is complete. Tell the patient that she will have a strong urge to void during

the examination. Discomfort caused by pressure applied over a full bladder may be experienced. If the bladder is not sufficiently filled, three to four 8-ounce glasses of water should be ingested, with rescanning done 30 to 45 minutes later.
3. See Chapter 1 guidelines for *intratest* care.

Clinical Implications

Abnormalities detected during fetal echocardiography include:

1. Cardiac arrhythmias
2. Septal defects, including tetralogy of Fallot
3. Hypoplastic heart syndrome
4. Valvular abnormalities, including Ebstein's anomaly (abnormality of the tricuspid valve)
5. Cardiac tumors
6. Vessel abnormalities, including coarctation of aorta, transposition, aortic stenosis, truncus arteriosus, and pulmonary stenosis

Interfering Factors

1. Artifacts may be produced when the transducer is moved out of contact with the skin. This can be resolved by adding more coupling agent to the skin and repeating the scan.
2. Artifacts (reverberations) may be produced by echoes emanating from the same surface several times. This can be avoided by careful positioning of the transducer.
3. A posterior placental site may be difficult to identify because of the angulation of the reflecting surface or insufficient penetration of the sound beam owing to the patient's size.

Interventions

Pretest Patient Care

1. A brief explanation of the procedure to be performed is given, emphasizing that it is not uncomfortable or painful and is not harmful to the mother or fetus. Explain that the procedure can be repeated without harm. Benefits of the procedure should also be explained.
2. Explain that a liberal coating of coupling agent must be applied to the skin so that there is no air between the skin and the transducer and to allow for easy movement of the transducer over the skin. A sensation of warmth or wetness may be felt. The couplant (ultrasound gel) does not stain or discolor clothing, but the patient may prefer to don a gown.
3. The woman may face the screen, and the sonographer may explain the images in basic terms. A photograph or video recording may be provided (per institution policy).
4. Follow guidelines in Chapter 1 for safe, effective, informed *pretest* care.

Posttest Patient Care

1. Review test results; report and record findings. Modify the nursing care plan as needed. Counsel the patient appropriately. Explain the possible need for follow-up testing and/or treatment: medical (to stimulate early onset of labor) or surgical (fetal surgery or immediate surgery for ectopic pregnancy).
2. Follow guidelines in Chapter 1 for safe, effective, informed *posttest* care.

● Pelvic Gynecologic Ultrasound; Pelvic (Uterine Mass) Ultrasound Diagnosis; Intrauterine Device (IUD) Localization

The pelvic gynecologic ultrasound study examines the area from the umbilicus to the pubic bone in women. It may be used in the evaluation of pelvic masses to determine the position of an IUD, to evaluate postmenopausal bleeding, or to aid in the diagnosis of cysts, tumors, abscess, fibroids, cancer, or thickened endometrium. Information can be provided on the size, location, and structure of masses. Spectral or color Doppler can be applied to pelvic vessels, demonstrating normal flow changes associated with the menstrual cycle, and can evaluate abnormal flow patterns to masses/tumors. The examination cannot provide a definitive diagnosis of pathology but can be used as an adjunct procedure when the diagnosis is not readily apparent. It is also used in treatment planning and follow-up radiation therapy for gynecologic cancer. Additionally, follicle development after infertility treatment can be monitored.

This test may be performed by a transvaginal method whereby a slim, covered, lubricated transducer is gently introduced into the vagina. A full bladder is not required. Because the sound waves do not need to transverse abdominal tissue, exquisite image detail is produced. This approach is most advantageous for examining the obese patient, the patient with a retroverted uterus, or the patient who has difficulty maintaining bladder distention. The transvaginal method is the approach of choice in monitoring follicular size during fertility workups and during aspiration of follicles for in vitro fertilization.

For pelvic sonograms using the transabdominal approach, a full bladder is necessary. The distended bladder serves four purposes: It acts as a "window" for transmission of the ultrasound beam; it pushes the uterus away from the pubic symphysis, thereby providing a less obstructed view; and it may be used as a reference for comparison in evaluating the internal characteristics of a mass under study.

Reference Values

Normal Sonogram

Normal pattern image of bladder, uterus, fallopian tubes, vagina, and surrounding structures
Normal Doppler flow patterns of major pelvic blood vessels

Procedure

Transabdominal Method

1. Have the patient lie on the back on the examining table during the test.
2. Apply a coupling agent to the area under study.
3. Place the active face of the transducer in contact with the patient's skin and sweep across the area being studied.
4. Tell the patient that the examination time is about 30 minutes.

Transvaginal (Endovaginal) Method

1. Have the patient lie on an examining table with hips slightly elevated in a modified lithotomy position. Drape the patient.
2. Lubricate and introduce a slim vaginal transducer, protected by a condom or sterile sheath, into the vagina. Some laboratories prefer that the patient insert the transducer herself.
3. Perform scans by using a slight rotation or movement of the handle and by varying the degree of transducer insertion. Typically, the transducer is inserted only a few inches into the vaginal vault.
4. Tell the patient that the examination time is about 15 to 30 minutes.
5. See Chapter 1 guidelines for *intratest* care.

PROCEDURAL ALERT

1. If the patient is taking nothing by mouth (NPO) or in certain emergency situations, the patient may be catheterized and the bladder filled through the catheter if a transabdominal approach is required.
2. Endovaginal studies, when indicated, typically involve the use of a latex condom to sheath the transducer before it is inserted into the vaginal vault. Contact the laboratory if the patient has a known or suspected latex sensitivity.

Clinical Implications

1. Uterine abnormalities such as fibroids, intrauterine fluid collections, and variations in structure such as bicornuate uterus can be detected. Uterine and cervical carcinomas may be visualized, although definitive diagnosis of cancer cannot be made by ultrasound alone.
2. Endometrial abnormalities such as polyps can be visualized by ultrasound. This procedure involves distention of the endometrial canal with saline and subsequent ultrasound scanning. Very small adnexal masses may not be demonstrated by ultrasound studies. Masses identified on ultrasound may be evaluated in terms of size and consistency.
3. Cysts
   a. Ovarian cysts (the most common ovarian mass detected by ultrasound) appear as smoothly outlined, well-defined masses. Cysts cannot be confirmed as either malignant or benign, but ultrasound studies can increase the suspicion that a particular mass is malignant.
   b. A corpus luteum cyst is a single, simple cyst commonly visualized in early pregnancy.
   c. Theca-lutein cysts are associated with hydatidiform mole, choriocarcinoma, or multiple pregnancy.
   d. Because normal ovaries often have numerous visible small cysts, the diagnosis of polycystic ovaries is difficult to make on the basis of ultrasound alone.
   e. Dermoid cysts or benign ovarian teratomas may be found in young adult women and have an extremely variable appearance. Because of their echogenicity, they are often missed on ultrasound. The only initial clue may be an indentation of the urinary bladder. When a dermoid cyst is suspected on ultrasound, a pelvic radiograph should be obtained.
4. Solid ovarian tumors such as fibromas, fibrosarcomas, Brenner's tumors, dysgerminomas, and malignant teratomas are not differentiated by diagnostic ultrasound. Ultrasound documents the presence of a solid lesion but can go no further in narrowing the diagnosis.
5. Metastatic tumors of the ovary may be solid or cystic in ultrasonic appearance. They are variable in size and are usually bilateral. Because ascites is often present, the pelvis and remainder of the abdomen should be scanned for fluid.
6. *Pelvic inflammatory disease*: Ultrasound differentiation between pelvic inflammatory disease and endometriosis is difficult. Evaluation of laboratory results and the clinical history leads to correct diagnosis. Other entities that may have similar ultrasonic presentation include appendicitis with rupture into the pelvis, chronic ectopic pregnancy, posttraumatic hemorrhage into the pelvis, and pelvic abscesses from various causes (e.g., Crohn's disease, diverticulitis).
7. *Bladder distortion*: Any distortion of the bladder raises the possibility of an adjacent mass. Tumor, infection, and hemorrhage are the major causes of increased thickness of the urinary bladder wall. Masses such as calculi and catheters may be seen within the bladder lumen. Urinary bladder calculi are highly echogenic. A urinary bladder diverticulum appears as a cystic mass adjacent to the urinary bladder. It may be mistaken for a cystic mass arising from some other pelvic structure, so attempts are made to demonstrate its communication to the bladder.
8. Ultrasound studies can help to determine whether a pelvic mass is mobile.
9. Solid pelvic masses such as fibroids and malignant tumors may be differentiated from cystic masses, which show sound patterns similar to those of the bladder.
10. Lesions may be shown to have metastasized.
11. Studies may aid in the planning of tumor radiation therapy.
12. The position of an IUD may be determined.

Interfering Factors

1. Severe obesity, intestinal gas, or barium in the intestine from recent procedures.
2. The success of a transabdominal scan depends on full bladder distention.

Interventions

Pretest Patient Care

1. Explain the purpose, benefits, and procedure of the test. Fasting is not required.
2. Have the patient drink four glasses of water or other liquid 1 hour before transabdominal scans. The patient should not void until the test is over.
3. Contact the laboratory performing the study to determine method to be used. If a transvaginal (endovaginal) approach is to be used, no patient preparation is required.
4. Explain that a liberal coating of coupling agent must be applied to the skin so that there is no air between the skin and the transducer and to allow for easy movement of the transducer over the skin. A sensation of warmth or wetness may be felt. The couplant (ultrasound gel) does not stain or discolor clothing, but the patient may prefer to don a gown.
5. Determine whether the patient has a latex sensitivity and communicate such sensitivities to the examining laboratory, if a transvaginal (endovaginal) approach is to be used. See latex precautions in Chapter 1.
6. Reassure the patient that the procedure is not painful.
7. Follow guidelines in Chapter 1 for safe, effective, informed *pretest* care.

Posttest Patient Care

1. Review test results; report and record findings. Modify the nursing care plan as needed. Counsel the patient appropriately about possible further testing (biopsy with cytologic and histologic exam) and/or treatment (medical, pharmacologic, or surgical interventions).
2. Follow guidelines in Chapter 1 for safe, effective, informed *posttest* care.

ABDOMINAL ULTRASOUNDS

● Kidney (Renal) Ultrasound

The kidney ultrasound is a noninvasive test used to visualize kidney parenchyma and associated structures, including renal blood vessels. This procedure is often performed after an intravenous pyelogram (IVP) to define and characterize mass lesions or the cause of a nonvisualized kidney. Because no contrast medium is administered, renal ultrasound is valuable for visualizing the kidneys of patients with iodine hypersensitivities. This procedure is also helpful in monitoring the status of a transplanted kidney, guiding stent and biopsy needle placement, and evaluating the progression of chronic conditions. Renal ultrasound is the preferred method for evaluating possible hydronephrosis in patients with spinal cord injury.

Reference Values

Normal

Normal pattern image indicating normal size and position of kidneys, appropriate blood flow in renal vessels

Procedure

1. Have the patient lie still on an examining table. Scans are often performed with the patient in the decubitus position.
2. Apply the coupling agent (ultrasound gel) to the patient's skin.
3. Ask the patient to inhale as deeply as possible for visualization of the upper parts of the kidney.
4. Tell the patient that the total study time varies from 15 to 30 minutes.
5. See Chapter 1 guidelines for *intratest* care.

PROCEDURAL ALERT

1. Scans cannot be done over open wounds or through dressings.
2. This examination must be performed before radiographic studies involving barium. If such scheduling is not possible, at least 24 hr must elapse between the barium procedure and the renal ultrasound.
3. Biopsies or drainage procedures are often done with ultrasound as a guide. If an invasive procedure is to be done, a signed, witnessed consent form must be obtained.

Clinical Implications

1. Abnormal pattern readings reveal:
   a. Cysts
   b. Solid masses
   c. Hydronephrosis
   d. Obstruction of ureters
   e. Calculi
2. Results provide information on the size, location, and internal structure of a nonfunctioning kidney.
3. Results differentiate between bilateral hydronephrosis, polycystic kidneys, and the small, end-stage kidneys of glomerulonephritis or pyelonephritis.
4. Results may be used to monitor kidney development in children with congenital hydronephrosis. This approach is considered safer than repeated IVP studies.
5. Perineal fluid collections such as those associated with complications of transplantation may be detected. These collections include abscesses, hematomas, urinomas, and lymphoceles.
6. Solid lesions may be differentiated from cystic lesions.
7. The spread of cancerous conditions from the kidney into the renal vein or inferior vena cava can be detected.
8. If ultrasound is combined with Doppler evaluations, the patency and flow characteristics of the renal vessels may be scrutinized.

Interfering Factors

1. Retained barium from radiology studies causes poor results.
2. Obesity adversely affects tissue visualization.

Interventions

Pretest Patient Care

1. Explain the purpose and procedure of the test.
2. Assure the patient that there is no pain involved and that the only discomfort is that caused by lying still for a long period.
3. Explain that a liberal coating of coupling agent must be applied to the skin so that there is no air between the skin and the transducer and to allow for easy movement of the transducer over the skin. A sensation of warmth or wetness may be felt. The couplant (ultrasound gel) does not stain or discolor clothing, but the patient may prefer to don a gown.
4. Explain that the patient will be instructed to control breathing patterns while the images are being made.
5. Check with your ultrasound department for guidelines about fasting. It usually is not necessary but may be required in certain laboratories.
6. Follow guidelines in Chapter 1 for safe, effective, informed *pretest* care.

Posttest Patient Care

1. Review test results; report and record findings. Modify the nursing care plan as needed. Counsel the patient appropriately about further testing (computerized axial tomography [CAT] scans, biopsies) and/or treatment of chronic conditions.
2. Follow guidelines in Chapter 1 for safe, effective, informed *posttest* care.

● Urinary Bladder Ultrasound

The urinary bladder ultrasound is done as part of the investigation of possible bladder tumor and provides a simple method of estimating postvoid residual urine volume. This test reduces the need for urinary catheterization and the risk of subsequent urinary tract infection. Portable bladder scans can be used at the bedside or in the doctor's office. This point-of-care testing allows for rapid, noninvasive measurement of bladder volume and postvoid residual urine volume. See Figure 13.1. Endourethral urologic ultrasound utilizing a transducer can be executed to place a stent.

Reference Values

Normal

Normal pattern image of the exact dimensions and contour of the bladder and little residual volume

Procedure

1. Instruct the patient to lie supine, with bladder fully distended, on an examination table.
2. Apply a coupling agent to the anterior pelvic region to allow maximum penetration of the ultrasound beam.
3. Place the active face of the transducer in contact with the patient's skin and sweep across the area being studied.
4. Instruct the patient to void. This is typically done when the full-bladder scans are completed. Then take additional images then to check for residual volume.

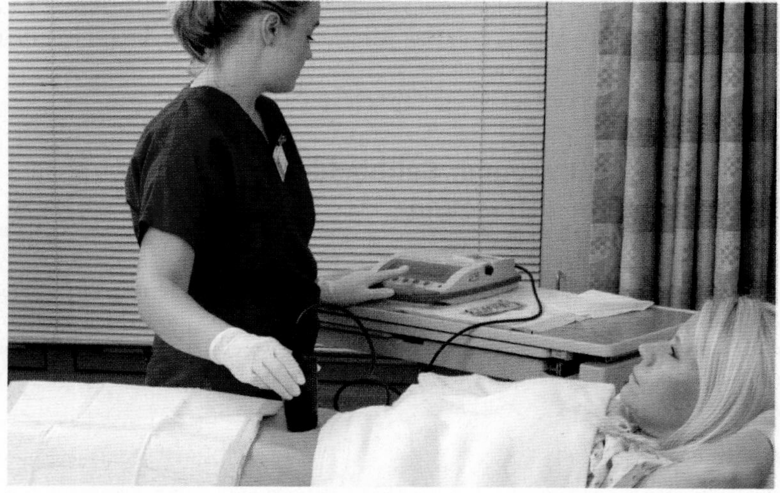

FIGURE 13.1. Placement of transducer during portable bladder scan. (From Craven R, Hirnle C, Henshaw CM: Fundamentals of Nursing, 8th ed. Philadelphia, Wolters Kluwer, 2017.)

5. Tell the patient that total examination time is about 10 to 20 minutes.
6. See Chapter 1 guidelines for *intratest* care.

Clinical Implications

Abnormal results reveal the following:

1. Tumors of the bladder
2. Cancerous extension to urinary bladder
3. Thickening of bladder wall
4. Masses posterior to bladder
5. Ureterocele

Interfering Factors

1. Residual barium from previous radiology studies affects test results.
2. Overlying gas or fat tissue affects test results.

Interventions

Pretest Patient Care

1. Explain the purpose, benefits, and procedure of the test.
2. Ask the patient to have a full bladder at the beginning, which is then emptied to complete the examination.
3. Assure the patient that there is no pain involved. Some discomfort may be experienced from maintaining a full urinary bladder.
4. Explain that a liberal coating of coupling agent must be applied to the skin so that there is no air between the skin and the transducer and to allow for easy movement of the transducer over the skin. A sensation of warmth or wetness may be felt. The couplant (ultrasound gel) does not stain or discolor clothing, but the patient may prefer to don a gown.
5. Follow guidelines in Chapter 1 for safe, effective, informed *pretest* care.

Posttest Patient Care

1. The patient may return to normal routines.
2. Review test results; report and record findings. Modify the nursing care plan as needed. Counsel the patient about bladder abnormalities and possible further tests (cystoscopy) and treatment: medical (drugs) or surgical interventions.
3. Follow guidelines in Chapter 1 for safe, effective, informed *posttest* care.

● Hepatobiliary Ultrasound; Gallbladder (GB) Ultrasound; Liver Ultrasound

These tests are helpful in differentiating hepatic disease from biliary obstruction. Unlike the oral cholecystogram, this procedure allows visualization of the GB and ducts in patients with impaired liver function. Stones and evidence of cholecystitis are readily visualized. This procedure is indicated as an initial study for patients with right upper quadrant pain. It is also useful as a guide for biopsy or other interventional procedures. Posttransplantation color Doppler sonography of the reconstructed vessels is an important diagnostic tool.

Reference Values

Normal

Normal size, position, wall thickness, and configuration of the GB and bile ducts
Normal adjacent liver tissue

Procedure

1. Ask the patient to lie still on an examination table. Scans usually are performed with the patient in the supine and decubitus positions.
2. Cover the skin with a layer of couplant (ultrasound gel).
3. Ask the patient to regulate breathing patterns as instructed during the examination.
4. Tell the patient that total examination time is about 10 to 30 minutes.
5. See Chapter 1 guidelines for *intratest* care.

PROCEDURAL ALERT

1. Scans cannot be done over open wounds or through dressings.
2. This examination must be performed before radiographic studies involving barium. If such scheduling is not possible, at least 24 hr must elapse between the barium procedure and the sonogram.
3. The GB's ability to contract may be tested by administering a fatty substance and rescanning.

Clinical Implications

1. *GB* abnormal patterns reveal:
   a. Size variations
   b. Thickened wall, indicative of cholecystitis, adenomyomatosis, or tumor and commonly seen as a manifestation of cholecystopathy in patients with AIDS
   c. Benign and malignant lesions such as polyps
   d. Gallstones
2. *Bile duct* abnormalities reveal:
   a. Dilation of ducts
   b. Duct obstruction by calculi, tumor, or parasites
   c. Congenital abnormalities such as choledochal cysts
3. Adjacent *liver* pathologies may include:
   a. Parenchymal disease such as cirrhosis
   b. Masses, including cysts, solid lesions, and metastatic tumors
4. If combined with Doppler evaluation, portal hypertension and hepatofugal (portal blood flow away from the liver) flow can be detected. Posttransplantation stenoses or flow variances can be monitored.

Interfering Factors

1. Intestinal gas overlying the area of interest interferes with sonographic visualization.
2. Barium from recent radiographic studies compromises the study.
3. Obesity adversely affects tissue visualization.

Interventions

Pretest Patient Care

1. Explain the purpose, benefits, and procedure of the test.
2. Instruct the patient to remain NPO at least 8 hours before the examination to fully dilate the GB and to improve anatomic visualization. Some laboratories prefer that the last meal before the study contain low quantities of fat.
3. Assure the patient that there is no pain involved. However, the patient may feel uncomfortable lying still for a long period.
4. Explain that a liberal coating of coupling agent must be applied to the skin so that there is no air between the skin and the transducer and to allow for easy movement of the transducer over the skin. A sensation of warmth or wetness may be felt. The couplant (ultrasound gel) does not stain or discolor clothing, but the patient may prefer to don a gown.

5. Explain that the patient will be instructed to control breathing patterns while the images are being made.
6. Follow guidelines in Chapter 1 for safe, effective, informed *pretest* care.

Posttest Patient Care

1. Review test results; report and record findings. Modify the nursing care plan as needed. Counsel the patient appropriately about further testing (biopsy).
2. Follow guidelines in Chapter 1 for safe, effective, informed *posttest* care.

CLINICAL ALERT

Results of ultrasounds alone cannot differentiate cancers from benign processes.

● Abdominal Aorta Ultrasound

The abdominal aorta ultrasound is a noninvasive examination used to evaluate the abdominal aorta and its major tributaries for structural abnormalities such as aneurysms and the presence of a thrombus. Many laboratories include Doppler evaluations to characterize blood flow through vessels. Typically, the path of the abdominal aorta is traced from its most proximal portion to the region of its bifurcation into the iliac arteries. The walls strongly reflect echoes, whereas the blood-filled lumen is echo free.

Reference Values

Normal

Normal pattern image showing regular contour and diameter of the aorta

Procedure

1. Ask the patient to lie still on an examination table. Scans are generally performed with the patient in the supine and decubitus positions.
2. Cover the skin with a layer of couplant (ultrasound gel).
3. Ask the patient to regulate breathing patterns as instructed during the examination.
4. Tell the patient that the total examination time is about 30 minutes.
5. See Chapter 1 guidelines for *intratest* care.

PROCEDURAL ALERT

1. **Scans cannot be done over open wounds or through dressings.**
2. **This examination must be performed before radiographic studies involving barium. If such scheduling is not possible, at least 24 hr must elapse between the barium procedure and the sonogram.**

Clinical Implications

1. The typical abnormal pattern reveals aortic aneurysms with or without thrombus. Intimal dissections and leaks also may be detected.
2. Barium from recent radiographic studies compromises the study.
3. Obesity adversely affects tissue visualization.

Interventions

Pretest Patient Care

1. Explain the purpose, benefits, and procedure of the test.
2. Instruct the patient to remain NPO for at least 8 hours before the examination to fully dilate the GB and to improve anatomic visualization of all structures.

3. Assure the patient that there is no pain involved. However, the patient may feel uncomfortable lying still for a long period.
4. Explain that a liberal coating of coupling agent must be applied to the skin so that there is no air between the skin and the transducer over the skin. A sensation of warmth or wetness may be felt. The couplant (ultrasound gel) does not stain or discolor clothing, but the patient may prefer to don a gown.
5. Explain that the patient will be instructed to control breathing patterns while the images are being made.
6. Follow guidelines in Chapter 1 for safe, effective, informed *pretest* care.

Posttest Patient Care

1. The patient may resume normal diet and fluids.
2. Review test results; report and record findings. Modify the nursing care plan as needed. Counsel the patient appropriately about possible further testing (arteriogram) and treatment (surgery).
3. Follow guidelines in Chapter 1 for safe, effective, informed *posttest* care.

● Abdominal Ultrasound

This noninvasive procedure visualizes all organs of the upper abdomen, including the liver, GB, bile ducts, pancreas, kidneys, spleen, and large abdominal blood vessels. Some diagnostic laboratories may perform organ-specific studies, such as renal or hepatobiliary ultrasound, together with abdominal ultrasound. This study is valuable in detecting a variety of pathologies, including fluid collections, masses, infections, and obstructions.

Reference Values

Normal

Normal size, position, and appearance of the liver, GB, bile ducts, pancreas, kidneys, adrenals, and spleen as well as the abdominal aorta and inferior vena cava and their major tributaries

Procedure

1. Ask the patient to lie still on the examination table. Scans are generally performed with the patient in the supine and decubitus positions.
2. Cover the skin with a layer of couplant (ultrasound gel).
3. Explain that the patient will be asked to regulate breathing patterns as instructed during the examination.
4. Tell the patient that total examination time is about 30 to 60 minutes.
5. See Chapter 1 guidelines for *intratest* care.

PROCEDURAL ALERT

1. Scans cannot be done over open wounds or through dressings.
2. This examination must be performed before radiographic studies involving barium. If such scheduling is not possible, at least 24 hr must elapse between the barium procedure and the sonogram.

Clinical Implications

1. *Liver* abnormalities reveal:
   a. Cysts, abscesses, tumors, and metastases
   b. Parenchymal disease (e.g., cirrhosis)
   c. Variations in portal venous flow
   d. Hepatic arterial and venous flow patterns

2. *GB* and *bile duct* abnormalities reveal:
    a. Duct dilation or obstruction
    b. Gallstones
    c. Cholecystitis
    d. Tumors
3. *Pancreas* abnormalities reveal:
    a. Pancreatitis
    b. Pseudocyst
    c. Cysts and tumors, including adenocarcinoma
4. *Kidney* abnormalities reveal:
    a. Hydronephrosis
    b. Cysts, tumors, abscesses
    c. Abnormal size, number, location of kidneys
    d. Calculi
    e. Perirenal fluid collections
    f. Patency and flow through renal artery; patency of renal vein
5. *Adrenal* abnormalities reveal:
    a. Pheochromocytoma
    b. Adrenal hemorrhage
    c. Metastases
6. *Spleen* abnormalities reveal:
    a. Splenomegaly
    b. Evidence of lymphatic disease, lymph node enlargement
    c. Evidence of trauma
7. *Vascular* abnormalities in the upper abdomen reveal:
    a. Aneurysm
    b. Thrombi
    c. Abnormal blood flow patterns
8. Miscellaneous pathologies include:
    a. Ascites
    b. Mesenteric or omental cysts or tumors
    c. Congenital absence or malplacement of organs
    d. Retroperitoneal tumors
    e. Hematomas

Interfering Factors

1. Intestinal gas overlying the area of interest interferes with ultrasound visualization.
2. Barium from recent radiology studies compromises the study.
3. Obesity adversely affects tissue visualization.

Interventions

Pretest Patient Care

1. Explain test purpose, benefits, and procedure.
2. Instruct the patient to remain NPO for a minimum of 8 hours before the examination to fully dilate the GB and to improve anatomic visualization of all structures. Some laboratories prefer that the last meal before the study contain low quantities of fat.
3. Assure the patient that there is no pain involved. However, the patient may feel uncomfortable lying still for a long period.
4. Explain that a liberal coating of coupling agent must be applied to the skin so that there is no air between the skin and the transducer and to allow for easy movement of the transducer over the

skin. A sensation of warmth or wetness may be felt. The couplant (ultrasound gel) does not stain or discolor clothing, but the patient may prefer to don a gown.

5. Explain that the patient will be instructed to control breathing patterns while the images are being made.
6. Follow guidelines in Chapter 1 for safe, effective, informed *pretest* care.

Posttest Patient Care

1. Normal diet and fluids are resumed.
2. Review test results; report and record findings. Modify the nursing care plan as needed. Counsel the patient appropriately.
3. Follow guidelines in Chapter 1 for safe, effective, informed *posttest* care.

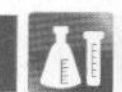

CLINICAL ALERT

The results of ultrasounds alone cannot differentiate malignant from benign conditions.

OTHER BODY STRUCTURE ULTRASOUNDS

● Breast Ultrasound

Breast ultrasound is useful for differentiating cystic, solid, and complex lesions; in the diagnosis of disease in women with very dense breasts; in the follow-up care of women with fibrocystic breast disease; and in evaluating axilla in the patient newly diagnosed with breast cancer. It is recommended as the initial method of examination in a young woman with a palpable mass and in a pregnant woman with a newly palpable mass. The pregnant patient presents a dilemma because malignancies in pregnancy grow rapidly and the increased glandular tissue causes difficulties in mammography. Ultrasound may be used to evaluate women who have silicone prostheses in their breasts. The prosthesis is readily penetrated by the ultrasound beam, and tissues behind the prosthesis can be examined. Such prostheses are known to obscure masses on physical examination; they also absorb x-ray beams, obscuring portions of the breast parenchyma.

Breast ultrasound is a valuable guide during breast biopsies and needle localization procedures. Although not optimal, ultrasound visualization of the breast is an alternative for women who refuse to have a radiographic mammogram and for those who should not be exposed to radiation. Breast ultrasound is not an appropriate method for visualizing microcalcifications.

Reference Values

Normal

Symmetric echo patterns in both breasts, including subcutaneous, mammary, and retromammary layers

Procedure

1. Ask the patient to lie on an examination table.
2. Apply a couplant (ultrasound gel) to the exposed breast to promote the transmission of sound.
3. Move a transducer slowly across the breast. In most laboratories, a handheld transducer is used, whereas in some, an automated breast scanner is used. The automated examination requires the patient to assume a position with the breast immersed in a tank of water. The tank contains transducers that are moved by remote control to image the breast.

4. Tell the patient that the total examining time is approximately 15 minutes.
5. See Chapter 1 guidelines for *intratest* care.

PROCEDURAL ALERT

1. If the breast ultrasound is to be performed on the same day as a radiographic mammogram, advise the patient not to apply any deodorant, powders, or lotions to the upper body on the day of the examination.
2. If the breast ultrasound is to be used for guidance during a biopsy, make certain that a signed, witnessed consent form is obtained.

Clinical Implications

Unusual and distinctive echo patterns may indicate the presence of:

1. Cysts
2. Benign solid growths
3. Malignant tumors
4. Tumor metastasis to muscles and lymph nodes
5. Ductal ectasia
6. Enlarged lymph nodes

Interventions

Pretest Patient Care

1. Explain the purpose and procedure of the examination. There is no discomfort involved. Many diagnostic departments show the patient a video that explains the test.
2. Ask that the patient wear a two-piece outfit on the day of examination because the garments on the torso are removed before the examination.
3. Explain that a liberal coating of a coupling agent must be applied to the skin so that there is no air between the skin and the transducer and to allow for easy movement of the transducer over the skin. A sensation of warmth or wetness may be felt. The couplant (ultrasound gel) does not stain or discolor clothing, but the patient may prefer to don a gown.
4. Follow guidelines in Chapter 1 for safe, effective, informed *pretest* care.

Posttest Patient Care

1. The breasts are cleaned and dried, and the patient is advised to contact the referring clinician for outcomes.
2. Answer the patient's questions regarding procedures and explain need for possible further testing (biopsy) and treatment.
3. Follow guidelines in Chapter 1 for safe, effective, informed *posttest* care.

● Prostate Ultrasound (Transurethral Ultrasound)

The prostate ultrasound is used to visualize the prostate gland, typically in response to an elevated concentration of prostate-specific antigen (PSA) on a blood test or as a complement to a digital rectal examination. Ultrasound of the prostate is also used to check for depth of transmural tumor involvement, as a guidance mechanism for biopsy procedures, and to assist in placement of radioactive implants. Carcinoma of the prostate is the second most common cause of cancer-related death in American men.

The patient typically is instructed to prepare by administering a Fleet enema before the procedure. The patient usually is examined with the use of a small endorectal transducer that is inserted while the patient is in the left lateral decubitus position with the knees flexed toward the chest. Multiple images of the prostate, rectal walls, prostate urethra, and ejaculatory ducts are taken. Prostatic volumes are calculated from 2D measurements. Doppler evaluation is used to assess blood flow through the prostate or any mass that might be detected.

Reference Values

Normal

Normal size, volume, shape, location, and echo texture or consistency of the prostate and adjacent structures

Procedure

1. Ask the patient to void and to remove clothing from the waist down.
2. Position the patient on an examination table in the left lateral decubitus position, with his knees flexed toward the chest. The patient is draped.
3. Perform a digital rectal examination before inserting the rectal transducer.
4. Carefully insert a slim endorectal transducer, lubricated and sheathed with a condom, a few centimeters into the rectum.
5. Perform scans by using a slight rotation of the probe handle. Total examination time is about 15 to 20 minutes.
6. See Chapter 1 guidelines for *intratest* care.

CLINICAL ALERT

1. If the prostate examination is performed in conjunction with a prostatic biopsy, be certain to obtain a signed, witnessed consent form.
2. If the patient is latex sensitive, contact the laboratory.

Clinical Implications

Abnormalities that may be detected include:

1. Prostatic enlargement—increased volume measurements may indicate:
   a. Benign prostatic hypertrophy (BPH)
   b. Space-occupying lesion (tumor, cyst, abscess)
2. Prostatic calcifications
3. Prostatitis
4. Prostate cancer, classically seen as a low-level echo structure within the outer gland (peripheral and central zones)

Interfering Factors

Excess fecal matter in the rectum compromises the study.

Interventions

Pretest Patient Care

1. Explain the purpose and procedure of the test.
2. Assure the patient that no pain is involved. However, a sensation of fullness within the rectum is to be expected. Because the transducer is typically draped within a condom, check for latex sensitivities.

3. Many laboratories require administration of a Fleet enema about 1 hour before the study.
4. Advise the patient to empty the bladder immediately before the study.
5. Follow guidelines in Chapter 1 for safe, effective, informed *pretest* care.

Posttest Patient Care

1. Review test results; report and record findings. Modify the nursing care plan as needed. Counsel the patient about any identified prostatic abnormalities and need for possible further testing (tissue biopsy with cytologic or histologic exam) and treatment.
2. Follow guidelines in Chapter 1 for safe, effective, informed *posttest* care.

● Scrotal Ultrasound

This noninvasive ultrasound study is useful in diagnosing testicular masses, varicoceles, hydroceles, spermatoceles, and diffuse processes. Doppler ultrasound or color-flow Doppler evaluation is helpful in demonstrating the presence of torsion of the testes. Testicular ultrasound is used to evaluate scrotal pain and to demonstrate the scope of scrotal trauma.

Reference Values

Normal

Normal scrotal structures, testicles, epididymis, and spermatic cord
Normal scrotal Doppler blood flow

Procedure

1. Tell the patient that total examination time is about 30 minutes.
2. Ask the patient to lie on his back. The penis is gently retracted, and the scrotum is supported on a rolled towel.
3. Apply a couplant (ultrasound gel) to the skin and then pass the transducer repeatedly over the scrotum. Sonographic images are generated.
4. Use color Doppler studies to assess presence, absence (as in torsion), or increase (as in infection and certain neoplasms) of blood flow in the testicle.
5. See Chapter 1 guidelines for *intratest* care.

Clinical Implications

Abnormal results are associated with:

1. Abscess
2. Infarcted testes (torsion)
3. Tumor (primary and metastatic)
4. Hydrocele
5. Spermatocele
6. Adherent scrotal hernia
7. Cryptorchidism
8. Epididymitis (chronic or acute), orchitis
9. Hematoma (associated with trauma)
10. Tuberculosis infection (associated with AIDS)
11. Testicular microlithiasis

Interventions

Pretest Patient Care

1. Explain the purpose, benefits, and procedure of the test.
2. Assure the patient that there is no pain involved.

3. Explain that a liberal coating of coupling media must be applied to the scrotum. A sensation of warmth or wetness may be felt. The couplant (ultrasound gel) does not stain or discolor clothing, but the patient may prefer to don a gown.
4. Follow guidelines in Chapter 1 for safe, effective, informed *pretest* care.

Posttest Patient Care

1. Review test results; report and record findings. Modify the nursing care plan as needed. Counsel the patient appropriately about further testing (nuclear scan) or surgery.
2. Follow guidelines in Chapter 1 for safe, effective, informed *posttest* care.

● Eye and Orbit Ultrasounds

Ultrasound can be used to describe both normal and abnormal tissues of the eye when no alternative visualization is possible because of opacities caused by inflammation or hemorrhage. This information is valuable in the management of eyes for keratoprosthesis. Orbital lesions can be detected and distinguished from inflammatory and congestive causes of exophthalmos with a high degree of reliability. An extensive preoperative evaluation before vitrectomy or surgery for vitreous hemorrhages is also done. In this case, the vitreous cavity is examined to rule out retinal and choroidal detachments and to detect and localize vitreoretinal adhesions and intraocular foreign bodies. Also, patients who are to have intraocular lens implants after removal of cataracts must be measured for the exact length of the eye (within 0.1 mm).

Reference Values

Normal

Pattern image indicating normal soft tissue of eye and retrobulbar orbital areas, retina, choroid, and orbital fat

Procedure

1. Tell the patient that if a lesion in the eye is detected, as much as 30 minutes may be required to differentiate the pathologic process accurately. Otherwise, orbital examinations can be done in 8 to 10 minutes.
2. Instill eye drops to anesthetize the eye area.
3. Ask the patient to close the eye, apply couplant (ultrasound gel), and place a small, very-high-frequency transducer on the eye directly, or position it over a water standoff pad placed onto the eye surface. Multiple images and measurements are taken.
4. Ask the patient to hold very still.
5. Place a probe gently on the corneal surface.
6. See Chapter 1 guidelines for *intratest* care.

Clinical Implications

1. Abnormal patterns are seen in:
   a. Alkali burns with corneal flattening and loss of anterior chamber
   b. Detached retina
   c. Keratoprosthesis
   d. Extraocular thickening in thyroid eye disease
   e. Pupillary membranes
   f. Cyclotic membranes
   g. Vitreous opacities
   h. Orbital mass lesions
   i. Inflammatory conditions
   j. Vascular malformations
   k. Foreign bodies

2. Abnormal patterns are also seen in tumors of various types based on specific ultrasonic patterns:
   a. Solid tumors (e.g., meningioma, glioma, neurofibroma)
   b. Cystic tumors (e.g., mucocele, dermoid, cavernous hemangioma)
   c. Angiomatous tumors (e.g., diffuse hemangioma)
   d. Lymphangioma
   e. Infiltrative tumors (e.g., metastatic lymphoma pseudotumor)

Interfering Factors

If at some time the vitreous humor in a particular patient has been replaced by a gas, no result can be obtained.

Interventions

Pretest Patient Care

1. Explain the purpose, benefits, and procedure of the test.
2. Instill topical anesthetic drops into the eyes before the examination is performed; this usually is done in the examining department.
3. Follow guidelines in Chapter 1 for safe, effective, informed *pretest* care.

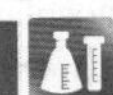

CLINICAL ALERT

When a ruptured globe is suspected, ophthalmic ultrasound should not be performed. Excessive pressure applied to the globe may cause expulsion of the contents and increases the risk of introduction of bacteria.

Posttest Patient Care

1. Instruct the patient to refrain from touching or rubbing the eyes until the effects of anesthetic have disappeared. This type of friction could cause corneal abrasions.
2. Advise the patient that minor discomfort and blurred vision may be experienced for a short time. Counsel regarding possible further testing and/or treatment for infection (medical or surgical for detached retina).
3. Follow guidelines in Chapter 1 for safe, effective, informed *posttest* care.

● Thyroid Ultrasound (Neck Ultrasound)

This ultrasound study is used to evaluate a neck mass, distinguish cysts from thyroid nodules, or to determine the size of the thyroid and reveal the depth and dimension of thyroid goiters and nodules. The response of a mass in the thyroid to suppressive therapy can be monitored by successive examinations. Theoretically, this technique offers the possibility of a good estimation of thyroid weight—information that is important in radioiodine therapy for Graves' disease.

The examination is easy to do, is often done before surgery, and gives 85% accuracy. Often, these studies are done in conjunction with radioactive iodine uptake tests. With pregnant patients, ultrasound studies are the method of choice because radioactive iodine is harmful to the developing fetus.

Reference Values

Normal

Normal, homogeneous pattern of thyroid and adjacent structures, including strap muscles and blood vessels

Normal size and anatomy of the thyroid

Procedure

1. Have the patient lie supine on the examining table, with the neck hyperextended.
2. Place a pillow under the shoulders for comfort and to bring the transducer into better contact with the thyroid.
3. Apply a couplant (ultrasound gel) to the patient's neck. This affords good contact between the transducer and the patient's skin and allows the transducer to be moved easily across the neck's surface. An alternate procedure involves separation of the neck surface from the transducer by a gel-filled pad that permits proper transmission of the ultrasound waves through the thyroid.
4. Tell the patient that the examination time is about 30 minutes.
5. See Chapter 1 guidelines for *intratest* care.

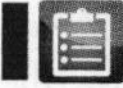

PROCEDURAL ALERT

Thyroid or neck biopsies are often performed with ultrasound guidance. If a biopsy is performed, a signed, witnessed consent form must be obtained.

Clinical Implications

1. An abnormal pattern may consist of a cystic, complex, or solid echo pattern.
2. Solitary "cold" nodules identified on radioisotope scans may appear as echo-free cysts on ultrasound. Most often, cysts are benign. Solid-appearing lesions may represent benign adenomas or malignant tumors. A biopsy is the only definitive method to determine the nature of such tumors.
3. Overall gland enlargement is indicative of goiter or thyroiditis.
4. Ultrasound studies of the neck may also reveal parathyroid lesions or evidence of changed lymph nodes.
5. Certain congenital deformities related to the embryologic development of neck structures may be detected, most commonly thyroglossal duct cyst, branchial cleft cyst, or cystic hygroma (congenital multiloculated lymphatic lesion).

Interfering Factors

1. Nodules <1 cm in diameter may escape detection.
2. Cysts not originating in the thyroid may show the same ultrasound characteristics as thyroid cysts.
3. Lesions >4 cm in diameter frequently contain areas of cystic or hemorrhagic degeneration and give a mixed echogram that is difficult to correlate with specific disease.

Interventions

Pretest Patient Care

1. Explain the purpose and procedure of the test.
2. Assure the patient that there is no pain involved. However, the patient may feel uncomfortable maintaining the neck position during the examination.
3. Explain that a liberal coating of coupling agent must be applied to the skin so that there is no air between the skin and the transducer and to allow for easy movement of the transducer over the skin. A sensation of warmth or wetness may be felt. The couplant (ultrasound gel) does not stain or discolor clothing, but the patient may prefer to don a gown.
4. Advise the patient to refrain from wearing necklaces to the laboratory.
5. Follow guidelines in Chapter 1 for safe, effective, informed *pretest* care.

Posttest Patient Care

1. Review test results; report and record findings. Modify the nursing care plan as needed. Counsel about follow-up testing (thyroid nuclear scans) or treatment for thyroid (surgical removal) or neck abnormalities.
2. Follow guidelines in Chapter 1 for safe, effective, informed *posttest* care.

VASCULAR ULTRASOUND STUDIES (DUPLEX SCANS)

The combination of anatomic imaging of blood vessels and hemodynamic information provided by Doppler ultrasound will result in duplex scans. These noninvasive studies can be performed on literally any area of human anatomy. Blood velocity is detected by positioning the Doppler sample gate within the lumen of the desired vessel. The resultant *spectral trace* (Fig. 13.1) also provides information as to the direction, phase, pulsatile rhythm, and resistivity of flow. *Antegrade* flow is demonstrated above the baseline. *Retrograde* flow (i.e., flow in the direction opposite that expected) is demonstrated by a spectral trace below the baseline. Flow that is antegrade through all phases (systole as well as diastole) demonstrates a *low-resistive* profile, which is normally associated with visceral blood vessels (e.g., renal artery, internal carotid artery). High-resistance, or *triphasic,* flow is typically associated with peripheral arteries (e.g., femoral artery, brachial artery) and shows a forward–backward–forward pattern in each cycle. *Spectral broadening* occurs when the sample contains blood cells moving at many velocities; this is generally associated with a flow disturbance. Mathematical ratios that contrast peak or mean velocities at various stages in the cycle can give further clues to the integrity of the vascular system examined. Color Doppler ultrasound generally is used to code flow velocities and direction with color and can readily differentiate the patency of vessels. B-flow is a technique that images the blood itself and has an enhanced ability to display plaque margins.

● Cerebrovascular Ultrasound (Carotid and Vertebral Arteries) Duplex Scans: Carotid Intima Media Thickness

Carotid duplex scans examine the major extracranial arteries supplying the brain to gain information about cerebrovascular blood flow. Carotid scans are used in the evaluation of ischemia, headache, dizziness, hemiparesis, paresthesias, and speech and visual disturbances. Testing is commonly performed before major cardiovascular surgery and as a follow-up to many surgeries. Carotid intima media thickness is used to predict heart disease risk in patients with no symptoms but who have a family history of heart disease.

Reference Values

Normal

Normal vascular anatomy and course of common carotid artery, internal and external carotids, and vertebral arteries

No evidence of stenosis or occlusion; normal flow patterns

Normal thickness of inner layers of arterial wall

Procedure

1. Ask the patient to lie supine on the examining table with the neck slightly extended. The head typically is turned away from the side being examined.
2. Apply a couplant (ultrasound gel) to the neck area to enhance the transmission of sound. During Doppler evaluation, an audible signal, representing blood flow, can be heard.
3. Move a handheld transducer gently up and down the neck while images of appropriate blood vessels are made. Examine both sides of the neck.

4. Tell the patient that the examination time is 30 to 60 minutes.
5. See Chapter 1 guidelines for *intratest* care.

Clinical Implications

Abnormal images and Doppler signals may provide evidence of the following:

1. Plaque
2. Stenosis
3. Occlusion
4. Dissection
5. Aneurysm
6. Carotid body tumor
7. Arteritis

Excess thickness or narrowing of carotid wall indicates the following:

1. Increased risk for heart disease
2. Sign of plaque buildup

Interfering Factors

1. Severe obesity and patient movement compromise examination quality.
2. Cardiac arrhythmias and disease may cause changes in hemodynamic patterns.

Interventions

Pretest Patient Care

1. Explain the test purpose, benefits, and procedure. The patient should refrain from smoking or consuming caffeine for at least 2 hours before the study. Assure the patient that no radiation is employed, typically no contrast medium is injected, and no pain is involved. Some slight discomfort may be experienced from lying with head extended.
2. Advise the patient that a liberal coating of coupling gel must be applied to the skin to promote sound transmission. A sensation of warmth or wetness may be felt during application. The couplant (ultrasound gel) does not stain or discolor clothing, but the patient may prefer to don a gown. Necklaces and earrings must be removed before the study.
3. Follow guidelines in Chapter 1 for safe, effective, informed *pretest* care.

Posttest Patient Care

1. Remind the patient to remove any residual gel from the skin.
2. Review test results; report and record findings. Modify the nursing care plan as needed. Provide support and counsel the patient appropriately should an abnormality be detected. Monitor for arterial disease and possible further testing (arteriogram) and treatment (surgery).
3. Follow guidelines in Chapter 1 for safe, effective, informed *posttest* care.

● Peripheral Arterial Doppler Studies; Lower Extremity Arterial and Upper Extremity Arterial Duplex Scans

Peripheral arterial studies visualize and document the arterial blood flow in the extremities. Duplex ultrasound scans can determine the presence, amount, and location of plaques and are helpful in assessing the cause of claudication. Graft patency and condition may also be evaluated. Ultrasound analysis is used to evaluate the site of a prior surgical or percutaneous intervention. Some institutions also incorporate *segmental blood pressure* readings into these examinations. Flow characteristics of upper versus lower extremities can be contrasted by calculating a mathematical ratio between pressures (see Ankle-Brachial Index [ABI] and Segmental Pressures).

Reference Values

Normal

Normal arterial anatomy of the extremity
Normal triphasic blood flow and flow velocities
No evidence of plaques or other pathologic processes

Procedure

1. Ask the patient to lie on the examining table with the leg or arm turned out slightly and the knee or elbow partially bent.
2. Apply a couplant (ultrasound gel) to the leg from groin down or to the arm from shoulder down to enhance the transmission of sound. During Doppler evaluation, an audible signal, representing blood flow, can be heard.
3. Move a handheld transducer gently up and down the limb while images of appropriate blood vessels are made.
4. Tell the patient that the examination time is about 60 minutes.
5. See Chapter 1 guidelines for *intratest* care.

Clinical Implications

Abnormal tracings (see Fig. 13.2) and Doppler signals may provide evidence of the following:

1. Plaque or calcification (particularly in the diabetic patient)
2. Stenosis
3. Occlusion
4. Arteritis
5. Aneurysm
6. Pseudoaneurysm
7. Graft diameter reduction
8. Abnormal communication between artery and vein

Interfering Factors

1. Severe obesity compromises examination quality.
2. Cardiac arrhythmias and disease may cause changes in hemodynamic patterns.

Interventions

Pretest Patient Care

1. Explain the test purpose, benefits, and procedure. Instruct the patient to refrain from smoking or consuming caffeine for at least 2 hours before the test. Assure the patient that no radiation is employed, typically no contrast medium is injected, and no pain is involved. Some slight discomfort may be experienced from lying with the extremity extended or if segmental blood pressures are taken.
2. Advise the patient that a liberal coating of coupling gel must be applied to the skin to promote sound transmission. A sensation of warmth or wetness may be felt during application. The couplant (ultrasound gel) does not stain or discolor clothing, but the patient may prefer to don a gown.
3. Follow guidelines in Chapter 1 for safe, effective, informed *pretest* care.

Posttest Patient Care

1. Remind the patient to remove any residual gel from the skin.
2. Review test results; report and record findings. Modify the nursing care plan as needed. Provide support and counsel appropriately should an abnormality be detected. Monitor and counsel for arterial disease and possible further testing (arteriogram or venogram) and treatment (surgery).
3. Follow guidelines in Chapter 1 for safe, effective, informed *posttest* care.

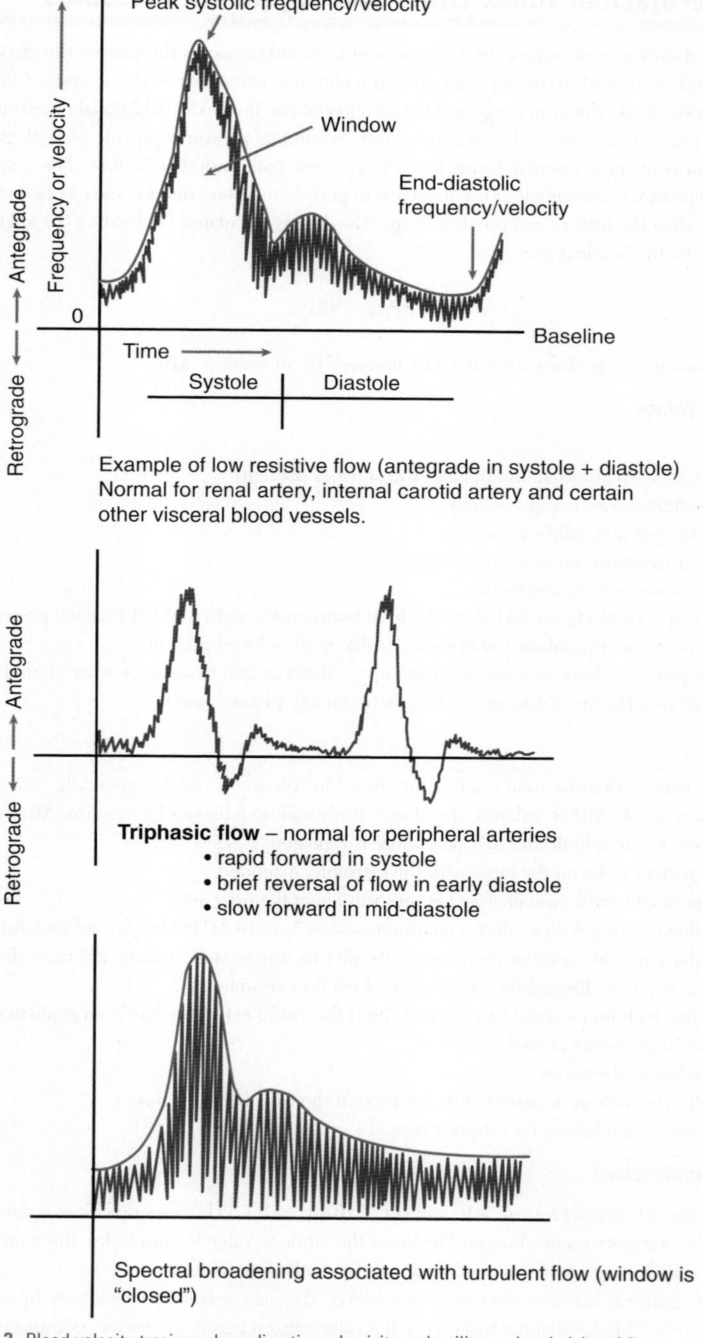

FIGURE 13.2. Blood velocity tracings show direction, phasicity, pulsatility, and resistivity of flow.

Ankle-Brachial Index (ABI) and Segmental Pressures

In some laboratories, as an adjunct to duplex scanning, blood pressures throughout the extremities are measured and contrasted. In the typical four-cuff technique, pneumatic cuffs are applied to the upper thigh, the lower thigh, the upper calf, and the area just above the ankle. Additionally, cuffs are applied to the upper arms to determine brachial pressures. Segmental pressures provide physiologic information that can confirm a vascular cause for ischemic rest pain and claudication. The ankle-brachial index (ABI) provides assessment of the presence of peripheral artery disease and can be more reliable and specific than the history and physical exam. The ABI is calculated by dividing the ankle pressure (in mm Hg) by the brachial pressure.

$$SBP_{ankle} / SBP_{arm}$$

Many laboratories perform a resting ABI followed by an exercise ABI.

Reference Values

Normal

ABI 0.9 to 1.3 (when a normal multiphasic waveform is present)

ABI >1.3 indicates poor compressibility

ABI 0.7 to 0.9 indicates mild obstruction

ABI 0.4 to 0.7 indicates moderate obstruction

ABI <0.4 indicates severe obstruction

A difference of 20 mm Hg (or 20 torr or 2.7 kPa) between the right and left brachial pressures may indicate proximal arterial obstruction on the side with reduced pressure.

The gradual pressure drop, as measured from upper thigh or arm to ankle or wrist, should not exceed 20 mm Hg (or 20 torr or 2.7 kPa) between any two segments.

Procedure

1. Tell the patient that the total examination time (for pressures only) is generally <15 minutes. If an exercise/stress ABI is ordered, the at-rest study will be followed by exercise. After walking for 5 minutes on a treadmill, the ABI procedure is repeated.
2. Ask the patient to lie on the table with the extremity extended.
3. Place pneumatic cuffs (usually four) at intervals along the extremity.
4. Place a flow-sensing device (often a continuous-wave 5- to 10-MHz Doppler device) distal to a cuff. Inflate the cuff (this is often done automatically) to suprasystolic values and then slowly deflate until flow resumes. Record the pressure at which flow resumes.
5. Repeat this technique, distal to each cuff, until the entire extremity has been evaluated. Measure the brachial pressures as well.
6. Examine both extremities.
7. Generally, the highest measurements are used in the calculation.
8. See Chapter 1 guidelines for *intratest* care.

Clinical Implications

1. Asymmetry in brachial pressure >10 mm Hg (>10 torr or >1.35 kPa) is suspicious for arterial disease.
2. ABI <1.0 is suspicious for disease. The lower the numeric value for this index, the more severe the disease may be (e.g., ABI <0, associated with impending tissue loss).
3. Pressure gradients between successive segments on the same extremity should vary by <20 mm Hg (<20 torr <2.7 kPa). Variations that exceed this value suggest significant disease (occlusion or stenosis).
4. A difference of >20 mm Hg (>20 torr or >2.7 kPa) between similar segments on opposite sides may suggest obstructive vascular disease.

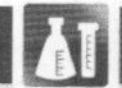

CLINICAL ALERT

1. **Segmental pressures are a screening tool that cannot distinguish stenosis from total occlusion and cannot be specific in determining the exact location of disease.**
2. **Vessel calcifications (commonly seen in the diabetic patient) can falsely elevate systolic pressures.**

Interfering Factors

1. Severe obesity compromises examination quality.
2. Cardiac arrhythmias and disease may cause changes in hemodynamic patterns.

Interventions

Pretest Patient Care

1. Explain the test purpose, benefits, and procedure. Instruct the patient to refrain from smoking or consuming caffeine for at least 2 hours before the study. Assure the patient that no radiation is employed, typically no contrast medium is injected, and no pain is involved. Some discomfort may be experienced from lying with the extremity extended or when pneumatic cuffs are inflated.
2. Follow guidelines in Chapter 1 for safe, effective, informed *pretest* care.

Posttest Patient Care

1. Review test results; report and record findings. Modify the nursing care plan as needed. Provide support and counsel the patient appropriately should an abnormality be detected. Monitor and counsel for arterial disease and explain need for possible further testing (arteriogram) and treatment (medical or surgical).
2. Follow guidelines in Chapter 1 for safe, effective, informed *posttest* care.

● Peripheral Venous Doppler Studies; Lower Extremity Venous and Upper Extremity Venous Duplex Scans

This procedure examines venous blood flow in the selected extremity (upper or lower). It is most commonly used to assess deep venous thrombosis and can also be used to map veins to be harvested and used for grafts. Peripheral ultrasound is also used to locate veins for venous access and to assess dialysis access grafts. This examination has replaced contrast venography in many institutions.

Reference Values

Normal Duplex Scan

Normal venous anatomy of the extremity
Spontaneous phasic flow pattern (rises and falls with respiration)
Normal venous augmentation (exhibits increased flow proximal to the site of venous compression)
Competent, intact valves, with no evidence of thrombi

Procedure

1. Ask the patient to lie on the examining table with the leg or arm turned out slightly and the knee or elbow partially bent.
2. Apply a couplant (ultrasound gel) to the leg from the groin down or to the arm from the shoulder area down to enhance the transmission of sound. During Doppler evaluation, an audible signal, representing blood flow, can be heard.
3. Move a handheld transducer gently up and down the limb while images of appropriate blood vessels are made. At intervals, apply gentle compression to the vessel. Examine both sides.

4. Tell the patient that the examination time is about 30 minutes.
5. See Chapter 1 guidelines for *intratest* care.

Clinical Implications

Abnormal images and Doppler signals may provide evidence of the following:

1. Acute or chronic deep venous thrombosis
2. Occlusive venous disease
3. Valvular incompetence
4. Clotted grafts

Interfering Factors

1. Severe obesity compromises examination quality.
2. Cardiac arrhythmias and disease may cause changes in hemodynamic patterns.

Interventions

Pretest Patient Care

1. Explain the test purpose, benefits, and procedure. Instruct the patient to refrain from smoking for at least 2 hours before the study. Assure the patient that no radiation is employed, typically no contrast medium is injected, and no pain is involved. Some slight discomfort may be experienced from lying with the extremity extended or when compression is applied.
2. Advise the patient that a liberal coating of couplant (ultrasound gel) must be applied to the skin to promote sound transmission. A sensation of warmth or wetness may be felt during application. Although the couplant (ultrasound gel) does not stain or discolor clothing, the patient may prefer to don a gown.
3. Follow guidelines in Chapter 1 for safe, effective, informed *pretest* care.

Posttest Patient Care

1. Remind the patient to remove any residual gel from the skin.
2. Review test results; report and record findings. Modify the nursing care plan as needed. Provide support and counsel appropriately should an abnormality be detected. Monitor and counsel for venous disease and need for possible further testing and/or treatment.
3. Follow guidelines in Chapter 1 for safe, effective, informed *posttest* care.

CARDIAC ULTRASOUND STUDIES

● Cardiac Ultrasound (Echocardiogram; Doppler Echocardiography)

This noninvasive technique for examining the heart can provide information about its position and size, movements of the valves and chamber, and velocity of blood flow. Echoes from pulsed high-frequency sound waves are used to locate and study the movements and dimensions of cardiac structures. Because the heart is a blood-filled organ, sound can be transmitted through it readily to the opposite wall and to the heart–lung interface. This test is commonly used to determine biologic and prosthetic valve dysfunction, to evaluate a pericardial effusion, to evaluate the velocity and direction of blood flow, to furnish direction for further diagnostic study, and to monitor cardiac patients over an extended period. Echocardiography is also used to monitor heart failure patients relying on a left ventricular assist device (LVAD). One of the advantages of this diagnostic technique is that it can be performed at the bedside with mobile equipment or can be done in the laboratory.

The various modes of echocardiography are capable of providing a great range of information concerning cardiac structure and function. The following are common types of echocardiograms:

Two-dimensional (2D): used to produce gray-scale, cross-sectional images of the heart's anatomy

M-mode: used to generate depictions of rapidly moving structures such as valves and for standardized dimensional measurements

Continuous-wave Doppler and pulsed-wave Doppler: used to determine velocity of blood flow

Color 2D: used for identifying areas of disturbed or eccentric blood flow

Color M-mode: used for evaluating movement of cardiac structures

Specialized types of echocardiography include:

Stress echocardiography: used to provide information relating to the function of heart structures during high cardiac output states. A treadmill or upright bicycle may be used, or the heart can be stressed by an infusion of dobutamine.

Transesophageal echocardiography (TEE): A small ultrasound transducer is placed at the end of a tube inserted into the esophagus to provide a closer view of cardiac structures without interference from superficial chest tissues.

Fetal echocardiography: performed through the pregnant woman's abdomen when there is a question of congenital cardiac defect.

Contrast echocardiography: A liquid containing nontoxic microbubbles is injected into a vein to opacify cardiac structures.

These special techniques may require a signed, witnessed consent form before performance and involve more complicated procedures. Check with the individual laboratory for specific guides and protocols.

Reference Values

Normal

Normal position, size, and movement of heart valves and chamber walls as visualized in 2D, M-mode, and Doppler mode

Color M-mode and color Doppler assessments of heart structures within normal limits

Procedures

1. Ensure that a specific diagnosis accompanies the request for the test (e.g., "rule out pericardial effusion," "determine severity of mitral stenosis"). If a stress echocardiogram is ordered, the patient's ability to perform exercise must be indicated.
2. Ask the patient to lie on the examining table in a slight side-lying position.
3. Apply a couplant (ultrasound gel) to the skin surface over the chest to permit maximum penetration of the ultrasound beam. Hold the transducer over various regions of the chest and upper abdomen to obtain the appropriate views of the heart.
4. Tell the patient that there should be no pain or discomfort involved. Leads may be attached for a simultaneous electrocardiogram reading during the ultrasound procedure.
5. Tell the patient that the examination time is 30 to 45 minutes.
6. See Chapter 1 guidelines for *intratest* care.

PROCEDURAL ALERT

Certain specialized echocardiographic procedures, such as stress echocardiography and TEE, may require individualized patient preparation. Check with the laboratory to determine specific protocols and preparation.

Clinical Implications

Abnormal values help to diagnose:

1. Acquired cardiac disease
   a. Valvular disease, stenosis, insufficiency, prolapse, and regurgitation
   b. Cardiomyopathies
   c. Evidence of coronary artery disease
   d. Pericardial disease, including effusion, tamponade, and pericarditis
   e. Endocarditis
   f. Cardiac neoplasm
   g. Intracardiac thrombi
2. Prosthetic valve function
3. Congenital heart disease

Interfering Factors

1. Dysrhythmias interfere with the test.
2. Hyperinflation of the lungs with mechanical ventilation, especially with positive end-expiratory pressure (PEEP) >10 cm H_2O, precludes adequate ultrasound imaging of the heart.
3. False-negative and false-positive diagnoses have been identified (especially in M-mode echocardiograms), including diagnoses of pleural effusion, dilated descending aorta, pericardial fat pad, tumors encasing the heart, clotted blood, and loculated effusions.
4. Doppler study results can vary greatly if the transducer position does not provide satisfactory angles for the beam.

Interventions

Pretest Patient Care

1. Explain the purpose, benefits, and procedure of the test.
2. Assure the patient that no pain is involved. However, some discomfort may be felt from lying quietly for a long period.
3. Explain that a liberal coating of coupling agent must be applied to the skin so that there is no air between the skin and the transducer and to permit easy movement of the transducer over the skin. A sensation of warmth or wetness may be felt. The couplant (ultrasound gel) does not stain or discolor clothing, but the patient may prefer to don a gown.
4. Follow guidelines in Chapter 1 for safe, effective, informed *pretest* care.

Posttest Patient Care

1. Review test results; report and record findings. Modify the nursing care plan as needed. Counsel the patient appropriately about cardiac disorders and explain need for possible further testing and/or treatment (medical, drugs, or surgical).
2. Follow guidelines in Chapter 1 for safe, effective, informed *posttest* care.

● Transesophageal Echocardiogram (TEE)

TEE permits optimal ultrasonic visualization of the heart when traditional transthoracic (noninvasive) echocardiography fails or proves inconclusive. A miniaturized high-frequency ultrasound transducer is mounted on an endoscope and coupled with an ultrasound instrument to display and record ultrasound images from the heart. Endoscope controls allow remote manipulation of the transducer tip. Various images of heart anatomy can be displayed by rotating the tip of the instrument and by varying the depth of insertion into the esophagus.

Indications for TEE include the following:

1. To assess function of prosthetic valves, diagnose endocarditis, evaluate valvular regurgitation and congenital abnormalities, and examine the aorta for dissecting aneurysms
2. To monitor left ventricular wall motion intraoperatively
3. To measure ejection fraction in selected patients
4. When a transthoracic echocardiogram has not been satisfactory (e.g., obesity, chest wall trauma, chronic obstructive pulmonary disease)
5. When results of traditional transthoracic echocardiography do not agree or correlate with other clinical findings

Reference Values

Normal

Normal position, size, and function of heart valves and heart chambers

Procedure

1. Apply a topical anesthetic to the pharynx. Insert a bite block into the mouth and secure it. This reduces the risk of damage to the patient's teeth and oral structures and accidental damage to the endoscope.
2. Ask the patient to assume a left lateral decubitus position while the lubricated endoscopic instrument is inserted to a depth of 30 to 50 cm. Ask the patient to swallow to facilitate advancement of the device.
3. Manipulate the ultrasound transducer to provide a number of image planes.
4. See Chapter 1 guidelines for *intratest* care.

CLINICAL ALERT

A variety of medications may be used during this procedure. Generally, these drugs are intended to sedate, anesthetize, reduce secretions, and serve as contrast agents for the ultrasound.

Clinical Implications

Abnormal TEE findings include:

1. Heart valve disease: stenosis, insufficiency, prolapse, and regurgitation
2. Pericardial effusion, pericarditis, tamponade
3. Congenital heart disease
4. Aortic dissection
5. Left ventricular dysfunction
6. Endocarditis
7. Intracardiac tumors or thrombi

Interventions

Pretest Patient Care

1. Explain the purpose, procedure, and the benefits and risks of the test.
2. The patient must remain NPO for at least 4 to 8 hours before the procedure to reduce the risk of aspiration. Pretest medication such as analgesics or sedatives may be ordered. Check with the laboratory or physician for specific instructions.
3. Obtain baseline vital signs.
4. Establish an intravenous access line to administer medications or contrast agents.

5. Remove dentures and any loose objects from the patient's mouth.
6. Follow guidelines in Chapter 1 for safe, effective, informed *pretest* care.

Patient Posttest Care

1. Review test results; report and record findings. Modify the nursing care plan as needed. Monitor vital signs and level of consciousness (if the patient is sedated). Ensure patent airway. Explain need for possible further testing and/or treatment: medical (drugs) or surgical (e.g., cardiac catheterization).
2. Position the patient on the side, if sedated, to prevent risk of aspiration.
3. Ascertain return of swallowing, coughing, and gag reflexes before allowing the patient to take oral food or fluids. Generally, the patient should remain NPO for at least 1 hour after the test.
4. Follow guidelines in Chapter 1 for safe, effective, informed *posttest* care.

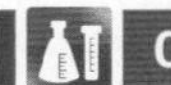

CLINICAL ALERT

Swallowing reflexes may be diminished for several hours because of the effects of the topical anesthetic.

BIBLIOGRAPHY

Ahuja AT, Griffith JF, Wong KT, et al: Diagnostic Imaging: Ultrasound. Philadelphia, Elsevier Mosby Saunders, 2007

Bluth EI, Benson CB, Ralls PW, et al: Ultrasound: A Practical Approach to Clinical Problems, 2nd ed. New York, Thieme, 2007

Case T: A Primer in Ultrasound and Vascular Physics. Philadelphia, Lippincott Williams & Wilkins, 2006

Fleischer AC, Toy EC, Lee W, et al: Sonography in Obstetrics and Gynecology, 7th ed. New York, McGraw-Hill, 2011

Goroll AH, Mulley AG: Primary Care Medicine, Office Evaluation and Management of Adult Patient, 7th ed. Philadelphia, Lippincott Williams & Wilkins, 2014

Hagen-Ansert SL: Textbook of Diagnostic Sonography, 7th ed. St. Louis, Mosby, 2012

Kremkau FW: Sonography Principles and Instruments, 8th ed. Philadelphia, Saunders, 2011

Kupesic S, Kurjak A: Clinical Application of 3D Sonography. New York, CRC Press, 2000

Lanfranchi ME: Breast Ultrasound. New York, Marban Books, 2000

Madden ME: Introduction to Sectional Anatomy, 3rd ed. Philadelphia, Lippincott Williams & Wilkins, 2012

Middleton WD, Kurtz AB, Hertzberg BS: Ultrasounds: The Requisites, 2nd ed. Maryland Heights, MO, Mosby, 2013

Perrino AC, Reeves ST: A Practical Approach to Transesophageal Echocardiography. Philadelphia, Lippincott Williams & Wilkins, 2013

Reuter KL, McGahan J: Obstetric and Gynecologic Ultrasound, 3rd ed. Philadelphia, Elsevier Mosby Saunders, 2013

Sanders RC: Ultrasound. Philadelphia, Lippincott Williams & Wilkins, 2001

Sanders RC, Dolk J, Miner NS: Exam Preparation for Diagnostic Ultrasound: Abdomen and OB/GYN. Philadelphia, Lippincott Williams & Wilkins, 2001

Sanders RC, Winter TC: Clinical Sonography: A Practical Guide, 5th ed. Philadelphia, Lippincott Williams & Wilkins, 2015

Tempkin BB: Ultrasound Scanning: Principles and Protocols, 3rd ed. Philadelphia, Elsevier Mosby Saunders, 2007

INTERNET SITES

- http://www.acr.org
- http://www.auntminnie.com
- http://www.intelihealth.com
- http://www.webmd.com

Pulmonary Function, Arterial Blood Gases (ABGs), and Electrolyte Studies

14

OVERVIEW OF PULMONARY FUNCTION TESTS

Pulmonary Physiology

There are three aspects of pulmonary function: perfusion, diffusion, and ventilation. *Perfusion* relates to blood flow through pulmonary vessels; *diffusion* refers to movement of oxygen and carbon dioxide across alveolar capillary membranes; and *ventilation* relates to air exchange between alveolar spaces and the atmosphere.

During breathing, the lung–thorax system acts as a bellows to provide air to the alveoli for adequate gas exchange to take place. Like a spring or rubber band, the lung tissue also possesses the property of elasticity. When the inspiratory muscles contract, the thorax and lungs expand; when the same muscles relax and the force is removed, the thorax and lungs return to their resting position. Also, when the thorax and lungs expand, the alveolar pressure is lowered below atmospheric pressure. This permits air to flow into the trachea, bronchi, bronchioles, and alveoli. Expiration is mainly passive. It occurs because the thorax and lungs recoil to their resting position. The alveolar pressure increases above atmospheric pressure, and air flows out through the respiratory tract. The major function of the lungs is to provide adequate ventilation to meet the metabolic demands of the body during rest and during exercise. The primary purpose of pulmonary blood flow is to conduct mixed venous blood through the capillaries of the alveoli so that oxygen (O_2) can be taken up by the blood and carbon dioxide (CO_2) can be removed from the blood.

Purpose of Tests

Pulmonary function tests determine the presence, nature, and extent of pulmonary dysfunction caused by obstruction, restriction, or both. When ventilation is disturbed by an increase in airway resistance (R_{aw}), the ventilatory defect is called an *obstructive* ventilatory impairment. When ventilation is disturbed by a limitation in chest wall excursion, the defect is referred to as a *restrictive* ventilatory impairment. When ventilation is altered by both increased R_{aw} and limited chest wall excursion, the defect is termed a *combined* or *mixed* defect. Table 14.1 presents the conditions that affect ventilation.

Pulmonary function studies may reveal locations of abnormalities in the airways, alveoli, and pulmonary vascular bed early in the course of a disease, when the physical examination and radiographic studies still appear normal.

Indications for Tests

1. Early detection of pulmonary or cardiogenic pulmonary disease (see Table 14.1)
2. Differential diagnosis of dyspnea
3. Presurgical assessment (e.g., ability to tolerate intraoperative anesthetics, especially during thoracic procedures)
4. Evaluation of risk factors for other diagnostic procedures
5. Detection of early respiratory failure
6. Monitoring progress of bronchopulmonary disease
7. Periodic evaluation of workers exposed to materials harmful to the respiratory system
8. Epidemiologic studies of selected populations to determine risks for or causes of pulmonary diseases
9. Workers' compensation claims
10. Monitoring after pharmacologic or surgical intervention

TABLE 14.1 Conditions That Affect Ventilation

Examples	Causes
Restrictive Ventilatory Impairments[a]	
Chest wall disease	Injury, kyphoscoliosis, spondylitis, muscular dystrophy, other neuromuscular diseases
Extrathoracic conditions	Obesity, peritonitis, ascites, pregnancy
Interstitial lung disease	Interstitial pneumonitis, fibrosis, pneumoconioses (e.g., asbestosis, silicosis), granulomatosis, edema, sarcoidosis
Pleural disease	Pneumothorax, hemothorax, pleural effusion, fibrothorax
Space-occupying lesions	Tumors, cysts, abscesses
Obstructive Ventilatory Impairments[b]	
Peripheral airway disease	Bronchitis, bronchiectasis, bronchiolitis, bronchial asthma, cystic fibrosis
Pulmonary parenchymal disease	Emphysema
Upper airway disease	Pharyngeal, tracheal, or laryngeal tumors; edema; infections; foreign bodies; collapsed airway; stenosis
Mixed-Defect Ventilatory Impairments[c]	
Pulmonary congestion	Both increased airway resistance and limited expansion of chest cavity and/or chest wall; obstruction caused by bronchial edema, compression of respiratory airway owing to increased interstitial (and intravenous fluid) pressure; restriction caused by impaired elasticity, anatomic deformity (e.g., kyphosis, lordosis, scoliosis)

[a]Characterized by interference with chest wall or lung movement, "stiff lung," and an actual reduction in the volume of air that can be inspired.

[b]Characterized by the need for increased effort to produce airflow; respiratory muscles must work harder to overcome obstructive forces during breathing; prolonged and impaired airflow during expiration; airway resistance increases and lungs become very compliant.

[c]Combined or mixed; exhibits components of both obstructive and restrictive ventilatory impairments.

Classification of Tests

Pulmonary function tests evaluate the ventilatory system and alveoli in an indirect, overlapping way. The patient's age, height, weight, ethnicity, and gender are recorded before testing because they are the basis for calculating predicted or normal reference values.

Pulmonary function tests are generally divided into three categories:

1. *Airway flow rates* typically include measurements of instantaneous or average airflow rates during a maximal forced exhalation to assess airway patency and resistance. These tests also assess responses to inhaled bronchodilators or bronchial provocations.
2. *Lung volumes and capacities* measure the various *air-containing compartments* of the lung to assess air trapping (hyperinflation, overdistention) or reduction in volume. These measurements also help to differentiate obstructive from restrictive ventilatory impairments.
3. *Gas exchange (diffusion capacity* or *transfer factor)* measures the rate of gas transfer across the alveolar capillary membranes to assess the diffusion process. It can also monitor for side effects of drugs, such as bleomycin (antineoplastic) or amiodarone (antiarrhythmic), which can cause interstitial pneumonitis or pulmonary fibrosis. Diffusion capacity in the absence of lung disease (e.g., anemia) can also be evaluated.

See Figure 14.1 for a sample Pulmonary Function Report.

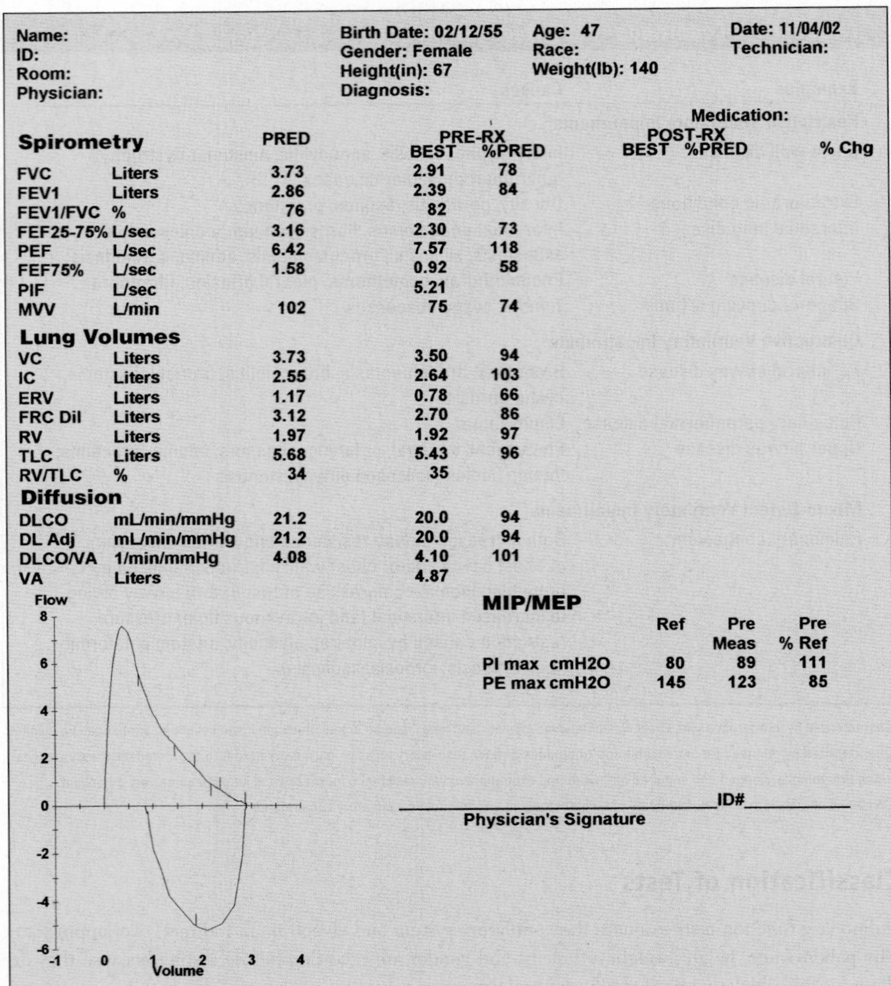

Name:
ID:
Room:
Physician:

Birth Date: 02/12/55
Gender: Female
Height(in): 67
Diagnosis:

Age: 47
Race:
Weight(lb): 140

Date: 11/04/02
Technician:

Medication:

Spirometry		PRED	PRE-RX BEST	PRE-RX %PRED	POST-RX BEST	POST-RX %PRED	% Chg
FVC	Liters	3.73	2.91	78			
FEV1	Liters	2.86	2.39	84			
FEV1/FVC	%	76	82				
FEF25-75%	L/sec	3.16	2.30	73			
PEF	L/sec	6.42	7.57	118			
FEF75%	L/sec	1.58	0.92	58			
PIF	L/sec		5.21				
MVV	L/min	102	75	74			
Lung Volumes							
VC	Liters	3.73	3.50	94			
IC	Liters	2.55	2.64	103			
ERV	Liters	1.17	0.78	66			
FRC Dil	Liters	3.12	2.70	86			
RV	Liters	1.97	1.92	97			
TLC	Liters	5.68	5.43	96			
RV/TLC	%	34	35				
Diffusion							
DLCO	mL/min/mmHg	21.2	20.0	94			
DL Adj	mL/min/mmHg	21.2	20.0	94			
DLCO/VA	1/min/mmHg	4.08	4.10	101			
VA	Liters		4.87				

MIP/MEP

	Ref	Pre Meas	Pre % Ref
PI max cmH2O	80	89	111
PE max cmH2O	145	123	85

Physician's Signature ID#

FIGURE 14.1. Pulmonary function report of a 47-year-old woman whose chief complaint is shortness of breath. The report includes spirometry, lung volumes, diffusion capacity, maximal voluntary ventilation, and maximal respiratory pressures. Note: The shape or configuration of the flow-volume loop (*lower left corner of report*) is significant for airflow obstruction (i.e., obstructive ventilatory impairment). The current flow-volume loop is essentially normal in appearance. (Reprinted with permission from Froedtert Hospital, Milwaukee, WI.)

Symbols and Abbreviations

Pulmonary function studies and blood gas analyses measure quantities of gas mixtures and their components, blood and its constituents, and various factors affecting these quantities. The symbols and abbreviations given here are based on standards developed by American physiologists. Familiarity with the major and secondary symbols facilitates interpretation of any combination of these symbols (Charts 14.1 through 14.4).

CHART 14.1 Gas Volumes: Symbols and Abbreviations

Large capital letters denote primary symbols for gases:

V = Gas volume

$\dot{V}$ = Gas volume per unit time (the dot over the symbol indicates the factor per unit time, as in flow)

P = Gas pressure or partial pressure of a gas in a gas mixture (exhaled air) or in a liquid (blood)

F = Fractional concentration of a gas

Small capital letters indicate the type of gas measured in relation to respiratory tract location or function:

A = Alveolar gas

D = Dead space gas

E = Expired gas

I = Inspired gas

T = Tidal gas

Chemical symbols for gases may be placed after the small capital letters:

O_2 = Oxygen

CO = Carbon monoxide

CO_2 = Carbon dioxide

N_2 = Nitrogen

Combinations of Symbols

The following are some examples of the ways these symbols may be combined:

F_ICO_2 = Fractional concentration of inspired oxygen

V_T = Tidal volume

V_E = Volume of expired gas

PACO = Partial pressure of carbon dioxide in alveolar gas

Blood Gas Symbols

Large capital letters are used as primary symbols for blood determinations:

C = Concentration of a gas in blood

S = Percent saturation of hemoglobin

Q = Volume of blood

$\dot{V}$ or $\dot{Q}$ = Volume of blood per unit time (blood flow)

To indicate whether blood is capillary, venous, or arterial, lowercase letters are used:

v = Venous blood

a = Arterial blood

c = Capillary blood

s = Shunted blood

bt = Brain tissue

CHART 14.2 Combinations of Symbols and Abbreviations

Blood gas symbols may be combined in the following ways:

Po_2 = Oxygen tension or partial pressure of oxygen
Pao_2 = Arterial oxygen tension or partial pressure of oxygen in arterial blood
$Pbto_2$ = Brain tissue oxygen tension or partial pressure
P_{AO_2} = Alveolar oxygen tension or partial pressure of oxygen in the alveoli
Pco_2 = Carbon dioxide tension or partial pressure of carbon dioxide
$Paco_2$ = Partial pressure of carbon dioxide in arterial blood
$Pvco_2$ = Partial pressure of carbon dioxide in venous blood
pH = Hydronium ion concentration
pHa = Hydronium ion concentration in arterial blood
So_2 = Oxygen saturation
Sao_2 = Percent saturation of oxygen in arterial blood as measured by hemoximetry (direct method)
Spo_2 = Percent saturation of oxygen in arterial blood as determined by pulse oximetry (indirect method)
Svo_2 = Percent saturation of oxygen in venous blood
Tco_2 = Total carbon dioxide content

AIRWAY FLOW RATES

Airway flow rates provide information about the severity of airway obstruction and serve as an index of dynamic function. The lung volume at which the flow rates are measured is useful for identifying a central or peripheral location of airway obstruction.

● Spirometry, Forced Expiratory Maneuver Volume-Time Spirogram (V-T Tracing); Flow-Volume Spirogram (F-V Loop)

Lung capacities, volumes, and flow rates are clinically measured by a mechanical device called a *spirometer*. The mechanical signal is converted to an electrical signal, which records the amounts of gas breathed in and out and produces a *spirogram*. Spirometers can be grouped into two major categories: (1) the mechanical or volume-displacement types (water-filled, dry-rolling seal, wedge, or bellows) and (2) the electronic or flow-sensing types (pneumotachometer or hot-wire anemometer [Fig. 14.2]). Spirometry determines the effectiveness of the various mechanical forces involved in lung and chest wall movement. The values obtained provide quantitative information about the degree of obstruction (obstructive ventilatory impairment) to expiratory airflow or the degree of restriction (restrictive ventilatory impairment) of inspired air. The forced expiratory maneuver (spirometry) is useful to quantify the extent and severity of airway obstruction. It measures the maximum amount of air that can be exhaled rapidly and forcibly after a maximal deep inspiration. The results are a measure of airway function and the patency of the airway.

Forced vital capacity (FVC) is the maximum amount of air that can be exhaled forcibly and completely after a maximal inspiration. The forced expiratory volumes exhaled within 1, 2, or 3 seconds are referred to as *timed vital capacities* (FEV_1, FEV_2, and FEV_3, respectively), whereas the FEF_{25-75} is the flow of air during the middle 50% (0.50) of the forced volume. These measurements are useful for evaluating a patient's response to bronchodilators. Generally, if the FEV_1 is <80% (<0.80) of predicted (reference value) or the FEF_{25-75} is <60% (<0.60) of predicted, bronchodilators (e.g., albuterol) are

CHART 14.3 Lung Volume Symbols: Pulmonary Function Terminology

This list indicates terms used in measuring lung volumes and the units that express these measurements.

FVC = Forced vital capacity: maximum amount of air that can be exhaled forcibly and completely after a maximal inspiration (liters)

FEV_t = Forced expiratory volume at specific time intervals (e.g., 1, 2, and/or 3 seconds): volume of air expired during the first, second, third, etc., seconds of FVC maneuver (liters)

FEV_t/FVC = Ratio of a timed forced expiratory volume to the forced vital capacity (e.g., FEV_1/FVC) (percent)

FEF_{25-75} = Forced expiratory flow between 25% and 75%: average flow of expired air measured between 25% and 75% of the FVC maneuver (liters/second)

PEFR = Peak expiratory flow rate: maximum flow of expired air attained during an FVC maneuver (liters/second or liters/minute)

PIFR = Peak inspiratory flow rate: maximum flow of inspired air achieved during a forced maximal inspiration (liters/second or liters/minute)

FEF_{25} = Forced instantaneous expiratory flow rate at 25% of lung volume achieved during an FVC maneuver (liters/second or liters/minute)

FEF_{50} = Forced instantaneous expiratory flow rate at 50% of lung volume achieved during an FVC maneuver (liters/second or liters/minute)

FEF_{75} = Forced instantaneous expiratory flow rate at 75% of lung volume achieved during an FVC maneuver (liters/second or liters/minute)

FRC = Functional residual capacity: volume of air remaining in the lung at the end of a normal expiration (i.e., end-tidal expiration) (liters)

IC = Inspiratory capacity: maximum amount of air that can be inspired from end-tidal expiration (liters)

IRV = Inspiratory reserve volume: maximum amount of air that can be inspired from end-tidal inspiration (liters)

ERV = Expiratory reserve volume: maximum amount of air that can be expired from end-tidal expiration (liters)

RV = Residual volume: volume of gas left in the lung after a maximal expiration (liters)

VC = Vital capacity: maximum volume of air that can be expired after a maximal inspiration (liters)

TLC = Total lung capacity: volume of gas contained in the lungs after a maximal inspiration (liters)

DLCO = Carbon monoxide diffusing capacity of the lung: rate of diffusion of carbon monoxide across the alveolar capillary membrane (i.e., rate of gas transfer across the alveolar capillary membrane) (milliliters/minute per millimeter of mercury)

CV = Closing volume: volume at which the lower lung zones cease to ventilate, presumably as a result of airway closure (percent of vital capacity)

MVV = Maximum voluntary ventilation: maximum number of liters of air a patient can breathe per minute by a voluntary effort (liters/minute)

VISO = Volume of isoflow: volume for which flow is the same with air and with helium during an FVC maneuver (percent)

CHART 14.4 Miscellaneous Symbols

This list shows some of the other symbols found in this chapter.

f = Frequency (of breathing)
CL = Compliance of the lung
COHb = Carboxyhemoglobin
D_{LO_2} = Oxygen diffusing capacity of the lung
$A\text{-}aDo_2$ = Alveolar-to-arterial oxygen gradient
BSA = Body surface area (square meters)
H_2CO_3 = Carbonic acid
HCO_3^- = Bicarbonate ion
TGV = Thoracic gas volume (also expressed as V_{TG})
R_{aw} = Airway resistance
G_{aw} = Airway conductance
F-V = Flow-volume
V-T = Volume-time

administered with a handheld nebulizer, and the spirometry is repeated. Studies have shown a better bronchodilator response with combined drugs (e.g., albuterol plus ipratropium) than either alone. An increase in these values of 20% or more (>0.20) above the pre-bronchodilator level suggests a significant response to the bronchodilator and is consistent with a diagnosis of reversible obstructive airway disease (e.g., asthma). Persons with emphysema typically do not demonstrate this type of response to bronchodilator. Measured (actual) spirometry values are compared with predicted values by means of regression equations using age, height, weight, ethnicity, and gender and are expressed as a percentage of the predicted value. Typically, a value >80% (>0.80) of predicted is considered within normal limits.

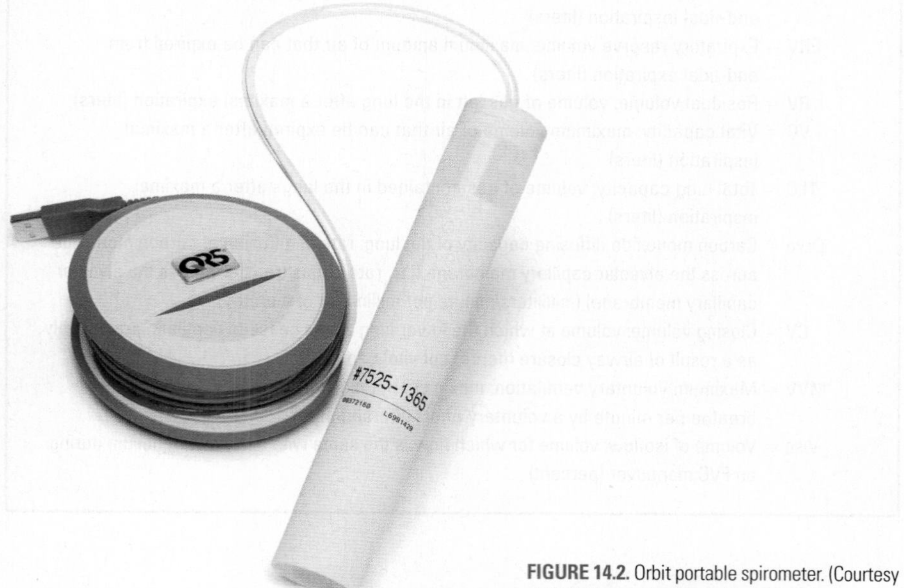

FIGURE 14.2. Orbit portable spirometer. (Courtesy of QRS Diagnostic, Maple Grove, MN.)

Reference Values

Normal

FVC: >80% (>0.80) of the predicted value

FEV_t: FEV_1, FEV_2, FEV_3, >80% (>0.80) of the predicted value

FEV_t/FVC:

FEV_1, 80% to 85% (0.80 to 0.85) of FVC

FEV_2, 90% to 94% (0.90 to 0.94) of FVC

FEV_3, 95% to 97% (0.95 to 0.97) of FVC

$FEF_{25–75}$: >60% (>0.60) of the predicted value

Predicted values are based on the patient's age, height, ethnicity, and gender.

Procedure

1. Have the patient either sit or stand. Place nose clips on the nose and instruct the patient to breathe normally through a mouthpiece/filter (bacterial/viral) combination into the spirometer.
2. Ask the patient to take a maximal inspiration and then forcibly and completely exhale into the spirometer.
3. Have the patient repeat this maneuver a minimum of three times. The two best tracings should compare within ±200 mL of one another, or additional forced expiratory efforts will be needed.
4. Administer bronchodilators with a handheld nebulizer and repeat spirometry if indicated.
5. See Chapter 1 guidelines for *intratest* care.

PROCEDURAL ALERT

1. Before testing, assess the patient's ability to comply with breathing requirements.
2. The patient may experience light-headedness, shortness of breath, or other slight discomforts. These symptoms are generally transitory. An appropriate rest period is usually all that is needed. If symptoms persist, testing is terminated.
3. Rarely, momentary loss of consciousness (caused by anoxia during forced expiration) may occur. Follow established protocols for testing under these circumstances.
4. Assess for contraindications such as pain or altered mental status.

Clinical Implications

1. With obstructive ventilatory impairments such as asthma, airway collapse occurs during the forced expiratory effort. This leads to decreases in airway flow rates and also, in the more severe forms, to apparent loss of volumes. Obstructive ventilatory impairments include the following:
   a. Emphysema
   b. Bronchitis
   c. Asthma
   d. Cystic fibrosis (CF)
   e. Byssinosis (rare lung disease caused by exposure to cotton dust)
2. With restrictive ventilatory impairments, the FVC is reduced; however, flow rates can be normal or elevated. Restrictive ventilatory impairments include the following:
   a. Pulmonary fibrosis
   b. Lung resection
   c. Thoracic cage deformities (e.g., pectus excavatum, kyphoscoliosis)
   d. Asbestosis (exposure to the asbestos fiber)
   e. Silicosis (exposure to crystalline silica dust)

Interfering Factors

1. Bronchodilators (e.g., albuterol) should be withheld for at least 4 hours if tolerated.
2. Respiratory infections may decrease airflow during the maneuver.
3. Patient noncompliance can adversely affect the results because this test is effort dependent.

Interventions

Pretest Patient Care

1. Explain the purpose and procedure of the spirometry test. Explain that the patient will be asked to perform a maximal forced inspiration in addition to the forced expirations.
2. Remind the patient that a light meal may be eaten before the test. However, no caffeine should be taken before testing. Specific instructions will be given regarding the use of bronchodilators or inhaler medications before the test.
3. Follow guidelines in Chapter 1 for safe, effective, informed *pretest* care.

Posttest Patient Care

1. Evaluate for dizziness, shortness of breath, or chest discomfort. Usually, these symptoms are transitory and subside after a short rest. If symptoms persist, use established follow-up protocols.
2. Treatment of pulmonary disorders includes bronchodilators, corticosteroids, supplemental oxygen, and surgery. In patients with CF, drugs (e.g., dornase sulfa [Pulmozyme]) can be used to thin secretions (i.e., reduce sputum viscosity).
3. Follow guidelines in Chapter 1 for safe, effective, informed *posttest* care.

● Peak Inspiratory Flow Rate (PIFR)

The peak inspiratory flow rate (PIFR) measures the function of the airways, identifies reduced breathing on inspiration, and is totally dependent on the effort the patient makes to inspire. The PIFR is the maximal flow of air achieved during a forced maximal inspiration.

Reference Values

Normal

Approximately 300 L/min or 5 L/sec
Predicted values are based on age, gender, and height.

Procedure

1. Have the patient either sit or stand. Place nose clips on the nose and instruct the patient to breathe normally through a mouthpiece/filter (bacterial/viral) combination into the spirometer.
2. Ask the patient to take a maximal inspiration forcibly and completely exhale into the spirometer and then inspire forcibly and completely again.
3. Have the patient repeat this maneuver a minimum of three times. Report the highest value.
4. The PIFR can also be measured with a handheld peak flow meter.

Clinical Implications

1. PIFR is *reduced* in neuromuscular disorders, with weakness or poor effort, and in extrathoracic airway obstruction (i.e., substernal thyroid, tracheal stenosis, and laryngeal paralysis).
2. The PIFR is decreased in upper airway obstruction.

Interfering Factors

1. Poor patient effort compromises the test.
2. Inability to maintain an airtight seal around the mouthpiece

Interventions

Pretest Patient Care

1. Explain the purpose and procedure of the test. Assess the patient's ability to follow verbal instructions.
2. Follow guidelines in Chapter 1 for safe, effective, informed *pretest* care.

Posttest Patient Care

1. Follow guidelines in Chapter 1 for safe, effective, informed *posttest* care.
2. See aftercare guidelines for V-T tracing (volume-time spirogram) on page 906.

● Peak Expiratory Flow Rate (PEFR)

The peak expiratory flow rate (PEFR) measurement is used as an index of large airway function. It is the maximum flow of expired air attained during a forced expiratory maneuver.

Reference Values

Normal

Approximately 450 L/min or 7.5 L/sec
Predicted values are based on age, gender, and height.

Procedure

1. Have the patient either sit or stand. Place nose clips on the nose and instruct the patient to breathe normally through a mouthpiece/filter (bacterial/viral) combination into the spirometer.
2. Ask the patient to take a maximal inspiration forcibly and completely exhale into the spirometer and then inspire forcibly and completely again.
3. Have the patient repeat this maneuver a minimum of three times. Report the highest value.
4. The PEFR can also be measured with a handheld peak flow meter.

Clinical Implications

1. The PEFR usually is *decreased* in obstructive disease (e.g., emphysema), during acute exacerbations of asthma, and in upper airway obstruction (e.g., tracheal stenosis).
2. The PEFR usually is *normal* in restrictive lung disease but is reduced in severe restrictive situations.

Interfering Factors

1. Poor patient effort compromises the test.
2. Inability to maintain an airtight seal around the mouthpiece

Interventions

Pretest Patient Care

1. Explain the purpose and procedure of the test. Assess the patient's ability to follow verbal instructions.
2. Follow guidelines in Chapter 1 for safe, effective, informed *pretest* care.

Posttest Patient Care

1. Monitor patient for dizziness, light-headedness, or chest pain following the test. Generally, these symptoms are transient and will subside quickly. If not, follow established protocols.
2. See aftercare guidelines for V-T tracings on page 906.
3. Follow guidelines in Chapter 1 for safe, effective, informed *posttest* care.

LUNG VOLUMES AND CAPACITIES

Lung volumes can be considered as basic subdivisions of the lung (not actual anatomic subdivisions). They may be subdivided as follows:

1. Tidal volume (V_T)
2. Inspiratory capacity (IC)
3. Inspiratory reserve volume (IRV)
4. Residual volume (RV)
5. Functional residual capacity (FRC)
6. Expiratory reserve volume (ERV)
7. Vital capacity (VC)

Combinations of two or more volumes are termed *capacities*. These volumes and capacities are shown graphically in Figure 14.3. Measurement of these values can provide information about the degree of air trapping or hyperinflation.

● Functional Residual Capacity (FRC)

FRC is used to evaluate both restrictive and obstructive lung defects. Changes in the elastic properties of the lungs are reflected in the FRC. The FRC is the volume of gas contained in the lungs at the end of a normal quiet expiration (see Fig. 14.3).

Reference Values

Normal

Approximately 2.50 to 3.50 L

Predicted values are based on age, height, weight, ethnicity, and gender.

The observed value should be 75% to 125% (0.75 to 1.25) of the predicted value.

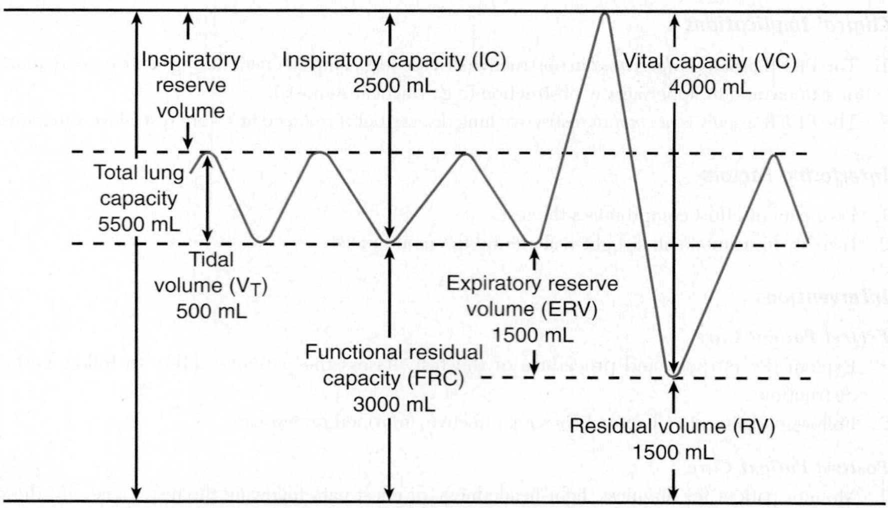

FIGURE 14.3. Subdivisions of lung volume in the normal adult male. (From Geschickter CF: The Lung in Health and Disease. Philadelphia, JB Lippincott, 1973.)

Procedure

1. Fit the patient with nose clips. Instruct the patient to breathe normally through the mouthpiece/filter (bacterial/viral) combination that is attached to the lung volume apparatus. The patient is generally in the seated position.
2. There are three methods, depending on the instrumentation used:
   a. Nitrogen washout or open-circuit technique
   b. Helium dilution or closed-circuit technique
   c. Whole-body plethysmography
3. Have the patient breathe normally for about 3 to 7 minutes.
4. Perform the test a second time. The FRC should vary by not more than 5% to 10% (0.05 to 0.10). Report the average of the test values.
5. See Chapter 1 guidelines for *intratest* care.

Clinical Implications

1. A value <75% (<0.75) of the predicted is consistent with restrictive ventilatory impairment.
2. A value >125% (>1.25) of predicted demonstrates air trapping (hyperinflation), consistent with obstructive airway disease (e.g., emphysema, asthma, bronchiolar obstruction).

Interventions

Pretest Patient Care

1. Explain the purpose and procedure of the test. Explain that this is a noninvasive test requiring patient cooperation. Assess the patient's ability to follow verbal instructions.
2. Record the patient's age, gender, weight, and height.
3. Follow guidelines in Chapter 1 for safe, effective, informed *pretest* care.

Posttest Patient Care

1. Explain test outcomes; allow the patient to rest if necessary.
2. Follow guidelines in Chapter 1 for safe, effective, informed *posttest*.

● Residual Volume (RV)

RV can help to distinguish between restrictive and obstructive ventilatory defects. It is the volume of gas remaining in the lungs after a maximal exhalation. Because the lungs cannot be completely emptied (i.e., a maximal expiratory effort cannot expel all of the gas), RV is the only lung volume that cannot be measured directly from the spirometer. It is calculated mathematically by subtracting the measured ERV from the measured FRC (see Fig. 14.3).

Reference Values

Normal

Approximately 1200 to 1500 mL

Predicted values are based on age, gender, and height.

Procedure

1. Remember that the RV is determined indirectly from other tests; that is, it is mathematically derived by subtracting the measured ERV from the FRC.
2. See Chapter 1 guidelines for *intratest* care.

Clinical Implications

1. An increase in the RV (>125% [>1.25] of predicted) indicates that, despite a maximal expiratory effort, the lungs still contain an abnormally large amount of gas (air trapping). This type of change occurs in young asthmatic patients and usually is reversible. In emphysema, the condition is permanent.
2. Increased RV is characteristic of emphysema, chronic air trapping, and chronic bronchial obstruction.
3. The RV and the FRC usually increase together but not always.
4. The RV sometimes decreases in diseases that occlude many alveoli.
5. An RV <75% (<0.75) of predicted is consistent with restrictive disorders (e.g., interstitial pulmonary fibrosis).

Interfering Factors

Residual volume normally increases with age.

Interventions

Pretest Patient Care

1. Explain the purpose of the test and how the results are calculated.
2. Follow guidelines in Chapter 1 for safe, effective, informed *pretest* care.

Posttest Patient Care

1. Review test results; report and record findings. Modify the nursing care plan as needed.
2. Follow guidelines in Chapter 1 for safe, effective, informed *posttest* care.

● Expiratory Reserve Volume (ERV)

ERV is the largest volume of gas that can be exhaled from end-tidal expiration. This measurement identifies lung or chest wall restriction. The ERV can be estimated mathematically by subtracting the IC from the VC. The ERV accounts for approximately 25% of the VC and can vary greatly in patients of comparable age and height (see Fig. 14.3).

Reference Values

Normal

Approximately 1200 to 1500 mL (1.20 to 1.50 L)
Predicted values are based on age, height, and gender.

Procedure

1. Have the patient either sit or stand. Place nose clips on the nose and instruct the patient to breathe normally through a mouthpiece/filter (bacterial/viral) combination into the spirometer.
2. Ask the patient to exhale completely and resume normal breathing. Record results on graph paper.
3. Ask the patient to repeat this maneuver at least twice. The measured volumes should be within ±60 mL of one another. Report the average value.

Clinical Implications

1. A decreased ERV indicates a chest wall restriction resulting from nonpulmonary causes.
2. Decreased values are associated with an elevated diaphragm (e.g., massive obesity, ascites, pregnancy). Decreased values also occur with massive enlargement of the heart, pleural effusion, kyphoscoliosis (abnormal curvature of the spine), or thoracoplasty (removal of one or more ribs).
3. Decreases in ERV also are seen in obstruction resulting from an increase in the RV impinging on the ERV.

Interventions

Pretest Patient Care

1. Explain the purpose and procedure of the spirometry test. Inform the patient that the test is noninvasive. Assess the patient's ability to comply with test procedures.
2. Follow guidelines in Chapter 1 for safe, effective, informed *pretest* care.

Posttest Patient Care

1. Review test results; report and record findings. Modify the nursing care plan as needed. Counsel the patient about respiratory abnormalities.
2. Follow guidelines in Chapter 1 for safe, effective, informed *posttest* care.

● Inspiratory Capacity (IC)

IC measures the largest volume of air that can be inhaled from the end-tidal expiratory level. This measurement is used to identify lung or chest wall restrictions. Mathematically, the IC is the sum of the VT and the IRV (see Fig. 14.3).

Reference Values

Normal

Approximately 3000 to 3300 mL (3.00 to 3.30 L)
Predicted values are based on age, height, and gender.

Procedure

1. Have the patient either sit or stand. Place nose clips on the nose and instruct the patient to breathe normally through a mouthpiece/filter (bacterial/viral) combination into the spirometer.
2. After several breaths, ask the patient to inhale maximally, expanding the lungs as much as possible from end-tidal expiration. Have the patient resume normal breathing. Record the results on graph paper.
3. Repeat step 2 two or more times until the two best values are within 5% of each other. Select the largest inspired volume value.

Clinical Implications

1. Changes in the IC usually parallel increases or decreases in the VC.
2. Decreases in IC can be related to either restrictive or obstructive ventilatory impairments.

Interventions

Pretest Patient Care

1. Instruct the patient about the purpose and procedure of the test and the need for patient cooperation.
2. Follow guidelines in Chapter 1 for safe, effective, informed *pretest* care.

Posttest Patient Care

1. Review test results; report and record findings. Modify the nursing care plan as needed.
2. Follow guidelines in Chapter 1 for safe, effective, informed *posttest* care.

● Vital Capacity (VC)

Measurement of the VC identifies defects of lung or chest wall restriction. The VC is the largest volume of gas that can be expelled from the lungs after the lungs are first filled to the maximum extent and then slowly emptied to the maximum extent. Mathematically, it is the sum of the IC and the ERV (see Fig. 14.3).

Reference Values

Normal

Approximately 4.50 to 5.00 L
Predicted values are based on age, gender, height, and ethnicity.

Procedure

1. Have the patient either sit or stand. Place nose clips on the nose and instruct the patient to breathe normally through a mouthpiece/filter (bacterial/viral) combination into the spirometer.
2. Instruct the patient then to inhale as deeply as possible and then to exhale completely, with no forced or rapid effort.
3. Record results on graph paper.
4. Repeat the procedure until the measurements are within about 5% of each other.

Clinical Implications

1. A reduced VC is defined as a value <80% (<0.80) of predicted.
2. The VC can be lower than expected in either a restrictive or an obstructive disorder. Inadequate patient effort causes lower VC values.
3. A decreased VC can be related to depression of the respiratory center in the brain, neuromuscular diseases, pleural effusion, pneumothorax, pregnancy, ascites, limitations of thoracic movement, scleroderma (autoimmune disease resulting in fibrosis), kyphoscoliosis, or tumors.
4. The VC increases with physical fitness and greater height.
5. The VC decreases after age 30 years.
6. The VC is generally less in women than in men of the same age and height.
7. The VC is decreased by approximately 15% in African Americans and by 20% to 25% in Asians compared with Caucasians of the same age, height, and gender.

Interventions

Pretest Patient Care

1. Explain the purpose and procedure of the test and need for patient cooperation. Assess for interfering factors.
2. Follow guidelines in Chapter 1 for safe, effective, informed *pretest* care.

Posttest Patient Care

1. Review test results; report and record findings. Modify the nursing care plan as needed. Monitor patient signs and symptoms and follow up if necessary.
2. Follow guidelines in Chapter 1 for safe, effective, informed *posttest* care.

● Total Lung Capacity (TLC)

Total lung capacity (TLC) is used mainly to evaluate obstructive defects and to differentiate restrictive from obstructive pulmonary disease. It measures the volume of gas contained in the lungs at the end of a maximal inspiration. Mathematically, it is the sum of the VC and the RV, or the sum of the primary lung volumes (see Fig. 14.3). This value is calculated indirectly from other tests.

Reference Values

Normal

Approximately 5.70 to 6.20 L
Predicted values are based on age, height, gender, and ethnicity.
All pulmonary volumes and capacities are about 20% to 25% less in women than in men.

Procedure

1. Have the patient either sit or stand. Place nose clips on the nose and instruct the patient to breathe normally through a mouthpiece/filter (bacterial/viral) combination into the spirometer.
2. Ask the patient to inspire maximally and exhale maximally. The total amount of air exhaled is the VC.
3. Use the following formula to derive the TLC mathematically: TLC = VC + RV.

Clinical Implications

1. Increased values are associated with:
   a. Emphysema
   b. CF
   c. Hyperinflation
2. Decreased values are associated with:
   a. Pulmonary edema
   b. Atelectasis
   c. Neoplasms
   d. Pulmonary congestion
   e. Pneumothorax
   f. Thoracic restriction

Interventions

Pretest Patient Care

1. Explain the purpose and procedure of the test. Even though it is noninvasive, it does require patient effort and cooperation.
2. Follow guidelines in Chapter 1 for safe, effective, informed *pretest* care.

Posttest Patient Care

1. Review test results; report and record findings (see Fig. 14.1). Modify the nursing care plan as needed.
2. Follow guidelines in Chapter 1 for safe, effective, informed *posttest* care.

GAS EXCHANGE (DIFFUSING CAPACITY), TRANSFER FACTOR

Gas exchange in the lungs is referred to as respiration, whereas the movement of gas in and out of the lung is ventilation. Gas exchange involves the movement of oxygen (O_2) from the alveolus (gas exchange units in the lung) to the blood (i.e., diffusion across the alveolar capillary membrane) and movement of carbon dioxide (CO_2) from the blood into the alveolus for subsequent removal.

● Carbon Monoxide Diffusing Capacity (DLCO, DL), Diffusing Capacity, Transfer Factor

The diffusing capacity measurement determines the rate of gas transfer across the alveolar capillary membranes. Carbon monoxide (CO) combines with hemoglobin about 210 times more readily than does O_2. If there is a normal amount of hemoglobin in the blood, the only other significant limiting factor to CO uptake is the state of the alveolar capillary membranes. Normally, the amount of CO in the blood is insufficient to affect the test. Two categories of factors (i.e., physical and chemical) determine the rate of gas (CO) transfer across the lung. The physical determinants are CO driving pressure, surface area, thickness of capillary walls, and diffusion coefficient for CO. The chemical determinants are red blood cell volume and reaction rate with hemoglobin.

This test is used to diagnose pulmonary vascular disease, emphysema, and pulmonary fibrosis and to evaluate the extent of functional pulmonary capillary bed in contact with functional alveoli. The alveolar volume (VA) can also be determined. The DLCO measures the diffusing capacity of the lungs for CO. The DLO_2 is obtained by multiplying the DLCO by 1.23.

Reference Values

Normal

Approximately 25 mL/min/mm Hg (8.4 mmol/min/kPa)
Predicted values are based on the patient's height, age, and gender.

Procedure

1. Have the patient either sit or stand. Place nose clips on the nose and instruct the patient to breathe normally through a mouthpiece/filter (bacterial/viral) combination into the diffusion instrument.
2. Ask the patient to expire maximally and then inspire maximally (a diffusion gas mixture), hold breath for 10 seconds, and then exhale, at which time a sample of exhaled gas is obtained.
3. Two techniques are used by laboratories:
   a. Single-breath or breath-holding technique
   b. Steady-state technique
4. See Chapter 1 guidelines for *intratest* care.

Clinical Implications

1. *Decreased* values are associated with:
   a. Multiple pulmonary emboli
   b. Emphysema
   c. Lung resection
   d. Pulmonary fibroses
      (1) Sarcoidosis (abnormal collection of inflammatory cells in multiple organs)
      (2) Systemic lupus erythematosus (SLE)
      (3) Asbestosis
      (4) Pneumonia
   e. Anemia
   f. Increased levels of carboxyhemoglobin (COHb)
   g. Pulmonary resection
   h. Scleroderma
2. *Increased* values are observed in polycythemia, left-to-right shunts, pulmonary hemorrhage, and exercise.
3. The value is relatively *normal* in chronic bronchitis.

Interfering Factors

Exercise (with an increased cardiac output) and polycythemia increase the value. Because increased levels of COHb (as seen in smokers) and anemia decrease the value, the DLCO is adjusted for COHb levels $>10\%$ (>0.10) and hemoglobin (Hb) values <8 g/dL (<80 g/L).

Interventions

Pretest Patient Care

1. Explain the purpose and procedure. Assess for interfering factors and explain that this noninvasive test requires patient cooperation. Assess the patient's ability to follow verbal instructions.
2. Follow guidelines in Chapter 1 for safe, effective, informed *pretest* care.

Posttest Patient Care

1. Review test results; report and record findings. Modify the nursing care plan as needed. Discuss with the patient the possible need for follow-up testing to monitor course of therapy (e.g., anti-inflammatory drugs, bronchodilators, and some antiarrhythmics and antineoplastics).
2. Follow guidelines in Chapter 1 for safe, effective, informed *posttest* care.

OTHER PULMONARY FUNCTION TESTS

● Maximum Voluntary Ventilation (MVV)

Maximum voluntary ventilation (MVV) measures several physiologic phenomena occurring at the same time, including thoracic cage compliance, lung compliance, R_{aw}, and available muscle force. It is the number of liters of air that the patient can breathe per minute with maximal voluntary effort.

Reference Values

Normal

Approximately 160 to 180 L/min

Predicted values are based on the patient's age, height, and gender. A healthy person may vary by as much as 25% to 35% from mean group values.

Procedure

1. Have the patient either sit or stand. Place nose clips on the nose and instruct the patient to breathe normally through a mouthpiece/filter (bacterial/viral) combination into the spirometer.
2. Instruct the patient to breathe into the spirometer as deeply and rapidly as possible for 10 to 15 seconds. Usually, the frequency reaches 40 to 70 breaths per minute, and the tidal volumes are about 50% of the VC.
3. The actual values are extrapolated from the 10- to 15-second time interval to a 1-minute time period.
4. Typically, the maneuver is performed twice and the largest value is reported.

Interfering Factors

Poor patient effort can be ruled out by using the following formula to predict the MVV of the patient: Predicted MVV $= 35 \times FEV_1$. This is a useful check to determine whether the recorded MVV is indicative of adequate patient effort. Low values can be related to patient effort and not to pathophysiology.

Clinical Implications

1. Obstructive ventilatory impairments of moderate to severe degree, abnormal neuromuscular control, and poor patient effort are causes of low values.
2. In restrictive disease, the value is usually normal; however, in more severe forms, MVV may be decreased.

Interventions

Pretest Patient Care

1. Explain the purpose and procedure of the test. Explain that it is a noninvasive test that requires patient cooperation. Assess the patient's ability to follow verbal instructions.
2. Record the patient's age, height, and gender.
3. Follow guidelines in Chapter 1 for safe, effective, informed *pretest* care.

Posttest Patient Care

1. Explain test outcome (see Fig. 14.1) and possible need for follow-up testing and treatment.
2. Follow guidelines in Chapter 1 for safe, effective, informed *posttest* care.

Maximal Respiratory Pressure (MRP), Maximal Expiratory Pressure (MEP), Maximal Inspiratory Pressure (MIP)

The maximal respiratory pressure (MRP) measurements assess ventilatory muscle strength in persons with neuromuscular disorders such as poliomyelitis, emphysema, and pulmonary fibroses. The maximal expiratory pressure (MEP) is the greatest pressure that can be generated at or near TLC after a maximal inspiration, whereas the maximal inspiratory pressure (MIP) is measured at or near the residual volume after a maximal expiration.

Reference Values

Normal

MEP: ~100 to 250 cm H_2O

MIP: ~40 to 125 cm H_2O

Predicted values (i.e., reference values) are based on the patient's age and gender.

Procedure

1. Instruct the patient, who should be in a seated position and wearing a nose clip, to inspire maximally. Place the mouthpiece of the handheld pressure manometer into the mouth and have the patient perform a forced expiration. Record this maximal sustained (1 to 3 seconds) pressure against the internal occlusion of the manometer as the MEP.
2. Repeat this same procedure to obtain the MIP, except that this time, the patient fully exhales before placing the mouthpiece of the manometer in the mouth. Have the patient then inspire forcefully, and record the maximal sustained (1 to 3 seconds) pressure.
3. Repeat each procedure and record the best of three measurements for each.
4. See Chapter 1 guidelines for *intratest* care.

Interfering Factors

The MIP and MEP measurements depend on patient effort; low values may be caused by poor effort rather than loss of respiratory muscle strength. If the patient does not inspire or expire maximally before performing the pressure measurement, the value may be low. Also, sustained efforts longer than 3 seconds should be avoided because they can cause a decrease in cardiac output as a result of increased intrathoracic pressures.

Clinical Implications

1. *Decreases in both MEP and MIP* are seen in neuromuscular disorders (e.g., myasthenia gravis, poliomyelitis).
2. *Decreased MEP* is common in both severe obstructive disease (e.g., emphysema) and severe restrictive ventilatory impairment (e.g., interstitial pulmonary fibrosis).
3. *Decreased MIP* is observed in patients with chest wall abnormalities (e.g., kyphoscoliosis) and in hyperinflation (e.g., emphysema).

Interventions

Pretest Patient Care

1. Explain the purpose and procedure of the test. Explain that it is a noninvasive, effort-dependent maneuver that requires patient cooperation.
2. Record the patient's age and gender.
3. Follow guidelines in Chapter 1 for safe, effective, informed *pretest* care.

Posttest Patient Care

1. Explain test outcomes (see Fig. 14.1) and possible need for follow-up testing and treatment.
2. Follow guidelines in Chapter 1 for safe, effective, informed *posttest* care.

● Closing Volume (CV)

In a healthy person, the concentration of alveolar nitrogen, after a single breath of 100% O_2, rapidly increases near the end of expiration. This rise is caused by closure of the small airways in the bases of the lung. The point at which this closure occurs is called the *closing volume* (CV). CV is used as an index of pathologic changes occurring within the small airways (those <2 mm in diameter). The conventional pulmonary function tests are not sensitive enough to make this determination. This test relies on the fact that the upper lung zones contain a proportionately larger residual volume of gas than the lower lung zones; there is a gradient of intrapleural pressure from the top to the bottom of the lung. Additionally, the uniformity of gas distribution within the lungs can be measured.

Reference Values

Normal

Average is 10% to 20% (0.10 to 0.20) of the patient's VC.

Predicted values are derived from mathematical regression equations and are based on the patient's age and gender.

Procedure

1. Have the patient assume a seated position. Place nose clips on the nose and instruct the patient to breathe normally through a mouthpiece/filter (bacterial/viral) combination into the spirometer.
2. Ask the patient to exhale completely, to inhale 100% O_2, and then to exhale completely at the rate of approximately 0.5 L/sec.
3. During exhalation, monitor simultaneously both the expired volume and percentage of alveolar nitrogen on an X-Y recorder. Remember that a sudden increase in nitrogen represents the CV.

Clinical Implications

1. Values are *increased* for those conditions in which the airways are narrowed (e.g., bronchitis, early airway obstruction, chronic smoking, old age).
2. A change in the *slope* of the nitrogen curve of >2% is indicative of maldistribution of inspired air (i.e., uneven alveolar ventilation).
3. Congestive heart failure, with subsequent edema, may also contribute to decreasing patency of the small airways leading to an increase in the CV.

Interfering Factors

1. The CV increases with age.
2. Patients in congestive heart failure may show an increased CV.

Interventions

Pretest Patient Care

1. Explain the purpose and procedure of the test. Explain that this is a noninvasive test that requires patient cooperation. Assess the patient's ability to comply with breathing requirement and instructions. Assess for interfering factors.
2. Follow guidelines in Chapter 1 for safe, effective, informed *pretest* care.

Posttest Patient Care

1. Explain the meaning of test outcomes and possible need for follow-up testing and treatment of early small airway disease.
2. Follow guidelines in Chapter 1 for safe, effective, informed *posttest* care.

Volume of Isoflow (V_{ISO} $\dot{V}$)

This test is designed to detect pathologic changes occurring in the small airways and may be more sensitive than conventional pulmonary function tests. Helium has the unique property of lowering gas density. Therefore, after the patient breathes a helium–oxygen gas mixture, the effects of convective acceleration and turbulence are negated. Any abnormality observed in the F-V loop, then, results from an increase in resistance to laminar (nonturbulent) flow, which indicates small airway abnormalities or lung disease.

Reference Values

Normal

Average is 10% to 25% of VC.
Predicted values are based on age.

Procedure

1. Have the patient assume a seated position. Place nose clips on the nose and instruct the patient to breathe normally through a mouthpiece/filter (bacterial/viral) combination into the spirometer.
2. Have the patient perform a baseline F-V loop, which is recorded by a spirometer on an X-Y recorder.
3. Have the patient next breathe a mixture of 80% He and 20% O_2 for several breaths and then perform another F-V loop maneuver; this is the heliox F-V loop.
4. Superimpose the F-V loop tracings, and measure the volume of isoflow at the point at which the two loops intersect.

Clinical Implications

An *increased* volume of isoflow is consistent with early small airway obstruction (e.g., asthma).

Interventions

Pretest Patient Care

1. Explain the purpose and procedure of the test.
2. Follow guidelines in Chapter 1 for safe, effective, informed *pretest* care.

Posttest Patient Care

1. Review test results; report and record findings. Modify the nursing care plan as needed. Explain the possible need for follow-up testing and treatment.
2. Follow guidelines in Chapter 1 for safe, effective, informed *posttest* care.

Body Plethysmography: Thoracic Gas Volume (V_{TG}), Lung Compliance (C_L), Airway Resistance (R_{aw}), Airway Conductance (G_{aw})

This test measures several parameters. Thoracic gas volume (V_{TG}) composes all the air contained within the thorax, whether or not it is in ventilatory communication with the rest of the lung. Compliance of the lung (C_L) is an indication of its elasticity, and R_{aw} is a measurement of the resistance to airflow in the tracheobronchial tree (which is a hyperbolic function). Airway conductance (G_{aw}) is the reciprocal of R_{aw}, decreasing in a linear fashion as R_{aw} increases.

The measurement of V_{TG} through body plethysmography is an application of Boyle's law, which states that for a gas at constant temperature, pressure and volume vary inversely ($P_1V_1 = P_2V_2$). R_{aw} increases with decreased lung volumes and decreases with higher lung volumes in a nonlinear, hyperbolic fashion. C_L increases in obstructive diseases (e.g., emphysema) and decreases in restrictive processes (e.g., interstitial lung disease).

Reference Values

Normal

VTG: ~2.50 to 3.50 L

CL: 0.2 L/cm H_2O (2.04 L/kPa)

R_{aw}: 0.6 to 2.4 L/sec/cm H_2O

G_{aw}: reciprocal of R_{aw}

Predicted values are based on the patient's age, height, weight, and gender.

Procedure

1. Have the patient sit in the plethysmograph (a glass-walled box-like chamber). Fit with nose clips and have the patient breathe through a mouthpiece/filter (bacterial/viral) combination connected to a transducer (Fig. 14.4).
2. Ensure that the plethysmograph door is secured. Delay the test for a few minutes to allow the box pressure to stabilize due to temperature changes.
3. Instruct the patient to perform a panting maneuver while holding the cheeks rigid and the glottis open against a closed shutter located within the transducer assembly. Plethysmograph box and mouth pressures are displayed on a monitor for subsequent determination of the VTG.
4. Ask the patient to breathe rapidly and shallowly. Plethysmograph box pressure changes versus flow are displayed on a monitor for subsequent determination of the R_{aw}.
5. To determine CL, pass a balloon catheter through the nose into the patient's esophagus. Typically, the balloon catheter is lightly coated with a topical anesthetic (e.g., lidocaine jelly) for patient comfort. Ensure that the inflated balloon is connected to a transducer and instruct the patient to breathe normally. Changes in intraesophageal pressure during normal respiration (which mimic changes in intrapleural pressure) are recorded for determination of the CL.
6. See Chapter 1 guidelines for *intratest* care.

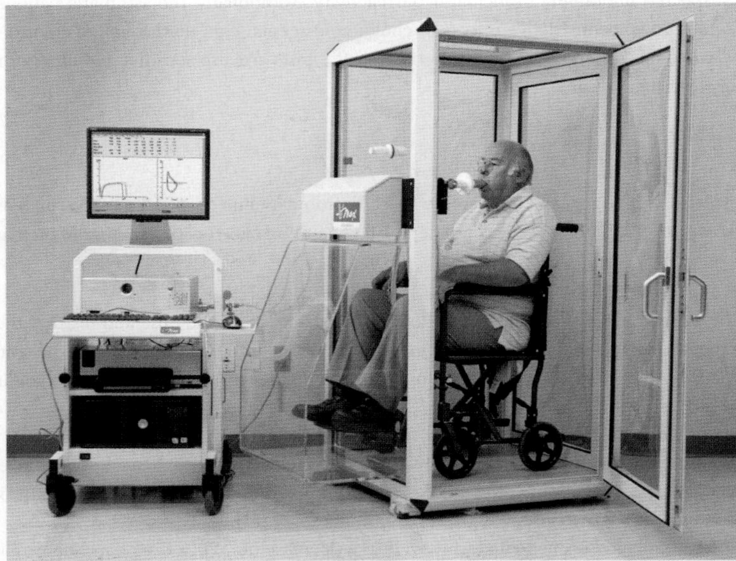

FIGURE 14.4. Vmax Autobox whole-body plethysmograph. (Becton Dickinson, Franklin Lakes, NJ.)

Clinical Implications

1. An *increased* VTG demonstrates air trapping, consistent with obstructive pulmonary disease (e.g., emphysema).
2. An *increased* R_{aw} or *decreased* G_{aw} demonstrates increased resistance to airflow through the tracheobronchial tree; this is seen in asthma, emphysema, bronchitis, and other forms of obstruction.
3. An *increase* in CL (i.e., lung is more distensible) is seen in obstructive diseases.
4. A *decrease* in CL (i.e., lung is more stiff) is seen in fibrotic diseases, restrictive diseases, pneumonia, congestion, and atelectasis.

Interventions

Pretest Patient Care

1. Explain the purpose and procedure of the test.
2. Assure the patient that although the chamber is airtight, the test only takes a few minutes. A technician will be in constant attendance to open the door should that be necessary. There is also a handle inside of the body box should the patient feel anxious and need to open the door. Assess for ability to comply with test requirements and instructions. Assess for predisposition to claustrophobia, panic attacks, or other similar responses.
3. Follow guidelines in Chapter 1 for safe, effective, informed *pretest* care.

Posttest Patient Care

1. Allow the patient time to rest quietly if necessary.
2. Explain the meaning of test outcomes.
3. Follow guidelines in Chapter 1 for safe, effective, informed *posttest* care.

● Bronchial Provocation: Methacholine Challenge, Histamine Challenge

Bronchial provocation challenge testing is performed in patients with normal pulmonary function tests who have suspected underlying bronchial hyperreactivity. Additionally, the asthmatic patient is more sensitive to the bronchoconstrictive effects of cholinergic agents (e.g., methacholine chloride) than is the healthy person as observed on a spirometry test. R_{aw} tests are also sensitive monitors of response to bronchoconstrictive agents.

Reference Values

Normal

Positive response: >20% (or >0.20) decrease in FEV_1 from baseline or >35% (>0.35) increase in R_{aw}
Negative response: <20% (or <0.20) decrease in FEV_1 from baseline or <35% (<0.35) increase in R_{aw}

Procedure

1. Have the patient assume the seated position. Place nose clips on the nose and instruct the patient to breathe normally through a mouthpiece/filter (bacterial/viral) combination into the spirometer.
2. Have the patient perform a forced expiratory maneuver and measure and record the baseline FEV_1 (or R_{aw} measurement).
3. The patient will inhale increasing concentrations of methacholine chloride (0.062 to 16.00 mg/mL) or histamine by nebulizer. Repeat the FVC or R_{aw} maneuver after each successive concentration is inhaled. A 20% reduction in the FEV_1 (primary outcome variable) or 35% increase in R_{aw} is considered a positive response.
4. Administer an inhaled bronchodilator when or if a decrease of >20% from baseline is reached.
5. If a patient goes through all dilution ratios and a 20% reduction in the FEV_1 or >35% increase in R_{aw} is not reached, the test is considered negative.

6. Remember that if the methacholine causes no change, histamine testing may be ordered.
7. See Chapter 1 for guidelines for *intratest* care.

Clinical Implications

A positive response to methacholine or histamine is consistent with bronchial hyperreactivity. Approximately 5% to 10% of asthmatic persons do not respond to the methacholine challenge test.

Interventions

Pretest Patient Care

1. Explain the purpose and procedure of the test and the need for patient cooperation. Assess the patient's ability to follow verbal instructions.
2. Withhold bronchodilators for 8 hours and antihistamines for 48 hours before testing, if tolerated.
3. Follow guidelines in Chapter 1 for safe, effective, informed *pretest* care.

Posttest Patient Care

1. Explain the meaning of test outcomes.
2. If the test is positive, advise the patient to avoid antigens that may be causing hypersensitivity reactions and bronchospasms.
3. Follow guidelines in Chapter 1 for safe, effective, informed *posttest* care.

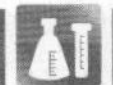

CLINICAL ALERT

1. Inhalation of methacholine can cause bronchospasm, chest pain, shortness of breath, and general discomfort.
2. These effects can be reversed with a bronchodilator.

● Carbon Dioxide (CO_2) Response

This test evaluates the respiratory response to increasing concentrations of inspired CO_2. As alveolar levels of CO_2 increase, so does arterial CO_2. The central chemoreceptors respond by initiating impulses to the respiratory control centers. In the healthy person, this causes the rate and depth of breathing to increase. The act of breathing successively greater concentrations of CO_2 should result in an increase in minute volume (VE), when compared with the VE during breathing of room air alone. (Room air contains ~0.03% CO_2.)

Reference Values

Normal

Increase in minute ventilation of 3 L/min/mm Hg increase of CO_2 (3 L/min/0.133 kPa)

Procedure

1. Remember that VE is determined while the patient breathes room air for several minutes into an instrument (e.g., spirometer) that records the frequency of breathing (f) and the depth of breathing or VT. Use the following formula to calculate the VE: VE = f × VT.
2. Have the patient breathe a gas mixture of 2% CO_2 in room air for 5 minutes. During the last 2 minutes, record f and VT and calculate the VE.
3. Have the patient breathe gas mixtures of 4% CO_2 and then 6% CO_2 in room air. Mixtures can be increased to as much as 8% CO_2. Repeat the entire process with each successive concentration.
4. Construct a graph to plot the changes in VE against the concentration of inspired CO_2 ($FICO_2$).
5. See Chapter 1 guidelines for *intratest* care.

Clinical Implications

Lack of response to increasing inspired CO_2 concentrations suggests a disturbance in the normal physiologic pathway of ventilatory changes to hypercapnia. This may result from ingestion of central nervous system depressants (e.g., anesthetics, barbiturates, narcotics) or from airflow obstruction (e.g., chronic obstructive pulmonary disease [COPD]).

Interventions

Pretest Patient Care

1. Explain the purpose and procedure of the test and need for patient cooperation. Assess the patient's ability to follow verbal instructions.
2. Follow guidelines in Chapter 1 for safe, effective, informed *pretest* care.

Posttest Patient Care

1. Review test results; report and record findings. Modify the nursing care plan as needed. Advise patient that pharmacologic intervention may be necessary to sensitize the chemoreceptors.
2. Follow guidelines in Chapter 1 for safe, effective, informed *posttest* care.

● Exercise Stress Testing, Maximum Oxygen Consumption (O_{2max}) Test

Respiratory disease reduces the ability to perform exercise. Dynamic exercise that involves large muscle groups produces increases in metabolic O_2 consumption (O_2) and CO_2 production (CO_2). This increase in metabolic demand leads to stresses on other mechanisms taking part in O_2 and CO_2 transport. Exercise testing measures the functional reserves of these mechanisms by testing under load. Analysis of ventilatory and cardiovascular disorders includes procedures that measure respiratory outcomes, blood gas values, and cardiovascular responses during exercise. Ventilation and gas exchange are altered during exercise in healthy persons; however, specific abnormalities are noted in the presence of cardiovascular or respiratory impairment. Exercise tests are valuable for assessing the severity and type of impairment in existing or undiagnosed conditions.

The normal response to graded exercise is an increase in ventilation and cardiac output such that alveolar and arterial gases (i.e., O_2 and CO_2) are maintained at optimal levels to meet metabolic demands. Measurement of the patient's ventilatory and alveolar–arterial gas responses during exercise is the primary objective of a pulmonary exercise stress test. No significant or abnormal changes in the electrocardiographic complex, blood pressure, airflow patterns during inspiration and expiration, arterial blood gases (ABGs) and chemistry, or hemodynamic pressures should occur. Exercise testing is done to evaluate fitness, functional capacity, and other limiting factors in persons with obstructive or restrictive diseases. The efficiency of the cardiopulmonary system may be altered during exercise; exercise testing assesses ventilation, gas exchange, and cardiovascular function during increased demands. Dyspnea on exertion due to cardiovascular causes can be differentiated from that due to respiratory causes. Precise information about mechanisms that influence O_2 and CO_2 transport during exercise can be obtained by using a staged approach.

An exercise test can detect or exclude many conditions even though the response may be nonspecific. For example, if the patient complains of severe shortness of breath despite a normal exercise response, a psychogenic cause is likely. However, a few conditions exhibit diagnostic responses—for example, exercise-induced asthma or myocardial ischemia. These tests can also reveal the degree of impairment in conditions affecting the respiratory and circulatory systems and may uncover unsuspected abnormalities (Table 14.2).

Most clinical problems can be assessed during the simple procedures included in *stage 1* (see Procedure section for description) that should be done before more complex tests. Abnormal results indicate that more precise information is required through *stage 2* protocols. If *stage 3* protocols are implemented, arterial blood analysis is necessary. In 75% of cases, stage 1 is sufficient. Oxygen titration can be done during graded exercise to determine the oxygen needs for improving exercise tolerance and increasing functional capacity.

TABLE 14.2 Ventilatory and Arterial Blood Gas Responses to Graded Exercise

Value	Change
O_2 consumption ($\dot{V}O_2$)	Increase
CO_2 production ($\dot{V}CO_2$)	Increase
Ventilatory equivalents for O_2 and CO_2	No change
Respiratory exchange ratio (RER) or RQ (respiratory quotient)	Increase
Minute ventilation (V_E)	Increase
Blood lactate	Increase
V_D/V_T ratio	Decrease
A-aDO_2	Slight increase
Arterial blood gas tensions (e.g., PaO_2, $PaCO_2$)	No change
Bicarbonate concentration (HCO_3^-)	Decrease
Oxygen saturation (SaO_2)	No change

Reference Values

Normal

Increase in ventilation, heart rate, and blood pressure appropriate to the level of exercise

No abnormal changes in the electrocardiogram (ECG; no arrhythmias), ABGs, or hemodynamic pressures

Procedure

1. *Stage 1*
   a. Record blood pressure readings, ECG analysis, and ventilation during incremental cycle ergometry or treadmill walking.
   b. Take measurements at the end of each minute. Remember that the test continues until maximal allowed symptoms occur (i.e., to a symptom-limited maximum). Measure O_2 uptake ($\dot{V}O_2$) and CO_2 output ($\dot{V}CO_2$) if possible.
   c. Alert the patient that total examination time is approximately 30 minutes.
2. *Stage 2*
   a. In this stage, more complex analytic methods are required.
   b. Have exercise build to a steady state, usually 3 to 5 minutes for each workload.
   c. In addition to stage 1 measurements, determine mixed venous CO_2 tension by means of rebreathing techniques.
3. *Stage 3*
   a. In this stage, blood gas sampling and analysis are required.
   b. Insert an indwelling catheter into the brachial or radial artery.
   c. In addition to stage 2 tests, determine measurements for cardiac output, alveolar ventilation, ratio of dead space to tidal volume (V_D/V_T), alveolar-to-arterial O_2 tension difference (A-aDO_2), venous admixture ratio, and blood lactate concentrations.
4. See Chapter 1 guidelines for *intratest* care.

Clinical Implications

Altered values may reveal:

1. Cardiac arrhythmias or ischemia
2. Degree of functional impairment caused by obstructive or restrictive ventilatory disease
3. Hypoventilation
4. Workload level at which metabolic acidosis (lactic acidosis) occurs

Interfering Factors

1. The exercise tolerance of any person is affected by the degree of impairment related to:
   a. Mechanical factors
   b. Ventilatory efficiency
   c. Gas exchange factors
   d. Cardiac status
   e. Physical condition
   f. Sensitivity of the respiratory control mechanism
2. Obese persons have a higher-than-normal oxygen consumption at any given work rate, even though muscular and work efficiency values are normal.

Interventions

Pretest Patient Care

1. Explain the purpose and procedure for exercise stress testing and assess for contraindications, interfering factors, and ability to follow verbal instructions.
2. Follow guidelines in Chapter 1 for safe, effective, informed *pretest* care.

CLINICAL ALERT

1. *Absolute contraindications* to exercise testing include:
   a. Acute febrile illness
   b. Pulmonary edema
   c. Systolic blood pressure >250 mm Hg (>33 kPa)
   d. Diastolic blood pressure >120 mm Hg (>16 kPa)
   e. Uncontrolled hypertension
   f. Uncontrolled asthma
   g. Unstable angina
2. *Relative contraindications* to exercise testing include:
   a. Recent myocardial infarction (<4 wk)
   b. Resting tachycardia (>120 beats per min)
   c. Epilepsy
   d. Respiratory failure
   e. Resting ECG abnormalities

Posttest Patient Care

1. Explain the meaning of test outcomes and possible need for lifestyle changes.
2. Follow guidelines in Chapter 1 for safe, effective, informed *posttest* care.

OVERVIEW OF BLOOD GASES, ACID–BASE BALANCE, AND OXYGENATION STATUS (TISSUE OXYGENATION, GAS EXCHANGE IN LUNGS)

Diagnostic evaluations of body fluid balance, electrolytes, blood gas exchange in the lungs, oxygen tissue saturation by pulse oximetry, and acid–base balance are important determinants of normal body function (homeostasis). Homeostatic mechanisms are affected by a variety of exogenous (originating from without; e.g., stress) and endogenous (originating from within; e.g., immune system) factors. Evidence supports a strong association between stress and altered immune function, which can subsequently lead to abnormal pathophysiology observable by a wide array of diagnostic tests. Abnormal test outcomes in hospitalized patients, as well as when complications of treatment occur (as in kidney and respiratory diseases, diabetes, anemia), gastric fluid loss, medication diuretics, sepsis, and fever, for this reason are discussed in this chapter. Other factors that need to be assessed include respiratory rate, fluid intake, urine output, amount of watery diarrhea, emesis, weight gain or loss, presence of burned or excoriated skin, food intake, and evidence of dehydration edema.

● Arterial Blood Gas (ABG) Tests

Measurements of ABGs are obtained to assess adequacy of oxygenation and ventilation, to evaluate acid–base status by measuring the respiratory and nonrespiratory components, and to monitor effectiveness of therapy (e.g., supplemental oxygen). They are also used to monitor critically ill patients, to establish baseline values in the perioperative and postoperative period, to detect and treat electrolyte imbalances, to titrate appropriate oxygen flow rates, to qualify a patient for use of oxygen at home, and in conjunction with pulmonary function testing. In the clinical setting (e.g., perioperative or intensive care environment), ABG studies usually include the following: pH, $Paco_2$, Sao_2, CO_2 content, O_2 content, Pao_2, base excess or deficit, HCO_3^-, hemoglobin, hematocrit, CO, Na^+, and K^+ (Table 14.3).

Reasons for using *arterial* rather than *venous* blood to measure blood gases include the following:

1. Arterial blood provides a better way to sample a mixture of blood from various parts of the body.
   a. Venous blood from an extremity gives information mostly about that extremity. The metabolism in the extremity can differ from the metabolism in the body as a whole. This difference is accentuated in the following instances:
      (1) In shock states, when the extremity is cold or underperfused
      (2) During local exercise of the extremity, as in opening and closing a fist
      (3) If the extremity is infected

TABLE 14.3 Normal Values[a] for Commonly Ordered Arterial Blood Gas and Electrolyte Studies

	Adults	Pediatrics
pHa	7.35–7.45	7.32–7.42
$Paco_2$	35–45 mm Hg (4.6–5.9 kPa)	30–40 mm Hg (4.0–5.3 kPa)
Pao_2	>80 mm Hg (>10.6 kPa)	80–100 mm Hg (10.6–13.3 kPa)
Sao_2	>94% (>0.94)	
CO_2 content	45–51 vol% (19.3–22.4 mmol/L)	
O_2 content	15–22 vol% (6.6–9.7 mmol/L)	
Base excess	>2 mEq/L (>2 mmol/L)	
Base deficit	<−2 mEq/L (<−2 mmol/L)	
HCO_3^-	22–26 mEq/L (22–26 mmol/L)	
Hb	12–16 g/dL or 120–160 g/L (women); 13.5–17.5 g/dL or 135–175 g/L (men)	
Hct	37%–47% (women); 40%–54% (men)	
COHb	<2% (<0.02)	
$[NA^+]$	135–148 mEq/L (135–148 mmol/L)	
$[K^+]$	3.6–5.2 mEq/L (3.6–5.2 mmol/L)	
$[Ca^{2+}]$	4.2–5.1 mEq/L (2.1–2.5 mmol/L)	
$[Cl^-]$	98–106 mEq/L (98–106 mmol/L)	

[a]Normal values vary greatly; check with your reference laboratory.

  b. Blood from a central venous catheter usually is an incomplete mix of venous blood from various parts of the body. For a sample to be completely mixed, the blood would have to be obtained from the right ventricle or pulmonary artery.
2. Arterial blood measurements indicate how well the lungs are oxygenating blood.
  a. If it is known that the arterial O_2 concentration is normal (indicating that the lungs are functioning normally) but the mixed venous O_2 concentration is low, it can be inferred that the heart and circulation are failing.
  b. Oxygen measurements of central venous catheter blood reveal tissue oxygenation but do not separate contributions of the heart from those of the lungs. If central venous catheter blood has a low O_2 concentration, it means either that the lungs have not oxygenated the arterial blood well or that the heart is not circulating the blood effectively. In the latter case, the body tissues must take on more than the normal amount of O_2 from each cardiac cycle because the blood is flowing slowly and permits this to occur; this produces a low venous O_2 concentration.
  c. ABG measurements do not indicate the degree of an abnormality. For this reason, the vital signs and mental function of the patient must be used as guides to determine adequacy of tissue oxygenation.
3. Arterial samples provide information about the ability of the lungs to regulate acid–base balance through retention or release of CO_2. Effectiveness of the kidneys in maintaining appropriate bicarbonate levels also can be gauged.

NOTE *Arterial puncture sites must satisfy the following requirements: (1) available collateral blood flow, (2) superficial or easily accessible location, and (3) relatively nonsensitive periarterial tissues.*

The radial artery is usually the site of choice, but brachial and femoral arteries can also be used. Samples can be drawn from direct arterial sticks or from indwelling arterial lines.

Reference Values

Normal

See Table 14.3.

Procedure

1. Observe standard precautions and follow agency protocols.
2. Have the patient assume a sitting or supine position.
3. Perform a modified Allen's test to assess collateral circulation before performing a radial puncture as follows:
  a. Use pressure to obliterate both radial and ulnar pulses.
  b. Make the hand blanch and then release pressure over only the ulnar artery. In a positive test, note flushing immediately; the radial artery may then be used for puncture.
  c. If collateral circulation from the ulnar artery is inadequate (negative test), choose another site.
4. Elevate the patient's wrist with a small pillow and ask the patient to extend the fingers downward (this flexes the wrist and positions the radial artery closer to the surface).
5. Palpate the artery and maneuver the patient's hand back and forth until a satisfactory pulse is felt.
6. Swab the area liberally with an antiseptic agent (e.g., an agent with an iodine base).
7. Optional: After assessing for allergy, inject the area with a small amount (<0.25 mL) of 1% lidocaine if necessary to anesthetize the site. This allows for a second attempt without undue pain.
8. Prepare a 20- or 21-gauge needle on a preheparinized self-filling syringe, puncture the artery, and collect a 3- to 5-mL sample. During the procedure, if the patient feels a dull or sharp pain radiating up the arm, withdraw the needle slightly and reposition it. If repositioning does not alleviate the pain, the needle should be withdrawn completely.

9. Withdraw the needle and place a 4 × 4-inch absorbent bandage over the puncture site. Maintain pressure over the site with two fingers for a minimum of 2 minutes or until no bleeding is evident; it may be necessary to use a pressure dressing, secured to the site with elastic tape, for several hours.
10. Meanwhile, ensure that all air bubbles in the blood sample are expelled as quickly as possible. Air in the sample changes ABG values. Cap the syringe and gently rotate to mix heparin with the blood.
11. Label the sample with patient's name, identification number, date, time, mode of O_2 therapy, and flow rate.
12. Place the sample on ice and transfer it to the laboratory. This prevents alterations in gas tensions resulting from metabolic processes that continue after blood is drawn.
13. See Chapter 1 guidelines for *intratest* care.

PROCEDURAL ALERT

1. Some patients experience light-headedness, nausea, or vasovagal syncope during arterial puncture. Respond according to established protocols.
2. Pressure must be applied to the arterial puncture site, and the site must be watched carefully for several hours for bleeding. Instruct the patient to report any bleeding from the site.
3. Information for the laboratory should include the patient's name, date, and test(s) ordered as well as the fraction of inspired oxygen (FIO_2), which is 0.21 (21%) for room air, and the time when the sample was obtained. Do not use blood for ABG measurements if the sample is >3 hr old.

Interventions

Pretest Patient Care

1. Explain the purpose and procedure for obtaining an arterial blood sample.
2. If the patient is apprehensive, explain that a local anesthetic can be used.
3. Follow guidelines in Chapter 1 for safe, effective, informed *pretest* care.

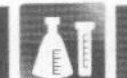

CLINICAL ALERT

1. Before obtaining an arterial blood sample, assess for the following contraindications to an arterial stick or indwelling line:
   a. Absent palpable radial artery pulse
   b. Negative modified Allen's test, indicating obstruction in the ulnar artery (i.e., compromised collateral circulation)—do not attempt to use radial artery for blood sample
   c. Cellulitis or infection in the area
   d. Arteriovenous fistula or shunt
   e. Severe thrombocytopenia
   f. Prolonged prothrombin or partial thromboplastin time (relative contraindication)
2. A Doppler probe or finger-pulse transducer may be used to assess circulation. This may be especially helpful with dark-skinned or uncooperative patients.
3. Before obtaining an arterial blood sample, record the most recent Hb concentration, the mode and flow of oxygen therapy, and the temperature. If the patient has recently undergone suctioning or been placed on mechanical ventilation, or if the inspired oxygen concentration has been changed, wait at least 15 min before drawing the sample. This waiting period allows circulating blood levels to return to baseline. Hyperthermia and hypothermia also influence oxygen release from hemoglobin at the tissue level.

Posttest Patient Care

1. Evaluate color, motion, sensation, degree of warmth, capillary refill time, and quality of pulse in the affected extremity or at the puncture site.
2. Monitor puncture site and dressing for arterial bleeding for several hours. No vigorous activity of the extremity should be undertaken for 24 hours.
3. Follow guidelines in Chapter 1 for safe, effective, informed *posttest* care.

● Alveolar-to-Arterial Oxygen Gradient (A-aDO_2); Arterial-to-Alveolar Oxygen Ratio (a/A Ratio)

This test gives an approximation of the difference in the partial pressure of O_2 between the alveoli and arteries. The alveolar-to-arterial oxygen gradient assesses oxygen delivery by comparing the arterial oxygen level to the theoretical maximal alveolar oxygen level. It identifies the cause of hypoxemia and intrapulmonary shunting as either (1) ventilated alveoli but no perfusion, (2) unventilated alveoli with perfusion, or (3) collapse of both alveoli and capillaries.

Reference Values

Normal

A-aDO_2: <10 mm Hg (<1.33 kPa) at rest (room air)
A-aDO_2: 20 to 30 mm Hg (2.7 to 4.0 kPa) at maximum exercise (room air)
a/A ratio: 75% (0.75)

Procedure

1. Obtain and analyze an arterial blood sample. This gives the *arterial* partial pressures of oxygen (PaO_2) and of carbon dioxide ($PaCO_2$). The barometric pressure (Pb) and water vapor pressure (PH_2O) are also known, as is the fractional concentration of inspired oxygen (FIO_2), which is 0.21 (21%) for room air.
2. From these, derive the *alveolar* oxygen tension (PAO_2), the arterial-to-alveolar oxygen ratio (a/A ratio), and the alveolar-to-arterial difference for PO_2 (A-aDO_2) by use of formulas.

Clinical Implications

1. *Increased* values may be caused by:
   a. Mucus plugs
   b. Bronchospasm
   c. Airway collapse, as seen in:
      (1) Asthma
      (2) Bronchitis
      (3) Emphysema
2. Hypoxemia (increased A-aDO_2) is caused by:
   a. Atrial septal defects
   b. Pneumothorax
   c. Atelectasis
   d. Emboli
   e. Edema

Interfering Factors

Values increase with age and increasing O_2 concentration (gradient increases by 5 to 7 mm Hg [0.6 to 0.9 kPa] for every 10% increase in oxygen).

Interventions

Pretest Patient Care

1. Explain the purpose, benefits, and risks of arterial blood sampling.
2. Follow guidelines in Chapter 1 for safe, effective, informed *pretest* care.

Posttest Patient Care

1. Review test results; report and record findings. Modify the nursing care plan as needed. Assess, monitor, and intervene appropriately for hypoxemia and ventilatory disturbances.
2. Frequently observe the puncture site for bleeding.
3. Follow guidelines in Chapter 1 for safe, effective, informed *posttest* care.

● Partial Pressure of Carbon Dioxide (PCO_2)

This test measures the pressure or tension exerted by dissolved CO_2 in the blood (10% [0.10] of CO_2 is carried in plasma and 90% [0.90] in red blood cells) and is proportional to the partial pressure of CO_2 in the alveolar air. The test is commonly used to detect a respiratory abnormality and to determine the alkalinity or acidity of the blood. To maintain CO_2 within normal limits, the rate and depth of respiration vary automatically with changes in metabolism. This test is an index of the effectiveness of alveolar ventilation; it is the most physiologically reflective blood gas measurement. An arterial sample directly reflects how well air is exchanged with blood in the lungs.

CO_2 tension in the blood and in cerebrospinal fluid is the major chemical factor regulating alveolar ventilation. When the CO_2 tension in arterial blood ($PaCO_2$) rises from 40 to 45 mm Hg (5.3 to 6.0 kPa), it causes a threefold increase in alveolar ventilation. A $PaCO_2$ of 63 mm Hg (8.4 kPa) increases alveolar ventilation 10-fold. When the $FICO_2$ is >0.05 (>5%), the lungs can no longer be ventilated fast enough to prevent a dangerous rise of CO_2 concentration in tissue fluids. Any further increase in CO_2 begins to depress the respiratory center, causing a progressive decline in respiratory activity rather than an increase.

Reference Values

Normal

$PaCO_2$ (arterial blood): 35 to 45 mm Hg (4.7 to 6.0 kPa)
$PvCO_2$ (venous blood): 41 to 57 mm Hg (5.4 to 7.6 kPa)

Procedure

1. Obtain an arterial blood sample (or venous sample if requested) according to protocols. See Procedure section in Overview of Blood Gases for collection of arterial blood sample and Chapter 2 for venous blood sample specimen collection.
2. Introduce a small amount of this blood into a blood gas analyzing instrument (Fig. 14.5) and measure the CO_2 tension.

Clinical Implications

1. An *increase* in $PaCO_2$ (hypercapnia) usually is associated with hypoventilation (CO_2 retention); a *decrease* is associated with hyperventilation ("blowing off" CO_2). A reduction in $PaCO_2$, through its effect on the plasma bicarbonate concentration, decreases renal bicarbonate reabsorption. For each 1–mm Hg (0.133 kPa) decrease in the $PaCO_2$, the plasma bicarbonate will decrease by approximately 1 mEq/L (1 mmol/L). Because HCO_3^- and $PaCO_2$ bear this close mathematical relationship, and this ratio, in turn, defends the hydrogen ion concentration, the outcome is that the steady-state $PaCO_2$ in simple metabolic acidosis is equal to the last two digits of the arterial pH (pHa). Also, addition of 15 to the bicarbonate level equals the last two digits of the pHa. Failure of the $PaCO_2$ to achieve predicted levels defines the presence of superimposed respiratory acidosis on alkalosis.

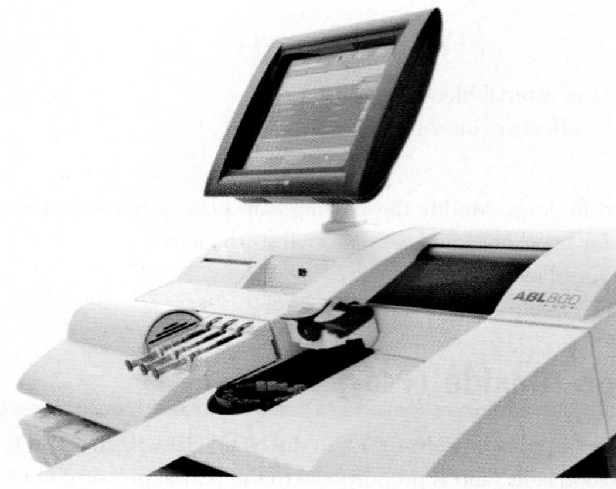

FIGURE 14.5. ABL800 FLEX blood gas analyzer. (Reprinted with permission from Radiometer America Inc., Westlake, OH.)

2. Causes of *decreased* $Paco_2$ include:
   a. Hypoxia
   b. Nervousness
   c. Anxiety
   d. Pulmonary emboli
   e. Pregnancy
   f. Pain
   g. Other cause of hyperventilation
3. Causes of *increased* $Paco_2$ include:
   a. Obstructive lung disease
      (1) Chronic bronchitis
      (2) Emphysema
   b. Reduced function of respiratory center
      (1) Overreaction
      (2) Head trauma
      (3) Anesthesia
   c. Other, less common causes of hypoventilation (e.g., pickwickian syndrome)

CLINICAL ALERT

Increased $Paco_2$ may occur, even with normal lungs, if the respiratory center is depressed. Always check laboratory reports for abnormal values. When interpreting laboratory reports, remember $Paco_2$ is a gas and is therefore regulated by the lungs, not the kidneys.

Interventions

Pretest Patient Care

1. Explain the purpose, benefits, and risks of the invasive arterial blood sampling procedure. Assess the patient's ability to cooperate.
2. Follow guidelines in Chapter 1 for safe, effective, informed *pretest* care.

Posttest Patient Care

1. Review test results; report and record findings. Modify the nursing care plan as needed. Assess, monitor, and intervene appropriately for hypoxemia and ventilatory disturbances.
2. Follow guidelines in Chapter 1 for safe, effective, informed *posttest* care.

● Oxygen Saturation (So_2)

This measurement is a ratio between the actual O_2 content of the hemoglobin and the potential maximum O_2-carrying capacity of the hemoglobin. The So_2 is a percentage indicating the relationship between O_2 and hemoglobin; it does not indicate the O_2 content. The maximum amount of O_2 that can be combined with hemoglobin is called the *oxygen capacity*. The combined measurements of So_2, Po_2, and Hb indicate the amount of O_2 available to tissues (tissue oxygenation). Pulse oximetry (Spo_2) (Fig. 14.6) is a noninvasive technique that permits continuous real-time monitoring and trending of arterial oxygen saturation. However, it cannot differentiate COHb. As a result, the Spo_2 is generally higher than the actual arterial oxygen saturation (Sao_2) by the amount of COHb, and a more direct measurement involves taking an arterial blood sample and measuring with a blood gas analyzer.

Reference Values

Normal

Sao_2 (arterial blood): >95% (>0.95)

Svo_2 (mixed venous blood): 70% to 75% (0.70 to 0.75)

Sao_2 (arterial) in newborns: 40% to 90% (0.40 to 0.90)

Procedure

1. Obtain an arterial blood sample (see Blood Specimen Collection Procedures, page 51, and Venipuncture and Arterial Puncture, pages 52 and 55, respectively, in Chapter 2). Two methods are used for determining So_2:
   a. *Direct method*: Introduce the blood sample into hemoximeter, a spectrophotometric device for direct determination of So_2.

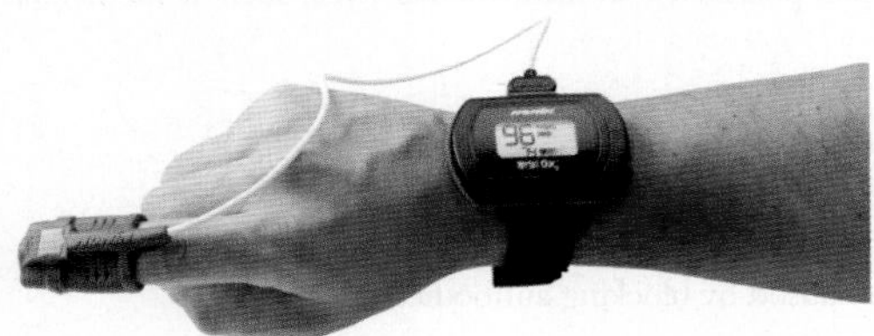

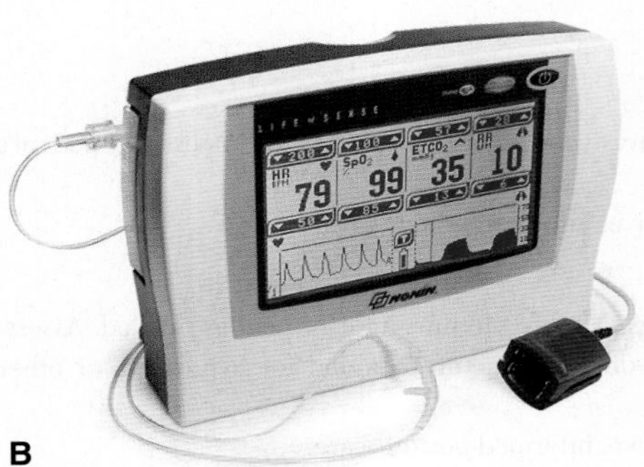

B

FIGURE 14.6. Pulse oximeters. **(A)** Nonin WristOx2 Model 3150. **(B)** Nonin LifeSense capnography/pulse oximeter with adult finger clip sensor. (Reprinted with permission from Nonin Medical, Inc., Plymouth, MN.)

b. *Calculated method*: Calculate So_2 from oxygen content (the volume of O_2 actually combined with hemoglobin) and oxygen capacity (the volume of O_2 to which hemoglobin could combine). Both of these values are expressed as volume percentages (vol%), or milliliters per deciliter of blood. Use the following formula:

$$So_2 = 100 \times \frac{O_2 \text{ content}}{O_2 \text{ capacity}}$$

2. *Pulse oximetry*: A small, clip-type sensor is placed on a digit over the fingernail (or toenail or earlobe, if necessary). The instrument, using transmitted light waves (in the infrared spectrum) and sensors, determines So_2 noninvasively and is referred to as the Spo_2.

Limitations

1. So_2 measures only the percentage of oxygen being carried by hemoglobin; it does not reveal the actual amount of oxygen available to the tissues (oxygen content).
2. Pulse oximetry equipment evaluates pulsatile blood flow. Many factors can interfere with the ability to measure flow:
   a. Digit motion
   b. A decrease in blood flow to the digit (e.g., cool extremity, decreased peripheral pulses, vasoconstriction, nail bed thickening, ambient light, digit malformation, vasoconstrictive drugs, localized obstruction)
   c. Decreased hemoglobin (anemia) or abnormal hemoglobin (COHb)
   d. Pulse rate and rhythm

Interfering Factors

Recent smoking or exposure to close secondhand smoke or to CO can increase the level of COHb, as can use of certain paint and varnish-type stripping agents, especially when they are applied in closed or poorly ventilated areas. The effect is to decrease the Sao_2 with little or no effect on the Pao_2. Other interfering factors include presence of fingernail polish; use of intravascular dyes, such as methylene blue; and exposure to ambient light.

Clinical Implications

1. Abnormal results occur in pulmonary diseases involving cyanosis and erythrocytosis.
2. Abnormal results occur with venous-to-arterial shunts.
3. Values are abnormal in Rh incompatibility caused by blocking antibodies.
4. Values usually are normal in polycythemia vera.
5. Values are decreased in ventilation-perfusion mismatching.
6. Values decrease with age.

Interventions

Pretest Patient Care

1. Explain the purpose, benefits, and risks of invasive arterial blood sampling. Assess the patient's ability to comply with the procedure.
2. Follow guidelines in Chapter 1 for safe, effective, informed *pretest* care.

Posttest Patient Care

1. Review test results; report and record findings. Modify the nursing care plan as needed. Assess, monitor, and intervene appropriately for bleeding at puncture site and for hypoxemia or other respiratory dysfunctions.
2. Follow guidelines in Chapter 1 for safe, effective, informed *posttest* care.

• Oxygen Content (Co_2)

The actual amount of O_2 in the blood is termed the *oxygen content* (Co_2). Blood can contain less O_2 than it is capable of carrying. About 98% of all O_2 delivered to the tissues is transported in chemical combination with hemoglobin. One gram of hemoglobin is capable of combining with 1.34 mL of O_2, whereas 100 mL of blood plasma can carry a maximum of only 0.3 mL of O_2 (under normoxic conditions or atmospheric conditions). The Co_2 measurement is determined mathematically.

Reference Values

Normal

Cao_2 (arterial blood): 15 to 22 vol% or 15 to 22 mL/dL of blood (6.6 to 9.7 mmol/L)
Cvo_2 (venous blood): 11 to 16 vol% or 11 to 16 mL/dL of blood (4.9 to 7.1 mmol/L)

Procedure

1. Obtain a blood sample. (See Chapter 2, pages 52 and 55, for venous and arterial blood collection, respectively.)
2. Measure the So_2, Po_2, and Hb concentration.
3. Use the following formulas for calculating O_2 content:

$$Cao_2 = 1.34(Sao_2 \times Hb) + 0.003(Pao_2)$$

$$Cvo_2 = 1.34(Svo_2 \times Hb) + 0.003(Pvo_2)$$

NOTE *0.003 = Bunsen solubility for oxygen in the blood.*

Clinical Implications

Decreased Cao_2 is associated with:
1. COPD
2. Postoperative respiratory complications
3. Flail chest
4. Kyphoscoliosis
5. Neuromuscular impairment
6. Obesity-caused hypoventilation
7. Anemia

Interventions

Pretest Patient Care

1. Explain the purpose, benefits, and risks of invasive arterial blood sampling (see Chapter 2, Arterial Puncture, pages 55 to 58).
2. Follow guidelines in Chapter 1 for safe, effective, informed *pretest* care.

Posttest Patient Care

1. Review test results; report and record findings. Modify the nursing care plan as needed. Assess, monitor, and intervene appropriately for bleeding at the puncture site and for hypoxemia or ventilatory disturbances.
2. Follow guidelines in Chapter 1 for safe, effective, informed *posttest* care.

Partial Pressure of Oxygen (Po_2), Brain Tissue ($Pbto_2$)

Oxygen is carried in the blood in two forms: dissolved in plasma (<2%) and combined with hemoglobin (98%). The partial pressure of a gas determines the force it exerts in attempting to diffuse through the pulmonary membrane. The Po_2 reflects the amount of O_2 passing from the pulmonary alveoli into the blood; it is directly influenced by the fraction of inspired oxygen (FIO_2).

This test measures the pressure exerted by the O_2 dissolved in the plasma. It evaluates the ability of the lungs to oxygenate the blood and is used to assess the effectiveness of oxygen therapy. The Po_2 indicates the ability of the lungs to diffuse O_2 across the alveolar membrane into the circulating blood.

Reference Values

Normal

Pao_2 (arterial blood): >80 mm Hg (>10.6 kPa)
$Pbto_2$ (brain tissue): 20 to 40 mm Hg (2.6 to 5.2 kPa)
Pvo_2 (venous blood): 30 to 40 mm Hg (4.0 to 5.3 kPa)

Procedure

1. Obtain an arterial (or venous, if ordered) blood sample (see Chapter 2, pages 55 and 58, for venous and arterial blood collection, respectively).
2. Introduce a small amount of this blood into a blood gas analyzing instrument (see Fig. 14.5) and measure the O_2 tension.

Clinical Implications

1. *Increased* Pao_2 is associated with:
   a. Polycythemia
   b. Increased FIO_2
   c. Hyperventilation
2. *Decreased* Pao_2 is associated with:
   a. Anemias
   b. Cardiac decompensation
   c. Insufficient atmospheric O_2
   d. Intracardiac shunts
   e. COPD
   f. Restrictive pulmonary disease
   g. Hypoventilation caused by neuromuscular disease
3. *Decreased* Pao_2 with normal or decreased $PACO_2$ is associated with:
   a. Diffuse interstitial pulmonary infiltration
   b. Pulmonary edema
   c. Pulmonary embolism
   d. Postoperative extracorporeal circulation

CLINICAL ALERT

In some persons with COPD, ventilatory efforts are stimulated by the hypoxic state, whereas for a healthy person, the respiratory stimulus is the buildup of CO_2. Administering a high concentration of supplemental oxygen may knock out the hypoxic drive, resulting in increased retention of CO_2. In persons with community-acquired pneumonia (CAP), arterial hypoxemia can signal impending respiratory failure.

Interventions

Pretest Patient Care

1. Explain the purpose, benefits, and risks of arterial blood sampling. Assess the patient's level of cooperation and understanding.
2. Follow guidelines in Chapter 1 for safe, effective, informed *pretest* care.

Posttest Patient Care

1. Review test results; report and record findings. Modify the nursing care plan as needed. Assess, monitor, and intervene appropriately for bleeding at the puncture site and for respiratory or ventilatory disturbances.
2. Follow guidelines in Chapter 1 for safe, effective, informed *posttest* care.

• Carbon Dioxide (CO_2) Content; Total Carbon Dioxide (Tco_2)

In normal blood plasma, >95% of the total CO_2 content (Tco_2) is contributed by bicarbonate ion (HCO_3^-), which is regulated by the *kidneys*. The other 5% is contributed by the dissolved CO_2 gas and by carbonic acid (H_2CO_3). Dissolved CO_2 gas, which is regulated by the *lungs*, therefore contributes little to the Tco_2, and the Tco_2 gives little information about the lungs.

The HCO_3^- in the extracellular spaces exists first as CO_2 and then as H_2CO_3; later, much of it is changed to sodium bicarbonate ($NaHCO_3$) by the buffers in the plasma and erythrocytes. This test is a general measure of the alkalinity or acidity of venous, arterial, or capillary blood. It measures the CO_2 contributions from dissolved CO_2 gas, total H_2CO_3, HCO_3^-, and carbaminohemoglobin (CO_2HHb).

Reference Values

Normal

23 to 30 mEq/L or 23 to 30 mmol/L

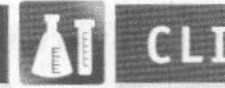

CLINICAL ALERT

Critical Value

Co_2 content: <6.0 mEq/L (<6.0 mmol/L)

Procedure

1. Collect a venous or arterial blood sample of 5 mL in a heparinized syringe. (See Chapter 2, pages 55 and 58, for venous and arterial blood collection, respectively.)
2. Measure the sample by a blood gas analyzer. If the collected blood sample cannot be studied immediately, place the syringe in an iced container.
3. Use the following formula: $Tco_2 = HCO_3^- + H_2CO_3$

Clinical Implications

1. *Increased* Tco_2 occurs in:
   a. Severe vomiting
   b. Emphysema
   c. Aldosteronism
   d. Use of mercurial diuretics

2. *Decreased* TCO_2 occurs in:
   a. Severe diarrhea
   b. Starvation
   c. Acute renal failure
   d. Salicylate toxicity
   e. Diabetic acidosis
   f. Use of chlorothiazide diuretics

NOTE *In diabetic acidosis, the supply of ketoacids exceeds the demands of the cell. Blood plasma acids rise. Blood plasma HCO_3^- decreases because it is used to neutralize these excess acids.*

Table 14.4 presents the changes in pH, HCO_3^-, and $PaCO_2$ that occur in various ventilatory disturbances and acid–base imbalances.

CLINICAL ALERT

1. A double use of the term CO_2 is one of the main reasons why understanding of acid–base problems may be difficult. Use the terms *CO_2 content* and *CO_2 gas* to avoid confusion. Remember the following:
   a. *CO_2 content* (i.e., TCO_2) is mainly bicarbonate and a base. It is a solution and is regulated by the kidneys.
   b. *CO_2 gas* is mainly acid. It is regulated by the lungs.

Interfering Factors

A number of drugs can either increase or decrease TCO_2.

Interventions

Pretest Patient Care

1. Explain the purpose, benefits, and risks of arterial blood sampling. Assess the patient's ability to comply with the procedure.
2. Follow guidelines in Chapter 1 for safe, effective, informed *pretest* care.

Posttest Patient Care

1. Review test results; report and record findings. Modify the nursing care plan as needed. Assess, monitor, and intervene appropriately for acid–base imbalances.
2. Monitor and intervene for bleeding at the puncture site and for respiratory or ventilatory disturbances.
3. Follow guidelines in Chapter 1 for safe, effective, informed *posttest* care.

● Blood pH

The pH is the negative logarithm of the hydrogen ion concentration in the blood. The sources of hydrogen ions are volatile acids, which can vary between a liquid and a gaseous state, and nonvolatile acids, which cannot be volatilized but remain fixed (e.g., dietary acids, lactic acids, ketoacids).

NOTE *A pH value of 7 is neutral; acidity increases as the pH falls from 7 to 1, and alkalinity increases as the pH rises from 7 to 14. Limits of pH compatible with life fall within the range of 6.9 to 7.8.*

TABLE 14.4 Summary of Ventilatory and Acid–Base Changes in Four Underlying Conditions of Acid–Base Imbalance[a]

Form of Disturbance	pHa[b]	Bicarbonate (HCO_3^-)[c]	$PaCO_2$[d]	Occurrence
Respiratory Acidosis				
Acute: caused by decreased alveolar ventilation and retention of CO_2	Decrease	Normal	Increase	*Depression of respiratory centers* Drug overdose Barbiturate toxicity Use of anesthetics *Interference with mechanical function of the thoracic cage* Deformity of thoracic cage Kyphoscoliosis *Airway obstruction* Extrathoracic tumors Asthma Bronchitis Emphysema *Circulatory disorders* Congestive heart failure Shock
Chronic: compensated via renal reabsorption of the bicarbonate ion	Normal	Increase	Increase	
Respiratory Alkalosis				
Acute: caused by increased alveolar ventilation and excessive blowing off of CO_2 and water	Increase	Normal	Decrease	*Hyperventilation* *Hysteria* *Lack of oxygen* *Toxic stimulation of the respiratory centers* High fever Cerebral hemorrhage Excessive artificial respiration Salicylates
Chronic: compensated via glomerular filtration of the bicarbonate ion	Normal	Decrease	Decrease	
Nonrespiratory or Metabolic Acidosis				
Acute: caused by accumulation of fixed body acids or loss of bicarbonate from the extracellular fluid	Decrease	Decrease	Normal	*Acid gain* Renal failure Diabetic ketoacidosis Lactic acidosis Anaerobic metabolism *Hypoxia* Base loss Diarrhea Renal tubular acidosis
Chronic: compensated via *hyperventilation* through stimulation of central chemoreceptors	Normal	Decrease	Decrease	

table continues on pg. 938 >

TABLE 14.4, continued

Form of Disturbance	pHa[b]	Bicarbonate (HCO_3^-)[c]	$PaCO_2$[d]	Occurrence
Nonrespiratory or Metabolic Alkalosis				
Acute: caused by loss of fixed body acids or gain in bicarbonate in extracellular fluid	Increase	Increase	Normal	*Acid loss* Loss of gastric juice Vomiting Potassium or chloride depletion Base gain Excessive bicarbonate or lactate administration
Chronic: compensated via *hypoventilation*	Normal	Increase	Increase	

[a]Although these four basic imbalances occur individually, a combination of two or more is observed more frequently. These disturbances may have an antagonistic or a synergistic effect on each other.

[b]Acid–base disturbances force kidney and lungs to compensate for changes in pH. Hyperventilation or hypoventilation can restore pH to normal within 15 minutes; the kidney, however, can take 2 to 3 days to compensate.

[c]The degree of hypoventilation is precisely related to the degree of hypobicarbonatemia. For each 1 mEq/L fall in bicarbonate, Pco_2 falls by 1 to 1.3 mm Hg. A close mathematical relationship prevails between bicarbonate and Pco_2; their ratio defines the prevailing hydrogen ion concentration. For this reason, the steady-state Pco_2 in simple metabolic acidosis is equal to the last two digits of the pH. Failure of the Pco_2 to reach predicted levels defines the presence of superimposed respiratory acidosis or alkalosis.

[d]Decreases in Pao_2 are interpreted separately and are referred to as *hypoxemia*.

Blood pH measures the body's chemical balance and represents a ratio of acids to bases. It is also an indicator of the degree to which the body is adjusting to dysfunctions by means of its buffering systems. It is one of the best ways to determine whether the body is too acidic or too alkaline and is an indicator of the patient's metabolic and respiratory status. The acid–base balance in the extracellular fluid is extremely delicate and intricate and must be kept within the very narrow range of 7.35 to 7.45 (slightly alkaline). Values <7.35 indicate an *acid state*, whereas pH values >7.45 indicate an *alkaline state*.

Reference Values

Normal

pHa (arterial blood): 7.35 to 7.45
pHv (venous blood): 7.31 to 7.41

Procedure

1. Obtain an arterial (or venous if ordered) blood sample. (See Chapter 2, pages 55 and 58, for venous and arterial blood collection, respectively.)
2. Use one of the following two methods to determine the pH:
   a. *Direct method*: Analyze a small amount of blood using a blood gas machine or analyzer (see Fig. 14.5).
   b. *Indirect method*: Solve the Henderson-Hasselbalch equation for the pH of a buffer system. In this equation, pK is the negative logarithm of the acid dissociation constant (the pH at which the associated and unassociated forms of an acid exist in equal concentrations). $[A^-]$ is the concentration of the ionized form (in this case HCO_3^-, the major blood base), and [HA] is the

concentration of the free acid (in this case H_2CO_3, the major blood acid) in milliequivalents per liter.

$$pH = pK + \log \frac{[A^-]}{[HA]}$$

$$pH = pK + \log \frac{[HCO_3^-]}{[H_2CO_3]}$$

$$pH = 6.1 = \log \frac{[HCO_3^-]}{0.03(PaCO_2)}$$

Clinical Implications

1. Generally speaking, the pH is *decreased* in acidemia (acidosis) because of increased formation of acids, and pH is *increased* in alkalemia (alkalosis) because of a loss of acids.
2. When interpreting an acid–base abnormality, certain steps should be followed:
   a. Check the pH to determine whether an acid or an alkaline state exists.
   b. Check the PCO_2 to determine whether a respiratory acidosis or alkalosis is present. (PCO_2 is the *breathing* component.)
   c. Check the HCO_3^- concentration to determine whether a metabolic acidosis or alkalosis is present. (HCO_3^- is the *renal* component.)
3. See Table 14.4 for a more complete explanation of the changes occurring in acute and chronic respiratory and metabolic acidosis and alkalosis.
4. Metabolic acidemia (acidosis) occurs in:
   a. Renal failure
   b. Ketoacidosis in diabetes and starvation
   c. Lactic acidosis
   d. Strenuous exercise
   e. Severe diarrhea
5. Metabolic alkalemia (alkalosis) occurs in:
   a. Hypokalemia
   b. Hypochloremia
   c. Gastric suction or vomiting
   d. Massive doses of steroids
   e. Sodium bicarbonate administration
   f. Aspirin intoxication
6. Respiratory alkalemia (alkalosis) occurs in:
   a. Acute pulmonary disease
   b. Myocardial infarction
   c. Chronic and acute heart failure
   d. Adult CF
   e. Third trimester of pregnancy and during labor and delivery
   f. Anxiety, neuroses, psychoses
   g. Pain
   h. Central nervous system diseases
   i. Anemia
   j. Carbon monoxide poisoning
   k. Acute pulmonary embolus
   l. Shock
7. Respiratory acidemia (acidosis) occurs in:
   a. Acute or chronic respiratory failure
   b. Ventilatory failure

c. Neuromuscular depression
d. Obesity
e. Pulmonary edema
f. Cardiopulmonary arrest

CLINICAL ALERT

1. *Ventilatory failure is a medical emergency. Aggressive and supportive measures must be taken immediately.*
2. Rate and depth of respirations may give a clue to blood pH.
   a. Acidosis usually *increases* respirations; this is the body's way of adjusting once the state is established.
   b. Alkalosis usually *decreases* respirations; this is the body's way of adjusting once the state is established.
3. Respiratory alkalosis may reflect hyperventilation in response to treatment for hypoxemia; however, correction of hypoxemia is essential.
4. Metabolic alkalosis, which is compensated through hypoventilation, may produce hypoxemia.

Interfering Factors

A number of drugs may alter the components of acid–base balance. See Appendix E.

Interventions

Pretest Patient Care

1. Explain the purpose, benefits, and risks of invasive blood sampling.
2. Follow guidelines in Chapter 1 for safe, effective, informed *pretest* care.

Posttest Patient Care

1. Review test results; report and record findings. Modify the nursing care plan as needed. Assess, monitor, and intervene appropriately for metabolic and respiratory acidosis and alkalosis (see Table 14.4).
2. Frequently observe the arterial puncture site for bleeding (see page 55, Chapter 2). Be prepared to initiate proper interventions in the event of life-threatening situations.
3. Follow guidelines in Chapter 1 for safe, effective, informed *posttest* care.

● Base Excess or Deficit

This test quantifies the patient's total base excess or deficit so that clinical treatment of acid–base disturbances (specifically those that are nonrespiratory in nature) can be initiated. It is also referred to as the *whole blood buffer base* and is the sum of the concentration of buffer anions (in milliequivalents per liter) contained in whole blood. These buffer anions are the bicarbonate ion (HCO_3^-) present in plasma erythrocytes and the hemoglobin, plasma proteins, and phosphates in plasma and red blood cells.

The total quantity of buffer anions is 45 to 50 mEq/L (45 to 50 mmol/L), or about twice that of HCO_3^- alone (22 to 26 mEq/L or 22 to 26 mmol/L). Therefore, the quantity of HCO_3^- ions accounts for only about half of the total buffering capacity of the blood. The base excess or deficit measurement provides a more complete picture of the buffering that is taking place and is a critical index of nonrespiratory versus respiratory changes in acid–base balance.

Reference Values

Normal

Normal values are ±2 mEq/L (±2 mmol/L).

A positive value indicates a base excess (i.e., nonvolatile acid deficit).

A negative value indicates a base deficit (i.e., nonvolatile acid excess).

Procedure

1. Make calculations from the measurements of pH, $PaCO_2$, and the hematocrit.
2. Plot these values on a nomogram and read the base excess or deficit.

Clinical Implications

1. A *negative* value (lower than −2 mEq/L or −2 mmol/L) reflects a nonrespiratory or metabolic disturbance or true base deficit or a nonvolatile acid accumulation caused by:
   a. Dietary intake of organic and inorganic acids
   b. Lactic acid
   c. Ketoacidosis
2. A *positive* value (higher than +2 mEq/L or +2 mmol/L) reflects a nonvolatile acid deficit or true base excess.

● Anion Gap (AG)

This test measures the difference between the sum of the sodium (Na^+) and potassium (K^+) ion concentrations (the measured cations) and the sum of the chloride (Cl^-) and bicarbonate (HCO_3^-) concentrations (the measured anions). This difference reflects the concentrations of other anions that are present in the extracellular fluid but are not routinely measured, the components of which include phosphates, sulfates, ketone bodies, lactic acid, and proteins. Increased amounts of these unmeasured anions are produced in the acidotic state.

Primary *hypobicarbonatemia* is brought about by any combination of three mechanisms: (1) overproduction of acids, which causes replacement of $NaHCO_3$ by the Na^+ salt of the offending acid (e.g., lactate replaces HCO_3^- in lactic acidosis); (2) loss of $NaHCO_3$ through diarrhea along with renal retention of dietary NaCl, which causes hyperchloremic metabolic acidosis; and (3) generalized renal failure or specific forms of renal tubular acidosis, which cause retention of acids that are normally produced by intermediary metabolism or by urinary excretion of alkali (Table 14.5).

Hyperbicarbonatemia with sustained increases in HCO_3^- levels is brought about by a source of *new* alkali or by the presence of factors that stimulate renal retention of excess HCO_3^-. These mechanisms include excessive gastrointestinal (GI) loss of acid exogenous alkali in persons whose kidneys avidly retain $NaHCO_3$, and renal synthesis of HCO_3^- in excess of daily consumption. Other pathophysiologic factors that affect renal reabsorption of >25 mEq/L (>25 mmol/L) of HCO_3^- and contribute to sustained hyperbicarbonatemia include extracellular fluid volume contraction, hypercapnia, hypokalemia, hyperaldosteronemia, and hypoparathyroidism (Table 14.6).

Reference Values

Normal

Normal values are 12 ± 4 mEq/L (12 ± 4 mmol/L).

If potassium concentration is used in the calculation, the normal value is 16 ± 4 mEq/L (16 ± 4 mmol/L).

TABLE 14.5 Subclassification of Anion Gap Metabolic Acidosis (Hypobicarbonatemia) into High- and Low-Potassium Forms[a]

High-Potassium Form	Low-Potassium Form
Acidifying agents	Diarrhea
Mineralocorticoid deficiency	Ureteral sigmoidostomy and malfunctioning ileostomy
Renal diseases such as systemic lupus erythematosus, interstitial nephritis, amyloidosis, hydronephrosis, and sickle cell nephropathy	Renal tubular acidosis, both proximal and distal
Early nonspecific renal failure	

[a]All metabolic acidoses can be classified on the basis of how they affect the anion gap.

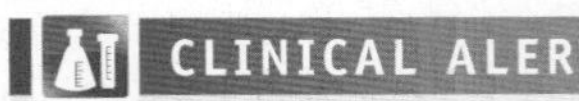

Critical Value
>16 mEq/L (>16 mmol/L)

Procedure

1. Obtain this measurement by calculating the difference between the measured serum cation concentrations (either with or without K^+) and the measured serum anion concentrations.
2. Use the following formulas:

$$AG = ([Na^+] + [K^+]) - ([Cl^-] + [HCO_3^-])$$

or

$$AG = [Na^+] - ([Cl^-] + [HCO_3^-])$$

Clinical Implications

1. An anion gap (AG) occurs in acidosis that is caused by excess metabolic acids and excess serum chloride levels. If there is no change in sodium content, anions such as phosphates, sulfates, and organic acids increase the AG because they replace bicarbonate.
2. *Increased* AG is associated with an increase in metabolic acid when there is excessive production of metabolic acids, as in:
   a. Alcoholic ketoacidosis
   b. Diabetic ketoacidosis
   c. Fasting and starvation
   d. Ketogenic diets
   e. Lactic acidosis
   f. Poisoning by salicylate, ethylene glycol (antifreeze), methanol, or propyl alcohol
3. *Increased* AG is also associated with decreased loss of metabolic acids as in renal failure. In the absence of renal failure or intoxication with drugs or toxins, an increase in AG is assumed to be caused by ketoacidosis or lactate accumulation.
   AG includes the determination of three gaps of toxicology (influence of drugs and heavy metals): (1) anion = type A lactic acidosis due to tissue hypoxia, (2) osmolar gap, and (3) oxygen saturation gap.

TABLE 14.6 Classification of Anion Gap Metabolic Alkalosis (Hyperbicarbonatemia) on the Basis of Urinary Excretion

Saline-Responsive Urinary Chloride Excretion of <10 mEq/d	Saline-Unresponsive Excretion of <10 mEq/d
Excess Body Bicarbonate Content	
Renal alkalosis	Renal alkalosis—normotensive conditions
Diuretic therapy	Bartter's syndrome
Poorly reabsorbable anion therapy (e.g., carbenicillin, penicillin, sulfate, phosphate)	Severe potassium depletion
	Refeeding alkalosis
Gastrointestinal alkalosis	Hypercalcemia and hypoparathyroidism
Gastric alkalosis	Hypertensive conditions—endogenous mineralocorticoids
Intestinal alkalosis (e.g., chloride diarrhea)	
Exogenous alkali	Primary aldosteronism
Baking soda	Hyperreninism
Sodium citrate, lactate, gluconate, acetate	Adrenal enzyme deficiency: 11- and 17-hydroxylase
Transfusions	
Antacids	Liddle's syndrome
	Exogenous mineralocorticoids
	Licorice
	Carbenoxolone
	Chewing tobacco
Normal Body Bicarbonate Content	
Contraction alkalosis—urinary loss of NaCl and water without bicarbonate loss causes extracellular fluid contraction around an unchanged body content of alkali, resulting in hyperbicarbonatemia (especially important in persons with edema and persons who have excess body stores of water, sodium, bicarbonate, and chloride).	

A list of drugs and toxic substances that cause *increased* AG (>12 mEq/L or >12 mmol/L) include the following:

Nonacidotic: carbenicillin and sodium salts

Metabolic acidosis: acetaminophen (ingestion of >75 to 100 g), acetazolamide, aluminum phosphate, amiloride, 4-aminopyridine, ammonium chloride, ascorbic acid, benzalkonium chloride, bialaphos, 2-butoxyethanol, carbon monoxide, cetrimonium bromide, chloramphenicol, clozapine, cobalt, colchicine, cyanide, dapsone, dimethyl sulfate, dinitrophenol, endosulfan, epinephrine (intravenous [IV] overdose), ethanol, ethylene dibromide, ethylene glycol, fenoprofen, fluoroacetate, formaldehyde, fructose (IV), funnel web spiders, glycol ethers, glyphosate, hydrogen sulfide, ibuprofen (ingestion of >300 mg/kg), inorganic acid, iodine, iron, isoniazid, ketamine, ketoprofen, lime sulfur, margosa (neem) oil, metaldehyde, metformin, methanol, methenamine mandelate, misoprostol, monochloracetic acid, nalidixic acid, naproxen, nefopam, niacin, papaverine, paraldehyde, pennyroyal oil, pentaborane, pentachlorophenol, phenelzine, phenformin (off the market), phenol, phenylbutazone, phosphoric acid, polyethylene glycol (low molecular weight), propofol, propylene glycol, salicylates, sodium azide, sorbitol (IV), strychnine, sublimed sulfur, sulthiame, surfactant herbicide, tetracycline (outdated), tienilic acid, toluene, tranylcypromine, Vacor, valproic acid, verapamil, zidovudine (chronic use >6 months), zinc phosphide

Toxins that cause osmolar gap >10 mOsm from baseline include ethanol, ethylene glycol, glycerol, hypermagnesemia (>9.5 mEq/L or >9.5 mmol/L), isopropanol (acetone), iodine (questionable), mannitol, methanol, and sorbitol.

Drugs and toxins that cause *decreased* AG (<6 mEq/L or <6 mmol/L) include the following: *acidosis*—acetazolamide, amiloride, ammonium chloride, amphotericin B, bromide, fialuridine (FIAU), iodide, Kombucha tea, lithium, polymyxin B, spironolactone, sulindac, toluene, and tromethamine.

Toxins that cause an oxygen saturation gap (>5% difference between measured and calculated value) include carbon monoxide, cyanide (questionable), hydrogen sulfide (possible), methemoglobin, and nitrates.

4. Increased bicarbonate loss with a *normal* AG is associated with:
   a. Decreased renal losses, as in:
      (1) Renal tubular acidosis
      (2) Use of acetazolamide
   b. Increased chloride levels, as in:
      (1) Altered chloride reabsorption by the kidney
      (2) Parenteral hyperalimentation
      (3) Administration of sodium chloride and ammonium chloride
   c. Loss of intestinal secretions, as in:
      (1) Diarrhea
      (2) Intestinal suction or fistula
      (3) Biliary fistula
5. *Low* AG is associated with:
   a. Multiple myeloma
   b. Hyponatremia caused by viscous serum
   c. Bromide ingestion (hyperchloremia)
6. The AG may provide evidence of a mixed rather than a simple acid–base disturbance.

Interventions

Pretest Patient Care

1. Explain the purpose and procedure of the test.
2. Follow guidelines in Chapter 1 for safe, effective, informed *pretest* care.

Posttest Patient Care

1. Review test results; report and record findings. Modify the nursing care plan as needed. Assess patient and monitor appropriately for acid–base disturbances.
2. Follow guidelines in Chapter 1 for safe, effective, informed *posttest* care.

● Lactic Acid (Lactate)

Lactic acid is produced during periods of anaerobic metabolism when cells do not receive adequate oxygen to allow conversion of fuel sources to CO_2 and water. Lactic acid is a weak acid that partially dissociates in water, resulting in production of lactate and hydrogen ions. Lactic acid accumulates because of excess production of lactate and decreased removal of lactic acid from blood by the liver. Measuring lactic acid is common in cases of suspected septic shock.

This measurement contributes to the knowledge of acid–base volume and is used to detect lactic acidosis in persons with underlying risk factors such as cardiovascular or renal disease that predispose them to this imbalance. Lactic acid is elevated in a variety of conditions in which hypoxia occurs due to shock or vascular occlusion and in liver disease. Lactic acidosis can occur in both diabetic and nondiabetic patients. It can be fatal.

Reference Values

Normal

In venous blood: 0.5 to 2.2 mEq/L (0.5 to 2.2 mmol/L)
In arterial blood: 0.5 to 1.6 mEq/L (0.5 to 1.6 mmol/L)

Procedure

1. Obtain a venous or arterial blood sample of at least 5 mL. (See Chapter 2 for venous and arterial blood collection.)
2. Label specimen with the patient's name, date, and test(s) ordered. Take the specimen to the laboratory immediately for analysis.

Clinical Implications

1. Values are *increased* in:
   a. Lactic acidosis
   b. Cardiac failure
   c. Pulmonary failure (sometimes defined as a PaO_2 <50 mm Hg [<6.7 kPa] and a $PaCO_2$ >50 mm Hg [>6.7 kPa])
   d. Hemorrhage
   e. Diabetes
   f. Shock
   g. Liver disease
2. Lactic acidosis can be distinguished from ketoacidosis by the absence of severe ketosis and hyperglycemia in this state.

Interfering Factors

Lactic acid levels normally rise during strenuous exercise, when blood flow and oxygen cannot keep pace with the increased needs of exercising muscle.

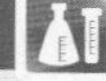

CLINICAL ALERT

An unexplained decrease in pH associated with a hypoxia-producing condition is reason to suspect lactic acidosis.

Interventions

Pretest Patient Care

1. Explain the purpose and procedure of arterial blood sampling. Assess patient cooperation.
2. Follow guidelines in Chapter 1 for safe, effective, informed *pretest* care.

Posttest Patient Care

1. Frequently observe the puncture site for bleeding. Manual pressure and a pressure dressing should be applied to the puncture site if necessary.
2. Base *posttest* assessments on patient outcomes; monitor and intervene appropriately for ventilatory and acid–base disturbances and hypoxemia.
3. Follow guidelines in Chapter 1 for safe, effective, informed *posttest* care.

ELECTROLYTE TESTS

Electrolytes (ions) are critical for cellular reactions. These electrolytes provide the necessary inorganic chemicals for a variety of cellular functions (e.g., nerve impulse transmission, muscular contraction, water balance). Typically, the concentration of cations (positively charged electrolytes; e.g., Na^+, K^+, Ca^{2+}, and Mg^+) is higher in the plasma than in the interstitial fluid owing to the *Donnan effect* (plasma proteins have a net negative charge), whereas the anions (negatively charged; e.g., Cl^-, HPO_4^-) tend to be higher in the interstitial fluid than the plasma.

Calcium (Ca^{2+})

The bulk of body calcium (99%) is stored in the skeleton and teeth, which act as huge reservoirs for maintaining blood levels of calcium. About 50% (0.50) of blood calcium is ionized; the rest is protein bound. Only ionized calcium can be used by the body in such vital processes as muscular contraction, cardiac function, transmission of nerve impulses, and blood clotting.

The amount of protein in the blood also affects calcium levels because 50% (0.50) of blood calcium is protein bound. Thus, a decrease in serum albumin will result in a decrease in total serum calcium. The decrease, however, does not alter the concentration of the ionized form of calcium. Measurements of ionized calcium are done during open heart surgeries, liver transplantations, and other operations in which large volumes of blood anticoagulated with citrate are given. These tests are also used to monitor renal disease, renal transplantation, hemodialysis, hyperparathyroidism, hypoparathyroidism, pancreatitis, and malignancy. Calcium levels are influenced by a variety of factors, including parathyroid hormone (PTH), calcitonin, vitamin D, and dietary calcium intake.

This test measures the concentration of total and ionized calcium in the blood to reflect parathyroid function, calcium metabolism, and malignancy activity.

CLINICAL ALERT

Hyperparathyroidism and cancer are the most common causes of hypercalcemia.
Hypoalbuminemia is the most common cause of decreased total calcium.

Reference Values

Normal

See Table 14.7.

TABLE 14.7 Normal Values[a] for Calcium

Total Calcium			Ionized Calcium		
Age	mg/dL	mmol/L	Age	mg/dL	mmol/L
0–10 d	7.6–10.4	1.90–2.60	Newborn	4.40–5.48	1.10–1.37
10 d–3 yr	6.7–9.8	2.24–2.75	1–18 yr	4.80–5.52	1.20–1.38
3–9 yr	8.8–10.1	2.20–2.70	Adult	4.65–5.28	1.16–1.32
4–11 yr	8.9–10.1	2.30–2.70			
11–13 yr	8.8–10.6	2.20–2.65			
13–15 yr	9.2–10.7	2.30–2.55			
15–18 yr	8.4–10.7	2.10–2.67			
Adult	8.8–10.4	2.20–2.60			

[a]Normal values vary greatly; check with your reference laboratory.

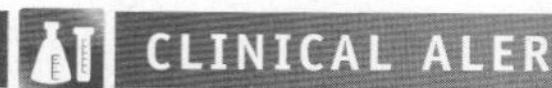

Critical Values

Total calcium

<4.4 mg/dL (<1.1 mmol/L) may produce tetany and convulsions.

>13 mg/dL (>3.25 mmol/L) may cause cardiotoxicity, arrhythmias, and coma.

Rapid treatment of hypercalcemia with calcitonin solution is indicated.

Ionized calcium

<2.0 mg/dL (<0.5 mmol/L) may produce tetany or life-threatening complications.

2.0–3.0 mg/dL (<0.5–0.75 mmol/L) in cases of multiple blood transfusions (this is an indication to administer calcium)

>7.0 mg/dL (>1.75 mmol/L) may cause coma.

Procedure

1. Obtain a 5-mL venous blood sample in a serum separator tube (SST) or red-topped tube; this will provide sufficient serum for this test.
2. Observe standard precautions. Be aware that heparinized samples are preferred for ionized calcium studies. Citrated ethylenediaminetetraacetic acid (EDTA) and oxalate give falsely low values and should not be used in the syringe.
3. Label specimen with the patient's name, date, and test(s) ordered. Place specimens on ice, keep tightly capped, and deliver immediately to the laboratory.

 PROCEDURAL ALERT

Excessive IV fluids decrease albumin levels and thus decrease calcium levels. Total serum protein and albumin should be measured at the same time as calcium for proper interpretation of calcium levels. Ionized calcium is not affected by albumin levels.

Clinical Implications

1. *Normal levels of total blood calcium*, combined with other findings, indicate the following conditions:
   a. Normal calcium levels with overall normal results in other tests indicate no problems with calcium metabolism.
   b. Normal calcium and abnormal phosphorus values indicate impaired calcium absorption owing to alteration of PTH activity or secretion (e.g., in rickets, the calcium level may be normal or slightly lowered and the phosphorus level depressed).
   c. Normal calcium and elevated blood urea nitrogen (BUN) levels indicate the following:
      (1) Possible secondary hyperparathyroidism: Initially, lowered serum calcium results from uremia and acidosis. The reduced calcium level stimulates the parathyroid to release PTH, which acts on bone to release more calcium.
      (2) Possible primary hyperparathyroidism: Excessive amounts of PTH cause elevation in calcium levels, but secondary kidney disease causes retention of phosphate and concomitant lower calcium levels.
   d. Normal calcium with decreased serum albumin indicates hypercalcemia. Normally, a decrease in calcium is associated with a decrease in albumin.
2. *Hypercalcemia* (increased total calcium levels [>12 mg/dL or >3 mmol/L]) is caused by or associated with the following conditions:
   a. Hyperparathyroidism due to parathyroid adenoma, hyperplasia of parathyroid glands, or associated hypophosphatemia

b. Cancer (PTH-producing tumors)
   (1) Metastatic bone cancers; cancers of lung, breast, thyroid, kidney, liver, and pancreas
   (2) Hodgkin's lymphoma, leukemia, and non-Hodgkin's lymphoma
   (3) Multiple myeloma with extensive bone destruction, Burkitt's lymphoma
   (4) Primary squamous cell carcinoma of lung, neck, and head
c. Granulomatous disease (e.g., tuberculosis, sarcoidosis)
d. Thyroid toxicosis
e. Paget's disease of bone (also accompanied by high levels of alkaline phosphatase)
f. Idiopathic hypercalcemia of infancy
g. Bone fractures combined with bed rest, prolonged immobilization
h. Excessive intake of vitamin D, milk, antacids
i. Renal transplantation
j. Milk-alkali syndrome (Burnett's syndrome)

3. *Hypocalcemia* (decreased total calcium levels [<4.0 mg/dL or <1.0 mmol/L]) is commonly caused by or associated with the following conditions:
   a. Pseudohypocalcemia, which reflects reduced albumin levels. The reduced protein is responsible for the low calcium level because 50% of the calcium total is protein bound.
   b. Hypoparathyroidism due to surgical removal of parathyroid glands, irradiation, hypomagnesemia, GI disorders, or renal wasting. The primary form is very rare.
   c. Hyperphosphatemia due to renal failure, laxative intake, or cytotoxic drugs
   d. Malabsorption due to sprue, celiac disease, or pancreatic dysfunction (fatty acids combine with calcium and are precipitated and excreted in the feces)
   e. Acute pancreatitis
   f. Alkalosis (calcium ions become bound to protein)
   g. Osteomalacia (advanced)
   h. Renal failure
   i. Vitamin D deficiency, rickets
   j. Malnutrition
   k. Alcoholism, hepatic cirrhosis
4. *Increased ionized calcium levels* occur in the following conditions:
   a. Hyperparathyroidism
   b. Ectopic PTH-producing tumors
   c. Increased vitamin D intake
   d. Malignancies
5. *Decreased ionized calcium levels* occur in the following conditions:
   a. Hyperventilation to control increased intracranial pressure (total Ca^{2+} may be normal)
   b. Administration of bicarbonate to control metabolic acidosis
   c. Acute pancreatitis (e.g., diabetic acidosis, sepsis)
   d. Hypoparathyroidism
   e. Vitamin D deficiency
   f. Magnesium deficiency
   g. Multiple organ failure
   h. Toxic shock syndrome

Interfering Factors

1. Thiazide diuretics may impair urinary calcium excretion and result in hypercalcemia (most common drug-induced factor).
2. For patients with renal insufficiency undergoing dialysis, a calcium-ion exchange resin is sometimes used for hyperkalemia. This resin may increase calcium levels.
3. Increased magnesium and phosphate uptake and excessive use of laxatives may lower blood calcium level because of increased intestinal calcium loss.

4. When decreased calcium levels are due to magnesium deficiency (as in poor bowel absorption), the administration of magnesium will correct the calcium deficiency.
5. If a patient is known to have or suspected of having a pH abnormality, a concurrent pH test with ionized calcium level should be requested.
6. Many drugs may cause increased or decreased levels of calcium. Calcium supplements taken shortly before specimen collection will cause falsely high values.
7. Elevated serum protein increases calcium; decreased protein decreases calcium.

Interventions

Pretest Patient Care

1. Explain purpose and procedure. Encourage relaxation.
2. Tourniquet application should be as brief as possible when drawing ionized calcium to prevent venous stasis and hemolysis.
3. Ensure that calcium supplements are not taken within 8 to 12 hours before the blood sample is drawn.
4. Follow guidelines in Chapter 1 for safe, effective, informed *pretest* care.

Posttest Patient Care

1. Have patient resume normal activities.
2. Review test results; report and record findings. Modify the nursing care plan as needed. Monitor patient appropriately for calcium abnormalities.
3. Follow guidelines in Chapter 1 for safe, effective, informed *posttest* care.

• Chloride (Cl^-)

Chloride, a blood electrolyte, is the major anion that exists predominantly in the extracellular spaces as part of sodium chloride or hydrochloric acid. Chloride maintains cellular integrity through its influence on osmotic pressure and acid–base and water balance. It increases or decreases in concentration in response to concentrations of other anions. In metabolic acidosis, there is a reciprocal rise in chloride concentration when the bicarbonate concentration drops. Similarly, when aldosterone directly causes an increase in the reabsorption of sodium (the positive ion), the indirect effect is an increase in the absorption of chloride (the negative ion).

Chlorides are excreted with cations (positive ions) during massive diuresis from any cause and are lost from the GI tract when vomiting, diarrhea, or intestinal fistulas occur.

Alteration of sodium chloride level is seldom a primary problem. Measurement of chlorides is helpful in diagnosing disorders of acid–base and water balance. Because of the relatively high chloride concentrations in gastric juices, prolonged vomiting may lead to considerable chloride loss and lowered serum chloride levels.

In an emergency, chloride is the least important electrolyte to measure. However, it is especially important in the correction of hypokalemic alkalosis. If potassium is supplied without chloride, hypokalemic alkalosis may persist.

Reference Values

Normal

Adults: 96 to 106 mEq/L (96 to 106 mmol/L)
Newborns: 96 to 113 mEq/L (96 to 113 mmol/L)

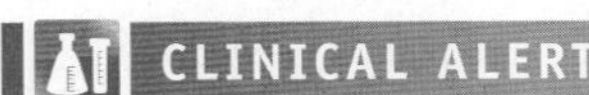

Critical Values
<70 or >120 mEq/L (<70 or >120 mmol/L)

Procedure

1. Obtain a 5-mL venous blood sample in a heparinized Vacutainer tube (see Chapter 2, page 52 for venous blood collection). Serum can also be used.
2. Observe standard precautions.

Clinical Implications

NOTE *Whenever serum chloride levels are much lower than 100 mEq/L (100 mmol/L), urinary excretion of chlorides is also low.*

1. *Decreased blood chloride levels* occur in the following conditions:
   a. Severe vomiting
   b. Gastric suction
   c. Chronic respiratory acidosis
   d. Burns
   e. Metabolic alkalosis
   f. Congestive failure
   g. Addison's disease (chronic adrenal insufficiency)
   h. Salt-losing diseases (syndrome of inappropriate antidiuretic hormone [SIADH])
   i. Overhydration or water intoxication
   j. Acute intermittent porphyria
   k. Salt-losing nephritis
2. *Increased blood chloride levels* occur in the following conditions:
   a. Dehydration
   b. Cushing's syndrome
   c. Hyperventilation, which causes respiratory alkalosis
   d. Metabolic acidosis with prolonged diarrhea
   e. Hyperparathyroidism (primary)
   f. Select kidney disorders (e.g., renal tubular acidosis)
   g. Diabetes insipidus
   h. Salicylate intoxication
   i. Head injury with hypothalamic damage
   j. Eclampsia

Interfering Factors

1. The plasma chloride concentration in infants is usually higher than that in children and adults.
2. Certain drugs may alter chloride levels.
3. Increases are associated with excessive IV saline infusions.

Interventions

Pretest Patient Care

1. Explain test purpose and blood collection procedure.
2. If possible, ensure that the patient fasts at least 8 to 12 hours before the test.
3. Follow guidelines in Chapter 1 for safe, effective, informed *pretest* care.

Posttest Patient Care

1. Resume normal activities and diet.
2. Review test results; report and record findings. Modify the nursing care plan as needed.
3. If an electrolyte disorder is suspected, daily weight and accurate fluid intake and output should be recorded.
4. Follow guidelines in Chapter 1 for safe, effective, informed *posttest* care.

Phosphate (P); Inorganic Phosphorus (PO_4)

Of the human body's total phosphorus content, 85% is combined with calcium in the bone and the remainder resides within the cells. Most of the phosphorus in the blood exists as phosphates or esters. Phosphate is required for generation of bony tissue and functions in the metabolism of glucose and lipids, in the maintenance of acid–base balance, and in the storage and transfer of energy from one site in the body to another. Phosphorus enters the red blood cells with glucose and therefore is lowered in the plasma after carbohydrate ingestion or infusion.

Phosphate levels are always evaluated in relation to calcium levels because there is an inverse relation between the two elements. When calcium levels are decreased, phosphorus levels are increased, and when phosphorus levels are decreased, calcium levels are increased. An excess of one electrolyte in serum causes the kidneys to excrete the other electrolyte. Many of the causes of elevated calcium levels are also causes of decreased phosphorus levels. As with calcium, the controlling factor is PTH.

Reference Values

Normal

Adults: 2.7 to 4.5 mg/dL (0.87 to 1.45 mmol/L)
Children: 4.5 to 5.5 mg/dL (1.45 to 1.78 mmol/L)
Newborns: 4.5 to 9.0 mg/dL (1.45 to 2.91 mmol/L)

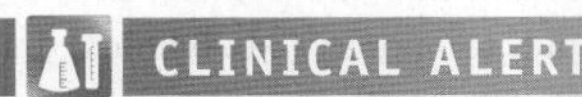

Critical Values
<1.0 mg/dL (<0.32 mmol/L)

Procedure

Obtain a fasting, 5-mL in an SST or red-topped tube, venous blood sample (see Chapter 2, page 52, for venous blood collection). Serum is preferred, but heparinized blood is acceptable. Serum should be removed from clot as soon as possible after collection.

Clinical Implications

1. *Hyperphosphatemia* (increased blood phosphorus levels) is most commonly found in association with kidney dysfunction and uremia. This is because phosphate is so minutely regulated by the kidneys. These conditions include the following:
   a. Renal insufficiency and severe nephritis (accompanied by elevated BUN and creatinine) and renal failure
   b. Hypoparathyroidism (accompanied by elevated phosphorus, decreased calcium, and normal renal function) and pseudohypoparathyroidism
   c. Hypocalcemia
   d. Milk-alkali syndrome (Burnett's syndrome; high levels of calcium and metabolic alkalosis)
   e. Excessive intake of vitamin D
   f. Fractures in the healing stage
   g. Bone tumors and metastases
   h. Addison's disease
   i. Acromegaly
   j. Liver disease and cirrhosis
   k. Cardiac resuscitation

2. *Hypophosphatemia* (decreased phosphorus level) occurs in the following conditions:
   a. Hyperparathyroidism
   b. Rickets (childhood) or osteomalacia (adult) and vitamin D deficiency
   c. Diabetic coma (increased carbohydrate metabolism)
   d. Hyperinsulinism
   e. Continuous administration of IV glucose in a nondiabetic patient (phosphorus follows glucose into the cells)
   f. Liver disease and acute alcoholism
   g. Vomiting and severe diarrhea
   h. Severe malnutrition and malabsorption
   i. Gram-negative septicemia
   j. Hypercalcemia of any cause
   k. Prolonged hypothermia
   l. Respiratory alkalosis due to cellular use of phosphorus for an accelerated glucose metabolism

Interfering Factors

1. Phosphorus levels are normally high in children.
2. Phosphorus levels can be falsely increased by hemolysis of blood; therefore, separate serum from cells as soon as possible.
3. Drugs can be the cause of decreases in phosphorus.
4. The use of laxatives or enemas containing large amounts of sodium phosphate will cause increased phosphorus levels. With oral laxatives, the blood phosphorus level may increase as much as 5 mg/dL (1.6 mmol/L) 2 to 3 hours after intake. This increased level is only temporary (5 to 6 hours), but this factor should be considered when abnormal levels are seen that cannot otherwise be explained.
5. Seasonal variations exist in phosphorus levels (maximal levels in May and June, lowest levels in winter).

Interventions

Pretest Patient Care

1. Explain test purpose and blood sampling procedures. The patient should fast before the test.
2. Note on test requisition if any catastrophic stressful events have taken place that may cause high phosphorus levels.
3. Note time of day test is drawn; levels are highest in the morning and lowest in the evening.
4. Follow guidelines in Chapter 1 for safe, effective, informed *pretest* care.

Posttest Patient Care

1. Have patient resume normal activities.
2. Review test results; report and record findings. Modify the nursing care plan as needed. Monitor patient as appropriate for calcium imbalances. When phosphorus rises rapidly, calcium drops; watch for arrhythmias and muscle twitching. The signs and symptoms of phosphate depletion may include manifestations in the neuromuscular, neuropsychiatric, GI, skeletal, and cardiopulmonary systems. Manifestations usually are accompanied by serum levels <1 mg/dL (<0.32 mmol/L).
3. Follow guidelines in Chapter 1 for safe, effective, informed *posttest* care.

● Magnesium (Mg^{2+})

Magnesium in the body is concentrated (40% to 60%) in the bone, 20% in muscle, 30% within the cell itself, and 1% in the serum and is required for the use of adenosine triphosphate (ATP) as a source of energy. It is therefore necessary for the action of numerous enzyme systems such as carbohydrate metabolism, protein synthesis, nucleic acid synthesis, and contraction of muscular tissue. Along with sodium, potassium, and calcium ions, magnesium also regulates neuromuscular irritability and the clotting mechanism.

Magnesium and calcium are intimately linked in their body functions, and deficiency of either one has a significant effect on the metabolism of the other because of magnesium's importance in the absorption of calcium from the intestines and in calcium metabolism. Magnesium deficiency will result in the drift of calcium out of the bones, possibly resulting in abnormal calcification in the aorta and the kidney. This condition responds to administration of magnesium salts. Normally, 95% of the magnesium that is filtered through the glomerulus is reabsorbed in the tubule. When there is decreased kidney function, greater amounts of magnesium are retained, resulting in increased blood serum levels.

Magnesium measurement is used to evaluate renal function, electrolyte status, and evaluate magnesium metabolism.

Reference Values

Normal

Adults: 1.8 to 2.6 mg/dL (0.74 to 1.07 mmol/L)
Children: 1.7 to 2.1 mg/dL (0.70 to 0.86 mmol/L)
Newborns: 1.5 to 2.2 mg/dL (0.62 to 0.91 mmol/L)

CLINICAL ALERT

Critical Values

1. Hypomagnesemia: <1.2 mg/dL (<0.49 mmol/L), tetany occurs
2. Hypermagnesemia: >5.0 mg/dL (>2.1 mmol/L)
   a. 5.0–10.0 mg/dL (2.1–4.1 mmol/L): central nervous system depression, nausea, vomiting, fatigue
   b. 10–15 mg/dL (4.1–6.2 mmol/L): coma, ECG changes, respiratory paralysis
   c. 30 mg/dL (12.3 mmol/L): complete heart block
   d. 34–40 mg/dL (14.0–16.0 mmol/L): cardiac arrest

Procedure

1. Obtain a fasting (4 hours), 5-mL in an SST or red-topped tube, venous blood sample (see Chapter 2, page 52, for venous blood collection).
2. Avoid hemolysis and separate serum from cells as soon as possible. Heparinized blood may be used.

PROCEDURAL ALERT

Blood sample should be drawn while the patient is in a prone position because an upright position increases the magnesium level by 4%.

Clinical Implications

1. *Reduced blood magnesium levels (<1.5 mg/dL or <0.62 mmol/L)* occur in the following conditions:
   a. Hypercalcemia of any cause
   b. Diabetic acidosis
   c. Hemodialysis
   d. Chronic renal disease (glomerulonephritis)
   e. Chronic pancreatitis
   f. Hyperaldosteronism
   g. Pregnancy (second and third trimester)

h. Hypoparathyroidism
i. Excessive loss of body fluids (due to sweating, lactation, diuretic abuse, chronic diarrhea)
j. Malabsorption syndromes
k. Chronic alcoholism (hepatic cirrhosis)
l. Long-term hyperalimentation
m. SIADH

2. *Increased blood magnesium levels* occur in the following conditions:
   a. Renal failure or reduced renal function (acute and chronic)
   b. Dehydration
   c. Hypothyroidism
   d. Addison's disease
   e. Adrenalectomy (adrenocortical insufficiency)
   f. Diabetic acidosis (severe)
   g. Use of antacids containing magnesium (e.g., milk of magnesia), administration of magnesium salts
   h. Oliguria

NOTE *In magnesium deficiency states, urinary magnesium decreases before the serum magnesium. Serum magnesium levels may remain normal even when total body stores are depleted up to 20%.*

Interfering Factors

1. Prolonged salicylate therapy, lithium, and magnesium products (e.g., antacids, laxatives) will cause falsely increased magnesium levels, particularly if there is renal damage.
2. Calcium gluconate, as well as a number of other drugs, can interfere with testing methods and cause falsely decreased results.
3. Hemolysis will invalidate results because about three fourths of the magnesium in the blood is found intracellularly in the red blood cells.

Interventions

Pretest Patient Care

1. Explain test purpose and blood-drawing procedure.
2. Ensure that patient is fasting for at least 4 hours if possible and is in a prone position when blood is drawn.
3. Follow guidelines in Chapter 1 regarding safe, effective, informed *pretest* care.

Posttest Patient Care

1. Review test results; report and record findings. Modify the nursing care plan as needed. Treatment of diabetic coma often results in low plasma magnesium levels. This change occurs because magnesium moves with potassium into the cells after insulin administration.
2. Measure serum magnesium in persons receiving aminoglycosides and cyclosporine. There is a known association between these therapies and hypermagnesemia. Treatment of hypermagnesemia involves withholding source of magnesium excess, promoting excretion, giving calcium salts, and performing hemodialysis.
3. Magnesium deficiency may cause apparently unexplained hypocalcemia and hypokalemia. In these instances, patients may have neurologic or GI symptoms. Observe for the following signs and symptoms:
   a. Muscle tremors, twitching, tetany
   b. Hypocalcemia
   c. Hyperactive deep-tendon reflexes

d. ECG: prolonged P-R and Q-T intervals; broad, flat T waves; premature ventricular tachycardia and fibrillation
e. Anorexia, nausea, vomiting
f. Insomnia, delirium, convulsions

4. Observe for signs of too much magnesium (which acts as a sedative):
   a. Lethargy, flushing, nausea, vomiting, slurred speech
   b. Weak or absent deep tendon reflexes
   c. ECG: prolonged P-R and Q-T intervals; widened QRS; bradycardia
   d. Hypotension, drowsiness, respiratory depression
5. Follow guidelines in Chapter 1 for safe, effective, informed *posttest* care.

● Potassium (K^+)

Potassium is the principal electrolyte (cation) of intracellular fluid and the primary buffer within the cell itself. Ninety percent of potassium is concentrated within the cell; only small amounts are contained in bone and blood. Damaged cells release potassium into the blood.

The body is adapted for efficient potassium excretion. Normally, 80% to 90% of the cells' potassium is excreted in the urine by the glomeruli of the kidneys; the remainder is excreted in sweat and in the stool. Even when no potassium is taken into the body (as in a fasting state), 40 to 50 mEq is still excreted daily in the urine. The kidneys do not conserve potassium, and when an adequate amount of potassium is not ingested, a severe deficiency will occur. Potassium balance is maintained in adults on an average dietary intake of 80 to 200 mEq/day (80 to 200 mmol/day). Normal intake, minimal needs, and maximum tolerance for potassium are almost the same as those for sodium.

Potassium plays an important role in nerve conduction, muscle function, acid–base balance, and osmotic pressure. Along with calcium and magnesium, potassium controls the rate and force of contraction of the heart and, thus, the cardiac output. Evidence of a potassium deficit can be noted on an ECG by flattening of the T wave and the presence of a U wave. Alternatively, an ECG may show a flattened P wave and a widened QRS complex with elevated potassium levels (Fig. 14.7).

Potassium and sodium ions are particularly important in the renal regulation of acid–base balance because hydrogen ions are substituted for sodium and potassium ions in the renal tubule. Potassium is more important than sodium because potassium bicarbonate is the primary intracellular inorganic buffer. In potassium deficiency, there is a relative deficiency of intracellular potassium bicarbonate, and the pH is relatively acid. The respiratory center responds to the intracellular acidosis by lowering PCO_2 through the mechanism of hyperventilation. The potassium concentration is greatly affected by the adrenal hormones. Potassium deficiency will cause a significant reduction in protein synthesis.

This test evaluates changes in body potassium levels and diagnoses acid–base and water imbalances. The level of potassium is not an absolute value; it varies with circulatory volume and other factors. Because a totally unsuspected potassium imbalance can suddenly prove lethal, its development must be anticipated. Thus, it is important to check the potassium level in severe cases of Addison's disease, uremic coma, intestinal obstruction, acute renal failure, GI loss in the administration of diuretics, steroid therapy, and cardiac patients on digitalis. Potassium levels should be monitored during treatment of acidosis, including ketoacidosis of diabetes mellitus.

Reference Values

Normal

Adults: 3.5 to 5.2 mEq/L (3.5 to 5.2 mmol/L)
Children (1 to 18 years): 3.4 to 4.7 mEq/L (3.4 to 4.7 mmol/L)
Infants (7 days to 1 year): 4.1 to 5.3 mEq/L (4.1 to 5.3 mmol/L)
Neonates (0 to 7 days): 3.7 to 5.9 mEq/L (3.7 to 5.9 mmol/L)

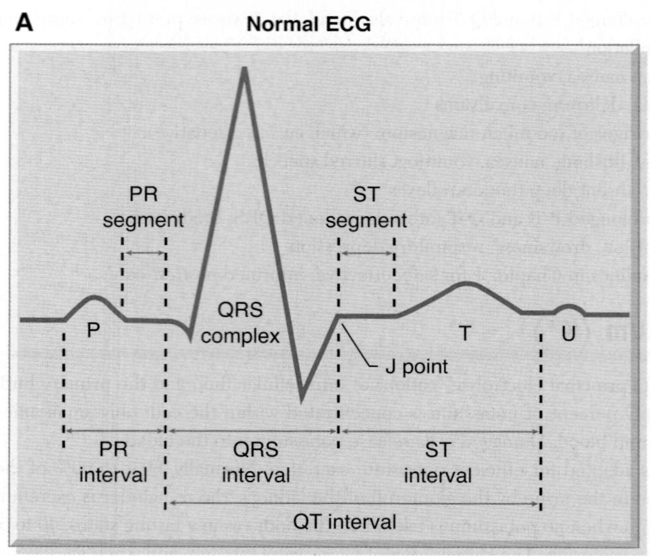

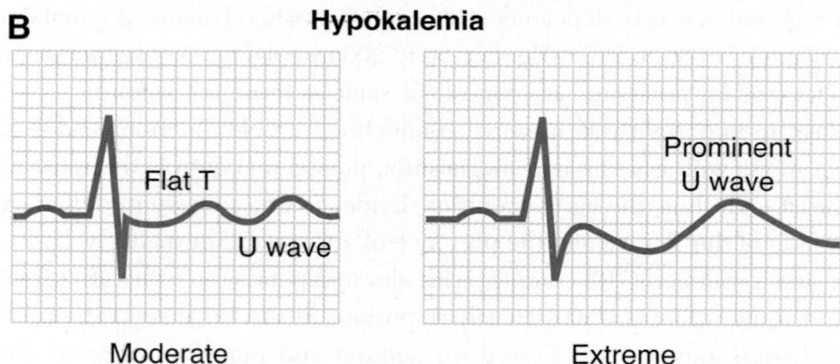

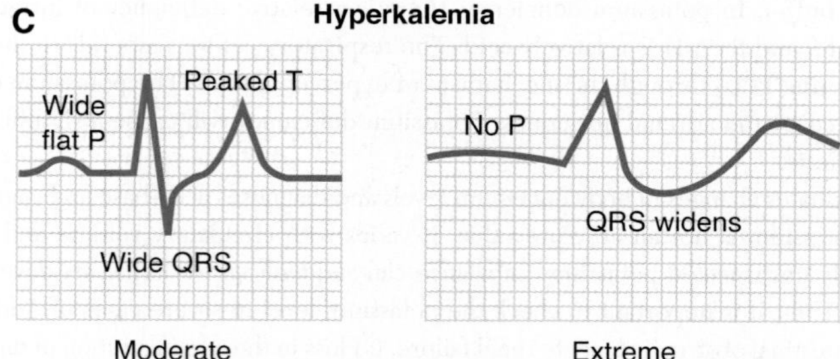

FIGURE 14.7. Potassium changes reflected on electrocardiogram. (From Pellico, LH: Focus on Adult Health. Philadelphia, Wolters Kluwer, 2013.)

CLINICAL ALERT

Critical Values

1. <2.5 mEq/L (<2.5 mmol/L) causes ventricular fibrillation.
2. >8.0 mEq/L (>8.0 mmol/L) causes muscle irritability, including myocardial irritability.

Procedure

1. General procedure for potassium (K^+)
   a. Collect a 5-mL venous blood sample using serum or heparinized Vacutainer tube (see Chapter 2, page 52, for venous blood collection). Observe standard/universal precautions. Avoid hemolysis in obtaining the sample.
   b. Label specimen with the patient's name, date, and test(s) ordered. Deliver the sample to the laboratory and centrifuge immediately to separate cells from serum. Potassium leaks out of the cell, and levels in the sample will be falsely elevated later than 4 hours after collection.
2. Procedure for hyperkalemia (excess K^+)
   a. Record fluid intake and output. Check blood volume and venous pressure, which will give clues to dehydration or circulatory overload. Identify ECG changes. In *hyperkalemia*, these include the following:
      (1) Elevated T-wave heart block
      (2) Flattened P wave
      (3) Cardiac arrest may occur without warning other than ECG changes.
   b. Observe for slow pulse, oliguria, neuromuscular alterations such as muscle irritability and impaired muscle function, flaccid paralysis, tremors, and twitching preceding actual paralysis.
   c. Hyperkalemia can be treated with sodium bicarbonate, glucose, and insulin. Kayexalate, a sodium–potassium exchange resin, can be administered orally, nasogastrically, or rectally.
3. Procedure for hypokalemia (deficiency of K^+)
   a. Record fluid intake and output. Check blood volume and venous pressure, which will give clues to circulatory overload or dehydration. Identify ECG changes. In *hypokalemia*, these include the following:
      (1) Depressed T waves
      (2) Peaking of P waves
   b. Observe for dehydration caused by severe vomiting, hyperventilation, sweating, diuresis, or nasogastric tube with gastric suction. Accurately record the state of hydration or dehydration.
   c. Observe for neuromuscular changes such as fatigue, muscle weakness, muscle pain, flabby muscles, paresthesia, hypotension, rapid pulse, respiratory muscle weakness leading to paralysis, cyanosis, respiratory arrest, anorexia, nausea, vomiting, paralytic ileus, apathy, drowsiness, tetany, and coma.
   d. Hypokalemia may be treated with a K^+ rice diet and K^+-sparing diuretics. Use salt substitutes containing potassium chloride and administer IV oral potassium chloride supplements.

Clinical Implications

1. *Decreased blood potassium (hypokalemia) levels* are associated with shifting of K^+ into cells, K^+ loss from GI and biliary tracts, renal K^+ excretion, and reduced K^+ intake, as can occur in the following conditions:
   a. Diarrhea, vomiting, sweating
   b. Starvation, malabsorption
   c. Bartter's syndrome (autosomal-recessive renal tubular disorders)
   d. Draining wounds
   e. CF
   f. Severe burns
   g. Primary aldosteronism
   h. Alcoholism, chronic
   i. Osmotic hyperglycemia
   j. Respiratory alkalosis
   k. Renal tubular acidosis
   l. Diuretic, antibiotic, and mineralocorticoid administration
   m. Barium chloride poisoning
   n. Treatment of megaloblastic anemia with vitamin B_{12} or folic acid

CLINICAL ALERT

1. The most common cause of *hypokalemia* in patients receiving IV fluids is water and sodium chloride administration without adequate replacement for K^+ lost in urine and drainage fluids. A patient receiving IV fluids needs K^+ every day. The minimum adult daily dose should be 40 mEq, but the optimal daily dose ranges between 60 and 120 mEq. (Pediatric dose, 0.5 to 1 mEq/kg of body weight/24 hr, not to exceed 40 mEq/d or 10 mEq/hr.) Potassium needs are greater in persons with tissue injury; wound infection; and gastric, intestinal, or biliary drainage. If adequate amounts of potassium (40 mEq/d) are not given in IV solution, hypokalemia will eventually develop. Patients receiving >10 mEq KCl in 100 mL of IV solution should be monitored by ECG for potential arrhythmia if the IV rate is ≥100/hr. Concentrated doses of IV potassium should always be administered through volume-controlled IV infusion devices. A burning sensation may be felt at the site of needle insertion. Normal saline can be infused along with the potassium, or the IV rate can be reduced. Some healthcare providers order a small dose of lidocaine to be added to IV potassium to eliminate the burning sensation that some patients experience. Always be sure to check for lidocaine allergies before administration of this local anesthetic.
2. Closely monitor for *hypokalemia* in patients taking digitalis and diuretics because cardiac arrhythmias can occur. Hypokalemia enhances the effect of digitalis preparations, creating the possibility of digitalis intoxication from even an average maintenance dose. Digitalis, diuretics, and hypokalemia are a potentially lethal combination.

2. Potassium levels of 3.5 mEq/L (3.5 mmol/L) are more commonly associated with deficiency than with normality. A falling trend (0.1 to 0.2 mEq/day or 0.1 to 0.2 mmol/day) is indicative of a developing potassium deficiency.
   a. The most frequent cause of potassium deficiency is GI loss.
   b. The most frequent cause of potassium depletion is IV fluid administration without adequate potassium supplements.
3. *Increased potassium levels (hyperkalemia)* occur when K^+ shifts from cells to intracellular fluid with inadequate renal excretion and with excessive K^+ intake, as can occur in the following conditions:
   a. Renal failure, dehydration, obstruction, and trauma
   b. Cell damage, as in burns, accidents, surgery, chemotherapy, disseminated intravascular coagulation (damaged cells release potassium into the blood)
   c. Metabolic acidosis (drives potassium out of the cells), diabetic ketoacidosis
   d. Addison's disease
   e. Pseudohypoaldosteronism
   f. Uncontrolled diabetes, decreased insulin
   g. Primary acquired hyperkalemia, such as in SLE, sickle cell disease, interstitial nephritis, and tubular disorders
   h. Kidney transplant rejection

CLINICAL ALERT

The following arrhythmias can occur with *hyperkalemia:*

1. Sinus bradycardia
2. Sinus arrest
3. First-degree atrioventricular block
4. Nodal rhythm

5. Idioventricular rhythm
6. Ventricular tachycardia
7. Ventricular fibrillation
8. Ventricular arrest

The following arrhythmias can occur with *hypokalemia:*

1. Ventricular premature beats
2. Atrial tachycardia
3. Nodal tachycardia
4. Ventricular tachycardia
5. Ventricular fibrillation

Interfering Factors

1. Hemolyzed blood may not be used; K^+ values are elevated to as much as 50% over normal with moderate hemolysis. Opening and closing the fist 10 times with a tourniquet in place results in an increase in potassium level by 10% to 20%. For this reason, it is recommended that the blood sample be obtained without a tourniquet or that the tourniquet be released after the needle has entered the vein.
2. Drug usage
   a. IV administration of potassium penicillin may cause hyperkalemia; penicillin sodium may cause increased excretion of potassium.
   b. Glucose administered during tolerance testing or the ingestion and administration of large amounts of glucose in patients with heart disease may cause a decrease of as much as 0.4 mEq/L (0.4 mmol/L) in potassium blood levels.
   c. A number of drugs raise potassium levels, especially potassium-sparing diuretics and nonsteroidal anti-inflammatory drugs, especially in the presence of renal disease.
   d. Excessive intake of licorice decreases potassium levels.
3. Leukocytosis, as occurs in leukemia, raises potassium levels.
4. Patients who have thrombocytosis due to polycythemia vera or a myeloproliferative disease may have spuriously high potassium levels. This falsely elevated level is caused by a high number of platelets, which release potassium during coagulation. Therefore, heparinized samples, rather than clotted serum samples, should be used in these patients.

Interventions

Pretest Patient Care

1. Explain test purpose and blood-drawing procedure. Do not have patient open and close fist while drawing blood.
2. Follow guidelines in Chapter 1 for safe, effective, informed *pretest* care.

Posttest Patient Care

1. Review test results; report and record findings. Modify the nursing care plan as needed. Monitor changes in body potassium and intervene as appropriate.
2. Recognizing signs and symptoms of hypokalemia and hyperkalemia is very important. Many of these originate in the nervous and muscular systems and are usually nonspecific and similar.
3. Remember that the potassium blood level increases 0.6 mEq/L (0.6 mmol/L) for every 0.1 decrease in blood pH.
4. Follow guidelines in Chapter 1 for safe, effective, informed *posttest* care.

● Sodium (Na^+)

Sodium is the most abundant cation (90% of the electrolyte fluid) and, as such, plays an important role in maintaining osmotic pressure and acid–base balance. Mechanisms for maintaining a constant sodium level in the plasma and extracellular fluid include renal blood flow, carbonic anhydrase enzyme activity, aldosterone, action of other steroids whose plasma level is controlled by the anterior pituitary gland, renin enzyme secretion, antidiuretic hormone (ADH), and vasopressin secretion.

Sodium levels are measured in order to determine acid–base balance and fluid balance (water intoxication and dehydration).

Reference Values

Normal

Adults: 136 to 145 mEq/L (136 to 145 mmol/L)
Children (1 to 16 years): 136 to 145 mEq/L (136 to 145 mmol/L)
Full-term infants: 133 to 142 mEq/L (133 to 142 mmol/L)
Premature infants: 132 to 140 mEq/L (132 to 140 mmol/L)

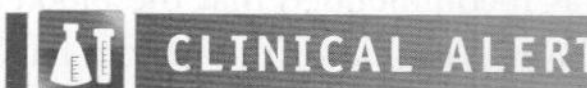

Critical Values

1. <125 mEq/L (<125 mmol/L) causes weakness and dehydration.
2. 90–105 mEq/L (90–105 mmol/L) causes severe neurologic symptoms and vascular problems.
3. >152 mEq/L (>152 mmol/L) results in cardiovascular and renal symptoms.
4. >160 mEq/L (>160 mmol/L) can cause heart failure.

Procedure

1. Obtain a 5-mL venous blood sample in an SST or red-topped tube. Heparinized blood can be used. Avoid hemolysis. Centrifuge for red-topped tube only and transfer serum to a plastic transport tube.
2. Observe standard/universal precautions.

Clinical Implications

1. *Hyponatremia* (decreased sodium levels) reflects a relative excess of body water rather than low total-body sodium. *Reduced* sodium levels (hyponatremia) are associated with the following conditions:
   a. Severe burns
   b. Congestive heart failure (predictor of cardiac mortality)
   c. Excessive fluid loss (e.g., severe diarrhea, vomiting, sweating)
   d. Excessive IV induction of nonelectrolyte fluids (e.g., glucose)
   e. Addison's disease (impairs sodium reabsorption)
   f. Severe nephritis (nephrotic syndrome)
   g. Pyloric obstruction
   h. Malabsorption syndrome
   i. Diabetic acidosis
   j. Drugs such as diuretics
   k. Edema (dilutional hyponatremia)
   l. Large amounts of water by mouth (water intoxication)

   m. Stomach suction accompanied by water or ice chips by mouth
   n. Hypothyroidism
   o. Excessive ADH production. Also known as vasopressin, ADH is secreted from the posterior pituitary gland.
2. *Hypernatremia* (increased sodium levels) is uncommon, but when it does occur, it is associated with the following conditions:
   a. Dehydration and insufficient water intake
   b. Primary aldosteronism (Conn's syndrome)
   c. Coma
   d. Cushing's disease
   e. Diabetes insipidus
   f. Tracheobronchitis

Interfering Factors

1. Many drugs affect levels of blood sodium.
   a. Anabolic steroids, corticosteroids, calcium, fluorides, and iron can cause increases in sodium level.
   b. Heparin, laxatives, sulfates, and diuretics can cause decreases in sodium level.
2. High triglycerides or low protein causes artificially low sodium values.

Interventions

Pretest Patient Care

1. Explain test purpose and procedure.
2. Follow guidelines in Chapter 1 for safe, effective, informed *pretest* care.

Posttest Patient Care

1. Review test results; report and record findings. Modify the nursing care plan as needed. Monitor for fluid and sodium imbalances.
2. Remember that IV therapy considerations are as follows:
   a. Sodium balance is maintained in adults with an average dietary intake of 90 to 250 mEq/day (90 to 250 mmol/day). The maximal daily tolerance to an acute load is 400 mEq/day (400 mmol/day). A patient who is given 3 L of isotonic saline in 24 hours will receive 465 mEq (465 mmol) of sodium. This amount exceeds the average, healthy adult's tolerance level. It will take a *healthy* person 24 to 48 hours to excrete the excess sodium.
   b. After surgery, trauma, or shock, there is a decrease in extracellular fluid volume. Replacement of extracellular fluid is essential if water and electrolyte balance is to be maintained. The ideal replacement IV solution should have a sodium concentration of 140 mEq/L (140 mmol/L).
3. Monitor for signs of edema or hypertension and record and report these if present.
4. Follow guidelines in Chapter 1 for safe, effective, informed *posttest* care.

● Osmolality and Water-Load Test (Water-Loading Antidiuretic Hormone [ADH] Suppression Test)

Osmolality, which is the measure of the number of dissolved solute particles in solution, increases with dehydration and decreases with overhydration. In general, the same conditions that reduce or increase serum sodium affect osmolality.

This test is used as an evaluation of water and electrolyte balance. It is helpful in assessing hydration status, seizures, liver disease, ADH function, and coma, and it is used in toxicology workups for ethanol, ethylene glycol, isopropanol, and methanol ingestions.

Reference Values

Normal

Serum Osmolality

Adults: 280 to 303 mOsm/kg H_2O (280 to 303 mmol/kg H_2O)
Newborns: as low as 266 mOsm/kg H_2O (266 mmol/kg H_2O)

Urine Osmolality

Adults

24-hour: 300 to 900 mOsm/kg H_2O (300 to 900 mmol/kg H_2O)
Random: 50 to 1400 mOsm/kg H_2O (50 to 1400 mmol/kg H_2O)
After 12-hour fluid restriction: >850 mOsm/kg H_2O (>850 mmol/kg H_2O)
Ratio of urine/serum osmolality: 0.2 to 4.7 (average, 1.0 to 3.0)
Ratio after fluid restriction: 3:1 or a range of 0.2 to 4.7:1

Osmolal Gap

Serum: 5 to 10 mOsm/kg H_2O (5 to 10 mmol/kg H_2O)
Urine: 80 to 100 mOsm/kg H_2O (80 to 100 mmol/kg H_2O)

NOTE *The simultaneous determination of urine and serum osmolalities facilitates interpretation of results. High urinary/serum (U/S) ratio is seen in concentrated urine. Normal ranges for the U/S ratio are 0.2 to 4.7 and may be >3.0 with overnight dehydration. With poor concentrating ability, the ratio is low but is still >1.0. In SIADH, sodium and urine osmolalities are high for the serum osmolality.*

NOTE *The determination of the urine osmolal gap is used to characterize metabolic acidosis and is described as the sum of urinary concentrations of sodium, potassium, bicarbonate, chloride, glucose, and urea compared with measured urine osmolality.*

CLINICAL ALERT

Critical Values

<240 or >321 mOsm/kg H_2O (<240 or >321 mmol/kg H_2O)
>385 mOsm/kg H_2O (>385 mmol/kg H_2O) is seen with symptoms of stupor in hyperglycemia.
400–420 mOsm/kg H_2O (400–420 mmol/kg H_2O) is associated with grand mal seizures.
>420 mOsm/kg H_2O (>420 mmol/kg H_2O) is often fatal.

Procedure

1. Determining osmolality
   a. Obtain a 5-mL venous blood sample in an SST or red-topped tube. Serum or heparinized plasma is acceptable. Observe standard/universal precautions. Label samples with the patient's name, date, and test(s) ordered.
   b. Collect a 24-hour urine specimen (see Chapter 3) concurrently and keep refrigerated.
   c. Determine osmolality in the laboratory using the freezing point depression methodology for both serum and urine.
2. Determining water-loading ADH suppression
   a. The ideal position during the testing period is the recumbent position because the response to water loading is reduced in persons in the upright position.
   b. One hour before testing, the patient is given 300 mL of water to replace fluid lost during the overnight fast. Do not count this water as part of the test load.

c. Have the patient drink a test load of water (20 mL/kg body weight) within 30 minutes.
d. After the test load of water is consumed, collect all urine for the next 4 to 5 hours, and check each voiding for volume osmolality and specific gravity. Obtain hourly blood samples for osmolality, and check the entire volume of urine obtained for osmolality.

3. Remember that normal values for water-loading ADH suppression test are excretion of >90% (>0.90) of water load within 4 hours. Urine osmolality falls to <100 mOsm/kg (<100 mmol/kg). Specific gravity falls to 1.001.
4. Determine plasma ADH at hourly intervals.

Clinical Implications

Decreased Renal Function

1. In *decreased renal function*, <80% of fluid is excreted, and urine specific gravity may not fall below 1.010. This phenomenon occurs in the following conditions:
   a. Adrenocortical insufficiency
   b. Malabsorption syndrome
   c. Edema
   d. Ascites
   e. Obesity
   f. Hypothyroidism
   g. Dehydration
   h. Congestive heart failure
   i. Cirrhosis
2. Disorders with *increased ADH secretion (SIADH)* give an inadequate response; <90% of water is excreted, and urine osmolality remains >100 mOsm/kg H_2O (>100 mmol/kg H_2O). Plasma ADH measured at 90 minutes confirms diagnosis of SIADH.

Hyperosmolality and Hypo-osmolality

1. *Increased values (hyperosmolality)* are associated with the following conditions:
   a. Dehydration
   b. Hypercalcemia
   c. Diabetes mellitus, hyperglycemia, diabetic ketoacidosis
   d. Hypernatremia
   e. Cerebral lesions
   f. Alcohol ingestion (ethanol, methanol, ethylene glycol)
   g. Mannitol therapy
   h. Azotemia (high levels of nitrogen-containing compounds; e.g., urea or creatinine)
   i. Inadequate water intake
   j. Chronic renal disease
2. *Decreased values (hypo-osmolality)* are associated with the following conditions:
   a. Loss of sodium with diuretics and low-salt diet (hyponatremia)
   b. Renal failure
   c. Adrenocortical insufficiency
   d. Inappropriate secretion of ADH, as may occur in trauma and lung cancer
   e. Excessive water replacement (overhydration, water intoxication)
   f. Panhypopituitarism
   g. Diabetes insipidus (central or nephrogenic)
   h. Pyelonephritis

Osmolal Gap

1. Abnormal levels (>10 mOsm/kg H_2O or >10 mmol/kg H_2O) can occur in the following conditions:
   a. Methanol
   b. Ethanol

c. Isopropyl alcohol
d. Mannitol
e. Severely ill patients, especially those in shock, lactic acidosis, and renal failure
2. Ethanol glycol, acetone, and paraldehyde have relatively small osmolal gaps, even at lethal levels.

Interfering Factors

Osmolal Gap

1. Decreases in osmolal gap are associated with altitude, diurnal variation with water retention at night, and some drugs.
2. Some drugs also cause increases in osmolal gap.
3. Hypertriglyceridemia and hyperproteinemia cause an elevated osmolal gap.
4. Radiographic contrast medium within 3 days

Interventions

Pretest Patient Care

Decreased Renal Function

1. Explain the test purpose and procedure. The test takes 5 to 6 hours to complete.
2. Do not allow food, alcohol, medications, or smoking for 8 to 10 hours before testing. No muscular exercise is allowed during the test.
3. The patient may experience nausea, abdominal fullness, fatigue, and desire to defecate.
4. Discard first morning urine specimen.
5. Follow guidelines in Chapter 1 for safe, effective, informed *pretest* care.

Hyperosmolality, Hypo-osmolality, Osmolar Gap

1. Explain test purpose and procedure.
2. Ensure that no alcohol is ingested during the 24 hours before the test.
3. Follow guidelines in Chapter 1 for safe, effective, informed *pretest* care.

Posttest Patient Care

Decreased Renal Function

1. Observe for adverse reactions to water-loading test such as extreme abdominal discomfort, shortness of breath, or chest pain.
2. Remember that if water clearance is impaired, the water load will not induce diuresis, and maximum urinary dilution will not occur.
3. Accurate results may not be obtained if nausea, vomiting, or diarrhea occurs or if a disturbance in bladder emptying is present. Note on chart if any of these effects occur.
4. Follow guidelines in Chapter 1 for safe, effective, informed *posttest* care.

CLINICAL ALERT

In patients with impaired ability to tolerate the water-loading test, seizures or fatal hyponatremia may occur.

Hyperosmolality, Hypo-osmolality, Osmolar Gap

1. Review test results; report and record findings. Modify the nursing care plan as needed. A patient receiving IV fluids should have a normal osmolality. If the osmolality increases, the fluids contain relatively more electrolytes than water. If it falls, relatively more water than electrolytes is present.
2. Remember that if the ratio of serum sodium to serum osmolality falls below 0.43, the outlook is guarded. This ratio may be distorted in cases of drug intoxication.
3. Follow guidelines in Chapter 1 for safe, effective, informed *posttest* care.

Sweat Test

This test is the *gold standard* for diagnosing CF. CF is a genetic disease affecting >30,000 children and adults in the United States, occurring in 1 out of every 3900 live births. More than 80% of cases are diagnosed by age 3 years, and 10% of diagnoses occur in persons older than 18 years. It has been recommended that the sweat test be performed in a laboratory accredited by the Cystic Fibrosis Foundation. It has been estimated that >10 million Americans are unknowing carriers of the defective CF gene.

Abnormally high concentrations of sodium and chloride appear in the secretions of eccrine sweat glands in persons with CF. This condition is present at birth and persists throughout life. This study uses sweat-inducing techniques (e.g., pilocarpine iontophoresis) followed by chemical analysis to determine sodium, chloride, and content of collected sweat.

Reference Values

Sweat Sodium
Normal: <70 mEq/L (<70 mmol/L)
CF: >90 mEq/L (>90 mmol/L)

Sweat Chloride
Normal: <40 mEq/L (<40 mmol/L)
Borderline: 40 to 60 mEq/L (40 to 60 mmol/L)
CF: >60 mEq/L (>60 mmol/L)

Procedure

1. The forearm is the preferred site for stimulation of sweating, but in thin or small babies, the thigh, back, or leg may be used. It may be necessary to stimulate sweating in two places to obtain sufficient sweat for testing, especially in young infants. At least 100 μL of sweat is necessary. In cold weather, or if the testing room is cold, a warm covering should be placed over the arm or other site of sweat collection.
2. Stimulate sweat production by applying gauze pads or filter paper saturated with a measured amount of pilocarpine and attachment of electrodes through which a current of 4 to 5 mA is delivered at intervals for a total of 5 minutes (a total of 5 to 12 minutes, according to the National Institutes of Health).
3. Remove the electrodes and pad, and thoroughly wash the area with distilled water; dry carefully.
4. Remember that successful iontophoresis is indicated by a red area about 2.5 cm in diameter that appears where the electrode was placed.
5. Scrub the skin thoroughly with distilled water and dry carefully. The area for sweat collection must be completely dry, free from contamination by powder or antiseptic, and free of any area that might ooze.
6. Collection of sweat occurs by applying preweighed filter paper or sweat collection cups that are taped securely over the red spot. The inside surfaces of the collecting device should never be touched.
7. Leave the paper on for at least 1 hour before removing and then place in a preweighed flask to avoid evaporation. Weigh the flask again. The desired volume of sweat is 200 mg; the minimum volume necessary is 100 mg.
8. If a cup is used, leave in place for 1 hour and then carefully remove by scraping it across the iontophoresed area. This "puddles" the sweat in the cup to reduce evaporation and to redissolve any salts left by the evaporation. Use suction capillary tubes to remove sweat from the collection cups.

Clinical Implications

1. Children with CF have sodium and chloride values >90 mEq/L and >60 mEq/L (>90 mmol/L and >60 mmol/L), respectively.
2. Borderline or gray-zone cases are those with values of 70 to 90 mEq/L (70 to 90 mmol/L) for sodium and 40 to 60 mEq/L (50 to 60 mmol/L) for chloride. These persons require retesting. Potassium values do not assist in differentiating borderline cases.

3. In adolescence and adulthood, chloride levels >80 mEq/L (>80 mmol/L) usually indicate CF.
4. Elevated sweat electrolytes also can be associated with the following conditions:
   a. Addison's disease
   b. Congenital adrenal hyperplasia
   c. Vasopressin-resistant diabetes insipidus
   d. Glucose-6-phosphatase dehydrogenase (G6PD) deficiency
   e. Hypothyroidism
   f. Familial hypoparathyroidism
   g. Alcoholic pancreatitis

Interfering Factors

1. The sweat test is not valuable after puberty because levels may vary over a very wide range among individuals.
2. Dehydration and edema, particularly of areas where sweat is collected, may interfere with test results.
3. A gap >30 mEq/L (>30 mmol/L) between sodium and chloride values indicates calculation or analysis error or contamination of the sample.
4. Sweat testing is not considered accurate until the third or fourth week of life because infants <3 weeks of age may not sweat enough to provide a sufficient sample.
5. Test may be falsely normal in patients with salt depletion, as in periods of hot weather.

CLINICAL ALERT

1. The test should always be repeated if the results, the clinical features, or other diagnostic tests do not fit together.
2. The test can be used to exclude the diagnosis of CF in siblings of diagnosed patients.
3. There have been reports of CF patients with normal sweat electrolyte levels.
4. Sweat potassium testing is not diagnostically valuable.

Interventions

Pretest Patient Care

1. Explain test purpose and procedure. The sweat test is indicated for the following persons:
   a. Infants who pass initial meconium late; who have intestinal obstruction, failure to thrive, steatorrhea, chronic diarrhea, rapid respiration and retraction with chronic cough, asthma, hypoproteinemia (especially on soybean formula), atelectasis, or hyperaeration on x-ray, hyperprothrombinemia, or rectal prolapse; who taste salty; or who are offspring of a parent with CF (i.e., the obligate heterozygote)
   b. Persons suspected of having CF or celiac disease, all siblings of patients with CF, or persons with disaccharide intolerance, recurrent pneumonia, chronic atelectasis, chronic pulmonary disease, bronchiolectasis, chronic cough, nasal polyposis, cirrhosis of the liver, and hypertension
   c. Any parents who request a sweat test on their child
2. Inform the patient that a slight stinging sensation is usually experienced, especially in fair-skinned persons.
3. Follow guidelines in Chapter 1 regarding safe, effective, informed *pretest* care.

Posttest Patient Care

1. After the cup is removed, carefully wash and dry the skin to prevent irritation caused by collection cups.
2. Have the patient resume normal activities.

3. Review test results; report and record findings. Modify the nursing care plan as needed. Counsel and monitor the patient as appropriate. Provide genetic counseling. CF is transmitted as an autosomal-recessive trait. The Caucasian carrier rate is 1 in 20, and the African American carrier rate is 1 in 60 to 1 in 100.
4. Treatment of CF includes chest physiotherapy to clear mucus secretions, antibiotics (e.g., aerosolized tobramycin or azithromycin), and mucus-thinning drugs (e.g., Pulmozyme).
5. Follow guidelines in Chapter 1 for safe, effective, informed *posttest* care.

BIBLIOGRAPHY

American Thoracic Society/European Respiratory Society Task Force: Interpretative strategies for lung function tests. Eur Respir J 26:948–968, 2005

American Thoracic Society/European Respiratory Society Task Force: Standardisation of spirometry. Eur Respir J 26:319–338, 2005

American Thoracic Society/European Respiratory Society Task Force: Standardisation of the measurement of lung volumes. Eur Respir J 26:511–522, 2005

American Thoracic Society/European Respiratory Society Task Force: Standardisation of the single-breath determination of carbon monoxide uptake in the lung. Eur Respir J 26:720–735, 2005

Crolla LJ, Maley T, Brunelle J: Blood gas measurements: It's all about quality control. Clin Lab News 31:12–13, 2005

Dunning MB: Respiratory physiology. In Raff H (ed): Physiology Secrets, 2nd ed. Philadelphia, Hanley & Belfus, 2003

Groer M: Advanced Pathophysiology: Applications to Clinical Practice. Philadelphia, Lippincott Williams & Wilkins, 2001

Grossman S, Porth C: Porth's Pathophysiology: Concepts of Altered Health States, 9th ed. Philadelphia, Lippincott Williams & Wilkins, 2013

Guyton AC, Hall J: Textbook of Medical Physiology, 13th ed. Philadelphia, Elsevier Saunders, 2015

Heitz UE, Horne MM: Pocket Guide to Fluid, Electrolyte, and Acid-Base Balance, 5th ed. Philadelphia, Elsevier Mosby Saunders, 2005

Huether SE, McCance KL: Understanding Pathophysiology, 6th ed. Philadelphia, Elsevier Mosby Saunders, 2016

Jardins TD: Clinical Manifestations & Assessment of Respiratory Disease, 7th ed. St. Louis, Mosby, 2015

Keefe S: Sufficient saturation: Cerebral and somatic oximetry provides noninvasive, real-time monitoring of regional saturation of oxygen. Advance for Nurses 4(26):21–22, 2006

Levin KP, Hanusa BH, Rotondi A, et al: Arterial blood gas and pulse oximetry in initial management of patients with community-acquired pneumonia. J Gen Intern Med 16:590–598, 2001

Malley WJ: Clinical Blood Gases: Assessment and Intervention, 2nd ed. Philadelphia, Elsevier Mosby Saunders, 2005

Medline Plus: Health Information. U.S. National Library of Medicine. Available at: www.nlm.nih.gov/medlineplus

Moloney ED, Kiely JL, McNicholas WT. Controlled oxygen therapy and carbon dioxide retention during exacerbations of COPD. The Lancet 357(9255):526–528, 2001

Mottram C: Ruppel's Manual of Pulmonary Function Testing, 10th ed. St. Louis, Mosby, 2012

Murphy R, Driscoll P, O'Driscoll R. Emergency oxygen therapy for the COPD patient. Emerg Med J 18:333–339, 2001

Porth CM: Essentials of Pathophysiology: Concepts of Altered Health States, 4th ed. Philadelphia, Lippincott Williams & Wilkins, 2014

Shapiro BA, Peruzzi WT, Templin RK: Clinical Application of Blood Gases, 5th ed. St. Louis, CV Mosby, 1994

Wasserman K, Hansen JE, Sue DY, et al: Principles of Exercise Testing and Interpretation: Including Pathophysiology and Clinical Applications, 5th ed. Philadelphia, Lippincott Williams & Wilkins, 2011

Prenatal Diagnosis and Tests of Fetal Well-Being

15

OVERVIEW OF PRENATAL DIAGNOSIS

Fetal well-being depends on maternal health (see Chapter 6, page 336 for gestational diabetes screening). Many routine prenatal tests assess maternal health and well-being. Prenatal testing usually includes a complete blood count or hemoglobin and hematocrit, Rh type and ABO blood group, red cell antibody screening, rubella immunity status, glucose challenge testing (see Chapter 6), urinalysis, maternal serum alpha$_1$-fetoprotein (MS-AFP) or maternal quadruple marker test or quad screen, hepatitis B testing, culture for sexually transmitted diseases, the syphilis immunoglobulin G (IgG) test, and surveillance for group B streptococci. Screening for HIV infection is recommended for all pregnant women to improve the care of HIV-positive women and to identify infants at risk; perinatal transmission is the primary route of HIV infection in children.

Tests in this chapter monitor the status of the maternal–fetal unit, identify the fetus at risk for intrauterine asphyxia, aid in the early diagnosis of infection, and identify genetic and biochemical disorders and major anomalies. (See Chapter 11 for more on genetic disorders.) Tests are also performed to predict normal fetal outcome or to identify the fetus at risk for asphyxia during labor (Table 15.1).

Noninvasive prenatal testing for fetal aneuploidy is available for women at increased risk of aneuploidy. Extraction of fetal cells from the maternal circulation (fetal cell sorting) is performed for screening of trisomy 21, 18, and 13, although it does not replace the need for diagnosis by chorionic villus sampling (CVS) or amniocentesis.

FIRST AND SECOND TRIMESTER SCREENING

First trimester screening provides early testing for aneuploidy between 11 and 13 weeks. Screening includes biochemical markers for pregnancy-associated plasma protein A (PAPP-A), free β human chorionic gonadotropin (hCG), and ultrasound measurement of fetal nuchal translucency (FNT). The detection rate for first trimester screening is 80%, with false-positive rate of 5%. First trimester combined screening can also screen for trisomy 18, and NT alone may detect trisomy 18, trisomy 13, and other chromosomal abnormalities. The maternal triple or quadruple screen tests are offered to pregnant women during their second trimester to identify risks for chromosome disorders such as Down syndrome (trisomy 21); major birth defects, including open neural tube defects such as spina bifida; placental insufficiency; and oligohydramnios. The evaluation consists of three or four separate blood protein tests done on maternal serum between 15 and 21 weeks of gestation: MS-AFP is decreased in Down syndrome and neural tube defects, unconjugated estriol (E_3) is decreased in Down syndrome, and β-hCG is increased in Down syndrome. Results are reported as *multiples of the median* (MoM). The triple screen detection rate for Down syndrome is approximately 69% (false-positive rate of 5%), 80% for neural tube defects, and 60% for trisomy 18 (false-positive rate of 0.2%). The detection rate for Down syndrome with quadruple screen is 81%. Combining first and second trimester screening improves the detection rate to 94% to 96%, with a 5% false-positive rate. Quad screen includes AFP, hCG, E_3, and inhibin A.

The maternal triple and quadruple tests are screening tests; therefore, an abnormal (positive) result is not diagnostic, and further testing with ultrasound, amniocentesis, and genetic counseling is indicated. The markers can be positive in normal variations such as multiple births or miscalculated gestational age.

Ultrasound testing is a method of assessing fetal well-being that has become a diagnostic tool for assessment of fetal age, health, growth, and identification of anomalies. Level I ultrasound assesses gestational age, number of fetuses, fetal death, and the condition of the placenta. Level II ultrasound assesses specific congenital anomalies or abnormalities. In some diagnostic centers, fetal echocardiography is also available. An additional ultrasound marker for Down syndrome is the absence or hypoplasia of nasal bones in fetuses at 11 to 14 weeks' gestation. When combining this marker

TABLE 15.1 Maternal Fetal Testing During Pregnancy

Tests and Procedures	Indications	Follow-Up and Interventions for Positive Test Results
First Trimester (1–14 wk)		
Human chorionic gonadotropin (hCG) levels	Confirm normal progress of pregnancy or if suspected for ectopic pregnancy, threatened or missed abortion, or to monitor success of insemination or in vitro fertilization	Levels increase 66% or double every 36–48 hr; if levels off or decline, may be ectopic or miscarriage. Usually, two tests are done 48 hr apart and often follow-up with ultrasound. Dramatic increase may indicate multiple fetuses.
Prenatal Profile		
Complete blood count (CBC) or hemoglobin/hematocrit (Hb/Hct)	Detection of anemia defined by the Centers for Disease Control and Prevention as below 11/33 in first trimester. CBC with red blood cell (RBC) indices for detection of carrier state of hemoglobinopathies	Anemia is treated with iron supplementation. Follow-up test is repeated at 28 wk and as indicated. Hb electrophoresis, Sickledex, or high-powered liquid chromatography and isoelectric focusing for those at risk for hemoglobinopathies: African Americans (sickle cell disease); Italian, Greek, or Corsican (β-thalassemia); and Southeast Asian (α-thalassemia)
ABO, Rh	Blood typing to identify Rh-negative women and ABO group for incompatibility	Intervention for Rh-negative women is to receive Rh immunoglobulin (RhoGAM) prophylaxis. Identification of type O women for consideration of ABO incompatibility in neonatal jaundice
Rubella immunity status	Identify nonimmune women to avoid possible exposure to rubella and report any possible exposure; considered immune if there is a documented dose of rubella vaccine or an immune serologic test result	Instruction to nonimmune women to report exposure to rubella for immunoglobulin prophylaxis; immunization is recommended postpartum.
HIV	All should be counseled for screening to reduce perinatal transmission to infant.	Positive results indicate need to recommend antiretroviral treatment and discussion about possible cesarean delivery to reduce perinatal transmission as well as avoidance of breast-feeding if indicated. Follow-up testing may be needed for high-risk individuals.
Syphilis antibody immunoglobulin G (IgG)	Identify syphilis infection in pregnant women to reduce fetal infection	Positive result indicates need for treatment with penicillin or other antibiotic if allergy exists.

table continues on pg. 971 >

TABLE 15.1, continued

Tests and Procedures	Indications	Follow-Up and Interventions for Positive Test Results
Venereal Disease Research Laboratory		Follow-up testing may be needed for high-risk individuals.
Hepatitis B surface antigen	All pregnant women should be screened to identify chronic disease carriers.	Follow-up includes immunization of those with negative test but considered high risk for acquiring hepatitis B during pregnancy, and positive results indicate need to immunize infant with hepatitis B immune globulin and hepatitis B vaccine as soon as possible after birth.
Antibody screen	All pregnant women should be screened to identify isoimmunized women.	If positive result, test is repeated to identify specific maternal antibody (e.g., anti-D, C, c, E, e, Kell, Duffy, Kidd).
Varicella status	All pregnant women unless reliable history of varicella as a measure of immunity	If nonimmune and with history of exposure, needs varicella titer within 24–48 hr; if needed, varicella-zoster immune globulin given within 96–144 hr of exposure. Varicella vaccine can be given postpartum.
Papanicolaou test	All pregnant women without a documented normal Pap test within the past 6 mo	Positive results may need follow-up with a colposcopy or repeat Pap test. Most often, treatment is delayed until postpartum.
Urinalysis, urine culture	All pregnant women are screened for asymptomatic bacteriuria.	Positive results of >100,000 colonies of single organism should be treated and high-risk patients screened each trimester.
For At-Risk Patients		
Wet prep	All pregnant women at risk for preterm birth	Positive clue cells, trichomonads, or *Candida* indicates need for treatment.
Gonorrhea	Pregnant women with risk factors	Positive results should be treated with appropriate antibiotic therapy, and test of cure should be obtained.
Chlamydia	Pregnant women with risk factors	Positive results should be treated with appropriate antibiotic therapy, and test of cure should be obtained.
Genital herpes culture if active lesion	All pregnant women with active lesion	Positive test may be treated with antiviral medication, and patient may be counseled regarding risks and benefits of cesarean delivery.
Tuberculosis test	High-risk pregnant women or symptomatic	Follow-up may include chest x-ray with shielding preferred after 12 wk and treatment with medications during pregnancy.

table continues on pg. 972 >

TABLE 15.1, continued

Tests and Procedures	Indications	Follow-Up and Interventions for Positive Test Results
Chorionic villus sampling (CVS)	Pregnant women at risk for fetal genetic or biochemical disorders or those with abnormal ultrasound	Positive test requires follow-up genetic counseling or discussion of treatment options.
Fetal nuchal translucency (FNT; may be combined with pregnancy-associated plasma protein A [PAPP-A], β-hCG to increase detection rate)	Any pregnant woman presenting by 11–13 wk can be screened, particularly desired screening for Down syndrome, trisomy 13, trisomy 18, Turner's syndrome.	Positive test follow-up with counseling regarding CVS or amniocentesis for definitive diagnosis. Positive test can be associated with other fetal conditions if no chromosomal abnormality.
Fetal cell-free nucleic acids—screening test to detect trisomy 13, 18, or 21	At-risk women include age 35 yr or older, ultrasound findings show increased risk for aneuploidy, history of a child with trisomy, or positive first or second trimester screening. Can be offered after 10 wk of gestation	Positive test indicates need for genetic counseling and further testing for confirmation of test results.
Carrier testing for cystic fibrosis (CF). American Congress of Obstetricians and Gynecologists (ACOG) recommends standard screening test should include 25 disease-causing mutations for CF	ACOG recommends that all pregnant women of northern European and Ashkenazi Jewish origin be offered carrier testing for CF as standard of care. Also, individuals with family history of CF, reproductive partners of individuals with CF, couples with one or both Caucasian partners who are pregnant or planning a pregnancy	Genetic counseling for positive test Those with a negative screening should be aware that they may be a carrier for mutation not included in the test.
Ultrasound	Pregnancy confirmation Viability, rule out (R/O) ectopic pregnancy, gestational age, fetal assessment	Follow-up ultrasound level I or II
PAPP-A	Screening for chromosomal abnormalities (can be used in combined testing with FNT and β-hCG based on maternal age)	Lower in pregnancies if fetus has Down syndrome
Preimplantation genetic diagnosis	Genetic testing of an early embryo at 6- to 8-cell stage (3 d after fertilization) examined for aneuploidy, structural chromosomal abnormalities, single-gene disorders, X-linked disorders	Embryos are implanted after genetic testing rules out abnormalities.
Gestational glucose screening—1 hr	Screening for gestational diabetes risk	Positive tests require a 3-hr oral (100 g) glucose tolerance test for diagnosis of gestational diabetes.

table continues on pg. 973 >

TABLE 15.1, continued

Tests and Procedures	Indications	Follow-Up and Interventions for Positive Test Results
Second Trimester (15–28 wk)		
Triple screen (hCG, unconjugated estriol [uE_3], maternal serum alpha-fetoprotein [AFP]) *Quadruple screen* adds inhibin A	Screening for Down syndrome, trisomy 18, and possibly Turner's syndrome, triploidy, Smith-Lemli-Opitz syndrome. Low inhibin A increases the detection of Down syndrome and trisomy 18.	Genetic counseling, evaluation by perinatologist, possibly level II ultrasound and amniocentesis
Amniocentesis	Amniotic fluid studies of fetal genetics to identify abnormalities, karyotyping to identify chromosomal disorders	Genetic counseling
Ultrasound 18–20 wk, level I or II	Facilitate amniocentesis, determine or confirm estimated date of delivery and fetal viability, R/O abnormal pregnancy, intrauterine growth retardation (IUGR), congenital anomalies, oligo- or polyhydramnios. Identify placental location, cervical length, multiple gestation, amniotic fluid index (AFI) Level II: assess specific anomalies in fetal anatomy such as congenital heart defects, omphalocele, anencephaly; identify ultrasound markers that increase risk for genetic abnormalities	Positive results may require repeat or serial ultrasound evaluations, MRI, 3D or 4D ultrasound, or genetic counseling.
Umbilical artery Doppler tests	Identify abnormal placental function in at-risk pregnancies such as pregnancy-induced hypertension, IUGR. Identify fetal acidosis, hypoxia.	Positive results may indicate need for further monitoring or need to deliver infant.
Fetoscopy	Identify fetal developmental defects, blood disorders such as hemophilia A and B, sickle cell anemia; perform therapeutic interventions, sample fetal tissue	Positive results may require interventions or need for care conference for plan of delivery of abnormal infant.
Percutaneous umbilical blood sampling	Need for fetal blood sampling with less risk than fetoscopy. Identify such disorders as hemophilia, hemoglobinopathies, infections, drug levels, chromosomal abnormalities, cord blood pH.	Positive results may indicate need for treatment, immediate delivery, or genetic counseling.

table continues on pg. 974 >

TABLE 15.1, continued

Tests and Procedures	Indications	Follow-Up and Interventions for Positive Test Results
Serum-Integrated Screening		
PAPP-A from first trimester screening Alpha fetoprotein monoclonal antibody (AFP3), inhibin A in second trimester	Prenatal screening for Down syndrome	Genetic counseling, evaluation by perinatologist, possibly level II ultrasound and amniocentesis
Fully Integrated Screening		
FNT and PAPP-A in first trimester AFP3, inhibin A in second trimester	Prenatal screening for Down syndrome	Genetic counseling, evaluation by perinatologist, possibly level II ultrasound and amniocentesis
Third Trimester (29–40 wk)		
Fetal fibronectin	With symptoms of preterm labor, if intact membranes and <3 cm dilation, may help to predict preterm delivery	Positive results predict probable delivery in next 7–14 d.
Nonstress test, contraction stress test, oxytocin challenge test, breast stimulation test, fetal activity acceleration determination	Assess fetal heart rate (FHR) in response to fetal movement or contractions to assess fetal well-being, fetal hypoxia, tolerance to labor	Positive result may indicate need for further testing, induction of labor, or immediate delivery.
Biophysical profile	Used in high-risk pregnancy to assess fetal well-being or diagnose fetal hypoxia or distress	Positive result may indicate need for further testing, induction of labor, or immediate delivery.
Amniocentesis	Determine fetal lung maturity, fetal infections or fetal hematologic disorders, previous history of erythroblastosis	Lecithin/sphingomyelin ratio of >2 indicates lung maturity and, if delivered, lessens chance of respiratory distress syndrome
Group B streptococcus screening	All pregnant women should be screened for anogenital group B streptococcus colonization between 35 and 37 wk.	Positive results indicate colonization and indication for antibiotic prophylaxis intrapartum.
Fetal oxygen saturation ($FSpo_2$) monitoring	Indicated if FHR monitoring is not reassuring or difficult to interpret; can be used if membranes are ruptured, vertex presentation, >36 wk	$FSpo_2$ <30% for >10 min is probably hypoxemia, indicating need for intervention or delivery.
Ultrasound	Indicated to determine fetal position, placenta previa, abruption or maturity, FHR if unable to Doppler fetal heart tones, assess fetal growth, AFI, estimate fetal weight, R/O multiple gestation, anomalies	To determine fetal well-being, need for immediate delivery or induction of labor, or need for follow-up ultrasounds

table continues on pg. 975 >

TABLE 15.1, continued

Tests and Procedures	Indications	Follow-Up and Interventions for Positive Test Results
Amniotic fluid fern test AmniSure detects human protein in amniotic fluid (PAMG-1)	Determine rupture of membranes	Positive results may indicate need to deliver within 24 hr or induction of labor if no spontaneous labor.
Human placental lactogen	High-risk pregnancies to evaluate placental function	Decreased or falling levels may indicate need for further testing of fetal well-being.
Electronic fetal monitoring	Indicated antepartum to evaluate fetal well-being for high-risk pregnancies, during or after procedures, for symptoms of preterm labor, decreased fetal movement, maternal drug administration. Indicated intrapartum intermittently for low-risk pregnancies or continuously for high-risk pregnancies, during oxytocin administration, epidural anesthesia, or other interventions	Signs of fetal distress warrant interventions to improve fetal oxygenation or immediate delivery.

with PAPP-A, β-hCG, and FNT, the detection rate for Down syndrome is significantly increased. Color-enhanced Doppler ultrasound is used to measure the velocity and direction of blood flow in fetal and uterine anatomy, to provide information about placental function, and as an especially good predictor of outcome for fetuses that are small for gestational age (see Chapter 13). American Congress of Obstetricians and Gynecologists (ACOG) guidelines support the use of umbilical artery Doppler surveillance in the management of intrauterine growth restriction. Middle cerebral artery Doppler assessment is used to predict fetal anemia in at-risk pregnancies. Ultrasound also includes three-dimensional (3D) and four-dimensional (4D) technologies. In fetal medicine, the use of these technologies may provide assessment of fetal anomalies of the limbs, thorax, spine, central nervous system, and face. Some centers use 4D ultrasound for guided needle procedures such as amniocentesis and cordocentesis to improve accuracy of the procedure. Three- and four-dimensional ultrasound is also used to evaluate fetal heart function and structure.

Although magnetic resonance imaging (MRI) is used at some prenatal centers, it is still under investigation for diagnostic evaluation in pregnancy, especially in the final trimester (see Chapter 16). MRI is most often used to define central nervous system defects. Some of the advantages of MRI during pregnancy are that it is a noninvasive technique, it permits easy differentiation between fat and soft tissue, it does not require a full bladder, and it can show the entire fetus in one scan. Currently, MRI confirms fetal abnormalities found by ultrasound and can be used for pelvimetry, placental localization, and determination of size. Fetal MRI is used at medical centers that specialize in fetal diagnosis and treatment (particularly those that perform fetal surgery). Ultrafast MRI is used for evaluation of congenital anomalies that are potentially correctable, such as congenital diaphragmatic hernia, neck masses that result in airway obstruction, myelomeningocele, and cleft lip and cleft palate. MRI is especially useful for definition of maternal anatomy in cases of suspected intra-abdominal or retroperitoneal disease.

● Maternal Serum Alpha-Fetoprotein (MS-AFP)

The measurement of MS-AFP is offered between 15 and 21 weeks' gestation when AFP concentration rises dramatically, and the test is used to screen for fetal abnormalities and neural tube defects. Approximately 90% of infants with neural tube defects are born to parents who have no recognized risk factors for the disorder. Maternal quadruple screen (MoM: AFP, hCG, and E_3 and inhibin A) aids in identifying Down syndrome risk. The test also detects complications of pregnancy, and AFP serves as a tumor marker in nonpregnant women. This test is also used to detect pregnancy complications such as intrauterine growth retardation, fetal distress, and fetal demise. It can also be used to diagnose and monitor hepatocellular, testicular, ovarian, and malignant liver diseases.

Reference Values

Normal

At 15 to 21 weeks' gestation: 10 to 150 ng/mL or 10 to 150 μg/L

Normal adult level: <10 ng/mL or <10 μg/L

MoM: 0.5 to 2.5 (calculated by dividing the patient's AFP by median AFP for a normal pregnancy at the same gestational age). An AFP MoM <2.5 is reported as screen negative. A screen negative result indicates that the calculated AFP MoM falls below the cutoff of 2.5 MoM. A negative screen does not guarantee absence of a neural tube defect.

Procedure

1. Obtain a 10-mL venous blood sample (red-topped tube). Observe standard precautions. Label specimen with the patient's name, date, and test(s) ordered and place specimen in a biohazard bag. Provide information for the laboratory about the duration of pregnancy, patient's weight, ethnicity, and presence of diabetes.
2. Plan the first screening at 15 to 18 weeks. If the result is normal, no further screening is necessary. If MS-AFP is low, consider ultrasound studies to determine exact fetal age. A second screening may be done after an initial elevated MS-AFP. If the result is normal, no further screening is necessary.

Clinical Implications

Abnormal levels should be followed by ultrasound and amniocentesis.

1. *Elevated* MS-AFP can indicate:
   a. Neural tube defects of spina bifida (a vertebral gap) or anencephaly (>2.5 MoM)
   b. Underestimation of gestational age
   c. Multiple gestation (>4.5 MoM)
   d. Threatened abortion
   e. Other congenital abnormalities
2. *Elevated* MS-AFP early in pregnancy is associated with:
   a. Congenital nephrosis
   b. Duodenal atresia
   c. Umbilical hernia or protrusion
   d. Sacrococcygeal teratoma
3. *Elevated* MS-AFP in the third trimester is associated with:
   a. Esophageal atresia
   b. Fetal teratoma
   c. Hydrencephaly
   d. Rh isoimmunization
   e. Gastrointestinal tract obstruction

4. *Low* MS-AFP is associated with:
   a. Long-standing fetal death
   b. Down syndrome (trisomy 21)
   c. Other chromosome abnormalities (trisomy 13, trisomy 18)
   d. Hydatidiform mole
   e. Pseudopregnancy

Interfering Factors

1. Obesity causes low MS-AFP.
2. Race is a factor: MS-AFP levels are 10% to 15% higher in African Americans and are lower in Asians than in Caucasians.
3. Insulin-dependent diabetes results in low MS-AFP levels.

CLINICAL ALERT

If the MS-AFP is elevated and no fetal defect is demonstrated (i.e., by ultrasound or amniocentesis), then the pregnancy is at an increased risk (e.g., premature birth, low-birth-weight infant, fetal death).

Interventions

Pretest Patient Care

1. Explain the reason for testing the patient's blood.
2. Determine the gestational age from the last menstrual period. If the last menstrual period is not known, determine gestational age with ultrasound.
3. Follow guidelines in Chapter 1 for safe, effective, informed *pretest* care.

Posttest Patient Care

1. Collaborate with the healthcare provider to interpret the outcome and counsel the patient about the results.
2. Explain the possible need for further testing.
3. Elevated maternal AFP levels should be followed by a second screening or ultrasound studies for fetal age.
4. Low maternal AFP levels should be followed by ultrasound studies and then by amniocentesis.
5. Follow guidelines in Chapter 1 for safe, effective, informed *posttest* care.

● Circulating Cell-Free DNA

Fetal "cell-free" nucleic acids (DNA and RNA) are found in the maternal circulation, are unique to the current pregnancy, and are thought to be from the placenta. Circulating cell-free DNA is taken from the plasma of maternal whole blood. Testing is available to detect fetal aneuploidies for chromosome 21, 18, and 13. The test can also determine X and Y chromosomes. This noninvasive test can be performed as early as 10 weeks' gestation with results available in 1 week. ACOG recommends that women, regardless of age, be offered prenatal screening for aneuploidy by screening or invasive testing. Cell-free DNA testing is one method of noninvasive screening for women at risk for aneuploidy. It is not recommended as a screening test for low-risk women at this time due to lack of testing in the low-risk population.

Indications for cell-free DNA testing for aneuploidy:

- Maternal age of 35 years or older at delivery
- Ultrasound findings of fetus indicating increased risk for aneuploidy

- Prior history of pregnancy with trisomy
- Positive first or second trimester sequential or integrated screen or quad screen
- Parental balanced Robertsonian translocation with increased risk of fetal trisomy 13 or trisomy 21
- Cell-free DNA testing can identify 99% of Down syndrome, 99.9% of trisomy 18, and 91.7% of trisomy 13.

Reference Values

Normal

Negative test indicates no evidence of aneuploidies for 21, 18, or 13.

Positive

Trisomy 21, trisomy 18, or trisomy 13 detected

Procedure

1. Explain that the test analyzes the relative amount of 21, 18, 13, and Y chromosomal material in circulating cell-free DNA from a maternal blood sample.
2. Obtain a blood draw with 2 × 10 mL mottled black/tan-topped cell-free DNA blood collection tubes. Label specimen with the patient's name, date, and test(s) ordered.

Clinical Implications

1. Test detects fetal chromosomal 21, 18, and 13 aneuploidies and the presence of the Y chromosome in singletons, twins, and higher order multiple pregnancies.
2. A negative test does not ensure an unaffected pregnancy.
3. A patient with a positive test should be referred to genetic counseling and offered invasive testing to confirm results.
4. Cell-free DNA testing does not replace diagnosis with CVS or amniocentesis.

Interventions

Pretest Patient Care

1. Discuss family history with the patient to determine whether patient should be offered other forms of prenatal screening or invasive testing depending on the genetic syndrome. Pretest counseling should include the discussion that cell-free DNA is not a diagnostic test but has a high sensitivity and specificity.
2. Follow guidelines in Chapter 1 for safe, effective, informed *pretest* care.

Posttest Patient Care

1. Refer to a genetics counselor and maternal fetal medicine provider for diagnostic testing and consultation if test is positive.
2. Follow guidelines in Chapter 1 for safe, effective, informed *posttest* care.

● Hormone Testing

Normally, the amounts of all steroid hormones increase as pregnancy progresses. The maternal unit responds to altered hormone levels even before the growing uterus is apparent. Serial testing may be done to monitor rising levels of a particular hormone over a period of time. Decreasing levels indicate that the maternal–placental–fetal unit is not functioning normally. Biochemical analyses of several hormones can be used to monitor changes in the status of the maternal-fetal unit (see Chapters 3 and 6).

1. In early pregnancy, hCG in maternal blood provides evidence of a viable pregnancy. The hCG in maternal serum is measured as a sensitive pregnancy test (the hCG level increases 66% to 100% every 48 hours during pregnancy). Also, it is used to monitor the success of in vitro fertilization or insemination, to diagnose trophoblastic tumor, to diagnose ectopic pregnancy (indicated by a

decrease in hCG over a 48-hour period), and to screen for Down syndrome in pregnancy. For further discussion of pregnancy tests, see Chapter 6.

2. Together with prolactin and luteinizing hormone (LH), hCG prolongs the life of the corpus luteum once the ovum is fertilized. It stimulates the ovary for the first 6 to 8 weeks of pregnancy, before placental synthesis of progesterone begins. Its function later in pregnancy (in maternal blood) is unknown.
3. PAPP-A, a circulating placental protein, has been shown to increase the stimulatory effects of placental insulin-like growth factors. Decreased serum levels in the maternal circulation in the first 10 weeks after conception are associated with uncomplicated full-term low birth weights. PAPP-A levels are detectable within 30 days after conception and slowly increase throughout the first 30 weeks of gestation. Maternal serum levels are 0.43 μg/L (12 pmol/L). Increased PAPP-A occurs in Down pregnancy.
4. Late in pregnancy, the levels of E_3 and human placental lactogen (hPL) in maternal blood reflect fetal homeostasis. hPL is a protein hormone produced by the placenta. Testing of hPL evaluates only placental functioning. Blood testing of the patient usually begins after the 30th week and may be done weekly thereafter. A concentration of 1 μg/mL (46 nmol/L) hPL may be detected at 6 to 8 weeks of gestation. The level slowly increases throughout pregnancy and reaches 7 μg/mL (324 nmol/L) at term before abruptly dropping to zero after delivery. hPL functions primarily as a fail-safe mechanism to ensure nutrient supply to the fetus, for example, at times of maternal starvation. However, it does not appear to be required for a successful pregnancy outcome (see Chapter 6).

● Estriol (E_3)

E_3 is the predominant estrogen in the blood and urine of pregnant women and is of fetal origin. Normal production serves as a measure of the integrity of the maternal–fetal unit and of fetal well-being.

This test is used during pregnancy to evaluate fetal disorders and is part of the maternal triple screen. Declining serial values indicate fetal distress, although in some high-risk pregnancies, E_3 is not reduced. A single determination cannot be interpreted in a meaningful fashion. E_3 is decreased in Down syndrome and in trisomy 18. An elevated serum or unconjugated E_3 above 3 multiples of the gestational age mean, or with an absolute value of >2.1 ng/mL, can indicate pending labor or fetal congenital adrenal hyperplasia.

Reference Values

Normal

Weeks of Gestation	E_3 (ng/mL)	SI Units (nmol/L)
28–30	38–140	132–485
32	35–330	121–1144
34	45–260	156–901
36	46–350	159–1277
38	59–570	214–1976
40	90–460	306–1595

Levels peak in the middle or late afternoon. The day-to-day variation is 12% to 15%.

Procedure

1. Obtain a 5-mL serum sample by venipuncture using a red-topped tube. Draw the specimen at same time of day on each visit. Observe standard precautions. Label specimen with the patient's name, date, and test(s) ordered. Record weeks of gestation on the requisition or computer screen. Serial measurements may be recommended to establish a trend.
2. Collect 24-hour urine specimens (E_3: 13 to 42 mg/24 hours or 46 to 164 nmol/day) during the third trimester.

Clinical Implications

1. *Decreased* E_3 is associated with risk for:
    a. Growth retardation
    b. Fetal death
    c. Fetal anomalies (Down syndrome, fetal encephalopathy)
    d. Fetus past maturity
    e. Preeclampsia
    f. Rh immunization
2. *Decreased* E_3 also occurs in:
    a. Anemia
    b. Diabetes
    c. Malnutrition
    d. Liver disease
    e. Hemoglobinopathy

Interfering Factors

Administration of radioactive isotopes within the previous 48 hours interferes with this test.
Estrogen or progesterone therapy can interfere with test results.
Drugs that can cause decreased levels include vitamins and some phenothiazines.
Tetracycline can increase levels.

Interventions

Pretest Patient Care

1. Explain test purpose and procedures. Serial testing may be required. See Hormone Testing.
2. No fasting is necessary.
3. Follow guidelines in Chapter 1 for safe, effective, informed *pretest* care.

Posttest Patient Care

1. Review test results; report and record findings. Modify the nursing care plan as needed. Continuously low E_3 values are sometimes seen in normal pregnancy. A decreasing trend is indicative of fetal distress. Provide counseling and support.
2. Follow guidelines in Chapter 1 for safe, effective, informed *posttest* care.

● Human Placental Lactogen (hPL) (Chorionic Somatomammotropin)

hPL is a growth-promoting hormone of placental origin and is similar to hCG (see Hormone Testing).

This test is used to evaluate placental function as an index of fetal well-being in at-risk pregnancies. Low hPL levels are associated with intrauterine growth retardation. Falling levels indicate a poor prognosis. The level of hPL correlates best with placental weight, but the clinical significance of this hormone is controversial.

Reference Values

Normal

Normal maternal serum: <0.5 µg/mL (<0.5 mg/L or <25 nmol/L)
1st Trimester: 0.2–2.1 µg/mL
2nd Trimester: 0.5–6.7 µg/mL
3rd Trimester: 4.5–12.8 µg/mL
Men and nonpregnant women: 0–0.1 µg/mL

Procedure

1. Obtain a serum sample of at least 1 mL in two separate vials (red-topped tube) by venipuncture. Observe standard precautions.
2. Record the week of gestation or last menstrual period on the test requisition or computer screen. These tests are usually done as serial measurements.

Clinical Implications

1. Normal values are associated with normal intrauterine growth but do not ensure lack of complications.
2. *Decreased* or *falling* values are associated with:
   a. Growth retardation
   b. Placental disease
   c. Fetal death
   d. Hypertensive state
   e. Toxemia
   f. Aborting hydatidiform mole
   g. Choriocarcinoma
   h. Placental insufficiency
3. Low levels are also associated with some normal pregnancies.
4. *Increased* values are found in:
   a. Multiple pregnancies (twins or more)
   b. Placental site trophoblastic tumor
   c. Intact molar pregnancy
   d. Diabetes
   e. Rh incompatibility

Interfering Factors

Administration of radiopharmaceuticals 24 hours before venipuncture interferes with this test.

Interventions

Pretest Patient Care

1. Explain the reason for testing the patient's blood.
2. Follow guidelines in Chapter 1 for safe, effective, informed *pretest* care.

Posttest Patient Care

1. Review test results; report and record findings. Modify the nursing care plan as needed. Explain possible need for serial blood testing if results are abnormal.
2. Use ultrasound studies to assess any abnormal results.
3. Follow guidelines in Chapter 1 for safe, effective, informed *posttest* care.

● Fetal Fibronectin (fFN)

Fetal fibronectin (fFN) is abundant in amniotic fluid and may be useful in the diagnosis of ruptured membranes. The detection of fFN in vaginal secretions before membrane rupture may be a marker for impending preterm labor within the next 7 to 14 days.

This test helps to predict a preterm delivery when the presenting symptoms are questionable so that early intervention (e.g., tocolytics, corticosteroids, transport to a tertiary center) can be initiated when indicated. This test is for women with intact membranes and cervical dilation <3 cm. fFN is secreted in early pregnancy to help attach the fertilized egg to the implantation site in the uterus, but it is not secreted after 22 weeks until near term. This test detects preterm labor from 24 until 34 weeks' gestation.

Reference Values

Normal

Negative: <0.05 μg/mL or <0.05 mg/L (delivery is unlikely to occur within 14 days)
Positive: >0.05 μg/mL or >0.05 mg/L (delivery within 7 to 14 days)

Procedure

1. Using a sterile speculum, obtain secretions from the cervix and vagina by rotating a sterile Dacron swab near the outside of the cervix and the posterior fornix of the vagina. Observe standard precautions.
2. Label the specimen with the patient's name, date and time of collection, and test(s) ordered. Place specimen in a biohazard bag and send the specimen to laboratory. Results may take 24 to 48 hours.

PROCEDURAL ALERT

Specimens for fFN should be obtained before digital cervical exam, collection of culture specimens, vaginal ultrasound exam, or any prior manipulation of the cervix because this can result in release of fFN and false results.

Clinical Implications

A level of fFN equal to or greater than a reference value (0.050 μg/mL) is considered positive and means that preterm labor is imminent. Transvaginal cervical ultrasonography may be used along with fFN to assess risk for preterm birth. A short cervix (<25 mm) with a positive fFN is a strong predictor of preterm delivery. The greatest value of this testing is a negative result in order to avoid unnecessary interventions.

Interfering Factors

1. Vaginal bleeding
2. Ruptured membranes
3. Sexual intercourse within 24 hours of collection

Interventions

Pretest Patient Care

1. Explain test purpose and procedure to the patient.
2. Follow guidelines in Chapter 1 for safe, effective, informed *pretest* care.

Posttest Patient Care

1. Counsel the patient regarding test results and need for follow-up medication, tocolysis (inhibition of contractions), or preparation for probable delivery.
2. Be sure the patient knows the warning signs of preterm labor.
   a. *Uterine contractions*—a hard feeling over the entire surface of the uterus that lasts 20 seconds or longer. The contractions can be painless. If more than four are felt per hour, notify healthcare provider.
   b. *Menstrual-like cramps* felt low in abdomen; may be constant or come and go
   c. *Pelvic pressure* or fullness in the pelvic area or back of the thighs
   d. *Backache*—a dull pain in the lower back, either constant or rhythmic, that is not relieved by changing positions
   e. *Persistent diarrhea*
   f. *Intestinal cramps* with or without diarrhea
   g. *Vaginal discharge* that is greater than normal or changes in consistency or color (especially if it is pink, bloody, or greenish)
   h. A general *feeling or sense that something is wrong*
3. Explain the possible causes and increased risks associated with preterm labor and birth:
   a. Past preterm birth
   b. Spontaneous abortion in second trimester

c. Uterine anomaly
d. Diethylstilbestrol exposure
e. Incompetent cervix
f. Hydramnios
g. Bleeding in second and third trimester
h. Preterm labor
i. Premature rupture of membrane
j. Multiple gestation
k. Preterm cervical dilation >2 cm (multipara) or >1 cm (primipara)
l. Pregnancy weight <115 pounds
m. Patient <15 years of age

4. Follow guidelines in Chapter 1 for safe, effective, informed *posttest* care.

TESTS TO PREDICT FETAL OUTCOME AND RISK FOR INTRAUTERINE ASPHYXIA

● Contraction Stress Test (CST)

This test is done in a hospital or clinic setting to assess fetal heart rate (FHR) in response to uterine contractions through electronic fetal monitoring.

Reference Values

Normal

The test result is negative if there are no late decelerations associated with at least three contractions within a 10-minute period.

A normal (negative) contraction stress test (CST) implies that placental support is adequate, that the fetus is probably able to tolerate the stress of labor should it begin within 1 week, and that there is a low risk for intrauterine death due to hypoxia.

Procedure

1. Obtain the FHR by using an external transducer.
2. Monitor uterine activity by a tocodynamometer.

Clinical Implications

A positive result indicates increased risk for intrauterine death due to hypoxia.

Interventions

Pretest Patient Care

1. Explain the reason for testing.
2. Follow guidelines in Chapter 1 for safe, effective, informed *pretest* care.

CLINICAL ALERT

Contraindications include the following:

1. Third-trimester bleeding (unexplained vaginal bleeding)
2. Preterm labor (premature)
3. Presence of classic uterine incision
4. Placenta previa

Posttest Patient Care

1. Review test results; report and record findings. Modify the nursing care plan as needed. Explain possible need for follow-up testing.
2. Follow guidelines in Chapter 1 for safe, effective, informed *posttest* care.

Oxytocin Challenge Test (OCT); Nipple Stimulation Test; Breast Stimulation Test (BST)

These tests are performed after 28 weeks of gestation, when a nonstress test (NST) is nonreactive or a CST is either positive or unsatisfactory. Continuous external fetal monitoring is used. Because uterine contractions are associated with a reduction in uteroplacental blood flow, spontaneous, oxytocin-induced, or nipple stimulation–induced contractions with a frequency of three in 10 minutes may be used clinically as a standard test of fetoplacental respiratory function. Stress of this magnitude has been proved clinically useful in separating fetuses with suboptimal oxygen reserve from those with adequate reserve (the vast majority), and it does not significantly compromise the normal fetus.

Reference Values

Normal

The test result is negative if there are no late decelerations associated with at least three contractions within a 10-minute period.

A normal (negative) result is reassuring; it implies that placental reserve is sufficient should labor begin within 1 week. There is a false-normal rate of 1 to 2 per 1000 pregnancies. The procedure is usually repeated weekly.

Procedure

1. Be aware that contractions may occur spontaneously, after breast stimulation test (BST), or after administration of intravenous oxytocin to produce three good-quality contractions of at least 40 seconds' duration each within a 10-minute period.
2. Monitor the FHR for reaction to this stress.

PROCEDURAL ALERT

With all methods of oxytocin challenge test (OCT), there is a risk for hyperstimulation, which could result in extended FHR decelerations that could be hypoxic for the fetus.

Clinical Implications

1. The presence of consistent and persistent late decelerations with most uterine contractions, regardless of their frequency, constitutes a positive (abnormal) OCT result. This is often associated with decreased baseline FHR variability, a lack of FHR acceleration with fetal movement, and a fetus at risk for intrauterine asphyxia.
2. The results of OCT can be categorized as follows:
   a. *Negative*: no late decelerations
   b. *Positive*: late decelerations following 50% or more of contractions, even if the frequency of the contractions is fewer than three in 10 minutes
   c. *Equivocal*: intermittent, late, or variable decelerations
   d. *Unsatisfactory*: fewer than three contractions within 10 minutes or a poor-quality tracing

Interventions

Pretest Patient Care

1. Explain test purpose and procedure.
2. Follow guidelines in Chapter 1 for safe, effective, informed *pretest* care.

> **CLINICAL ALERT**
>
> Contraindications for OCT include:
>
> a. Third-trimester bleeding (unexplained vaginal bleeding)
> b. Preterm labor (premature)
> c. Presence of classic uterine incision
> d. Placenta previa

Posttest Patient Care

1. Review test results; report and record findings. Modify the nursing care plan as needed. Counsel the patient accordingly about the meaning of fetal heart activity and movement.
2. Follow guidelines in Chapter 1 for safe, effective, informed *posttest* care.

● Nonstress Test (NST)

The NST can be performed in a hospital, a clinic, or possibly a home care setting. The NST is a screening test and can be safely done once a week. Test results reflect the functions of the fetal brainstem, autonomic nervous system, and heart.

Reference Values

Normal

Negative result: reactive NST

ACOG criteria for a reactive NST (with or without stimulation): two or more accelerations of FHR, peaking at least 15 beats/minute above the baseline FHR and lasting at least 15 seconds from baseline to baseline, within a 20-minute period

Procedure

1. Assess maternal vital signs, last oral intake (including medicines or street drugs), smoking history, and fetal movement history.
2. Apply external fetal monitor with the woman positioned off her back in lateral tilt position.
3. After 26 weeks of gestation, this assessment of the FHR pattern without contractions evaluates fetal oxygenation. Fetal movement may or may not be identified by the woman during the test. If gestation is <26 to 30 weeks, the fetus may not meet the criteria for a reactive NST yet may be a healthy fetus.
4. It is no longer recommended to feed the woman before this test because of the possibility of emergency delivery. Glucose does not alter the FHR pattern.
5. If unable to elicit FHR accelerations during NST, acoustic stimulation of a fetus that is not acidotic may evoke FHR accelerations that seem to predict fetal well-being. An artificial larynx (vibroacoustic stimulator) that is designed for fetal monitoring is placed on the patient's abdomen, and the stimulus is activated for 1 to 2 seconds. The stimulus may be repeated up to three times for gradually increased durations up to 3 seconds to bring about FHR accelerations. Use of acoustic stimulation can shorten the time needed for reactive NST and reduce false-positive test results.

PROCEDURAL ALERT

1. A nonreactive NST (positive test) should be followed by a CST.
2. Ultrasound studies and a fetal biophysical profile (FBP) may be needed after a nonreactive NST.

Clinical Implications

A nonreactive NST (positive test) consists of fewer than two accelerations of FHR (ACOG criteria). If the fetus does not react within the first 20 minutes, stimulation should be applied. The test is considered nonreactive if, after extension to 40 minutes, the ACOG criteria are not met. This extended testing minimizes the possibility of lack of activity owing to fetal sleep. If the FHR pattern is unclear, the test is considered inconclusive or unsatisfactory.

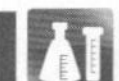

CLINICAL ALERT

1. Nonrepetitive, brief (<30 s) variable decelerations may be noted in up to 50% of NSTs and do not indicate a compromised fetus or a need for interventions.
2. Repetitive variable decelerations (three in 20 min) or decelerations that last 60 s or longer indicate nonreassuring FHR pattern and increased risk for cesarean delivery.

Interfering Factors

A false-positive result may be caused by fetal sleep, preterm gestation, smoking before the NST, congenital anomalies, or maternal use of drugs such as central nervous system depressants or β blockers.

Interventions

Pretest Patient Care

1. Explain test purpose and procedure.
2. Follow guidelines in Chapter 1 for safe, effective, informed *pretest* care.

Posttest Patient Care

1. Review test results; report and record findings. Modify the nursing care plan as needed.
2. Advise the patient regarding the need for weekly or twice-weekly testing according to the healthcare provider's orders if pregnancy history indicates risk factors for antepartum fetal demise. If NST is performed for a single occurrence of decreased fetal movement in uncomplicated pregnancy and reactive NST results, reassure the patient that the test need not be repeated.
3. Follow guidelines in Chapter 1 for safe, effective, informed *posttest* care.

● Fetal Activity Acceleration Determination (FAD)

The fetal activity acceleration determination (FAD) test often is not distinguished from NST, but it is different. In the FAD test, both acceleration of FHR and fetal movement are evaluated.

Reference Values

Normal

Negative result: reactive test

Criteria are similar to those for NST, but fetal movement is also required: more than three discrete body or limb movements within 30 minutes. In a reactive test (well-oxygenated fetus), spontaneous accelerations of FHR begin at about the time of onset of fetal movement. This effect expresses the condition of the neurologic system and its effect on fetal movement and FHR.

Procedure

1. The procedure is the same as for the NST.
2. Give the woman a button to push when fetal movement occurs; pushing the button causes a mark to appear on the monitor strip.

Clinical Implications

1. A nonreactive FAD test (positive result) is ascertained in the same manner as is the NST. Results are of questionable validity before 30 weeks' gestation. Follow-up for a nonreactive test should include an ultrasound study to assess fetal movement and tone.
2. A nonreactive FAD test (positive result) is associated with greater risk for hypoxia.

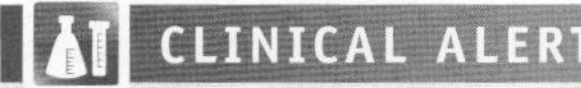

Fetal movement tends to decrease as gestation progresses.

Interventions

Pretest Patient Care

1. Explain reason for testing and FHR monitoring.
2. This test may be performed in a hospital or clinic setting.
3. Follow guidelines in Chapter 1 for safe, effective, informed *pretest* care.

Posttest Patient Care

1. Review test results; report and record findings. Modify the nursing care plan as needed. Explain need for possible follow-up ultrasound.
2. Follow guidelines in Chapter 1 for safe, effective, informed *posttest* care.

● Continuous Fetal Heart Rate (FHR) Monitoring

Continuous FHR monitoring is done (both before and during labor) to evaluate postterm pregnancy (>42 weeks); after a nonreactive stress or nonstress test; and in the presence of diabetes, preeclampsia, chronic hypertension, or intrauterine growth retardation. Normally, the rate is 100 to 150 beats/minute; accelerations occur with fetal movement, and a return of variable decelerations to baseline occurs with no evidence of decreasing baseline variability or increasing baseline rate.

● Fetal Biophysical Profile (FBP) (Biophysical Profile [BPP])

The biophysical profile (BPP) measurements, used in the later stages of pregnancy, assess fetal well-being. The BPP or FBP is more accurate and provides more information than does the NST alone. It can identify the fetus affected by hypoxia that is at risk for intrauterine distress or death. In high-risk pregnancies, testing usually begins by 32 to 34 weeks of gestation; those with severe complications may require earlier testing at 26 to 28 weeks.

The FBP uses ultrasound imaging to evaluate five distinct parameters: (1) evidence of FHR (cardiac rate) accelerations (NST), (2) muscle tone, (3) fetal movement, (4) fetal breathing, and (5) volume of amniotic fluid. Based on sonographic evidence during a typical 20- to 30-minute survey, each parameter is assigned a value of 0 to 2 points (2 is optimal). The maximum number of points obtainable is 10; a score of 10 indicates a normal test without evidence of fetal distress. Generally, a score >8 indicates fetal well-being. The FBP also provides the healthcare provider with valuable information regarding fetal size and position, number of fetuses, placental location and grade, and evidence of specific fetal activities such as micturition and eye movements.

Another version of the FBP, termed the *modified biophysical profile*, has become a primary mode of antepartum fetal testing. The modified version includes the NST as a measure of fetal acid–base status and the amniotic fluid index (AFI) as a long-term placental function assessment. The modified FBP is normal if the NST is reactive and if the AFI is >5. Abnormal results include nonreactive NST and AFI ≥5.

In some laboratories, Doppler examinations of the umbilical vessels assess uterofetal blood flow. Abnormal Doppler blood flow studies (umbilical artery velocimetry) may be detected before changes in NST, CST, or FBP are detectable. Abnormal Doppler umbilical artery waveforms become indicative of acidosis, hypoxia, and intrauterine growth retardation, which result in a poor outcome. Doppler velocimetry has demonstrated benefits for fetuses with suspected intrauterine growth retardation.

Reference Values

Normal

Fetal well-being score: >8 points, based on normal NST; normal fetal muscle tone, movement, and breathing; and normal volume of amniotic fluid

Procedure

1. Explain test purpose and procedure.
2. Position the patient on her back and apply a gel (coupling agent) to the skin of the lower abdomen. Then, move the ultrasound transducer across the lower abdominal area to visualize the fetus and surrounding structures.
3. Examining time is usually 30 minutes but may vary because of fetal age or fetal state.
4. A CST or NST is also done at this time.

PROCEDURAL ALERT

To assess the fetal state properly, a sonographic determination of eye movement and respiration must be done. If no eye movements and no respirations are evident, the fetus is most likely asleep. On the other hand, if rapid eye movement is evident but breathing is absent, the fetus is probably in distress.

Clinical Implications

1. Variables that influence FBP include fetal age, fetal behavioral states, maternal or fetal infection, hypoglycemia, hyperglycemia, and postmaturity.
2. If a fetus <36 weeks of gestation does not have stable behaviors, a longer test may be needed. Infection may cause absence of FHR reactivity and fetal breathing movements. Frequency of fetal breathing increases during maternal hyperglycemia and decreases with maternal hypoglycemia. Other variables that influence FBP include use of therapeutic or nontherapeutic chemicals. Magnesium sulfate may decrease or eliminate fetal breathing movements and decrease FHR variability. Nicotine can decrease the profile parameters, and cocaine may also decrease the FBP score.
3. When the five major BPP parameters can be observed, the fetus is considered to be free of distress. Generally, a score of 8 points indicates fetal well-being.
4. A score of 6 points is equivocal, and retesting should be done in 12 to 24 hours.
5. A score of <4 indicates the potential for or the existence of fetal distress. This warrants further testing or the consideration of delivery.

Interventions

Pretest Patient Care

1. Explain the test purpose and procedure and include information regarding each part of the test and how it relates to fetal well-being.
2. Follow guidelines in Chapter 1 for safe, effective, informed *pretest* care.

Posttest Patient Care

1. Review test results; report and record findings. Modify the nursing care plan as needed. Counsel the patient appropriately and inform about further testing.
2. Instruct the patient regarding need for weekly or twice-weekly testing if pregnancy history indicates risk for antepartum fetal demise.
3. Follow guidelines in Chapter 1 for safe, effective, informed *posttest* care.

● Fetoscopy

Fetoscopy allows direct observation of the fetus and facilitates fetal blood sampling, skin or muscle biopsy, or fetal therapy. It provides direct visualization of the fetus in 2- to 4-cm segments so that developmental defects can be more accurately identified. The fetal blood sample allows early diagnosis of disorders such as hemophilia A and B that are not amenable to detection through other means. Fetoscopy can also be used for therapeutic interventions in conditions such as abnormal vascular connection in twin–twin transfusion, congenital diaphragmatic hernia, fetal bladder outlet obstruction, and amniotic band syndrome. Because there are risks associated with fetoscopy, it is only offered when there is a significant risk of a major birth defect that can be diagnosed or treated by this method.

Reference Values

Normal

Normal fetal development; no evidence of fetal developmental defects
Negative for hemophilia types A and B and sickle cell anemia

Procedure

1. Obtain a properly signed and witnessed consent form.
2. Apply a local anesthetic to the patient's abdominal wall. Sedation may be given to the patient to quiet the fetus.
3. Use real-time ultrasound to locate the proper maternal abdominal area through which to make a small incision and then insert the cannula and the trocar into the uterus.
4. After cannulation into the uterus, insert an endoscope (fetoscope), consisting of a fiberoptic light source and a self-focusing lens, and then manipulate for optimal views and fetal tissue sampling (e.g., skin, blood, amniotic fluid).

PROCEDURAL ALERT

Fetoscopy poses an increased risk for spontaneous abortions (5%–10%), preterm delivery (10%), amniotic fluid leakage (1%), and intrauterine fetal death.

Clinical Implications

Abnormal results reveal:

1. Fetal malformation
2. Neural tube defects
3. Sickle cell anemia
4. Hemophilia

Interventions

Pretest Patient Care

1. Genetic counseling and a thorough explanation of the procedure and its benefits, risks, and limitations should be provided.

2. Antibiotics may be ordered before the procedure to prevent amnionitis. Assess for possible allergies to the drug.
3. Follow guidelines in Chapter 1 for safe, effective, informed *pretest* care.

Posttest Patient Care

1. Monitor the patient and fetus for several hours after the procedure. Institute proper protocols for dealing with maternal blood pressure and pulse changes, FHR abnormalities, uterine activity, vaginal bleeding, or amniotic fluid leakage. Rh-negative patients should receive human Rho(D) immune globulin (RhoGAM) unless the fetus is also known to be Rh negative. Repeat ultrasound studies should be done to check amniotic fluid volume and fetal viability.
2. Instruct the patient to report any pain, bleeding, infected cannulation site, amniotic fluid leakage, or fever (amnionitis).
3. Review test results; report and record findings. Modify the nursing care plan as needed.
4. Follow guidelines in Chapter 1 for safe, effective, informed *posttest* care.

● Percutaneous Umbilical Blood Sampling (PUBS) (Cordocentesis)

Percutaneous umbilical blood sampling (PUBS) is a diagnostic procedure in which fetal blood is drawn from the vein in the umbilical cord. PUBS may be used if ultrasound, amniocentesis, and CVS do not provide adequate information about the fetus. PUBS has somewhat replaced fetoscopy because of the risk factors associated with the latter test. PUBS, for which research is ongoing, is probably a safer and easier way to sample blood from the umbilical cord of the fetus in utero. Fetal blood can be examined for hemophilia, hemoglobinopathies, fetal infections, chromosomal abnormalities, fetal distress, fetal drug levels, and other blood studies. Other common indications include rapid karyotype evaluation, fetal platelet abnormalities, and fetal growth restriction. PUBS is usually performed after 18 weeks' gestation.

Reference Values

Normal

No abnormalities noted (see explanation of test)

Procedure

1. Scan with a real-time ultrasound transducer (placed into a sterile glove) to provide landmarks as a 20- to 25-gauge spinal needle is first inserted into the maternal abdomen and then guided into the fetal umbilical vein, 1 to 2 cm from the cord insertion site on the placenta.
2. Aspirate the fetal blood sample into a syringe containing anticoagulant to prevent clotting of the sample.

PROCEDURAL ALERT

Risks include transient fetal bradycardia, maternal infection, premature labor, and a 1%–2% incidence of fetal loss.

Clinical Implications

Abnormal blood results reveal:

1. Hemoglobinopathies
2. Hemophilia A or B; other coagulation disorders

3. Fetal infection
4. Chromosome abnormalities, genetic diseases
5. Isoimmunization
6. Metabolic disorders
7. Fetal hypoxia

Interventions

Pretest Patient Care

1. Explain the procedure and its purpose, benefits, and risks. Obtain a properly signed and witnessed consent form.
2. Assist with relaxation exercises during the procedure. Antibiotics may be given before the test to prevent infection.
3. Follow guidelines in Chapter 1 for safe, effective, informed *pretest* care.

Posttest Patient Care

1. Monitor maternal vital signs and perform external fetal monitoring or an NST. Observe for signs of fetal distress.
2. Perform an ultrasound 1 hour after the procedure to ensure that there is no bleeding at the puncture site.
3. Review test results; report and record findings. Modify the nursing care plan as needed. Counsel the patient appropriately about fetal therapy (e.g., red blood cell and platelet transfusion and drug treatment).
4. Follow guidelines in Chapter 1 for safe, effective, informed *posttest* care.

● Chorionic Villus Sampling (CVS)

CVS can provide very early diagnosis of fetal genetic or biochemical disorders. Some specialists advise that this procedure be reserved for evaluation of conditions that present relatively high genetic risks, such as hemoglobinopathies. CVS involves extraction of a small amount of tissue from the villi of the chorion frondosum. This tissue is composed of rapidly proliferating trophoblastic cells that ultimately form the placenta. Although not a part of the fetus, these villus cells are genetically identical to the fetus and are considered fetal rather than maternal in origin.

CVS differs from amniocentesis in several respects and therefore is not considered an alternative. In amniocentesis, the cells examined are desquamated fetal cells; the cells sampled in CVS divide rapidly and are easier to culture. For this reason, karyotyping (see Chapter 11) can be performed much more rapidly, and diagnostic information can be provided within 24 hours, much faster than with amniotic fluid cells. Also, CVS can be performed much earlier in pregnancy, typically at 7 to 11 gestational weeks, whereas amniocentesis usually is performed after 15 weeks' gestation, with results available several weeks later. CVS, therefore, has the advantage of providing first-trimester diagnosis, which is of particular value when the choice is made to abort an affected fetus because first-trimester terminations of pregnancy are medically safer.

CVS reveals chromosome abnormalities and fetal metabolic or blood disorders. However, because CVS cannot be used to measure AFP, it cannot detect neural tube defects or other disorders associated with increased AFP levels.

Prenatal chromosomal microarray analysis (CMA) is a diagnostic test that can detect genetic abnormalities in a fetus using CVS cells or amniocytes. The sensitivity and specificity of prenatal CMA is much higher than the standard technique of karyotype analysis. It is possible to identify abnormalities such as DiGeorge syndrome, Miller-Dieker syndrome, Telomere deletion syndromes, 22q11 syndrome, Smith-Magenis syndrome, Angelman syndrome, and Prader-Willi syndrome.

Indications for CVS include the following:

1. Abnormal ultrasound test
2. Fetus at risk for detectable Mendelian disorders
   a. Tay-Sachs disease
   b. Hemoglobinopathies
   c. Cystic fibrosis
   d. Muscular dystrophy
3. Birth of previous child with evidence of chromosome abnormality
4. Parent with known structural chromosomal rearrangement
5. Diagnosis of fetal infection

Reference Values

Normal

Negative for chromosomal and DNA abnormalities
No fetal metabolic enzyme or blood disorders

Procedure

1. Position the patient on her back to permit ultrasound documentation of the number of fetuses in utero and their viability and localization of trophoblastic tissue. Ask the patient either to maintain a full bladder or to empty the bladder so as to optimize the sampling path. A bimanual pelvic examination is often performed concurrently with this preliminary ultrasound examination.
2. Have the patient assume a lithotomy position. Insert a sterile speculum after the vagina has been cleansed with an iodine-based antiseptic.
3. Introduce a sterile flexible catheter with a stainless-steel obturator into the vaginal canal and advance through the cervical canal into the trophoblastic tissue. The catheter is visually tracked by the ultrasound device.
4. Once the catheter is in place, attach a syringe to the end of the catheter to extract approximately 5 mL of tissue. Immediately examine the tissue sample under a low-power microscope to determine that both quantity and tissue quality are acceptable.
5. Make up to three passes of the catheter. Use a new, sterile catheter each time. After sufficient tissue has been gathered, use ultrasound again to monitor fetal viability. Use the tissue sample for chromosome and enzyme analysis and for other tests.
6. Be aware that a transabdominal method may also be used. This method is similar to amniocentesis except that the thin-walled needle is inserted into the chorionic bed.

PROCEDURAL ALERT

1. The safety of the CVS procedure is related to the experience and skill of the examiner. In experienced hands, the rates of complications and fetal loss are only slightly greater than for amniocentesis. Risks include leakage of amniotic fluid, bleeding, intrauterine infection, spontaneous abortion, maternal tissue contamination of specimen, Rh isoimmunization, and fetal death (5%).
2. Transcervical CVS is difficult in patients who have a fundal placental implantation site or an extremely retroflexed or anteflexed uterus. In such patients, a transabdominal approach similar to that used for amniocentesis is employed.
3. An increased risk for severe limb deformities is associated with this procedure, especially if performed before 10 weeks' gestation.

Clinical Implications

Abnormal CVS results indicate:

1. Abnormal fetal tissue
2. Chromosome abnormalities
3. Fetal metabolic and blood disorders
4. Fetal infection

Interventions

Pretest Patient Care

1. Be aware that genetic counseling typically precedes any CVS procedure.
2. Explain the purpose, procedure, and risks of the test.
3. Ensure that a signed, witnessed informed consent document is obtained.
4. Have the patient drink four 8-oz glasses of water about 1 hour before the examination. The patient should not void until instructed to do so.
5. Obtain baseline measurements of maternal vital signs and FHR.
6. Advise the patient that she may experience cramping as the catheter passes through the cervical canal.
7. Help the patient to relax.
8. Follow guidelines in Chapter 1 for safe, effective, informed *pretest* care.

Posttest Patient Care

1. Monitor maternal vital signs and FHR every 15 minutes for the first hour after test completion.
2. Instruct the patient to notify her healthcare provider if she experiences abdominal pain, vaginal bleeding or abnormal discharge, elevated temperature, chills, or amniotic fluid leakage.
3. Review test results; report and record findings. Modify the nursing care plan as needed. Counsel the patient appropriately. Rh-negative women usually receive RhoGAM.
4. Support the patient and her significant others during decision making. Provide opportunity for questions and discussion.
5. Follow guidelines in Chapter 1 for safe, effective, informed *posttest* care.

AMNIOTIC FLUID STUDIES

The fluid filling the amniotic sac serves several important functions. It provides a medium in which the fetus can readily move, cushions the fetus against possible injury, helps maintain an even temperature, and provides useful information concerning the health and maturity of the fetus. The origin of amniotic fluid is not completely understood. In early pregnancy, it is produced by the amniotic membrane covering the placenta and the cord. As the pregnancy progresses, it is believed to be primarily a byproduct of fetal pulmonary secretions, urine, and metabolic products from the intestinal tract.

Initially, amniotic fluid is produced from the amniotic membrane cells. Later, most of it is derived from the maternal blood. The volume increases from about 30 mL at 2 weeks' gestation to 350 mL at 20 weeks. After 20 weeks, the volume ranges from 500 to 1000 mL. The volume of amniotic fluid changes continuously because of fluid movement in both directions through the placental membrane. Later in pregnancy, the fetus contributes to amniotic fluid volumes through excretion of urine and swallowing of amniotic fluid. The fetus also absorbs up to 400 mL of amniotic fluid every 24 hours through its gastrointestinal tract, bloodstream, and umbilical artery exchanges across the placenta. Probably, some fluid is also absorbed by direct contact with the fetal surface of the placenta. Amniotic fluid contains castoff cells from the fetus and resembles extracellular fluid with suspended, undissolved material. It is slightly alkaline and contains albumin, urea, uric acid, creatinine, lecithin, sphingomyelin, bilirubin, fat, fructose, epithelial cells, leukocytic enzymes, and lanugo hair.

When amniocentesis is advised early in pregnancy (15 to 18 weeks), the purpose is to study the fetal genetic makeup and to determine developmental abnormalities. Fetal cells are separated from the amniotic fluid by centrifugation and are placed in a tissue culture medium so that they can be grown and harvested for subsequent karyotyping to identify chromosome disorders. Testing in the third trimester is done to determine fetal age and well-being, to study blood groups, or to detect amnionitis.

• Amniocentesis

Amniotic fluid is aspirated by means of a needle guided through the patient's abdominal and uterine walls into the amniotic sac. Amniocentesis is preferably performed after the 15th week of pregnancy. By this time, amniotic fluid levels have expanded to 150 mL, so that a 10-mL specimen can be aspirated. If the purpose of amniocentesis is to ascertain fetal maturity, it should be done after the 35th week of gestation.

Amniocentesis provides a method to detect fetal abnormalities in situations in which the risk for an abnormality may be high. The test can evaluate fetal hematologic disorders, fetal infections, inborn errors of metabolism, and sex-linked disorders. It is not done to determine the sex of the fetus simply out of curiosity.

Chromosomal abnormalities and neural tube defects such as anencephaly, encephalocele, spina bifida, and myelomeningocele can be determined, as can estimates of fetal age, fetal well-being, and pulmonary maturity. Fluorescence in situ hybridization (FISH) technology is useful in the diagnosis of chromosomal abnormalities or deletion disorders. FISH can identify translocations, inversions, or deletions on chromosomes 13, 18, 21, and X and Y. This technique is most helpful if results are needed quickly for management of pregnancy.

The development of significant maternal Rh antibody titers or a history of previous erythroblastosis can be an indication for amniocentesis.

High-Risk Parents Who Should Be Offered Prenatal Diagnosis

1. Women of advanced maternal age (>35 years) who are at risk for having a child with a chromosome abnormality, especially trisomy 21. At maternal age 35 to 40 years, the risk for Down syndrome is 1% to 3%; at age 40 to 45, it is 4% to 12%; and at >45 years, the risk is ≥12%
2. Women who have previously borne a trisomic child or a child with another kind of chromosome abnormality
3. Parents of a child with spina bifida or anencephaly or a family history of neural tube disorders
4. Couples in which either parent is a known carrier of a balanced translocation chromosome for Down syndrome
5. Couples in which both partners are carriers for a diagnosable metabolic or structural autosomal recessive disorder; more than 70 inherited metabolic disorders can be diagnosed by amniotic fluid analysis.
6. Couples in which either partner or a previous child is affected with a diagnosable metabolic or structural dominant disorder
7. Women who are presumed carriers of a serious X-linked genetic disorder
8. Couples from families whose medical history reveals mental retardation, ambiguous genitalia, or parental exposure to toxic environmental agents (e.g., drugs, irradiation, infections)
9. Couples whose personal and family medical history reveals multiple miscarriages, stillbirths, or infertility
10. Parents with anxiety about the health status of potential offspring
11. Women with abnormal ultrasound results

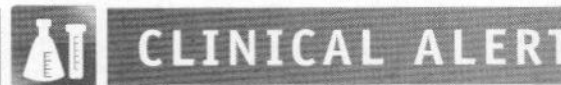

The in utero diagnosis of many genetic disorders may lead the parents to consider abortion as an option for dealing with an unfavorable situation. Because this can be a very difficult and controversial choice, communication between the parents and the healthcare team must take place in a nonjudgmental, nonthreatening manner.

Reference Values

Normal

Normal amniotic fluid constituents and properties vary according to the age of the fetus and the laboratory methods used; pH is slightly alkaline. See descriptions of individual tests.

Procedure

1. Position the patient on her back with her arms behind her head to prevent touching of the abdomen and the sterile field during the procedure (see Obstetric Sonogram in Chapter 13).
2. Perform ultrasound scanning before the procedure to assess fetal number, viability, and position. An appropriate pocket of amniotic fluid is localized in the scan. The tap site should be located away from the fetus, from the site of umbilical cord insertion, and from any thick placental segments.
3. Cleanse the skin thoroughly with an appropriate antiseptic solution and properly drape with sterile drapes. Inject a local anesthetic slowly at the puncture site.
4. Advance a 3.5- or 5-inch spinal needle (20- to 22-gauge) with stylet through the abdominal and uterine walls into the amniotic sac but away from the fetus and, when possible, from the placenta. Use continuous ultrasound surveillance to track the position of the fetus. Should the fetus move close to the needle, withdraw the needle.
5. Once the needle is properly positioned, remove the stylet and attach a syringe to the needle to permit aspiration of a 20- to 30-mL specimen. Discard the first 0.5 mL of aspirated fluid to prevent contamination by maternal cells or blood.
6. Withdraw the needle and place an adhesive bandage over the puncture site. Postprocedure ultrasound scanning confirms fetal viability.
7. Label specimen with the patient's name, date, and test(s) ordered. Place the amniotic fluid specimen in a sterile brown or foil-covered silicone container to protect it from light and thereby prevent breakdown of bilirubin. Label the container properly. Include the estimated weeks of gestation and the expected delivery date. Deliver the sample to the laboratory immediately.
8. Be aware that the laboratory workup for genetic diagnoses usually takes 2 to 4 weeks to complete. However, specimens obtained for determination of fetal age (e.g., creatinine) take 1 to 2 hours; determinations of the lecithin-to-sphingomyelin (L/S) ratio and phosphatidylglycerol (PG) take 3 to 4 hours; Gram stain to rule out infection takes 30 minutes, and cultures take 48 to 72 hours.
9. The procedure may have to be repeated if no amniotic fluid is obtained or if there is failure of cell growth or culture results are negative.
10. Techniques have been developed for performing amniocentesis in the presence of twin fetuses. Amniotic fluid is aspirated from one of the amniotic sacs, and a small amount of contrast material is injected into the sac. When the adjacent sac is tapped and produces clear amniotic fluid, the healthcare provider is assured that each sac has been tapped and each fetus will be accurately assessed.
11. Record the type of procedure done, date, time, name of healthcare provider performing the test, maternal-fetal response, and disposition of specimen.

PROCEDURAL ALERT

1. Accurate and optimally safe results from amniocentesis are possible only if the following protocols are observed:
   a. Gestation ≥15 wk
   b. Ultrasound monitoring to locate suitable pools of amniotic fluid, outline the placenta, exclude the presence of a multiple pregnancy, and accurately estimate fetal maturity. These considerations are necessary to correctly interpret AFP values in amniotic fluid and maternal blood.
   c. Precise and meticulous amniocentesis technique, including use of 20- or 22-gauge needle
   d. Maximum of two needle insertion attempts for a single tap
   e. Administration of RhoGAM for the Rh-negative woman
2. Fetal loss attributable to the procedure is <0.5%. Repeat amniocentesis is necessary in 0.1% of cases.
3. Fetal complications include:
   a. Spontaneous abortion
   b. Injury to the fetus (fetal puncture)
   c. Hemorrhage
   d. Infection
   e. Rh sensitization if fetal blood enters the patient's circulation
4. Maternal complications include:
   a. Hemorrhage
   b. Hematomas

This test is contraindicated in women with a history of premature labor or incompetent cervix and in the presence of placenta previa or abruptio placentae. Women who are carriers of hepatitis B or C should be informed of the limited information regarding transmission with invasive procedures. HIV-positive women should avoid invasive testing. If the amniotic fluid is bloody (blood is usually of maternal origin) and if a significant number of fetal cells (Kleihauer-Betke–positive smear) are present in the amniotic fluid of an Rh-negative patient, administration of RhoGAM should be considered. Some doctors prefer to administer RhoGAM to all Rh-negative patients for amniocentesis, unless they are already sensitized at that time.

Clinical Implications

1. Elevated amniotic fluid AFP can indicate possible neural tube defects as well as multiple gestations, fetal death, abdominal wall defects, teratomas, Rh sensitization, and fetal distress.
2. Decreased AFP is associated with fetal trisomy 21 (Down syndrome).
3. Creatinine levels are reduced in fetal prematurity. At 37 weeks of gestation, creatinine in amniotic fluid should be >2 mg/dL (>15 μmol/L).
4. Increased or decreased total amniotic fluid volumes are associated with certain types of arrested fetal development.
5. Increased bilirubin levels are associated with impending fetal death.
6. Amniotic fluid color changes are associated with fetal distress and other disorders such as chromosome abnormalities.
7. Sickle cell anemia and thalassemia can be detected through analysis of amniotic fibroblast DNA.
8. X-linked disorders are not routinely diagnosed in utero. However, because these disorders affect only men, the fetal sex may need to be determined when the patient is a known carrier of the X-linked gene in question (e.g., hemophilia, Duchenne's muscular dystrophy).
9. Screening for carrier state or affected fetus is done through chromosomal testing.

10. The presence of some of the >100 detectable metabolic disorders can be detected in the amniotic fluid sample. Examples include Tay-Sachs disease, Lesch-Nyhan syndrome, Hunter's syndrome, Hurler's syndrome, and various hemoglobinopathies. Hereditary metabolic disorders are caused by absence of an enzyme due to deletion or by alteration of the structure or synthesis of an enzyme due to gene mutation. If the enzyme in question is expressed in amniotic fluid cells, it can potentially be used for prenatal diagnosis. An unaffected fetus would have a normal enzyme concentration, a clinically normal carrier of the gene defect would have perhaps half of the normal enzyme level, and an affected fetus would have a very small amount or none of the enzyme.
11. For disorders in which an abnormal protein is not expressed in amniotic fluid cells, other test procedures are necessary, such as *DNA restriction endonuclease analysis*.

Interfering Factors

1. Fetal blood contamination can cause false-positive results for AFP.
2. False-negative and false-positive errors in karyotyping can occur.
3. Polyhydramnios may falsely lower bilirubin values as a result of dilution.
4. Hemolysis of the specimen can alter test results.
5. Oligohydramnios may falsely increase some amniotic fluid analysis values, especially bilirubin; this can lead to errors in predicting the clinical status of the fetus.

Interventions

Pretest Patient Care

1. Ensure that elective genetic counseling includes a discussion of the risk for having a child with a genetic defect and problems (e.g., depression, guilt) associated with selective abortion. The father should be present and should be a partner in the decision-making process. In genetic counseling, do not coerce the parents into undergoing abortion or sterilization; this should be an individual choice.
2. Explain test purpose, procedure, and risks; assess for contraindications.
3. Ensure that a properly signed and witnessed legal consent form is obtained.
4. Instruct the patient to empty her bladder just before the test.
5. Obtain baseline measurements of fetal and maternal vital signs. Monitor fetal signs for 15 minutes.
6. Alert the patient to the possibility that transient feelings of nausea, vertigo, and mild cramping may occur during the procedure. Help the patient to relax.
7. Follow guidelines in Chapter 1 for safe, effective, informed *pretest* care.

Posttest Patient Care

1. Check maternal blood pressure, pulse, respiration, and fetal heart tone every 15 minutes for the first half hour after test completion. Palpate the uterine fundus to assess fetal and uterine activity; monitor for 20 to 30 minutes with an external fetal monitor, if one is available.
2. Position the patient on her left side to counteract supine hypotension and to increase venous return and cardiac output.
3. Instruct the patient to notify her healthcare provider if she experiences amniotic fluid loss, signs of onset of labor, redness and inflammation at the insertion site, abdominal pain, bleeding, elevated temperature, chills, unusual fetal activity, or lack of fetal movement.
4. Follow guidelines in Chapter 1 for safe, effective, informed *posttest* care.

CLINICAL ALERT

1. Families need to know that prenatal diagnoses based on amniotic fluid assay are not infallible; sometimes, results do not reflect the true fetal status. Findings from amniocentesis cannot guarantee a normal or abnormal child; they can only determine the relative likelihood of

specific disorders within the limits of laboratory measurements. Some conditions cannot be predicted by this method, including nonspecific mental retardation, cleft lip and palate, and phenylketonuria (PKU).

2. Cytogenetic analysis can produce results that are 99.8% accurate.
3. An anteriorly located placenta does not preclude amniocentesis. A thin portion of placenta can be traversed during amniocentesis with no apparent increase in postamniocentesis complications.

Amniotic Fluid Alpha$_1$-Fetoprotein (AFP)

AFP is synthesized by the embryonic liver and is the major protein (glycoprotein) found in fetal serum. It resembles albumin in molecular weight, amino acid sequence, and immunologic characteristics. However, it is not normally detectable after birth. Ordinarily, high levels of fetoproteins are found in the developing fetus, and low levels exist in maternal serum and amniotic fluid.

The amniotic fluid AFP test is used to diagnose fetal neural tube defects (malformations of the central nervous system); fetoprotein leaks into the amniotic fluid during such pregnancies. The causes of neural tube defects are not known; however, a genetic component is assumed because an increased risk for recurrence exists. Neural tube defects usually exhibit polygenic traits (added effects of genes at multiple loci). In cases of anencephaly and open spina bifida, both MS-AFP and amniotic fluid AFP concentrations are abnormal by the 18th week of gestation.

In addition, AFP measurements have been used as indicators of fetal distress; in such cases, both amniotic fluid AFP and MS-AFP may be increased. However, final confirmation must come from further studies.

Reference Values

Normal

12 to 16 weeks

Peak at 12 to 16 weeks is 14.5 μg/L or 196 pmol/L.

Values vary considerably according to age of fetus and laboratory methods used.

Values peak at 12 to 16 gestational weeks and then gradually decline to term.

Procedure

In the laboratory, amniotic fluid is analyzed for concentration of AFP.

Clinical Implications

Increased amniotic AFP levels are associated with:

1. Neural tube defects such as anencephaly (100% reliable), encephalocele, spina bifida, and myelomeningocele (90% reliable)
2. Congenital nephrosis
3. Omphalocele
4. Turner's syndrome with cystic hydromas
5. Gastrointestinal tract obstruction
6. Missed abortion
7. Fetal distress
8. Imminent or actual fetal death
9. Severe Rh immunization
10. Esophageal or duodenal atresia
11. Fetal liver necrosis secondary to herpesvirus infection
12. Sacrococcygeal teratoma

13. Spontaneous abortion
14. Trisomy 13
15. Urinary obstruction (e.g., fetal bladder neck obstruction with hydronephrosis)
16. Cystic fibrosis

Interfering Factors

1. Fetal blood contamination causes increased AFP.
2. Increased AFP is associated with multiple pregnancies.
3. False-positive (0.1% to 0.2%) results may be associated with fetal death, twins, or genetic anomalies, but sometimes, no explanation can be given for the results.

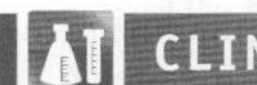 **CLINICAL ALERT**

Any parents who have already produced a child with a neural tube defect should be offered antenatal studies in anticipation of future pregnancies. If one parent has spina bifida, the pregnancy should be closely monitored.

Interventions

Pretest Patient Care

1. Explain the test purpose and the meaning of positive and negative test results.
2. Provide for genetic counseling.
3. Follow guidelines in Chapter 1 for safe, effective, informed *pretest* care.

Posttest Patient Care

1. Review test results; report and record findings. Modify the nursing care plan as needed. Counsel the patient and monitor appropriately.
2. Follow guidelines in Chapter 1 for safe, effective, informed *posttest* care.

● Amniotic Fluid Total Volume

Measurement of amniotic fluid total volume is helpful for estimating the changes in total amounts of certain substances that circulate in the amniotic fluid, including bilirubin, creatinine, and surface-active agents. Knowledge of total amniotic fluid volume is important because marked changes in the amount of amniotic fluid can decrease the predictive value of serial concentration measurements of specific substances. This measurement is most important when test results do not agree with the clinical picture.

Reference Values

Weeks of Gestation	Average Volume (mL)
12	~50
15	350
20	450
25	750
30–35	1500

After 35 weeks, values decrease to 1250 mL at term.

Procedure

1. Study a sample of amniotic fluid with the use of a solution of para-aminohippuric acid (PAH) for absorbency and dilution to calculate the probable amniotic fluid volume in milliliters.
2. Correct amniotic fluid total volume by multiplying the measured levels of specific substance by the actual fluid volume divided by average volume (for gestation age).
3. If either polyhydramnios or oligohydramnios is suspected, the fetus should be screened with ultrasound to detect physical anomalies.

Clinical Implications

1. Polyhydramnios (increased amniotic fluid, >2000 mL) is suggested by a total intrauterine volume >2 standard deviations (SD) above the mean for a given gestational age. It is estimated that 18% to 20% of fetuses in such pregnancies have congenital anomalies, the two most common being anencephaly and esophageal atresia (fetal swallowing is greatly impaired). The remainder have involvement secondary to Rh disease, diabetes, or other unknown causes. Polyhydramnios is also associated with multiple births (e.g., twins).
2. Oligohydramnios (reduced volume of amniotic fluid, <300 mL) is suggested by a total intrauterine volume >2 SD below the mean occurring before the 25th week of gestation. A disturbance of kidney function caused by renal agenesis or kidney atresia can result in oligohydramnios (fetal urination is impaired). After 25 weeks, the suspected causes of decreased amniotic fluid volume are premature rupture of membranes, intrauterine growth retardation, and postterm pregnancy.

Interventions

Pretest Patient Care

1. Explain the reason for amniotic fluid testing and the meaning of results.
2. Follow guidelines in Chapter 1 for safe, effective, informed *pretest* care.

Posttest Patient Care

1. Review amniotic fluid test results; report and record findings. Modify the nursing care plan as needed.
2. Follow guidelines in Chapter 1 for safe, effective, informed *posttest* care.

● Amniotic Fluid Index (AFI)

Reference Values

Normal

At term, the AFI is usually between 8 and 18 cm. Values <5 cm indicate oligohydramnios, and those >24 cm indicate polyhydramnios.

Procedure

1. The pregnant woman lies supine with displacement of the uterus to the left. The abdomen is divided into four quadrants.
2. Ultrasound is used to locate the largest pocket of amniotic fluid in each of the four quadrants, and each pocket is measured vertically. The four values are added together to obtain the AFI. The advantage of this test is that serial follow-up measurements can be done.

Clinical Implications

1. Oligohydramnios and polyhydramnios are indicators of poor outcome in pregnancy.
2. Oligohydramnios can indicate chronic uteroplacental insufficiency or renal anomaly.
3. An AFI higher than the 97.5 percentile for a certain gestational age is considered to indicate polyhydramnios. Polyhydramnios is associated with upper gastrointestinal tract obstruction or malformation (e.g., tracheoesophageal fistula, hydrops fetalis).

Interfering Factors

False-positive results can occur in a severely dehydrated woman.

Interventions

Pretest Patient Care

1. Explain the reason for the AFI procedure.
2. Follow guidelines in Chapter 1 for safe, effective, informed *pretest* care.

Posttest Patient Care

1. Explain the test results to the patient. Prepare the patient for follow-up procedures or need for delivery of the infant.
2. Follow guidelines in Chapter 1 for safe, effective, informed *posttest* care.

• Amniotic Fluid Creatinine

Creatinine, a byproduct of muscle metabolism found in amniotic fluid, reflects increased fetal muscle mass and the ability of the maturing kidney (i.e., glomerular filtrating system) to excrete creatinine into the amniotic fluid. The amniotic fluid creatinine concentration progressively increases as pregnancy advances. The patient's blood creatinine level should be known before the amniotic fluid creatinine value is interpreted.

Creatinine indicates fetal physical maturity and correlates reasonably well with the level of lung maturity. Normal lung development is dependent on normal kidney development. As pregnancy progresses, the amniotic fluid creatinine level increases. A value of 2 mg/dL (177 μmol/L) is accepted as an indicator that gestation is at 37 weeks or more. However, the use of this value alone to assess maturity is not advised for several reasons. A high creatinine concentration may reflect fetal muscle mass but not necessarily kidney maturity. For example, a large fetus of a patient with diabetes may have high creatinine levels because of increased muscle mass. Conversely, a hypertensive patient who has a small infant with growth retardation may have low creatinine levels because of decreased muscle mass. Creatinine levels can be misleading if they are used without other supporting data. So long as maternal blood creatinine levels are not increased, amniotic fluid creatinine measurements have a certain degree of reliability if they are interpreted in conjunction with other maturity studies.

Reference Values

Normal

A value >2 mg/dL or >177 μmol/L indicates fetal maturity (at 37 weeks) if maternal creatinine is normal.

Procedure

1. Obtain an amniotic fluid sample of at least 0.5 mL.
2. Protect the specimen from direct light.
3. Obtain a maternal venous blood sample.

Clinical Implications

Creatinine levels lower than expected may occur in the following situations:

1. Early in the gestational cycle (not yet at 37 weeks)
2. Fetus smaller than normal (growth retardation)
3. Fetal kidney abnormalities
4. Prematurity

Interfering Factors

Causes of elevated amniotic fluid creatinine concentrations that are not consistent with gestational age include abnormal maternal creatinine, diabetes, and preeclampsia.

Interventions

Pretest Patient Care

1. Explain the purpose of the test.
2. Follow guidelines in Chapter 1 for safe, effective, informed *pretest* care.

Posttest Patient Care

1. Review test results; report and record findings. Modify the nursing care plan as needed.
2. Follow guidelines in Chapter 1 for safe, effective, informed *posttest* care.

● Amniotic Fluid Lecithin-to-Sphingomyelin (L/S) Ratio, Surfactant-to-Albumin (S/A) Ratio, Phosphatidylglycerol (PG) (Surfactant Components), Lamellar Body Counts

These tests are used to assess fetal lung maturity (FLM). FLM tests can be grouped into either biochemical tests (e.g., L/S ratio or measurement of PG) or biophysical tests (e.g., lamellar body counts or surfactant/albumin [S/A] ratio). Lecithin and sphingomyelin, produced by lung tissue, have detergent-like action (pulmonary surfactant), which stabilizes the neonatal alveoli to prevent their collapse on expiration and consequent atelectasis. The amount of lecithin in amniotic fluid is less than the amount of sphingomyelin until 26 weeks of gestation; at 30 to 32 weeks of gestation, the two lipid values are about equal. At 35 weeks, lecithin level rises abruptly but sphingomyelin stays constant or decreases slightly. Saturated phosphatidylcholine, a subfraction of total lecithin, is a major surface-active component of lung surfactant.

The relationship between the phospholipids and the surface-active agents, L/S ratio, is used as an index of FLM. If early delivery is anticipated because of conditions such as diabetes, premature rupture of membranes, maternal hypertension, placental insufficiency, or erythroblastosis (Rh disease), the L/S ratio can be used to predict whether the fetal lung will function properly at birth. When early delivery is necessary for fetal viability, the result may be prematurity, pulmonary immaturity, or perinatal mortality. The L/S ratio should be determined on all repeat cesarean sections before delivery to ascertain when fetal lungs are functionally mature. Sphingomyelin exhibits surface-active properties in the lung but plays no role in the surfactant system except to be used as a convenient marker. The S/A ratio also indicates FLM.

Typically, screening for FLM is unnecessary if gestational age is >39 weeks. However, complications of maternal diabetes or Rh isoimmunization can retard fetal lung development; therefore, assessment of FLM may be indicated. Rapid screening tests, such as AmnioStat-FLM-PG (Irvine Scientific, Santa Ana, CA), are available for assessing FLM. The AmnioStat-FLM-PG is a semiquantitative, immunologic, card-agglutination test that can determine the presence of PG, a component of pulmonary surfactant, to assess FLM. Another rapid screening test, the TDx FLM II system (Abbott Diagnostics, Abbott Park, IL), uses fluorescence polarization technology to determine the S/A ratio. These rapid tests seem to be highly reliable in uncomplicated pregnancies.

Lamellar body counts are measures of the phospholipid that represents the storage form of surfactant. The count is used to assess for FLM.

Reference Values

Normal

L/S ratio: >2.0

S/A ratio: >55 mg/g (indicates lung maturity)

PG

Presence of PG indicates mature fetal lung.

Absence of PG indicates high risk for developing respiratory fetal distress.

Lamellar body counts: >60,000 particles/μL

Procedure

1. Withdraw at least 3 mL of amniotic fluid, or collect from a free flow of fluid from the vagina in cases of ruptured membranes.
2. Centrifuge the fluid and prepare for analysis and read the results in a reflectance densitometer. Calculate the L/S ratio.

Clinical Implications

1. A decreased L/S ratio (<1.5) is often associated with pulmonary immaturity and respiratory distress syndrome (RDS).
2. An L/S ratio >2.0 signifies FLM. The occurrence of RDS is extremely unlikely.
3. An L/S ratio between 1.5 and 1.9 indicates possible mild-to-moderate RDS (50% risk).
4. Fetuses of women with insulin-dependent diabetes develop RDS at higher ratios. The L/S ratio should be >3.5 for these infants.
5. A decreased S/A ratio (<40 mg/g) is consistent with immature fetal lungs.
6. An S/A ratio of 40 to 55 mg/g is considered indeterminate of FLM status.
7. Lamellar body counts of <15,000 particles/μL indicate fetal lung immaturity, whereas 15,000 to 60,000 particles/μL indicates transitional lung.

CLINICAL ALERT

1. If the L/S ratio is <1.5, it is preferable to delay induced delivery until the fetal lung becomes more mature.
2. FLM appears to be regulated by hormonal factors, some stimulatory and others possibly inhibitory. For this reason, hormones such as betamethasone (Celestone) are given in two doses, administered 24 hr apart, if premature labor occurs.
3. Under certain stressful conditions, premature fetal lung maturation may be seen. This accelerated fetal lung maturation is thought to be a protective mechanism for the preterm fetus should delivery actually occur.
   a. Premature rupture of the membranes. Prolonged rupture of the membranes (after 72 hr) has an acute negative effect on lung maturation.
   b. Acute placental function
   c. Placental insufficiency
   d. Chronic abruptio placentae
   e. Renal hypertensive disease caused by degenerative forms of diabetes
   f. Cardiovascular hypertensive disease associated with drug abuse
   g. Severe pregnancy-induced hypertension
4. Delayed fetal lung maturation may be seen in the following conditions; in these instances, a higher L/S ratio (>3.5) may be necessary to ensure adequate FLM:
   a. Infants born to patients with insulin-dependent diabetes
   b. Infants born to patients with nonhypertensive glomerulonephritis
   c. Hydrops fetalis
5. A *lung profile* of amniotic fluid to evaluate lung maturity looks not only for lecithin but also for two other phospholipids—PG and phosphatidylinositol (PI). PI increases in the amniotic fluid after 26–30 wk of gestation, peaks at 35–36 wk, and then decreases gradually. PG appears after 35 wk and continues to increase until term; measurements are classified as positive PG or negative PG. The lung profile is a useful adjunct in evaluating the L/S ratio. It appears that lung maturity can be confirmed in most pregnancies if PG is present (positive) in conjunction with an L/S ratio >2.0. PG may provide stability that makes the infant less susceptible to RDS when experiencing hypoglycemia, hypoxia, or hypothermia. The PG measurement is especially useful in borderline cases and in class A, B, and C diabetes when pulmonary maturation is delayed.

Interfering Factors

1. High false-negative result rates
2. Unpredictability or borderline values
3. Unpredictability of contaminated blood specimens
4. Occasional false-positive values associated with conditions such as Rh disease, diabetes, or severe birth asphyxia

Interventions

Pretest Patient Care

1. Explain the reason for testing and the meaning of results.
2. Follow guidelines in Chapter 1 for safe, effective, informed *pretest* care.

Posttest Patient Care

1. Review test results; report and record findings. Modify the nursing care plan as needed.
2. Follow guidelines in Chapter 1 for safe, effective, informed *posttest* care.

● Amniotic Fluid Shake Test (Foam Stability Test)

The shake test is a qualitative measurement of the amount of pulmonary surfactant contained in the amniotic fluid. It is quick and inexpensive. It is a "bedside test" of lung maturity. In an obstetric emergency, an immediate decision about delivery can be made. The advantages of this test over the L/S ratio are that a physician, technician, or nurse can perform it and the results are highly reliable. The L/S ratio usually is not determined when the shake test is positive because the shake test also indicates fetal maturity. A table of dilutions is used to determine the stage of lung maturity.

Reference Values

Normal

Positive: Persistence of a foam ring for 15 minutes after shaking (at an amniotic fluid–alcohol dilution of 1:2) indicates lung maturity.

Procedure

1. The test is based on the ability of amniotic fluid surfactant to form a complete ring of bubbles on the surface of the amniotic fluid in the presence of 95% ethanol.
2. Place a mixture of 95% ethanol and amniotic fluid in an appropriate container and shake for 15 seconds. A commercial kit may be used.

Clinical Implications

1. If a complete ring of foam forms and persists for 15 minutes, the test is positive.
2. If no ring of bubbles forms, the test is negative.
3. The test has a high false-negative rate but a low false-positive rate. The L/S ratio must be >4:1 for this test to be positive.

Interfering Factors

1. Blood or meconium contamination
2. Contamination of glassware or reagents

Interventions

Pretest Patient Care

1. Explain the reason for testing and the meaning of results.
2. Follow guidelines in Chapter 1 for safe, effective, informed *pretest* care.

Posttest Patient Care

1. Review test results; report and record findings. Modify the nursing care plan as needed.
2. Follow guidelines in Chapter 1 for safe, effective, informed *posttest* care.

● Amniotic Fluid Foam Stability Index (FSI)

The foam stability index (FSI) is a modification of the shake test. It provides a functional measurement of FLM based on the surface tension properties of surfactant phospholipids.

Reference Values

Normal

FSI: >0.47

Procedure

1. Mix a fixed amount of undiluted amniotic fluid with increasing volumes of ethanol.
2. Shake the sample and observe for foam.
3. Document the largest column of ethanol in which the amniotic fluid can form and support foam. This test is almost as reliable as the L/S ratio in normal pregnancies, and it appears to have a lower false-positive rate than the shake test.

Clinical Implications

An FSI of >0.48 is termed *mature*; a value of <0.46 is termed *immature*.

Interfering Factors

1. Blood or meconium contamination can produce a false mature result.
2. The test is not reliable for amniotic fluid collected from the vagina.

Interventions

Pretest Patient Care

1. Explain the reason for testing and the meaning of results.
2. Follow guidelines in Chapter 1 for safe, effective, informed *pretest* care.

Posttest Patient Care

1. Review test results; report and record findings. Modify the nursing care plan as needed.
2. Follow guidelines in Chapter 1 for safe, effective, informed *posttest* care.

● Amniotic Fluid Fern Test

Fern production is a result of the concentration of electrolytes, especially sodium chloride, in the cervical glands; it is under the control of estrogen. Close to term, amniotic fluid shows a typical fern pattern similar to that seen in cervical mucus; this indicates a predominantly estrogen effect rather than progesterone.

This study differentiates urine from amniotic fluid. It is done to determine whether the fluid passed is urine or prematurely leaked amniotic fluid. Urine can be differentiated from amniotic fluid if the fluid is tested for the presence of urea, nitrogen, potassium, and creatinine and the absence of AFP. This is a relatively fast and inexpensive test that can be easily done.

Reference Values

Normal

Positive test for presence of amniotic fluid

Procedure

1. Perform a vaginal examination with the use of a sterile speculum.
2. Place a few drops of fluid on a slide and allow it to dry.
3. Look for a fern or palm leaf pattern (arborization) under the microscope.

Clinical Implications

1. A positive test shows the fern pattern indicative of amniotic fluid.
2. A negative test shows no ferning or crystallization; this indicates little or no estrogen effect.
3. No fern pattern is seen if the specimen is urine.

Interfering Factors

Blood contaminating the specimen inhibits fern formation.

Interventions

Pretest Patient Care

1. Explain test purpose and procedure.
2. Follow guidelines in Chapter 1 for safe, effective, informed *pretest* care.

Posttest Patient Care

1. Review test results; report and record findings. Modify the nursing care plan as needed.
2. Follow guidelines in Chapter 1 for safe, effective, informed *posttest* care.

● Placental Alpha Macroglobulin-1 Protein Assay (AmniSure)

Immunochromatography is used to detect trace amounts of placental alpha macroglobulin-1 protein in the vaginal fluid to detect ruptured membranes. The advantages of this test include that it is not affected by semen or trace amounts of blood. Sensitivity is 94.4% to 98.9%; specificity, 87.5% to 100%. This test is used to confirm fern or Nitrazine testing.

Procedure

1. Insert a sterile swab into the vagina for 1 minute.
2. Place the swab into a vial that contains a solvent for 1 minute.
3. Insert an AmniSure test strip into the vial.

Clinical Indications

1. A negative test for amniotic fluid shows one visible line after 5 to 10 minutes.
2. A positive test for amniotic fluid shows two visible lines after 5 to 10 minutes.
3. No visible line is an invalid result.

Interventions

Pretest Patient Care

1. Explain test purpose and procedure.
2. Follow guidelines in Chapter 1 for safe, effective, informed *pretest* care.

Posttest Patient Care

1. Review test results; report and record findings. Modify the nursing care plan as needed.
2. Follow guidelines in Chapter 1 for safe, effective, informed *posttest* care.

● Amniotic Fluid Color

Amniotic fluid specimens should be visually inspected for color. The range of color may vary from clear to a pale straw-yellow color. White particles of vermin cases from fetal skin and lanugo hair may be present. In certain disorders such as missed abortion, chromosomally abnormal fetus, and fetal anencephaly, the amniotic fluid color is altered.

Reference Values

Normal

Sound: colorless or pale straw-yellow color

Procedure

1. Observe color changes and staining through amnioscopy before the amniotic membranes have ruptured.
2. Place an amnioscope into the vagina and against the fetal presenting part. Visualize the amniotic fluid through the amniotic membranes. Problems with amnioscopy include inadvertent rupture of membranes, insufficient dilation of the cervix and consequent difficulty inserting the amnioscope, intrauterine infection, and occasional difficulty in interpreting amniotic fluid color.
3. Be aware that the test may also be difficult to perform if the patient is in active labor.

PROCEDURAL ALERT

1. Meconium staining may also be observed when an amniocentesis is done. After the membranes have ruptured, meconium staining may be observed in the vaginal discharge. Once meconium staining is identified, more assessments (e.g., FHR patterns) must be made before delivery is contemplated to determine whether the fetus is experiencing ongoing episodes of hypoxia.
2. The presence of meconium in the amniotic fluid is normal in breech presentations.

Clinical Implications

1. *Yellow* amniotic fluid indicates blood incompatibility, erythroblastosis fetalis, or presence of bile pigment released by red blood cell hemolysis (fetal bilirubin).
2. *Dark yellow* aspirate indicates probable fetal involvement.
3. *Red* color indicates blood, in which case it must be determined whether the blood is from the patient or the fetus. Fetal blood in the amniotic fluid is of grave concern.
4. *Green, opaque* fluid indicates meconium contamination. The fetus passes meconium because of hyperperistalsis in response to a stressor that may be very transient or may be more serious and protracted (e.g., hypoxia). A very good correlation states that the more meconium present, the more severe and immediate the stressor. Additional assessments, such as amnioscopy and amniography, must be made to determine whether the fetus is experiencing ongoing episodes of hypoxia or other stressors. Green color can also indicate erythroblastosis but is not necessarily indicative of it.
5. *Yellow-brown, opaque* fluid may indicate intrauterine death and fetal maceration (although not necessarily from erythroblastosis), oxidized hemoglobin, or maternal trauma.

Interventions

Pretest Patient Care

1. Explain the purpose of the test and the procedure if amnioscopy is done.
2. Follow guidelines in Chapter 1 for safe, effective, informed *pretest* care.

Posttest Patient Care

1. Review test results; report and record findings. Modify the nursing care plan as needed. Counsel the patient and monitor appropriately.
2. Follow guidelines in Chapter 1 for safe, effective, informed *posttest* care.

● Amniotic Fluid Bilirubin Optical Density (OD)

Bilirubin is a pigment acquired by the amniotic fluid during its circulation through the gastrointestinal tract. Bilirubin may be found in amniotic fluid as early as the 12th week of gestation. It reaches its highest concentration between 16 and 30 weeks. As the pregnancy continues, the amount of bilirubin progressively decreases until it finally disappears near term. Bilirubin levels increase in the presence of erythroblastotic fetuses and fetuses with anencephaly or intestinal obstruction.

This measurement is used to monitor the fetal state in an Rho-negative pregnant women who has a rising anti-Rho antibody titer. The rising titer is synonymous with Rh erythroblastosis fetalis or hemolytic disease of the newborn (HDN). This determination usually is not made before 20 to 24 weeks' gestation because no therapy is available to the fetus before that time. Close to term, the amniotic fluid bilirubin pigment concentration normally decreases in the absence of Rh sensitization.

Determination of optical density (OD) is only one of several laboratory methods used to measure bilirubin. The degree of hemolytic disease falls into three zones (zones 1, 2, and 3) using OD measurement and a wavelength (absorbance) of 450 nm (the Liley or Diazo method). Difficulty in interpretation occurs frequently. Findings must be interpreted by a knowledgeable person who can recognize pitfalls. Pertinent clinical information and other laboratory data also may be taken into consideration. After 30 weeks' gestation, the Liley test result is usually combined with an assessment of FLM (L/S ratio) to assist in the decision of whether to induce delivery.

Reference Values

Normal

OD <0.02 mg/dL or <0.34 μmol/L at 450-nm absorbance wavelength by the Liley method, or 0.025 mg/dL (0.43 μmol/L) by the Diazo method, indicates maturity.

Procedure

1. Collect 5 to 10 mL of amniotic fluid in a lightproof container. Label specimen with the patient's name, date, and test(s) ordered.
2. Send the fluid to the laboratory immediately.
3. Be aware that the specimen may be refrigerated for up to 24 hours. It can be frozen if a longer time will elapse before analysis.
4. Avoid blood in the specimen. If initial aspiration produces a bloody fluid, the needle should be repositioned to obtain a specimen free of red cells. If a blood-free specimen cannot be obtained, the specimen must be examined at once before hemolysis occurs.
5. Indicate weeks of gestation on the laboratory request form.

Clinical Implications

1. If OD = 0.28 to 0.46 (zone 1, low zone, 2+ OD) at 28 to 31 weeks, the fetus will not be affected or will have very mild hemolytic disease.
2. If OD = 0.47 to 0.90 (zone 2, middle zone, 3+ OD), there is a moderate effect on the fetus. The fetal age and the trend in OD indicate the need for intrauterine transfusion and early delivery.
3. If OD = 0.91 to 1.0 (zone 3, high zone, 4+ OD), the fetus is severely affected, and fetal death is a possibility. In this case, a decision concerning delivery or intrauterine transfusion, depending on the age of the fetus, should be made. After 32 to 33 weeks of gestation, early delivery and extrauterine treatment are preferred.

4. An OD <0.04 indicates fetal maturity and well-being.
5. *Increased* OD is found in:
   a. Erythroblastosis fetalis
   b. Other fetal hemolytic diseases
   c. Maternal infectious hepatitis
   d. Maternal sickle cell crisis

Interfering Factors

1. Blood, hemoglobin, or meconium in the specimen can produce inaccurate results.
2. Maternal use of steroids interferes with the test.
3. Exposure of the amniotic fluid to light compromises the test.
4. Fetal acidosis interferes with the test.

CLINICAL ALERT

A bilirubin level that fails to decline as expected or increases indicates that the fetal status is deteriorating.

Interventions

Pretest Patient Care

1. Explain the test purpose and the meaning of test results.
2. Follow guidelines in Chapter 1 for safe, effective, informed *pretest* care.

Posttest Patient Care

1. Review test results; report and record findings. Modify the nursing care plan as needed. Monitor the patient and counsel appropriately.
2. Follow guidelines in Chapter 1 for safe, effective, informed *posttest* care.

● Amniotic Fluid and Desaturated Phosphatidylcholine (DSPC)

Desaturated phosphatidylcholine (DSPC) is the major component (50%) of fetal pulmonary surfactant. The concentration in amniotic fluid can be measured by separating DSPC from unsaturated lecithin. Phosphatidylcholine is the second most surface-active component of surfactant.

This test is a direct measure of primary phospholipid in surfactant and is used in the assessment of FLM.

Reference Values

Normal

Presence of DSPC is evidence that fetus is at least 36 to 37 weeks in development.

Procedure

Obtain and examine amniotic fluid for the primary phospholipid (DSPC).

Clinical Implications

1. Normal levels are consistent with FLM and indicate a negligible risk for RDS.
2. Low levels are associated with immaturity and a high risk for RDS.

Interfering Factors

Results may be altered by changes in amniotic fluid volume (oligohydramnios or polyhydramnios).

Interventions

Pretest Patient Care

1. Explain test purpose and the amniotic fluid sampling procedure.
2. Follow guidelines in Chapter 1 for safe, effective, informed *pretest* care.

Posttest Patient Care

1. Review test results; report and record findings. Modify the nursing care plan as needed. Monitor the patient and counsel appropriately.
2. Follow guidelines in Chapter 1 for safe, effective, informed *posttest* care.

ADDITIONAL MEASUREMENTS

● Group B Streptococcus (GBS) Screening

Group B Streptococcus (GBS) is a frequent cause of newborn pneumonia. Sepsis and meningitis are also common problems of GBS infection. Preterm infants are more susceptible to GBS disease, but it occurs most often in full-term infants.

The Centers for Disease Control and Prevention guidelines recommend that all pregnant women should be screened for anogenital group B streptococcal colonization at 35 to 37 weeks' gestation.

Reference Values

Normal

A negative vaginal and anorectal culture indicates GBS has not colonized in the cultured sites.

A positive culture indicates a GBS carrier, and results should be recorded on the prenatal record so that it is available to the healthcare providers at the time and place of delivery.

Procedure

1. Use a single standard culture swab for the distal vagina and anorectum, or two separate swabs can be used. See Chapter 7 for more information. Place swabs in transport medium if laboratory is off-site.
2. Report results on prenatal record and ensure that a copy is available at the hospital where delivery of the infant is anticipated.

Clinical Implications

1. Intrapartum antibiotic prophylaxis should be considered with positive culture results by weighing the risks and benefits of treatment with each GBS carrier who is pregnant.
2. Intravenous penicillin G is the preferred treatment, but ampicillin is an alternative. Antimicrobial susceptibility testing should be ordered for antenatal GBS cultures performed on penicillin-allergic women at high risk for anaphylaxis because of a history of anaphylaxis, angioedema, respiratory distress, or urticaria following administration of a penicillin or a cephalosporin (AII). To ensure proper testing, healthcare providers must inform laboratories of the need for antimicrobial susceptibility testing in such cases (AIII). Penicillin-allergic women at high risk for anaphylaxis should receive clindamycin if their GBS isolate is susceptible to clindamycin and erythromycin as determined by antimicrobial susceptibility testing; if the isolate is sensitive to clindamycin but resistant to erythromycin, clindamycin may be used if testing for inducible clindamycin resistance is negative (CIII). Penicillin-allergic women at high risk for anaphylaxis should receive vancomycin if their isolate is intrinsically resistant to clindamycin as determined by antimicrobial susceptibility testing, if the isolate demonstrates inducible resistance to clindamycin, or if susceptibility to both agents is unknown.
3. Prophylaxis should be continued throughout active labor until delivery.

4. Women with GBS isolated from the urine at any time during the current pregnancy, or who had a previous infant with invasive GBS disease, should receive intrapartum antibiotic prophylaxis and do not need third trimester screening for GBS colonization (AII). Women with symptomatic or asymptomatic GBS urinary tract infection detected during pregnancy should be treated according to current standards of care for urinary tract infection during pregnancy and should receive intrapartum antibiotic prophylaxis to prevent early-onset GBS disease (AIII).
5. If GBS status is unknown at the onset of labor, intrapartum chemoprophylaxis should be given to women with the following risk factors:
   a. <37 weeks' gestation
   b. Ruptured membranes ≥18 hours
   c. Temperature ≥100.4°F (>38°C)

Interventions

Pretest Patient Care

1. Explain the screening test to the patient, including the risks of GBS disease to newborn.
2. Follow guidelines in Chapter 1 for safe, effective, informed *pretest* care.

Posttest Patient Care

1. Review test results; report and record findings. Modify the nursing care plan as needed. Monitor the patient and counsel appropriately.
2. Oral antibiotics should not be used to treat pregnant women with a positive anogenital GBS culture because they are not effective in eliminating the carrier status or preventing neonatal disease. Treatment should take place intrapartum.
3. If symptomatic or asymptomatic GBS bacteria are detected in pregnancy, treatment should be considered at the time of diagnosis because this usually indicates a heavily colonized individual. Intrapartum treatment is also indicated for this individual.
4. If GBS status is unknown at the onset of labor (culture not done, incomplete, or results unknown) and any of the following are present—delivery will be at <37 weeks of gestation, amniotic membrane rupture ≥18 hours, intrapartum temperature ≥100.4°F (≥38.0°C), or intrapartum rapid test is positive for GBS—then GBS prophylaxis is indicated (ACOG Committee Opinion No. 485: Prevention of early-onset group B streptococcal disease in newborns).
5. Follow guidelines in Chapter 1 for safe, effective, informed *posttest* care.

● Fetal Oxygen Saturation ($FSpo_2$) Monitoring

Fetal oxygen saturation ($FSpo_2$) monitoring is used with external fetal monitoring (EFM) as an additional means of assessment when the FHR is not reassuring or not interpretable. The $FSpo_2$ monitoring system involves a single-use sterile disposable sensor that is inserted through the cervix into the uterus and rests against the fetal temple, cheek, or forehead. The sensor is a reflectance sensor in which a light source and a photodetector are placed next to each other. Backscatter of light (light absorption by pulsing arterial blood) is measured from a vascular bed under the sensor, and when it is reflected back to photodetector, reflected light is analyzed and displayed on the monitor and on the FHR paper tracing. $FSpo_2$ monitoring should only be used after maternal membranes have ruptured and on a singleton fetus in vertex presentation with a gestational age of ≥36 weeks.

Reference Values

Normal

With $FSpo_2$ of ≥30% between uterine contractions with a nonreassuring FHR, the fetus can be assumed to be adequately oxygenated.

Normal range for $FSpo_2$ is 30% to 70%. Continued $FSpo_2$ readings of <30% for >10 minutes are likely to lead to progressive fetal hypoxemia, acidemia, and deterioration in fetal well-being.

Procedure

1. Be aware that $FSpo_2$ is indicated if there is a nonreassuring FHR pattern.
2. Perform Leopold's maneuvers to determine fetal position and sterile vaginal exam to assess dilation, station, and presentation.
3. Apply sensors when membranes are ruptured and cervical dilation of $\geq$2 cm has been achieved with the fetus at station of −2 or below and vertex presentation.
4. Insert a single-use sterile sensor (proficiency in fetal scalp electrode insertion or intrauterine pressure catheter insertion is necessary). Insert the sensor perpendicularly to sagittal suture. Insertion should be done between uterine contractions.
5. Attach the sensor to the $FSpo_2$ monitor. This monitor may be able to interface with a FHR monitor and record as a continuous line with uterine activity.
6. Document $FSpo_2$ on labor flow sheet as a range (e.g., 40% to 45%), and follow standard documentation intervals of other fetal assessments such as FHR.

Clinical Implications

1. Single measurements of $FSpo_2$ are not useful; need to track trends
2. $FSpo_2$ monitoring, along with the use of other fetal monitoring, provides the ability to detect a compromised fetus and a healthy fetus with nonreassuring FHR.
3. Provides data that a fetus with a nonreassuring FHR pattern can safely continue in labor and reduce unnecessary interventions during labor and birth, therefore improving maternal-fetal outcomes and decreasing costs

Interfering Factors

1. Vernix can cause interruption in $FSpo_2$ monitoring if present in significant quantity. Meconium does not interfere.
2. Strong uterine contractions may cause temporary loss of the signal from sensor at peak of uterine contractions.
3. Fetal and maternal movement can displace sensor.

Interventions

Pretest Patient Care

1. Explain the reason for monitoring and the procedure involved.
2. Follow guidelines in Chapter 1 for safe, effective, informed *pretest* care.

CLINICAL ALERT

Contraindications include the following:

1. Documented or suspected placenta previa
2. Ominous FHR pattern requiring immediate intervention
3. Need for immediate delivery not related to FHR pattern
4. Active genital herpes, hepatitis B or E, or other infections that preclude internal monitoring
5. Seropositivity for HIV

Posttest Patient Care

1. Review test results; report and record findings. Modify the nursing care plan as needed. Counsel the patient and monitor appropriately during labor. Treat accordingly.
2. Follow guidelines in Chapter 1 for safe, effective, informed *posttest* care.

● Fetal Nuchal Translucency (FNT)

FNT is a noninvasive prenatal screening tool used to alert healthcare providers of potential fetal abnormalities. Ultrasonography is used to assess for a fluid collection at the nape of the fetal neck. An abnormal fluid collection may be due to genetic disorders or fetal physical abnormalities. The test is most accurate at 11 to 13 weeks' gestation. This screening test cannot identify fetal abnormalities; it is used as a screening tool for pregnancies that need diagnostic testing. If the FNT exceeds the normal range, then diagnostic genetic testing is recommended. There is a relationship between increased fluid in the nuchal area and cardiac abnormalities. The nuchal edema is thought to be a compensation factor in the fetus. It may indicate trisomy 18, trisomy 21 (Down syndrome), or fetal cardiac anomalies.

Reference Values

Abnormal

FNT during 11 to 13 weeks' gestation that is >2.5 mm of fluid in the fetal neck is considered abnormal.

A nuchal translucency measurement of ≥3 mm is highly suggestive of fetal abnormalities.

Procedure

FNT screening is performed by specially trained practitioners.

1. Explain the test purpose and the procedure.
2. Position the patient on her back as you would for obstetric ultrasound. A coupling gel is applied to the skin of the lower abdomen, and the ultrasound transducer is moved across the abdomen to visualize the fetal neck for fluid accumulation.
3. FNT is determined by ultrasound measurement of fluid in the nape of the neck between 10 and 14 weeks' gestation.

Clinical Implications

1. FNT screening can alert healthcare providers to potential fetal abnormalities.
2. Analyzing maternal serum level of β-hCG and PAPP-A levels, along with FNT, increases accuracy of testing for pregnancy that is at risk for fetal abnormalities.

Interfering Factors

1. There is a small but significant difference in FNT of some ethnic groups (Caucasian and Asian fetuses have larger measurements than African and Caribbean fetuses).
2. Nuchal cord will decrease accuracy. Color Doppler ultrasound needs to be used in these cases to differentiate cord from fluid.
3. Improper caliper placement during ultrasound

Interventions

Pretest Patient Care

1. Explain the test purpose and procedure to the patient.
2. Follow guidelines in Chapter 1 for safe, effective, informed *pretest* care.

Posttest Patient Care

1. Review test results; report and record findings. Modify the nursing care plan as needed. Monitor the patient and counsel appropriately. Educate the patient about further testing (genetic) and genetic counseling.
2. Follow guidelines in Chapter 1 for safe, effective, informed *posttest* care.

Fetal Alcohol Syndrome (FAS), Alcohol in Pregnancy

Fetal alcohol syndrome (FAS), a constellation of growth, mental, and physical birth defects, is a result of alcohol consumption by the pregnant woman. Because a safe level of alcohol consumption has not been established, a pregnant woman consuming any amount places the developing fetus at risk. Although studies have shown that alcohol consumed during the first trimester can cause more defects than alcohol consumed during subsequent trimesters, consumption at any time during fetal development poses a risk. The prevalence of FAS is about 1 per 1000 live births worldwide. Early recognition of FAS can result in better treatment, counseling, and referral.

CHART 15.1 Characteristics for Diagnosing Fetal Alcohol Syndrome

Facial Dysmorphia

On the basis of racial norms (i.e., those appropriate for a person's race), the person exhibits all three of the following characteristic facial features:

- Smooth philtrum (University of Washington Lip-Philtrum Guide[a] rank 4 or 5[a])
- Thin vermilion border (University of Washington Lip-Philtrum Guide rank 4 or 5)
- Small palpebral fissures (≤10th percentile)

Growth Problems

Confirmed, documented prenatal or postnatal height, weight, or both ≤10th percentile, adjusted for age, sex, gestational age, and race or ethnicity

Central Nervous System Abnormalities

Structural

- Head circumference ≤10th percentile, adjusted for age and sex
- Clinically meaningful brain abnormalities observable through imaging (e.g., reduction in size or change in shape of the corpus callosum, cerebellum, or basal ganglia)

Neurologic

- Neurologic problems (e.g., motor problems or seizures) not resulting from a postnatal insult or fever or other soft neurologic signs outside normal limits

Functional

Test performance substantially below that expected for a person's age, schooling, or circumstances, as evidenced by either:

- Global cognitive or intellectual deficits representing multiple domains of deficit (or substantial developmental delay in younger children) with performance below the 3rd percentile (i.e., 2 standard deviations [SD] below the mean for standardized testing)
- Functional deficits <16th percentile (i.e., 1 SD below the mean for standardized testing) in at least three of the following domains:
  — Cognitive or developmental deficits or discrepancies
  — Executive functioning deficits
  — Motor functioning delays
  — Problems with attention or hyperactivity
  — Social skills
  — Other (e.g., sensory problems, pragmatic language problems, memory deficits)

[a]Astley SJ: Diagnostic Guide for Fetal Alcohol Spectrum Disorders: The 4-Digit Diagnostic Code. 3rd ed. Seattle, WA, University of Washington Publication Services, 2004.

Source: Bertrand J, Floyd RL, Weber MK, et al: Fetal alcohol syndrome: Guidelines for referral and diagnosis. Atlanta, GA: U.S. Department of Health and Human Services, 2004. Available at: http://www.cdc.gov/ncbddd/fas/documents/FAS_guidelines_accessible.pdf

Reference Values

Normal

No abnormalities seen on ultrasound
No abnormalities seen on fetal echocardiography
Negative for blood alcohol

Procedure

1. Ultrasound may be performed to assess intrauterine growth (see Chapter 13).
2. Fetal echocardiography may be performed to assess cardiac abnormalities (see Chapter 13).
3. Blood alcohol level testing may be performed on the pregnant patient (see Chapter 6).

Clinical Implications

1. Criteria for diagnosing FAS requires three findings: (1) three specific facial abnormalities, (2) documented growth deficit, and (3) central nervous system abnormalities (Chart 15.1).
2. Other disorders, such as autism, conduct disorder, or oppositional defiant disorder, can coexist with FAS.
3. Central nervous system abnormalities are difficult to evaluate within FAS; therefore, a differential diagnosis should be made by healthcare providers trained in FAS and the broad array of birth defects.

Interventions

Pretest Patient Care

1. Explain the testing procedures to the patient and the meaning of the results.
2. Follow guidelines in Chapter 1 for safe, effective, informed *pretest* care.

Posttest Patient Care

1. Review test results; report and record findings. Modify the nursing care plan as needed. Counsel the patient and provide referral as needed. Referrals could include medical, educational, and social services.
2. Encourage the pregnant woman to refrain from alcohol consumption.
3. Follow guidelines in Chapter 1 for safe and informed *posttest* care.

BIBLIOGRAPHY

American Congress of Obstetricians and Gynecologists: Antepartum fetal surveillance. Washington, DC, ACOG Practice Bulletin, No. 145, July 2014; Obstet Gynecol 124:182–192, 2014

American Congress of Obstetricians and Gynecologists: Cell-free DNA Screening for Fetal Aneuploidy. Committee Opinion No. 640. Washington, DC, ACOG, 2015

American Congress of Obstetricians and Gynecologists Committee on Practice Bulletins: Obstetrics, and Committee on Genetics: Screening for fetal chromosomal abnormalities. ACOG Practice Bulletin No. 77. Washington, DC, ACOG, January 2007; reaffirmed 2008. Replaced by Practice Bulletin No. 163, Screening for Fetal Aneuploidy, May 2016

American Congress of Obstetricians and Gynecologists, Committee Opinion No. 485: Prevention of early-onset group B streptococcal disease in newborns. Obstet Gynecol 117(4):1019–1027, 2011

Baylor College of Medicine: Prenatal chromosomal microarray analysis. Available at: http://www.bcm.edu/geneticlabs/index.cfm?pmid=16837, 2012

Beamer LC: Fetal nuchal translucency: A prenatal screening tool. J Obstet Gynecol Neonat Nurs 30(4):376–384, 2001

Bertrand J, Floyd RL, Weber MK: Guidelines for identifying and referring persons with fetal alcohol syndrome. MMWR Recomm Rep 54(RR-11):1–14, 2005

Bubb JA, Matthews AL: What's new in prenatal screening and diagnosis? Prim Care 31:561–582, 2004

Centers for Disease Control and Prevention: Prevention of perinatal group B streptococcal disease. MMWR 59(RR10):1–32, 2010

Centers for Disease Control and Prevention: Pinkbook: Rubella. Available at: http://www.chop.edu/service/fetal-diagnosis-and-treatment/home.html

Children's Hospital of Philadelphia: Center for Fetal Diagnosis and Treatment. Available at: http://fetalsurgery.chop.edu/fetalnews.shtml

Cunningham FG, Leveno KJ, Bloom SL, et al: Williams' Obstetrics, 24th ed. New York, McGraw-Hill, 2014

Harvey D: Fetal MRI: Seeing what ultrasound doesn't. Radiol Today 6(2):18, 2005

Henney JE: New system for monitoring intrapartum fetal oxygen saturation. JAMA 284:33, 2000

Hubbard AM, Harty MP, States LS: A new tool for prenatal diagnosis: Ultrafast MRI. Semin Perinatol 6:437–447, 1999

Lopez RL, Francis JA, Garite TJ, et al: Fetal fibronectin detection as a predictor of preterm birth in actual clinical practice. Am J Obstet Gynecol 182:1103–1106, 2000

McPherson RA, Pincus MR: Henry's Clinical Diagnosis and Management by Laboratory Methods, 23rd ed. Philadelphia, Saunders Elsevier, 2016

Neerhof MG, Dohnal JC, Ashwood ER, et al: Lamellar body counts: A consensus on protocol. Obstet Gynecol 97(2):318–320, 2001

Ralston SJ, Craigo SD: Ultrasound-guided procedures for prenatal diagnosis and therapy. Obstet Gynecol Clin North Am 31:101–123, 2004

Simpson JL, Richards DS, Otano L, et al: Prenatal genetic diagnosis. In Gabbe SG, Niebyl JR, Simpson JL, et al (eds.): Obstetrics: Normal and Problem Pregnancies, 7th ed. Philadelphia, Elsevier Saunders, 2016

Soldin SJ, Wong EC, Brugnara C, et al: Pediatric Reference Intervals, 7th ed. Washington, DC, AACC Press, 2011

Wisconsin Association for Perinatal Care: Laboratory Testing During Pregnancy, 5th ed. Madison, WI, WAPC Perinatal Testing Committee, 2015.

Special Diagnostic Studies

16

OVERVIEW OF SPECIAL DIAGNOSTIC STUDIES

These special studies have been selected for discussion because of their great diagnostic value in identifying diseases and disorders of certain organs and systems. Tests after death serve to identify previously undiagnosed disease; evaluate accuracy of predeath diagnosis; provide information about sudden, suspicious, or unexplained deaths; assist in organ donation and postmortem legal investigations; and promote quality control in healthcare settings.

THE EYE

● Visual Field Testing

This procedure is used in conjunction with a basic eye examination in order to quantify the sensitivity of the peripheral vision. The test can be used to evaluate and rule out glaucoma and to evaluate the integrity of the visual pathway. Small blind spots in the visual field begin to appear early in glaucoma. The visual field exam may detect diseases that affect the eye, optic nerve, or brain and screen for visual sequelae of cerebrovascular accident or head or eye trauma.

Reference Values

Normal

Negative for depressions of sensitivity other than the physiologic blind spot

Procedure

1. The patient is seated in front of the visual field analyzer with the forehead resting against the machine.
2. The patient is instructed to stare at the fixation light.
3. The patient is asked to click a button when he or she sees lights of varying intensity that are displayed at intervals.
4. Check one eye at a time.
5. Inform the patient that the procedure time is about 5 to 10 minutes for each eye.

Clinical Implications

1. Abnormal findings show the depressions of sensitivity that appear in glaucoma or pathology affecting the optic nerve (i.e., ischemic neuropathy).
2. Positive results should be confirmed with a repeat examination.
3. Repeat testing for positive findings will show larger spots and progression of disease (Fig. 16.1).

Interventions

Pretest Patient Care

1. Explain the purpose and procedure of the test.
2. Although there may be some slight discomfort during the procedure, assure the patient that there is no pain involved. The only discomfort is related to feeling sleepy, similar to being hypnotized.
3. If evaluating for glaucoma, explain that risk factors include age, race, family history, and elevated intraocular pressure.
4. Follow guidelines in Chapter 1 for safe, effective, informed *pretest* care.

Posttest Patient Care

1. Review test results (Fig. 16.2) and counsel the patient regarding abnormal findings; explain the need for possible follow-up testing and treatment. Modify the nursing care plan as needed.
2. Follow guidelines in Chapter 1 for safe, effective, informed *posttest* care.

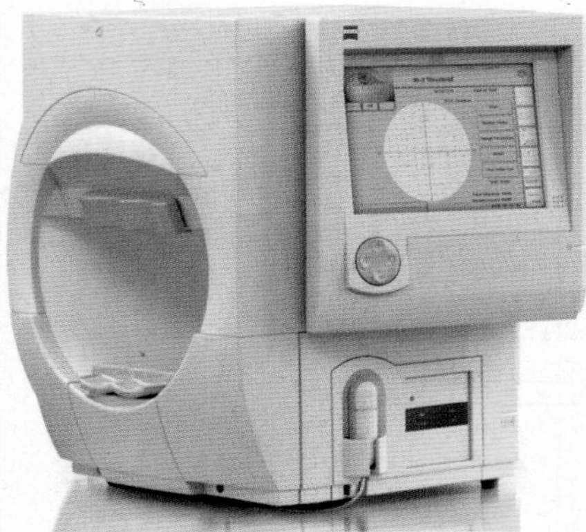

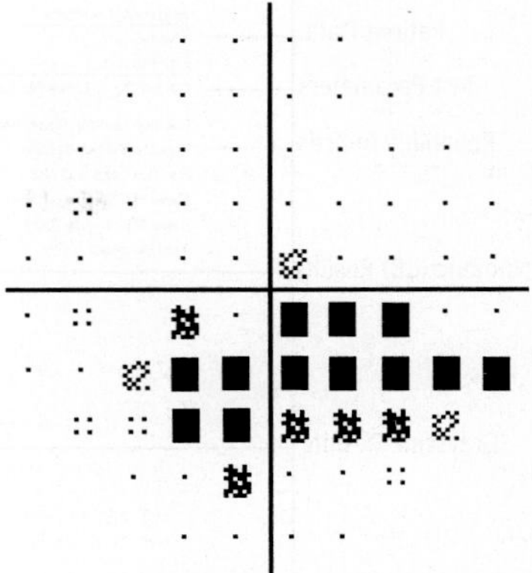

FIGURE 16.1. Humphrey Field Analyzer II-*i* and visual field grid. The darker the symbol (from a single dot to a black square), the less likely the field is normal in that location. (Courtesy of Humphrey Field Analyzer II-*i* User Manual, Carl Zeiss Meditec, Inc., Dublin, CA.)

NOTE *For the previous section, information was produced by the Eye Clinic of Wisconsin. Laser Diagnostic Technologies of San Diego, California, supplied the technical information.*

● Retinal Nerve Fiber Analysis

This procedure evaluates glaucoma by use of microscopic laser technology to precisely measure the thickness of the retinal nerve fiber of the eye and is recorded in computerized data for analysis. It is this nerve layer that receives and transmits images and gives us vision.

Reference Values

Normal

No abnormalities of retinal nerve fiber
Normal thickness of retinal nerve layer

Procedure

1. Dilation of the eye is not necessary.
2. Have the patient sit upright in the examining chair.
3. Place the patient's forehead and chin in cuplike holders and check one eye at a time. Twenty sectional images are obtained in <1 second and then analyzed to determine thickness of the nerve layer.

Clinical Implications

Abnormal appearance of the optic nerve is associated with changes in the eye that occur in glaucoma. Changes may be associated with vision loss.

Interventions

Pretest Patient Care

1. Explain test purpose and procedure. No pain or discomfort is associated with this test. There are no bright flashes of light.
2. Contact lenses may be left in place.
3. Follow guidelines in Chapter 1 for safe, effective, informed *pretest* care.

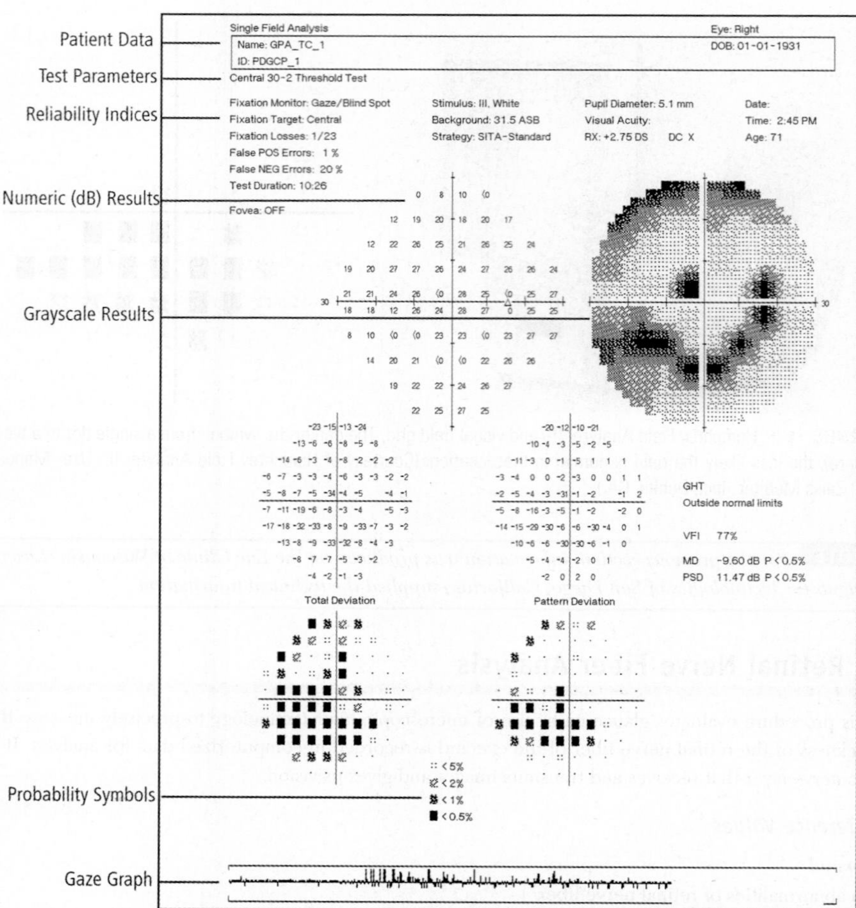

FIGURE 16.2. Patient report of a single visual field analysis of the right eye. The darker the symbol (from a single dot to a black square), the less likely the field is normal in that location. For example, $P < 0.5\%$ means that the deviation from normal at that location occurs in $<0.5\%$ of normal patients. (Courtesy of Humphrey Field Analyzer II-*i* User Manual, Carl Zeiss Meditec, Inc., Dublin, CA.)

Posttest Patient Care

1. Evaluate outcomes, counsel appropriately, and explain if there is need for further testing and possible treatment of abnormal outcomes. Modify the nursing care plan as needed.
2. Follow guidelines in Chapter 1 for safe, effective, informed *posttest* care.

● Fluorescein Angiography (FA)

The purpose of this test is to detect vascular disorders of the retina that may be the cause of poor vision. Fluorescein, a yellow-red contrast substance, is injected intravenously over a 10- to 15-second period. Under ideal conditions, retinal capillaries 5 to 10 μm in diameter can be visualized using fluorescein angiography (FA). Images of the eye, taken by a special camera, are studied to detect the presence of retinal disorders. Choroidal circulation is not seen with color photographs.

Reference Values

Normal

Normal retinal vessels, retina, and circulation

Procedure

1. Give a series of three drops to dilate the pupil of the eye. Complete dilation occurs within 30 minutes of giving the last drop.
2. When dilation is complete, take a series of color photographs of both eyes.
3. Have the patient sit with the head immobilized in a special headrest in front of a fundus camera.
4. Inject fluorescein dye intravenously.
5. Take a series of photographs as the dye flows through the retinal blood vessels over a period of 3 to 4 minutes.
6. Take a final series of photographs 8 to 10 minutes after the injection.

PROCEDURAL ALERT

1. Some patients may experience nausea for a short period of time following the injection.
2. The eyedrops may sting or cause a burning sensation.

Clinical Implications

Abnormal results reveal:

1. Diabetic retinopathy
2. Aneurysm
3. Macular degeneration
4. Diabetic neovascularization
5. Blocked blood vessels
6. Leakage of fluid from vessels

Interventions

Pretest Patient Care

1. Determine whether the patient has any known allergies to medications or contrast agent.
2. Instruct the patient about the purpose, procedure, and side effects of the test.
3. Follow guidelines in Chapter 1 for safe, effective, informed *pretest* care.

Posttest Patient Care

1. Inform the patient that he or she may experience color changes in the skin (yellowish) and urine (bright yellow or green) for 36 to 48 hours after the test.
2. Advise the patient to wear dark glasses and not to drive while the pupils remain dilated (4 to 8 hours). During this time, patients are unable to focus on nearby objects and react abnormally to changes in light intensity.
3. Review test results; report and record findings. Modify the nursing care plan as needed.
4. Follow guidelines in Chapter 1 for safe, effective, informed *posttest* care.

● Electroretinography (ERG)

Electroretinography (ERG) is used to study hereditary and acquired disorders of the retina, including partial and total color blindness (achromatopia), night blindness, retinal degeneration, and detachment of the retina in cases in which the ophthalmoscopic view of the retina is prohibited by some opacity, such as vitreous hemorrhage, cataracts, or corneal opacity. When these disorders exclusively involve either the rod system or the cone system to a significant degree, the ERG shows corresponding abnormalities.

In this test, an electrode is placed on the eye to obtain the electrical response to light. When the eye is stimulated with a flash of light, the electrode will record potential (electric) change that can be displayed and recorded on an oscilloscope. The ERG is indicated when surgery is considered in cases of questionable retinal viability.

Reference Values

Normal

Normal A and B waves

NOTE *"A" waves are produced by photoreceptor cells and "B" waves by Müller radial cells.*

Procedure

1. Have the patient hold eyes open during the procedure.
2. The patient may be sitting up or lying down.
3. Instill topical anesthetic eyedrops.
4. Place bipolar cotton wick electrodes, saturated with normal saline, on the cornea.
5. Use two states of light adaptation to detect rod and cone disorders along with different wavelengths of light to separate rod and cone function. Normally, the more intense the light, the greater the electrical response.
   a. Room (ambient) light
   b. Room darkened for 20 minutes and then a white light is flashed
   c. Bright flash (In cases of trauma, when there is vitreous hemorrhage, a much more intense flash of light must be used.)
6. Use chloral hydrate or a general anesthesia for infants and small children who are being tested for a congenital abnormality.
7. Total examining time is about 1 hour.

Clinical Implications

1. Changes in the ERG are associated with:
   a. Diminished response in ischemic vascular diseases, such as arteriosclerosis and giant cell arteritis
   b. Siderosis (poisoning of the retina when copper is embedded intraocularly [this is not associated with stainless steel foreign bodies])
   c. Drugs that produce retinal damage, such as chloroquine and quinine
   d. Retinal detachment
   e. Opacities of ocular media
   f. Decreased response, such as in vitamin A deficiency or mucopolysaccharidosis
2. Diseases of the macula do not affect the standard ERG. Macular disorder can be detected using a focal ERG.

Interventions

Pretest Patient Care

1. Explain the purpose and procedure of the test. For the most part, the patient will experience little or no discomfort. The electrode may feel like an eyelash in the eye.
2. Follow guidelines in Chapter 1 for safe, effective, informed *pretest* care.

Posttest Patient Care

1. Review test results; report and record findings. Modify the nursing care plan as needed.
2. Follow guidelines in Chapter 1 for safe, effective, informed *posttest* care.

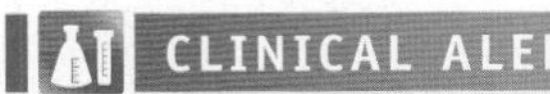

CLINICAL ALERT

Caution the patient not to rub the eyes for at least 1 hr after testing to prevent accidental corneal abrasion.

● Eye and Orbit (Ophthalmic) Ultrasound

Ultrasound can be used to describe both normal and abnormal tissues of the eyes when no alternative visualization is possible because of opacities caused by corneal edema, vitreal hemorrhage, or cataracts. This information is valuable in the management of eyes with large corneal leukomas or conjunctival flaps and in the evaluation of the eyes for keratoprosthesis. Orbital lesions can be detected and distinguished from inflammatory and congestive causes of exophthalmus with a high degree of reliability. An extensive preoperative evaluation before vitrectomy or surgery for vitreous hemorrhages is also done. In this case, the vitreous cavity is examined to rule out retinal and choroidal detachments and to detect and localize vitreoretinal adhesions, choroidal lesions, and intraocular foreign bodies. It can also be used to detect optic nerve drusen. Persons who are to have intraocular lens implants after removal of cataracts must be measured for the length of the eye (within 0.1 mm). The ophthalmic ultrasound can produce biometric readings for lens calculation prior to cataract surgery.

Reference Values

Normal

Normal image pattern indicating normal soft tissue of eye, retrobulbar orbital areas, retina, choroid, and orbital fat

Procedure

1. Anesthetize the eye area by instilling eyedrops.
2. Ask the patient to fix the gaze and hold very still. If imaging a lesion, movement is required for a retinal detachment evaluation.
3. Place a small, very-high-frequency transducer directly on the eye or position over a water standoff pad placed onto the eye surface.
4. Take multiple images.
5. If a lesion in the eye is detected, as much as 30 minutes may be required to differentiate the pathologic process accurately.
6. Orbital examination can be done in 8 to 10 minutes.
7. Follow guidelines in Chapter 1 for safe, effective, informed *intratest* care.

PROCEDURAL ALERT

1. **When a ruptured globe is suspected or surgery has been performed, ophthalmic ultrasound can be performed over a closed eyelid.**
2. **Caution must be used to avoid excessive pressure applied to the globe causing expulsion of the contents and increased risk for introduction of bacteria.**

Clinical Implications

1. Abnormal patterns are seen in:
   a. Alkali burns with corneal flattening and loss of anterior chamber
   b. Detached retina

c. Keratoprosthesis
d. Extraocular thickening in thyroid eye disease
e. Pupillary membranes
f. Cyclotic membranes
g. Vitreous opacities
h. Orbital mass lesions
i. Inflammatory conditions
j. Vascular malformations
k. Foreign bodies
l. Hypotony
m. Optic nerve drusen
n. Congenital cataract
o. Posterior vitreous detachment
p. Retinoschisis
q. Choroidal hemorrhage or detachment
r. Trauma

2. Abnormal patterns are also seen in tumors of various types based on specific ultrasonic patterns:
   a. Solid tumors (e.g., meningioma, glioma, neurofibroma)
   b. Cystic tumors (e.g., mucocele, dermoid, cavernous hemangioma)
   c. Angiomatous tumors (e.g., diffuse hemangioma)
   d. Lymphangioma
   e. Infiltrative tumors (e.g., metastatic lymphoma, pseudotumor)

Interfering Factors

If, at some time, the vitreous humor in a particular patient was replaced by gas or silicone oil, no result may be obtained.

Interventions

Pretest Patient Care

1. Explain the purpose and procedure of the test. For the most part, the patient will experience little to no discomfort.
2. Follow guidelines in Chapter 1 for safe, effective, informed *pretest* care.

Posttest Patient Care

1. Review test results; report and record findings. Modify the nursing care plan as needed.
2. Caution the patient not to rub the eyes until the effects of the anesthesia have disappeared to prevent accidental corneal abrasion. Minor blurred vision may be experienced for a short time.
3. Follow guidelines in Chapter 1 for safe, effective, informed *posttest* care.

BRAIN AND NERVOUS SYSTEM

Electroencephalogram (EEG) and Epilepsy/Seizure Monitoring

The electroencephalogram (EEG) measures and records electrical impulses from the brain cortex. It is used to investigate causes of seizures, to diagnose epilepsy, and to evaluate brain tumors, brain abscesses, subdural hematomas, cerebral infarcts, and intracranial hemorrhages, among other conditions. It can be a tool for diagnosing narcolepsy, Parkinson's disease, Alzheimer's disease, and certain psychoses. It is common practice to consider the EEG pattern, along with other clinical procedures, drug levels, body temperature, and thorough neurologic examinations, to establish electrocerebral silence, otherwise known as "brain death." The American Clinical Neurophysiology Society sets guidelines for obtaining these recordings. When an electrocerebral silence pattern is recorded in the absence of any hope for neurologic recovery, the patient may be declared brain dead despite cardiovascular and respiratory support.

Epilepsy/seizure monitoring using simultaneous video and EEG recordings (online computer) is done to verify a diagnosis of epilepsy, when seizures begin, and how they appear. The results differentiate and define seizure type, localize region of seizure onset, quantify seizure frequency, and identify candidates for medical implantation of vagus nerve stimulator or surgical treatment of seizures. Hospital admission is required.

Reference Values

Normal

1. Normal, symmetric patterns of electrical brain activity
2. Range of alpha: 8 to 11 Hz (cycles per second)
3. Seizure monitoring: expected outcome of at least three typical recorded seizures that may be different from what the patient usually experiences because medications have been reduced; also, onset area and type of seizures
4. No cross-circulation of internal carotid arteries
5. Evidence of hemispheres to support language and memory

Procedure for Electroencephalogram

1. Scalp hair should be recently washed.
2. Fasten electrodes containing conduction gel to the scalp with a special skin glue or paste. Seventeen to 21 electrodes are used according to an internationally accepted measurement known as the *10–20 System*. This system correlates electrode placement with anatomic brain structure.
3. Place the patient in a recumbent position, instruct to keep the eyes closed, and encourage the patient to sleep during the test (resting EEG). (seizure activating procedure [see numbers 4 to 6])
4. Before beginning the test, some patients may be instructed to breathe deeply through the mouth 20 times per minute for 3 minutes. This hyperventilation may cause dizziness or numbness in the hands or feet but is nothing to be alarmed about. This activating breathing procedure induces alkalosis, which causes vasoconstriction, which in turn may activate a seizure pattern.
5. Place a light flashing at frequencies of 1 to 30 times per second close to the face. This technique, called *photic stimulation*, may cause an abnormal EEG pattern not normally recorded.
6. Be aware that certain persons may be intentionally sleep deprived before the test to promote sleep during the test. Administer an oral medication to promote sleep (e.g., diazepam [Valium] or chloral hydrate). The sleep state is valuable for revealing abnormalities, especially different forms of epilepsy. Make recordings while the patient is falling asleep, during sleep, and while the patient is waking.
7. Remove electrodes, glue, and paste after the test. The patient may then wash the hair.
8. Follow guidelines in Chapter 1 for safe, effective, informed *intratest* care.

Procedure for Seizure Monitoring

1. Apply electrodes, take the EEG, and explain video and EEG monitoring (for up to 6 days). An electrode panel is applied and must be covered when the patient eats. The patient remains in bed except to use the bathroom; a helmet is worn when out of bed.
2. Perform neuropsychological testing to evaluate memory (remember objects), language (circles, squares), and problem solving (4 to 6 hours of testing).
3. A cerebral angiogram to assess cross-circulation in carotids is followed by a Wada test to determine the dominant hemisphere for language and whether the opposite hemisphere can support memory. An intravenous line is started and a catheter is threaded through the femoral artery to the internal carotid to inject sodium amobarbital to "put the brain to sleep" for 5 minutes in each half of the

brain. The Wada test is also known as the *amobarbital study* or *intracarotid Amytal test*, or the *Brevital test* when sodium methohexital is used.

4. Perform a functional brain magnetic resonance imaging (MRI) study. Procedure time is about 90 minutes. The patient wears earphones and is asked to respond to questions, sounds, and pictures by pressing a special button.
5. A combined positron emission tomography/computed tomography (PET/CT) scan is often done to provide further information about brain hemispheres.

Clinical Implications

1. Abnormal EEG pattern readings reveal seizure activity (e.g., grand mal epilepsy, petit mal epilepsy) if recorded during a seizure. If a patient suspected of having epilepsy shows a normal EEG, the test may have to be repeated using sleep deprivation or special electrodes. The EEG may also be abnormal during other types of seizure activity (e.g., focal [psychomotor], infantile myoclonic, or jacksonian seizures); between seizures, 20% of patients with petit mal epilepsy and 40% with grand mal epilepsy show a normal EEG pattern, and the diagnosis of epilepsy can be made only by correlating the clinical history with the EEG abnormality, if one exists.
2. An EEG may often be normal in the presence of cerebral pathology. However, most brain abscesses and glioblastomas produce EEG abnormalities.
3. Electroencephalographic changes due to cerebrovascular accidents depend on the size and location of the infarcts or hemorrhages.
4. Following a head injury, a series of EEGs may be helpful in predicting the likelihood of posttraumatic epilepsy, especially if a previous EEG is available for comparison.
5. In cases of dementia, the EEG may be normal or abnormal.
6. In early stages of metabolic disease, the EEG is normal; in the later stages, it is abnormal.
7. The EEG is abnormal in most diseases or injuries that alter the level of consciousness. The more profound the change in consciousness, the more abnormal the EEG pattern.
8. Abnormal procedure results (e.g., identification of major connections between the anterior and posterior circulation, or abnormal connection between the internal carotid arteries, or isolation of seizure onset and number and types of seizures)

Interfering Factors

1. Sedative drugs, mild hypoglycemia, or stimulants can alter normal EEG tracings.
2. Oily hair, hair spray, and other hair care products interfere with the placement of EEG patches and the procurement of accurate EEG tracings.
3. Artifacts can appear in technically well-performed EEGs. Eye and body movements cause changes in brain wave patterns and must be noted so that they are not interpreted as abnormal brain waves.

Interventions

Pretest Patient Care

1. Explain test purpose and procedure to allay patient fears and concerns. Emphasize that electroencephalography is not painful, that it is not a test of thinking or intelligence, that no electrical impulses pass through the body, and that it is not a form of shock therapy. The transmitted impulses are magnified at least 1 million times and transcribed to permanent hard copy for further study.
2. Explain seizure monitoring procedures, purposes, and risks. Risks of angiogram and Wada test include allergy to sodium amobarbital, cross-circulation leading to respiratory arrest, and stroke related to allergy to contrast agent used in angiography.
3. Allow food if the patient is to be sleep deprived. However, no coffee, tea, or cola is permitted within 12 hours of the test. Emphasize that food should be eaten to prevent hypoglycemia.
4. Allow, but do not encourage, smoking before the test.

5. Have the patient wash and thoroughly rinse hair with clear water the evening before the test so that the EEG patches remain firmly in place during the test. Tell the patient to not apply conditioners or oils after shampooing.
6. If a sleep study is ordered, the adult patient should sleep as little as possible the night before (i.e., stay up past midnight) so that sleep can occur during the test.
7. Call the electroencephalography department for special instructions if a sleep deprivation study is ordered for a child.
8. Medications are generally reduced before the Wada test. A liquid breakfast is permitted.
9. EEG and video monitoring of seizures occur for up to 6 days, with medications gradually reduced by one third for 3 days.
10. Follow guidelines in Chapter 1 regarding safe, effective, informed *pretest* care.

Posttest Patient Care

1. Wash the hair after the test. Application of oil to the adhesive before shampooing can ease its removal.
2. Allow the patient to rest after the test if a sedative was given during the test. Put bedside rails in the raised position for safety. Resume medications (if reduced preprocedure).
3. Skin irritation from the electrodes usually disappears within a few hours.
4. Review test results; report and record findings. Modify the nursing care plan as needed. If a repeat testing is necessary, provide explanations and support to the patient. Explain possible treatment of uncontrolled seizures (e.g., newer antiseizure medications, surgical implantation of vagus nerve stimulator). Explain role of female hormones in epilepsy: Seizures may be worsened by hormones; adult epilepsy involves areas of the brain sensitive to reproductive hormones; and, at menopause, seizures tend to increase, worsen, or lessen.
5. Follow guidelines in Chapter 1 for safe, effective, informed *posttest* care.

● Evoked Responses/Potentials: Brainstem Auditory Evoked Response (BAER); Visual Evoked Response (VER); Somatosensory Evoked Response (SSER)

These tests use conventional EEG recording techniques with specific electrode site placement for each procedure and include computer data processing to evaluate electrophysiologic integrity of the auditory, visual, and sensory pathways. These are brain responses "time locked" to some event. See Chart 16.1 for wave and standard deviation (SD) measurements.

Brainstem auditory evoked response (BAER). This study allows evaluation of suspected peripheral hearing loss, cerebellopontine angle lesions, brainstem tumors, infarcts, multiple sclerosis, and comatose states. Special stimulating techniques permit recording of signals generated by subcortical structures in the auditory pathway. Stimulation of either ear evokes potentials that can reveal lesions in the brainstem involving the auditory pathway without affecting hearing. Evoked potentials of this type are also used to evaluate hearing in newborns, infants, children, and adults through electrical response audiometry.

Visual evoked response (VER). This test of visual pathway function is valuable for diagnosing lesions involving the optic nerves and optic tracts, multiple sclerosis, and other disorders. Visual stimulation excites retinal pathways and initiates impulses that are conducted through the central visual path to the primary visual cortex. Fibers from this area project to the secondary visual cortical areas on the brain's occipital convexity. Through this path, a visual stimulus to the eyes causes an electrical response in the occipital regions, which can be recorded with electrodes placed along the vertex and the occipital lobes. It is also used to assess development of blue-yellow pathway in infants.

Somatosensory evoked response (SSER). This test assesses spinal cord lesions, stroke, and numbness and weakness of the extremities. It studies impulse conduction through the somatosensory pathway. Electrical stimuli are applied to the median nerve in the wrist or peroneal nerve near the knee at a level near that which produces thumb or foot twitches. The milliseconds it takes

CHART 16.1 Wave and Standard Deviation Measurements for Evoked Response/Potential

Normal Potentials, Brainstem Auditory Evoked Response, and Visual Evoked Response

Absolute latency, measured in milliseconds (msec), of the first five waveforms at a sound stimulation rate of 11 clicks/second

Wave	Mean ± Standard Deviation (SD)
I	1.7 ± 0.15
II	2.8 ± 0.17
III	3.9 ± 0.19
IV	5.1 ± 0.24
V	5.7 ± 0.25

Normal Visual Evoked Response

Absolute latency, measured in milliseconds of the first major positive peak (P_{100})

Wave	Mean ± Standard Deviation	Range
P_{100}	102.3 ± 5.1	89–114

Normal Somatosensory Evoked Response

Absolute latency of major waveforms, measured in milliseconds at a stimulation rate of 5 impulses/second

Wave	Mean ± Standard Deviation
EP	9.7 ± 0.7
A	11.8 ± 0.7
B	13.7 ± 0.8
II	11.3 ± 0.8
III	13.9 ± 0.9
N_2	19.1 ± 0.8
P_2	22.0 ± 1.2

for the current to travel along the nerve to the cortex of the brain is then measured. SSERs can also be used to monitor sensory pathway conduction during surgery for scoliosis or spinal cord decompression and/or ischemia. Loss of the sensory potential can signal impending cord damage.

Procedures

1. Obtain BAERs through electrodes placed on the vertex of the scalp and on each earlobe. Stimuli in the form of clicking noises or tone bursts are delivered to one ear through earphones. Because sound waves delivered to one ear can be heard by the opposite ear, a continuous masking noise is simultaneously delivered to the opposite ear.
2. Place electrodes used in VER on the scalp along the vertex and occipital lobes. Ask the patient to watch a checkerboard pattern flash for several minutes, first with one eye and then with the other, while brain waves are recorded.
3. Record SSERs through several pairs of electrodes. Apply electrical stimuli to the median nerve at the wrist or to the peroneal nerve at the knee. Scalp electrodes placed over the sensory cortex of the opposite hemisphere of the brain pick up the signals and measure, in milliseconds, the time it takes for the current to travel along the nerve to the cortex of the brain.
4. Follow guidelines in Chapter 1 for safe, effective, informed *intratest* care.

Clinical Implications

1. Abnormal BAERs are associated with the following conditions:
   a. Acoustic neuroma
   b. Cerebrovascular accidents
   c. Multiple sclerosis
   d. Lesions affecting any part of the auditory nerve or brainstem area
2. Abnormal VERs are associated with the following conditions:
   a. Demyelinating disorders such as multiple sclerosis
   b. Lesions of the optic nerves and eye (prechiasmal defects)
   c. Lesions of the optic tract and visual cortex (postchiasmal defects)
   d. Abnormal visual evoked potentials may also be found in persons without a history of retrobulbar neuritis, optic atrophy, or visual field defects. However, many patients with proven damage to the postchiasmal visual path and known visual field defects may have normal visual evoked potentials.
3. Abnormal SSERs are associated with the following conditions:
   a. Spinal cord lesions
   b. Cerebrovascular accidents
   c. Multiple sclerosis
   d. Cervical myelopathy accident

Interfering Factors

1. Some difficulty in interpreting brainstem evoked potentials may arise in persons with peripheral hearing defects that alter evoked potential results (i.e., subthreshold stimulation of peripheral nerves and inadequate skin preparation).
2. Maximum depolarization stimulation is divided into two protocols:
   a. Brachial plexus (BP) protocol involves stimulation of the median, ulnar, and superficial sensory radial nerves just proximal to the wrist.
   b. Lumbosacral (LS) protocol involves stimulating the posterior tibial and common peroneal nerves, which are the primary divisions of the LS plexus forming the sciatic nerve.

Interventions

Pretest Patient Care

1. Explain test purpose and procedure.
2. Have the patient wash and rinse hair before testing. Instruct the patient not to apply any other hair preparations.
3. Follow guidelines in Chapter 1 for safe, effective, informed *pretest* care.

Posttest Patient Care

1. Allow the patient to wash his or her hair (assist if necessary). Remove gel from other skin areas.
2. Review test results; report and record findings. Modify the nursing care plan as needed.
3. Monitor the patient for neurologic changes.
4. Follow guidelines in Chapter 1 for safe, effective, informed *posttest* care.

● Cognitive Tests: Event-Related Potentials (ERPs)

Event-related potentials (ERPs) are used as objective measures of mental function in neurologic diseases that produce cognitive defects. These measurements use the method of auditory evoked response testing in which sound stimuli are transmitted through earphones. A rare tone is associated with a prominent endogenous P_3 component that reflects the differential cognitive processing of that tone. Although a systematic neurologic increase in P_3 component latency occurs as a function of increasing age in normal persons, in many instances of neurologic diseases associated with dementia, the latency of the P_3 component has been reported to exceed substantially the normal age-matched value.

This test is useful in evaluating persons with dementia or decreased mental functioning. It is also helpful in differentiating persons with real organic brain defects affecting cognitive function from those who are unable to interact with the examiner because of motor or language defects or those unwilling to cooperate because of problems such as depression or schizophrenia.

Reference Values

Normal

No shift of P_3 components to longer latencies
ERP: absolute latency of P_3 waveform
P_3 wave mean and SD 294 ± 21 msec

Procedure

1. This procedure is the same as that for auditory brainstem response.
2. Ask patients to count the occurrences of audible rare tones they hear through the earphones.
3. Follow guidelines in Chapter 1 for safe, effective, informed *intratest* care.

Clinical Implications

An increased or abnormal P_3 latency is associated with neurologic diseases producing dementia, such as the following:

1. Alzheimer's disease
2. Metabolic encephalopathy such as that associated with hypothyroidism or alcoholism with severe electrolyte disturbances
3. Brain tumor
4. Hydrocephalus

Interfering Factors

Latency of P_3 component normally increases with age.

Interventions

Pretest Patient Care

1. Explain the purpose and procedure of the test.
2. Follow guidelines in Chapter 1 regarding safe, effective, informed *pretest* care.

Posttest Patient Care

1. Review test results; report and record findings. Modify the nursing care plan as needed.
2. Monitor for neurologic disease.
3. Follow guidelines in Chapter 1 for safe, effective, informed *posttest* care.

● Brain Mapping: Computed Tomography (CT)

Brain mapping uses transitional EEG data and specialized computer digitization to display the diagnostic information as a topographic map of the brain and spinal cord. The computer analyzes EEG signals for amplitude and distribution of alpha, beta, theta, and delta frequencies and displays the analysis as a color map. Specific or minute abnormalities are enhanced and allow comparison with normal data. This methodology is used for assessing cognitive function and for evaluating patients with migraine headaches, trauma, or episodes of vertigo or dizziness. Persons who lose periods of time and select patients with generalized seizures, dementia of organic origin, ischemic abnormalities, or certain psychiatric disorders are also candidates for this testing. With this procedure, it is possible to localize a specific area of the brain that may otherwise show up as a generalized area of deficit in the conventional EEG. Children or adults who demonstrate hyperactivity, dyslexia, dementia, or Alzheimer's disease may benefit from evaluation through brain mapping.

Reference Values

Normal

Normal frequency signals and evoked responses presented as a color-coded map of electrical brain activity

Procedure

1. Ensure that the patient is rested and awake for the test so that no sleep signals appear as indicators of beta wave activity.
2. After the skin of the scalp is cleansed with an abrasive solution, place 42 electrodes at designated areas on the scalp and hold in place with adhesive or paste formulated for this purpose.
3. Place the patient in a recumbent position and instruct him or her to keep the eyes closed and to refrain from any movement.
4. Follow guidelines in Chapter 1 for safe, effective, informed *intratest* care.

Clinical Implications

Abnormal brain maps can pinpoint the following conditions:

1. Areas of focal seizure discharge in persons who experience generalized seizures
2. Areas of focal irritation in persons with migraine
3. Areas of ischemia
4. Areas of dysfunction in states of dementia
5. Areas of possible brain abnormalities associated with schizophrenia or other psychotic states

Interfering Factors

1. Tranquilizers may alter results.
2. Unwashed hair or the use of hair preparations can interfere with electrode placement.
3. Eye and body movements cause changes in signals and wave patterns.

Interventions

Pretest Patient Care

1. Explain test purpose and procedure. There are no known risks. Emphasize the fact that electrical impulses pass from the patient to the machine and not the opposite.
2. Tell the patient that food and fluids can be taken before testing. However, no coffee, tea, or caffeinated drinks should be ingested for at least 8 hours before test.
3. Ensure that hair has been recently washed.
4. Ensure that tranquilizers are not taken before testing (check with healthcare provider). Other prescribed medications such as antihypertensives and insulin may be taken. If in doubt, contact the testing laboratory for guidelines.
5. Follow guidelines in Chapter 1 for safe, effective, informed *pretest* care.

Posttest Patient Care

1. Remove the conduction gel and encourage the patient to wash his or her hair. Provide supplies if possible.
2. Review test results; report and record findings. Modify the nursing care plan as needed.
3. Monitor the patient for seizure activity and other neurologic changes.
4. Follow guidelines in Chapter 1 for safe, effective, informed *posttest* care.

• Electromyography (EMG); Electroneurography; Electromyoneurogram (EMNG)

Electromyoneurography combines electromyography (EMG) and electroneurography. These studies, done to detect neuromuscular abnormalities, measure nerve conduction and electrical properties of skeletal muscles. Together with evaluation of range of motion, motor power, sensory defects, and reflexes, these tests can differentiate between neuropathy and myopathy. The electromyogram can define the site and cause of muscle disorders such as myasthenia gravis, muscular dystrophy, and myotonia; inflammatory muscle disorders such as polymyositis; and lesions that involve the motor neurons in the anterior horn of the spinal cord. EMG can also localize the site of peripheral nerve disorders such as radiculopathy and axonopathy. Skin and needle electrodes measure and record electrical activity. Electrical sound equivalents are amplified and recorded for later studies.

Reference Values

Normal

Normal EMG and electromyoneurogram (EMNG)

Procedure

1. The test is done in a copper-lined room to screen out outside interference.
2. The patient may lie down or sit during the test.
3. Apply a surface disk or lead strap to the skin around the wrist or ankle to ground the patient. Choose the muscles and nerves examined according to the patient's signs and symptoms, history, and physical condition (select nerves innervate specific muscles).
4. Encourage the patient to relax (massage certain muscles to get the patient to relax) or to contract certain muscles (e.g., to point to toes) at specific times during the test.
5. Testing is divided into two parts.

   The first test determines nerve conduction.
   a. Coat metal surface electrodes with electrode paste and firmly place over a specific nerve area. Pass electrical current (maximum, 100 mA for 1 msec) through the area to cause sensations, similar to shock from carpeting or static electricity or the equivalent of an AA battery, that are directly proportional to the time the current is applied. Patients with mild forms of neuromuscular disorders may feel mild discomfort, whereas those with polyneuropathies may experience moderate discomfort.
   b. Read the amplitude wave on an oscilloscope and record on magnetic tape for later studies.
   c. Electrical current leaves no mark but can cause unusual sensations that are not usually considered unpleasant. How fast and how well a nerve transmits messages can be measured. Nerves in the face, arms, or legs are appropriate for testing in this way.

   The second test determines muscle potential.
   a. Insert a monopolar electrode (a 1.25- to 7.5-cm-long small-gauge needle) and incrementally advance into the muscle. Manipulate the needle without actually removing it to see if readings change, or place the needle in another muscle area.
   b. The electrode usually causes no pain unless the tip is near a terminal nerve. Ten or more needle insertions may be necessary. The needle electrode detects electricity normally present in muscle.
   c. Observe the oscilloscope for normal wave forms and listen for normal quiet sounds at rest. A "machine-gun popping" sound or a rattling sound like hail on a tin roof is normally heard when the patient contracts the muscle.
   d. If the patient reports pain, remove the needle because the pain stimulus yields false results.
   e. Total examining time is 45 to 60 minutes if testing is confined to a single extremity; testing may take up to 3 hours for more than one extremity. There is no completely "routine" EMG. The length of the test depends on the clinical problem.
6. Follow guidelines in Chapter 1 regarding safe, effective, informed *intratest* care.

PROCEDURAL ALERT

1. Enzyme levels that reflect muscle activity (e.g., aspartate aminotransferase, lactate dehydrogenase, creatine phosphokinase) must be determined before actual testing because the EMG causes elevation of these enzymes for up to 10 d postprocedure.
2. Although rare, hematomas may form at needle insertion sites. Take measures, such as application of pressure to the site, to control bleeding. Notify the healthcare provider. Ascertain whether the patient is taking anticoagulants or aspirin-like drugs.

Clinical Implications

1. Abnormal neuromuscular activity occurs in diseases or disturbances of striated muscle fibers or membranes in the following conditions:
   a. Muscle fiber disorders (e.g., muscular dystrophy)
   b. Cell membrane hyperirritability; myotonia and myotonic disorders (e.g., polymyositis, hypocalcemia, thyrotoxicosis, tetanus, rabies)
   c. Myasthenia (muscle weakness states) caused by the following conditions:
      (1) Myasthenia gravis
      (2) Cancer due to nonpituitary adrenocorticotropic hormone (ACTH) secretion by the tumor
         (a) Bronchial cancer
         (b) Sarcoid
      (3) Deficiencies
         (a) Familial hypokalemia
         (b) McArdle's phosphorylase
      (4) Hyperadrenocorticism
      (5) Acetylcholine-blocking agents
         (a) Curare
         (b) Botulin
         (c) Kanamycin
         (d) Snake venom
2. Disorders or diseases of lower motor neurons
   a. Lesions involving motor neuron on anterior horn of spinal cord (myelopathy)
      (1) Tumor
      (2) Trauma
      (3) Syringomyelia
      (4) Juvenile muscular dystrophy
      (5) Congenital amyotonia
      (6) Anterior poliomyelitis
      (7) Amyotrophic lateral sclerosis
      (8) Peroneal muscular atrophy
   b. Lesions involving the nerve root (radiculopathy)
      (1) Guillain-Barré syndrome
      (2) Entrapment of the nerve root
         (a) Tumor
         (b) Trauma
         (c) Herniated disk
         (d) Hypertrophic spurs
         (e) Spinal stenosis

c. Damage to or disease of peripheral or axial nerves
    (1) Entrapment of the nerve
        (a) Carpal or tarsal tunnel syndrome
        (b) Facial, ulnar, radial, or peroneal palsy
        (c) Neuralgia paresthetica
    (2) Endocrine
        (a) Hypothyroidism
        (b) Diabetes
    (3) Toxic
        (a) Heavy metals
        (b) Solvents
        (c) Antiamebicides
        (d) Chemotherapy
        (e) Antibiotics
d. Early peripheral nerve degeneration and regeneration

Interfering Factors

1. Conduction can vary with age and normally decreases with increasing age.
2. Pain can yield false results.
3. Electrical activity from extraneous persons and objects can produce false results as a result of movement.
4. The test is ineffective in the presence of edema, hemorrhage, or thick subcutaneous fat.

Interventions

Pretest Patient Care

1. Explain test purpose and procedure. There is a risk for hematoma if the patient is on anticoagulant therapy.
2. Sedation or analgesia may be ordered.
3. Follow guidelines in Chapter 1 for safe, effective, informed *pretest* care.

Posttest Patient Care

1. If the patient experiences pain, provide pain relief through appropriate interventions. Obtain an order for an analgesic if necessary.
2. Promote rest and relaxation.
3. Review test results; report and record findings. Modify the nursing care plan as needed.
4. Monitor the patient for nerve and muscle disease. Provide assistance as necessary.
5. Follow guidelines in Chapter 1 for safe, effective, informed *posttest* care.

● Electronystagmogram (ENG)

This study aids in the differential diagnosis of lesions in the brainstem and cerebellum. It can confirm the causes of unilateral hearing loss of unknown origin, vertigo, or ringing in the ears. Evaluation of the vestibular system and the muscles controlling eye movement is based on measurements of the nystagmus cycle. In health, the vestibular system maintains visual fixation during head movements by means of nystagmus, the involuntary back-and-forth eye movement caused by initiation of the vestibular-ocular reflex.

Reference Values

Normal

Vestibular-ocular reflex: Normal nystagmus accompanying head turning is expected.

Procedure

1. The test is usually done in a darkened room with the patient sitting or lying down.
2. Remove any earwax before testing.
3. Tape five electrodes at designated positions around the eye.
4. During the study, ask the patient to look at different objects, to open and close his or her eyes, and to change head position.
5. Toward the end of the test, gently blow air into each external ear canal, starting on the affected side. Instill cold water and then warm water into the ears during the test to record eye movement in response to various stimuli.
6. Follow guidelines in Chapter 1 for safe, effective, informed *intratest* care.

 **PROCEDURAL ALERT**

Water irrigation of the ear canal should not be done when there is a perforated eardrum. Instead, a finger cot may be inserted into the ear canal to protect the middle ear.

Clinical Implications

Prolonged nystagmus and postural instability following a head turn is abnormal and can be caused by lesions of the vestibular or ocular system, as in the following conditions:

1. Cerebellar disease
2. Brainstem lesion
3. Peripheral lesion occurring in elderly persons; head trauma; middle ear disorders
4. Congenital disorders
5. Ménière's disease

Interfering Factors

1. Test results are altered by the inability of the patient to cooperate, poor eyesight, blinking of the eyes, or poorly applied electrodes.
2. The patient's anxiety or medications such as central nervous system depressants, stimulants, or antivertigo agents can cause false-positive test results.

Interventions

Pretest Patient Care

1. Explain test purpose and procedure. No pain or known risks are associated with the test. The procedures to stimulate involuntary rapid eye movements are uncomfortable.
2. Have the patient remove makeup.
3. Have the patient abstain from all caffeinated and alcoholic beverages for at least 48 hours. Heavy meals should be avoided before testing.
4. In most cases, medications such as tranquilizers, stimulants, or antivertigo agents should be withheld for 5 days before the test. If in doubt, consult the healthcare provider who ordered the test.
5. Follow guidelines in Chapter 1 for safe, effective, informed *pretest* care.

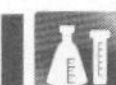 **CLINICAL ALERT**

The test is contraindicated in persons who have pacemakers.

Posttest Patient Care

1. Allow the patient to rest as necessary.
2. If present, nausea, vertigo, and weakness may require treatment and medication. Check with the healthcare provider who ordered the test.
3. Review test results; report and record findings. Modify the nursing care plan as needed.
4. Monitor the patient for brain disease, which may manifest as loss of balance, or middle ear disease, which may cause spasmodic eye movement, vertigo, or hearing loss.
5. Follow guidelines in Chapter 1 for safe, effective, informed *posttest* care.

HEART

● Electrocardiogram (ECG or EKG) and Vectorcardiogram

An electrocardiogram (ECG) records the electrical impulses that stimulate the heart to contract. It also records dysfunctions that influence the conduction ability of the myocardium. The ECG is helpful in diagnosing and monitoring the origins of pathologic rhythms; myocardial ischemia; myocardial infarction; atrial and ventricular hypertrophy; atrial, atrioventricular, and ventricular conduction delays; and pericarditis. It can be helpful in diagnosing systemic diseases that affect the heart, determining cardiac drug effects (especially digitalis and antiarrhythmic agents), evaluating disturbances in electrolyte balance (especially potassium and calcium), and analyzing cardiac pacemaker or implanted defibrillator functions.

An ECG provides a continuous picture of electrical activity during a complete cycle. Heart cells are charged or polarized in the resting state, but they depolarize and contract when electrically stimulated. The intracellular body fluids are excellent conductors of electrical current and are an important component of this process. When the depolarization (stimulation) process sweeps in a wave across the cells of the myocardium, the electrical current generated is conducted to the body's surface, where it is detected by special electrodes placed on the patient's limbs and chest. An ECG tracing shows the voltage of the waves and the time duration of waves and intervals. By studying the amplitude of the waves and measuring the duration of the waves and intervals, disorders of impulse formation and conduction can be diagnosed.

NOTE *The LightSpeed (GE Healthcare, Waukesha, WI) volume computed tomography (VCT) allows for imaging of an organ (e.g., heart, brain) and display of a three-dimensional anatomic view. Clinical applications include comprehensive views of heart and coronary vessels, ability to rule out (or in) aortic dissection and pulmonary embolism, and dynamic acquisition of perfusion of the brain.*

Reference Values

Normal

Normal positive and negative deflections in an ECG recording

Normal cardiac cycle components (one normal cardiac cycle is represented by the P wave, QRS complex, and T wave; additionally, a U wave may be observed). This cycle is repeated continuously and rhythmically (Fig. 16.3).

The P wave indicates atrial depolarization; QRS complex indicates ventricular depolarization; T wave indicates ventricular repolarization/resting stage between beats; and U wave indicates nonspecific recovery after potentials.

Normal Waves

1. The P wave is normally upright; it represents atrial depolarization and indicates electrical activity associated with the original impulse that travels from the sinus node through the atrial sinus.

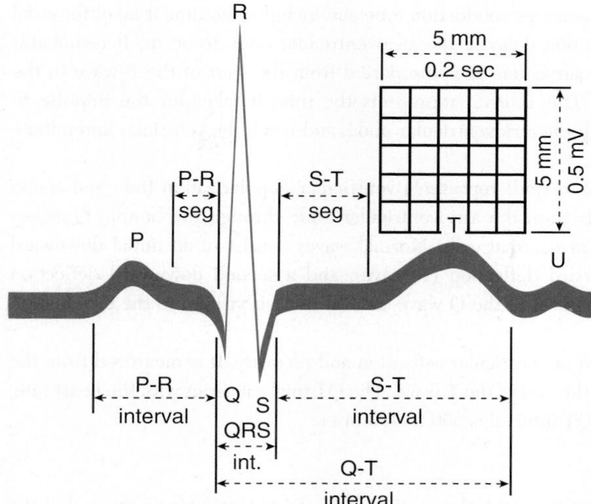

FIGURE 16.3. Commonly measured complex components. (From Smeltzer SC, Bare BG: Brunner and Suddarth's Textbook of Medical-Surgical Nursing, 8th ed. Philadelphia, Lippincott-Raven, 1996.)

If P waves are present; are of normal size, shape, and deflection; have normal conduction intervals to the ventricles; and demonstrate rhythmic timing variances between cardiac cycles, it can be assumed that they began in the sinoatrial node.

2. The T_a or T_p designation is used to differentiate atrial repolarization, which ordinarily is obscured by the QRS complex, from the more conventional T wave, which signifies ventricular repolarization (see number 8 below).
3. The Q(q) wave is the first downward/negative deflection in the QRS complex; it results from ventricular depolarization. The Q(q) wave may not always be apparent.
4. The R(r′) wave is the first upright/positive deflection after the P wave (or in the QRS complex); it results from ventricular depolarization.
5. The S(s′) wave is the downward/negative deflection that follows the R wave.
6. The Q and S waves are negative deflections that do not normally rise above the baseline.
7. The T wave is a deflection produced by ventricular repolarization. There is a pause after the QRS complex, and then a T wave appears. The T wave is a period of no cardiac activity before the ventricles are again stimulated. It represents the recovery phase after the ventricular contraction.
8. The U wave is a deflection (usually positive) following the T wave. It represents late ventricular repolarization of Purkinje's fibers or the intraventricular papillary muscles. This wave may or may not be present on an ECG. If it appears, it may be abnormal, depending on its configuration.

NOTE *In some cases, capital letters are used to refer to relatively large waves (>5 mm) and small letters to refer to relatively small waves (<5 mm). For example, qRS rather than QRS.*

Normal Intervals

1. The RR interval (normally, 0.83 second at a heart rate of 72 beats/minute) is the distance between successive R waves. In normal rhythms, the interval, in seconds or fractions of seconds, between two successive R waves divided into 60 seconds provides the heart rate per minute.
2. The PP interval (normally, 0.83 second at a heart rate of 72 beats/minute) will be the same as the RR interval in normal sinus rhythm. The responsiveness of the sinus node to physiologic activity (e.g., exercise, rest, respiratory cycling) produces a rhythmic variance in PP intervals.

3. The PR interval (~0.16 second) measures conduction tone and includes the time it takes for atrial depolarization and normal conduction delay in the atrioventricular node to occur. It terminates with the onset of ventricular depolarization. It is the period from the start of the P wave to the beginning of the QRS complex. This interval represents the time it takes for the impulse to traverse the atria, proceed through the atrioventricular node, and reach the ventricles and initiate ventricular depolarization.
4. The QRS interval (normally, 0.12 second) represents ventricular depolarization time and tracks the electrical impulse as it travels from the atrioventricular node through the bundle branches to Purkinje's fibers and into the myocardial cells. Normal waves consist of an initial downward deflection (Q wave), a large upward deflection (R wave), and a second downward deflection (S wave). It is measured from the onset of the Q wave (or R if no Q is visible) to the termination of the S wave.
5. QT interval measures the duration of ventricular activation and recovery. It is measured from the beginning of the QRS complex to the end of the T wave. The QT interval varies with the heart rate, gender, and time of day. Normal QT interval is 350 to 430 msec.

Normal Segments and Junctions

1. The PR segment is normally isoelectric and is the portion of the ECG tracing from the end of the P wave to the onset of the QRS complex.
2. The J junction (or J point) is the point at which the QRS complex ends and the ST segment begins.
3. The ST segment is that part of the ECG from the J point to the onset of the T wave. Elevation or depression is determined by comparing its location with the portion of the baseline between the end of the T wave and the beginning of the P wave or relating it to the PR segment. This segment represents the period between the completion of depolarization and onset of repolarization (i.e., recovery) of the ventricular muscles.
4. The TP segment (~0.25 second) is the portion of the ECG record between the end of the T wave and the beginning of the next P wave. It is usually isoelectric.

Normal Voltage Measurements

1. Voltage from the top of the R wave to the bottom of the S wave is 1 mV. Voltage of the P wave is ~0.1 to 0.3 mV. Voltage of the T wave is ~0.2 to 0.3 mV. Upright deflection voltage is measured from the upper part of the baseline to the peak of the wave.
2. Negative deflection voltage is measured from the lower portion of the baseline to the nadir of the wave.

Recording the Electrical Impulses

1. Because cardiac electrical forces extend in several directions at the same time, a comprehensive view of heart activity is possible only if the flow of current in several different planes is recorded.
2. For a 12-lead ECG, 12 leads are simultaneously used to present this comprehensive picture:
   Limb leads (I, II, III, AVL, AVF, AVR) record events in the frontal plane of the heart.
   Chest leads (V_1, V_2, V_3, V_4, V_5, and V_6) record a horizontal view of the heart's electrical activity.
3. Occasionally, an esophageal lead, which is swallowed or placed in the esophagus, can supply additional information. This type of lead is frequently used during surgical procedures.
4. His bundle electrography is a very specialized procedure that requires placement of an intravenous catheter, which is then advanced into the heart. An ECG is simultaneously being recorded while the electrical activity of the bundle of His is measured by a sensor at the end of the catheter. This test measures the electrical activity between contractions (Fig. 16.4).

Electrocardiogram Versus Vectorcardiogram

The vectorcardiogram, like the ECG, records the electrical forces of the heart. The major difference between these two methods is the way in which these forces are displayed (Table 16.1).

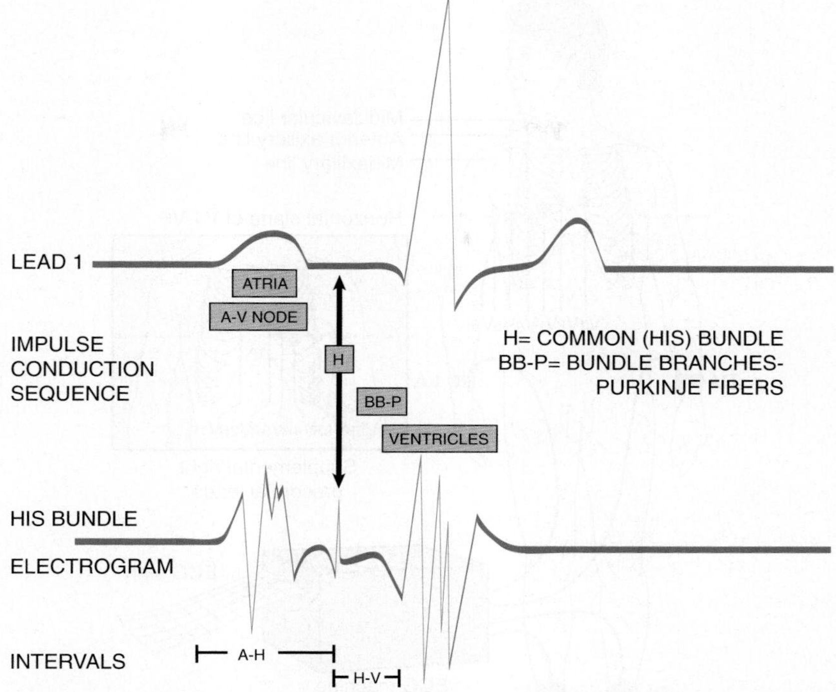

FIGURE 16.4. His bundle electrogram. Note that electrophysiologic events are presented in relation to the surface electrocardiogram. (From Phillips RE, Feeney MK: The Cardiac Rhythms, 3rd ed. Philadelphia, WB Saunders, 1990.)

A vectorcardiogram records a three-dimensional display of the heart's electrical activity, whereas the ECG is a single-plane representation. The following are the three planes of the vectorcardiogram:

1. Frontal plane (combines the Y and X axes)
2. Sagittal plane (combines the Y and Z axes)
3. Horizontal plane (combines the X and Z axes)

Procedure

The following steps apply to both the ECG and the vectorcardiogram:

1. Have the patient assume a supine position; however, recordings can be taken during exercise.
2. Prepare the skin sites and, if necessary, shave, and place electrodes on the four extremities and on specific chest sites. Ensure that the right leg is the ground (Fig. 16.5).

TABLE 16.1 Comparison of the Electrocardiogram and Vectorcardiogram

Electrocardiogram	Vectorcardiogram
Records electrical forces as positive or negative deflections on a scale	Depicts electrical forces as vector[a] loops, which show the direction of electrical flow
Records activity in the frontal and horizontal planes	Records activity in the frontal, horizontal, and sagittal planes

[a]The term *vector* indicates the directional flow of electrical activity.

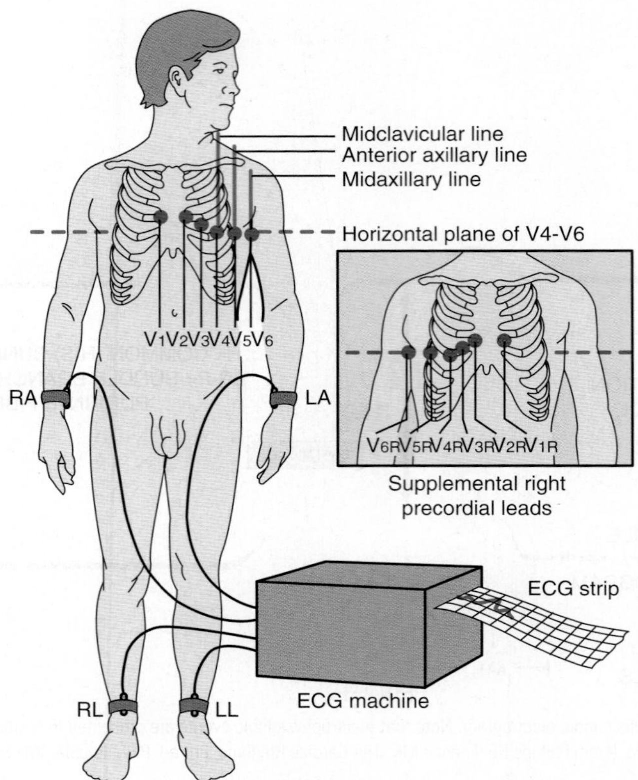

FIGURE 16.5. Electrocardiogram electrode placement. (From Smeltzer SC, Bare BG: Brunner and Suddarth's Textbook of Medical-Surgical Nursing, 8th ed. Philadelphia, Lippincott-Raven, 1996.)

3. A typical rhythm strip is a 2-minute recording from a single lead, usually lead II. It is frequently used to evaluate dysrhythmias.
4. Follow guidelines in Chapter 1 for safe, effective, informed *intratest* care.

PROCEDURAL ALERT

1. Chest pain, if present, should be noted on the ECG strip.
2. The presence of a pacemaker and the use of a magnet in testing should be documented.
3. Marking the position on the chest wall in ink ensures a reproducible precordial lead placement.

Clinical Implications

1. ECG
   a. The ECG does not depict the actual mechanical state of the heart or functional status of the valves.
   b. An ECG may be normal in the presence of heart disease unless the pathologic process disturbs the electrical forces. It cannot predict future cardiac events.

c. An ECG should be interpreted and treatment ordered within the context of a comprehensive clinical picture.
d. ECG abnormalities are categorized according to five general areas:
  (1) Heart rate
  (2) Heart rhythm
  (3) Axis or position of the heart
  (4) Hypertrophy
  (5) Infarction/ischemia
e. Typical abnormalities include the following:
  (1) Pathologic rhythms
  (2) Conduction system disturbances
  (3) Myocardial ischemia
  (4) Myocardial infarction
  (5) Hypertrophy of the heart
  (6) Pulmonary infarction
  (7) Altered potassium, calcium, and magnesium levels
  (8) Pericarditis
  (9) Effects of drugs
  (10) Ventricular hypertrophy

2. Vectorcardiogram
   a. The vectorcardiogram is more sensitive than the ECG for diagnosing myocardial infarction; it is probably not any more specific.
   b. Vectorcardiography is more specific than the ECG in determining hypertrophy or ventricular dilation.
   c. Differentiation of intraventricular conduction abnormalities is possible.

Interfering Factors

1. Race: ST elevation with T-wave inversion is more common in African Americans but disappears with maximal exercise effort.
2. Food intake: High carbohydrate content is especially associated with an intracellular shift of potassium in association with intracellular glucose metabolism. Nondiagnostic ST depression and T-wave inversion are evident with hypokalemia.
3. Anxiety: Episodic anxiety and hyperventilation are associated with prolonged PR interval, sinus tachycardia, and ST depression with or without T-wave inversion. This may be due to autonomic nervous system imbalances.
4. Deep respiration: The position of the heart in the chest shifts more vertically with deep inspiration and more horizontally with deep expiration.
5. Exercise/movement: Strenuous exercise before the test can produce misleading results. Muscle twitching can also alter the tracing.
6. Position of heart within the thoracic cage: There may be an anatomic cardiac rotation in both horizontal and frontal planes.
7. Position of precordial leads: Inaccurate placement of the bipolar chest leads and the transposition of right and left arm and left leg electrodes will affect test results. In normal persons, lead reversal produces the typical ECG findings of dextrocardia (congenital anomaly resulting in the heart being on the right side of the chest) in frontal plane leads and can mimic a myocardial infarction pattern.
8. A leftward shift in the QRS axis occurs with excess body weight, ascites, and pregnancy.
9. Age: At birth and during infancy, the right ventricle is hypertrophied because the fetal right ventricle performs more work than the left ventricle. T-wave inversion in leads V_1 to V_3 persists into the second decade of life and into the third decade in African Americans.
10. Gender: Women exhibit slight ST-segment depression.

11. Chest configuration and dextrocardia: In this congenital anomaly in which the heart is transposed to the right side of the chest, the precordial leads must also be placed over the right side of the chest.
12. Severe drug overdose, especially with barbiturates, and many other medications can influence ECG configuration. Antiarrhythmics, antihistamines, and antibiotics can widen QT intervals.
13. The serious effects of electrolyte imbalances show up on the ECG as follows:
    a. Increased Ca^{2+}: shortened QT; less frequently, prolonged PR interval and QRS complex
    b. Decreased Ca^{2+}: prolonged QT
    c. Alterations in K^+ may produce cardiac arrhythmias.

Interventions

Pretest Patient Care

1. Explain test purpose, procedure (ECG is a graphic record of electric pulses associated with the contraction and relaxation of heart), and interfering factors. Emphasize that ECG is painless and does not deliver electrical current to the body. A resting ECG is no more than a 1-minute record of the heart's electrical activity (the amount of voltage generated by the heart and the time required for that voltage to travel through the heart).
2. Have the patient completely relax to ensure a satisfactory tracing.
3. Be aware that, ideally, the person should rest for 15 minutes before ECG recording. Have the patient avoid heavy meals and smoking for at least 30 minutes before the ECG and longer if possible.
4. Follow guidelines in Chapter 1 for safe, effective, informed *pretest* care.

Posttest Patient Care

1. Recognize the limitations of an ECG. A normal ECG does not rule out coronary artery disease or areas of cardiac ischemia. Conversely, an abnormal ECG in and of itself does not always signify heart disease.
2. Review test results and counsel the patient regarding abnormal findings; explain the need for possible follow-up testing and treatment. Modify the nursing care plan as needed. A resting ECG is usually normal in those patients who experience only angina. It can provide evidence of prior heart damage. The ECG is one diagnostic tool within a repertoire of diagnostic modalities and should be viewed as such. The presence or absence of heart disease should not be presumed solely on the basis of the ECG.
3. Follow guidelines in Chapter 1 for safe, effective, informed *posttest* care.

CLINICAL ALERT

1. When an ECG shows changes that indicate ischemia, injury, or infarction, these changes must be reported and acted on immediately. The goal of diagnosis and treatment is to increase myocardial blood supply and reduce oxygen demand.
    a. When ECG changes represent stages of ischemia, injury, or necrosis and symptoms of possible myocardial infarction appear, the primary concern is balancing myocardial oxygen supply and demand as follows:
        (1) Nitroglycerin dilates blood vessels.
        (2) Narcotics relieve pain and anxiety.
        (3) Calcium channel blockers relieve coronary spasm.
        (4) Oxygen increases O_2 supply available to the myocardium.
        (5) β-Blocking drugs slow rapid heart rates.
        (6) Antiarrhythmic agents correct abnormal rhythms.
        (7) Frequent reassurances alleviate patient anxiety.

b. Monitoring for cardiac rhythm disturbances is an essential component of care. Potentially lethal dysrhythmias, especially ventricular tachyarrhythmias, require immediate intervention and may signal the need for possible cardiopulmonary resuscitation.

2. Serious diagnostic errors can be made if the ECG is not interpreted in the broader context of the patient's history, signs, and symptoms.
3. The electrical axis is not synonymous with the anatomic position of the heart.

● Signal-Averaged Electrocardiogram (SAE)

The signal-averaged ECG (SAE) is a noninvasive tool for identifying patients at risk for malignant ventricular dysrhythmias, particularly after myocardial infarction. During the later phase of the QRS complex and ST segment, the myocardium produces high-frequency, low-amplitude signals termed *late potentials*. These late potentials correlate with delayed activation of certain areas within the myocardium, a condition that predisposes to reentrant forms of ventricular tachycardia.

Indications

SAEs are performed to evaluate the etiology of ventricular dysrhythmias or as a precursor to electrophysiologic studies. Disorders that may produce regions of delayed myocardial conduction include myocardial infarction, nonischemic dilated cardiomyopathy, left ventricular aneurysm, and some forms of healed ventricular incisions (e.g., scar from tetralogy of Fallot surgical intervention).

Reference Values

Normal

Normal QRS complexes and ST segments

Procedure

1. The SAE, which is a modification of the conventional ECG, uses computerized techniques to provide signal averaging, amplification, and filtering of electrical potentials.
2. Place electrodes on the abdomen and anterior and posterior thorax. The signals received are converted to a digital signal. A typical QRS complex is used as a template against which subsequent cardiac cycles are compared. Typically, several hundred beats are averaged to analyze for late potentials.
3. Data collection usually takes about 20 minutes. Optimal recordings require that the patient be in a comfortable position and remain quiet, the proper application of electrodes, and elimination of interference from other electrical equipment.
4. Follow guidelines in Chapter 1 for safe, effective, informed *intratest* care.

Clinical Implications

1. SAE provides predictive values for potential ventricular tachycardias in patients who have a history of myocardial infarction or coronary artery disease.
2. Late potentials are stronger predictors of sudden death or sustained ventricular tachycardias than are ventricular dysrhythmias from a Holter monitor recording.
3. Evidence shows that late potentials associated with ventricular tachycardias are abolished following successful surgical intervention.
4. Patients who experience late potentials have a 17% incidence of sustained ventricular tachycardia or sudden death, compared with a 1% incidence in patients without late potentials. The incidence is even greater in the presence of decreased ejection fractions.
5. SAE may explain the cause of syncope subsequently identified as ventricular tachycardia during electrophysiologic study.

Interfering Factors

1. Increased time is required for recording beats in the presence of slow heart rates or frequent ventricular ectopics. Patient movement, talking, and restlessness also delay data procurement.
2. Bundle branch block can interfere with impulse averaging.
3. SAE does not provide information about antiarrhythmic drug effectiveness.
4. Late potentials do not occur in every patient with ventricular tachycardia.
5. Ventricular pacing prolongs ventricular activation time and obscures late potentials. Conversely, atrial pacing, even at rapid rates, does not alter ventricular late potentials.

Interventions

Pretest Patient Care

1. Explain test purpose and procedure.
2. Follow guidelines in Chapter 1 for safe, effective, informed *pretest* care.

Posttest Patient Care

1. Review test results; report and record findings. Modify the nursing care plan as needed.
2. Follow guidelines in Chapter 1 for safe, effective, informed *posttest* care.

● Cardiac Event Monitoring; Electrocardiogram (ECG) Continuous Monitoring; Holter Monitoring; 30-Day Event Monitoring; Implantable Monitor

Cardiac event monitoring refers to continuous ECG recording of cardiac rhythms, unusual cardiac events, and patient activity. The patient wears a special monitor (Holter) using a loop magnetic tape recording for 24 to 48 hours or a memory loop battery-operated ECG recorder. These tracings are used to record onset and termination of rhythm disturbances and to diagnose the cause of dizziness, palpitations, fainting (syncope), light-headedness, and unexplained fatigue. These procedures are also used to check pacemaker function and automatic implantable defibrillator function status and to trace drug and treatment effectiveness.

Reference Values

Normal

Normal tracings of cardiac ECG sinus rhythms and heart rate
No hypoxic or ischemic ECG changes

Procedure

1. Holter, 24- to 48-hour ECG monitor
   a. Prepare the site and apply the leads. Areas may need to be shaved, cleansed with rubbing alcohol, and abraded with gauze.
   b. If and when the patient experiences symptoms, ask the patient to push an indicator marked to save the current ECG tracing. The tracings are transmitted by telephone for analysis.
2. Thirty-day cardiac event ECG monitoring
   a. Prepare the site appropriately (e.g., shaving, cleansing).
   b. Apply two-channel electrodes, place leads, and connect to the monitor.
   c. Ask the patient to press a record marker when any symptoms (events) occur and also to keep a diary of symptoms.
3. Implantable monitor
   a. Surgically inserted just beneath the skin in the upper chest area
   b. Following a symptom (e.g., dizziness, fainting spell), a pager-sized device is placed over the implanted monitor to capture and save the data.
   c. Data are then analyzed by the healthcare provider.

Interfering Factors

1. Incomplete diary or event marker not pushed during symptoms
2. Mechanical ineffectiveness
3. Smoking, certain drugs

Clinical Implications

1. Abnormal tracings and record may indicate unsuspected disturbances, such as arrhythmias, friction, scratching, and tachycardia (atrial and ventricular).
2. Brachycardia and bradycardia-tachycardia syndrome
3. Premature atrial and bradycardia-tachycardia syndrome
4. Heart blocks
5. Junctional rhythms
6. Flutter or fibrillation
7. Premature atrial or ventricular contractions
8. Hypoxic/ischemic changes

Interventions

Pretest Patient Care

1. Explain monitoring purpose and procedure. Holter monitor is usually worn for 24 to 48 hours and then removed. The loop recorders are usually worn for 1 to 2 weeks and up to 1 month. Implantable monitors can be used for several days up to several months.
2. If the patient experiences symptoms such as dizziness or palpitations, ask the patient to push an indicator and record time of event in a diary.
3. Encourage the patient to continue normal daily events; do not get the recorder wet.
4. Instruct the patient to avoid magnets, metal detectors, high-voltage environments, and electric blankets.
5. An itching sensation under electrodes is common. Instruct patients not to adjust placement sites unless they call in and receive proper procedure.
6. Follow guidelines in Chapter 1 for safe, effective, informed *pretest* care.

Posttest Patient Care

1. Remove recorder and chart the time that the monitor is discontinued.
2. Clean electrode sites with mild soap and water and dry thoroughly.
3. Evaluate outcomes and counsel the patient appropriately about further testing and possible treatment. Modify the nursing care plan as needed.
4. Follow guidelines in Chapter 1 for safe, effective, informed *posttest* care.

● Stress Test/Exercise Testing (Graded Exercise Tolerance Test), Submaximal Effort

This test measures the efficiency of the heart during a dynamic exercise stress period on a motor-driven treadmill or ergometer. It is valuable for diagnosing ischemic heart disease and investigating physiologic mechanisms underlying cardiac symptoms such as angina, dysrhythmias, inordinate blood pressure elevations, and functionally incompetent heart valves. Exercise testing can also measure functional capacity for work, sports, or participation in rehabilitation programs, and it can be a predictor of potential response to medical or surgical treatment. Additionally, upper limits of physiologically responsive pacemakers can be evaluated.

Systolic blood pressure normally increases with exercise, and diastolic pressure normally remains essentially unchanged. Stress exercise testing takes place under controlled conditions that include low temperatures (20°C) and low humidity.

Reference Values

Normal

Negative when the patient does not exhibit significant symptoms, arrhythmias, or other ECG abnormalities at 85% of maximum heart rate predicted for age and gender

Procedure

There are many different types of stress tests. Most include the following steps:

1. Place recording electrodes on the patient's chest (see description of ECG) and attach to a monitor. Place a blood pressure recording device appropriately.
2. As the patient walks on a motor-driven treadmill, or pedals an ergometer if walking is not possible, computerized ECG and heart monitoring devices record performance. The patient walks at progressively greater speeds and higher levels of elevation to increase both heart rate and workload.
3. Record the initial or resting ECG, heart rate, and blood pressure. Ask the patient to report any symptoms such as chest pain or shortness of breath experienced during the test. Normal persons are symptom free at submaximal efforts; however, at peak or maximal efforts, symptoms expected in normal persons include exhaustion, fatigue, and, sometimes, nausea or dizziness.
4. Have the patient undergo stress testing in stages. Each stage consists of a predetermined treadmill speed (in miles or kilometers per hour) and a treadmill grade elevation (in percentage grade or degrees).
5. Monitor the ECG, heart rate, and blood pressure continually for abnormalities and any unusual symptoms such as intolerable dyspnea, chest pain, or severe cramping (claudication) in the legs.
6. Record vital signs, together with other abnormalities and complaints, at 1- to 3- minute intervals for 6 to 8 minutes posttest as the patient rests. The test is terminated if ECG abnormalities, fatigue, weakness, abnormal blood pressure changes, or other intolerable symptoms occur during the test.
7. The common criteria for terminating a test include the following:
   a. Achieving maximum possible performance
   b. Emerging signs or symptoms that indicate an existing disease process
   c. Recording a predetermined end point, such as 85% of age-related maximal heart rate, arbitrary workload (one that raises heart rate to 150 beats/minute), or diagnostic ECG change
8. Total examination time is about 30 minutes; however, ask the patient to plan to be in the laboratory for 1 to 1.5 hours.
9. Follow guidelines in Chapter 1 for safe, effective, informed *intratest* care.

Clinical Implications

Abnormal responses to exercise testing include the following:

1. Alterations in blood pressure, such as:
   a. Failure of systolic pressure to rise
   b. Progressive fall in systolic pressure
   c. Elevation of diastolic blood pressure
2. Alterations in heart rate, such as:
   a. Tachycardia above that which is predetermined
   b. Brachycardia
3. Changes in ECG, such as:
   a. Depression or elevation of ST segments caused by ischemia
   b. Dysrhythmias, ventricular tachycardia, multifocal premature ventricular contractions, atrial tachycardia, second- or third-degree atrioventricular block
   c. Pacemaker failure to perform within set rate limits
4. Ventricular or supraventricular ectopics are considered abnormal responses not necessarily ischemic in origin.

5. Ischemic ST-segment depression >0.2 mm or elevation >1.0 mm is the most common abnormality. Men ages 40 to 59 years who develop ST depression during exercise that is not present at rest have 5 times the risk for overt coronary heart disease compared with men without this ST depression.
6. Unusual symptoms such as:
   a. Anginal pain
   b. Severe breathlessness
   c. Faintness, dizziness, lightheadedness, confusion
   d. Claudication, leg pain
7. Unusual signs such as:
   a. Cyanosis, pallor, skin mottling
   b. Cold sweats, piloerection
   c. Ataxia, glassy stare
   d. Gallop heart sounds
   e. Valvular regurgitation

Interfering Factors

Common causes of false-positive exercise ECG responses include the following:

1. Left ventricular hypertrophy
2. Digitalis toxicity
3. ST-segment abnormality
4. Hypertension
5. Valvular heart disease
6. Left bundle branch block
7. Anemia
8. Hypoxia
9. Vasoregulatory asthenia
10. Lown-Ganong-Levine syndrome
11. Panic or anxiety attack
12. Wolff-Parkinson-White syndrome

Interventions

Pretest Patient Care

1. Explain test purpose and procedure. No food, coffee, or cigarettes are allowed for 2 hours before testing. Water may be taken.
2. Ensure that a legal consent form is signed by the patient or patient's designee.
3. Ask the patient to wear flat walking shoes or tennis shoes (no slippers). Men should wear gym shorts or light, loose-fitting trousers. Women should wear a bra, a short-sleeved blouse that buttons in front, and slacks, shorts, or pajama pants (no one-piece undergarments, pantyhose, or slips).
4. Certain medications should be withheld or discontinued before testing. Dosages of β-adrenergic blocking agents (e.g., propranolol) should be reduced or tapered gradually. The healthcare provider should write orders regarding management of the patient's drug regimen well before the test.
5. Follow guidelines in Chapter 1 regarding safe, effective, informed *pretest* care.

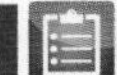

PROCEDURAL ALERT

Stress exercise testing can be risky for patients with recent onset of chest pain associated with significantly elevated blood pressures or with frequent attacks of angina. Testing may require a 4- to 6-wk delay in these situations.

Posttest Patient Care

1. Review test results; report and record findings. Modify the nursing care plan as needed.
2. Monitor the patient for abnormal responses to exercise. Immediately report significant events or symptoms.
3. Do not discharge the patient until acceptable levels for vital signs and ECG monitoring have been met.
4. Follow guidelines in Chapter 1 for safe, effective, informed *posttest* care.

● Cardiac Catheterization and Angiography (Angiocardiography, Coronary Arteriography)

These procedures are performed to evaluate the coronary vessels and function of the heart. The method chosen—that is, a left heart and/or right heart catheterization—is determined by the cardiologist in order to study and diagnose defects of the chambers of the heart, the heart valves, and certain blood vessels. Special sheathed catheters, which can carry contrast material into the right and left sides of the heart and measure pressures, are inserted into an artery. As these catheters are introduced and advanced toward the heart, fluoroscopy and high-speed x-ray pictures projected onto monitors show actual heart function and motion. Injected contrast medium provides a visual definition of cardiac structures. Coronary artery patency and circulation is filmed as well. The patient's heart rate, rhythm, and pressures are monitored continuously.

Coronary arteriograms are useful for evaluating abnormal stress tests, diagnosing heart disease, assessing the complications of a myocardial infarction, diagnosing congenital abnormalities, identifying cardiac structure and function, and measuring hemodynamic pressures within heart chambers and great vessels. They are used to measure cardiac output using contrast dilution, thermodilution, and Fick's method and to obtain cardiac blood samples for measuring oxygen content and oxygen saturation.

Cardiac catheterization combined with angiography is indicated for patients who exhibit angina, chest pain, syncope, valve problems, ischemic heart disease, cholesterolemia, symptoms with history of familial heart disease, abnormal resting or exercise ECGs, and recurring cardiac symptoms after revascularization. Other indications include young patients with a history of coronary insufficiency or ventricular aneurysm and patients who experience coronary neurosis and need assurance that their cardiac status is normal. This test can be performed during the acute stage of myocardial infarction, and, if necessary, surgical intervention can be accomplished without significant delay. Although cardiac catheterization poses some risk, it is highly accurate diagnostic resource.

Reference Values

Normal Cardiac Catheterization

Normal heart valves, chamber size, and patent coronary arteries
Normal ventricular wall and valve motion
Normal cardiac output (CO): 4 to 8 L/minute
Normal percentage of oxygen content (15 to 22 vol%) and oxygen saturation (95% to 100% of capacity, or 0.95 to 1.00)

Normal Cardiac Volumes

End-diastolic volume (EDV): 50 to 90 mL/m^2 (body surface area)
End-systolic volume (ESV): 25 mL/m^2
Stroke volume (SV): 45 ± 12 mL/m^2
Ejection fraction (EF): 0.67 ± 0.07

Normal Hemodynamic Pressure (mm Hg)

	Average	Range
Right atrium		
A wave	6	1–10
U wave	5	
Mean	3	0–8
Right ventricle		
Peak systolic	25	15–30
End diastolic	4	1–7
PAP		
Peak systolic	25	15–30
End diastolic	9	3–12
Mean	15	9–19
PCWP	9	4–12
Left atrium		
A wave	10	3–15
U wave	12	6–21
Mean	8	2–12
Left ventricle		
Peak systolic	130	100–140
End diastolic	8	3–12
Complete aortic		
Peak systolic	130	100–140
End diastolic	70	60–90
Mean	85	70–105

PAP, pulmonary artery pressure; PCWP, pulmonary capillary wedge pressure.

Procedure

1. The test is normally done in a special, darkened procedure room.
2. To decrease anxiety, explain the procedure and provide information about sensations the patient may experience.
   a. For right heart catheterization, the medial cubital, brachial, or femoral vein is accessed and catheterized. The catheter is threaded through the vena cava to the right atrium, through the tricuspid valve and right ventricle, to the pulmonary artery. Take pressure measurements and O_2 saturations from these areas as you manipulate the catheter.
   b. For left heart catheterization procedure, the femoral or brachial artery is accessed and catheterized. The catheter is advanced through the femoral or brachial artery, the aortic valve, and to the left ventricle. Again, take pressure readings. Introduction of contrast material, if done, provides data about left ventricular contractility, contour size, and presence of mitral regurgitation.
   c. Observe sterile surgical conditions. Prepare the skin with an antiseptic solution scrub. Inject a local anesthetic into the catheter insertion site area (e.g., groin [femoral artery], antecubital [brachial artery]). Small incisions may be made to facilitate insertion. Once inserted, gently advance the catheters to the heart and great vessels.
3. If left-to-right shunt is suspected, also obtain blood samples from the superior and inferior vena cava.
4. Have the patient lie on a special x-ray table and monitor the ECG continuously. Use intravenous sedation if necessary. During the procedure, the patient is placed in several different positions. The patient may be asked to exercise to evaluate heart changes associated with activity. Atrial pacing can also be done as part of the procedure in persons who cannot walk (e.g., paraplegics) or use a

treadmill. In these instances, there is a sequence of events that stress the heart followed by a rest period; then, measurements are taken. The heart is paced again, followed by another rest period.

5. The patient may be able to observe the procedure on a television monitor if it happens to be positioned properly.
6. After x-ray films have been taken from all angles, remove the catheters and apply manual pressure to the site for 20 to 30 minutes. Apply a sterile pressure bandage for several additional hours, if necessary. Some facilities no longer use pressure bandages. There are several devices on the market to close the access site (vascular closure devices) following the procedure. These devices can be separated into two categories: self-adsorbing sutures and hemostasis-promoting pads or patches. Less pressure and less time may be required for venous sites. Give protamine sulfate to reverse the effects of heparinization.
7. Reassure the patient frequently.
8. Follow guidelines in Chapter 1 for safe, effective, informed *intratest* care.

PROCEDURAL ALERT

1. Left atrial function and measurements are usually calculated from other measurements. If direct measurements are necessary, a transseptal approach must be done by advancing the catheter through the saphenous leg vein into the right atrium and then passing a needle through the catheter to puncture the atrial septum so that direct pressure readings may be obtained. The patient may be asked to exercise during the procedure to evaluate consistent changes; atrial pacing may be done during the procedure to incrementally stress and rest the heart for those patients unable to move normally (e.g., paraplegic patients).
2. Complications include the following:
   a. Dysrhythmias
   b. Allergic reactions to contrast agent (evidenced by urticaria, pruritus, conjunctivitis, or anaphylaxis)
   c. Thrombophlebitis
   d. Insertion site infection
   e. Pneumothorax
   f. Hemopericardium
   g. Embolism
   h. Liver lacerations, especially in infants and children
   i. Excessive bleeding at the catheter site
3. Notify the healthcare provider immediately if increased bleeding, hematoma, dramatic fall or elevation in blood pressure, or decreased peripheral circulation and abnormal or changed neurovascular findings are noted. Rapid treatment may prevent more severe complications.
4. The following equipment should always be available to treat complications of angiography:
   a. Resuscitation equipment
   b. Direct current defibrillator
   c. External pacemaker
   d. EEG monitor
   e. Emergency drugs

Clinical Implications

1. Abnormal results include the following:
   a. Altered hemodynamic pressures
   b. Injected contrast agent reveals altered ventricular structure and dynamics of occluded coronary arteries.
   c. Blood gas analysis confirms cardiac, circulatory, or pulmonary problems.

CHART 16.2 Grading of Coronary Occlusions

1. Normal, no decrease in lumen diameter
2. 25%: decrease in the lumen diameter of up to 25%
3. 50%: decrease in the lumen diameter of 26%–50%
4. 75%: decrease in the lumen diameter of 51%–75%
5. 90%: decrease in the lumen diameter of 76%–90%
6. 99%: hair-width lumen with >90% narrowing
7. 100%: total occlusion

2. Abnormal hemodynamic pressures indicate the following conditions:
   a. Valve stenosis or insufficiency
   b. Left and/or right ventricular failure
   c. Idiopathic hypertrophic subaortic stenosis (IHSS)
   d. Rheumatic fever sequelae
   e. Cardiomyopathies
3. Abnormal blood gas results indicate the following conditions:
   a. Congenital or acquired circulatory shunting
   b. Septal defects
   c. Other cardiac and pulmonary defects or pathology
4. When a contrast agent is injected into the ventricles, abnormalities (of size, function, structure, ejection fractions), aneurysms, leaks, stenosis, and altered contractility can be detected.
5. When contrast is injected into coronary arteries, occluded vessels and circulatory function can be recorded. See Chart 16.2.

Interventions

Pretest Patient Care

1. Explain test purpose (determine whether arteries are obstructed and show evidence of lesions, grade the occlusions, and assess left ventricular function), procedure, benefits, and risks. A consent form must be signed before the examination. Always check for allergies, especially to iodine and contrast media. Extensive teaching may be necessary.
2. Have the patient fast for 6 to 8 hours before the procedure. Give routine, scheduled medications, such as cardiac drugs or insulin, before the procedure unless directed otherwise. Discontinue anticoagulants at least 1 to 2 days before the procedure.
3. Give analgesics, sedatives, or tranquilizers before the procedure.
4. Ask the patient to void before the procedure.
5. The patient may wear dentures; have the patient remove jewelry and other accessories.
6. Instruct the patient regarding the need to perform deep breathing and coughing during the test and inform the patient that he or she may feel certain sensations.
   a. Catheter insertion through antecubital or groin sites may produce significant pressure sensations when the sheath, through which the catheter is inserted and advanced, is introduced.
   b. A slight shock or "funny bone" sensation may be felt if the nerve adjacent to the artery is touched. A tiny "bump" in the neck may be felt as the catheter is inserted into the heart. Normally, pain is not felt.
   c. When the contrast agent is injected into the catheter, a pumping sensation with feelings of palpitations and hot flashes may last 30 to 60 seconds. Skin vessels vasodilate, and blood rises to the skin surface for a short time.

   d. Patients may experience nausea, vomiting, headache, and cough.
   e. Angina may occur with exercise or with the contrast agent injection. Nitroglycerin or narcotics may be given.
7. Follow guidelines in Chapter 1 for safe, effective, informed *pretest* care.

CLINICAL ALERT

This procedure is contraindicated in patients with gross cardiomegaly.

Posttest Patient Care

1. Bed rest is usually maintained for 6 hours after the test based on the nature of the procedure, healthcare provider's protocols, and patient status. The patient is usually not permitted to raise his or her head more than 30 degrees during this time because greater angles put strain on the insertion site. Conversely, movement of the uninvolved extremities should be promoted.
2. Check vital signs frequently according to institution protocols. At the same time, check catheter insertion site for hematomas, swelling, bleeding, or bruits. Normal or other mechanical pressure to the catheter insertion site may be necessary if bleeding or hematoma develops. A bruised appearance around the site is normal. Swelling or lumps should be promptly reported to the healthcare provider. Neurovascular checks should be done along with assessment of vital signs in bilateral extremities and results compared. Assess color, motion, sensation, capillary refill times, temperature, and pulse quality. *Report significant changes immediately.*
3. Administer prophylactic antibiotics as necessary.
4. Encourage fluid intake. Unless contraindicated, an intravenous infusion site may be maintained while the patient is on bed rest in the event that rapid intravenous access is needed.
5. Keep the affected extremity extended, not elevated or flexed. Immobilize the legs with sandbags if necessary. Apply ice packs or sandbags to the catheter site, if ordered; this pressure can be very painful. Prescribed analgesics can be administered for pain of hematomas or discomfort.
6. Sutures, if used, are removed per healthcare provider's instructions.
7. Review test results; report and record findings. Modify the nursing care plan as needed.
8. Monitor the patient for cardiac, circulatory, neurovascular, and pulmonary problems. Figure 16.6 shows a sample cardiac catheterization report.
   a. Risk factors for complications following cardiac catheterization include >60 years of age, hypertension, peripheral vascular disease, and procedure done on an emergency basis or at same time as angioplasty. Risk factors for complications may be as high as 10% when more than three factors are present.
   b. Complications associated with risk factors include myocardial infarction, cerebrovascular accidents, or death within 24 hours of procedure; hemorrhage requiring transfusion; presudoaneurysm; fistula; or femoral thromboses.
9. Treatment may include percutaneous transluminal coronary angioplasty (PTCA), coronary artery stent placement, coronary rotablation, or medications (see Chart 16.3).
10. Follow guidelines in Chapter 1 for safe, effective, informed *posttest* care.

● Electrophysiology (EP) Studies; His Bundle Procedure

Electrophysiology (EP) studies are accomplished through an invasive test for diagnosis and treatment of ventricular and supraventricular arrhythmias. This is similar to cardiac catheterization, the difference being that EP studies measure cardiac electrical conduction system activity through

Hospital Name and Address: ______________________________
Patient Name: ______________ MRN: ______________ Date: ____________
Cardiologist: ______________

EF% (LV ejection fraction): 45%

Valve Regurgitation: AO: mild Mean Gradient: 21 mmHg Valve Area: 1.13 cm^2

Findings:

LAD: moderate size vessel, mid 60% after D1
D1: w/mild LI; D2 without obstructive disease
LCX: moderate size vessel, small disease prox-mid LIs, distally diffuse 6%–70%
OM1 and OM2 small vessels
OM3 moderate diffuse disease
RCA: 80% prox w/distal full bridging and extensive L>R collaterals

Impression:

Three vessels CAD (coronary artery disease):
1) 80% in the proximal RCA (right coronary artery)
2) 60% in the mid area of the LAD (left anterior descending) after the D1 branch, with extensive blood flow distally using left to right collateral arteries between the distal RCA and LAD
3) Luminal irregularities (LIs) (<20%) in the D1 and in the proximal left circumflex (LCX), with diffuse 60%–70% disease in the distal portion of the LCX
Mildly depressed left ventricular systolic function with an ejection fraction of 45%
Calcified aortic valve; mild aortic insufficiency (AI); moderate aortic stenosis (AS)

FIGURE 16.6. Sample of a cardiac catheterization report.

solid electrode catheters instead of the open-lumen catheters used to measure circulatory system pressures. Chest electrode catheters are almost always inserted into veins because of the greater risk they pose in the arterial system (spasms, occlusion). Using fluoroscopy as a visual guide, the catheters are advanced into the right atrium and right ventricle. An x-ray monitor tracks the catheter location, and a physiologic monitor shows ECG rhythms as well as intracardiac catheter electrograms.

An EP study is highly useful for diagnosing diseases of the cardiac conduction system and provides indications for optimal treatment. In addition to measuring baseline values, the electrode catheters are used to pace the heart in an attempt to induce the same arrhythmia causing the problem. When the patient is taking antiarrhythmic drugs, the EP study can determine how well the medication is working by how easily the arrhythmia can be induced. This is in contrast to the trial-and-error method, in which there is no way to know that a particular drug is ineffective until that drug has failed to resolve the problem, frequently over a significant period of time.

EP is indicated to differentiate disorders of impulse formation (supraventricular versus ventricular rhythms). EP studies also provide diagnostic insight into the etiology and mechanism of conduction disorders. EP studies are often part of the workup for syncope, sick sinus syndrome, or tachyarrhythmias. Finally, EP studies are indicated for testing the effectiveness of antiarrhythmic drugs. Each antiarrhythmic drug has certain effects that must be anticipated during the loading phase (e.g., hypotension with quinidine and procainamide, abdominal cramping with quinidine, venous pain with phenytoin). A state of "happy drunkenness" may also occur. Intravenous saline is normally used to support blood pressure in the event hypotension occurs.

CHART 16.3 Cardiac Treatment Procedures

These procedures are performed by a cardiologist in the cardiac catheterization laboratory. Typically, the procedure is performed similarly to a cardiac catheterization (i.e., a sheath is inserted into a femoral, brachial, or radial artery, and a guide catheter is then advanced into the coronary arteries).

Percutaneous Transluminal Coronary Angioplasty

PTCA is a nonsurgical procedure of dilating significantly occluded arteries, thus allowing more blood flow and, subsequently, an increase in oxygen being delivered to the heart. It is primarily performed as an alternative to the medical or surgical management of coronary heart disease. This procedure can be done at the same time as an initial catheterization, electively at some time after the catheterization, or urgently during an acute myocardial infarction.

The procedure involves passing a small catheter, tipped with a balloon, through the groin or brachial artery to the narrowed artery. The balloon is then inflated several times against the narrowed area in an attempt to reduce the occlusion and enlarge the inner lumen of the artery. During the procedure, nitroglycerin is frequently administered into the coronary artery to help dilate the artery and to prevent coronary spasms. Intravenous anticoagulation with heparin is also maintained throughout the procedure to prevent thrombus formation on the catheters and at the areas of vascular damage.

Coronary Artery Stent

A coronary artery stent is a coiled metal device permanently embedded into the coronary artery. The stent can be balloon-inflated or self-expanding. A balloon-inflated–type stent is fluoroscopically guided to the occluded artery and subsequently embedded into the artery upon inflation of the balloon. Self-expanding stents are covered by a retaining sheath, which is removed at the site of occlusion. Patients are maintained on antiplatelet agents for 4–6 wk after the procedure.

Directional Atherectomy

Directional atherectomy is a technique in which a portion of the blockage is mechanically shaved off and removed from inside the artery. This procedure uses a balloon-tipped catheter with a special cutting blade on one side. As the catheter is placed against the stenotic lesion, the balloon is inflated at a low pressure on the opposite side of the artery to stabilize the catheter. The blade is then passed through the plaque (works best on noncalcified lesions).

Rotational Atherectomy

Rotational atherectomy (Rotablator [Boston Scientific, Marlborough, MA], rotational ablation) is used when the blockages are long and hard. This system uses a high-speed, rotating, diamond-studded burr. When the burr is spun at a high speed (140,000 to 200,000 rpm), the plaque is pulverized, and the debris is then released into the bloodstream as microparticles. This procedure is particularly effective on heavily calcified lesions.

Reference Values

Normal

Normal EP/His bundle procedure

Normal conduction intervals, refractory periods, and recovery times

Controlled, induced arrhythmias

Procedure

1. Darken the room.
2. To decrease anxiety, keep the patient informed of what is being done as the procedure evolves.
3. Position the patient on an x-ray table and attach the ECG leads to specific locations.
4. Maintain sterile, aseptic surgical conditions. Usually, one or two sites are chosen and prepared for catheter insertion (right and/or left antecubital area, right and/or left groin). The sites chosen depend on where in the heart the catheters have to be placed and the patency and size of the patient's veins. Inject the insertion site with local anesthetic before catheter insertion.
5. As the catheters are advanced toward the desired location, record baseline information. Sometimes, cardiac pacing may be necessary; for example, measuring sinus node recovery times requires pacing atrium until the sinus is fatigued and then measuring the time the sinus takes to recover.
6. After baseline values have been determined, use pacing to induce arrhythmias. If a sustained arrhythmia is induced, make an attempt to terminate the arrhythmia through pacing. Should the patient lose consciousness, use an external cardioverter-defibrillator to terminate the arrhythmia.
7. Hold a continuous, quiet conversation to assess the patient's level of consciousness.
8. After the procedure, remove the catheters and apply a sterile pressure bandage to the catheter insertion site. Manual pressure on the site may be necessary if bleeding occurs.

Clinical Implications

1. Abnormal EP results will reveal the following conditions:
   a. Conduction intervals longer or shorter than normal
   b. Refractory periods longer than normal
   c. Prolonged recovery times
   d. Induced dysrhythmia in a normal subject
2. Abnormal results indicate the following conditions:
   a. Long atrial His (AH) bundle intervals indicate disease in the atrioventricular (AV) node if sympathetic and vagal influences on the AV node have been eliminated.
   b. Long ventricular His (VH) bundle intervals indicate disease in the His-Purkinje system.
   c. Prolonged sinus node recovery times indicate sinus node dysfunction such as sick sinus syndrome.
   d. Prolonged sinoatrial conduction times can indicate sinus exit block.
   e. A wide or split His bundle deflection indicates a His bundle lesion.
   f. Induction of a sustained ventricular and supraventricular tachycardia confirms the diagnosis of recurrent ventricular tachycardia (Chart 16.4).

CHART 16.4 Features of Interventional or Therapeutic Electrophysiology (EP) Studies

1. Endocardial catheter ablation
2. Placement of implantable cardioverter-defibrillators for management of ventricular tachycardia (VT) or ventricular fibrillation (VF)
3. Radiofrequency (RF) transcatheter ablation has become the treatment of choice to obliterate pathways within the atrioventricular (AV) node and accessory pathways causing palpitations.
4. Intracardiac transcatheter ablation is used to destroy accessory bypass tracks, reentrant pathways, or pathways within the AV node. A special catheter is used to produce an injury to the target site(s) using RF energy.

From Van Riper S, Van Riper J: Cardiac Diagnostic Tests. Philadelphia, WB Saunders, 1997, p. 320.

Interventions

Pretest Patient Care

1. Explain test purpose, procedure, benefits, and risks. Describing possible physical sensations that may be felt helps to reduce patient anxiety. These sensations may include the following:
   a. The sensation of a bug crawling in the arm and neck as the catheter is advanced
   b. Palpitations or racing heart during pacing
   c. Light-headedness or dizziness (these must be reported when felt)
2. Obtain a signed consent form before the procedure.
3. Draw blood samples for potassium levels and other drug levels if the effectiveness of a drug is to be determined.
4. Perform a standard 12-lead ECG before testing.
5. Ensure that nothing is consumed for at least 3 hours before testing.
6. Be aware that analgesics, sedatives, or tranquilizers are usually withheld before the procedure.
7. Ask the patient to void before the procedure is initiated.
8. Allow the patient to wear dentures.
9. Follow guidelines in Chapter 1 for safe, effective, informed *pretest* care.

CLINICAL ALERT

Relative contraindications to EP: Although an acute myocardial infarction may limit detailed and prolonged EP procedures, brief but clinically useful procedures can be performed in this situation.

Posttest Patient Care

1. Have the patient remain on flat bed rest for 4 to 8 hours postprocedure and do not allow flexion or bending of the extremity used for the catheter insertion because this may lead to bleeding or vascular occlusion. A pillow may be placed under the head.
2. Check vital signs, neurovascular status of extremity used, and insertion site for swelling, bleeding, hematoma, or bruit every 15 minutes for 4 hours, 30 minutes for 2 hours, and every hour for 2 hours postprocedure or according to institutional protocols. Neurovascular checks include assessing for pulses, color, motion, sensation, temperature, and capillary refill times.
3. Keep the affected extremity extended, not elevated or flexed, to decrease discomfort and risk for bleeding. Prescribed analgesics can be administered.
4. Encourage range-of-motion exercise of uninvolved limbs.
5. If an electrode catheter is left in place for sequential studies, ensure that it is sutured in place and covered with sterile dressings. Care for the site using sterile, aseptic technique.
6. Review test results; report and record findings. Modify the nursing care plan as needed.
7. Stress the importance of compliance with prescribed therapies, including drugs.
8. Follow guidelines in Chapter 1 regarding safe, effective, informed *posttest* care.

CLINICAL ALERT

1. Complications can include the following conditions:
   a. Rapid, dramatic hemorrhage at the catheter insertion site (apply manual pressure to the site and notify the healthcare provider immediately)
   b. Thrombosis at the puncture site; thromboembolism
   c. Phlebitis
   d. Hemopericardium

e. Atrial fibrillation (usually transient)
f. Ventricular fibrillation or ventricular ectopy

2. Notify the healthcare provider of bleeding, hypotension, altered neurovascular status, decrease in distal perfusion, or life-threatening arrhythmias. Be aware of drug studies performed and monitor for effects of that drug. Have cardiopulmonary resuscitation equipment and drugs readily available for emergency use.

● Transesophageal Echocardiography (TEE)

This test permits optimal ultrasonic visualization of the heart when traditional transthoracic (noninvasive) echocardiography fails or proves inconclusive. A miniaturized high-frequency ultrasound transducer is mounted on an endoscope and coupled with an ultrasound instrument to display and record ultrasound images from the heart. Endoscope controls allow remote manipulation of the transducer tip. Various images of heart anatomy can be displayed by rotating the tip of the instrument and by varying the depth of insertion into the esophagus.

Indications for Transesophageal Echocardiography

1. To assess function of prosthetic valves, diagnose endocarditis, evaluate valvular regurgitation and congenital abnormalities, and examine the aorta for dissecting aneurysms
2. To monitor left ventricular wall motion intraoperatively
3. To measure ejection fraction in selected patients
4. Situations in which a transthoracic echocardiogram has not been satisfactory (e.g., obesity, chest wall trauma, chronic obstructive pulmonary disease)
5. When results of traditional transthoracic echocardiography do not agree or correlate with other clinical findings

Reference Values

Normal

Normal position, size, and function of heart valves and heart chambers

Procedure

1. Explain test purpose, procedure, benefits, and risks.
2. Apply a topical anesthetic to the pharynx. Insert a bite block into the mouth to reduce the risk for damage to the teeth and other oral structures as well as the endoscope itself (see Chapter 12).
3. Have the patient assume a left lateral decubitus position before the lubricated endoscopic instrument is inserted to a depth of 30 to 50 cm. The patient may be asked to swallow so that the scope advances more easily.
4. Manipulation of the ultrasound transducer allows a number of image planes to be visualized.
5. Follow guidelines in Chapter 1 for safe, effective, informed *intratest* care.

Clinical Implications

Abnormal TEE findings may reveal the following conditions:

1. Heart valve diseases
2. Pericardial effusion
3. Congenital heart disease
4. Endocarditis
5. Intracardiac tumors or thrombi
6. Left ventricular dysfunction

Interventions

Pretest Patient Care

1. Explain test purpose, procedure, benefits, and risks.
2. Ensure that the patient fasts from food and fluids at least 8 hours before the procedure to reduce the risk for aspiration. Premedications such as analgesics or sedatives may be ordered. Prescribed oral medications may be taken with small sips of water.
3. Follow guidelines in Chapter 1 for safe, effective, informed *pretest* care.

Posttest Patient Care

1. Review test results; report and record findings. Modify the nursing care plan as needed.
2. Monitor vital signs and level of consciousness (if sedated). Ensure patent airway at all times.
3. Position the patient on his or her side if sedated to prevent risk for aspiration.
4. Swallowing reflexes may be diminished for several hours because of topical anesthetic effects. Ingesting food or fluids may result in aspiration if these reflexes are not intact. Evaluate return of swallow, cough, and gag reflexes before introducing food or fluids orally.
5. Follow guidelines in Chapter 1 for safe, effective, informed *posttest* care.

OTHER ORGANS AND BODY FUNCTIONS

● Magnetic Resonance Imaging (MRI); Magnetic Resonance Angiography (MRA); Magnetic Resonance Spectroscopy (MRS)

Magnetic resonance (MR) is a diagnostic modality that employs a superconducting magnet and radiofrequency (RF) signals to cause hydrogen nuclei to emit their own signal; computers use these signals to construct detailed, sectional images of the body. Unlike CT, no ionizing radiation is used. Additionally, the ability of MR to discern anatomy is most closely linked to the molecular nature of tissue. For example, MR spectroscopy (MRS) provides information about the chemical composition of tissue and is commonly used to evaluate brain function. Special techniques primarily based on the magnetic reactions of hydrogen nuclei can influence the MR signal to enhance certain types of tissue (e.g., fat is accentuated in T1-weighted images, cerebrospinal fluid and other pure fluids are highlighted in T2-weighted images). Computer reconstruction techniques allow images to be produced in any plane as well as in the three-dimensional views.

During the procedure, the patient lies on a specially designed table, which is moved into a gantry. "Conventional cylindrical bore" systems, typically of higher magnetic strength, are the most commonly used magnets and can range from 0.5 to 3.0 T (international unit of magnetic flux density). To improve the patient experience, "wide bore" magnets have been introduced which feature a slightly more spacious gantry and are often used when claustrophobia or obesity is a problem (Fig. 16.7). "Extremity" magnets allow for scanning of one's extremities and only require the area in question to be positioned inside the bore. These systems are particularly useful with sports injuries (Fig. 16.8). Chart 16.5 lists the advantages of open MRI. Older open magnets employed low-field magnets (3.2 T), but today, high-field open magnets (0.7 to 1.0 T) are available. Generally speaking, a higher tesla strength magnet is associated with improved image quality. For certain procedures, surface coils are placed over the body area to be imaged. During the test, loud, rhythmic knocking sounds are produced; less noise is associated with the open-design scanner. To relieve patient anxiety and the potential for claustrophobia, some laboratories provide music for relaxation. Two-way communication systems and pulse oximeters are commonly used to monitor patient responses to the procedure. MR applications are continually evolving and improving.

The 3 Tesla (3T) MRI has moved from the research setting to the clinical setting. This shift has come about with innovative methods to reduce RF deposition, ambient noise levels, and chemical shift effects in return for a higher quality diagnostic image.

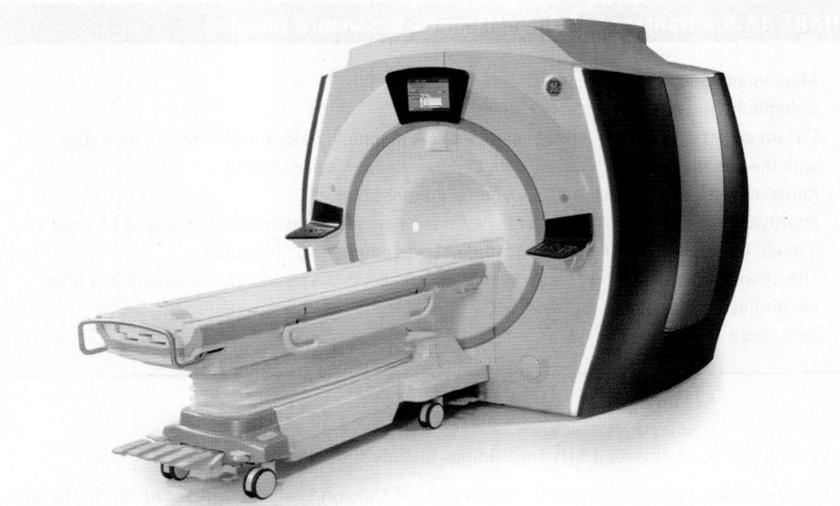

FIGURE 16.7. Discovery MR750w wide-bore scanner. (Used with permission from GE Healthcare, a business of the General Electric Company.)

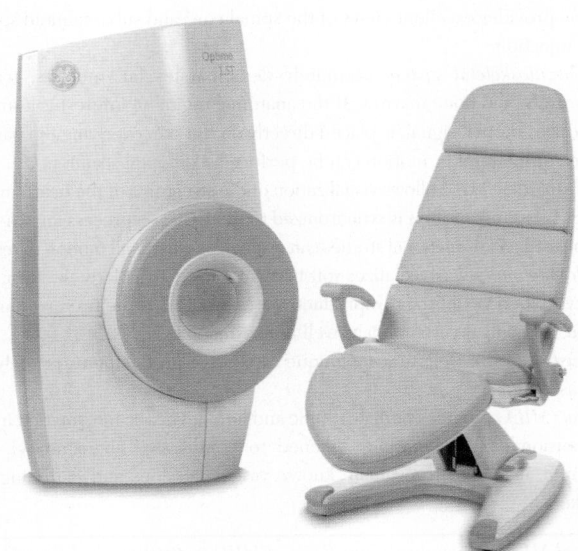

FIGURE 16.8. Optima MR430s extremity scanner. (Used with permission from GE Healthcare, a business of the General Electric Company.)

CHART 16.5 Advantages of Open Magnetic Resonance Imaging

- May not need to sedate the claustrophobic patient
- Suitable for the extremely obese patient
- Enhances patient comfort—Because of the low magnetic field, another person may stay with the patient (especially useful with children or confused patients).
- Kinematic studies of joints (e.g., shoulders) are possible.
- Improved accessibility to the patient allows open magnetic resonance imaging to be used as a guide for interventional and select surgical procedures (e.g., biopsies).
- The open head coil features a unique mirror that allows the patient to see outside the magnet during the procedure.
- Less noise

In general, the most common MR applications include the following:

1. *MRI of the brain* provides exquisite visualization of the soft tissue structures of the brain. Some laboratories perform neurofunctional imaging, which maps the brain's response to the stimuli. Although bony anatomy is seen using MRI, CT is the test of choice to evaluate bone lesions and fractures. A newer MRI technology referred to as *whole-brain T1 mapping* can detect damage to the white and gray matter of the brain in patients with multiple sclerosis. T1 mapping measures "proton relaxation" following exposure to a magnetic field and an RF pulse. Patients with multiple sclerosis show a reduction in brain volume, that is, brain atrophy. Another form of MRI, functional MRI (fMRI), uses MR to measure metabolic changes in the active parts of the brain. fMRI is used quite extensively to study the diseased or injured brain.
2. *MRI of the spine* provides excellent views of the spinal cord and subarachnoid space without intrathecal contrast injection.
3. *MRI of the musculoskeletal system* accurately demonstrates fat, muscles, tendons, ligaments, nerves, blood vessels, and bone marrow. If the anatomic region of interest is a small area, a surface coil, which produces the RF signal, is placed directly on the skin overlying the part to be examined. Dynamic studies of the joint in motion can be performed on open scanners.
4. *MRI of the heart* (cardiac MRI) allows visualization of the structures of the heart, including valves and coronary vessels. Image acquisition is synchronized to the ECG—a process known as *gating*—to help eliminate motion artifacts. Functional studies can evaluate cardiac wall motion in response to exercise.
5. *MRI of the abdomen and pelvis* visualizes soft tissue organs, particularly the liver, pancreas, spleen, adrenals, kidneys, blood vessels, and reproductive organs. This is the preferred method for staging uterine, cervical, and vulvar carcinoma as well as prostate cancer.
6. *MRI of the breast* is a promising new technique capable of producing exquisitely detailed analysis of complex breast lesions.
7. *MR angiography (MRA)* provides both anatomic and hemodynamic information in two-dimensional and three-dimensional representations (likened to noninvasive angiography). MRA is becoming more common; it is used to evaluate known vascular lesions and is finding greater utility in evaluating stroke.

NOTE *Functional MRI with an uppercase F (i.e., FMRI) is distinguished from fMRI in its use for monitoring brain tumors.*

MRS uses a conventional MR scanner to detect chemicals in all body tissues to evaluate tumors, muscle disease, or ischemic heart disease; to differentiate causes of coma; to rule out Alzheimer's disease; to monitor cancer treatment; to differentiate the diagnosis of multiple sclerosis, HIV infection, and adrenoleukodystrophy; to prepare for temporal lobe epilepsy surgery; and to assess the extent of stroke and head injury.

Intravenous MR contrast agents, all primarily containing water-soluble gadolinium complex (most commonly gadolinium-50-diethylenetriamine pentaacetate [DTPA] or 1,4,7,10-tetraazacyclododecane-1,4,7,10-tetraacetic acid [DOTA]) or other metals such as manganese dipyridoxyl diphosphate (MN-DPDP), iron (monocrystalline iron oxide nanoparticle [MION]), and ultrasmall superparamagnetic iron oxide (USPIO) are often used in evaluating the central nervous system. These agents have been approved as safe for patients, including those <2 years of age, and are available in oral, intravenous (most common), and inhalation formulations. Gadolinium presents with very low toxicity and fewer side effects than traditional x-ray contrast agents because of its rapid renal clearance. Other agents used include gadodiamide (nonionic) and gadopentetate, which are used for body scanning. MR contrast agents have lower toxicity and fewer side effects than x-ray contrast agents. However, because these MR contrast agents are primarily excreted through the kidneys, renal failure is a contraindication for use. Other potential contraindications include pregnancy, allergies or asthma, anemia, hypotension, epilepsy, and sickle cell disease.

CLINICAL ALERT

1. Adverse effects, although rare, of Gd-DOTA include vomiting, sensations of local warmth or coldness, headache, dizziness, urticaria, paresthesias, unusual mouth sensations, and respiratory problems.
2. MR contrast agents allow for better basic contrast and tissue signals; most abnormal tissues show regions of increased T1 and T2 (relaxation time, RF signals) regardless of the nature of tumors, edema, hemorrhage, inflammation, and necrosis.
3. Some open MRI systems use only a fraction of the traditional high-field magnets (e.g., 0.2 to 0.3 T compared with 1.0 to 1.5 T). This results in a slimmer profile and much less intimidating appearance for the magnet. Although extremely appealing in certain instances, the open-design magnet is not always the best choice for MRI testing, and careful consideration to magnetic field strength should be given. Certain types of studies can only be performed with a high-field magnet. Some scans performed on an open-design, low-field magnet must be repeated.

Reference Values

Normal

Soft tissue structures: normal brain, spinal cord, subarachnoid spaces, fat, muscles, tendons, ligaments, nerves, blood vessels, marrow of limbs and joints, heart, abdomen, and pelvis

Blood vessels: normal size, anatomy, and hemodynamics

Procedure

1. Have the patient lie supine on a movable examination couch after a thorough medical history is obtained.
2. Sedation may be necessary if the patient is claustrophobic or restless. Earplugs with music are another option. A two-way communication system between the patient and the operator allows continual monitoring and vocal feedback and somewhat reduces the patient's sense of isolation. Many MR laboratories routinely use a pulse oximeter to monitor the patient's arterial oxygenation during the study.
3. For examining many superficial structures (e.g., knee, neck, shoulder, breast), apply a surface coil over the skin. Obtain improved images of the prostate or reproductive organs by using a transrectal coil.

4. Once the patient is positioned and instructed to remain still, move the couch into the scanner.
5. In some instances, inject a noniodinated contrast agent into a vein for better anatomic visualization. For abdominal or pelvic scans, administer glucagon to reduce bowel peristalsis.
6. Examination time varies and averages between 30 and 90 minutes.
7. Follow guidelines in Chapter 1 for safe, effective, informed *intratest* care.

NOTE *The closed-gantry design is narrow and may upset some individuals. Reassure patients that there is sufficient air to breathe and that they will be monitored and given voice contact during the entire procedure.*

PROCEDURAL ALERT

Usually, no special dietary restrictions or preparations are necessary before MRI, unless conscious sedation is to be used. However, numerous safety factors must be considered.

1. Absolute contraindications to MRI include the following conditions:
   a. Implanted devices, including pacemakers, automatic cardiac defibrillators, cochlear implants, certain prosthetic devices (consult with MR laboratory for specific information), implanted drug infusion pumps, neurostimulators, bone growth stimulators, cardioverters, certain intrauterine contraceptive devices, and metal artificial heart valves. Most new surgical implants are MRI compatible; however, most labs will not scan a patient with compatible implants until approximately 2 wk after placement. The exact brand, style, and serial number of the device are needed in order for the MRI department to verify compatibility.
   b. Internal metallic objects such as bullets or shrapnel and certain surgical clips, pins, plates, screws, metal sutures, or wire mesh
2. MRI is generally not advised for pregnant patients (increase in amniotic fluid temperature may be harmful) or individuals with epilepsy. All patients having an MRI need to remove hearing aids, dentures, jewelry, hair pins, wigs, hairpieces, and other accessories.
3. Patients unable to remain still and those who are claustrophobic may require intravenous conscious sedation before MRI.
4. Certain types of eye makeup and permanent eye liners that contain metallic fragments sometimes cause discomfort during MRI. Assess for these cosmetic enhancements.
5. A thorough patient history is mandatory before any MR study. Commonly, radiology services perform conventional x-ray imaging to confirm or rule out the presence of metallic fragments before MRI. This is particularly important for metal or foundry workers, who may have tiny metallic fragments in their eyes.
6. Common metallic equipment (e.g., scissors, oxygen tanks, electronic devices) can become lethal projectiles when exposed to the strong magnetic fields. Therefore, a thorough screening of all patients, visitors, and staff before entering the scan room is mandatory.
7. Local burns from ECG leads, other wires, and surface coils have been reported. It is imperative that the patient describe any burning sensation to the technologist during the procedure.
8. In the event of respiratory or cardiac arrest, the patient must be removed from the scanning room before resuscitation. Most general hospital equipment (e.g., oxygen tanks, intravenous pumps, monitors) is not permitted in the MR suite.

Special Pediatric Considerations for Magnetic Resonance Testing

Pediatric cautions related to MR testing include the following considerations:

1. Age, ability to understand and cooperate, physical condition, and reasons for testing
2. MRI body imaging: Most of the adult guidelines apply. Sedatives, tranquilizers, or modified restraints may be necessary if the child is uncooperative or fearful.
3. MRI for blood flow studies in extremities: Simple restraints may be used to restrict motion of arms or legs. No tranquilizers or sedatives may be used because blood flow will be affected.

Interfering Factors

1. Respiratory motion causes severe artifacts with abdominal and thoracic imaging.
2. Morbidly obese persons may not fit into the gantry opening or surface coil configurations.

Clinical Implications

1. MRI and MRS of the brain demonstrate the following conditions:
   a. White matter disease (e.g., multiple sclerosis)
   b. Infectious disorders affecting the brain (e.g., toxoplasmosis in AIDS, vasculitis, tuberculosis)
   c. Neoplasms (primary and metastatic brain tumors, pituitary adenomas)
   d. Ischemia, cerebrovascular accident
   e. Aneurysms, hemorrhage
   f. Hydrocephalus
   g. Vascular abnormalities (aneurysm, angiomas)
   h. Congenital central nervous system defects (Chiari malformation, Dandy-Walker syndrome)
   i. Alzheimer's disease
2. MRI and MRS of the spine demonstrate the following conditions:
   a. Disk herniation or degeneration
   b. Neoplasm (primary and metastases)
   c. Inflammatory disease
   d. Demyelinating disease
   e. Congenital abnormalities (e.g., tethered cord, spinal dysraphism)
3. MRI of the heart demonstrates the following conditions:
   a. Abnormal chamber size or myocardial thickness
   b. Cardiac tumors
   c. Congenital heart disorders
   d. Pericarditis
   e. Graft patency
   f. Thrombotic disorders
   g. Aortic dissection or aneurysm
   h. Cardiac ischemia
   i. Anomalous pulmonary venous connection
4. MRI and MRS of the limbs, joints, and soft tissue demonstrate the following conditions:
   a. Neoplasms of soft tissue and bone
   b. Ligament or tendon damage
   c. Osteonecrosis, occult fracture
   d. Bone marrow disorders
   e. Muscle fatigue
   f. Changes in blood flow
      (1) Atherosclerosis
      (2) Aneurysm
      (3) Thrombus

(4) Embolism
(5) Bypass grafts
(6) Endocarditis
(7) Shunt placement

5. MRI of the abdomen and pelvis demonstrates the following conditions:
   a. Neoplasms (especially useful in staging tumors)
   b. Retroperitoneal structures
   c. Status of renal transplants
6. MRA demonstrates the following conditions:
   a. Aneurysms
   b. Stenosis or occlusions
   c. Graft patency
   d. Vascular malformations

Interventions

Pretest Patient Care

1. Explain test purpose, procedure, benefits, and risks. Safety concerns for the patient and staff during MRI procedures are based on interaction of strong magnetic fields with body tissues and metallic objects. These potential hazards are mainly due to projectiles (metallic objects can be displaced, giving rise to potentially dangerous projectiles); torquing of metallic objects (implanted surgical clips and other metallic structures or implants can be torqued or twisted within the body when exposed to strong magnetic fields); local heating (exposure to RF pulses can cause heating of tissues or metallic objects within the patient's body; for this reason, pregnant women are not routinely scanned because an increase in the temperature of the amniotic fluid or fetus may be harmful); interference with electromechanical implants (electronic device implants are at risk for damage from both magnetic fields and the RF pulses; consequently, patients with cardiac pacemakers, implanted drug infusion pumps, cochlear implants, and similar devices should not be exposed to MR procedures); and allergic reactions to MR contrast agents.
2. Assess for contraindications to testing. Obtain a relevant history regarding any implanted devices such as heart valves, surgical and aneurysm clips, plates, internal orthopedic screws and rods, and pacemakers, among other objects.
3. Ensure that the following materials are removed before the procedure: removable dental bridges and oral appliances, credit cards, keys, hair clips, shoes, belts, jewelry, clothing with metal fasteners, wigs, hairpieces, and removable prostheses
4. Claustrophobic feelings can be avoided if the patient keeps his or her eyes closed during the test. Recommend that the patient not eat a large meal within 1 hour of testing to reduce physiologic demands and possible emesis while in the scanner.
5. Encourage the patient to relax and instruct him or her to remain as motionless as possible during testing. Reassure the patient that this is a painless procedure.
6. Ask patients having blood flow testing to abstain from alcohol, nicotine, caffeine, and prescription drugs for iron. The patient should fast for 2 hours before testing to avoid unexpected blood vessel vasoconstrictions or dilation. No smoking is permitted before the test. Promote rest in the supine position for 10 minutes before the test.
7. Fasting or drinking only clear liquids may be necessary for several hours before an abdominal pelvic MR.
8. Follow guidelines in Chapter 1 for safe, effective, informed *pretest* care.

Posttest Patient Care

1. Review test results; report and record findings. Modify the nursing care plan as needed.
2. Monitor the patient for side effects of the MR contrast agent. Common side effects include coldness at the injection site, dizziness, and headache. Treatment is usually not needed unless symptoms are bothersome or prolonged. Rare side effects include convulsions, irregular or rapid

heart rate, itching and watery eyes, skin rash or hives, facial swelling, thickening of tongue, fatigue or weakness, wheezing, chest tightness, and difficulty breathing. Alert the healthcare provider if any of these occur and initiate treatment as indicated.

3. Assess the contrast dye injection site for signs of inflammation, bruising, irritation, or infection.
4. Follow guidelines in Chapter 1 for safe, effective, informed *posttest* care.

SLEEP STUDIES

Excessive daytime sleepiness (hypersomnolence) is a classic symptom of inadequate nocturnal sleep, which manifests itself pathologically in various ways. Typically, much of the daytime sleepiness in today's society is a result of irregular sleep patterns and times (e.g., shift work), lack of adequate sleep, poor nutrition, and certain medications. Sleep disorders are grouped into eight major categories:

1. Insomnias, including psychophysiologic insomnia and inadequate sleep hygiene
2. Sleep-related breathing disorders, including central or obstructive sleep apnea
3. Hypersomnias, including narcolepsy and recurrent hypersomnia
4. Circadian rhythm sleep disorders, including jet lag disorder and shift work disorder
5. Parasomnias, including sleep terrors, sleep walking, and nightmare disorder
6. Sleep-related movement disorders, including restless legs syndrome and sleep-related bruxism
7. Apparently normal variations, including long or short sleeper and sleep talking
8. Other sleep disorders, including physiologic sleep disorder and environmental sleep disorder

The insomnias are sleep disorders characterized by difficulty initiating or maintaining sleep or problems with sleep duration, consolidation, or quality. Sleep-related breathing disorders are characterized by problems associated with ventilation, such as partial (hypopnea) or complete (apnea) cessation of airflow during sleep, or alveolar hypoventilation. The hypersomnias include those disorders in which the primary complaint is excessive daytime sleepiness; however, it is not due to nocturnal disturbed sleep or a circadian rhythm disorder. The circadian rhythm disorders result from a misalignment of the endogenous rhythm and the exogenous factors that affect the timing of sleep. The parasomnias are a group of disorders that occur during initiation or within sleep as a result of some undesirable experience or physical event. Movements that disturb the normal sleep architecture fall into the category of sleep-related movement disorders. These disorders are marked by relatively simple, stereotyped body movements that range from leg jerks to teeth grinding. The "short" and "long" sleepers are classified under the category of apparently normal variants. A short sleeper, also referred to as a *healthy hyposomniac*, sleeps substantially less in a 24-hour period than is expected (sleep duration <5 hours in a 24-hour period before age 60 years). A longer sleeper, also referred to as a *healthy hypersomniac*, consistently sleeps more in a 24-hour period than is expected (sleep duration >10 hours in a 24-hour period). Finally, there are those sleep disorders that fall into a category, other sleep disorders, for lack of a clear underlying cause or insufficient background to make a diagnosis. There are other disorders, such as fibromyalgia or gastroesophageal reflux, that may affect sleep or may be affected by sleep but do not fall into any of the categories as listed in *The International Classification of Sleep Disorders*, 3rd edition, published in 2014 by the American Academy of Sleep Medicine. This group of disorders, nonetheless, should be considered in the differential diagnosis.

Types and Indications of Tests

Sleep studies, or polysomnography (PSG), can be divided into two types: standard, in-laboratory, technician-attended, overnight PSG (gold standard) (Fig. 16.9), and portable monitoring (PM) PSG (limited) studies. Standard PSG is indicated in any of the previously described sleep disorders, whereas PM is limited to the evaluation of suspected obstructive sleep apnea (OSA). A portable, battery-powered sleep-screening device (ApneaLink, ResMed Corp., Poway, CA) can also be used to identify patients at risk for OSA.

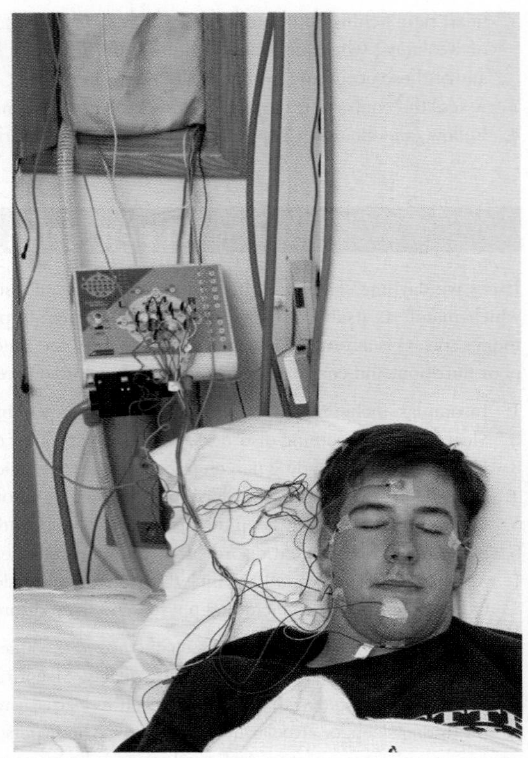

FIGURE 16.9. Polysomnography study in a laboratory environment. (Photo by Hank Morgan/ Photo Researchers, Inc.)

Classification of Tests

The standard PSG includes the following channels:

1. EEG: At least two channels are recorded to determine sleep onset, sleep stages, and sleep offset.
2. Electro-oculogram (EOG): documents both slow, rolling and rapid eye movements seen at sleep onset and in rapid eye movement sleep (REM sleep), respectively
3. EMG: The chin EMG is used as a criterion for REM sleep; the leg EMG is used to evaluate periodic leg movements or leg jerks.
4. ECG: monitors heart rate and rhythm
5. Chest impedance: monitors respiratory effort by use of cardiopneumotachographs, strain gauges, or piezoelectric crystal belts
6. Airflow monitors: Thermistors or thermocouples are used to monitor oral and nasal airflow.
7. Capnography end-tidal CO_2 ($ETCO_2$): continuous monitoring of carbon dioxide
8. Pulse oximetry (Spo_2): continuous monitoring of arterial oxygen saturation by noninvasive means
9. Snoring sensor: microphone placed just below the jaw and lateral to the trachea
10. pH meter: pH probe placed in the lower third of the esophagus transnasally to monitor episodes of gastric reflux
11. Audio and video recordings: document restless sleep, sleep walking, sleep talking, and night terrors, among other conditions

The limited PM includes the following channels:

1. ECG
2. Chest impedance

3. Airflow monitoring
4. Pulse oximetry

● Polysomnography (PSG)

The PSG determines underlying sleep disorder pathology, provides qualitative and quantitative measurements associated with the disorder, and provides information on which to base the proper course of treatment. PSG is indicated for persons complaining of daytime sleepiness, fatigue, inability to stay on task, falling asleep at inappropriate times, insomnia, nocturnal awakenings, waking with gasping or choking feelings, witnessed sleep-related apneas, abnormal snoring patterns, and any other unexplained symptoms associated with disruption of normal sleeping patterns that have persisted for 6 to 12 months.

Reference Values

Normal

EEG: normal sleep onset time, sleep stages, and sleep offset (going from sleepfulness to wakefulness [i.e., awakening])
Airflow monitors: evidence of sustained airflow throughout the night
EOG: normal slow, rolling movements at sleep onset; rapid eye movement during REM sleep
$ETCO_2$: normocapnic (35 to 45 mm Hg during the awake state, increasing a couple of mm Hg during sleep)
EMG: absence of periodic leg movements or jerks
Spo_2: >90%
Snoring sensor: absence of abnormal patterns of snoring
ECG: absence of rhythmic disturbances, bradycardias, or tachycardias
Audio and video recordings: absence of restless sleep, sleep walking, sleep talking, and night terrors, among other conditions
Chest impedance: evidence of sustained respiratory effort throughout night
Apnea/hypopnea index (AHI): adults <5 apneas/hypopneas per hour (after age 60 years, <10 apneas/hypopneas per hour)
Oxygen desaturation index (ODI): adults, <5 per hour (Spo_2 <90%)

Stages of Sleep[a]

Term	Electroencephalogram (EEG) Definition
Sleep onset	Transition from wakefulness to sleepfulness; usually takes at least 10 minutes (i.e., nonrapid eye movement [nREM] stage I)
Stage I nREM	Occurs at sleep onset, consists of low-voltage EEG with mainly theta and alpha activity; 4%–5% of sleep
Stage II nREM	Follows stage I; low-voltage EEG with sleep spindles and K complexes; 45%–55% of sleep
Stage III nREM	Consists of 20%–50% high-amplitude delta waves, referred to as *delta* or *slow-wave sleep*; 4%–6% of sleep
Stage IV nREM	Consists of 50% high-amplitude delta waves and is also called *slow-wave sleep;* 12%–15% of sleep
Stage REM	Low-voltage, mixed frequency, nonalpha activity with rapid eye movements, called *paradoxical sleep*; 20%–25% of sleep
Sleep offset	Transition from sleepfulness to wakefulness, alpha and beta activity, also called *awakening*

[a]Sleep staging is done in 30-second epochs.

Procedure

1. Instruct the patient to keep a sleep log for 1 to 2 weeks before the PSG.
2. Remind the patient that on the day of the study, caffeinated beverages, alcohol, and sedatives are not permitted.
3. Extra time is needed to set up and attach equipment to the patient. Typically, the PSG is recorded during the patient's normal sleep time; however, partial or extended periods of sleep deprivation may be necessary if seizure activity is suspected.
4. The sleep technologist records the patient's history and factors such as age, height, weight, current medications, visual problems, and history of seizures, head injuries, headaches, or strokes. The sleep log is reviewed, and a bedtime questionnaire is completed. The patient wears normal bedtime attire.
5. Use the following list to identify the monitoring equipment used:
   a. Two sets of scalp electrodes to monitor sleep stages (EEG)
   b. One electrode to the outer canthus of each eye (EOG)
   c. One electrode to the chin (submental)
   d. Electrodes to the legs (anterior tibialis; EMG)
   e. ECG leads for heart rhythms and rates
   f. Impedance monitor (respiratory effort)
   g. Oral/nasal thermistor between nose and upper lip (airflow)
   h. Pulse oximeter (SpO_2; O_2 sensor)
6. After application, interface all electrode leads with a "jack box," which contains the preamplifiers and impedance meter. From the jack box, signals are sent through additional amplifiers and filters and finally to a multichannel recorder or polygraph. The polygraph can provide a hard-copy recording of all channels and signals that can be computer processed and displayed on a monitor. Electrode connections are subsequently tested for integrity and adjustments made before the patient retires.
7. During the recording, both audio and infrared camera video recordings are made.
8. Provide a bedside commode because the leads are relatively short.
9. When the test is completed and equipment removed from the patient, ask the patient to complete another questionnaire; score related to the patient's sleep experience during the test.
10. Follow guidelines in Chapter 1 for safe, effective, informed *intratest* care.

NOTE *If seizures are a factor, up to 16 additional scalp electrodes are applied according to the International 10–20 System of Electrode Placement. The International 10–20 System of Electrode Placement is the conventional system (established in 1958) used to identify and place scalp surface electrodes for the recording of brain electrical potentials. The 10–20 System nomenclature is used to indicate that the distance between electrodes is either 10% or 20% of the front to back or right-side to left-side distance of the skull.*

PROCEDURAL ALERT

A home sleep study is an alternative for patients who have trouble falling asleep in a laboratory. Sensors are applied in the clinic, and the patient is shown how to attach the mobile monitoring unit.

Interfering Factors

1. Caffeinated beverages and alcohol can delay sleep onset or exacerbate some types of sleep disorders.
2. Sedatives (hypnotics) shorten sleep onset and reduce nocturnal awakenings, which may skew the results of the PSG.
3. Changes in daily routine on the day of the sleep study may cause false-positive or false-negative results.
4. During the PSG, environmental noise, lights, and temperature may have an adverse effect on the patient's ability to fall asleep.

Clinical Implications

1. Abnormal EEG recordings indicate problems with either sleep architecture (e.g., sleep onset, stages, offset) or seizure disorders.
2. Abnormal leg EMG is consistent with movement disorders (e.g., restless-leg syndrome, nocturnal myoclonus, leg jerks).
3. An AHI >5 indicates sleep-disordered breathing. OSA is characterized by absence of airflow for >10 seconds despite continued respiratory effort (e.g., thoracic breathing or snoring accompanied by periods of apnea). Central sleep apnea (CSA) is characterized by absence of both airflow and respiratory effort; airflow ceases because respiratory effort is absent. Mixed sleep apnea (MSA) generally begins as a central apnea and becomes obstructive apnea.

   Sleep apnea has been linked with cardiac arrest, strokes, pulmonary hypertension, brainstem lesions, and head trauma.
4. An ODI >5 is associated with oxygen desaturation, which generally occurs with an apneic event but can also occur with hypoventilation.

Interventions

Pretest Patient Care

1. Explain test purpose and procedure. These tests are done when signs and symptoms have persisted for at least 6 to 12 months. Caution the patient not to change his or her daily routine the day before the test.
2. Reassure the patient that lead wires, monitors, and sensors will not interfere with changes of position during sleep.
3. Record the patient's age, height, weight, and gender. A brief history and before- and after-bedtime questionnaires are taken.
4. Have the patient prepare for sleep at the normal time according to routine and discontinue any medications used to help with sleep.
5. Follow guidelines in Chapter 1 for safe, effective, informed *pretest* care.

Posttest Patient Care

1. Have the patient resume usual activities and routines.
2. Review test results; report and record findings. Modify the nursing care plan as needed.
3. Explain the need for possible follow-up treatment—for example, surgery (uvulopalatopharyngoplasty) for OSA, medications for restless legs syndrome (Requip), nocturnal supplemental oxygen in patients with low oxygen levels, continuous or bilevel positive airway pressure (CPAP or BiPAP) devices for OSA, or variable positive airway pressure (VPAP) for CSA. Treatment for insomnia may involve a combination of approaches, including cognitive behavioral therapy (CBT) and pharmacologic intervention.
4. Maintaining good sleep hygiene (e.g., getting a good night's sleep) has been shown to increase levels of leptin (a hormone produced by adipose tissue), which decreases appetite and increases metabolism. As most patients with OSA are obese, sleeping 7 to 8 hours nightly will promote weight loss as well.
5. Follow guidelines in Chapter 1 for safe, effective, informed *posttest* care.

● Sleepiness Test; Multiple Sleep Latency Test (MSLT); Maintenance of Wakefulness Test (MWT)

The multiple sleep latency test (MSLT) is used as an objective measure of excessive daytime sleepiness and determines its severity. Typically, the MSLT is administered the morning following sleep study. An alternative to this test is the maintenance of wakefulness test (MWT), which measures the ability of an individual to stay awake rather than to fall asleep. Both the MSLT and MWT are used to diagnose narcolepsy and to evaluate the effectiveness of pharmacologic interventions in the treatment of daytime hypersomnolence. Indications for these tests include falling asleep at inappropriate times, daytime hypersomnolence, suspected narcolepsy, and evaluation of drug effectiveness in treating various sleep disorders.

The MSLT is an objective measure of a patient's sleepiness and is done to evaluate the severity of daytime sleepiness, to diagnose narcolepsy or falling asleep at inappropriate times, and to evaluate effectiveness of drug therapy for daytime hypersomnolence. The MSLT is administered after a sleep study to rule out any sleep-related pathology that might affect the results and to assess the quality of sleep. An alternative to the MSLT is the MWT, which measures the ability of a person to stay awake rather than to fall asleep.

The MSLT includes the following tests:

1. EEG: At least two channels are recorded to determine sleep onset, sleep stages, and sleep offset.
2. EOG: to document both slow and rapid eye movements present at sleep onset and during REM sleep, respectively
3. EMG: The chin EMG is used as a criterion for REM sleep.
4. ECG: to monitor heart rate and rhythm

The MWT includes the following tests:

1. EMG: The chin EMG is used as a criterion for REM sleep.
2. ECG: to monitor heart rate and rhythm

Reference Values

Normal

MSLT: Average sleep latency is 10 to 20 minutes.
MWT

Average sleep latency on the 40-minute test is 35 minutes.
Average sleep latency on the 20-minute test is 18 minutes.

Procedure

1. Typically, the MSLT or MWT is administered the morning following a sleep study. Following the sleep study, have the patient dress, eat (avoiding caffeine), and report back to the sleep laboratory.
2. Reapply the electrodes if necessary.
3. The first nap (for the MSLT) or first session (for the MWT) will begin 1.5 to 2 hours after morning awakening, with a minimum of four additional naps or sessions at 2-hour intervals throughout the day.
4. Terminate the nap or session after 20 minutes for the MSLT or after 20 to 40 minutes for the MWT. With the MSLT test, if the patient falls asleep, continue the recording for 15 minutes after sleep onset.
5. Instruct the patient to allow him- or herself to fall asleep or not to resist the urge to fall asleep for the MSLT, whereas for the MWT, instruct the patient to resist the urge to sleep or to attempt to remain awake.
6. Between the naps or sessions, ensure that the patient remains awake and encourage moving around.
7. Following the testing, disconnect all equipment and discharge the patient.
8. Have the technologist score the MSLT or MWT in conjunction with the PSG test results.
9. Follow guidelines in Chapter 1 for safe, effective, informed *intratest* care.

NOTE *The term* nap *indicates a short intentional or unintentional episode of subjective sleep taken during habitual wakefulness, whereas the term falling* asleep *or* sleep onset *is defined objectively by EEG recordings (i.e., stage 1 of nREM sleep).*

Interfering Factors

Caffeinated beverages can delay sleep, whereas sedatives (hypnotics) shorten sleep onset. Additionally, sleep deprivation may result in a false-positive MSLT result. During naps, environmental noise, lights, and temperature can have an adverse effect on the patient's ability to fall asleep.

Clinical Implications

1. An average sleep onset of 6 to 9 minutes in the MSLT is considered a "gray area" diagnostically because these tests are done in a laboratory setting and not in the patient's home environment. Reevaluation may be necessary if the patient complains and symptoms persist.
2. An average sleep onset <5 minutes and two or more REM periods in the five to six naps during the MSLT is diagnostic for narcolepsy. This indicates a disturbance of the normal sleep architecture pattern, although the REM periods are not unlike nocturnal REM periods. These REM episodes, however, occur prematurely in the cycle and are termed *sleep-onset REMs* (SOREMs).

Interventions

Pretest Patient Care

1. Explain MSLT or MWT purpose and procedure. Remind the patient not to change daily routines on the day of testing.
2. Reassure the patient that lead wires, monitors, and sensors will not interfere with sleep.
3. Record the patient's age, height, weight, and gender.
4. The patient should not consume alcohol or caffeinated beverages the day of the test.
5. Administer standard sleep questionnaires or scales (e.g., Epworth Scale, Stanford Scale) and evaluate.
6. Follow guidelines in Chapter 1 regarding safe, effective, informed *pretest* care.

Posttest Patient Care

1. Explain test outcome and possible need for follow-up testing. Modify the nursing care plan as needed.
2. Pharmacologic treatment for narcolepsy with cataplexy (an attack of extreme weakness) includes medications (e.g., sodium oxybate [Xyrem]); for narcolepsy without cataplexy, modafinil (Provigil) is prescribed.
3. Follow guidelines in Chapter 1 for safe, effective, informed *posttest* care.

● Nasal Continuous Positive Airway Pressure (nCPAP) Titration

Following the diagnosis of OSA, this test is done before treatment is begun. The nasal continuous positive airway pressure (nCPAP) machine supplies air under pressure, acting as a pneumatic splint that keeps the upper airway open during sleep. The pressure required depends on the severity of the OSA and can vary; therefore, the patient is typically required to return to the sleep laboratory on a second night to repeat the sleep study (PSG) while wearing an nCPAP mask. Positive airway pressures are increased until the apneas "break." This procedure is referred to as *nCPAP titration*. Under some circumstances (e.g., severe sleep apnea), titration can be done on the same night as the PSG. In that case, it is termed a *split-night study*. The nCPAP machine provides continuous positive pressure during both inspiration and expiration. Conversely, nasal bilevel positive airway pressure (nBiPAP) uses two separate pressures: one during inspiration and a lower pressure during expiration. In cases in which nCPAP is not well tolerated, nBiPAP may be a better alternative. An nCPAP unit may be used in the home and is preset to the test pressures that ameliorated the apneas.

Reference Values

Normal

EEG: normal time to sleep onset, sleep stages, and sleep offset
Chest impedance: evidence of continuous respiratory effort throughout the night
EOG: normal slow, rolling movements at sleep onset and rapid eye movement during REM sleep
Airflow monitors: evidence of continuous airflow throughout the night
EMG: submental chin placement used as a criterion for REM sleep
$ETCO_2$: normocapnic (35 to 45 mm Hg during wakefulness, which may increase a couple of millimeters of Hg during sleep)
ECG: absence of rhythmic disturbances or bradycardias/tachycardias
Spo_2: >90%
Respiratory disturbance index (RDI): <5 apneas/hypopneas per hour
ODI: <5 per hour (Spo_2 <90%)

Procedure

1. On the day of the titration, instruct the patient to avoid caffeinated beverages, alcohol, and sedatives and to keep a sleep log.
2. Allow sufficient time before testing to attach the patient to the monitoring devices and other equipment, including the nCPAP machine. A brief orientation to nCPAP should take place before the actual day of titration to relieve the patient's anxiety.
3. The sleep technologist takes a brief patient history. The sleep log is reviewed, and a bedtime questionnaire is completed. The patient then prepares for sleep.
4. Have the technologist apply the electrodes, monitors, sensors, microphone, and interface with the polygraph.
5. Fit the patient with an nCPAP mask and ensure that it can be easily removed in case of discomfort, shortness of breath, or claustrophobia.
6. Provide a bedside commode because the leads are relatively short.
7. Adjust CPAP pressures throughout the sleep period, beginning with 3 to 5 cm H_2O and increasing in 2.5-cm H_2O increments until the apneas "break." Time increments can vary from 15 minutes to 2 hours per pressure setting. Decisions are based on protocols being used, severity of sleep apnea, and patient tolerance for testing. If nBiPAP is being performed, inspiratory and expiratory pressures are adjusted separately, keeping the inspiratory pressure at least 2 to 4 cm H_2O above the expiratory pressure.
8. After the test, remove the equipment and have the patient complete another questionnaire, which the sleep technologist evaluates and scores.
9. Follow guidelines in Chapter 1 for safe, effective, informed *intratest* care.

Interfering Factors

1. Caffeinated beverages and alcohol can delay sleep onset or exacerbate OSA, which may interfere with determining optimal pressure settings.
2. Changes in the patient's daily routine on the day of titration can alter results.
3. Patients with a deviated nasal septum or chronic sinusitis may have problems tolerating the nCPAP. The use of nCPAP is contraindicated in persons with severe bullous emphysema or chronic perforated tympanic membrane.
4. Skin irritations from tight-fitting masks (especially on the bridge of the nose), nasal congestion, and headaches are occasional complaints with the use of nCPAP.
5. The benefit of nCPAP to patients with CSA has not been well documented.

Clinical Implications

1. An AHI >5 indicates OSA, which is characterized by the absence of airflow for >10 seconds in the presence of continued respiratory effort. nCPAP used in treating OSA has been shown to be clinically beneficial.
2. Following even short-term nCPAP use, there is documented evidence of rapid symptomatic improvement, with restoration of nocturnal sleep and subsequent lessening of daytime sleepiness and improved quality of life.

Interventions

Pretest Patient Care

1. Explain test purpose and nCPAP titration procedure.
2. Reassure patients that the mask can easily be removed if anxiety or claustrophobia develops.
3. Record the patient's age, height, weight, and gender. A brief history is taken, and before- and after-bedtime questionnaires are filled out.
4. Have the patient prepare for sleep at the normal time in the usual manner.
5. Follow guidelines in Chapter 1 for safe, effective, informed *pretest* care.

Posttest Patient Care

1. Explain test outcome and possible need for follow-up testing and treatment. Depending on the test outcome, an nCPAP unit may be ordered for home use. Modify the nursing care plan as needed.
2. Follow guidelines in Chapter 1 for safe, effective, informed *posttest* care.

BIBLIOGRAPHY

American Academy of Sleep Medicine: Practice parameters for the indications for polysomnography and related procedures: An update for 2005. Sleep 28(4):499–521, 2005

American Academy of Sleep Medicine: Practice parameters for the treatment of narcolepsy and other hypersomnias of central origin. Sleep 30(12):1705–1711, 2007

American Academy of Sleep Medicine: The International Classifications of Sleep Disorders, 3rd ed. Westchester, IL, ASDA, 2014

American Clinical Neurophysiology Society: Guideline 6: Minimum Technical Standards for EEG Recording in Suspected Cerebral Death, 2016

American Speech-Language Hearing Association: The Prevalence and Incidence of Hearing Loss in Children. 2005. Available at: www.asha.org

Bontrager KL, Lampignano J: Textbook of Radiographic Positioning and Related Anatomy, 8th ed. St. Louis, Elsevier Saunders, 2013

Brown K: Evidence collection and preservation, health care setting. Nursing Spectrum in a Health Care Setting, 4(5):22–27, 2003

Bushong SC: Magnetic Resonance Imaging: Physical and Biological Principles, 4th ed. Philadelphia, Elsevier Mosby, 2014

Bushong SC: Radiologic Science for Technologists: Physics, Biology, and Protection, 11th ed. St. Louis, Mosby, 2016

Darty SN, Thomas MS, Neagle CM, et al: Cardiovascular magnetic resonance imaging. Am J Nurs 102(12):34–39, 2002

Edelman RR, Hesselink JR, Zlatkin MB, et al: Clinical Magnetic Resonance Imaging, 3rd ed. Philadelphia, Elsevier Mosby Saunders, 2006

Frank ED, Long BW, Smith BJ: Merrill's Atlas of Radiographic Positioning and Procedures, 12th ed. Philadelphia, Elsevier Mosby, 2013

Groer MW: Advanced Pathophysiology: Applications to Clinical Practice. Philadelphia, Lippincott Williams & Wilkins, 2001

Grossman S, Porth C: Porth's Pathophysiology: Concepts of Altered Health States, 9th ed. Philadelphia, Lippincott Williams & Wilkins, 2013

Guyton AC, Hall JE: Textbook of Medical Physiology, 13th ed. Philadelphia, Elsevier Saunders, 2015

Hampton JR: The ECG in Practice, 5th ed. New York, Churchill Livingstone, 2008

International Association of Forensic Nurses. Available at: www.forensicnurse.org

Jacobs DS, Demott UR, Oxley DK: Laboratory Test Handbook, 5th ed. Hudson, OH, Lexi Comp, 2001

Jemal A, Murray T, Ward W, et al: Cancer statistics, 2005. CA Cancer J Clin 55:10–30, 2005

Kanal E, Borgstede JP, Barkovich AJ, et al: American College of Radiology White Paper on MR Safety. Am J Roentgenol 178(6):1335–1347, 2002

Kryger MM, Roth T, Dement WC: Principles and Practice of Sleep Medicine, 6th ed. Philadelphia, Elsevier Saunders, 2016

Olshaker JS, Jackson MC, Smock WS: Forensic Emergency Medicine, 2nd ed. Philadelphia, Lippincott Williams & Wilkins, 2006

Ostler HB, Maibach HI, Hoke AW, Schwab IR: Diseases of the Eye and Skin. Philadelphia, Lippincott Williams & Wilkins, 2003

Oxorn D, Otto CM: Atlas of Intraoperative Transesophageal Echocardiography: Surgical and Radiologic Correlations. Philadelphia, Elsevier Mosby Saunders, 2007

Pavan-Langston D: Manual of Ocular Diagnosis and Therapy, 6th ed. Philadelphia, Lippincott Williams & Wilkins, 2008

Saferstein R: Criminalistics: An Introduction to Forensic Science, 10th ed. Englewood Cliffs, NJ, Prentice Hall, 2011

Siegel R, Naishadham D, Jemal A: Cancer statistics, 2013. CA Cancer J Clin 63:1–30, 2013

U.S. Preventive Services Task Force: Newborn hearing screening: Recommendations and rationale. Am J Nurs 102(11):83–89, 2002

Varghese A, Pennell DJ: Cardiovascular Magnetic Resonance Made Easy. Philadelphia, Elsevier Mosby Saunders, 2008

Von Schulthess GK: Molecular Anatomic Imaging: PET-CT and SPECT-CT Integrated Modality Imaging, 3rd ed. Philadelphia, Elsevier Mosby Saunders, 2015

Whittman-Price RA, Pope KA: Universal newborn hearing screening. Am J Nurs 102(11):71–77, 2002

Woodard P: MRI for Technologists, 2nd ed. New York, McGraw-Hill, 2000

Appendices

A Standard Precautions for Prevention and Control of Infection

"Infectious diseases are caused by microscopic organisms—including bacteria, viruses, fungi and animal parasites—that penetrate the body's natural barriers and multiply to create symptoms that can range from mild to deadly" (Infectious Diseases Society of America, 2010; www.idsociety.org/factsaboutid.html). Examples of infections include measles, yellow fever, the common cold, tuberculosis, mumps, hepatitis, influenza, and so forth. The sites of infection include lungs, eyes, ears, and urinary and digestive tracts, among others. The Centers for Disease Control and Prevention (CDC) defines infectious disease as "a disease caused by a microorganism and therefore potentially infinitely transferable to new individuals," which may or may not be communicable. The CDC further defines communicable disease as "an infectious disease that is contagious (capable of spreading either by contact or close proximity) and which can be transmitted from one source to another by infectious bacteria or viral organisms" (www.bt.cdc.gov/preparedness/quarantine). Prevention of infection thus includes activities by patients, physicians, nurses, and public health professionals that are aimed at ensuring safety and reducing the likelihood of microbial invasion and multiplication as well as eliminating the possibility of a preventable adverse event. Toxins from food poisoning or infection caused by toxins in the environment, such as tetanus, are examples of noncommunicable diseases.

The term *standard precautions* refers to a system designed to reduce the risk for transmission of microorganisms from both recognized (e.g., environment) and unrecognized sources of infections. Standard precautions direct safe practice and are designed to protect healthcare workers, patients, and others from exposure to blood-borne pathogens or other potentially infectious materials from *any* body fluid or *unfixed* human tissue from any person, *living or dead*. The term *universal precautions* was replaced in 1996 with the term *standard precautions*.

Guidelines are based on information about infectious disease patterns, modes of transmission (e.g., skin contact, inhalation, ingestion, insect bites), and safe practice interventions. The guidelines are designed to be user-friendly, to control nosocomial infections, and to reduce the risk for transmission of both known and suspected infections and include airborne, droplet, and contact precautions to prevent the spread of known or suspected transmissible and virulent pathogens. Isolation and quarantine may be needed to stop the spread of disease.

COMMON CATEGORIES OF BODY SUBSTANCES, SECRETIONS, AND FLUIDS ENCOUNTERED DURING INVASIVE PROCEDURES, PROCURING AND HANDLING SPECIMENS, AND LAB TESTING

1. Blood and blood products
2. Urine
3. Vaginal secretions
4. Saliva
5. Pericardial fluid
6. Peritoneal fluid
7. Pleural fluid
8. Cerebrospinal fluid
9. Gastric fluid
10. Respiratory secretions
11. Semen
12. Synovial fluid
13. Vomitus
14. Wound or ulcer drainage
15. Ascites
16. Amniotic fluid
17. Sweat

NOTE *Standard precautions should also be used before and after death, when handling amputated limbs, and during removal of body parts (surgery, autopsy, or donation).*

IF A BLOOD EXPOSURE OCCURS

Immediately after an exposure to blood, wash needlesticks and cuts with soap and water; flush splashes to the nose, mouth, or skin with water; and irrigate eyes with clean water, saline, or sterile irrigants. Report the exposure to the department (e.g., occupational health, infection control) responsible for managing exposures. Prompt reporting is essential because, in some cases, postexposure treatment may be recommended and should be started as soon as possible.

RISK FOR INFECTION AFTER OCCUPATIONAL EXPOSURE

Hepatitis B Virus

Healthcare personnel who have received hepatitis B vaccine and developed immunity to the virus are at virtually no risk for infection. For a susceptible person, the risk from a single needlestick or cut exposure to hepatitis B virus (HBV)–infected blood ranges from 6% to 30% and depends on the hepatitis Be antigen (HBeAg; this is an extracellular form of the core antigen, HBcAg) status of the source individual. Hepatitis B surface antigen (HBsAg)–positive individuals who are HBeAg positive have more virus in their blood and are more likely to transmit HBV than those who are HBeAg negative. Although there is a risk for HBV infection from exposures of mucous membranes or non-intact skin, there is no known risk for HBV infection from exposure to intact skin.

Hepatitis C Virus

The average risk for infection after a needlestick or cut exposure to hepatitis C virus (HCV)–infected blood is approximately 1.8%. The risk following a blood exposure to the eye, nose, or mouth is unknown but is believed to be very low; however, HCV infection from blood splash to the eye has been reported. HCV transmission may result from exposure to non-intact skin, but there is no known risk from exposure to intact skin.

HIV

The average risk for HIV infection after a needlestick or cut exposure to HIV-infected blood is 0.3% (i.e., three tenths of 1%, or about 1 in 300). Stated another way, 99.7% of needlestick and cut exposures do not lead to infection. The risk after exposure of the eye, nose, or mouth to HIV-infected blood is estimated to be, on average, 0.1% (1 in 1000). The risk after exposure of non-intact skin to HIV-infected blood is estimated to be <0.1%. A small amount of blood on intact skin probably poses no risk at all. There have been no documented cases of HIV transmission due to an exposure involving a small amount of blood on intact skin (a few drops of blood on skin for a short period of time).

SAFE PRACTICE

When handling specimens and performing or assisting with diagnostic procedures, it is important for all healthcare workers to protect and *always* take care of themselves *first*. Presume that all patients have HBV, HCV, HIV, or other potential pathogens, and practice standard precautions consistently. Healthcare personnel are at risk for occupational exposure to blood-borne pathogens, including HBV, HCV, and HIV. Exposures occur through needlesticks or cuts from other sharp instruments contaminated with an infected patient's blood or through contact of the eye, nose, mouth, or skin with a patient's blood. Important factors that influence the overall risk for occupational exposures to blood-borne pathogens include the number of infected individuals in the patient population and the type and number of blood contacts. Most exposures do not result in infection. Following a specific exposure, the risk for infection may vary with factors such as pathogen involved, type of exposure, amount of blood involved in the exposure, and amount of virus in the patient's blood at the time of exposure. Use special care when collecting, handling, packaging, transporting, storing, and receiving specimens. Practice needle safety. Initial observations and specimen handling in the laboratory are to be performed under a laminar flow hood and protective clothing, which includes, but is not limited to, gloves, gowns, facemasks or shields, and eye protection. These same precautions prevail in the performance of invasive diagnostic procedures. Evidence-based practices for infection control and prevention are directed toward hygiene, intravenous therapy, nutrition and the gastrointestinal system, the environment, and treatment with medications.

STANDARD PRECAUTIONS, GUIDELINES, AND PRACTICES FOR SPECIFIC SITUATIONS

Personal Protection Equipment (PPE)

1. Use appropriate barrier precautions when exposure of skin and mucous membranes to blood, blood droplets, or other body fluids is anticipated.
2. Use personal protective equipment devices to protect eyes, face, head, extremities, air passages, and clothing. This equipment must always be used during invasive procedures. Ensure proper fit.

Gloves

1. Wear gloves when collecting and handling specimens; touching blood, urine, other body fluids, mucous membranes, or non-intact skin; or performing vascular access procedures or other invasive procedures.
2. Wear gloves when handling items or surfaces soiled with blood, urine, or body fluids.
3. Mandate wearing of gloves when the healthcare worker's skin is cut, abraded, or chapped during examination of a patient's oropharynx, gastrointestinal or genitourinary tract, non-intact or abraded skin, or active bleeding wounds and when cleaning specimen containers or engaged in decontaminating procedures.
4. *Possible exceptions to use of gloves*
   a. When gloves impede palpation of veins for venipuncture (e.g., neonates, morbidly obese patients)
   b. In a life-threatening situation in which delay could be fatal (wash hands and wear gloves as soon as possible)
5. Disposable gloves *must* be changed:
   a. When moving between patients
   b. When moving from a contaminated to a cleaner site on a patient or on an environmental surface
   c. When gloves are torn or punctured or their barrier function is compromised (do so as soon as feasible)

CLINICAL ALERT

Gloves, barrier gowns, aprons, and masks are worn only at the site of use. They are disposed of appropriately at the site of use.

Gowns, Masks, and Eye Protection

1. Wearing of gowns, aprons, or fluid-impervious lab coats to cover all exposed skin is necessary whenever there is a potential for splashing onto clothing.
2. Gowns or aprons may *not* be hung and reused.
3. Wear masks correctly situated over nose and chin and tied at the crown of the head and the nape of the neck. Do not hang the mask around the neck. Change the mask when it becomes moist.
4. Wear mask, face shields, and goggles (or prescription glasses with side shields) when contamination of eye, nose, or mouth from fluid is most likely to occur.
5. Shoe covers should be worn in areas where contamination might occur (e.g., operating room, obstetrics or emergency department). These are disposed of at the site of care.
6. Provide masks, Ambu bags, or other ventilation devices as part of emergency resuscitation equipment kept in strategic locations.

Disposal of Medical Wastes

1. Pour fluids slowly and close to the receptacle to prevent splash, spray, or aerosol effect.
2. Take precautions to prevent injuries caused by needles, lancets, scalpels, and other sharp instruments and devices during and after procedures and when disposing of used needles. Do *not* recap needles under normal circumstances.
3. Dispose all disposable sharp instruments in specially designed, puncture-resistant containers. Do not recap, bend, break by hand, or remove needles from disposable syringes (Fig. A.1). Use forceps or cut intravenous tubing if necessary. Use care when transferring "sharps" to another person. Use forceps or put the "sharp" in a receptacle.
4. Place, transport, and store specimens in leak-proof receptacles with solid, tight-fitting covers. Cap ports of containers. Before transport, specimens must be placed in a tightly sealed bag marked with a "biohazard" tag. Biohazard symbols warn of biologic hazards and must be displayed in the presence of these hazardous biologic agents or locations.
5. Place soiled linens and similar items in leak-proof bags before transport.

Placement of Warning Tags and Signs

1. Properly place warning tags to prevent accidental injury to or illness in healthcare providers who are exposed to equipment or procedures that are hazardous, unexpected, or unusual.
2. Require warning tags to contain a *signal word* or symbol, such as "Biohazard" or "Biochemical Material," along with the major message, such as "Blood Banking Specimen Inside." All specimens are placed in biohazard bags.

General Environmental Cautions

1. Use approved antimicrobial soaps between care of individual patients.
2. Wash hands immediately after removing gloves.
3. Wash hands and other skin surfaces immediately and thoroughly if contaminated with blood or other body fluids.
4. Consider saliva when blood is visible to be potentially infectious, even though it has not been implicated in HIV transmission.
5. Transmission of AIDS is possible from stool specimens, especially if there is a possibility of blood existing in the stool.
6. Healthcare workers with open skin lesions or skin conditions should not engage in direct care until the condition clears up or does not present a risk to the patient.
7. Development of an HIV infection during pregnancy may put the fetus at risk for infection.

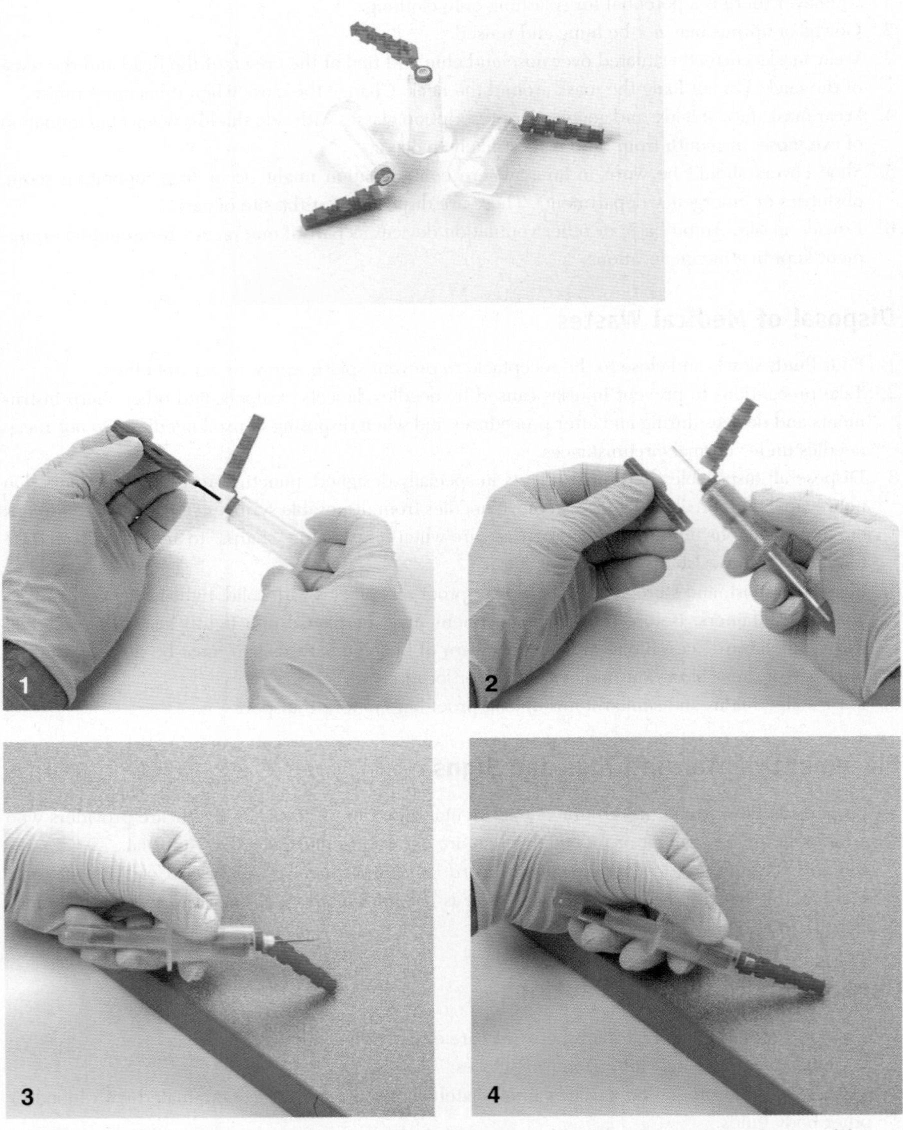

FIGURE A.1. Needle safety device. **(1)** Attach any brand of needle. **(2)** Remove cap and draw patient. **(3)** Press sheath on flat surface. **(4)** Snap closed and dispose. (Photo courtesy of MarketLab Inc., Kentwood, MI.)

CLINICAL ALERT

The healthcare facility environment is rarely implicated in disease transmission, except among patients who are immunocompromised. Nonetheless, inadvertent exposures to environmental pathogens (e.g., *Aspergillus* and *Legionella* species) or airborne pathogens (e.g., *Mycobacterium tuberculosis* and varicella-zoster virus) can result in adverse patient outcomes and cause illness among healthcare workers. Environmental infection can be minimized by increased appropriate use of cleaners and disinfectants, appropriate maintenance of medical equipment (e.g., automated endoscope reprocessors or hydrotherapy equipment), adherence to water-quality standards for hemodialysis and to ventilation standards for specialized care environments (e.g., airborne infection isolation rooms, protective environments, or operating rooms), and prompt management of water intrusion into the facility. Routine environmental sampling is not usually advised except for water-quality determinations in hemodialysis settings and other situations where sampling is directed by epidemiologic principles and results can be applied directly to infection control decisions.

In Case of Exposure to HIV or Hepatitis B Virus

1. Identify, obtain consent, and test source of exposure immediately for evidence of HIV, HBV, and HCV. If the patient refuses consent, a nonconsenting form must be signed. If nonconsenting testing is done on the source, the exposed staff member must also have testing.
2. Advise the HIV-negative worker to seek medical evaluation of any acute febrile illness that occurs within 12 weeks after exposure to HIV and be retested 6 weeks, 12 weeks, and 6 months after exposure.
3. Vaccine is available at no cost to healthcare workers to prevent HBV infection. There is *no* vaccine for HIV or HCV.

Handwashing Protocols

Hands must *always* be washed:

1. Before surgical or obstetric procedures
2. Before direct contact with an immunocompromised patient
3. Before and after care activities that involve direct contact
4. Before and after endoscopy
5. Before and after invasive procedures
6. After contact with body fluids or tissues or with soiled equipment, supplies, or surfaces
7. After direct contact with patients in isolation units

SAFE PRACTICE DOMAINS FOR SPECIFIC SITUATIONS

1. Hygiene
   - Handwashing is the single most important nursing intervention to prevent infection and may be accomplished with antimicrobial soap and water.
   - When hands are not visibly soiled, alcohol-based hand rubs that come in contact with all surfaces of the hand are acceptable substitutes. Alcohol-based hand rubs cannot be used when caring for patients with *Clostridium difficile* diarrhea, norovirus infection, and when hands are visibly soiled.
   - Avoid urinary catheterization. If not clinically feasible, intermittent catheterization—using sterile technique and a closed drainage system—is preferred to continuous catheterization.

- When long-term catheterization is necessary, suprapubic catheters may be considered.
- Document insertion and care of urinary catheters.
- To prevent infection in malignant cutaneous wounds, irrigate thoroughly between dressing changes, debride necrotic material, and dress appropriately to absorb exudate.
- Give neutropenic patients with cancer frequent oral care (toothbrushing and gentle flossing as tolerated). Oral rinses should be "palatable," and antimicrobial rinses should be considered when gingivitis or poor hygiene is noted.

2. Intravenous therapy
   - Select intravascular catheter type and site for insertion that considers risk for complications related to the planned type and duration of intravenous therapy.
   - Avoid placement of permanent or semipermanent catheters when patients are functionally or quantitatively neutropenic.
   - Insert central venous catheters using full barrier precautions (i.e., sterile field, caps, gowns, masks, sterile gloves).
   - Always aseptically place catheters, regardless of site.
   - Two percent chlorhexidine preparation is the preferred cleansing agent of catheter sites.
   - Remove catheters promptly when deemed unnecessary.
   - Cleanse injection ports and diaphragms of multidose vials with 70% alcohol before accessing.
   - Replace catheter dressings promptly when damp, soiled, or loosened.
   - Replace intravenous administration sets, extensions, and secondary sets no more frequently than 96 hours, unless infection is suspected or documented.
3. Nutrition and gastrointestinal system
   - When clinically appropriate, enteral nutrition is preferred to the parenteral route in the cancer patient population.
   - Appropriate dietary restrictions for the neutropenic cancer patient include fruits and vegetables well washed with tap water and avoidance of raw and unwashed meat, eggs, fish, and shellfish.
   - Outcomes related to other dietary restrictions popular in clinical care are not supported by the literature.
4. Environment
   - No systematic evidence exists for the practice of protective isolation of the neutropenic patient with cancer. Such measures may be substituted with aggressive hygienic measures.
   - Neutropenic patients with cancer should not be in contact with fresh flowers or plants.
5. Drug prevention
   - To prevent oral candidiasis in the cancer patient, the use of prophylactic antifungals that are entirely or partially absorbed in the gastrointestinal tract (e.g., fluconazole, clotrimazole) is preferable to use of nonabsorbed agents mycostatin [Nystatin].
   - Prophylactic anti-infectives are indicated in specific situations:
     - Allogeneic bone marrow transplantation against
       - Mycoses: fluconazole, itraconazole, amphotericin B
       - Herpes simplex virus: acyclovir, famciclovir, or valacyclovir
       - *Pneumocystis carinii*: trimethoprim-sulfamethoxazole
     - Acute leukemia undergoing induction against
       - Mycoses: fluconazole, itraconazole, amphotericin B
       - Herpes simplex virus: acyclovir, famciclovir, or valacyclovir
6. Protocols for prevention of catheter-related infections
   - Obtain paired blood cultures: one peripherally, the second set obtained from the distal port of the catheter.
   - Obtain the peripheral culture first; both sets should contain the same volume of blood.
   - The time to positivity (the time between obtaining culture and a positive result) should be compared for set obtained by the catheter versus peripherally. If the culture obtained by the

catheter is positive first, the difference between the two is greater than 120 minutes, and colonization is focused within the catheter, catheter-related infection should be strongly suspected.

7. Protocol for obtaining blood cultures for central venous catheter–related infections
   - Obtain cultures within 30 minutes of the order.
   - One peripheral set of blood cultures is obtained at the first fever.
   - One set of cultures is obtained from each lumen of a central venous catheter, with no blood discarded.
   - Subsequent cultures are drawn from central lines only. Only one set of central line cultures is obtained after the fever has occurred outside the initial 48-hour period.

PROTOCOLS FOR FIRST RESPONDERS

Examples of protocols for suspected serious infectious disease with signs and symptoms classified as high risk (e.g., skin rash or skin involvement and high fever); high fever prodrome (early symptom), as in possible smallpox (classic lesions); yellow fever (jaundice); and plague (buboes, which is a swelling of the lymph nodes) are stated as follows: When any of these other serious infectious diseases cannot be ruled out and there is uncertain diagnosis or no diagnosis, the patient is classified as high risk. Institute airborne and contact precautions, report immediately, and notify the appropriate health department. If rash is present, obtain a dermatology consult and collect specimens by specially trained personnel. Testing is done at the CDC.

Some of these diseases may be the result of possible bioterrorism and can only be diagnosed by the febrile stage and classic signs. A diagnosis of smallpox (a serious disease that kills 30% of infected people) is based on tests for variola virus and recognition of the febrile stage, classic smallpox lesions, and lesions in same stage of development.

CLINICAL ALERT

1. **All first responders and response teams need to be vaccinated before exposure to high-risk serious infectious disease (smallpox) or any other disease for which vaccines are available within 3 days to a week after exposure.**
2. **Anyone directly exposed and those at risk for exposure should be vaccinated. For additional information, go to the CDC website (www.cdc.gov/smallpox).**

PANDEMIC PREPAREDNESS

Pandemic preparedness includes:

1. Using point-of-care testing (POCT) for influenza
2. Maintaining surveillance and tracking of new types of influenza
3. Collecting respiratory samples from patient with flu-like symptoms and exposed to virus using swabs and bronchial exudates for laboratory testing. A gene-based screening test can detect H5N1 viruses in less than 2 hours.
4. Performing tests that confirm and determine subtype for changes in strains. Variances in flu strains confirmed by the CDC become candidates for the next year's vaccine.
5. Using *isolation* to stop spread of next year's communicable diseases; applies to persons who are known to be ill with a contagious disease; may be conducted on voluntary or mandatory basis
6. Using *quarantine* to stop spread of virulent communicable infectious diseases; applies to those who have been exposed but who may or may not become ill; may be conducted on a voluntary or mandatory basis

CLINICAL ALERT

Quarantine may last for one incubation period. In an annual influenza, the incubation period is as long as 4 days.

Quarantinable diseases and potentially pandemic (worldwide) influenza viruses (e.g., avian or bird flu, H5N1), re-emergent influenza viruses, and novel viruses include cholera, diphtheria, infectious tuberculosis, plague, smallpox, yellow fever, viral hemorrhagic fevers, and severe acute respiratory syndrome (SARS). Reporting of infectious and virulent communicable diseases is required under state and federal laws.

Future pandemics will be assigned to one of five discrete categories of increasing severity (Fig. A.2). The Pandemic Severity Index (Chart A.1) provides communities with a tool for scenario-based contingency planning to guide local pre-pandemic preparedness efforts. Accordingly, communities facing the imminent arrival of pandemic disease will be able to use the pandemic severity assessment to define which pandemic mitigation interventions are indicated for implementation.

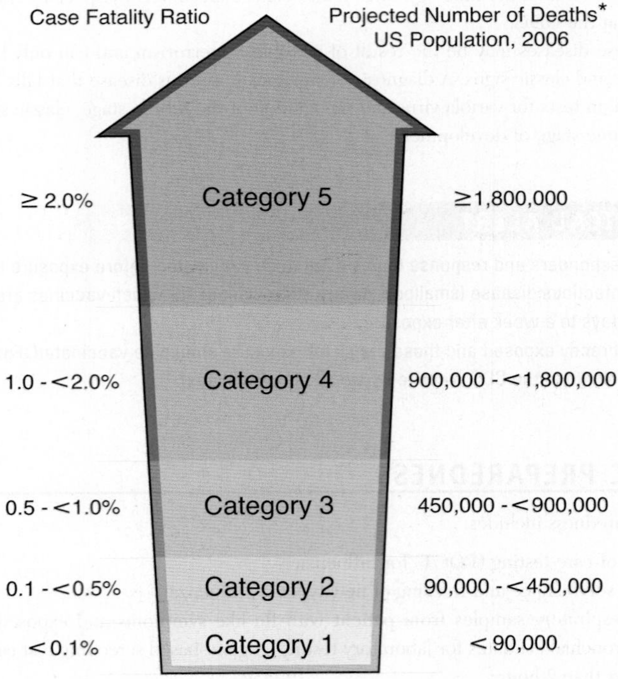

FIGURE A.2. Pandemics are assigned one of five categories of increasing severity (category 1 to 5). (From http://www.flu.gov/planning-preparedness/community/community_mitigation.pdf, page 10.)

CHART A.1 Pandemic Severity Index

Interventions[a] by Setting	Pandemic Severity Index 1	2 and 3	4 and 5
Home			
Voluntary isolation of ill at home (adults and children): combine with use of antiviral treatment as available and indicated.	Recommend[b,c]	Recommend[b,c]	Recommend[b,c]
Voluntary quarantine of household members in homes with ill persons[d] (adults and children): consider combining with antiviral prophylaxis if effective, feasible, and quantities sufficient.	Generally not recommended	Consider[e]	Recommend[e]
School			
Child social distancing: dismissal of students from school and school-based activities and closure of child care activities. Reduce out-of-school social contacts and community mixing.	Generally not recommended	Consider ≤4 weeks[f]	Recommend ≤12 weeks[g]
Workplace and Community			
Adult social distancing: decrease number of social contacts (e.g., encourage teleconferences, alternatives to face-to-face meetings). Increase distance between persons (e.g., reduce density in public transit, workplace). Modify, postpone, or cancel selected public gatherings to promote social distance (e.g., stadium events, theater performances). Modify workplace schedules and practices (e.g., telework, staggered shifts).	Generally not recommended	Consider	Recommend

Generally not recommended: Unless there is a compelling rationale for specific populations or jurisdictions, measures are generally not recommended for entire populations because the consequences may outweigh the benefits.

Consider: It is important to consider these alternatives as part of a prudent planning strategy, considering characteristics of the pandemic, such as age-specific illness rate, geographic distribution, and the magnitude of adverse consequences. These factors may vary globally, nationally, and locally.

Recommended: Generally recommended as an important component of the planning strategy.

[a]All these interventions should be used in combination with other infection control measures, including hand hygiene, cough etiquette, and personal protective equipment such as facemasks.

[b]This intervention may be combined with the treatment of sick individuals using antiviral medications and with vaccine campaigns, if supplies are available.

[c]Many sick individuals who are not critically ill may be managed safely at home.

[d]The contribution made by contact with asymptomatically infected individuals to disease transmission is unclear. Household members in homes with ill persons may be at increased risk for contracting pandemic disease from an ill household member. These household members may have asymptomatic illness and may be able to shed influenza virus that promotes community disease transmission. Therefore, household members of homes with sick individuals would be advised to stay home.

[e]To facilitate compliance and decrease risk for household transmission, this intervention may be combined with provision of antiviral medications to household contacts, depending on drug availability, feasibility of distribution, and effectiveness; policy recommendations for antiviral prophylaxis are addressed in a separate guidance document.

[f]Consider short-term implementation of this measure—that is, <4 weeks.

[g]Plan for prolonged implementation of this measure—that is, 1 to 3 months; actual duration may vary depending on transmission in the community as the pandemic wave is expected to last 6 to 8 weeks.

From http://www.flu.gov/planning-preparedness/community/community_mitigation.pdf, page 12.

BIBLIOGRAPHY

Centers for Disease Control and Prevention: Guideline for hand hygiene in healthcare settings: Recommendations of the Healthcare Infection Control Practices Advisory Committee. MMWR Recomm Rep 51(RR-16): 1–44, 2002

Centers for Disease Control and Prevention: Guidelines for preventing opportunistic infections among hematopoietic stem cell transplant recipients. MMWR Recomm Rep 49(RR-10):1–128, 2000

Centers for Disease Control and Prevention: Prevention Strategies for Seasonal Influenza in Healthcare Settings. Recommendations of the Advisory Committee on Immunization Practices-United States, 2016-17 Influenza Season. Available at: https://www.cdc.gov/flu/professionals/acip/index.htm

Centers for Disease Control and Prevention: Prevention Strategies for Seasonal Influenza in Healthcare Settings. Guidelines and Recommendations. Available at: http://www.cdc.gov/flu/professionals/infectioncontrol/healthcaresettings.htm

Centers for Disease Control and Prevention: Guidelines for environmental infection control in health-care facilities: Recommendations of CDC and the Healthcare Infection Control Advisory Committee (HICPAC). MMWR 2003; 52(No. RR-10):1–48. Updates to Part II recommendations in MMWR 2003 as "Errata: Vol. 52 (No. RR-10)" (MMWR Vol. 52 [42]: 1025–1026)

Centers for Disease Control and Prevention: Updated U.S. Public Health Service guidelines for the management of occupational exposures to HIV and recommendations for postexposure prophylaxis. MMWR 2005; 54(No. RR-9):1–17

Centers for Disease Control and Prevention: Emergency Preparedness and Response. Available at: http://www.bt.cdc.gov/preparedness/quarantine. Current as of February 10, 2014

Gould CV, Umscheid CA, Agarwal RK, et al: Guideline for prevention of catheter-associated urinary tract infections 2009. Infect Control Hosp Epidemiol 31(4):319–326, 2010

Infectious Diseases Society of America: www.idsociety.org/factsaboutid.html

Institute of Medicine: Preventing transmission of pandemic influenza and other viral respiratory diseases: Personal protective equipment for healthcare personnel. Update 2010. Washington, DC, The National Academies Press, 2011

Needlestick Safety and Prevention Act. Pub.L. 106-430; November 6, 2000

Occupational Safety & Health Administration: Healthcare wide hazards. Available at: www.osha.gov/SLTC/etools/hospital/harzards/univprec/univ.html

Occupational Safety & Health Administration: Revision to OSHA's Bloodborne Pathogens Standard (29 C.F.R. 1910.1030); Technical Background and Summary; Published January 18, 2001; effective April 18, 2001

O'Grady NP, Alexander M, Burns LA, et al: Guidelines for the prevention of intravascular catheter-related infections. Am J Infect Control 39(4, Suppl. 1):S1–S34, 2011

Siegel JD, Rhinehart E, Jackson M, et al: Guideline for Isolation Precautions: Preventing Transmission of Infectious Agents in Healthcare Settings. Available at: http://www.cdc.gov/ncidod/dhqp/pdf/isolation2007.pdf

Wisconsin HIV Act 209: http://www.dhs.wiscosnin.gov/aids-hiv/ClinicianResources/09Act209Memo.pdf

World Health Organization: WHO Guidelines on Hand Hygiene in Health Care. Geneva, Switzerland, World Health Organization, 2009

B Guidelines for Specimen Transport and Storage

Routines for collection and handling of specimens and reporting of specific patient information vary depending on agency protocols, the clinical setting, and specialty laboratory requirements. Chart B.1 defines various substances and diagnostic specimens that can be encountered in a clinical setting for possible transport. The primary objective in the transport of diagnostic specimens is to maintain the sample as near to its original state as possible with minimum deterioration and to minimize hazards to specimen handlers. Specimens should be collected and transported as quickly as possible to the laboratory for analysis. For urine transport, a small amount of boric acid may be used; a holding or transport medium can be used for most other specimen types. Follow carefully the instructions for handling and transport of specimens provided on the kit by the manufacturer or by the laboratory that has provided these collection kits. Infectious substances must be handled with the utmost care. Chart B.2 lists the current classifications of substances and diagnostic specimens. Chart B.3 lists examples of Category A infectious substances.

1. When the patient delivers the specimen directly, provide a biohazard bag and include clearly written directions about the specific handling precautions, storage conditions, and specific directions for locating the physical facility.
2. Specimens may be mailed or transported to specialty laboratories located in other cities or distant areas. To avoid delays in specimen analysis, it is important to follow specific instructions for collection, packaging, labeling, and transporting of specimens. Some specimens must be received in the laboratory within an exact time frame, under specified storage conditions. Regulatory agencies (e.g., the Department of Transportation [DOT], or the International Air Transport Association [IATA]) require training to ensure that samples are properly packaged. The DOT requires training every 3 years, whereas IATA requires every 2 years.
   a. When packaging a specimen for shipping to a specialty laboratory, place the specimen in a securely closed, watertight container (e.g., a test tube, vial, or other primary container), and then enclose the entire primary container in a second durable, watertight container (secondary container). Each set of primary and secondary containers should then be enclosed in a sturdy, strong outer shipping container (Fig. B.1).
   b. Follow appropriate labeling for etiologic agents and biomedical materials (Figs. B.2 and B.3). If the package becomes damaged or leaks, the carrier is required, by federal regulations, to isolate the package and notify the Biohazards Control Office, Centers for Disease Control and Prevention, in Atlanta, Georgia. The carrier must also notify the sender that (improper) packaging not meeting regulatory requirements can cause a significant delay in specimen analysis, reporting of results, and medical diagnosis and treatment of the patient's problem. Examples of specialty laboratory requirements for transporting, packaging, and mailing of specific specimens are shown in Table B.1.

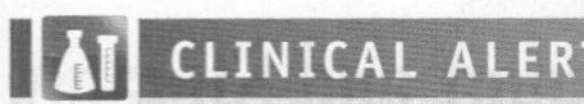

The Code of Federal Regulations governing the shipment of etiologic agents (*42 C.F.R. 72.2 Transportation of Diagnostic Specimens, Biological Products, and Other Materials; Minimum Packaging Requirements*) reads as follows:

> No person may knowingly transport or cause to be transported in interstate traffic, directly or indirectly, any material, including, but not limited to, diagnostic specimens and biological products which such persons reasonably believe may contain an etiologic agent unless such material is packaged to withstand leakage of contents, shocks, pressure changes, and other conditions incident to ordinary handling in transportation.

CHART B.1 Definitions of Substances and Diagnostic Specimens

Infectious substances are defined as substances known to contain, or reasonably expected to contain, pathogens.

Pathogens are defined as microorganisms (including bacteria, viruses, rickettsiae, parasites, fungi) and other proteinaceous infectious particles (e.g., prions) that can cause disease in humans or animals.

Cultures are the result of a process by which pathogens are intentionally propagated. (Note: Cultures do not include human or animal specimens.)

Patient specimens are those collected directly from humans or animals, including, but not limited to, excreta, secreta, blood and its components, tissue and tissue fluid swabs, and body parts being transported for purposes such as research, diagnosis, investigational activities, disease treatment, and prevention.

From Transporting infectious substances safely. Federal Register Hazardous Materials: Infectious Substances. October 1, 2006.

CHART B.2 Classification of Substances and Specimens

Exempt human specimen: Substances with minimal likelihood that pathogens are present; for example, blood or urine for screening tests such as glucose and cholesterol screens.

Infectious substances are now classified as category A infectious substances (UN2814) affecting humans or affecting animals or affecting animals only (UN2900) and biologic substances category B (UN3373).

Infectious substances category A: Substances in a form that, when exposure to it occurs, is capable of causing permanent disability or life-threatening or fatal disease in otherwise healthy humans or animals (see Chart B.3). Refer to the most current edition of the *IATA Dangerous Goods Regulations* manual for a complete list.

Biological substances category B: Substances that do not meet the criteria for inclusion in category A, for example, blood or urine samples for detection of pathogens such as HIV and HBV.

It is recommended to work with the reference laboratory to:

1. Obtain the correct shipping containers and labels.
2. Obtain the needed training to meet compliance.

From Transporting infectious substances safely. Federal Register Hazardous Materials: Infectious Substances. October 1, 2006.

CHART B.3 Examples of Category A Infectious Substances[a]

African swine fever virus (cultures only)
Avian paramyxovirus type 1—velogenic Newcastle disease virus (cultures only)
Bacillus anthracis (cultures only)
Brucella abortus (cultures only)
Brucella melitensis (cultures only)
Brucella suis (cultures only)
Burkholderia mallei (*Pseudomonas mallei*)—glanders (cultures only)
Burkholderia pseudomallei (*Pseudomonas pseudomallei*) (cultures only)
Chlamydia psittaci—avian strains (cultures only)
Classical swine fever virus (cultures only)
Clostridium botulinum (cultures only)
Coccidioides immitis (cultures only)
Coxiella burnetii (cultures only)
Crimean–Congo hemorrhagic fever virus
Dengue virus (cultures only)
Eastern equine encephalitis virus (cultures only)
Escherichia coli, verotoxigenic (cultures only)
Ebola virus
Flexal virus
Foot and mouth disease virus (cultures only)
Francisella tularensis (cultures only)
Goatpox virus (cultures only)
Guanarito virus
Hantaan virus
Hantaviruses causing hemorrhagic fever with renal syndrome
Hendra virus
Herpes B virus (cultures only)
HIV (cultures only)
Highly pathogenic avian influenza virus (cultures only)
Japanese encephalitis virus (cultures only)
Junin virus
Kyasanur Forest disease virus
Lassa virus
Lumpy skin disease virus (cultures only)
Machupo virus
Marburg virus
Monkeypox virus
Mycobacterium tuberculosis (cultures only)
Mycoplasma mycoides—contagious bovine pleuropneumonia (cultures only)
Nipah virus
Omsk hemorrhagic fever virus
Pestes bovines et des petits ruminants virus (cultures only)
Poliovirus (cultures only)
Rabies virus (cultures only)
Rickettsia prowazekii (cultures only)
Rickettsia rickettsii (cultures only)
Rift Valley fever virus (cultures only)
Rinderpest virus (cultures only)
Russian spring-summer encephalitis virus (cultures only)
Sabia virus
Sheep-pox virus (cultures only)
Shigella dysenteriae type 1 (cultures only)
Swine vesicular disease virus (cultures only)
Tick-borne encephalitis virus (cultures only)
Variola virus
Venezuelan equine encephalitis (cultures only)
Vesicular stomatitis virus (cultures only)
West Nile virus (cultures only)
Yellow fever virus (cultures only)
Yersinia pestis (cultures only)

[a]List is not exhaustive.

From the International Air Transportation Dangerous Goods Regulations, January 2015.

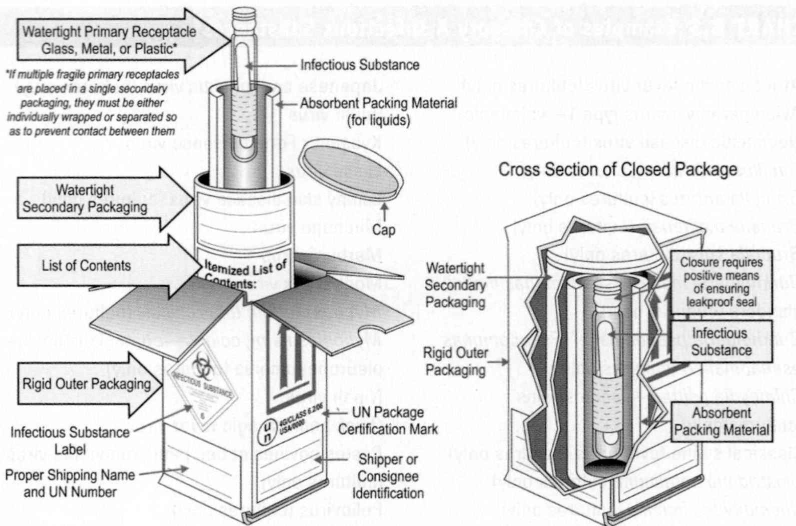

FIGURE B.1. Proper technique for packaging and shipping clinical specimens using triple packaging system (primary sealable contained wrapped in absorbent material, within a secondary watertight, leakproof container, within a shipping package). (From CDC Guidance for Collection, Transport, and Submission of Specimens for Ebola Virus Testing in the United States, updated January 30, 2015).

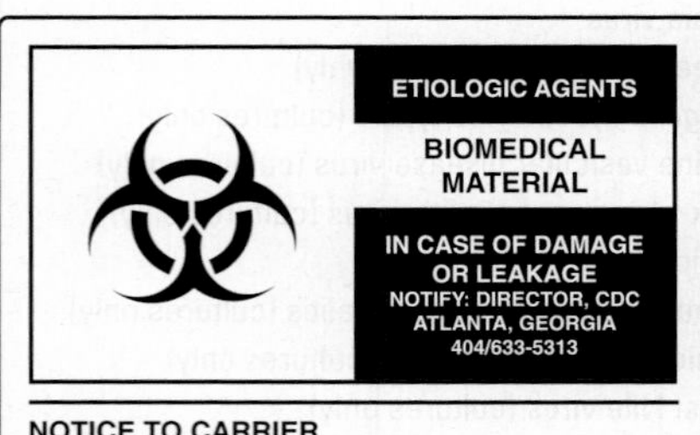

NOTICE TO CARRIER

This package contains LESS THAN 50 ml of AN ETIOLOGIC AGENT, N. O. S., is packaged and labeled in accordance with the U.S. Public Health Service Interstate Quarantine Regulations (42 CFR, Section 72.25[c], [1] and [4]) and MEETS ALL REQUIREMENTS FOR SHIPMENT BY MAIL AND ON PASSENGER AIRCRAFT.

This shipment is EXEMPTED FROM ATA RESTRICTED ARTICLES TARIFF 6-D (see General Requirements 386 ([d] [1]) and from DOT HAZARDOUS MATERIALS REGULATIONS (see 49 CRF, Section 173, 386 [d] [3]). SHIPPERS CERTIFICATES, SHIPPING PAPERS, AND OTHER DOCUMENTATION OR LABELING ARE NOT REQUIRED.

Date Signature of Shipper

CENTERS FOR DISEASE CONTROL
ATLANTA, GEORGIA 30333

FIGURE B.2. Etiologic agents logo and "notice to carrier" that must be affixed to the outside of any package containing potentially hazardous and infectious biologic materials. Refer to packaging instructions in the event that additional paperwork is required to accompany the package.

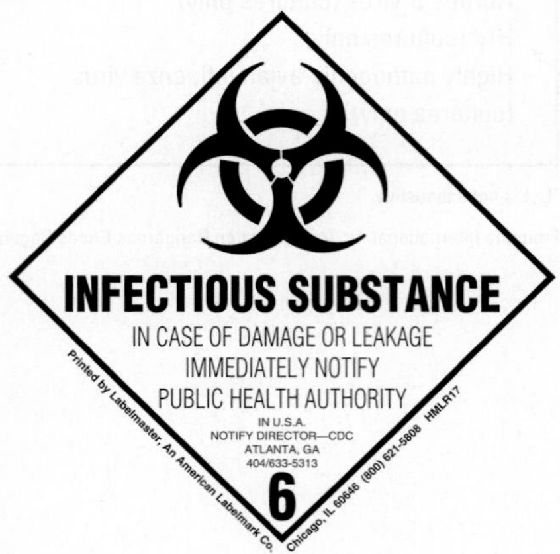

FIGURE B.3. Infectious substance label.

TABLE B.1 Transporting, Packaging, and Mailing Specimens

Specimen	Cautions (Also Include Packaging and Mailing Instructions)
Blood for trace metals	Observe contamination control in sample collection. For example, most blood tubes are contaminated with trace metals, and all plastic syringes with black rubber seals contain aluminum, varying amounts of zinc, and all heavy metals (lead, mercury, cadmium, nickel, chromium, and others). The trace metal sample should be collected first. Once the needle has punctured the rubber stopper, it is contaminated and should not be used for trace metal collection. Use alcohol swabs to cleanse sets; avoid iodine-containing disinfectants, use only stainless steel phlebotomy needles. Blood for serum testing of trace elements should be collected in a royal-blue top (sodium heparin anticoagulant) trace element blood collection tube. After collecting and centrifuging, place in a 5-mL, metal-free, screw-capped polypropylene vial; transfer 5 mL using sterile polypropylene pipette. Cap vial tightly, attach specimen label, and send to lab cool or frozen. All specimens stored >48 hr should be frozen and sent on dry ice. (Keep specimen cool with *frozen* coolant April to October, *refrigerated* coolant November to March.)
Blood for photosensitive analysis	Avoid exposure to any type of light (artificial or sunlight) for any length of time. These specimens need aluminum foil wrap or brown plastic vial. Specimens for vitamin A, vitamin B_6, β-carotene, porphyrins, vitamin D, and bilirubin are examples of substances that need to be protected from light.
Routine urinalysis, random, midstream	Preferred transport container is a yellow plastic screw-capped tube that contains a tablet that preserves any formed element (crystals, casts, or cells) and prevents alteration of chemical constituents caused by bacterial overgrowth. Pour urine into tube, cap tube securely, and invert to dissolve the tablet.
Urine culture	Use a culture and sensitivity (C&S) transport kit containing a sterile plastic tube and transfer device for collection. This tube contains a special urine maintenance formula that prevents rapid multiplication of the bacteria in the urine. Pour the urine specimen into the tube and seal properly.
Urine for calcium, magnesium, and oxalate	Use acid-washed plastic containers for collection and transport of specimen. If urine pH is >4, the results may be inaccurate. Do not collect urine in metal-based containers such as metal bedpans or urinals.
Stool	Use a special 1000-mL container, such as Nalgene, for total sample collection and a 100-mL white polypropylene container for a portion of a large sample (aliquot) for feces collection. Each container should have a similar label affixed before it is given to the patient. When the container is given to the patient, provide the following instructions: test to be done, specimen requirements, diet requirements, collection and storage of specimen; two 1000-mL Nalgene containers provided for timed collection and one 100-mL container for a random collection specimen; information on how to obtain additional containers if necessary; and *do not* fill any container more than three fourths full (indicated by line on label). At the time that the patient returns the container to the clinic, the healthcare worker fills in the label with the correct information. If "Other" is checked, enter duration on line on label. If more than one container is sent, be sure to indicate total number sent on the line.

table continues on pg. 1092 >

TABLE B.1, continued

Specimen	Cautions (Also Include Packaging and Mailing Instructions)
Stool, homogenized	For a homogenized (blended) specimen, the required mailed specimen is an 80-mL portion of homogenized feces. Homogenize and weigh according to laboratory protocol. Pour the homogenate into the container as soon as possible to avoid settling. On the request form, indicate specimen total weight and amount of water added. Include length of period of collection on request form. Send the homogenized specimen at the preferred transport temperature listed in agency specimen requirements protocol. This test is usually performed at a special reference laboratory.
Infectious substance	A biohazard ("Etiologic Agent") label must be affixed (or preprinted on bags) to all patient specimens for transport. Body fluids have been recognized by the Centers for Disease Control and Prevention as being directly linked to the transmission of HIV (AIDS) and hepatitis B virus (HBV). Standard precautions apply to these fluids and include special handling requirements of blood, semen, blood products, vaginal secretions, cerebrospinal fluid, synovial fluid, pleural fluid, peritoneal fluid, pericardial fluid, amniotic fluid, and concentrated HIV and HBV. Also, a "Biohazard" label must be affixed to all microbiology specimens, including anaerobic and aerobic bacteria, mycobacteria, fungi, and yeast. The specimen must be sent on an agar slant tube in a special transport container (a pure culture, actively growing); do *not* send on culture plates. The outer shipping container of all etiologic agents transported via interstate traffic must be labeled as illustrated in Figure B.2.
Specimens requiring exceptional handling	Clearly and accurately label each specimen with patient's full name, sex, birth date, unique identification number, time and date of specimen collection, name of practitioner ordering specimen, and signature of person collecting specimens. The test order form and sample should be checked for a match and transported in a single package.
Frozen	If a delay of >4 d before specimen examination is expected, freezing of the specimen is preferred. Place the specimen in a plastic vial (not glass); the container should not be more than three fourths full to allow for expansion when frozen. Store in freezer or on dry ice until specimen is picked up by carrier or transported to the laboratory. Label vial with patient's name, date, and type of specimen (e.g., ethylenediaminetetraacetic acid [EDTA] plasma, serum, urine).
Refrigerated (iced or cooled)	Urine, respiratory exudates, and stool or feces (transport medium is not used) must all be refrigerated before transport. Specimens that must be kept at room temperature (ambient) before inoculation of media include spinal fluids and other body fluids, specimen for *Neisseria gonorrhoeae* isolation, and blood and wound cultures. Place specimen in the refrigerator for storage before pickup by courier. When packaging, place the specimen container in the zip-top portion of bag and the required coolant in the outer pouch. If dry ice or a refrigerant is used, it must be placed outside the secondary container and the outer shipping container; the shock-absorbant material should be placed so that the secondary container does not become loose inside the outer shipping container as the dry ice evaporates.

table continues on pg. 1093 >

TABLE B.1, continued

Specimen	Cautions (Also Include Packaging and Mailing Instructions)
Anaerobic	Aspiration with a needle and syringe, rather than a swab, is the preferred method of collection of a specimen for recovery of anaerobic bacteria; once collected, the specimen must be protected from ambient oxygen and kept from drying until it can be processed in the laboratory. Transport container for anaerobic specimen includes: a. Syringe and needle for aspiration—valid *only* if specimen can be transported without delay. Remove needle cap before transporting. (Organism will survive in the aspirated material.) b. Port-a-cult (tube or vial)—tubes are used primarily for insertion of swab specimens; vials are used for inoculation of liquid specimen. c. Anaerobic culturette—plastic tube or jacket is fitted with a swab and contains either transport or pre-reduced medium. The culturette system also includes a vial or chamber separated by a membrane that contains chemicals that generate CO_2 catalysts and desiccants to eliminate any residual O_2 that may get into the system. The ampule must be crushed to activate this system. d. Bio-bag or plastic pouch system—transparent plastic bag that contains a CO_2-generating system, palladium catalyst cups, and an anaerobic indicator. Bag is sealed after inoculated plates have been inserted and the CO_2-generating system is activated. The advantage of this system is that the plates can be directly observed for early growth of colonies.

Consult with reference laboratory for any special handling, labeling, collection, or packaging of samples. Laboratories may have special requirements or courier arrangements dictated by testing methods.

CENTERS FOR DISEASE CONTROL AND PREVENTION SHIPPING INSTRUCTIONS FOR SPECIMENS COLLECTED FROM PEOPLE WHO MAY HAVE BEEN EXPOSED TO CHEMICAL-TERRORISM AGENTS

Collecting Specimens

Whole Blood

- Collect a minimum of 12 mL of blood.
- Use three 4-mL or larger vacuum-fill only (unopened), non-gel, purple-topped (ethylenediamine-tetraacetic acid [EDTA]) tubes; use four tubes if using 3-mL tubes.
- Using indelible ink, mark each purple-topped tube of blood *in the order collected* (e.g., #1, #2, #3, #4 [if using 3-mL tubes]).

Urine

- Collect at least 25 to 50 mL from potentially exposed adults and children.
- Use a screw-capped plastic container; do not overfill.
- Freeze specimen as soon as possible (−70°C or dry ice preferred).

Blanks

For each lot number of tubes and urine cups used for collection, provide the following to be used as blanks for measuring background contamination:

- Two (2) empty, unopened purple-topped tubes.
- Two (2) empty, unopened green- or gray-topped tubes.
- Two (2) empty, unopened urine cups.

Labeling Specimens

In addition to unique patient identifiers (e.g., medical records number, specimen identification number), labels should convey the collector's initials and date and time of collection so that law enforcement officials may trace the specimen to the collector should investigations lead to legal action and the collector has to testify that he or she collected the specimen.

Maintain a list of names with corresponding specimen identification numbers at the collection site so that results can be reported to patients. It is recommended to record additional data for use in the interpretation of results. Additional data may include time of potential exposure, method of urine collection if other than "clean-catch," indication if sample was collected postmortem, and antidotes administered prior to sample collection.

Packaging Specimens

Packaging consists of primary receptacles (blood tubes or urine cups), secondary packaging (materials used to protect primary receptacles), and outer packaging (polystyrene foam–insulated, corrugated fiberboard shipper).

Shipping Specimens

Follow the guidance provided in each state's chemical-terrorism comprehensive response plan.

BIBLIOGRAPHY

Centers for Disease Control and Prevention: Guidance for Collection, Transport, and Submission of Specimens for Ebola Virus Testing in the United States; updated January 30, 2015. Available at: https://www.cdc.gov/vhf/ebola/healthcare-us/laboratories/shipping-specimens.html

Code of Federal Regulations. Title 49; Transportation, Part 172. Hazardous materials table, special provisions, hazardous materials communication, emergency response information, training requirements, and security plans, revised 7/2011

Code of Federal Regulations. Title 49; Transportation, Part 173, 199-Category B infectious substances

International Air Transportation Association: www.iata.org

United States Department of Transportation: www.dot.gov

C Vitamins in Human Nutrition

VITAMIN TESTING

Vitamins are organic substances found in minute quantities in food that are essential for metabolism. Both fat-soluble (which dissolve in fat and thus can be stored by the body) and water-soluble (which dissolve in water and thus cannot be stored by the body) vitamins play a variety of physiologic roles in the body. Vitamin concentrations in blood, urine, and certain body tissues can be measured and reflect the nutritional status of the patient.

Vitamins have varying modes of action. For instance, vitamin E is an antioxidant, vitamin C is an enzyme cofactor, and vitamin A is an anti-infection agent.

Sources of *fat-soluble* vitamins include dietary substances and biologic or intestinal microorganisms. Fat-soluble vitamins include vitamin A (retinol or carotene), vitamin D (calciferol), vitamin E (tocopherol), and vitamin K (consisting of phylloquinones or K_1, menaquinones or K_2, and menadiones or K_3).

The sources of *water-soluble* vitamins are dietary substances and intestinal microorganisms. Water-soluble vitamins include vitamin C (ascorbic acid) and the B-complex vitamins, such as biotin, vitamin B_{12} (cobalamin), folate (folic acid), vitamin B_3 (niacin), vitamin B_6 (pyridoxine), vitamin B_2 (riboflavin), vitamin B_1 (thiamine), and pantothenic acid.

These tests are measurements of nutritional status. Low levels indicate recent inadequate oral intake, poor nutritional status, and/or malabsorption problems. They may not reflect tissue stores. High levels indicate excessive intake, intoxication, or absorption problems.

Reference Values

Dietary Reference Intakes (DRIs), adopted by the Food and Nutrition Board, Institute of Medicine, and National Academy of Sciences, provide estimates of vitamin intake. The DRIs look beyond deficiency disease and include the role of nutrients and food components in long-term health.

The DRIs consist of four reference intakes:

- Recommended Dietary Allowances (RDAs)
- Tolerable Upper Intake Levels (ULs)
- Estimated Average Requirements (EARs)
- Adequate Intake (AI)

When an RDA cannot be set, an AI is given as a normal value; both are to be used as goals for the patient. Levels are given for each individual vitamin. The RDAs are the amounts of ingested vitamins needed by a healthy person to meet daily metabolic needs, allow for biologic variation, maintain normal blood serum values, prevent depletion of body stores, and preserve normal body functions. The EARs are the amount of ingested vitamins needed by 50% of healthy persons in a particular age group. ULs are the highest amount that can be consumed on a daily basis and not cause side effects.

Procedure

1. Examine blood, urine, and hair or nail samples for vitamin levels. The types of specimens needed are listed in the table.
2. Test for vitamins by both direct and indirect methods.

Clinical Implications

Increased and decreased levels and critical ranges are shown in Table C.1.

Interfering Factors

Factors that affect vitamin levels include age, season of the year, diarrhea or vomiting, certain drugs, various diseases, and long-term hyperalimentation.

Interventions

Pretest Patient Care

1. Assess overall nutritional status and address potential deficiencies. Often, one deficiency is accompanied by several nutrient deficiencies.
2. Evaluate signs and symptoms of disrupted vitamin-related metabolic reactions that indicate the need for testing.
3. Be cognizant that the cost of testing (high) and time frames for obtaining test results (slow) may be issues for some individuals. Samples for vitamin tests are usually sent to specialty laboratories, which increases cost and turnaround time dramatically.
4. Explain the purpose of the test before collecting blood, urine, hair, or nail specimens.
5. Inform the patient that vitamins are micronutrients that can be detected in the blood and urine as an indication of overt nutritional deficiency states, toxic levels, or subclinical hypovitaminosis. The potential for toxicity from excessive intake exists.
6. Follow the guidelines in Chapter 1 for safe, effective, informed *pretest* and *intratest* care.

Intratest Care

Collect required specimens.

Posttest Patient Care

1. Verify and report reference ranges (RR) and critical ranges (CR). Take appropriate action when values are too high or too low. Treat nutrient deficiencies and toxicities immediately.
2. In collaboration with other healthcare providers (e.g., pharmacist, dietitian), counsel the patient about abnormal results, follow-up tests, dietary changes, and treatment. Water-soluble vitamins are needed on a daily basis. RRs vary and are method dependent. Check with your laboratory.
3. Follow guidelines in Chapter 1 for safe, effective, informed *posttest* care.

BIBLIOGRAPHY

Dietary Reference Intakes Tables and Application. Available at: http://www.nationalacedemies.org/hmd/Activities/Nutrition/SummaryDRIs/DRI-Tables.aspx. Last updated November 4, 2016

Institute of Medicine: Dietary Reference Intakes: Essential Guide Nutrient Requirements. Washington, DC, The National Academies Press, 2006

Institute of Medicine: Dietary Reference Intakes for Calcium and Vitamin D. Washington, DC, The National Academies Press, 2011

Institute of Medicine: Front-of-Package Nutrition Rating Systems and Symbols: Promoting Healthier Choices. Washington, DC, The National Academies Press, 2012

Institute of Medicine: The Development of DRIs 1994–2004: Lessons Learned and New Challenges—Workshop Summary. Washington, DC, The National Academies Press, 2008

The National Academies Press: www.nap.edu

USDA National Agricultural Library, Food and Nutrition Information Center. Dietary Reference Intakes. Available at: https://www.nal.usda.gov/fnic/dietary-reference-intakes

Wu AHB: Tietz Clinical Guide to Laboratory Tests, 4th ed. Philadelphia, Saunders Elsevier, 2006

TABLE C.1 Vitamin Levels and Ranges

Substance Tested (Specimen Needed), Reference Range (RR), and Critical Toxic Range (CR) and DRIs When Available	Patient Preparation, Substance Function, and Indications for Test	Clinical Significance of Values	
		Increased	Decreased
Fat-Soluble Vitamins			
Vitamin A			
Retinol (serum) RR: 360–1200 μg/L or 0.70–1.75 μmol/L CR: <10 μg/dL or <0.35 μmol/L indicates severe deficiency, >100–2000 μg/dL or >3.49–69.8 μmol/L indicates hypervitaminosis A Carotene (serum) RR: 50–300 μg/dL or 1.5–7.4 μmol/L CR: >250 μg/dL or >4.65 μmol/L indicates carotenemia RR: Retinyl esters <10 μg/L when selected Relative dose response (%) RR: >20; CR: >50 deficiency Children show an age-related rise in serum retinol, and values lower before puberty. Levels in adults increase slightly with age. Premenopausal women have slightly lower values than men. After menopause, values are similar.	Fasting; no alcohol 24 hr before blood draw Prevents night blindness and other eye problems and skin disorders (acne) Enhances immunity, protects against pollution and cancer formation Needed for maintenance repair of epithelial tissues Aids fat storage Protects against colds, infections Acts as antioxidant (protects cells against cancer and other diseases) Evaluate night blindness, malabsorption disorders, chronic nephritis, acute protein deficiency, Bitot's spots, intestinal parasites, acute infections, chronic intake of >10 mg of retinol equivalent (RE)	Activation of phagocytes and/or cytotoxic T cells Alopecia Amenorrhea Arthralgia (gout) Birth defects Carotenodermia/aurantiasis Cheilosis Chronic nephritis Cortical hyperostoses Excessive dietary or supplement intake Hepatosplenomegaly Hypercholesterolemia Hyperlipemia Peeling of skin Permanent learning disabilities Pregnancy Premature epiphyseal closure Pseudotumor cerebri Spontaneous abortions Nyctalopia (night blindness) Oral contraceptives (carotene) Pancreatic surgery	Acute infections Arthralgia (gout) Bile duct obstruction Bitot's spots Celiac disease Cirrhosis of the liver Congenital obstruction of the jejunum Cystic fibrosis Duodenal bypass Fat malabsorption syndrome Giardiasis Immunity compromised (cell-mediated response, antibody response) Insufficient dietary intake Keratinization of lung, gastrointestinal tract, and urinary epithelia Keratomalacia Measles

table continues on pg. 1098 >

TABLE C.1, continued

Substance Tested (Specimen Needed), Reference Range (RR), and Critical Toxic Range (CR) and DRIs When Available	Patient Preparation, Substance Function, and Indications for Test	Clinical Significance of Values	
		Increased	Decreased
DRI: Men: 900 μg/retinol equivalent (RE)/d Women: 700 μg/retinol equivalent (RE)/d		Protein-energy malnutrition (marasmus or kwashiorkor) Perifollicular hyperkeratosis (Darier's disease) Sprue Xerophthalmia Xerosis of the conjunctiva and cornea	
Vitamin D			
1,25-Dihydroxycholecalciferol, calciferol (serum) RR: 60 ng/mL or 150 nmol/L Toxic: >150 ng/mL or >375 nmol/L Deficient: <10 ng/mL or <25 nmol/L CR: Serum calcium levels of 12–16 mg/dL or 3.0–4.0 mmol/L (vitamin D toxicity) DRI: Adults: Cholecalciferol 15 μg/d or 600 IU of vitamin D	Fasting Synthesized by skin exposure to the sunshine Required for absorption of calcium and phosphorus by the intestinal tract Necessary for normal development of bones in children Protects against muscle weakness, involved in regulation of heartbeat Important in treatment of osteoporosis and hypocalcemia Evaluate rickets, osteomalacia, fat malabsorption; disorders of parathyroid, liver, or kidney; prolonged supplement intake of 2000 IU/d	Gastrointestinal symptoms (anorexia, nausea, vomiting, constipation) Infants: "elfin facies," hypercalcemia with failure to thrive, mental retardation, stenosis of the aorta Metastatic extraosseous calcification Renal colic Supplements Williams' syndrome	Anticonvulsants Familial hypophosphatemic rickets (diabetes mellitus, Fanconi's syndrome, hypoparathyroidism, renal osteodystrophy, renal tubular acidosis) High phosphate or phytate intake Inadequate diet Inadequate exposure to sunlight (especially in the elderly) Liver disease Malabsorption syndromes Osteomalacia (adults) Rachitic tetany Rickets (children)

Vitamin E Serum α-tocopherol, tocopherol equivalent (TE) (most active) RR (serum): Adults: 0.5–1.8 mg/dL or 12–42 μmol/L NOTE: Concentration of vitamin E in newborns is less than half that of adults. DRI: Adults: 15 mg of α-TE	Fasting. No alcohol 24 hr before draw Antioxidant Important in prevention of cancer and cardiovascular diseases Promotes normal blood clotting, healing Reduces wound scarring Improves circulation necessary for tissue repair; maintains healthy nerves and muscles while strengthening capillary walls Prevents cell damage by inhibiting the oxidation of lipids and formation of free radicals (antioxidants) Aids utilization of vitamin A Retards aging and may prevent age spots Evaluate premature-birth-weight infants, abetalipoproteinemia, malabsorption	Low-birth-weight infants (sepsis, necrotizing enterocolitis) Vitamin E supplementation Increased bleeding tendency Impaired leukocyte formation Reduced cataract formation (with high β-carotene and ascorbic acid levels)	Menstrual problems Infertility (men and women) Biliary atresia Carotid deposits in muscle Cholestasis Dermatitis (flaky) Edema Malabsorption syndromes with steatorrhea Neurologic syndromes affecting the spinal posterior columns and the retina (abeta- or hyperlipoproteinemia), blind loop syndrome, chronic pancreatitis, cystic fibrosis, inborn errors of metabolism, obstructive liver disease, short bowel syndrome Premature infants (bronchopulmonary dysplasia, intraventricular hemorrhage, platelet dysfunction, low retinopathy) Protein-energy malnourished children Reperfusion injury Platelet hyperaggregation, decreased erythrocyte survival and increased susceptibility to hemolysis

table continues on pg. 1100 >

TABLE C.1, continued

Substance Tested (Specimen Needed), Reference Range (RR), and Critical Toxic Range (CR) and DRIs When Available	Patient Preparation, Substance Function, and Indications for Test	Clinical Significance of Values: Increased	Clinical Significance of Values: Decreased
Vitamin K			
Phylloquinone (K_1), plants; menaquinone (K_2 series), bacterial; menadione (K_2), synthetic RR: 1.3–1.9 ng/mL, PIVKA 11 test (proteins induced in vitamin K absence). This test is superior. Plasma prothrombin concentration 10.5–12.5 s DRI: Men: 120 μg/d Women: 90 μg/d	Fasting Needed for the production of prothrombin (blood clotting) Essential for bone formation and repair Necessary for synthesis of osteocalcin (the protein in bone tissue on which calcium crystalizes) Therefore, prevents osteoporosis Plays role in converting glucose into glycogen for storage in liver Antibiotics interfere with absorption of vitamin K Evaluate renal insufficiency and chronic antibiotic treatment	Glucose-6-phosphate dehydrogenase deficiency Increased dietary intake or administered vitamin K preparation Low-birth-weight infants (increased menadione) Anemia with Heinz bodies Hyperbilirubinemia Kernicterus (bilirubin encephalopathy) Loss of sucking reflex Post-kernicterus syndrome	Breast-fed infants (no vitamin K received) Conditions limiting for absorption or synthesis of vitamin K Coumadin (warfarin) Excessive oral mineral oil Hypoprothrombinemia Dietary lack Lack of bile salts (external biliary fistulas, obstructive jaundice) Liver disease Nonabsorbable sulfonamides Salicylate therapy Megadoses of fat-soluble vitamins A or E are known to antagonize vitamin K. Long-term total parenteral nutrition Chronic fat malabsorption, pancreatic disease, gastrointestinal disease

Water-Soluble Vitamins *Ascorbic Acid (Vitamin C)*			
RR: 0–114 μmol/L plasma, 0–2.0 mg/dL plasma, 114–301 nmol/10^3 cells (mixed leukocytes), 20–53 μg/10^3 cells (mixed leukocytes) CR: <11 μmol/L plasma ascorbate, <0.2 mg/dL plasma ascorbate, <57 nmol/10^3 cells (mixed leukocytes), <10 μg/10^3 cells (mixed leukocytes) Women consistently show higher vitamin C levels in tissues and fluids than men. Plasma values are the best indicator of recent dietary intake. Leukocyte vitamin C levels are indicative of cellular stores and body pool. NOTE: Salivary vitamin C levels are not consistent; urinary vitamin C levels are not useful. DRI: Men: 90 mg/d Women: 75 mg/d	Antioxidant needed for tissue growth and repair, adrenal gland function, and healthy gums Aids in production of antistress hormones and interferon; needed for metabolism of folic acid, tyrosine, and phenylalanine Increases absorption of iron; reduces cholesterol levels and high blood pressure Essential in neurotransmitter synthesis and metabolism Essential in the formation of collagen; promotes wound healing; protects against infection Enhances immunity Evaluate scurvy, poor diet, and nephrolithiasis	Decreased anticoagulant effect of heparin and warfarin (Coumadin) Diarrhea Overabsorption of iron Supplementation (alteration of tests for diabetes and occult blood) Nausea Some patients with history of kidney stones are at an increased risk for oxalate stones with too much vitamin C intake.	Adult scurvy (acne, listlessness, deep muscle hemorrhages, swan-neck deformity, gingivitis, perifollicular hemorrhages, hyperkeratosis, and hypochondriasis) Alcoholism and drug abuse Anemia (microcytic hypochromic) Burns Cold or heat stress Edema, lower extremities Gastric ulcers Impaired iron absorption Inadequate diet (especially elderly men) Infantile scurvy (Barlow's disease, "pithed frog" position) Inflammatory diseases, oxidative damage (proteins, DNA, human sperm DNA) Lactation Petechiae and total ecchymoses Pregnancy Risk for cancer (esophagus, oral cavity, uterine, cervix) Smokers (decreased ascorbic acid half-life) Thyrotoxicosis Toxicity from chemical carcinogens (anthracene, benzpyrene, organochlorine pesticides, heavy metals, nitrosamines) Poor wound healing Bleeding gums, dyspnea, edema, and weakness

table continues on pg. 1102 >

TABLE C.1, continued

Substance Tested (Specimen Needed), Reference Range (RR), and Critical Toxic Range (CR) and DRIs When Available	Patient Preparation, Substance Function, and Indications for Test	Clinical Significance of Values: Increased	Clinical Significance of Values: Decreased
Biotin			
Plasma RR: 0.82–2.87 nmol/L CR: <1.02 nmol/L deficiency Whole blood or serum RR: 200–500 pg/mL or 0.82–2.05 nmol/L Prenatal diagnosis of multiple carboxylase deficiency (MCD) by direct analysis of amniotic fluid for methylcitric acid or 3-hydroxyisovaleric acid DRI: 30 μg/d	Biotin is produced by the gut flora. Aids in cell growth; fatty acid production; metabolism of fats, carbohydrates, and proteins; and utilization of other complex vitamins Promotes healthy sweat glands, nerve tissue, and bone marrow Needed for healthy hair and skin Assess for ingestion of raw eggs, inflammatory bowel disease, alcoholism, sulfonamide therapy, and depression.		Alopecia Anorexia with nausea Antibiotics Biotin responsive MCD syndromes Changes in mental status (depression) Glossitis (magenta hue) High fetal resorption rate Hyperesthesia (algesia) Immunodeficiency Increased serum cholesterol and bile pigments Ingestion of large amounts of (6/d) of *raw* egg white, ingestion of raw avidin Localized paresthesia Papulosquamous dermatitis of the extremities Myalgia Pallor Long-term total parenteral nutrition after gut resection, if not supplemented High blood sugar

Cobalamin (Vitamin B_{12}) Serum RR: >200–835 pg/mL or 148–616 pmol/L CR: <100 pg/mL or <74 pmol/L deficiency DRI: Adults: 2.4 μg/d	Overnight fast. Avoid heparin, ascorbic acid, fluoride, and alcohol before testing. Aids folic acid in formation of iron; prevents anemia Required for proper digestion, absorption of food, synthesis of protein, and metabolism of fats and carbohydrates Prevents nerve damage, maintains fertility, production of acetylcholine (neurotransmitter that assists memory and learning) Found mostly in animal sources, so strict vegetarians may need supplements Regional enteritis Evaluate strict vegetarian diet spanning 20–30 yr, alcoholism, after gastrectomy, and parasitic infections	Improved mental function in elderly receiving B_{12} supplements Toxicity to vitamin B_{12} has not been reported.	Deficiency caused by malabsorption—common in elderly and those with digestive disorders Alcoholism Addisonian pernicious anemia Thalassemia Diet lacking microorganisms and animal foods (sole B_{12} sources) Distal sensory neuropathy ("glove and stockings" sensory loss) Gastrectomy Gastric atrophy (superficial gastritis, hereditary—degenerative congenital) Liver disease Pigmentation of skin creases and nail beds (brownish) Polyendocrinopathy Pregnancy Renal disease Small intestine disorders (cancer, gluten-induced enteropathy, celiac disease, granulomatous lesions, intestinal resections, "stagnant bowel" syndrome, tropical sprue) Subacute combined degeneration of the cord Tapeworms Tinnitus and noise-induced hearing loss Tongue—red, smooth, shining, painful Vegans (and their breast-fed infants) Visual loss from optic atrophy Zollinger-Ellison syndrome

table continues on pg. 1104 >

TABLE C.1, continued

Substance Tested (Specimen Needed), Reference Range (RR), and Critical Toxic Range (CR) and DRIs When Available	Patient Preparation, Substance Function, and Indications for Test	Clinical Significance of Values	
		Increased	Decreased
Folate (Folic Acid) Pteroylglutamate, pteroylglutamic acid, 5-methyltetrahydrofolate Red blood cell (RBC) folate (best indicator of status): RR: 150–800 ng/mL or 340–18,120 nmol/L whole blood, corrected to packed cell volume of 45% Tissue folate depletion (serum dietary fluctuations): <160 ng/mL or <360 nmol/L RR: 3–21 ng/mL or 6.7–47.5 nmol/L CR: <1.5 ng/mL or <3.4 nmol/L deficiency Negative folate balance: <3 ng/mL or <7 nmol/L DRI: Adults: 400 µg/d Children: <13 yr 300 µg/d Pregnant women: 600 µg/d Other methods (infrequently used): Deoxyuridine suppression test (DU or dUST), a functional indicator of folate status; in vitro laboratory test that defines presence of megaloblastosis and identifies which nutrient deficiency is responsible (folate or vitamin B_{12}) Formiminoglutamic acid (FIGLU)—after histidine loading	Fasting Needed for energy production and formation of RBCs Strengthens immunity by aiding white blood cell functioning Important for healthy cell division and replication (DNA and RNA synthesis) Protein metabolism Prevention of folic acid anemia In pregnancy, regulates embryonic and fetal nerve cell formation, prevents premature birth Works best when combined with vitamins B_{12} and C Cooking destroys folic acid Evaluate megaloblastic anemia, cancer, inflammatory bowel disease, alcoholism, drug treatment with phenytoin, cholestyramine, sulfasalazine, oral contraceptives Detect folate deficiency	Folacin is dominant form in serum and RBC Loss of seizure control Acute renal failure Active liver disease RBC hemolysis Supplemental folate (400 µg/4 mg/d—side effects)	Alcohol, alcoholics Liver disease Elderly Breast-fed infants of mothers taking estrogen-progesterone contraceptives Cervical dysplasia Cigarette smoking Drug therapy (phenytoin, primidone, barbiturates, methotrexate, metformin, cholestyramine, cycloserine, azathioprine, oral contraceptives, antacids) Increased requirements Hematopoiesis (thalassemia major) Increased metabolism Infancy Lactating women Malignancy (lymphoproliferative) Pregnancy HPV-16 infection Inadequate dietary intake Malabsorption syndromes (celiac disease, sprue, blind loop syndrome) Megaloblastosis Neural tube defects (spina bifida, anencephaly) Pancytopenia Protection from malaria

Urine—24 hr after initial dose RR: <35 mg/d or <201 μmol/d Folate deficiency: <35 mg/d or <201 μmol/d			Psoriasis Renal dialysis Scurvy Tongue papillae atrophy (shiny, smooth) Vitamin B_{12} deficiency Increased mean corpuscular volume Depression Methotrexate-treated patients Hyperhomocysteinemia Long-term unsupplemented total parenteral nutrition Rheumatoid arthritis
Riboflavin (Vitamin B_2) Serum or plasma RR: 4–24 μg/dL or 106–638 nmol/L Urine—much more sensitive to nutritional status RR: >80 μg/dL or >213 nmol/dL erythrocyte; 10–50 μg/dL or 266–1330 nmol/L Creatinine indicates deficiency <27 μg/g creatinine (urine) or <8 μmol/mol creatinine Erythrocyte glutathione reductase assay, expressed in activity coefficients (AC) test cannot be used in persons with glucose-6-phosphate deficiency RR: 10–50 μg/dL or 266–1330 nmol/L DRI: Men: 1.3 mg/d Women: 1.1 mg/d	Fasting Necessary for RBC formation, antibody production, cell respiration, and growth Alleviates eye fatigue and important in treatment and prevention of cataracts Aids metabolism of fat, carbohydrates, and protein With vitamin A, maintains and improves mucous membranes in digestive tract Helps absorption of iron and B_6 Pure, uncomplicated riboflavin deficiency is rare—if seen, it is usually accompanied by multiple nutrient deficiencies.	None	Alcoholism Angular stomatosis Ariboflavinosis Barbiturate use (long-term) Cheilosis Chronic diarrhea Dyssebacia (shark skin) Glossitis Inadequate consumption of milk and other animal products Irritable bowel syndrome Liver disease Normocytic anemia Nutritional amblyopia Oroaggulogenital syndrome Perlèche (*Candida albicans* infection with cheilosis)

table continues on pg. 1106 >

TABLE C.1, continued

Substance Tested (Specimen Needed), Reference Range (RR), and Critical Toxic Range (CR) and DRIs When Available	Patient Preparation, Substance Function, and Indications for Test	Clinical Significance of Values	
		Increased	Decreased
	Needed for metabolism of amino acid tryptophan, which is converted to niacin in the body Easily destroyed by light, antibiotics, and alcohol Increased need for B_2 with use of oral contraceptives or strenuous exercise Assess poor dietary intake, as in congenital heart disease and some cancers.		Photophobia and lacrimation of eye Sore throat Tongue (magenta hue) Use of phenothiazine derivatives
Niacin (Vitamin B_3) Nicotinic acid, niacinamide (urinary *N'*-methylnicotinamide [NMN]) 24-hr urine RR: 2.4–6.4 mg/d or 17.5–46.7 μmol/d CR: <0.8 mg/d or <5.8 μmol/d deficiency DRI: Men: 16 mg/d Women: 14 mg/d	24-hr urine collection Essential for proper circulation and healthy skin Aids functioning of nervous system and metabolism of carbohydrates, fats, and protein in the production of hydrochloric acid for digestion Involved in normal secretion of bile and stomach fluids and synthesis of sex hormones Lowers cholesterol Helpful for schizophrenia and other mental diseases Evaluate antituberculosis drug therapy (isoniazid), malabsorptive disorders, and alcoholism	Abnormal liver function Hypocholesterolemia Use as hypolipidemic drug Atrial fibrillation Cystoid maculopathy Epigastric discomfort Glucose intolerance Gout Hyperglycemia Hypotension Pruritus Smooth, swollen tongue Upper body flushing	Alcoholism Carcinoid syndrome Casal's necklace Cirrhosis of the liver Diarrheal disease Diet lacking in niacin and tryptophan Dyssebacia Hartnup's disease Isoniazid therapy Pellagra dermatosa; glossitis (scarlet, raw beef) Gastrointestinal dysfunction Central nervous system dysfunction Organic psychosis Encephalopathic syndrome

Pyridoxine (Vitamin B_6) RR (direct) Plasma vitamin B_6: 5–24 ng/mL or 20–97 nmol/L Plasma pyridoxal 5 phosphate: >7 ng/mL or >30 nmol/L Plasma total vitamin B_6: >10 ng/mL or >40 nmol/L Urinary 4-pyridoxic acid (4rPA): <3.0 μmol/d (useful short-term index) Urinary total vitamin B_6 antagonists: B_6 >0.5 μmol/day (isoniazid, penicillamine, cycloserine) RR (indirect) Erythrocyte alanine transaminase index (EALT/EGPT) >1.25 (EALT is a better indicator than erythrocyte aspartate aminotransferase (EAST); standardized approach needed to compare tests)	Fasting or urine collection Needed for production of hydrochloric acid and absorption of fats and protein, sodium and potassium balance, and RBC formation Required by nervous system for normal brain function Tryptophan metabolism Niacin formation Gluconeogenesis Synthesis of nucleic acids, RNA and DNA; activates many enzymes and aids in absorption of vitamin B_{12} Cancer immunity, prevents arteriosclerosis Mild diuretic—reduces premenstrual syndrome Diuretics and cortisone drugs block absorption of B_6. Antidepressants, estrogen therapy, and oral contraceptives increase need for B_6. Evaluate groups at risk, including newborn infants with low B_6, some cancers, excess alcohol	Infants: neurologic symptoms and abdominal distress Peripheral neuropathy; progressive sensory ataxia; lower limb impairment Photosensitivity Neurotoxicity	Alcoholism Anemias Asthma Breast cancer Cheilosis Coronary heart disease Depression and confusion Diabetes Drugs (isoniazid, cycloserine, penicillamine, ethinyl estradiol, mestranol) Glossitis Hodgkin's disease Impaired interleukin-2 production Increased metabolic activity Infants (abnormal electroencephalogram pattern, confusions) Irritability Lymphopenia Peripheral neuropathy Premenstrual syndrome Seborrheic dermatosis Sickle cell anemia Smokers Stomatitis

table continues on pg. 1108 >

TABLE C.1, continued

Substance Tested (Specimen Needed), Reference Range (RR), and Critical Toxic Range (CR) and DRIs When Available	Patient Preparation, Substance Function, and Indications for Test	Clinical Significance of Values: Increased	Clinical Significance of Values: Decreased
Thiamine (Vitamin B_1) RR: 0.2–0.4 μg/dL or 5.9–11.8 nmol/L (serum or plasma) 2.5–7.5 μg/dL or 74–222 nmol/L (whole blood) Late changes: <50 μg/d or <148 nmol/d urine with elevated blood pyruvate RBC transketolase measurement (most reliable method) Enzyme assays—using thiamine pyrophosphate (TPP): 79–178 nmol/L RR (stimulation): 0%–25%; deficiency, >20% DRI: Men: 1.2 mg/d Women: 1.1 mg/d	Fasting Enhances circulation and blood formation, carbohydrate metabolism, and production of hydrochloric acid Optimizes cognitive activity and brain function Has a positive effect on energy, growth, normal appetite, and learning capacity Needed for muscle tone of intestines, stomach, and heart Acts as antioxidant, protecting body from degenerative effects of aging, alcohol consumption, and smoking Evaluate alcoholism, impaired absorption, excess intravenous glucose infusion, in diets primarily of refined, unenhanced grain products	Parenteral dosages High-carbohydrate diet increases need for B_1. Thiamine is poorly absorbed in adults with folate or protein.	Antibiotics, sulfa drugs, oral contraceptives Alcoholism Beriberi—dry beriberi (peripheral neurologic changes; i.e., symmetric foot drop); infantile beriberi; wet beriberi Cardiovascular (high-output congestive heart failure, low-output Shoshin disease) Wernicke-Korsakoff syndrome (acute hemorrhagic polioencephalitis) Cerebral beriberi Dependency states (thiamine-responsive megaloblastic anemia, lactic acidosis, ketoaciduria, subacute necrotizing encephalopathy, Leigh's disease) Dextrose infusions (frequent, long-continued or highly concentrated) Folate deficiency High-carbohydrate diet (mainly from milled [polished] rice) Hyperthyroidism Impaired absorption (i.e., long-term diarrheas) Impaired utilization (i.e., severe liver disease) Inadequate calorie or protein intake Increased requirements (fever, lactation, pregnancy, strenuous physical exertion) Poor memory Renal dialysis Long-term total parenteral nutrition Unsupplemented

DRIs, Dietary Reference Intakes.

D Minerals in Human Nutrition

MINERAL TESTING

Minerals are nutrients needed in relatively small amounts. Unlike vitamins, the source for minerals comes from naturally occurring elements, such as mineral salts in the soil that become a part of the chemical constituents of food or minerals that are dissolved in ocean water and ingested in seafood. Mineral concentrations in blood, urine, and certain body tissues can be measured and reflect the nutritional status of the patient.

Minerals can be classified as either macronutrients (major minerals) or micronutrients (trace or ultratrace). If the body requires a significant amount of the mineral (>100 mg/day) and a Recommended Dietary Allowance (RDA) has been established, it is a macronutrient; if the body requires less (<100 mg/day) and an RDA or Estimated Safe and Adequate Daily Dietary Intake (ESADDI) has been established, it is a micronutrient trace mineral; if the body requires <1 mg/day and no RDA or ESADDI has been established, it is a micronutrient ultratrace mineral.

Macronutrients (major minerals) include calcium, chloride, magnesium, phosphorus, potassium, sodium, and sulfur. Macronutrients are not listed in this table. See Chapter 6 for additional information.

Micronutrients (trace minerals) include chromium, cobalt, copper, fluorine, iodine, iron, manganese, molybdenum, selenium, and zinc. *Ultratrace minerals* include the micronutrients arsenic, boron, bromine, cadmium, lead, lithium, nickel, silicon, tin, and vanadium.

Minerals found in the body without an assigned metabolic role include aluminum, antimony, beryllium, bismuth, cyanide, gold, mercury, silver, lead, thallium, and many others.

These measurements of minerals are used to assess environmental or occupational exposure and toxicity (sometimes referred to as "heavy metals"), monitor effectiveness of treatment, and evaluate mineral status along with other laboratory levels to verify deficiencies.

Reference Values

Dietary Reference Intakes (DRIs), adopted by the Food and Nutrition Board, Institute of Medicine, and National Academy of Sciences, provide estimates of mineral intake. The DRIs look beyond deficiency disease and include the role of nutrients and food components in long-term health and prevention of chronic disease (i.e., calcium balance and calcium retention).

The DRIs consist of four reference intakes:

- RDAs
- Tolerable Upper Intake Levels (ULs)
- Estimated Average Requirements (EARs)
- Adequate Intake (AI)

The RDAs reflect the amounts of ingested vitamins needed by a healthy person to meet daily metabolic needs, allow for biologic variation, maintain normal blood serum values, prevent depletion of body stores, and preserve normal body functions. The EARs reflect the amount of ingested vitamins needed by 50% of healthy persons in a particular age group. ULs are the highest amount that can be consumed on a daily basis and not cause side effects. The RDA and EAR levels have been established for some minerals, including those with and without an assigned role in the human body.

Procedure

1. Examine blood, urine, hair, or nail samples for mineral levels by indirect and direct methods.
2. Types of specimens required are listed in Table D.1.

Clinical Implications

Increased and decreased levels and critical toxic ranges are found in Table D.1.

Interfering Factors

Factors that affect mineral levels include:

1. Genetic makeup
2. Age or stage of life cycle
3. Environmental factors
4. Drugs
5. Intestinal malabsorption
6. Stress
7. Strenuous physical activity
8. Smoking
9. Alcohol consumption
10. Dietary intake

Interventions

Pretest Patient Care

1. Evaluate overall nutritional status, dietary intake, and supplement usage to determine overconsumption.
2. Evaluate signs and symptoms of occupational and environmental toxicity and mineral deficiencies that indicate the need for testing.
3. Explain the purpose of the test before collecting blood, urine, hair, or nail specimens.
4. Inform the patient that minerals are nutrients that can be detected in the blood and urine as an indication of toxicity or exposure and nutritional status. The amounts needed are determined by what is necessary for optimal function and health and to prevent disease.
5. Follow guidelines in Chapter 1 for safe, effective, informed *pretest* and *intratest* care.

Intratest Patient Care

Collect the specimen sample.

Posttest Patient Care

1. Verify and report reference ranges (RR) and critical toxic ranges (CR). Take appropriate action when values are too high or too low.
2. Counsel the patient appropriately about abnormal results, follow-up testing, occupational and lifestyle changes, treatment, and diet. RRs vary and are method dependent. Check with your laboratory. Notify employer, workplace, and physician about exposure results.
3. Follow the guidelines in Chapter 1 for safe, effective, informed *posttest* care.

BIBLIOGRAPHY

Moghadaszadeh B, Beggs AH: Selenoproteins and their impact on human health through diverse physiologic pathways. Physiology 21:307–315, 2006

Institute of Medicine: Dietary Reference Intakes for Energy, Carbohydrate, Fiber, Fat, Fatty Acids, Cholesterol, Protein, and Amino Acids. Washington, DC, National Academies Press, 2005

Institute of Medicine: Dietary Reference Intakes for Vitamin A, Vitamin K, Arsenic, Boron, Chromium, Copper, Iodine, Iron, Manganese, Molybdenum, Nickel, Silicon, Vanadium, and Zinc. Washington, DC, National Academies Press, 2001

Wu AHB: Tietz Clinical Guide to Laboratory Tests, 4th ed. Philadelphia, Saunders Elsevier, 2006

TABLE D.1 Mineral Levels and Ranges

Substance Tested (Specimen Needed), Reference Range (RR), and Critical Toxic Range (CR) and DRIs When Available	Patient Preparation, Substance Function, and Indications for Test	Clinical Significance of Values	
		Increased	Decreased
Aluminum (Al)			
Serum RR: <6 μg/L or <0.22 μmol/L (dialysis patients) RR: 20–550 μg/L or 0.74–20.4 μmol/L Urine RR: 5–30 μg/L or 0.19–1.11 μmol/L	Collect urine in acid-washed polypropylene container. No metabolic role Metal used in other forms as an astringent (Burow's solution) and as an antacid Assess for occupational exposure and toxicity from antacids; monitor dialysis patients.	Aluminum absorption with citrate-containing drugs (effervescent or analgesics) Use of aluminum-containing astringents, hydroxide gels, aluminum-containing phosphate binders Excessive occupational exposure *Toxicity:* Aluminosis (lung disease) Aluminum-induced encephalopathy Hypophosphatemia Dialysis dementia Iron-resistant microcytic anemia Aluminum-related osteomalacia In renal failure, when aluminum containing antacids are used; long-term intermittent dialysis NOTE: Aluminum is a neurotoxin. The primary symptom is motor dysfunction leading to dysarthria, myoclonus, or epilepsy. Aluminum toxicity is not related to Alzheimer's disease. Aluminum can be found in laboratory solutions used with tissue samples and in laboratory dust. New testing methods are being adopted to rule out contamination.	

table continues on pg. 1112 >

TABLE D.1, continued

Substance Tested (Specimen Needed), Reference Range (RR), and Critical Toxic Range (CR) and DRIs When Available	Patient Preparation, Substance Function, and Indications for Test	Clinical Significance of Values: Increased	Clinical Significance of Values: Decreased
Antimony (Sb) 24-hr urine RR: <10 μg/L or <82.1 nmol/L CR: >1 mg/L or >8.2 μmol/L Plasma RR: 0.03–0.07 μg/dL or 2.5–5.7 nmol/L	No metabolic role Compounds used in alloys, medicines, poisons Assess for occupational exposure and toxicity.	Excessive occupational exposure (ore from mining, bronze ceramics) Ingested compounds (drugs used in parasitic infections) *Toxicity*: acid metallic taste, burning gastrointestinal pain (as in arsenic poisoning), throat constriction, dysphagia, pulmonary edema, liver and renal failure *Lethal dose*: 5–50 mg/kg body weight	
Arsenic (As) Hair or nails <1.0 μg/g of hair or nails Serum ≥5 μg/mL or 0.07 μmol/L Normal concentration 100–500 μg/L or 1.33–6.65 μmol/L Toxic concentration ≥5000 μg/specimen Chronic poisoning 50–5,000 μg/L or 0.67–66.5 μmol/L Acute poisoning, 1,000–20,000 μg/L or 13.3–266 μmol/L	Ultratrace mineral; no function Found in pesticides and paints Used as a homicidal poison High selectivity Assess for occupational exposure, exposure from pesticides and herbicides, and intentional poisoning.	Dermatoses (hyperpigmentation, hyperkeratosis, desquamation, and hair loss); hematopoietic for hair and nails Depression Liver damage characterized by jaundice Peripheral neuropathy Accidental or intentional poisoning Excessive occupational exposure (ceramics, agriculture) *Toxicity*: metallic taste and odor of garlic on breath, burning pain in gastrointestinal tract, shock syndrome, bloody diarrhea, pulmonary edema, liver failure *Lethal dose*: 5–50 mg/kg body weight	

Whole blood 2–23 μg/L or 0.03–0.31 μmol/L 24-hr urine 5–50 μg/d or 0.07–0.67 μmol/L		
Beryllium (Be)		
24-hr urine RR: negative, none detected CR: >20 μg/L or >2.22 μmol/L	No metabolic role; a metallic element Assess for occupational exposure and toxicity.	Acute beryllium disease (a chemical pneumonitis) Excessive occupational exposure (metal extraction, refinery, rocket base, nuclear plant, extensive coal burning); secondary polycythemia Historical—beryllium mining, electronics, chemical plants, manufacture of fluorescent lights (inhalation, introduction into or under skin and/or conjunctiva): berylliosis or granulomatosis NOTE: Almost impossible to distinguish from sarcoidosis
Bismuth (Bi)		
24-hr urine RR: 0.3–4.6 μg/L or 1.4–22.0 nmol/L Plasma 0.1–3.5 μg/L or 0.5–16.7 nmol/L	Collect urine in metal-free container. No metabolic role; workers exposed in cosmetics, disinfectants, pigments, and solder industries Used in some drugs; poisoning as a consequence of therapy for syphilis Assess for occupational exposure, toxicity, and medication levels.	Bismuth used as treatment for syphilis in a growing child when mother has been treated during pregnancy Treatment of peptic ulcer with bismuth-containing drug (zolimidine, colloidal bismuth subcitrate) Bismuth subcarbonate, subgallate, and subnitrate compounds (used as antiseptics, astringents, sedatives, and to treat diarrhea and inflamed skin) *Toxicity*: ulcerative stomatitis, anorexia, headache, rash, renal tubular damage, bluish line at gum margin, albuminuria; resembles lead poisoning, without the blood changes and paralysis; rheumatic-like pain

table continues on pg. 1114 >

TABLE D.1, continued

Substance Tested (Specimen Needed), Reference Range (RR), and Critical Toxic Range (CR) and DRIs When Available	Patient Preparation, Substance Function, and Indications for Test	Clinical Significance of Values	
		Increased	Decreased
Boron (Bo)			
Blood, 4-mL serum Total RR: <2 mg/L or <33 μmol/L CR: >20 mg/L or >330 μmol/L	Ultratrace mineral; a nonmetallic element, found as a compound such as boric acid or borax (sodium borate) Assess for exposure and toxicity, ingestion of boric acid, and unexpected absorption of boric acid from diapers or infant pacifier dipped in borax preparation and honey.	Increase in total plasma calcium concentrations and urinary excretions of calcium and magnesium *Toxicity*: riboflavinuria; lethargy; gastrointestinal symptoms; bright, red rash; shock. *Infants*: reports of scanty hair; patchy, dry, erythema; anemia; seizure disorders *Lethal dose* (adults): boric acid or borate salts, 50–500 mg/kg body weight	Decreased serum concentrations of 17β-estradiol, testosterone, and iodized calcium Depressed mental alertness
Bromine (Br), Bromide			
Serum RR: 20–120 mg/dL or 2.5–15.0 mmol/L Plasma RR: 1,000–2,000 mg/L or 12.5–25.0 mmol/L	Ultratrace mineral; a central nervous system depressant. Bromine is a liquid, nonmetallic element obtained from natural brines from wells and sea water; compounds used in medicine and photography. Assess for occupational exposure to bromide in medicine or photography.	Bromide acne Neurologic disturbances Increased spinal fluid pressure *Toxicity*: bromism or brominism *Lethal dose*: 500–5000 mg/kg body weight	Recent findings support incidence of depressed growth, conception rate, milk fat production, and hemoglobin. Central nervous system depressant
Cadmium (Cd)			
Blood RR: 0–5 μg/L or 0–44 nmol/L Urine—preferred 0–5.0 μg/24 hr or 0–44 nmol/d Toxic: 100–3,000 μg/L or 0.9–26.7 μmol/L	Ultratrace mineral, a metallic element in zinc ores Used in electroplating and in atomic reactors Its salts are poisonous. Assess for occupational exposure, and environmental poisoning.	In tissue, in prostatic and renal cancer In urine, in hypertension, industrial exposure (electroplating—atomic reactors, zinc ores, cadmium solder) In blood, poisoning from foods prepared in cadmium-lined vessels, inhalation of cadmium dust and fumes, softened drinking water, goods grown in soil heavily fertilized with superphosphate	

		Toxicity: severe gastroenteritis, mild liver damage, acute renal failure, pulmonary edema, cough, duck-like gait, brown urine *Lethal dose*: several hundred mg/kg body weight	
Chromium (Cr)			
Whole blood RR: 0.7–28.0 μg/L or 13.4–538 nmol/L 24-hr urine 0.1–2.0 μg/d or 1.9–38.4 nmol/d	Required for normal glucose metabolism; affects cholesterol synthesis Assess for occupational exposure, poor diet, and elderly at risk. Severe trauma and stress increase need.	Excessive industrial exposure (carcinogenic) Renal damage	Insulin resistance (hyperinsulinemia) Impaired glucose Increased risk for congestive heart disease Hypercholesterolemia Decreased fertility
Cobalt (Co)			
Part of the vitamin B_{12} molecule Serum RR: 0.11–0.45 μg/L or 1.9–7.6 nmol/L	Essential element in vitamin B_{12}—stimulates production of red blood cells Assess for occupational exposure and monitor dialysis.	Cardiomyopathy after industrial exposure, during maintenance dialysis, and after drinking beer contaminated with cobalt during processing	Cobalamin (vitamin B_{12}) deficiency
Copper (Cu)			
Serum RR (total): 85–180 μg/dL or 13.3–28.3 μmol/L 24-hr urine RR: 3–35 μg/d or 0.047–0.55 μmol/d Plasma RR: 62–140 μg/dL or 9.7–21.9 μmol/L	Required for hemoglobin synthesis, essential component of several enzyme systems; present in the liver and excreted by the kidneys and in bile Assess for excessive antacid intake, nephronic malabsorptive disorder, hemodialysis, and consumption of water high in copper by infants.	T-cell proliferation Hepatic glutathione Wilson's disease (hepatolenticular degeneration) Ingestion of solutions of copper salts Contaminated water or dialysis fluids Native-American childhood cirrhosis Female rheumatoid arthritis Oral contraceptive use Inflammatory conditions Cancer at injection sites or muscles *Toxicity*: hepatic or renal failure *Lethal dose*: 50–500 mg/kg body weight	Rheumatoid arthritis Menkes' steely hair disease: lack of pigmentation of skin and hair Collagen abnormalities, osteoporosis Ataxia Hypochromic anemia unresponsive to iron therapy Hypercholesterolemia Impaired cardiovascular system

table continues on pg. 1116 >

TABLE D.1, continued

Substance Tested (Specimen Needed), Reference Range (RR), and Critical Toxic Range (CR) and DRIs When Available	Patient Preparation, Substance Function, and Indications for Test	Clinical Significance of Values: Increased	Clinical Significance of Values: Decreased
Ceruloplasmin is an indirect test for copper. RR: 21–53 mg/dL, 210–530 mg/L (neonate: 5–18 mg/dL, 50–180 mg/L)			Oversupplementation of zinc Altered interleukin-2 production Neutropenia, leukopenia Liver disease, kidney disease
Cyanide (Cn Radical)			
Blood Nonsmokers RR: <0.02 mg/L or <0.61 μmol/L Smokers RR: <0.04 mg/L or <1.57 μmol/L Nonsmokers Toxic: >1.0 mg/L or >38.4 μmol/L Serum Nonsmokers RR: 0.004 mg/L or 0.15 μmol/L Smokers RR: 0.006 mg/L or 0.23 μmol/L	No metabolic role The most common and most deadly poison—stops cellular respiration by inhibiting the actions of cytochrome oxidase, carbonic anhydrase, and other enzyme systems Toxicity comes from inhalation or ingestion—a hazard to firefighters. Assess for industrial exposure, inhalation, or accidental poisoning from ingestion.	Industrial exposure (pesticides, metallurgy) Inhalation of hydrocyanic acid and fumes from burning nitrogen-containing products Ingestion of salts and laetrile (derived from broken seeds of apricots, peaches, jetberry bush, toyon, bitter almonds, and some apple seeds) *Toxicity*: Lethal dose is <5 mg/kg body weight (small child), fatal dose = 5–25 seeds. Death within 5 min of ingestion/inhalation. Adverse effects are dizziness, weakness, mental and motor impairment, and sudden death.	
Fluoride DRI: Men: 4 mg/d Women: 3 mg/d			

Fluorine (F)			
Plasma RR: 0.01–0.2 μg/mL or 0.5–10.5 μmol/L Urine RR: 0.02–3.2 μg/mL or 1.05–168.3 μmol/L	Gaseous chemical found in soil in combination with calcium Used as a compound (fluoride) in toothpaste Assess for excess ingestion; evaluate dental caries or mottling.	Fluorosis (excess fluorine use; >4 million ppm in water; treatment of osteoporosis, multiple myeloma, or Paget's disease) Osteosclerosis Exostoses of spine and genu valgum Excess ingestion from swallowing fluoridated toothpaste *Toxicity*: peculiar taste with salivation and thirst (salty-soapy); hemorrhagic gastroenteritis; hypoglycemia; central nervous system depression; renal failure *Lethal dose*: 50–500 mg/kg body weight; 5–10 g sodium fluoride	Marginal to deficient dietary intake from deficiencies in geochemical environments Dental caries Skeletal changes, especially in long bones
Gold (Au)			
Colloidal gold in cerebrospinal fluid RR: minute amount Serum RR: <10 mg/dL or <0.5 μmol/L Therapeutic range, 100–200 mg/dL or 5.1–10.2 μmol/L Whole blood RR: <0.5 μg/L or <0.0026 μmol/L 24-hr urine RR: <1.0 μg/d or <5.1 mmol/d	Collect in metal-free container. No metabolic role; a metallic element Salts used in early rheumatoid arthritis and in nondisseminated lupus erythematosus Detectable in serum 10 mo after cessation of treatment Assess for toxicity in treatment of rheumatoid arthritis.	Rheumatoid arthritis if gold sodium thiomalate or gold thioglucose (aurothioglucose) is given parenterally; oral gold compound *Toxicity*: At least 35% of patients undergoing chrysotherapy develop some degree of toxicity. Pruritus, dermatitis, stomatitis, albuminuria with or without nephrotic syndrome, agranulocytosis, thrombocytopenic purpura, and aplastic anemia *Adverse reactions*: enterocolitis, intrahepatic cholestasis, skin hyperpigmentation, peripheral neuropathy, and pulmonary infiltrates	

table continues on pg. 1118 >

TABLE D.1, continued

Substance Tested (Specimen Needed), Reference Range (RR), and Critical Toxic Range (CR) and DRIs When Available	Patient Preparation, Substance Function, and Indications for Test	Clinical Significance of Values	
		Increased	Decreased
Iodine (I)			
Plasma RR: 2–4 μg/dL, 60 ng/mL Deficiency: iodine deficiency disorders (IDD) Daily urine Mild IDD, RR: 50–100 μg/d (median urine, 3.5 μg/dL) Moderate IDD, RR: 25–49 μg/d (median urine, 2–3.4 μg/dL) Severe IDD, RR: <25 μg/d (median urine, 0–1.9 μg/dL) DRI: adults 150 μg/d	Nonmetallic element belonging to the halogen group Aids in the development and function of the thyroid gland, formation of thyroxine, and prevention of goiter Assess for goiter.	Prolonged excessive intake of iodine leading to iodide-goiter and myxedema (common with preexisting Hashimoto's thyroiditis) Excessive consumption of seaweed, kelp supplements; caffeine High dietary intake of known goitrogens (rutabagas, turnips, cabbages) Hypothyroidism in autoimmune thyroid diseases, inhibition of thionamide drugs Dysgeusia Acne-like skin lesions *Toxicity*: mucous membranes stained brown; burning pain in mouth and esophagus, laryngeal edema, shock, nephritis, circulatory collapse *Lethal dose*: 5–50 mg/kg body weight	Simple, endemic, colloid, or euthyroid goiter Endemic cretinism (neurologic and/or myxedematous) Fetus: abortions, stillbirths, congenital anomalies Child/teen: impaired mental function, retarded physical development Adult: hypo- or hyperthyroidism, impaired mental function
Iron (Fe)			
Serum (5 mL, diurnal; morning specimen shows higher values), toxic >300 μg/dL or >53.7 μmol/L	Essential to hemoglobin formation, transportation of oxygen, and cellular respiration Plays a role in the nutrition of epithelial tissues and the development of red blood cells	Diets high in heme iron or high in promoters of nonheme iron absorption	Iron deficiency anemia: inadequate diet (grossly iron deficient, high in cereals, low in animal protein and vitamin C) Koilonychia (spoon-shaped nails) Excessive menstrual loss Pregnancy, lactation Blood donors

Iron RR values Males: 65–175 μg/dL or 11.6–31.3 μmol/L Females: 50–170 μg/dL or 9.0–30.4 μmol/L Newborn: 100–250 μg/dL or 17.9–44.8 μmol/L Child: 50–120 μg/dL or 9.0–21.5 μmol/L *Total iron binding capacity (TIBC)* RR: 250–425 μg/dL or 44.8–76.1 mmol/L Infants: RR: 100–400 μg/dL or 17.9–71.6 mmol/L (Also see Chapter 6) *Transferrin* RR values Adult: 250–425 mg/dL or 44.8–76.1 μmol/L Newborn (0–4 d): 130–275 mg/dL or 1.30–2.75 g/L Child: 203–360 mg/dL or 2.03–3.60 g/L DRI: Adults: 10–15 mg/d	Assess for ingestion of iron pills or vitamin and mineral pills (toxicity). Populations at risk for deficiency are infants and children 0.5–4.0 yr, early adolescents, and women who are pregnant.	Excessive iron absorption in hereditary hemochromatosis (African or "Bantu" siderosis); prolonged therapeutic administration of iron to subjects not iron deficient; chronic alcoholism or liver disease; pancreatic insufficiency potential; "shunt hemochromatosis"; severe anemia with ineffective erythropoiesis and increased hemolysis; diabetes in 80% of patients Transfusional hemosiderosis, β-thalassemia major, some chronic sideroblastic anemias, hypoplastic or other refractory anemias *Other*: cancers (primary hepatic carcinoma, acute leukemia, early breast cancer), demyelinating disease, Alzheimer's disease, increased risk of congestive heart disease, listeriosis	Premature infants Intestinal helminthiasis (especially hookworm disease) Malabsorption syndromes, chronic diarrhea, gastrectomy, patients with atrophic gastritis and achlorhydria, occult gastrointestinal bleeding Hereditary hemorrhagic telangiectasia Turner's syndrome Angiodysplasia (vascular ectasis or arteriovenous anomaly) Blue rubber bleb nevi (hereditary cutaneous hemangiomas) Ménière's disease Zollinger-Ellison syndrome, pseudo-Zollinger-Ellison syndrome (hypersecretion of gastric hydrochloric acid [HCl]) Drugs (aspirin and ethanol), adrenocorticosteroids or nonsteroidal anti-inflammatory agents Sports anemia Paterson-Kelly (Plummer-Vinson) syndrome Factitious iron-deficiency anemia (Lasthénie de Ferjol syndrome—self-induced bloodletting) Poor dietary intake

table continues on pg. 1120 >

TABLE D.1, continued

Substance Tested (Specimen Needed), Reference Range (RR), and Critical Toxic Range (CR) and DRIs When Available	**Patient Preparation, Substance Function, and Indications for Test**	**Clinical Significance of Values**	
		Increased	Decreased
			Transferrin: severe protein-energy malnutrition Iron sequestration (idiopathic pulmonary hemosiderosis, paroxysmal nocturnal hemoglobinuria, chronic disease with inability to metabolize iron from reticuloendothelial cell deposits, congenital atransferrinemia [rare]) Vitamin A deficiency—lack in developmental periods causes deficits in neural functioning and behavior.
Lead (Pb)			
Blood, preferred specimen 2 mL, collect with oxalate–fluoride mixture Adult: RR: <25 μg/dL or <1.21 μmol/L (in most adults without occupational exposure) Child: RR: <10 μg/dL or <0.48 μmol/L CR: ≥ 100 μg/dL or ≥ 4.8 μmol/L in adults	Collect specimen in lead-free container and avoid airborne contaminants. For blood, use specifically manufactured tubes for blood lead collection. Ultratrace mineral; a metallic element—its compounds are poisonous, and any level of lead in blood is abnormal. Lead oxides are used in paint pigment; lead additives in gasoline provide air pollutants.	Children: irreversible cognitive deficits, acute encephalopathy Adults: progressive, irreversible renal disease; toxic psychosis from inhalation of tetraethyl or tetraethyllead Children and adults, hypochromic microcytic anemia	Depressed growth, altered iron metabolism

24-hr urine RR: <80 μg/L or <0.39 μmol/L Hair RR: <155 μg/g dry weight or <0.75 μmol/g dry weight CR: >200 μg/g dry weight	Earthenware made of clay rich in lead salts, lead in some insecticides Assess for environmental or occupational contaminants and toxic exposure.	*Lead sources*: ingested or inhaled leaded paint (renovation dust); contaminated soil; contaminated water (lead pipes, lead solder on copper pipes, softened water); retention of a lead object in the stomach or joint (shot, curtain weight, fishing weight, bauble); contaminated acidic foods and beverages (storage in lead-glazed ceramics, leaded crystal, galvanized or non–stainless steel pots); inhalation (burning lead-painted wood or battery casings in home fireplaces or stoves); leaded gas fumes; occupational exposure *Lethal dose*: 30 g/kg body weight	
Lithium (Li)			
Serum RR: 0.5–0.9 mg/dL or 0.7–1.3 mmol/L 24-hr urine 0.8 mg/24 hr or 115 μmol/d	Ultratrace mineral; a metallic element Lithium carbonate is used as drug to treat manic phase of manic-depressive illness. Decreased dietary sodium intake lowers the excretion rate of lithium. Assess psychotherapeutic drug monitoring.	Therapy for bipolar disorder Diabetes insipidus Renal failure, weight gain Diminished taste perception High "hard water" levels	High dietary caffeine and/or sodium intake
Manganese (Mn)			
Serum, fasting RR: 1.6–2.6 mg/dL or 0.66–1.07 mmol/L CR: >100 ng/mL 24-hr urine RR: 6.0–10.0 mEq/d or 3.0–5.0 mmol/d CR: Urine: >10 μg per specimen	Essential for lipid and carbohydrate metabolism, bone and tissue formation, and reproductive processes Assess for occupational exposure and evaluate certain diseases.	Chronic inhalation of airborne manganese (mines, steel mills, chemical industries) "Manganese madness," permanent crippling neurologic disorder of the extrapyramidal system (similar to lesions in Parkinson's disease) Increased urine levels in acute hepatitis, myocardial infarction, and rheumatoid arthritis Low tissue values in children with maple syrup urine disease and phenylketonuria	High in nonheme iron; certain types of epilepsy; impaired bone metabolism; weak bone in association with low concentrations of copper and zinc, possibly in alcohol abuse

table continues on pg. 1122 >

TABLE D.1, continued

Substance Tested (Specimen Needed), Reference Range (RR), and Critical Toxic Range (CR) and DRIs When Available	Patient Preparation, Substance Function, and Indications for Test	Clinical Significance of Values	
		Increased	Decreased
Mercury (Hg)			
24-hr urine RR: <20 μg/L or <0.10 mmol/L Whole blood—dark-blue–topped container, refrigerate RR: 0.6–59.0 μg/L or 3.0–294.4 mmol/L Toxic >150 μg/L or >0.75 mmol/L Lethal >800 μg/L or >4.0 mmol/L	Use acid-washed, leakproof container; keep specimen on ice. No metabolic role. Mercury is the only metal that is liquid at ordinary temperatures. Primarily absorbed by inhalation but can also be absorbed through the skin and gastrointestinal tract. It is then distributed to the central nervous system and kidneys and excreted in the urine. Evaluate for mercury toxicity, neurologic findings related to inorganic or organic mercurials, inhalation of mercury vapors. Assess for occupational exposure, toxicity, and poisoning from contaminated fish.	Mercury poisoning; occupational activities (smelters, miners, gilders, hatters, and factory workers), hobbies (painting, ceramics, target shooting), home renovation, auto repair Most common nonindustrial mercury poisoning is the consumption of methyl mercury–contaminated fish. Blood is recommended specimen for organic mercury, and urine is recommended specimen for inorganic mercury measurement. Iodine-containing drugs may cause false low levels. Organic mercury poisoning is more serious because it develops quickly. Inhalation of mercury vapors may lead to pneumonitis, cough, fever, and other pulmonary symptoms. Acute and chronic mercury poisoning affects kidneys, central nervous system, and gastrointestinal tract.	

Molybdenum (Mo)			
Serum RR: 0.1–3.0 μg/L or 1.0–31.3 nmol/L Whole blood RR: 0.8–3.3 μg/L or 8.3–34.4 nmol/L	A trace element, associated with inborn error of molybdenum metabolism Assess for genetic and dietary molybdenum deficiency.	Massive ingestion of tungsten (W) Occupational and high dietary intake (elevated uric acid blood concentration, gout) Sulfur amino acid toxicity Growth depression and anemia similar to copper deficiency	Sulfite oxidase deficiency (lethal inborn error of metabolism deranges cysteine metabolism) Prolonged total parenteral nutrition ("acquired molybdenum deficiency") Interference with copper metabolism
Nickel (Ni)			
Serum or plasma RR: 0.14–1.0 μg/L or 2.4–17.0 nmol/L 24-hr urine RR: 0.1–10 μg/d or 2–170 nmol/d	Ultratrace mineral; metallic element Nickel carbonyl is an industrial chemical used in plating metals—toxic when inhaled, causes pulmonary edema. Assess for occupational exposure.	Consistent in alcoholic liver disease Nickel dermatitis Inhalation of nickel carbonyl (promotes lung cancer)	Lack in diet, depressed iron absorption
Selenium (Se)			
Component of the enzyme glutathione peroxidase, isolated from human red blood cells Serum RR: 46–143 μg/L or 0.58–1.82 μmol/L DRI: Adults: 55 μg/d Hair RR: 0.12–1.4 μg/g dry weight or 2.5–17.8 nmol/g dry weight	A chemical element resembling sulfur, found in soil Has a role in the metabolism of enzymes As a sulfide, used in treating dandruff and tinea versicolor (i.e., Selsun Blue) Determine cause for loss of pigmentation of hair and skin.	Endemic selenosis Nail and hair loss Increased dietary intake owing to high soil concentrations (North Dakota, USA; Venezuela), excessive intake from "health store" tablets (skin lesions, polyneuritis) Hair and nail loss, changes in nail beds, inhibition of protein synthesis	Keshan disease (endemic cardiomyopathy) Kashin-Beck disease (endemic osteoarthritis) Parenteral nutrition Decreased dietary intake owing to low soil concentrations (New Zealand, China, Finland); aspermatogenesis Long-term total parenteral nutrition (cardiomyopathy)

table continues on pg. 1124 >

TABLE D.1, continued

Substance Tested (Specimen Needed), Reference Range (RR), and Critical Toxic Range (CR) and DRIs When Available	Patient Preparation, Substance Function, and Indications for Test	Clinical Significance of Values	
		Increased	Decreased
			Duchenne's muscular dystrophy, cataracts, tumor development Whitening of nail beds, loss of pigmentation of hair and skin, muscle pain and weakness
Silicon (Si)—silicic acid (H_2SiO_3) Plasma RR: 0.13–0.15 mg/L or 4.63–5.43 μmol/L 24-hr urine RR: 6.0–15.0 mg/d or 214–534 μmol/d	Ultratrace mineral; nonmetallic element in soil Occurs in traces in skeletal structures (bones and teeth) Necessary for the formation of collagen, bones, and connective tissue; healthy nails, skin, and hair; and calcium absorption in early stages of bone formation Needed to maintain flexible arteries and major role in cardiovascular disease Important in prevention of Alzheimer's disease and osteoporosis; inhibits aging process in tissues Evaluate renal stone etiology.	Long-term antacid therapy (magnesium trisilicate) Siliceous renal calculi	

Silver (Ag)		
Serum RR: 2.1 ± 1.5 μg/L, 19.5 ± 13.90 nmol/L Plasma RR: 0.68 ± 0.63 μg /L or 6.3 ± 5.8 nmol/L 24-hr urine <1 μg/d or <9.3 nmol/d	Collect in metal-free container. No metabolic role; salts used as antiseptic and bacteriostatic agents In normal individuals, silver slowly accumulates in body tissue with age but causes no apparent harm. Assess for occupational exposure or toxicity from medicinal uses of silver.	Chemical conjunctivitis from silver nitrate Gastroenteritis (dose by mouth), grayish discoloration of mucous membranes Argyria (bluish gray skin discoloration) from nose/eyedrops over time or industrial exposure Silvadene topically for burns Silver picrate (antiseptic) *Lethal dose*: 3.5–35 g total dose
Thallium (Tl)		
Blood RR: <0.5 μg/dL or <24.5 nmol/L CR: 10–800 μg/dL or 0.5–39.1 μmol/L 24-hr urine RR: <2 μg/L or 9.8 nmol/L CR: 1.0–20.0 μg/L or 4.9–97.8 μmol/L	Collect in metal-free container. No metabolic role Used in medications, cosmetics, and pesticides Poisoning occurs from ingestion or from absorption through intact skin and mucous membranes; accumulates in liver, kidneys, bone, and muscle tissue. Assess for toxicity from either accidental ingestion or exposure.	Formerly used in ant, rat, and roach poisons *Toxicity*: thallotoxicosis (ingestion of pesticides); vomiting, hair loss, delirium, coma, ataxia, pulmonary edema, paralysis, death Poisoning results in blindness, facial paralysis, paresthesias, peripheral neuropathy, liver and renal damage. *Lethal dose*: 5–50 mg
Tin (Sn)		
Serum RR: 0.40–0.64 μg/L or 3.4–5.4 nmol/L Whole blood RR: 140 μg/L or 1176 nmol/L	Collect in metal-free container. Ultratrace mineral; used in manufacturing of alloys, plating, food containers Assess for industrial exposure.	Diet high in canned fruits/juices Zinc balance negatively affected at 50-mg intake; industrial exposure to organic tin compounds and dust Tin salts used in calico printing Organic compounds found in polyvinyl plastics, chlorinated rubber paints, fungicides, insecticides, and anthelmintics

table continues on pg. 1126 >

TABLE D.1, continued

Substance Tested (Specimen Needed), Reference Range (RR), and Critical Toxic Range (CR) and DRIs When Available	Patient Preparation, Substance Function, and Indications for Test	Clinical Significance of Values	
		Increased	Decreased
Vanadium (V)			
Serum RR: 0.01–0.23 μg/L or 0.20–4.51 nmol/L Blood RR: 0.06–0.87 μg/L or 1.2–17.1 nmol/L Hair RR: 0.10–0.16 μg/g dry weight or 1.96–3.14 nmol/g dry weight Urine RR: <0.24 μg/L or <4.7 nmol/L	Collect in metal-free container. Ultratrace mineral Used in the steel industry and to a lesser degree in photography and in the manufacturing of insecticides, dyes, inks, paints, and varnish Assess for occupational exposure.	Occupational inhalation (fuel combustion for electricity), hemorrhagic endotheliotoxin with leukocytotactic and hematotoxic components *Toxicity*: industrial processes (sore eyes and bronchi), dermatitis, depletion of ascorbic acid, gastrointestinal distress, cardiac palpitation, kidney damage, central nervous system disturbances, green tongue, and disturbances of mental function	
Zinc (Zn)			
Serum RR: 70–120 μg/dL or 10.7–18.4 μmol/L 24-hr urine RR: 150–1,200 μg/d or 2.3–18.4 μmol/d	Fasting morning specimen Plays a role in protein synthesis; critical for growth and sexual maturation Important in wound healing and sensory perception (particularly taste and smell) Important in activating certain serum enzymes and in insulin and porphyrin metabolism	Zinc therapy for Wilson's disease Ingestion of food or beverage contaminated by storage in a galvanized container Long-term ingestion of excessive zinc supplements >150 mg/d (secondary copper deficiency) Low serum high-density lipoprotein Gastric erosion	Decreased intake (chronic alcoholics, vegetarians, young women with anorexia nervosa), diarrhea Decreased circulatory and splenic T lymphocytes Prolonged bed rest

	Assess population that may have increased needs for intake—alcoholism, chronic illness, stress, trauma, surgery, malabsorption, lactovegetarians, children consuming vegetarian diets, decubitus ulcers, anorexics.	Depressed immune system Lethargy in dialysis patients Hyperzincuria increasing with the severity of diabetes Inhalation of zinc oxide fumes causing neurologic damage (metal fume fever, brass-founders' ague, zinc shakes), metallic taste, bloody diarrhea	Decrease in absorption of tetracycline Rheumatic diseases Infection Growth retardation Male hypogonadism and hypospermism Nyctalopia (night blindness) Hypogeusia (blunting of sense of taste) Impaired wound healing, long-term total parenteral nutrition without zinc supplement Chronic liver disease Acrodermatitis enteropathica (dermatitis of the extremities seen in children between 3 wk and 18 mo) Dwarfism Parasitism (Egypt) Compromised immune function Low facteur thymique serique (FTS) (thymulin, hormone secreted by the thymus) Impaired embryogenesis Behavioral disturbances (impaired hedonic tone) Skeletal abnormalities, defective collagen synthesis, alopecia, impaired protein synthesis Some cancers

DRIs, Dietary Reference Intakes.

E Effects of Drugs on Laboratory Tests (Blood, Whole Plasma, Serum, Stool, and Urine)

DRUGS AND LABORATORY TEST OUTCOMES

Many prescription medications, over-the-counter medications, vitamins, minerals, and herbal preparations can influence the results of laboratory tests. Mechanisms of drug effects are either pharmacologic (e.g., furosemide usually increases the excretion of potassium, resulting in a low serum potassium level) or analytic (e.g., when a drug in a patient's body fluid or tissue interferes with a chemical step in a laboratory test, resulting in an erroneous test result). The drug classes that cause the majority of analytical interferences include antibiotics, antihypertensives, anticonvulsants, hormones, and antidepressants.

Accurate and complete medication histories, including prescription medications, over-the-counter medications, vitamins, minerals, and herbal preparations, are essential to interpret laboratory test results that fall out of the normal range.

Table E.1 is not an exhaustive list, and whenever laboratory results are suspected of being spurious, further research is necessary. There are many references available, including drug monographs in *American Hospital Formulary Service* (AHFS), *Drug Information* (published by the American Society of Health-System Pharmacists), drug package inserts, and the *Physician's Desk Reference* (PDR), which contains official product information. Services that maintain this information include the Iowa Drug Information Service (IDIS) and DRUGDEX.

Discoloration of Feces Caused by Drugs

1. **Black**—acetazolamide, aluminum hydroxide, aminophylline, 5-aminosalicylic acid, amphetamine, amphotericin B, antacids, anticoagulants, aspirin, betamethasone, bismuth, charcoal, chloramphenicol, chlorpropamide, clindamycin, corticosteroids, cortisone, cyclophosphamide, cytarabine, digitalis, ethacrynic acid, ferrous salts, floxuridine, fluorides, fluorouracil, halothane, heparin, hydralazine, hydrocortisone, ibuprofen, indomethacin, iodine, levarterenol, levodopa, manganese, melphalan, methotrexate, methylene blue, methylprednisolone, paraldehyde, phenolphthalein, phosphorus, potassium salts, prednisolone, procarbazine, reserpine, salicylates, sulfonamides, tetracycline, theophylline, thiotepa, triamcinolone, warfarin
2. **Gray**—colchicine
3. **Green**—indomethacin, iron, medroxyprogesterone
4. **Dark brown**—dexamethasone
5. **Blue**—chloramphenicol, methylene blue
6. **Pink**—anticoagulants, aspirin, salicylates
7. **Red**—anticoagulants, aspirin, phenolphthalein, salicylates, tetracycline
8. **Orange**—phenazopyridine, rifampin
9. **Tarry**—warfarin, ergot preparations, ibuprofen, salicylates
10. **White/speckling**—aluminum hydroxide, indocyanine green
11. **Yellow**—senna

Discoloration of Urine Caused by Drugs

1. **Black**—cascara, co-trimoxazole, ferrous salts, levodopa, methocarbamol, methyldopa, naphthalene, quinine, sulfonamides
2. **Dark**—cascara, levodopa, metronidazole, primaquine, quinine, senna
3. **Brown**—cascara, chloroquine, levodopa, methocarbamol, methyldopa, metronidazole, nitrofurantoin, primaquine, quinine, rifampin, senna, sulfonamides
4. **Blue**—indigo blue, methylene blue, mitoxantrone, nitrofurantoin, triamterene
5. **Blue/green**—amitriptyline, Doan's pills, indigo blue, indomethacin, magnesium salicylate, methylene blue, propofol
6. **Orange**—chlorzoxazone, dihydroergotamine, heparin, phenazopyridine, rifampin, sulfasalazine, warfarin
7. **Pink**—anthraquinone dyes, aspirin, cascara, deferoxamine, methyldopa, phenytoin, salicylates, senna, phenothiazines
8. **Purple**—phenolphthalein
9. **Red**—cascara, chlorpromazine, daunorubicin, deferoxamine, dihydroergotamine, dimethylsulfoxide, doxorubicin, heparin, ibuprofen, methyldopa, phenazopyridine, phenolphthalein, phenothiazines, phenytoin, rifampin, senna
10. **Red-purple**—chlorzoxazone, ibuprofen, senna

BIBLIOGRAPHY

American Society of Health-System Pharmacists: AHFS Drug Information, Bethesda, MD, American Society of Health-System Pharmacists, 2017

Drug Facts and Comparisons 2017. Philadelphia, Wolters Kluwer, 2017

Drug Information Handbook: A clinically relevant resource for all healthcare professionals, 25th ed. Hudson, OH, Lexicomp, 2016

Lee M (ed): Basic Skills in Interpreting Laboratory Data, 5th ed. Bethesda, MD, American Society of Health System Pharmacists, 2013

Roach SS, Ford SM: Introductory Clinical Pharmacology, 10th ed. Philadelphia, Lippincott Williams & Wilkins, 2013

Young DS: Effects of Drugs on Clinical Laboratory Tests, 5th ed. Washington, DC, AACC Press, 2000

TABLE E.1 Effects of the Most Commonly Used Drugs on Frequently Ordered Laboratory Tests

Test	Increased Can Lead to a False-Positive Value Decreased Can Lead to a False-Negative Value
Acid Phosphatase (Serum)	**Increased by:** *p*-aminosalicylic acid **Decreased by:** clofibrate, mirtazapine
Alanine Aminotransferase (Serum)	**Increased by:** abacavir, acarbose, acebutolol, acetaminophen, acetohexamide, acyclovir, adefovir, albendazole, aldesleukin, allopurinol, alprazolam, aminoglutethimide, aminosalicylic acid, amiodarone, amitriptyline, amoxapine, amphotericin B, ampicillin, anabolic steroids, anastrazole, anticonvulsants, antifungal agents, aprepitant, ardeparin, aripiprazole, arsenic trioxide, asparaginase, aspirin, atomoxetine, atorvastatin, atovaquone, auranofin, azathioprine, azithromycin, aztreonam, barbiturates, barium, bacillus Calmette-Guérin (BCG) vaccine, benazepril, bepridil, betaxolol, bicalutamide, bismuth subsalicylate, bisoprolol, bromocriptine, bupropion, busulfan, calcitriol, candesartan, capecitabine, carbenicillin, carmustine, cephalosporin antibiotics, cetirizine, chloral hydrate, chlorambucil, chloramphenicol, chlordiazepoxide, chlorothiazide, chlorpheniramine, chlorpromazine, chlorpropamide, chlorthalidone, chlorzoxazone, cholestyramine, choline magnesium trisalicylate, cidofovir, cimetidine, cinoxacin, ciprofloxacin, cladribine, clarithromycin, clindamycin, clofarabine, clofazimine, clofibrate, clomiphene, clomipramine, clonidine, clopidogrel, clorazepate, cloxacillin, clozapine, colchicine, colestipol, conjugated estrogens, cortisone, cyclobenzaprine, cyclophosphamide, cyproheptadine, cytarabine, dacarbazine, dactinomycin, dalteparin, danazol, dantrolene, dapsone, demeclocycline, desipramine, desmopressin, diazepam, diazoxide, diclofenac, didanosine, diflunisal, diltiazem, disopyramide, disulfiram, docetaxel, doxorubicin, doxycycline, dronabinol, eletriptan, enalapril, enoxacin, enoxaparin, eplerenone, erlotinib, erythromycin, esterified estrogens, estropipate, ethacrynic acid, ethambutol, ethchlorvynol, ether, etodolac, etoposide, famotidine, felbamate, fenofibrate, fenoprofen, flecainide, fluconazole, flucytosine, fluorouracil, fluoxymesterone, fluphenazine, flurazepam, flutamide, fluvastatin, fluvoxamine, foscarnet, fosinopril, fosphenytoin, furosemide, gamma-globulin, ganciclovir, garlic, gemcitabine, gemfibrozil, gentamicin, glimepiride, glyburide, glycopyrrolate, gold, goserelin, granisetron, griseofulvin, guanethidine, haloperidol, heparin, hepatitis A vaccine, hepatitis B vaccine, hydralazine, hydrochlorothiazide, ibuprofen, idarubicin, ifosfamide, imipenem/cilastin, imipramine, indinavir, indomethacin, infliximab, interferon, interleukin, iron, isoniazid, isosorbide dinitrate, isotretinoin, isradipine, itraconazole, kanamycin, ketamine, ketoconazole, ketoprofen, ketorolac, labetalol, lamotrigine, lansoprazole, leflunomide, levodopa, levothyroxine, lincomycin, lisinopril, lomefloxacin, loracarbef, loratadine, losartan, lovastatin, low-molecular-weight (LMW) heparins, loxapine, maprotiline, mechlorethamine, meclofenamate, medroxyprogesterone, mefenamic acid, mefloquine, melphalan, meperidine,

table continues on pg. 1131 >

TABLE E.1, continued

Test	Increased Can Lead to a False-Positive Value Decreased Can Lead to a False-Negative Value
	meprobamate, mercaptopurine, meropenem, mesalamine, metaxalone, methenamine, methimazole, methotrexate, methoxsalen, methyldopa, methylphenidate, methyltestosterone, metoclopramide, metolazone, metoprolol, mexiletine, minocycline, mirtazapine, mitomycin, mitoxantrone, moexipril, molindone, monoamine oxidase (MAO) inhibitors, montelukast, moricizine, morphine, muromonab-CD3, mycophenolate, nabumetone, nafarelin, nafcillin, nalidixic acid, naltrexone, nandrolone, naproxen, nelfinavir, netilmicin, nevirapine, niacin, niacinamide, nicardipine, nifedipine, nilutamide, nisoldipine, nitazoxanide, nitisinone, nitrofurantoin, nizatidine, norethandrolone, norfloxacin, nortriptyline, octreotide, ofloxacin, olmesartan, olsalazine, omeprazole, ondansetron, oral contraceptives, oxacillin, oxaprozin, oxazepam, oxymetholone, palivizumab, palonosetron, papaverine, paroxetine, pegaspargase, pegvisomant, penicillamine, pentamidine, pentoxifylline, perphenazine, phenazopyridine, phenelzine, phenobarbital, phenothiazines, phenytoin, phosphorus, pindolol, pioglitazone, piperacillin, piroxicam, pravastatin, prazosin, probenecid, procainamide, prochlorperazine, propafenone, propranolol, propylthiouracil, pyrazinamide, pyrimethamine, quazepam, quinapril, quinidine, ramipril, ranitidine, rifampin, riluzole, risperidone, ritonavir, rosiglitazone, saquinavir, sargramostim, sildenafil, simvastatin, sodium oxybate, sparfloxacin, spectinomycin, stanozolol, stavudine, streptokinase, streptomycin, streptozocin, sulfadiazine, sulfamethoxazole, sulfanilamide, sulfasalazine, sulfisoxazole, sulfonylureas, sulindac, sumatriptan, tacrine, tacrolimus, tadalafil, tamoxifen, terbinafine, terbutaline, tetracycline, thiabendazole, thiazides, thioguanine, thiopental, thioridazine, thiothixene, thiouracil, ticarcillin, ticlopidine, timolol, tinzaparin, tobramycin, tocainide, tolazamide, tolazoline, tolbutamide, tolmetin, topotecan, tramadol, trandolapril, tranylcypromine, trastuzumab, tretinoin, triazolam, trichlormethiazide, trifluoperazine, trimethoprim, trimetrexate, trimipramine, triptorelin, troleandomycin, uracil mustard, ursodiol, valproic acid, valsartan, venlafaxine, verapamil, vidarabine, vitamin A, vitamin C, warfarin, zalcitabine, zidovudine, zileuton, zolmitriptan, zolpidem **Decreased by:** aspirin, carvedilol, cyclosporine, interferon, ketoprofen, phenothiazines, simvastatin, toremifene, ursodiol
Albumin (Urine)	**Increased by:** amikacin, basiliximab, calcitriol, carbamazepine, carvedilol, cisplatin, diazoxide, doxorubicin, eplerenone, gentamicin, lansoprazole, lithium, mesalamine, mycophenolate, nabumetone, naproxen, nifedipine, norfloxacin, ofloxacin, oral contraceptives, pregabalin, radiographic agents, sevoflurane, sodium oxybate, triazolam, venlafaxine, verapamil, zalcitabine **Decreased by:** atenolol, captopril, cilostazol, dipyridamole, enalapril, fosinopril, furosemide, ibuprofen, indapamide, perindopril, quinapril, ramipril

table continues on pg. 1132 >

TABLE E.1, continued

Test	Increased Can Lead to a False-Positive Value Decreased Can Lead to a False-Negative Value
Aldolase (Serum)	**Increased by:** corticotropin, diclofenac, itraconazole, lovastatin, niacin, quinidine (intramuscular [IM] injection), simvastatin, thiabendazole, vasopressin **Decreased by:** probucol
Aldosterone (Plasma)	**Increased by:** amiloride, ammonium chloride, chlorthalidone, corticotropin, dobutamine, fenoldopam, fosinopril, furosemide, hydralazine, hydrochlorothiazide, indomethacin, laxatives, metoclopramide, nifedipine, opiates, pravastatin, spironolactone, triamterene, verapamil **Decreased by:** atenolol, candesartan, captopril, carvedilol, clonidine, cyclosporine, dexamethasone, enalapril, ergoloid mesylates, etomidate, finasteride, fosinopril, furosemide, indomethacin, ketoconazole, lisinopril, LMW heparins, losartan, nicardipine, nifedipine, nisoldipine, nonsteroidal anti-inflammatory drugs, perindopril, ramipril, ranitidine, verapamil
Alkaline Phosphatase (Serum)	**Increased by:** acebutolol, acetaminophen, acetohexamide, acyclovir, albumin, albendazole, aldesleukin, allopurinol, alprazolam, altretamine, aluminum hydroxide, amantadine, aminoglutethimide, aminoglycosides, aminosalicylic acid, amiodarone, amitriptyline, amoxapine, amphotericin B, amrinone, anabolic steroids, anastrazole, anticonvulsants, antifungal agents, arsenicals, asparaginase, aspirin, atovaquone, auranofin, azathioprine, azithromycin, aztreonam, baclofen, barbiturates, BCG vaccine, bicalutamide, bismuth subsalicylate, bleomycin, bromocriptine, budesonide, bumetanide, bupropion, busulfan, candesartan, capecitabine, capreomycin, captopril, carbamazepine, carbenicillin, carmustine, carvedilol, cephalosporin antibiotics, cetirizine, chloramphenicol, chlordiazepoxide, chloroform, chlorothiazide, chlorpromazine, chlorpropamide, chlorzoxazone, cidofovir, cimetidine, ciprofloxacin, clindamycin, clofibrate, clonidine, clorazepate, clozapine, cocaine, colchicine, colestipol, conjugated estrogens, cyclobenzaprine, cyclophosphamide, cycloserine, cyclosporine, cyproheptadine, cytarabine, dactinomycin, danazol, dantrolene, dapsone, daunorubicin, demeclocycline, desipramine, diazepam, diazoxide, diclofenac, didanosine, diltiazem, disopyramide, disulfiram, docetaxel, doxorubicin, doxycycline, enalapril, eplerenone, erythromycin, estrogens, estropipate, ethacrynic acid, ethambutol, ether, ethionamide, etoposide, factor IX complex, famotidine, felodipine, fenoprofen, filgrastim, flecainide, fluconazole, flucytosine, fluorouracil, fluoxymesterone, fluphenazine, flurazepam, flutamide, fluvastatin, foscarnet, fosphenytoin, furosemide, ganciclovir, gemcitabine, gemfibrozil, gentamicin, glimepiride, glyburide, glycopyrrolate, gold, granulocyte colony-stimulating factor (GCSF), griseofulvin, haloperidol, hepatitis A vaccine, hepatitis B vaccine, human growth hormone, hydralazine, ibandronate, ibuprofen, idarubicin, ifosfamide, imipenem/cilastin, imipramine, indomethacin, insulin, interferon, interleukin, irinotecan, isoniazid, isotretinoin, isradipine, itraconazole,

table continues on pg. 1133 >

TABLE E.1, continued

Test	Increased Can Lead to a False-Positive Value Decreased Can Lead to a False-Negative Value
	itraconazole, kanamycin, ketamine, ketoconazole, ketoprofen, ketorolac, labetalol, lamotrigine, lansoprazole, leflunomide, levodopa, levothyroxine, lincomycin, lisinopril, lithium, lomefloxacin, loracarbef, loratadine, lovastatin, MAO inhibitors, mechlorethamine, meclofenamate, medroxyprogesterone, melphalan, meprobamate, mercaptopurine, meropenem, mesalamine, metaxalone, methimazole, methotrexate, methoxsalen, methyldopa, methyltestosterone, metoclopramide, metolazone, metoprolol, minocycline, mirtazapine, misoprostol, mitoxantrone, moexipril, molindone, morphine, moxalactam, mycophenolate, nabumetone, nafarelin, nalidixic acid, nandrolone, naproxen, nelfinavir, netilmicin, niacin, niacinamide, nicardipine, nifedipine, nilutamide, nitrofurantoin, nizatidine, norethindrone, norfloxacin, nortriptyline, octreotide, ofloxacin, oleandomycin, olsalazine, omeprazole, oral contraceptives, oral hypoglycemics, oxacillin, oxaprozin, oxazepam, oxymetholone, papaverine, pargyline, paroxetine, pegaspargase, penicillamine, perphenazine, phenazopyridine, phenobarbital, phenothiazines, phenytoin, phosphorus, pindolol, piperacillin, piroxicam, plicamycin, polythiazide, procainamide, prochlorperazine, progesterone, promazine, promethazine, propafenone, propylthiouracil, protriptyline, pyrazinamide, pyrimethamine, quazepam, quinapril, quinidine, ramipril, ranitidine, rifampin, riluzole, risperidone, sargramostim, sildenafil, spectinomycin, stanozolol, streptokinase, sulfadiazine, sulfamethoxazole, sulfanilamide, sulfasalazine, sulfisoxazole, sulfonylureas, sulindac, tacrolimus, tamoxifen, terbinafine, tetracycline, thiabendazole, thiazides, thiethylperazine, thioguanine, thiopental, thioridazine, thiothixene, thiouracil, ticarcillin, ticlopidine, timolol, tocainide, tolazamide, tolazoline, tolbutamide, tolmetin, topotecan, toremifene, tramadol, trastuzumab, tretinoin, triazolam, trichlormethiazide, trifluoperazine, trimethoprim, trimetrexate, trimipramine, troleandomycin, uracil mustard, ursodiol, valproic acid, venlafaxine, verapamil, vidarabine, vitamin D, warfarin, zalcitabine, zidovudine, zolmitriptan, zolpidem **Decreased by:** acyclovir, alendronate, aluminum antacids, arsenicals, azathioprine, calcitonin, calcitriol, carvedilol, clofibrate, colchicine, cyclosporine, danazol, estrogens, etidronate, norethindrone, oral contraceptives, pamidronate, penicillamine, prednisolone, prednisone, tamoxifen, trifluoperazine, ursodiol, vitamin D
Amino Acids (Total/Fractions) (Urine)	**Increased by:** acetaminophen, amikacin, aminocaproic acid, amphetamine, ampicillin, aspirin, bismuth subsalicylate, brompheniramine, carbenicillin, cefaclor, cefadroxil, cephalexin, cephradine, cisplatin, cytarabine, doxorubicin, ephedrine, erythromycin, gentamicin, hydrocortisone, ifosfamide, Isomil (Similac), insulin, kanamycin, levarterenol, levodopa, mafenide, methamphetamine, methyldopa, neomycin, nystatin, penicillamine, parathyroid extract, phenobarbital, phenylephrine, primidone, ProSobee (Enfamil), pseudoephedrine, streptozocin, tetracycline, triamcinolone, tromethamine **Decreased by:** insulin

table continues on pg. 1134 >

TABLE E.1, continued

Test	Increased Can Lead to a False-Positive Value Decreased Can Lead to a False-Negative Value
Ammonia (Plasma)	**Increased by:** acetazolamide, asparaginase, chlorothiazide, chlorthalidone, ethacrynic acid, felbamate, furosemide, hydroflumethiazide, ion exchange resins, isoniazid, pegaspargase, tetracycline, thiazides, valproic acid **Decreased by:** cefotaxime, diphenhydramine, kanamycin, *Lactobacillus acidophilus*, levodopa, MAO inhibitors, neomycin, tetracycline, tromethamine
Amylase (Serum)	**Increased by:** acetaminophen, aminosalicylic acid, amoxapine, amphotericin B, asparaginase, aspirin, atazanavir, atovaquone, azathioprine, azithromycin, benzthiazide, bethanechol, calcitriol, chloride salts, chlorothiazide, chlorthalidone, cholinergics, cidofovir, cimetidine, cisplatin, clozapine, codeine, conjugated estrogens, corticosteroids, cyclosporin A, cyproheptadine, cytarabine, demeclocycline, desipramine, dexamethasone, diazoxide, didanosine, donepezil, doxorubicin, enalapril, enfuvirtide, estropipate, ethacrynic acid, felbamate, fentanyl, fludrocortisone, fluvastatin, foscarnet, furosemide, glucocorticoids, hetastarch, human growth hormone, hydrochlorothiazide, hydroflumethiazide, ibuprofen, indinavir, indomethacin, isoniazid, lamivudine, lisinopril, meperidine, mercaptopurine, mesalamine, methacholine, methyclothiazide, methylprednisolone, metolazone, metronidazole, minocycline, mirtazapine, morphine, nabumetone, naproxen, narcotics, nelfinavir, niacin, nitrofurantoin, norfloxacin, octreotide, opium alkaloids, oral contraceptives, palifermin, pegaspargase, penicillamine, piroxicam, polythiazide, potassium iodide, prazosin, prednisolone, prednisone, quinapril, radiographic agents, simvastatin, sulfamethoxazole, sulindac, tamoxifen, tetracycline, thiazides, trastuzumab, tretinoin, triamcinolone, trichlormethiazide, valproic acid, zalcitabine, zidovudine, zolmitriptan **Decreased by:** anabolic steroids, cefotaxime, lamivudine, propylthiouracil, somatostatin, zidovudine
Angiotensin-Converting Enzyme (Serum)	**Increased by:** nicardipine, triiodothyronine **Decreased by:** benazepril, captopril, cilazapril, enalapril, fosinopril, lisinopril, magnesium sulfate, methylprednisolone, nicardipine, perindopril, prednisolone, prednisone, propranolol, quinapril, ramipril, trandolapril
Antidiuretic Hormone (Plasma)	**Increased by:** chlorthalidone, cisplatin, ether, furosemide, hydrochlorothiazide, lithium methyclothiazide, polythiazide **Decreased by:** chlorpromazine, clonidine, guanfacine
Antinuclear Antibody Test (ANA) (Serum)	**Increased by:** acebutolol, amitriptyline, anticonvulsants, bisoprolol, captopril, chlorpromazine, etanercept, ethosuximide, fluvastatin, gemfibrozil, hydralazine, interferon alfa-2a, isoniazid, labetalol, methyldopa, mexiletine, nitrofurantoin, oral contraceptives, penicillamine, phenytoin, piroxicam, procainamide, propafenone, propylthiouracil, quinidine, rosuvastatin, sodium oxalate, sulfasalazine, tocainide, valproic acid

table continues on pg. 1135 >

TABLE E.1, continued

Test	Increased Can Lead to a False-Positive Value Decreased Can Lead to a False-Negative Value
Aspartate Aminotransaminase or Aspartate Aminotransferase (AST) (Serum)	**Increased by:** abecarnil, acarbose, acebutolol, acetaminophen, acetohexamide, acetylcysteine, acyclovir, adefovir, albendazole, aldesleukin, allopurinol, alprazolam, amantadine, aminocaproic acid, aminoglutethimide, aminosalicylic acid, amiodarone, amitriptyline, amoxapine, amoxicillin, amphotericin, ampicillin, anabolic steroids, anastrazole, anticonvulsants, antifungals, aprepitant, ardeparin, aripiprazole, arsenicals, ascorbic acid, asparaginase, aspirin, atomoxetine, atorvastatin, atovaquone, auranofin, azathioprine, azithromycin, aztreonam, baclofen, barbiturates, barium, BCG vaccine, benazepril, bepridil, betaxolol, bethanechol, bicalutamide, bismuth subsalicylate, bisoprolol, bleomycin, bupropion, busulfan, calcitriol, candesartan, canola oil, capreomycin, captopril, carbamazepine, carbenicillin, carmustine, carvedilol, cetuximab, cephalosporin antibiotics, cetirizine, chloral hydrate, chlorambucil, chloramphenicol, chlordiazepoxide, chloroform, chlorothiazide, chlorpheniramine, chlorpromazine, chlorpropamide, chlorthalidone, chlorzoxazone, cholestyramine, choline magnesium trisalicylate, cholinergics, cidofovir, cimetidine, ciprofloxacin, cisplatin, cladribine, clarithromycin, clindamycin, clofarabine, clofazimine, clofibrate, clomiphene, clomipramine, clonidine, clopidogrel, clorazepate, clotrimazole, clozapine, codeine, colchicine, colestipol, conjugated estrogens, cortisone, cyclobenzaprine, cyclophosphamide, cycloserine, cyclosporine, cyproheptadine, cytarabine, dacarbazine, dactinomycin, dalteparin, danazol, dantrolene, dapsone, demeclocycline, desipramine, desmopressin, diazepam, diazoxide, diclofenac, dicloxacillin, didanosine, diflunisal, diltiazem, disopyramide, disulfiram, docetaxel, doxorubicin, doxycycline, dronabinol, eletriptan, enalapril, enoxaparin, epirubicin, eplerenone, erlotinib, erythromycin, estazolam, esterified estrogens, estropipate, ethacrynic acid, ethambutol, ethchlorvynol, ether, ethionamide, ethosuximide, ethyl chloride, etodolac, etoposide, factor IX, famotidine, felbamate, fenofibrate, fenoprofen, flecainide, fluconazole, flucytosine, fluoxymesterone, fluphenazine, flurazepam, flutamide, fluvastatin, fluvoxamine, foscarnet, fosinopril, fosphenytoin, furazolidone, furosemide, ganciclovir, gemcitabine, gemfibrozil, gemtuzumab, gentamicin, glimepiride, glutamine, glyburide, glycopyrrolate, gold, goserelin, granisetron, griseofulvin, guanethidine, haloperidol, halothane, heparin, hepatitis A vaccine, hepatitis B vaccine, hydralazine, hydrochlorothiazide, ibuprofen, idarubicin, ifosfamide, imatinib, imipenem/cilastin, imipramine, indinavir, indomethacin, infliximab, interferon, interleukin, irinotecan, iron, isoniazid, isoproterenol, isosorbide dinitrate, isotretinoin, isradipine, itraconazole, kanamycin, ketamine, ketoconazole, ketoprofen, ketorolac, labetalol, lamivudine, lamotrigine, lansoprazole, leflunomide, lepirudin, levodopa, levothyroxine,

table continues on pg. 1136 >

TABLE E.1, continued

Test	Increased Can Lead to a False-Positive Value Decreased Can Lead to a False-Negative Value
	lincomycin, lisinopril, LMW heparins, lomefloxacin, loracarbef, losartan, lovastatin, loxapine, MAO inhibitors, maprotiline, mechlorethamine, medroxyprogesterone, mefenamic acid, mefloquine, melphalan, meperidine, meprobamate, mercaptopurine, meropenem, mesalamine, mesoridazine, metaxalone, methacholine, methenamine, methimazole, methotrexate, methoxsalen, methyldopa, methylphenidate, methyltestosterone, metoclopramide, metolazone, metoprolol, mexiletine, milk thistle, minocycline, mirtazapine, mitomycin, mitoxantrone, moexipril, molindone, montelukast, moricizine, morphine, moxalactam, muromonab-CD3, mycophenolate, nabumetone, nafarelin, nafcillin, nalidixic acid, naltrexone, nandrolone, naproxen, narcotics, nelfinavir, netilmicin, nevirapine, niacin, niacinamide, nicardipine, nicotinic acid, nifedipine, nilutamide, nisoldipine, nitisinone, nitrofurantoin, nizatidine, norfloxacin, nortriptyline, octreotide, ofloxacin, oleandomycin, olmesartan, omeprazole, ondansetron, opium alkaloids, oral contraceptives, oxacillin, oxaprozin, oxazepam, oxymetholone, palonosetron, papaverine, pargyline, paroxetine, pegaspargase, pegvisomant, penicillamine, penicillin, pentamidine, pentoxifylline, perphenazine, phenazopyridine, phenelzine, phenobarbital, phenothiazines, phenytoin, phosphorus, pindolol, pioglitazone, piperacillin, piroxicam, plicamycin, polythiazide, pralidoxime, pravastatin, prazosin, probenecid, procainamide, prochlorperazine, progesterone, promazine, promethazine, propafenone, propranolol, propylthiouracil, protriptyline, pyrazinamide, quazepam, quinapril, quinidine, quinolones, ramipril, ranitidine, rifampin, riluzole, risperidone, ritonavir, rosiglitazone, salicylate, saquinavir, sildenafil, simvastatin, sirolimus, sodium oxybate, sparfloxacin, stanozolol, stavudine, streptokinase, streptomycin, streptozocin, sulfadiazine, sulfamethoxazole, sulfanilamide, sulfasalazine, sulfisoxazole, sulfonylureas, sulindac, sumatriptan, tacrine, tacrolimus, tadalafil, tamoxifen, telithromycin, terbinafine, terbutaline, tetracycline, thiabendazole, thiazides, thiethylperazine, thioguanine, thiopental, thioridazine, thiothixene, ticarcillin, ticlopidine, timolol, tinzaparin, tobramycin, tocainide, tolazamide, tolazoline, tolbutamide, tolmetin, topotecan, toremifene, tramadol, tranylcypromine, trastuzumab, tretinoin, triazolam, trichlormethiazide, trifluoperazine, trimethoprim, trimetrexate, trimipramine, triptorelin, troleandomycin, uracil mustard, ursodiol, valproic acid, valsartan, vasopressin, venlafaxine, verapamil, vidarabine, vincristine, vinorelbine, vitamin A, vitamin C, warfarin, zalcitabine, zidovudine, zileuton, zolmitriptan, zolpidem **Decreased by:** allopurinol, ascorbic acid, cyclosporine, eletriptan, ibuprofen, ketoprofen, metronidazole, naltrexone, pindolol, prednisone, progesterone, rifampin, simvastatin, toremifene, trifluoperazine, ursodiol

table continues on pg. 1137 >

TABLE E.1, continued

Test	Increased Can Lead to a False-Positive Value Decreased Can Lead to a False-Negative Value
Apolipoprotein A (Serum)	**Increased by:** carbamazepine, furosemide, gemfibrozil, nisoldipine, oral contraceptives, phenobarbital, phenytoin, prednisolone **Decreased by:** lovastatin
Apolipoprotein B (Serum)	**Increased by:** amiodarone, atenolol, chlorthalidone, conjugated estrogens, cyclosporine, estrogen/progestin therapy, furosemide, gemfibrozil, isotretinoin, levonorgestrel, methyclothiazide, metoprolol, oral contraceptives, phenobarbital, radioactive iodine, simvastatin, stanozolol **Decreased by:** atorvastatin, bisoprolol, captopril, cholestyramine, colestipol, conjugated estrogens, doxazosin, fenofibrate, gemfibrozil, indomethacin, interferon alfa-2a, interferon beta-1b, ketoconazole, levothyroxine, lisinopril, LMW heparins, losartan, lovastatin, neomycin, niacin, nicotinic acid, nifedipine, phenytoin, pravastatin, prazosin, prednisolone, probucol, psyllium, raloxifene, simvastatin, tacrolimus
Atrial Natriuretic Peptide (Plasma)	**Increased by:** atenolol, captopril, carteolol, cyclosporine, dipyridamole, doxorubicin, morphine, nifedipine, oral contraceptives, vasopressin, verapamil **Decreased by:** benazepril, chlorthalidone, clonidine, erythropoietin, methimazole, prazosin, ramipril
Basophils	**Increased by:** desipramine, paroxetine, tretinoin, triazolam, venlafaxine **Decreased by:** procainamide, thiopental
Bilirubin (Serum)	**Increased by:** acarbose, acebutolol, acetaminophen, acetazolamide, acetohexamide, acyclovir, albendazole, aldesleukin, allopurinol, alprazolam, amiloride, aminoglutethimide, amiodarone, amitriptyline, amoxapine, amphotericin, amrinone, amyl nitrate, anabolic steroids, antifungal agents, antimalarials, antipyretics, ascorbic acid, asparaginase, aspirin, atazanavir, atomoxetine, atorvastatin, auranofin, azathioprine, azithromycin, barbiturates, BCG vaccine, benazepril, bevacizumab, bicalutamide, bismuth subsalicylate, bleomycin, bortezomib, bupropion, busulfan, candesartan, captopril, carbamazepine, carmustine, carvedilol, cefazolin, cefdinir, cefoperazone, cefoxitin, cefpodoxime, ceftazidime, ceftibuten, ceftizoxime, ceftriaxone, cefuroxime, cephalothin, cetirizine, chloral hydrate, chlorambucil, chloramphenicol, chlordiazepoxide, chloroform, chloroquine, chlorothiazide, chlorpromazine, chlorpropamide, chlortetracycline, chlorzoxazone, cidofovir, cimetidine, cisplatin, cladribine, clindamycin, clofarabine, clofazimine, clofibrate, clonidine, clopidogrel, clozapine, colchicine, conjugated estrogens, Coumadin, cyclobenzaprine, cyclophosphamide, cycloserine, cyclosporine, cyproheptadine, cytarabine, dacarbazine, dactinomycin, dantrolene, dapsone, desipramine, diazepam, diclofenac, dicloxacillin, didanosine, diflunisal, diltiazem, dimercaprol, diphenhydramine, disopyramide, disulfiram, docetaxel, doxepin, doxorubicin, doxycycline, duloxetine, enalapril, enoxaparin, epinephrine, erlotinib, erythromycin, escitalopram,

table continues on pg. 1138 >

TABLE E.1, continued

Test	Increased Can Lead to a False-Positive Value Decreased Can Lead to a False-Negative Value
	estramustine, estropipate, ethacrynic acid, ethambutol, ether, ethionamide, ethosuximide, etoposide, factor IX, famotidine, fenoprofen, fluconazole, flucytosine, fluorouracil, fluoxymesterone, fluphenazine, flurazepam, flutamide, fluvastatin, fluvoxamine, fosinopril, fosphenytoin, furosemide, ganciclovir, gemcitabine, gemfibrozil, gentamicin, glimepiride, glyburide, glycopyrrolate, gold, griseofulvin, haloperidol, halothane, hepatitis A vaccine, hepatitis B vaccine, hydralazine, hydrochlorothiazide, hydroxyurea, ibuprofen, idarubicin, imipramine, indapamide, indinavir, indomethacin, interferon, interleukin, irinotecan, iron, iron dextran, isoniazid, isotretinoin, isradipine, itraconazole, kanamycin, ketoconazole, ketoprofen, ketorolac, labetalol, lamivudine, lamotrigine, lansoprazole, laronidase, levodopa, lincomycin, lisinopril, lomefloxacin, losartan, lovastatin, loxapine, Lugol's iodine, MAO inhibitors, medroxyprogesterone, mefenamic acid, melphalan, meprobamate, mercaptopurine, meropenem, mesalamine, mesoridazine, metaxalone, methacholine, methimazole, methotrexate, methoxsalen, methsuximide, methyclothiazide, methyldopa, methylene blue, methylphenidate, methyltestosterone, metoclopramide, metolazone, minocycline, mirtazapine, mitoxantrone, molindone, moricizine, morphine, moxalactam, nabumetone, nalidixic acid, naproxen, netilmicin, nevirapine, niacin, niacinamide, nicardipine, nitrofurantoin, nitrofurazone, nizatidine, norethandrolone, norethindrone, nortriptyline, novobiocin, octreotide, ofloxacin, oleandomycin, olmesartan, omeprazole, oral contraceptives, oxacillin, oxaliplatin, oxazepam, oxymetholone, papaverine, pargyline, paroxetine, pegaspargase, penicillamine, penicillin, pentoxifylline, perphenazine, phenazopyridine, phenelzine, phenobarbital, phenothiazines, phenytoin, phosphorus, piperacillin, piroxicam, polythiazide, prazosin, primaquine, probenecid, procainamide, procarbazine, prochlorperazine, progesterone, promazine, promethazine, propafenone, propranolol, propylthiouracil, pyrazinamide, quazepam, quinapril, quinethazone, quinidine, quinine, quinupristin, radiographic agents, ramipril, ranitidine, reserpine, rifampin, riluzole, salicylate, saquinavir, sargramostim, spironolactone, stanozolol, stavudine, streptomycin, sulfacetamide, sulfadiazine, sulfadoxine, sulfamethoxazole, sulfasalazine, sulfinpyrazone, sulfisoxazole, sulfonylureas, sulindac, tacrine, tacrolimus, tamoxifen, telithromycin, terbinafine, testosterone, tetracycline, thiabendazole, thiazides, thiethylperazine, thioguanine, thiopental, thioridazine, thiothixene, thiouracil, ticarcillin, ticlopidine, timolol, tobramycin, tocainide, tolazamide, tolazoline, tolbutamide, tolmetin, topotecan, toremifene, tramadol, trandolapril, tranylcypromine, trastuzumab, tretinoin, triazolam, trichlormethiazide, trifluoperazine, trimethobenzamide, trimethoprim, trimetrexate, trimipramine, trioxsalen, troleandomycin, uracil mustard, valproic acid, venlafaxine, verapamil, vidarabine, vinorelbine, vitamin K, voriconazole, zafirlukast, zalcitabine, zidovudine, zinc, ziprasidone, zolmitriptan, zolpidem

table continues on pg. 1139 >

TABLE E.1, continued

Test	Increased Can Lead to a False-Positive Value Decreased Can Lead to a False-Negative Value
	Decreased by: amikacin, anticonvulsants, aspirin, barbiturates, carbamazepine, cyclosporine, hydroxyurea, isotretinoin, penicillin, pindolol, prednisone, sulfisoxazole, theophylline, thioridazine, ursodiol, valproic acid
Bilirubin (Urine)	**Increased by:** acetohexamide, aminosalicylic acid, chlorpromazine, dapsone, etodolac, fluphenazine, imipramine, isoniazid, methyldopa, nabumetone, norethandrolone, perphenazine, phenothiazines, tolmetin **Decreased by:** ascorbic acid, chlorhexidine
Bleeding Time (Blood)	**Increased by:** acetylsalicylic acid, aminocaproic acid, ampicillin, aspirin, canola oil, carbenicillin, clopidogrel, dextran, diflunisal, diltiazem, flurbiprofen, fluoxetine, gabapentin, hetastarch, ketorolac, moxalactam, nafcillin, naproxen, nifedipine, nonsteroidal anti-inflammatory drugs, oxaprozin, penicillin, piroxicam, plicamycin, propafenone, propranolol, streptokinase, sulindac, ticarcillin, ticlopidine, tolmetin, valproic acid, warfarin **Decreased by:** conjugated estrogens, desmopressin, epoetin alfa, erythropoietin
Blood Cells and Red Casts (Urine)	**Increased by:** abciximab, aldesleukin, alprostadil, alteplase, ardeparin, auranofin, aurothioglucose, basiliximab, BCG vaccine, bicalutamide, candesartan, carvedilol, cefuroxime, chlorothiazide, cidofovir, clofibrate, clopidogrel, danazol, donepezil, doxorubicin, ethosuximide, fenoprofen, gabapentin, ganciclovir, gemcitabine, gold, goserelin, ibuprofen, indinavir, indomethacin, isotretinoin, itraconazole, ketoprofen, ketorolac, lansoprazole, leuprolide, lomefloxacin, mefenamic acid, mesalamine, metyrosine, mirtazapine, misoprostol, mycophenolate, naproxen, nisoldipine, octreotide, ofloxacin, olsalazine, omeprazole, oxaprozin, oxycodone, paroxetine, pegaspargase, penicillamine, piroxicam, probenecid, pyrimethamine, rifampin, risperidone, sargramostim, somatotropin, sulfasalazine, sulfisoxazole, sulindac, thiabendazole, ticlopidine, tolazoline, tolmetin, trastuzumab, urokinase, venlafaxine **Decreased by:** ascorbic acid, captopril, finasteride, lamotrigine
Blood Urea Nitrogen (BUN)	**Increased by:** acetaminophen, acetazolamide, acyclovir, albendazole, aldesleukin, alkaline antacids, allopurinol, altretamine, amantadine, amikacin, amiloride, amino acids, aminocaproic acid, amiodarone, amphotericin B, amyl nitrite, anabolic steroids, angiotensin-converting enzyme (ACE) inhibitors, aprepitant, aripiprazole, arsenicals, asparaginase, aspirin, atenolol, azathioprine, azithromycin, bacitracin, benazepril, benzthiazide, betaxolol, bismuth subsalicylate, bisoprolol, busulfan, calcitriol, candesartan, cannabis, capreomycin, captopril, carbamazepine, carvedilol, castor oil, cefaclor, cefamandole, cefazolin, cefixime, cefonicid, cefoperazone, cefotaxime, cefotetan, cefoxitin, cefpodoxime, ceftazidime, ceftibuten, ceftizoxime, ceftriaxone, cefuroxime, cephalexin, cephalothin, cetirizine, chemotherapy, chloroform, chlorothiazide,

table continues on pg. 1140 >

TABLE E.1, continued

Test	Increased Can Lead to a False-Positive Value Decreased Can Lead to a False-Negative Value
	chlorpheniramine, chlortetracycline, chlorthalidone, cimetidine, cinoxacin, ciprofloxacin, cisplatin, clarithromycin, clindamycin, clonidine, clorazepate, codeine, colistin, co-trimoxazole, cyclosporin, demeclocycline, dexamethasone, dextran, diazepam, diazoxide, diclofenac, disopyramide, diuretics, doxorubicin, doxycycline, enalapril, eplerenone, epoetin alfa, eprosartan, ergot preparations, ethacrynic acid, ethambutol, ether, ethosuximide, etidronate, fenoprofen, flucytosine, fludarabine, flutamide, foscarnet, furosemide, gabapentin, ganciclovir, gemcitabine, gentamicin, gold, griseofulvin, guanethidine, hydralazine, hydrochlorothiazide, hydroxyurea, ibuprofen, idarubicin, ifosfamide, imipramine, immune globulin, indomethacin, interleukin, irbesartan, iron, isosorbide, kanamycin, ketoprofen, ketorolac, labetalol, leuprolide, levodopa, levorphanol, lisinopril, lithium, lomefloxacin, loracarbef, losartan, meclofenamate, mefenamic acid, melphalan, meropenem, mesalamine, methotrexate, methsuximide, methyclothiazide, methyldopa, methysergide, metolazone, metoprolol, Micardis, minocycline, misoprostol, mitomycin, mitoxantrone, moexipril, molindone, nabumetone, nalidixic acid, naproxen, neomycin, netilmicin, nifedipine, nilutamide, nisoldipine, nitrofurantoin, norfloxacin, ofloxacin, olsalazine, oxacillin, oxaprozin, oxytetracycline, pamidronate, pargyline, paromomycin, paroxetine, pegaspargase, penicillamine, penicillin, pentamidine, pentostatin, phenazopyridine, phosphorus, piperacillin, piroxicam, plicamycin, probenecid, propafenone, propranolol, propylthiouracil, quazepam, quinapril, quinine, radiographic agents, ramipril, rifampin, risperidone, sargramostim, semustine, silver, spectinomycin, spironolactone, streptokinase, sulfamethoxazole, sulfasalazine, sulfisoxazole, sulindac, suprofen, tacrolimus, tetracycline, thallium, thiazides, ticarcillin, ticlopidine, timolol, tinzaparin, tobramycin, tolmetin, trandolapril, tretinoin, triamterene, trimethoprim, trimetrexate, vancomycin, vasopressin, venlafaxine, vitamin D, zalcitabine, zolpidem **Decreased by:** amikacin, ascorbic acid, capreomycin, cefotaxime, chloramphenicol, levodopa, phenothiazines, streptomycin
C3 Complement (Serum)	**Increased by:** cimetidine, cyclophosphamide, oral contraceptives **Decreased by:** danazol, hydralazine, methyldopa, phenytoin
C4 Complement (Serum)	**Increased by:** cyclophosphamide, danazol, oral contraceptives **Decreased by:** dextran, methyldopa, penicillamine
C-Peptide (Plasma)	**Increased by:** betamethasone, deferoxamine, glimepiride, glyburide, indapamide, isoproterenol, oral contraceptives, prednisone, terbutaline **Decreased by:** atenolol, calcitonin, miglitol
Calcitonin (Plasma)	**Increased by:** estrogen/progestin therapy, pentagastrin **Decreased by:** estrogens, octreotide, phenytoin

table continues on pg. 1141 >

TABLE E.1, continued

Test	Increased Can Lead to a False-Positive Value Decreased Can Lead to a False-Negative Value
Calcium (Serum)	**Increased by:** aldesleukin, alkaline antacids, aluminum, anabolic steroids, antacids, basiliximab, calcitriol, calcium gluconate, captopril, cefotaxime, chlorothiazide, chlorpropamide, chlorthalidone, dihydrotachysterol, doxorubicin, estramustine, estropipate, fluoxymesterone, hydralazine, hydrochlorothiazide, iron, leuprolide, lithium, magnesium, methyclothiazide, methyltestosterone, metolazone, mycophenolate, nandrolone, nisoldipine, oral contraceptives, oxymetholone, parathyroid hormone, paroxetine, pentostatin, phenobarbital, polystyrene sulfonate, polythiazide, progesterone, propranolol, riluzole, sirolimus, spironolactone, tamoxifen, teriparatide, theophylline, thiazides, toremifene, trastuzumab, tretinoin, trichlormethiazide, vitamin D, zalcitabine **Decreased by:** acetazolamide, aldesleukin, alendronate, amifostine, amlodipine, amphotericin B, anticonvulsants, arsenic trioxide, asparaginase, aspirin, basiliximab, bisphosphonates, calcitonin, carbamazepine, chloroquine, chlorothiazide, cidofovir, cinacalcet, cisplatin, corticosteroids, cortisone, diuretics, doxorubicin, erythropoietin, estrogen/progestin therapy, estropipate, etidronate, felbamate, foscarnet, furosemide, gallium, gentamicin, glucocorticoids, hydrochlorothiazide, insulin, interferon, iron dextran, isoniazid, ketoconazole, laxatives, magnesium salts, mycophenolate, oral contraceptives, pamidronate, paroxetine, pentamidine, phenobarbital, phenytoin, plicamycin, polystyrene sulfonate, prednisone, probucol, raloxifene, sargramostim, streptozocin, tacrolimus, tamoxifen, tetracycline, theophylline, tobramycin, trimetrexate, zalcitabine, zoledronic acid
Calcium (Urine)	**Increased by:** acetazolamide, aluminum hydroxide, amiloride, ammonium chloride, ascorbic acid, asparaginase, bumetanide, calcitonin, chlorothiazide, cholestyramine, corticosteroids, corticotropin, dexamethasone, diltiazem, dimercaprol, diuretics, ergocalciferol, ethacrynic acid, fenoldopam, furosemide, glucocorticoids, interferon, mannitol, methyclothiazide, metolazone, nandrolone, plicamycin, prednisolone, spironolactone, torsemide, triamcinolone, triamterene, vitamin D, vitamin K **Decreased by:** alendronate, bicarbonate, bisphosphonates, bortezomib, calcitonin, chloroquine, chlorothiazide, etidronate, gallium nitrate, hormone replacement therapy, hydrochlorothiazide, ketoconazole, lithium, mestranol, methyclothiazide, neomycin, octreotide, oral contraceptives, pamidronate, parathyroid extract, phenytoin, polythiazide, quinapril, sodium oxybate, spironolactone, thiazides, trichlormethiazide, vitamin K, zoledronic acid
Chloride (Serum)	**Increased by:** acetazolamide, acetylcysteine, ammonium chloride, aspirin, cannabis, carbamazepine, carvedilol, cefotaxime, chloride salts, chlorothiazide, cholestyramine, corticosteroids, cyclosporine, diazoxide, guanethidine, hydrochlorothiazide, hydrocortisone, iodide, ion exchange resins, lithium, methyclothiazide, methyldopa, methyltestosterone, neostigmine, triamterene

table continues on pg. 1142 >

TABLE E.1, continued

Test	Increased Can Lead to a False-Positive Value Decreased Can Lead to a False-Negative Value
	Decreased by: allopurinol, amiloride, ascorbic acid, bicarbonate, bumetanide, cefotaxime, chlorpropamide, chlorthalidone, corticosteroids, corticotropin, cortisone, diuretics, furosemide, hydrochlorothiazide, hydrocortisone, hydroflumethiazide, laxatives, mannitol, metolazone, polythiazide, prednisone, silver, thiazides, triamterene, trimethoprim
Cholesterol (Serum)	**Increased by:** acebutolol, acetohexamide, adalimumab, alitretinoin, aminoglutethimide, amiodarone, amphotericin B, amprenavir, anabolic steroids, anastrozole, antibiotics, antihypertensives, aripiprazole, ascorbic acid, asparaginase, aspirin, atazanavir, atenolol, azathioprine, basiliximab, bicalutamide, beclomethasone, betaxolol, beta-blockers, bisoprolol, calcitriol, captopril, carbamazepine, carvedilol, cefotaxime, chenodiol, chlorothiazide, chlorpromazine, chlorpropamide, chlorthalidone, clofibrate, clonidine, clopidogrel, conjugated estrogens, corticosteroids, cortisone, cyclophosphamide, cyclosporine, danazol, dantrolene, dapsone, dextran, diazepam, diclofenac, disulfiram, efavirenz, enalapril, epinephrine, eplerenone, escitalopram, ethanol, ether, fluoxymesterone, fluvoxamine, fosinopril, furosemide, gabapentin, glyburide, gold, heparin, hydrochlorothiazide, ibandronate, ibuprofen, imipramine, indapamide, isotretinoin, lansoprazole, levarterenol, lisinopril, lithium, medroxyprogesterone, meprobamate, methimazole, methyltestosterone, miconazole, mirtazapine, mycophenolate, nafarelin, nandrolone, naproxen, norethandrolone, norfloxacin, Norplant, ofloxacin, olmesartan, oral contraceptives, oxymetholone, paroxetine, penicillamine, phenobarbital, phenothiazines, phenytoin, pindolol, polythiazide, pravastatin, prednisolone, prednisone, prochlorperazine, promazine, propranolol, quetiapine, radioactive iodine, riluzole, ritonavir, rosiglitazone, sargramostim, sirolimus, sodium oxybate, sotalol, spironolactone, sulfadiazine, tamoxifen, testosterone, tetracycline, theophylline, thiabendazole, thiazides, thiouracil, ticlopidine, tretinoin, trifluoperazine, venlafaxine, vitamin A, vitamin C, vitamin D, vitamin E, zolpidem **Decreased by:** acarbose, acebutolol, albuterol, aldesleukin, allopurinol, aluminum hydroxide, amikacin, amiloride, aminosalicylic acid, amiodarone, amlodipine, ampicillin, ascorbic acid, asparaginase, aspirin, atenolol, atorvastatin, azathioprine, bisoprolol, captopril, carvedilol, chlorambucil, chloroform, chlorpropamide, chlorthalidone, cholestyramine, cilazapril, clofibrate, clomiphene, clonidine, coenzyme Q10, colchicine, colestipol, conjugated estrogens, diltiazem, dobutamine, doxazosin, enalapril, erythromycin, esterified estrogens, estrogen therapy, fenofibrate, fluoxymesterone, fluvastatin, fosinopril, GCSF, gemfibrozil, glyburide, green tea, guanabenz, haloperidol, heparin, hydralazine, hydroxychloroquine, hydroxymethylglutaryl coenzyme A (HMG CoA)-reductase inhibitors, indomethacin, insulin, isoniazid, isosorbide dinitrate,

table continues on pg. 1143 >

TABLE E.1, continued

Test	Increased Can Lead to a False-Positive Value Decreased Can Lead to a False-Negative Value
	isosorbide mononitrate, isotretinoin, isradipine, kanamycin, ketoconazole, lansoprazole, levonorgestrel, levothyroxine, lincomycin, lisinopril, LMW heparin, losartan, MAO inhibitors, medroxyprogesterone, metformin, methyldopa, metoprolol, metronidazole, nandrolone, neomycin, niacin, nicotinic acid, nifedipine, nitroglycerin, Norplant, oral contraceptives, orlistat, oxandrolone, oxymetholone, pentamidine, perindopril, phenytoin, pindolol, pravastatin, prazosin, prednisolone, probucol, progesterone, psyllium, raloxifene, ramipril, rifampin, simvastatin, spironolactone, statins, streptokinase, tacrolimus, tamoxifen, terazosin, tetracycline, thiazides, thyroid, tolbutamide, trazodone, ursodiol, valproic acid, verapamil
Chorionic Gonadotropin (Plasma)	**Decreased by:** octreotide
Coagulation Time (Blood)	**Increased by:** anticoagulants, carbenicillin, pegaspargase, plicamycin, tetracycline, ticarcillin
Coombs' Test	**Decreased by**: aminophylline, oral contraceptives **Positive result by:** aminosalicylic acid, aztreonam, ceftazidime, ceftizoxime, cefuroxime, chlorpromazine, chlorpropamide, ethosuximide, hydralazine, ibuprofen, imipenem/cilastatin, isoniazid, levodopa, mefenamic acid, melphalan, methyldopa, moxalactam, penicillamine, phenytoin, procainamide, quinidine, quinine, streptomycin, sulfonylureas, tetracycline
Cortisol (Plasma)	**Increased by:** anticonvulsants, aspirin, atropine, benzodiazepines, citalopram, clomipramine, corticotropin, corticotropin-releasing hormone, cortisone, diazoxide, diclofenac, estrogens, ether, ethinyl estradiol, fenoprofen, furosemide, gemfibrozil, glyburide, hydrocortisone, insulin, interferon, interleukin, lithium, methadone, methoxamine, metoclopramide, naloxone, octreotide, opiates, oral contraceptives, prednisolone, prednisone, ranitidine, spironolactone, tumor necrosis factor, vasopressin **Decreased by:** aminoglutethimide, barbiturates, beclomethasone, budesonide, clonidine, corticosteroids, danazol, dexamethasone, dextroamphetamine, diazoxide, ephedrine, etomidate, fluocinolone, indomethacin, ketoconazole, labetalol, levodopa, lithium, magnesium sulfate, medroxyprogesterone, megestrol, mesalamine, methylprednisolone, midazolam, morphine, nifedipine, nitrous oxide, norethindrone, oxazepam, phenobarbital, phenytoin, pravastatin, prednisolone, ranitidine, rifampin, sumatriptan, triamcinolone, trimipramine
Creatinine (Serum)	**Increased by:** ACE inhibitors, acebutolol, acetaminophen, acetohexamide, acyclovir, adefovir, albendazole, aldesleukin, alkaline antacids, allopurinol, alprazolam, alprostadil, altretamine, amikacin, amiloride, amiodarone, ammonium chloride, amoxapine, amphotericin B, aprepitant, ascorbic acid, asparaginase, aspirin, azathioprine, azithromycin, aztreonam, barbiturates, benazepril, betaxolol, bicalutamide, bisoprolol, candesartan, capreomycin, captopril, carbamazepine, carvedilol,

table continues on pg. 1144 >

TABLE E.1, continued

Test	Increased Can Lead to a False-Positive Value Decreased Can Lead to a False-Negative Value
	caspofungin, cefaclor, cefadroxil, cefamandole, cefazolin, cefepime, cefixime, cefoperazone, cefotaxime, cefotetan, cefoxitin, cefpodoxime, cefprozil, ceftazidime, ceftibuten, ceftizoxime, ceftriaxone, cefuroxime, cephalexin, cephalothin, cephradine, cetirizine, chlorothiazide, chlorpropamide, chlorthalidone, cidofovir, cimetidine, ciprofloxacin, cisplatin, clarithromycin, clindamycin, clofarabine, clofibrate, clonidine, clorazepate, codeine, colistimethate, cyclosporine, danazol, demeclocycline, dexrazoxane, dextran, diclofenac, didanosine, disopyramide, diuretics, dopamine, doxorubicin, doxycycline, enalapril, eplerenone, epoetin alfa, eprosartan, ethambutol, etidronate, fenoprofen, flucytosine, fludarabine, fluoxymesterone, foscarnet, furosemide, gabapentin, ganciclovir, GCSF, gemcitabine, gemfibrozil, gentamicin, glycerin, griseofulvin, hetastarch, hydralazine, hydrochlorothiazide, hydroxychloroquine, hydroxyurea, ibuprofen, idarubicin, imatinib, imipramine, immune globulin, indomethacin, interleukin alfa-2, irbesartan, isotretinoin, kanamycin, ketoprofen, ketorolac, labetalol, lactulose, lamotrigine, lansoprazole, leuprolide, levodopa, lidocaine, lisinopril, lithium, loracarbef, losartan, lovastatin, mannitol, meclofenamate, mefenamic acid, meropenem, mesalamine, methotrexate, methyldopa, methylprednisolone, metoprolol, mitomycin, mitoxantrone, moexipril, moxalactam, mycophenolate, nalidixic acid, nandrolone, naproxen, neomycin, netilmicin, nifedipine, nilutamide, nisoldipine, nitazoxanide, nitrofurantoin, nonsteroidal anti-inflammatory drugs, norfloxacin, ofloxacin, olsalazine, oxacillin, oxaprozin, pamidronate, paromomycin, pegaspargase, penicillamine, penicillin, pentamidine, pentostatin, phenazopyridine, phosphorus, piperacillin, piroxicam, plicamycin, prednisone, propafenone, propranolol, quazepam, quinapril, radiographic agents, ramipril, ranitidine, risperidone, salsalate, sargramostim, sevoflurane, sirolimus, sodium oxybate, spironolactone, streptokinase, streptomycin, streptozocin, sulfamethoxazole, sulfasalazine, sulfisoxazole, sulindac, tacrolimus, telmisartan (Micardis), tetracycline, thiazides, ticarcillin, ticlopidine, timolol, tobramycin, tolazoline, tramadol, trandolapril, tretinoin, triamterene, triazolam, trimethoprim, trimetrexate, ursodiol, valsartan, vancomycin, vasopressin, venlafaxine, vitamin D, zoledronic acid **Decreased by:** alprazolam, amikacin, ascorbic acid, atenolol, cannabis, captopril, chlorambucil, dobutamine, dopamine, ibuprofen, interferon alfa-2a, ketoprofen, lisinopril, methyldopa, nicardipine, prednisone, quinapril, terazosin, triazolam, tromethamine, valproic acid, zidovudine
Creatinine Phosphokinase (CPK) (Serum)	**Increased by:** albuterol, aminocaproic acid, amoxapine, amphotericin B, ampicillin, ampicillin (IM injection), analgesics (IM injection), aripiprazole, aspirin, atorvastatin, azithromycin, candesartan, captopril, carbenicillin, carteolol, cefotaxime, ceftizoxime, chlorpromazine, chlorthalidone, cholestyramine,

table continues on pg. 1145 >

TABLE E.1, continued

Test	Increased Can Lead to a False-Positive Value Decreased Can Lead to a False-Negative Value
	clindamycin, clofibrate, clonidine, clozapine, cyclosporin, danazol, dantrolene, diclofenac, didanosine, digoxin, diltiazem, diuretics (IM injection), donepezil, ethchlorvynol, fenofibrate, 5-fluorouracil, fluvastatin, foscarnet, ganciclovir, gemfibrozil, haloperidol, hydrocortisone, insulin, interleukin, isotretinoin, itraconazole, labetalol, lamivudine, lidocaine, lithium, lovastatin, loxapine, meperidine, morphine (IM injection), nelfinavir, niacin, nifedipine, nisoldipine, olanzapine, oral contraceptives, paroxetine, penicillamine, penicillin, phenelzine, phenothiazines, phenytoin, pindolol, pioglitazone, pramipexole, pravastatin, probucol, promethazine, propranolol, quinidine, risperidone, ritonavir, simvastatin, sirolimus, streptokinase, succinylcholine, trimethoprim, tubocurarine, vasopressin, zalcitabine, zidovudine **Decreased by:** acetylsalicylic acid, amikacin, ascorbic acid, calcium, dantrolene, dexamethasone, droperidol, phenothiazines, pindolol, prednisone, sulfamethoxazole
Creatinine (Urine)	**Increased by:** ascorbic acid, cefoxitin, cephalothin, corticosteroids, fluoxymesterone, methotrexate, methyldopa, nandrolone, nitrofurantoin, nitrofurazone, oxymetholone, prednisone **Decreased by**: anabolic steroids, captopril, ketoprofen, nandrolone, prednisone, quinapril, thiazides
Eosinophils (Blood)	**Increased by:** aldesleukin, allopurinol, alprazolam, aminosalicylic acid, amoxapine, amoxicillin, amphotericin B, ampicillin, auranofin, aztreonam, benazepril, capreomycin, captopril, carbamazepine, carbenicillin, carisoprodol, caspofungin, cefamandole, cefdinir, cefonicid, cefoperazone, cefotaxime, cefotetan, cefoxitin, cefpodoxime, ceftazidime, ceftizoxime, ceftriaxone, cephalexin, cephalothin, chloramphenicol, chlorpromazine, cinoxacin, ciprofloxacin, clindamycin, clofibrate, clonazepam, cloxacillin, cyclobenzaprine, danazol, dantrolene, dapsone, demeclocycline, desipramine, diazoxide, diclofenac, donepezil, doxepin, doxorubicin, doxycycline, enalapril, ethosuximide, felbamate, flucytosine, fluorouracil, fluphenazine, famciclovir, GCSF, gemfibrozil, gentamicin, haloperidol, hepatitis A vaccine, ibuprofen, imipenem/cilastin, interleukin, isoniazid, ketorolac, lamotrigine, lansoprazole, levodopa, loracarbef, maprotiline, mefenamic acid, methsuximide, minocycline, moxalactam, nafarelin, nafcillin, naproxen, netilmicin, nitrofurantoin, nizatidine, nonsteroidal anti-inflammatory drugs, norfloxacin, ofloxacin, paroxetine, penicillamine, pentazocine, perphenazine, piperacillin, piroxicam, procarbazine, propafenone, quinolones, ramipril, ranitidine, rifampin, spironolactone, streptomycin, sulfamethoxazole, sulfasalazine, tetracycline, thioridazine, thiothixene, ticarcillin, ticlopidine, tobramycin, topiramate, triazolam, trifluoperazine, trimipramine, valproic acid, venlafaxine, zalcitabine, zolmitriptan

table continues on pg. 1146 >

TABLE E.1, continued

Test	Increased Can Lead to a False-Positive Value Decreased Can Lead to a False-Negative Value
	Decreased by: amitriptyline, aspirin, captopril, clozapine, corticotropin, desipramine, ethosuximide, indomethacin, niacin, niacinamide, nortriptyline, olsalazine, procainamide, rifampin, sulfamethoxazole, triazolam
Erythrocytes (Blood)	**Increased by:** alglucerase, antithyroid therapy, basiliximab, corticotropin, danazol, erythropoietin, glucocorticoids, hydrochlorothiazide, mycophenolate, pilocarpine **Decreased by:** acetaminophen, acetazolamide, acetohexamide, acyclovir, allopurinol, aminoglutethimide, amitriptyline, amphetamine, amphotericin B, ampicillin, amyl nitrate, antimalarials, antineoplastics, aspirin, auranofin, azathioprine, barbiturates, benazepril, benzocaine, bismuth subsalicylate, bupropion, busulfan, capecitabine, captopril, carbamazepine, carbenicillin, carvedilol, ceftazidime, ceftizoxime, cephaloridine, cephalothin, chloramphenicol, chlordiazepoxide, chloroquine, chlorothiazide, chlorpheniramine, chlorpromazine, chlortetracycline, chlorthalidone, cimetidine, clomipramine, clonazepam, colchicine, corticosteroids, cyclophosphamide, cycloserine, cyclosporin A, cytarabine, dactinomycin, dapsone, demeclocycline, desipramine, digitalis, dimercaprol, diphenhydramine, donepezil, doxapram, doxorubicin, eflornithine, ethosuximide, etidronate, etoposide, fenoprofen, flucytosine, fludarabine, fluorouracil, fluphenazine, fluvastatin, furosemide, gentamicin, glimepiride, haloperidol, hydralazine, hydrochlorothiazide, hydroxychloroquine, hydroxyurea, ibuprofen, idarubicin, indomethacin, iodoquinol, isoniazid, isotretinoin, levodopa, Lipomul, local anesthetics, MAO inhibitors, mechlorethamine, meclofenamate, melphalan, mephobarbital, meprobamate, mercaptopurine, mesoridazine, methazolamide, methicillin, methimazole, methotrexate, methsuximide, methyclothiazide, methyldopa, methylene blue, mitomycin, mitoxantrone, nalidixic acid, naproxen, neomycin, nitrofurantoin, nitrofurazone, norfloxacin, omeprazole, oral contraceptives, orphenadrine, oxacillin, penicillamine, penicillin, pentamidine, pentoxifylline, phenazopyridine, phenobarbital, phenothiazines, phenytoin, phytonadione, piperazine, piroxicam, primaquine, primidone, probenecid, procainamide, procarbazine, propylthiouracil, pyrimethamine, quinidine, radioactive compounds, ramipril, rifampin, streptomycin, sulfadiazine, sulfamethoxazole, sulfanilamide, sulfasalazine, sulfinpyrazone, tetracycline, thiazides, thioridazine, thiotepa, thiothixene, ticlopidine, tocainide, tolazamide, tolmetin, trastuzumab, trazodone, triamterene, trichlormethiazide, trifluoperazine, trimethoprim, tripelennamine, uracil mustard, vinblastine, zidovudine
Erythrocyte Sedimentation Rate (Blood)	**Increased by:** anticonvulsants, aspirin, carbamazepine, cephalothin, cephapirin, clozapine, cyclosporine A, dexamethasone, fluvastatin, hydralazine, indomethacin, isotretinoin, lomefloxacin, misoprostol, ofloxacin, oral contraceptives, procainamide, propafenone, quinidine, sulfamethoxazole, zolpidem

table continues on pg. 1147 >

TABLE E.1, continued

Test	Increased Can Lead to a False-Positive Value Decreased Can Lead to a False-Negative Value
	Decreased by: aspirin, corticotropin, cortisone, cyclophosphamide, dexamethasone, gold, hydroxychloroquine, leflunomide, methotrexate, minocycline, nonsteroidal anti-inflammatory drugs, penicillamine, prednisolone, prednisone, quinine, sulfasalazine, tamoxifen, trimethoprim
Erythropoietin (Serum)	**Increased by:** anabolic steroids, daunorubicin, erythropoietin, fluoxymesterone, hydroxyurea, theophylline, zidovudine **Decreased by:** acetazolamide, amphotericin B, cisplatin, enalapril, furosemide, theophylline
Ethanol (Serum)	**Increased by:** aspirin, chloral hydrate, cimetidine, metoclopramide, ranitidine **Decreased by:** ascorbic acid, atropine, phenobarbital, propantheline
Euglobulin Clot Lysis Time (Blood)	**Increased by:** cyclosporine A **Decreased by:** asparaginase, clofibrate, dextran, gemfibrozil, streptokinase
Fatty Acids (Free) (Serum)	**Increased by:** aminophylline, amphetamine, chlorpromazine, clonidine, desipramine, diazoxide, enoxaparin, growth hormone–releasing hormone, human growth hormone, isoproterenol, levarterenol, levodopa, mescaline, molindone, oral contraceptives, prazosin, reserpine, ritodrine, terbutaline, theophylline, trichlormethiazide, valproic acid **Decreased by:** acarbose, acebutolol, amino acids, asparaginase, aspirin, atenolol, clofibrate, glyburide, insulin, isoproterenol, levothyroxine, metformin, metoprolol, neomycin, niacin, nicotinic acid, nifedipine, prazosin, propranolol, propylthiouracil, simvastatin, sotalol
Ferritin (Blood)	**Increased by:** ferrous sulfate, iron preps, oral contraceptives, theophylline **Decreased by:** antithyroid therapy, ascorbic acid, deferoxamine, methimazole
Fibrinogen (Plasma)	**Increased by:** aspirin, bicalutamide, chemotherapy, estropipate, fluvastatin, gemfibrozil, lovastatin, norethandrolone, oral contraceptives, oxandrolone, oxymetholone, pyrazinamide, simvastatin **Decreased by:** anabolic steroids, asparaginase, atenolol, cefamandole, clofibrate, danazol, dextran, estrogen/progestin therapy, estrogens, factor VIIa, fenofibrate, 5-fluorouracil, gemfibrozil, iron, kanamycin, lamotrigine, lovastatin, medroxyprogesterone, oral contraceptives, pegaspargase, pentoxifylline, phosphorus, pravastatin, prednisone, raloxifene, reteplase, simvastatin, streptokinase, sulfisoxazole, ticlopidine, valproic acid
Folic Acid (Serum)	**Decreased by:** aminosalicylic acid, ampicillin, antacids, anticonvulsants, aspirin, barbiturates, chloramphenicol, cholestyramine, cycloserine, erythromycin, estropipate, iron, isoniazid, levodopa, lincomycin, metformin, methotrexate, nitrofurantoin, oral contraceptives, penicillin, pentamidine, phenobarbital, phenytoin, primidone, pyrimethamine, rifampin, sulfasalazine, sulfisoxazole, tetracycline, triamterene, trimethoprim

table continues on pg. 1148 >

TABLE E.1, continued

Test	Increased Can Lead to a False-Positive Value Decreased Can Lead to a False-Negative Value
Follicle-Stimulating Hormone (FSH) (Plasma)	**Increased by:** bicalutamide, bromocriptine, cimetidine, clomiphene, danazol, erythropoietin, finasteride, follicle-stimulating hormone, gonadotropin-releasing hormone, growth hormone–releasing hormone, hydrocortisone, ketoconazole, leuprolide, levodopa, metformin, naloxone, nilutamide, phenytoin, pravastatin, tamoxifen **Decreased by:** anabolic steroids, anticonvulsants, carbamazepine, conjugated estrogens, corticotropin-releasing hormone, danazol, estrogen/progestin therapy, finasteride, goserelin, leuprolide, medroxyprogesterone, megestrol, octreotide, oral contraceptives, phenothiazines, pimozide, pravastatin, prednisone, stanozolol, tamoxifen, toremifene, valproic acid
Free Thyroxine Index (Serum)	**Increased by:** amiodarone, carbamazepine, furosemide, levothyroxine, oral contraceptives, orphenadrine, phenobarbital, propranolol **Decreased by:** amiodarone, aspirin, clomiphene, co-trimoxazole, corticosteroids, ferrous sulfate, iodide, isotretinoin, lovastatin, methimazole, phenobarbital, phenytoin, primidone, radioactive iodine, salsalate
Glucagon (Plasma)	**Increased by:** aspirin, calcitonin, danazol, glucocorticoids, guanabenz, hydrochlorothiazide, insulin, interferon alfa-2a, nifedipine, prednisolone, propranolol **Decreased by:** atenolol, insulin, metoprolol, octreotide, pindolol, propranolol, verapamil
Glucose (Cerebrospinal Fluid)	**Increased by:** cefotaxime, dexamethasone **Decreased by:** cefotaxime
Glucose (Serum)	**Increased by:** abacavir, acetaminophen, acetazolamide, adenosine, albuterol, aldesleukin, aminophylline, aminosalicylic acid, amiodarone, amitriptyline, amoxapine, amphotericin B, ampicillin, ampicillin/sulbactam, aripiprazole, asparaginase, aspirin, atazanavir, atenolol, atropine, azathioprine, azithromycin, baclofen, basiliximab, benazepril, betamethasone, betaxolol, bicalutamide, bisoprolol, budesonide, calcitonin, candesartan, cannabis, captopril, carvedilol, cefdinir, cefotaxime, cefpodoxime, cefuroxime, chloramphenicol, chlorothiazide, chlorthalidone, cholestyramine, cidofovir, clonidine, clozapine, colchicine, corticotropin, cortisone, cyclobenzaprine, cyclophosphamide, cyclosporine, daclizumab, desipramine, dexamethasone, dextran, dextroamphetamine, diazoxide, diclofenac, didanosine, diltiazem, dimercaprol, diphenoxylate, dobutamine, donepezil, dopamine, doxepin, doxorubicin, enalapril, enfuvirtide, ephedra, ephedrine, epinephrine, escitalopram, ethacrynic acid, ethionamide, felbamate, fludrocortisone, fluoxymesterone, fluvoxamine, fosamprenavir, foscarnet, fosinopril, fosphenytoin, furosemide, ganciclovir, gemfibrozil, glimepiride, glucagon, glucosamine, goserelin, haloperidol, hydralazine, hydrochlorothiazide, imipramine, indapamide, indinavir, indomethacin, interferon alfa, interferon gamma-1b, irinotecan, iron dextran, isoniazid, isoproterenol, isotretinoin,

table continues on pg. 1149 >

TABLE E.1, continued

Test	Increased Can Lead to a False-Positive Value Decreased Can Lead to a False-Negative Value
	ketoprofen, labetalol, lactose, lansoprazole, L-asparaginase, leuprolide, levalbuterol, levodopa, levodopa/carbidopa, levofloxacin, levonorgestrel, liothyronine, lisinopril, loperamide, maprotiline, medroxyprogesterone, megestrol, meperidine, mercaptopurine, methimazole, methyclothiazide, methyldopa, metolazone, metoprolol, metronidazole, mirtazapine, molindone, morphine, mycophenolate, nabumetone, nalidixic acid, naproxen, nelfinavir, niacin, nicardipine, nifedipine, nilutamide, nisoldipine, norethindrone, norfloxacin, nortriptyline, octreotide, ofloxacin, olanzapine, oxazepam, palonosetron, pancreozymin, paraldehyde, paroxetine, pegaptanib, pegaspargase, pentamidine, perindopril, perphenazine, phenazopyridine, phenelzine, phenylephrine, phenytoin, piroxicam, polythiazide, pravastatin, prazosin, prednisolone, prednisone, probenecid, propafenone, propranolol, propylthiouracil, protriptyline, quinapril, ramipril, reserpine, rifampin, riluzole, risperidone, ritonavir, saquinavir, sargramostim, sildenafil, sodium oxybate, somatostatin, streptozocin, sulfisoxazole, sulindac, sumatriptan, tacrine, tacrolimus, terbutaline, tetracycline, theophylline, thiabendazole, thiothixene, thyroid, timolol, tolbutamide, triamcinolone, triamterene, trichlormethiazide, trifluoperazine, trimipramine, ursodiol, valproic acid, venlafaxine, verapamil, vidarabine, vitamin C, zalcitabine, zidovudine, ziprasidone, zolmitriptan, zolpidem **Decreased by:** acarbose, acetaminophen, acetaminophen/codeine, acetazolamide, acetohexamide, aldesleukin, allopurinol, amikacin, amino acids, aminoglutethimide, amiodarone, amitriptyline, amphetamine, aspirin, atenolol, atropine, basiliximab, benazepril, butalbital/acetaminophen/caffeine, butalbital/acetaminophen/caffeine/codeine, calcium gluconate, cannabinol, captopril, carvedilol, cefdinir, cefpodoxime, cefuroxime, chloramphenicol, chloroquine, chlorpromazine, chlorpropamide, cholestyramine, cimetidine, ciprofloxacin, clofibrate, desipramine, dextroamphetamine, diazepam, diazoxide, diltiazem, dimercaprol, disopyramide, doxazosin, doxepin, doxorubicin, duloxetine, enalapril, erythromycin, ethacrynic acid, felbamate, fenofibrate, flucytosine, fluoxymesterone, flurazepam, fluvoxamine, foscarnet, fosinopril, furosemide, ganciclovir, gemfibrozil, glimepiride, glipizide, glucosamine, glyburide, GCSF, green tea, guanethidine, guar, haloperidol, hydralazine, hydrocodone/acetaminophen, imipramine, indomethacin, interferon beta-1b, isocarboxazid, isoniazid, lansoprazole, leuprolide, levodopa, levofloxacin, lisinopril, lomefloxacin, maprotiline, megestrol, metformin, methyldopa, methyltestosterone, metronidazole, midazolam, miglitol, mycophenolate, nadolol, nandrolone, nelfinavir, niacin, nifedipine, norfloxacin, nortriptyline, octreotide, ofloxacin, oxandrolone, oxycodone/acetaminophen, oxytetracycline, oxymetholone, paroxetine, pegaspargase, penicillamine, pentamidine,

table continues on pg. 1150 >

TABLE E.1, continued

Test	Increased Can Lead to a False-Positive Value Decreased Can Lead to a False-Negative Value
	perindopril, perphenazine, phenazopyridine, phentolamine, phosphorus, pioglitazone, piroxicam, prednisone, probenecid, progesterone, promethazine, propranolol, protriptyline, psyllium, quinapril, quinine, ramipril, repaglinide, rosiglitazone, saquinavir, selegiline, sildenafil, simvastatin, somatostatin, St. John's wort, sulfamethoxazole/trimethoprim, sulfisoxazole, sumatriptan, terbutaline, tetracycline, thiabendazole, tolazamide, tolbutamide, trastuzumab, trimipramine, tromethamine, valproic acid, verapamil, vitamin C
Glucose (Urine)	**Increased by:** acetazolamide, aminosalicylic acid, ampicillin, ampicillin/sulbactam, ascorbic acid, asparaginase, aspirin, azlocillin, benzthiazide, betamethasone, bicalutamide, bismuth subsalicylate, bupropion, captopril, carbamazepine, carbenicillin, carvedilol, cefaclor, cefadroxil, cefamandole, cefazolin, cefdinir, cefepime, cefixime, cefoperazone, cefuroxime, cephalexin, cephalosporin antibiotics, chloral hydrate, chlorothiazide, chlorpromazine, chlorthalidone, cidofovir, corticosteroids, corticotropin, dexamethasone, dextroamphetamine, diazoxide, dicloxacillin, doxorubicin, enalapril, ephedrine, ethacrynic acid, ether, ethionamide, fludrocortisone, foscarnet, furosemide, gabapentin, glucagon, histrelin, hydrochlorothiazide, hydrocortisone, ifosfamide, indomethacin, isoniazid, lansoprazole, levodopa/carbidopa, lisinopril, lithium, methyclothiazide, methylprednisolone, metolazone, mirtazapine, misoprostol, nalidixic acid, naproxen, niacin, nitrofurantoin, norfloxacin, ofloxacin, penicillin, perphenazine, phenazopyridine, phenothiazines, phenytoin, piperacillin, polythiazide, probenecid, quinethazone, reserpine, sevoflurane, somatropin, streptomycin, streptozocin, sulfonamides, tacrine, tetracycline, theophylline, thiazides, thiothixene, ticarcillin, timolol, triamcinolone, trichlormethiazide, trifluoperazine, venlafaxine, zalcitabine **Decreased by:** acarbose, aminosalicylic acid, ampicillin, ampicillin/sulbactam, ascorbic acid, aspirin, bisacodyl, carbidopa, chloral hydrate, cholestyramine, demeclocycline, diazepam, digoxin, doxycycline, ferrous sulfate, flurazepam, furosemide, hydroquinone, insulin, levodopa, minocycline, oxytetracycline, phenazopyridine, phenobarbital, radiographic agents, secobarbital, tetracycline, vitamin preparations
Glucose Tolerance (Serum)	**Increased by:** acarbose, atenolol, clofibrate, fluoxymesterone, glyburide, guanethidine, lisinopril, MAO inhibitors, metformin, metoprolol, nandrolone, norethindrone, octreotide, pargyline, phenytoin, prazosin, terazosin **Decreased by:** acebutolol, atenolol, beclomethasone, betamethasone, calcitonin, cannabis, chlorothiazide, chlorpromazine, chlorthalidone, clofibrate, conjugated estrogens, cortisone, danazol, dexamethasone, diazoxide, estropipate, ethacrynic acid, felodipine, fludrocortisone, foscarnet, furosemide, human growth hormone, hydrochlorothiazide, imipramine,

table continues on pg. 1151 >

TABLE E.1, continued

Test	Increased Can Lead to a False-Positive Value Decreased Can Lead to a False-Negative Value
	interferon alfa-2a, iron, levonorgestrel, lithium, medroxyprogesterone, mefenamic acid, mestranol, methylprednisolone, metoprolol, naproxen, niacin, niacinamide, nicotinic acid, nifedipine, nitrofurantoin, norethindrone, octreotide, oral contraceptives, perphenazine, phenytoin, pindolol, polythiazide, prednisolone, prednisone, promethazine, quinethazone, spironolactone, streptozocin, thiazides, triamcinolone, triamterene, verapamil
Glycosylated Hemoglobin (HBA_{1c}) (Blood)	**Increased by:** aspirin, atenolol, beta-blockers, gemfibrozil, glimepiride, hydrochlorothiazide, indapamide, lovastatin, niacin, nicardipine, nicotinic acid, propranolol **Decreased by:** acarbose, deferoxamine, diltiazem, enalapril, glipizide, glyburide, insulin, lisinopril, metformin, nisoldipine, pravastatin, ramipril, terazosin, verapamil
μ-Glutamyltransferase (μGTT) (Serum)	**Increased by:** acetaminophen, allopurinol, alprazolam amiodarone, amphotericin B, anastrazole, anticonvulsants, azithromycin, barbiturates, captopril, carbamazepine, cefdinir, cefonicid, cefpodoxime, ceftazidime, cetirizine, chloramphenicol, chlorpromazine, chlorpropamide, cimetidine, cisplatin, clomipramine, clozapine, cyclosporin A, dactinomycin, dantrolene, diclofenac, disopyramide, disulfiram, doxorubicin, doxycycline, enalapril, esterified estrogens, estropipate, etoposide, famotidine, fluconazole, flucytosine, fluoxymesterone, flutamide, fluvastatin, fosphenytoin, gold, griseofulvin, haloperidol, hepatitis A vaccine, hydrochlorothiazide, ibuprofen, interferon alfa-n3, isoniazid, isotretinoin, isradipine, ketamine, ketoprofen, labetalol, lansoprazole, levothyroxine, lisinopril, lomefloxacin, loratadine, lovastatin, medroxyprogesterone, meropenem, mesalamine, methotrexate, methyldopa, metoprolol, moexipril, mycophenolate, nabumetone, naproxen, nelfinavir, nevirapine, niacin, nicardipine, nisoldipine, nitrofurantoin, nortriptyline, octreotide, ofloxacin, olsalazine, omeprazole, oral contraceptives, papaverine, pegaspargase, phenazopyridine, phenobarbital, phenothiazines, phenytoin, piroxicam, prazosin, probenecid, prochlorperazine, propafenone, quinapril, quinidine, rifampin, riluzole, ritonavir, sibutramine, stanozolol, streptokinase, sulfamethoxazole, sulfasalazine, sulfisoxazole, sulindac, terbinafine, thiabendazole, thiethylperazine, thiopental, thioridazine, tocainide, tolmetin, trifluoperazine, troleandomycin, valproic acid, warfarin, zalcitabine, zidovudine **Decreased by:** azathioprine, clofibrate, conjugated estrogens, methotrexate, ursodiol
Growth Hormone (Plasma)	**Increased by:** amino acids, anabolic steroids, citalopram, clomipramine, clonidine, desipramine, dexamethasone, diazepam, ethinyl estradiol, growth hormone–releasing hormone, indomethacin, insulin, interferon, interleukin, methamphetamine, metoclopramide, midazolam, niacin, oral contraceptives, phenytoin, propranolol, pyridostigmine, tumor necrosis factor, vasopressin

table continues on pg. 1152 >

TABLE E.1, continued

Test	Increased Can Lead to a False-Positive Value Decreased Can Lead to a False-Negative Value
	Decreased by: bromocriptine, chlorpromazine, corticosteroids, hydrocortisone, medroxyprogesterone, methyldopa, octreotide, prednisone, propantheline, valproic acid
5-Hydroxyindoleacetic Acid (Urine)	**Increased by:** acetaminophen, chlordiazepoxide, cisplatin, diazepam, ephedrine, flurazepam, fluorouracil, guaifenesin, melphalan, methocarbamol, naproxen, phenobarbital, phentolamine, rauwolfia, reserpine, sulfasalazine **Decreased by:** aspirin, chlorpromazine, corticotropin, imipramine, interferon alfa-2a, isoniazid, levodopa, MAO inhibitors, methyldopa, octreotide, phenothiazines, promazine, streptozocin
Complement CH_{50} (Serum)	**Increased by:** chlorpropamide, cyclophosphamide **Decreased by:** hydralazine
High-Density Lipoprotein (HDL) Cholesterol (Serum)	**Increased by:** acarbose, ACE inhibitors, albuterol atorvastatin, beclomethasone, captopril, carbamazepine, carvedilol, cholestyramine, cimetidine, clofibrate, coenzyme Q10, colestipol, corn oil, diltiazem, doxazosin, estrogen therapy, estrogen/progestin therapy, efavirenz, fenofibrate, fluvastatin, furosemide, gemfibrozil, glyburide, goserelin, hydroxychloroquine, indapamide, insulin, isradipine, ketoconazole, levonorgestrel (Norplant), lovastatin, medroxyprogesterone, metformin, methimazole, minoxidil, nafarelin, niacin, nicardipine, nicotinic acid, nifedipine, nisoldipine, oral contraceptives, perindopril, phenobarbital, phenytoin, pindolol, pravastatin, prazosin, prednisone, ramipril, rosiglitazone, simvastatin, terazosin, terbutaline, theophylline, verapamil **Decreased by:** acebutolol, ascorbic acid, atenolol, azathioprine, beta-blockers, bisoprolol, carvedilol, chenodiol, chlorpropamide, clofibrate, cyclosporin A, danazol, estrogen/progestin therapy, gemfibrozil, hydrochlorothiazide, indapamide, indomethacin, interferon alfa-2a, isotretinoin, levonorgestrel (Norplant), levothyroxine, linseed oil, lisinopril, medroxyprogesterone, methimazole, methyldopa, metoprolol, nadolol, nandrolone, neomycin, oral contraceptives, prednisolone, probucol, propranolol, psyllium, raloxifene, sotalol, spironolactone, stanozolol, tamoxifen, thiazides, timolol, trichlormethiazide, ursodiol, verapamil
Hydroxyproline (Urine)	**Increased by:** anticonvulsants, corticosteroids, cyclosporine, danazol, hormone replacement, interferon, levothyroxine, nafarelin, parathyroid hormone, phenobarbital, phenytoin, somatotropin, thyroid, tolbutamide, vitamin D **Decreased by:** antineoplastic agents, ascorbic acid, aspirin, bisphosphonates, budesonide, calcitonin, conjugated estrogens, corticosteroids, estrogen/progestin therapy, etidronate, gallium nitrate, glucocorticoids, medroxyprogesterone, pamidronate, plicamycin, prednisolone, prednisone, propranolol
Immunoglobulin E Antibody (Serum)	**Increased by:** aztreonam, penicillin G **Decreased by:** phenytoin

table continues on pg. 1153 >

TABLE E.1, continued

Test	Increased Can Lead to a False-Positive Value Decreased Can Lead to a False-Negative Value
Insulin (Plasma)	**Increased by:** acetohexamide, adenosine, albuterol, amino acids, aspirin, beclomethasone, calcium gluconate, cannabis, captopril, chlorpropamide, chlorthalidone, deferoxamine, glimepiride, glipizide, glyburide, human growth hormone, hydrochlorothiazide, insulin, interferon alfa-2a, isoproterenol, levodopa, lisinopril, medroxyprogesterone, megestrol, methylprednisolone, metoprolol, niacin, nicotinic acid, norethindrone, oral contraceptives, perindopril, prazosin, prednisolone, prednisone, quinine, rifampin, ritodrine, secretin, spironolactone, streptozocin, terbutaline, tolazamide, tolbutamide, trichlormethiazide, verapamil **Decreased by:** acarbose, acetohexamide, calcitonin, chlorpropamide, cimetidine, clofibrate, conjugated estrogen, diazoxide, diltiazem, doxazosin, enalapril, ethacrynic acid, ether, furosemide, hydrochlorothiazide, metformin, midazolam, morphine, niacin, nifedipine, octreotide, phenytoin, prazosin, propranolol, psyllium, tolazamide, tolbutamide
Iron (Blood)	**Increased by:** acetylsalicylic acid, cefotaxime, chemotherapeutic agents, chloramphenicol, cisplatin, ferrous sulfate, iron, iron dextran, methicillin, methimazole, methotrexate, multivitamin, oral contraceptives, pyrazinamide **Decreased by:** allopurinol, aspirin, cholestyramine, corticotropin, cortisone, deferoxamine, metformin, oxymetholone, pyrazinamide, risperidone
Ketones (Urine)	**Increased by:** acetylcysteine, aminosalicylic acid, aspirin, captopril, cefdinir, cefixime, dimercaprol, ether, etodolac, ifosfamide, isoniazid, levodopa, mesna, metformin, methyldopa, niacin, paraldehyde, penicillamine, phenazopyridine, phenolphthalein, phenothiazines, streptozocin, valproic acid **Decreased by:** aspirin, phenazopyridine
Lactate Dehydrogenase (LD) (LDH) (Serum)	Increased by: acebutolol, amiodarone, amphotericin B, anabolic steroids, aripiprazole, aspirin, auranofin, azithromycin, betaxolol, captopril, carbenicillin, cefdinir, cefonicid, cefotaxime, cefotetan, cefoxitin, cefpodoxime, ceftazidime, cefuroxime, chloramphenicol, chlorpromazine, chlorpropamide, chlorthalidone, cimetidine, ciprofloxacin, clindamycin, clofibrate, codeine, dapsone, diclofenac, diltiazem, donepezil, doxorubicin, estramustine, fenoprofen, fluphenazine, fluvoxamine, foscarnet, furosemide, ganciclovir, GCSF, gentamicin, gold, hydralazine, ibuprofen, imipramine, interferon alfa-2a, interleukin-2, isotretinoin, itraconazole, levodopa, meperidine, mesalamine, methotrexate, methyldopa, metoprolol, morphine, mycophenolate, nefazodone, nelfinavir, nifedipine, nitrofurantoin, norfloxacin, ofloxacin, oxacillin, oxaprozin, paroxetine, pegfilgrastim, penicillamine, pindolol, piperacillin, propranolol, propylthiouracil, quinidine, quinupristin/dalfopristin, riluzole, simvastatin, streptokinase, streptozocin, sulfamethoxazole, sulfasalazine, sulfisoxazole, sulindac, tacrolimus, tetracycline, thiopental, ticarcillin, tobramycin, tolmetin, valproic acid, vasopressin, verapamil

table continues on pg. 1154 >

TABLE E.1, continued

Test	Increased Can Lead to a False-Positive Value Decreased Can Lead to a False-Negative Value
	Decreased by: amikacin, anticonvulsants, ascorbic acid, cefotaxime, clofibrate, enalapril, hydroxyurea, metronidazole, naltrexone
Luteinizing Hormone (LH) (Plasma)	**Increased by:** bicalutamide, bromocriptine, clomiphene finasteride, gonadotropin-releasing hormone, goserelin, growth-releasing hormone, hydrocortisone, ketoconazole, leuprolide, naloxone, nilutamide, spironolactone, tamoxifen, valproic acid **Decreased by:** anabolic steroids, anticonvulsants, carbamazepine, conjugated estrogens, corticotropin-releasing hormone, danazol, digoxin, estrogen/progestin therapy, ethinyl estradiol, finasteride, goserelin, ketoconazole, leuprolide, medroxyprogesterone, megestrol, metformin, octreotide, oral contraceptives, phenothiazines, phenytoin, pimozide, pravastatin, prednisone, progesterone, stanozolol, tamoxifen, thioridazine, toremifene, valproic acid
Lipase (Serum)	**Increased by:** acetaminophen, asparaginase, azathioprine, bethanechol, calcitriol, chlorothiazide, cholinergic agents, cidofovir, cimetidine, clozapine, codeine, conjugated estrogens, cyclosporine, demeclocycline, desipramine, diazoxide, didanosine, donepezil, doxorubicin, enalapril, estropipate, fluvastatin, furosemide, human growth hormone, hydrocortisone, ibuprofen, indomethacin, interferon, lisinopril, meperidine, mercaptopurine, mesalamine, methacholine, methylprednisolone, metolazone, metronidazole, minocycline, mirtazapine, morphine, nabumetone, naproxen, narcotics, nitrofurantoin, norfloxacin, octreotide, oral contraceptives, oxaprozin, pegaspargase, penicillamine, pentazocine, piroxicam, prazosin, prednisone, quinapril, secretin, simvastatin, sulfamethoxazole, sulindac, trastuzumab, tretinoin, valproic acid, zalcitabine, zolmitriptan **Decreased by:** calcium, hydroxyurea, mesalamine, protamine, somatostatin
Lymphocytes (Blood)	**Increased by:** aminosalicylic acid, cefaclor, cefdinir, ceftazidime, chlorambucil, chlorpropamide, dexamethasone, gabapentin, GCSF, griseofulvin, haloperidol, levodopa, narcotics, niacinamide, ofloxacin, paroxetine, propylthiouracil, quazepam, spironolactone, triazolam, valproic acid, venlafaxine **Decreased by:** alprazolam, aripiprazole, asparaginase, azacitidine, benzodiazepines, bevacizumab, bupropion, cefdinir, cefpodoxime, ceftriaxone, cetuximab, chlorambucil, cyclosporine, dexamethasone, eprosartan, etanercept, fludarabine, folic acid, fulvestrant, furosemide, gabapentin, glucocorticoids, hydrocortisone, ibuprofen, infliximab, irinotecan, levetiracetam, levofloxacin, lithium, mechlorethamine, mirtazapine, muromonab-CD3, nelfinavir, niacin, nitisinone, ofloxacin, olsalazine, oxaliplatin, pamidronate, pentostatin, phenytoin, quazepam, rabeprazole, sirolimus, telithromycin, terbinafine, thiamine, trastuzumab, triazolam, voriconazole

table continues on pg. 1155 >

TABLE E.1, continued

Test	Increased Can Lead to a False-Positive Value Decreased Can Lead to a False-Negative Value
Magnesium (Serum)	**Increased by:** alkaline antacids, amiloride, aminoglycosides, aspirin, calcitriol, cefotaxime, felodipine, hydroflumethiazide, lithium, magnesium salts, medroxyprogesterone, progesterone, sodium bicarbonate, tacrolimus, triamterene, zoledronic acid **Decreased by:** albuterol, aldesleukin, amphotericin B, arsenic trioxide, azathioprine, basiliximab, calcitriol, calcium gluconate, cefotaxime, chlorothiazide, chlorthalidone, cisplatin, cyclosporine, digoxin, doxorubicin, ethacrynic acid, foscarnet, furosemide, gentamicin, haloperidol, hydrochlorothiazide, hydroflumethiazide, insulin, metolazone, neomycin, oral contraceptives, pamidronate, pentamidine, prednisolone, sirolimus, tacrolimus, theophylline, thiazides, tobramycin, trastuzumab, voriconazole, zalcitabine, zoledronic acid
Magnesium (Urine)	**Increased by:** acetazolamide, ammonium chloride, amphotericin B, bumetanide, calcitonin, chlorothiazide, cisplatin, cyclosporin A, ethacrynic acid, furosemide, gentamicin, hydrochlorothiazide, lithium, magnesium hydroxide, methyclothiazide, thiazides, torsemide, triamterene **Decreased by:** acetazolamide, amiloride, calcium gluconate, interferon alfa-2a, oral contraceptives, parathyroid extract
Methemoglobin (Blood)	**Increased by:** acetaminophen, aminosalicylic acid, amyl nitrite, analgesics, antimalarials, aspirin, benzocaine, bismuth nitrate, chloramphenicol, chlorpheniramine, co-trimoxazole, dapsone, dimercaprol, furazolidone, isoniazid, isosorbide, local anesthetics, methicillin, methylene blue, metoclopramide, nitrofurantoin, nitrofurazone, nitroglycerin, phenazopyridine, phenytoin, potassium chloride, primaquine, probenecid, quinidine, quinine, sulfacetamide, sulfamethizole, sulfanilamide, sulfisoxazole **Decreased by:** sulfamethoxazole, sulfasalazine, trimethoprim
Monocytes (Blood)	**Increased by:** alprazolam, ampicillin, carbenicillin, chlorpromazine, GCSF, griseofulvin, haloperidol, lomefloxacin, methsuximide, paroxetine, penicillamine, piperacillin, prednisone, propylthiouracil, quazepam **Decreased by:** alprazolam, GCSF, glucocorticoids (transient), triazolam
Oxalate (Urine)	**Increased by:** ascorbic acid, bumetanide, ethylene glycol **Decreased by:** ascorbic acid, calcium carbonate
Parathyroid Hormone Assay (Plasma)	**Increased by:** chemotherapy, cyclosporine, estrogen/progestin therapy, foscarnet, human growth hormone, hydrocortisone, isoniazid, ketoconazole, lithium, nifedipine, octreotide, pamidronate, phenytoin, prednisone, tamoxifen, verapamil **Decreased by:** aluminum hydroxide, calcitriol, cimetidine, diltiazem, famotidine, gallium nitrate, gentamicin, magnesium sulfate, oral contraceptives, parathyroid hormone, pindolol, prednisone, thiazides, vitamin D

table continues on pg. 1156 >

TABLE E.1, continued

Test	Increased Can Lead to a False-Positive Value Decreased Can Lead to a False-Negative Value
Phosphate (Serum)	**Increased by:** aldesleukin, aluminum hydroxide, anabolic steroids, aspirin, azithromycin, basiliximab, bisoprolol, cefdinir, cefotaxime, dipyridamole, epoetin alfa, erythropoietin, etidronate, foscarnet, furosemide, human growth hormone, hydrochlorothiazide, mannitol, medroxyprogesterone, methicillin, methyltestosterone, methotrexate, minocycline, nafarelin, naproxen, nifedipine, nitrofurantoin, oral contraceptives, paroxetine, Phospho-Soda (Fleet), pindolol, rifampin, risedronate, risperidone, sirolimus, tacrolimus, tetracycline, theophylline, timolol, venlafaxine, vitamin D **Decreased by:** acetazolamide, albuterol, aldesleukin, alendronate, alkaline antacids, aluminum salts, amino acids, amlodipine, anesthetic agents, anticonvulsants, azathioprine, calcitonin, calcitriol, carbamazepine, cefdinir, cisplatin, doxorubicin, foscarnet, hydrochlorothiazide, insulin, isoniazid, lithium, mannitol, mestranol, mycophenolate, niacin, nicardipine, oral contraceptives, pamidronate, phenothiazines, phenytoin, plicamycin, raloxifene, sirolimus, sucralfate, tacrolimus, theophylline, venlafaxine, zoledronic acid
Plasminogen (Blood)	**Increased by:** anabolic steroids, danazol, fluoxymesterone, norethandrolone, oral contraceptives, oxandrolone, oxymetholone, stanozolol **Decreased by:** alteplase, anistreplase, asparaginase, chemotherapy, dextran, gemfibrozil, streptokinase
Platelet (Blood)	**Increased by:** alglucerase, amoxapine, auranofin, cefazolin, cefdinir, cefonicid, cefotetan, cefpodoxime, ceftibuten, ceftriaxone, cidofovir, clindamycin, clozapine, danazol, diltiazem, dipyridamole, donepezil, epoetin alfa, ertapenem, erythropoietin, estropipate, fludarabine, gemfibrozil, glucocorticoids, imipenem/cilastin, immune globulin, indinavir, interferon alfa-2a, isotretinoin, lansoprazole, lithium, lomefloxacin, megestrol, meropenem, mesalamine, methylprednisolone, metoprolol, metyrosine, miconazole, moxalactam, netilmicin, ofloxacin, oral contraceptives, paroxetine, penicillamine, pergolide, propranolol, steroids, telithromycin, ticlopidine, venlafaxine, zalcitabine, zidovudine **Decreased by:** abciximab, acetaminophen, acetazolamide, adalimumab, albendazole, albuterol, aldesleukin, alemtuzumab, allopurinol, altretamine, aminocaproic acid, aminoglutethimide, amiodarone, amitriptyline, amoxicillin, amphotericin B, ampicillin, amrinone, anagrelide, anticonvulsants, antineoplastic agents, aprepitant, ardeparin, aripiprazole, arsenic trioxide, asparaginase, aspirin, auranofin, aurothioglucose, azathioprine, azithromycin, barbiturates, basiliximab, BCG vaccine, benazepril, benzthiazide, betaxolol, bevacizumab, bicalutamide, bismuth subsalicylate, bleomycin, bortezomib, bupropion, candesartan, capecitabine, capreomycin, captopril, carbamazepine, carbenicillin, carmustine, carvedilol, cefaclor, cefamandole, cefazolin, cefditoren, cefixime, cefonicid, cefotetan,

table continues on pg. 1157 >

TABLE E.1, continued

Test	Increased Can Lead to a False-Positive Value Decreased Can Lead to a False-Negative Value
	cefoxitin, cefpodoxime, ceftibuten, ceftizoxime, ceftriaxone, cefuroxime, cetirizine, chlorambucil, chloramphenicol, chlordiazepoxide, chloroquine, chlorothiazide, chlorpheniramine, chlorpromazine, chlorpropamide, chlortetracycline, chlorthalidone, cimetidine, cladribine, clemastine, clindamycin, clofibrate, clomipramine, clonazepam, clopidogrel, co-trimoxazole, codeine, colchicine, cyclobenzaprine, cyclophosphamide, cyproheptadine, cytarabine, dacarbazine, dactinomycin, dalteparin, danazol, demeclocycline, desipramine, dextroamphetamine, diazoxide, diclofenac, didanosine, diethylpropion, digitalis, digitoxin, diltiazem, diphenhydramine, disopyramide, docetaxel, donepezil, doxepin, doxorubicin, doxycycline, duloxetine, eflornithine, enalapril, enoxaparin, epirubicin, eprosartan, erythromycin, escitalopram, esomeprazole, estramustine, etanercept, ethacrynic acid, ethchlorvynol, ethosuximide, etidronate, etoposide, factor VIIa, famotidine, fenoprofen, flecainide, fluconazole, flucytosine, fludarabine, fluorouracil, fluphenazine, fluvastatin, fluvoxamine, fomivirsen, fondaparinux, fosphenytoin, furosemide, gabapentin, galantamine, ganciclovir, gatifloxacin, gemcitabine, gentamicin, glimepiride, glyburide, gold, granisetron, hepatitis B vaccine, hydralazine, hydrochlorothiazide, hydroxychloroquine, hydroxyurea, ibritumomab, ibuprofen, idarubicin, ifosfamide, imatinib, imipenem/cilastin, imipramine, immunoglobulin, indinavir, indomethacin, infliximab, interferon alfa-2a, interleukin-2, irinotecan, isoniazid, isosorbide dinitrate, isotretinoin, itraconazole, ketoprofen, lamivudine, lamotrigine, lansoprazole, laronidase, lepirudin, levodopa, lincomycin, lisinopril, lomefloxacin, lomustine, loracarbef, lovastatin, loxapine, maprotiline, measles virus vaccine, mechlorethamine, mefenamic acid, mefloquine, meloxicam, melphalan, meprobamate, mercaptopurine, meropenem, mesalamine, mesoridazine, metformin, methazolamide, methicillin, methimazole, methotrexate, methsuximide, methyclothiazide, methyldopa, methylphenidate, methysergide, metoprolol, metronidazole, metyrosine, mexiletine, milrinone, minocycline, mirtazapine, misoprostol, mitomycin, mitoxantrone, moricizine, morphine, moxalactam, mumps virus vaccine, muromonab-CD3, mycophenolate, nabumetone, nalidixic acid, naproxen, netilmicin, nevirapine, niacin, nicardipine, nitisinone, nitrofurantoin, nitroglycerin, nizatidine, norfloxacin, nortriptyline, nystatin, ofloxacin, olsalazine, omeprazole, orphenadrine, oxacillin, oxaliplatin, oxytetracycline, paclitaxel, pamidronate, pegaspargase, peginterferon alfa-2a, penicillamine, penicillin, pentamidine, pentostatin, pentoxifylline, perphenazine, phenobarbital, phenothiazines, pindolol, piroxicam, polio virus vaccine, polythiazide, potassium iodide, pravastatin, prednisone, pregabalin, primidone, probenecid, procainamide, procarbazine, promazine, promethazine, propafenone, propranolol, propylthiouracil, protriptyline,

table continues on pg. 1158 >

TABLE E.1, continued

Test	Increased Can Lead to a False-Positive Value Decreased Can Lead to a False-Negative Value
	pyrazinamide, pyrimethamine, quazepam, quinidine, quinupristin/dalfopristin, rabeprazole, raloxifene, ramipril, reserpine, rifampin, rifapentine, risperidone, rivastigmine, rubella virus vaccine, saquinavir, sargramostim, sirolimus, smallpox vaccine, spironolactone, stavudine, streptomycin, streptozocin, sulfamethoxazole, sulfasalazine, sulfisoxazole, sulfonylureas, sulindac, tacrolimus, tamoxifen, telithromycin, temozolomide, tetracycline, thiabendazole, thiazides, thioguanine, thioridazine, thiotepa, thiothixene, ticarcillin, ticlopidine, timolol, tinzaparin, tobramycin, tocainide, tolazamide, tolazoline, tolbutamide, tolmetin, topotecan, toremifene, tranylcypromine, trastuzumab, trichlormethiazide, trifluoperazine, trimethoprim, trimetrexate, trimipramine, tripelennamine, uracil mustard, valganciclovir, valproic acid, vancomycin, vinblastine, vincristine, vinorelbine, voriconazole, zidovudine, zoledronic acid, zolmitriptan
Porphobilinogen (Urine)	**Increased by:** aminosalicylic acid, anticonvulsants, barbiturates, cascara, chlordiazepoxide, chlorpromazine, chlorpropamide, griseofulvin, imipenem/cilastin, meprobamate, oral contraceptives, phenothiazines, pentazocine, phenytoin, procaine, tolbutamide **Decreased by:** actinomycin, ascorbic acid, cimetidine, oral contraceptives
Porphyrins (Urine)	**Increased by:** antipyretics, barbiturates, chloral hydrate, chlordiazepoxide, chlorpropamide, ciprofloxacin, diazepam, ergot preparations, griseofulvin, nalidixic acid, hydantoin derivatives, norfloxacin, meprobamate, methyldopa, hydroxychloroquine, ofloxacin, oxytetracycline, pentazocine, phenazopyridine, progestin derivatives, sulfamethoxazole, tetracycline, vitamin K **Decreased by:** oral contraceptives
Potassium (Serum)	**Increased by:** ACE inhibitors, aldesleukin, amiloride, aminocaproic acid, aminoglutethimide, ammonium chloride, amphotericin B, aripiprazole, atenolol, azathioprine, azithromycin, basiliximab, benazepril, betaxolol, bisoprolol, candesartan, cannabis, captopril, cefdinir, cefotaxime, cisplatin, clofibrate, cyclosporine, danazol, dexamethasone, digoxin, doxorubicin, enalapril, eplerenone, epoetin alfa, erythropoietin, felodipine, fosphenytoin, heparin, indomethacin, isoniazid, ketoconazole, ketorolac, labetalol, lisinopril, lithium, LMW heparin, lovastatin, mannitol, methicillin, methyltestosterone, metoprolol, moexipril, mycophenolate, naproxen, netilmicin, nifedipine, nonsteroidal anti-inflammatory drugs, norfloxacin, ofloxacin, palonosetron, paroxetine, penicillin, pentamidine, perindopril, pindolol, piroxicam, potassium chloride, procainamide, propranolol, quinapril, quinupristin/dalfopristin, ramipril, risedronate, somatotropin, spironolactone, succinylcholine, sulfamethoxazole, sulindac, tacrolimus, telmisartan (Micardis), timolol, trandolapril, triamterene, trimethoprim, tromethamine, valsartan, venlafaxine, zalcitabine

table continues on pg. 1159 >

TABLE E.1, continued

Test	Increased Can Lead to a False-Positive Value Decreased Can Lead to a False-Negative Value
	Decreased by: acetazolamide, albuterol, aldesleukin, aminosalicylic acid, amlodipine, ammonium chloride, amphotericin, aprepitant, aripiprazole, arsenic trioxide, aspirin, azathioprine, basiliximab, benzthiazide, betamethasone, betaxolol, bevacizumab, bisacodyl, bortezomib, bumetanide, candesartan, capreomycin, captopril, carbamazepine, carbenicillin, carvedilol, cascara, cathartics, cephalexin, chloroquine, chlorothiazide, chlorthalidone, cidofovir, cisplatin, corticosteroids, corticotropin, cortisone, dexamethasone, digoxin immune fab, diuretics, dobutamine, donepezil, doxazosin, doxorubicin, enalapril, epoprostenol, ethacrynic acid, felbamate, fluconazole, flucytosine, fludrocortisone, fluvoxamine, formoterol, foscarnet, fosinopril, fosphenytoin, furosemide, ganciclovir, gentamicin, glucose, hydrochlorothiazide, imatinib, indapamide, insulin, itraconazole, ketoprofen, laxatives, levalbuterol, levodopa, lithium, lomefloxacin, methazolamide, methyclothiazide, methylprednisolone, metoclopramide, metolazone, mifepristone, milrinone, moxalactam, mycophenolate, nabumetone, nafcillin, naproxen, neomycin, nifedipine, nisoldipine, ondansetron, oxaliplatin, pamidronate, paroxetine, penicillin, piperacillin, plicamycin, polystyrene sulfonate, polythiazide, prednisolone, prednisone, quinethazone, riluzole, risperidone, ritodrine, sirolimus, sodium bicarbonate, streptozocin, sulfasalazine, tacrolimus, terbutaline, tetracycline, theophylline, thiazides, ticarcillin, tobramycin, triamterene, trichlormethiazide, trimethoprim, venlafaxine, vidarabine, voriconazole, zalcitabine, ziconotide, zoledronic acid
Potassium (Urine)	**Increased by:** acetazolamide, ammonium chloride, antibiotics, aspirin, betamethasone, bumetanide, calcitonin, carbenicillin, cathartics, chlorthalidone, corticosteroids, corticotropin, cortisone, dexamethasone, diuretics, ethacrynic acid, fenoldopam, fludrocortisone, gentamicin, hydrochlorothiazide, hydrocortisone, indomethacin, isosorbide, levodopa, lithium, mafenide, methyclothiazide, metolazone, niacinamide, oral contraceptives, parathyroid extract, prednisolone, quinethazone, streptozocin, thiazides, torsemide, triamcinolone, viomycin **Decreased by:** amiloride, anesthetic agents, carbamazepine, cyclosporin A, diazoxide, felodipine, ketoconazole, levarterenol, niacin, ramipril, sulfamethoxazole, trimethoprim
Pregnanediol (Urine)	**Increased by:** corticotropin, phenazopyridine, tamoxifen **Decreased by:** medroxyprogesterone, oral contraceptives, phenothiazines, progesterone
Progesterone (Plasma)	**Increased by:** corticotropin, ketoconazole, progesterone, tamoxifen **Decreased by:** ampicillin, carbamazepine, danazol, goserelin, leuprolide, medroxyprogesterone, oral contraceptives, pentobarbital, phenytoin, pravastatin, valproic acid

table continues on pg. 1160 >

TABLE E.1, continued

Test	Increased Can Lead to a False-Positive Value Decreased Can Lead to a False-Negative Value
Prolactin (Serum)	**Increased by:** amitriptyline, amoxapine, butorphanol, carbidopa, chlorpromazine, cimetidine, citalopram, clomipramine, danazol, desipramine, enalapril, fenoldopam, fluphenazine, fluvoxamine, furosemide, gonadotropin-releasing hormone, growth hormone–releasing hormone, haloperidol, imipramine, insulin, interferon, interleukin, labetalol, loxapine, megestrol, mestranol, methyldopa, metoclopramide, molindone, morphine, nitrous oxide, oral contraceptives, parathyroid hormone, perphenazine, phenytoin, prochlorperazine, promazine, ranitidine, reserpine, risperidone, thioridazine, thiothixene, thyrotropin-releasing hormone, trifluoperazine, trimipramine, tumor necrosis factor, verapamil **Decreased by:** anticonvulsants, bromocriptine, calcitonin, carbamazepine, conjugated estrogens, cyclosporine, dexamethasone, finasteride, levodopa, metoclopramide, morphine, nifedipine, octreotide, phenytoin
Protein (Cerebrospinal Fluid)	**Increased by:** ampicillin, aspirin, cefotaxime, chloramphenicol, ibuprofen, imipramine, methicillin, methotrexate, oxytetracycline, penicillin, perphenazine, phenothiazines, procaine, radiographic agents, streptomycin, sulfadiazine, sulfanilamide, sulfisoxazole, tetracycline, tolbutamide, trifluoperazine, vancomycin **Decreased by:** acetaminophen, cytarabine, cefotaxime, dexamethasone, ranitidine, rifampin, ropinirole, tamoxifen, toremifene, valproic acid
Protein (Urine)	**Increased by:** acetaminophen, acetazolamide, aldesleukin, aminophylline, aminosalicylic acid, amphotericin B, ampicillin, arsenicals, ascorbic acid, asparaginase, aspirin, auranofin, aurothioglucose, bacitracin, benazepril, betaxolol, bicarbonate, bismuth subsalicylate, capreomycin, carbamazepine, castor oil, cefaclor, cefamandole, cefdinir, cephaloridine, cephalothin, chloral hydrate, chlorhexidine, chloroform, chlorpheniramine, chlorpromazine, chlorpropamide, chlorthalidone, cidofovir, cisplatin, clindamycin, clofibrate, codeine, colistin, corticosteroids, corticotropin, cyclosporine, dantrolene, demeclocycline, dihydrotachysterol, doxapram, doxycycline, enalapril, ergot preparations, ether, ethosuximide, fenoprofen, foscarnet, furosemide, gabapentin, gemcitabine, gentamicin, glyburide, glycerin, gold, griseofulvin, hepatitis A vaccine, hydralazine, ibuprofen, ifosfamide, indomethacin, interferon alfa-2a, iodine-containing drugs, iron, isoniazid, isotretinoin, kanamycin, ketorolac, Lipomul, lithium, mefenamic acid, mercury compounds, mesalamine, metaxalone, methenamine, methicillin, mitomycin, mitotane, naproxen, neomycin, netilmicin, nifedipine, nonsteroidal anti-inflammatory drugs, norfloxacin, olsalazine, oxacillin, oxaprozin, paraldehyde, paramethadione, paromomycin, pegaspargase, penicillamine, penicillin, phenazopyridine, phenolphthalein, phosphorus, piperacillin, piroxicam, probenecid, promazine, quinine, radiographic agents, ramipril, ranitidine, rifampin, salsalate, silver,

table continues on pg. 1161 >

TABLE E.1, continued

Test	Increased Can Lead to a False-Positive Value Decreased Can Lead to a False-Negative Value
	sodium bicarbonate, streptokinase, streptomycin, sulfadiazine, sulfamethoxazole, sulfasalazine, sulfisoxazole, sulindac, tacrolimus, tetracycline, thallium, theophylline, thiabendazole, ticarcillin, ticlopidine, tobramycin, tolbutamide, tolmetin, tramadol, trifluoperazine, vancomycin
Renin (Plasma)	**Elevated by:** captopril, furosemide
	Decreased by: oral contraceptives
Sodium (Serum)	**Increased by:** aldesleukin, amiloride, amino acids, ampicillin, anabolic steroids, betamethasone, cannabis, carbamazepine, carbenicillin, cefotaxime, chlorthalidone, cholestyramine, clonidine, corticosteroids, cortisone, diazoxide, doxorubicin, estrogens, fludrocortisone, fosphenytoin, guanethidine, human growth hormone, hydrocortisone, isosorbide, ketoprofen, mannitol, methyclothiazide, methyldopa, methyltestosterone, nitrofurantoin, oral contraceptives, penicillin G sodium, phenelzine, polystyrene sulfonate, prednisolone, prednisone, progesterone, ramipril, sildenafil, sodium bicarbonate, sodium phenylbutyrate, tetracycline, ticarcillin/clavulanate, valproic acid, vitamin E, zalcitabine
	Decreased by: acetaminophen, acetazolamide, aldesleukin, amiloride, aminoglutethimide, ammonium chloride, amphotericin, atovaquone, benazepril, captopril, carbamazepine, carvedilol, cathartics, chlorothiazide, chlorpropamide, chlorthalidone, cisplatin, clofibrate, clonidine, clozapine, cyclophosphamide, cytarabine, dapsone, desmopressin, diclofenac, diuretics, doxepin, doxorubicin, eplerenone, esomeprazole, ethacrynic acid, fluoxetine, fluvoxamine, foscarnet, furosemide, gentamicin, glimepiride, glyburide, glycerin, haloperidol, hydrochlorothiazide, hydroflumethiazide, indomethacin, isosorbide dinitrate, itraconazole, ketoconazole, ketorolac, laxatives, lisinopril, lithium, mannitol, methyclothiazide, methylprednisolone, metolazone, miconazole, morphine, nicardipine, nicotine, nifedipine, nisoldipine, nonsteroidal anti-inflammatory drugs, olanzapine, omeprazole, oxycodone, oxytocin, paroxetine, pentostatin, phenoxybenzamine, pimozide, polythiazide, propafenone, quinethazone, ramipril, riluzole, risperidone, sertraline, sirolimus, spironolactone, sulfonylureas, tacrolimus, theophylline, thiazides, ticlopidine, tobramycin, trastuzumab, triamterene, trimethoprim, trimetrexate, valproic acid, vasopressin, venlafaxine, vidarabine, vincristine, zalcitabine
Sodium (Urine)	**Increased by:** ACE inhibitors, acetazolamide, amiloride, ammonium chloride, aspirin, atenolol, benzthiazide, bumetanide, calcitonin, captopril, carvedilol, chlorothiazide, chlorthalidone, cisplatin, clofibrate, cyclothiazide, dexamethasone, digitalis, doxepin, enalapril, ethacrynic acid, felodipine, fenoldopam, furosemide, hydrochlorothiazide, hydrocortisone, hydroflumethiazide, ifosfamide, indomethacin, insulin, isosorbide, levodopa, lithium, losartan, mannitol, methyclothiazide, metoprolol,

table continues on pg. 1162 >

TABLE E.1, continued

Test	Increased Can Lead to a False-Positive Value Decreased Can Lead to a False-Negative Value
	metolazone, niacin, niacinamide, oral contraceptives, paramethasone, parathyroid extract, polythiazide, progesterone, quinethazone, secretin, spironolactone, tetracycline, thiazides, torsemide, triamcinolone, triamterene, trichlormethiazide, trimethoprim, verapamil, vincristine **Decreased by:** anesthetic agents, carbamazepine, corticosteroids, cortisone, cyclosporine, diazoxide, etodolac, fluoxetine, ibuprofen, indomethacin, insulin, ketorolac, levarterenol, lithium, methylprednisolone, naproxen, nifedipine, octreotide, omeprazole, propranolol, ramipril
Somatomedin C (Insulin-like, Growth Factor I) (Plasma)	**Elevated by:** aminoglutethimide, clonidine, dexamethasone goserelin, human growth hormone, medroxyprogesterone, prednisolone, somatropin, tamoxifen **Decreased by:** estrogens, ethinyl estradiol, methimazole, octreotide, oral contraceptives, tamoxifen
Testosterone (Serum)	**Increased by:** anabolic steroids, barbiturates, bromocriptine, Casodex, cimetidine, clomiphene, danazol, estrogen/progestin, finasteride, flutamide, goserelin, leuprolide, levonorgestrel, mifepristone, nafarelin, nalmefene, naloxone, nilutamide, oral contraceptives, phenytoin, pravastatin, rifampin, tamoxifen, valproic acid **Decreased by:** carbamazepine, cimetidine, cinacalcet, conjugated estrogens, cyclophosphamide, danazol, dexamethasone, diazoxide, digoxin, estradiol valerate, fenoldopam, finasteride, follicle-stimulating hormone, gemfibrozil, goserelin, interleukin, ketoconazole, letrozole, leuprolide, magnesium, medroxyprogesterone, metformin, methylprednisolone, nafarelin, octreotide, oral contraceptives, pravastatin, prednisone, spironolactone, stanozolol, tamoxifen, tetracycline, verapamil
Thrombin Time (Blood)	**Increased by:** asparaginase, streptokinase, urokinase **Decreased by:** dextran, LMW heparin
Thyroglobulin (Serum)	**Increased by:** amiodarone **Decreased by:** neomycin, thyroxine
Thyroid-Stimulating Hormone (TSH) (Serum)	**Increased by:** amiodarone, aripiprazole, atenolol, calcitonin, carbamazepine, chlorpromazine, clomiphene, conjugated estrogens, ferrous sulfate, iodide, levothyroxine, lithium, lovastatin, methimazole, metoclopramide, morphine, phenytoin, potassium iodide, prazosin, prednisone, propranolol, radiographic agents, rifampin, sumatriptan, tamoxifen, thyrotropin-releasing hormone, valproic acid **Decreased by:** amiodarone, anabolic steroids, aspirin, carbamazepine, clofibrate, corticosteroids, danazol, fenoldopam, growth-releasing hormone, hydrocortisone, interferon alfa-2, levothyroxine, nifedipine, octreotide, peginterferon alfa-2a, somatostatin, thyroxine, troleandomycin
Thyroxine-Binding Globulin (TBG) (Serum)	**Increased by:** carbamazepine, clofibrate, erythropoietin estrogens, mestranol, oral contraceptives, perphenazine, phenothiazines, progesterone, raloxifene, tamoxifen

table continues on pg. 1163 >

TABLE E.1, continued

Test	Increased Can Lead to a False-Positive Value Decreased Can Lead to a False-Negative Value
	Decreased by: anabolic steroids, asparaginase, colestipol, corticosteroids, corticotropin, cortisone, danazol, fluoxymesterone, methyltestosterone, nandrolone, norethandrolone, norethindrone, oxymetholone, phenytoin, prednisone, propranolol, stanozolol
Triiodothyronine Uptake (Serum)	**Increased by:** aminoglutethimide, aminosalicylic acid, amiodarone, anabolic steroids, aspirin, barbiturates, chlorpropamide, cobalt, corticosteroids, Coumadin, fluoxymesterone, furosemide, levonorgestrel (Norplant), levothyroxine, methyltestosterone, metoprolol, mitotane, nandrolone, orphenadrine, oxymetholone, penicillin, phenytoin, propranolol, stanozolol, sulfonylureas, tamoxifen, thyroid, tolbutamide, warfarin (Coumadin) **Decreased by:** amiodarone, chlordiazepoxide, clofibrate, diazepam, diflunisal, estropipate, fluoxymesterone, lithium, medroxyprogesterone, methimazole, oral contraceptives, perphenazine, phenothiazines, thiazides
Triiodothyronine (T_3) (Serum)	**Increased by:** amiodarone, amphetamine, clofibrate, erythropoietin, estropipate, fluorouracil, insulin, levothyroxine, mestranol, methadone, opiates, oral contraceptives, phenothiazines, phenytoin, propylthiouracil, ranitidine, tamoxifen, terbutaline, thyrotropin-releasing hormone, valproic acid **Decreased by:** amiodarone, anabolic steroids, asparaginase, aspirin, atenolol, carbamazepine, cholestyramine, cimetidine, clomiphene, clomipramine, co-trimoxazole, corticosteroids, danazol, dexamethasone, diclofenac, furosemide, glucocorticoids, hydrocortisone, interferon alfa-2, iodide, isotretinoin, lithium, methimazole, metoprolol, mitotane, naproxen, netilmicin, oral contraceptives, penicillamine, phenobarbital, phenytoin, potassium iodide, prednisone, propranolol, propylthiouracil, radiographic agents, salsalate, somatostatin, stanozolol, sulfonylureas, theophylline
Thyroxine (T_4) Free (Serum)	**Increased by:** amiodarone, aspirin, carbamazepine, danazol, enoxaparin, erythropoietin, furosemide, levothyroxine, phenytoin, propranolol, propylthiouracil, radiographic agents, tamoxifen, thyroxine, valproic acid **Decreased by:** amiodarone, anabolic steroids, carbamazepine, clofibrate, corticosteroids, estrogen therapy, isotretinoin, levothyroxine, lithium, mestranol, methadone, methimazole, norethindrone, octreotide, oral contraceptives, phenobarbital, phenytoin, ranitidine
Triglycerides (Serum)	**Increased by:** abarelix, acetylsalicylic acid, amiodarone, ardeparin, ascorbic acid, atenolol, beta-blockers, bisoprolol, carbamazepine, carvedilol, Casodex, chlordane, chlorothiazide, chlorthalidone, cholestyramine, colchicine, cyclosporine, danazol, didanosine, enalapril, enfuvirtide, estrogen/progestin therapy, estrogens, fluconazole, fluvastatin, fosamprenavir, furosemide, glucocorticoids, glycerin, goserelin, hydrochlorothiazide, interferon alfa-2a, isotretinoin, itraconazole, labetalol, levothyroxine, methyclothiazide, methyldopa, metoprolol,

table continues on pg. 1164 >

TABLE E.1, continued

Test	Increased Can Lead to a False-Positive Value Decreased Can Lead to a False-Negative Value
	miconazole, mirtazapine, nadolol, nafarelin, norfloxacin, ofloxacin, olmesartan, oral contraceptives, pindolol, polythiazide, prazosin, prednisolone, prednisone, propranolol, radioactive iodine, risperidone, ritonavir, simvastatin, sotalol, spironolactone, tamoxifen, tenofovir, thiazides, ticlopidine, timolol, tretinoin, trichlormethiazide, warfarin, zalcitabine
	Decreased by: acarbose, ACE inhibitors, acetylsalicylic acid, amiodarone, amlodipine, anabolic steroids, ascorbic acid, asparaginase, atorvastatin, azathioprine, bisoprolol, captopril, carvedilol, chlorthalidone, cholestyramine, clofibrate, colestipol, danazol, diltiazem, doxazosin, enalapril, estrogen therapy, fenofibrate, flaxseed oil, fluvastatin, gemfibrozil, glyburide, HMG CoA-reductase inhibitors, hydroxychloroquine, hydroxyurea, indomethacin, insulin, ketoconazole, levodopa, levonorgestrel, levothyroxine, LMW heparins, lovastatin, medroxyprogesterone, metformin, methimazole, niacin, nicardipine, nicotinic acid, nifedipine, nisoldipine, norethindrone, oxandrolone, pentoxifylline, pindolol, pravastatin, prazosin, prednisolone, probucol, psyllium, simvastatin, stanozolol, terazosin, unfractionated heparin, verapamil
Uric Acid (Serum)	**Increased by:** acetaminophen, acetazolamide, aldesleukin, amiloride, ampicillin, anabolic steroids, antineoplastic agents, aripiprazole, asparaginase, ascorbic acid, aspirin, atenolol, azathioprine, basiliximab, benzthiazide, betaxolol, bisoprolol, bortezomib, bumetanide, busulfan, calcitriol, candesartan, capreomycin, carvedilol, chloral hydrate, chlorambucil, chlorothiazide, chlorthalidone, cimetidine, cisplatin, clopidogrel, clozapine, cyclosporine, cytarabine, dantrolene, dextran, diazoxide, diclofenac, didanosine, diltiazem, diuretics, donepezil, doxazosin, doxorubicin, epoetin alfa, ethacrynic acid, ethambutol, etoposide, fludarabine, furosemide, GCSF, gentamicin, goserelin, hydralazine, hydrochlorothiazide, hydroflumethiazide, hydroxyurea, ibuprofen, indomethacin, irbesartan, isoniazid, isosorbide dinitrate, isotretinoin, lansoprazole, leuprolide, levarterenol, levodopa, lisinopril, lomefloxacin, losartan, mechlorethamine, mercaptopurine, mesalamine, methotrexate, methyclothiazide, metolazone, misoprostol, mitomycin, mycophenolate, nabumetone, naproxen, nelfinavir, niacin, niacinamide, nicotinic acid, nisoldipine, nizatidine, olmesartan, oxytetracycline, pancrelipase, paroxetine, pegaspargase, pegfilgrastim, pentostatin, phenelzine, phenothiazines, pindolol, piroxicam, polythiazide, prednisone, propranolol, propylthiouracil, pyrazinamide, quinethazone, radioactive agents, ramipril, rifampin, rifapentine, riluzole, risperidone, ritonavir, salicylates, sildenafil, sodium oxybate, spironolactone, sulfanilamide, tacrolimus, theophylline, thiazides, thioguanine, thiotepa, timolol, triamterene, trichlormethiazide, trimetrexate, venlafaxine, vincristine, warfarin, zalcitabine

table continues on pg. 1165 >

TABLE E.1, continued

Test	Increased Can Lead to a False-Positive Value Decreased Can Lead to a False-Negative Value
	Decreased by: acetohexamide, allopurinol, amiloride, amlodipine, ascorbic acid, aspirin, azathioprine, cannabis, canola oil, chlorothiazide, chlorpromazine, cidofovir, clofibrate, corticosteroids, corticotropin, cortisone, diflunisal, dobutamine, doxazosin, enalapril, ethacrynic acid, etodolac, fenofibrate, griseofulvin, guaifenesin, ibuprofen, indomethacin, levodopa, lisinopril, lithium, mannitol, mechlorethamine, mefenamic acid, methotrexate, methyldopa, phenothiazines, prednisolone, probenecid, radiographic agents, salicylate, sertraline, spironolactone, sulfamethoxazole, sulfinpyrazone, ticarcillin/clavulanate, verapamil, vinblastine, warfarin (Coumadin)
Uric Acid (Urine)	**Increased by:** acetaminophen, acetohexamide, ascorbic acid, asparaginase, aspirin, busulfan, chlorothiazide, clofibrate, corticotropin, cortisone, ethacrynic acid, ifosfamide, lithium, mannitol, mercaptopurine, methotrexate, niacinamide, nifedipine, pancrelipase, phenothiazines, prednisolone, probenecid, salicylates (large doses), sulfamethoxazole, sulfinpyrazone, thioguanine, triamterene, verapamil, warfarin (Coumadin) **Decreased by:** acetazolamide, allopurinol, aspirin (low dose), azathioprine, bumetanide, chlorothiazide, chlorthalidone, diazoxide, ethacrynic acid, ethambutol, furosemide, hydrochlorothiazide, levarterenol, niacin, probenecid, pyrazinamide, salicylates (low doses), thiazides
Urine Specific Gravity	**Increased by:** dextran, isotretinoin, penicillin, radiographic agents **Decreased by:** lithium
Urobilinogen (Stool)	**Increased by:** amyl nitrate **Decreased by:** antibiotics, aspirin, chloramphenicol, chlordiazepoxide, chlorpromazine, erythromycin, methimazole, nalidixic acid, neomycin, oral contraceptives, oxymetholone, prochlorperazine, promazine, sulfamethoxazole, sulfisoxazole, tetracycline, thiabendazole, thiazides, tolbutamide, trifluoperazine
Vanillylmandelic Acid (VMA) (Urine)	**Increased by:** aminosalicylic acid, chlorpromazine, disulfiram guaifenesin, guanethidine, insulin, isoproterenol, labetalol, levarterenol, levodopa, lithium, methocarbamol, methyldopa, nalidixic acid, nifedipine, nitroglycerin, oxytetracycline, phenazopyridine, prazosin, prochlorperazine, rauwolfia, reserpine **Decreased by:** clonidine, disulfiram, fluvoxamine, guanethidine, guanfacine, imipramine, levodopa, MAO inhibitors, methyldopa, morphine, phenelzine, phenothiazines, radiographic agents, reserpine
Vitamin B_{12} (Serum)	**Increased by:** chloral hydrate, omeprazole **Decreased by:** anticonvulsants, ascorbic acid, chlorpromazine, cholestyramine, colchicine, metformin, neomycin, octreotide, oral contraceptives, ranitidine, rifampin

Index

Note: Test names are in blue type. Page numbers followed by "*c*" indicate charts; those followed by "*f*" indicate figures; those followed by "*t*" indicate tables.

B

D

G

I

J

K

M

O

P

S

T

U

V

W